Imaging of Soft Tissue Tumors

SECOND EDITION

Imaging of Soft Tissue Tumors

SECOND EDITION

■ **MARK J. KRANSDORF, M.D.**

Professor, Department of Radiology
Mayo Clinic College of Medicine
Rochester, Minnesota
Consultant, Department of Radiology
Mayo Clinic
Jacksonville, Florida

■ **MARK D. MURPHEY, M.D.**

Chief, Musculoskeletal Radiology
Department of Radiologic Pathology
Armed Forces Institute of Pathology
Department of Radiology
Walter Reed Army Medical Center
Washington, DC

Lippincott Williams & Wilkins
a Wolters Kluwer business

Philadelphia · Baltimore · New York · London
Buenos Aires · Hong Kong · Sydney · Tokyo

Acquisition Editor: Lisa McAllister
Managing Editor: Kerry Barrett
Project Manager: Fran Gunning
Marketing Manager: Angela Panetta
Manufacturing Coordinator: Kathleen Brown
Design Coordinator: Risa Clow
Production Services: TechBooks
Printer: Edwards Brothers

Library of Congress Cataloging-in-Publication Data

Kransdorf, Mark J.
   Imaging of soft tissue tumors / Mark J. Kransdorf, Mark D. Murphey.—2nd ed.
      p. ; cm.
   Includes bibliographical references and index.
   ISBN 0-7817-4771-6 (case)
   1. Soft tissue tumors—Imaging. I. Murphey, Mark D. II. Title.
   [DNLM: 1. Soft Tissue Neoplasms—diagnosis. 2. Diagnostic Imaging.
3. Soft Tissue Neoplasms—pathology. WD 375 K89i 2006]
RC280.S66K73 2006 616.99′40754—dc22

2005033281

10 9 8 7 6 5 4 3 2

To our families:
    Judy, Pam, Evan, and Kaity
    Jill, Matthew, and Lucas
    . . . . . . our strength and inspiration

                                MJK
                                MDM

Contents

Preface

This book was written to provide a systematic approach to the radiologic evaluation and diagnosis of soft tissue tumors and tumorlike masses. We have illustrated the full spectrum of lesions encountered in a clinical practice, emphasizing lesions with a characteristic or relatively characteristic radiologic appearance, while not neglecting those with a nonspecific appearance. As our knowledge and experience with the imaging of soft tissue expands, we truly expect the number of those lesions designated as nonspecific to continue to decrease (perhaps to 15% to 20% of masses).

Following a brief introductory chapter, we present the results of a retrospective analysis of more than 31,000 soft tissue tumors that were seen in consultation over 10 years by the Department of Soft Tissue Pathology, Armed Forces Institute of Pathology, to determine the relative prevalence, age at presentation, sex distribution, and skeletal distribution of soft tissue tumors, and the relative frequency of those tumors in specific anatomic locations and age groups. These data were collected prior to the nomenclature changes incorporated into the 2002 World Health Organization Classification of Soft Tissue Tumors, and we have chosen to present it with the original tumor designations. We have, however, incorporated the current nomenclature throughout the text, emphasizing applicable changes in each chapter.

Tumor population data are followed by an overview of the imaging evaluation of soft tissue tumors, highlighting advantages and limitations of the various modalities available. The imaging evaluation of patients following treatment is also reviewed. An algorithm for the evaluation of patients presenting with a soft tissue mass is provided, as are considerations to be used in the differentiation of benign from malignant soft tissue lesions. The chapter concludes with a review of the criteria required for tumor staging.

The following chapters review lipomatous, vascular and lymphatic, fibrous and fibrohistiocytic, muscle, neurogenic, synovial, extraskeletal osseous, and cartilaginous tumors, and tumors of uncertain histogenesis. The final imaging chapter discusses a collection of tumorlike masses of soft tissue arising from a variety of causes. These do not represent a comprehensive review of tumorlike masses but rather our experience with lesions that may clinically present as musculoskeletal tumors. Individual discussions highlight magnetic resonance imaging and computed tomography imaging appearances. Radiography, angiography, scintigraphy, ultrasound, and positron emission tomography are covered where appropriate. In addition to imaging appearance, discussions include a summary of general information, clinical presentation, pathology, treatment, and prognosis. The text concludes with a review compartmental anatomy required for local tumor staging.

MARK J. KRANSDORF
MARK D. MURPHEY

Acknowledgments

Mark and I greatly appreciate the privilege of serving as members of the Department of Radiologic-Pathology at the Armed Forces Institute of Pathology (AFIP). Our affiliation with the AFIP has allowed us to be both teachers and students.

We are grateful to all of those who have contributed material to the AFIP, and we would particularly like to thank the radiology residents who attend the Radiologic-Pathology Course and our musculoskeletal fellows (past, present, and future), for:

their dedication to knowledge—which inspires us,
their enthusiasm—which gives us the energy to
    continue, and
their penetrating questions—*which keep us humble!*

I am particularly indebted to my orthopedic oncology colleagues and would especially like to thank Mary I. O'Connor, H. Thomas Temple, G. Douglas Letson, William C. Foster, and B. Hudson Berrey for allowing me to assist them in the care of their patients.

Special thanks must also be extended to Jeanne M. Meis-Kindblom, for her assistance and guidance in the conception of this project, and to Richard P. Moser, for his continued help over the years. Finally, I would like to thank Joseph A. Utz and James S. Jelinek, for their encouragement and counsel, and, more importantly, for teaching and reminding me just how much fun radiology can be.

MJK

I want to acknowledge the importance of the section of Orthopedic Surgery and the Department of Radiology (particularly James R. Neff, Arthur A. DeSmet, and Arch W. Templeton) while I was at the University of Kansas Medical Center, for fostering my initial interest in musculoskeletal radiology. A special thank you to Mark J. Kransdorf, for inviting me to participate in this project and for putting up with me during the book's production.

I am also particularly indebted to both musculoskeletal and orthopedic colleagues who have shared their valuable knowledge and allowed me to assist in the care of their patients, including Howard G. Rothenthal, H. Thomas Temple, Fred Gilkey, Francis H. Gannon, Albert J. Aboulafia, Alan M. Levine, Donald Gajewski, Richard Schaefer, John F. Fetsch, Julie C. Fanburg-Smith, and Markku Miettinen. Special thanks to my closest musculoskeletal colleagues for their help in teaching me through my academic career: James S. Jelinek, Mark J. Kransdorf, and Donald J. Flemming.

I am grateful to my parents, Douglas K. Murphey and Joyce M. Murphey, for their unwavering support and love and their ability to instill within me a thirst for knowledge without which this book would not be possible. Finally, and most importantly, I want to thank my family, sons Matthew Travis and Lucas Ryan, and Jill (my much better half, a fact that anybody who knows me will thoroughly agree with). They provide my foundation and strength through their love and support and put up with my often early morning hours of work.

MDM

Special Acknowledgment

We would like to acknowledge our personal indebtedness to Donald E. Sweet and Lent C. Johnson for their inspiration in the pursuit of knowledge. They taught us substance over style and concept over doctrine. They may be gone, but their teachings are incorporated into the fundamental fabric of what we know as radiologic-pathology.

MJK
MDM

Origin and Classification of Soft Tissue Tumors

Soft tissue sarcomas, unlike benign soft tissue lesions, are relatively uncommon and are estimated to represent about 1% of all malignant tumors (1–3). Hajdu (1) noted that in the United States, the incidence of soft tissue sarcomas is about the same as that of multiple myeloma or carcinoma of the thyroid. Soft tissue sarcomas are three to four times as common as primary malignant bone tumors (1). An analysis of soft tissue sarcomas by Baldursson et al. (4) in Iceland, between 1955 and 1988, revealed an age-standardized incidence rate of 2.7 per 100,000 of population. Rydholm (5) noted an age-standardized incidence rate of 1.4 per 100,000 of population in Sweden. The incidence of soft tissue sarcoma increases markedly with age; the age-specific annual incidence for patients 80 years and older is 8 per 100,000 (5). It is difficult to estimate the annual incidence of benign soft tissue tumors, because many lipomas, hemangiomas, and other benign lesions do not undergo biopsy; however, the annual clinical incidence of benign soft tissue tumors is estimated at 300 per 100,000 (5).

CLASSIFICATION

The soft tissue is derived primarily from mesenchyme and, by convention, comprises the skeletal muscle, fat, fibrous tissue, peripheral nervous system, and the serving vascular structures (6). Soft tissue tumors are classified histologically on the basis of the adult tissues that they resemble (6,7). The designations of *lipoma* and *liposarcoma*, for example, do not indicate that these lesions arise from fat, but that they "recapitulate to a varying degree normal fatty tissue" (6). Many sarcomas are poorly differentiated; consequently, they lack the microscopic features that are required to make a specific diagnosis. In such cases, immunohistochemical staining and genetic analysis have aided pathologists in further classifying tumors. These techniques are well established and are used routinely. Despite the pathologist's best efforts, a small number of soft tissue sarcomas can not be further classified. This group of sarcomas that cannot be further subclassified previously comprised approximately 5% to 15% of soft tissue sarcomas (4,8), although current immunochemical and genetic techniques will continue to reduce this number.

The histological classification of soft tissue tumors used in this text reflects the new World Health Organization (WHO) classification adopted in 2002 (9). This new classification includes a revised categorization of biological behavior that now allows for two designations of intermediate malignancy: locally aggressive and rarely metastasizing (9). This new classification also redefines certain existing lesions; for example, the term *malignant fibrous histiocytoma* (MFH) has been replaced with the term *undifferentiated pleomorphic sarcoma* (9). The current WHO classification is summarized in Table 1.1. This table does not include tumors of the peripheral nervous system, which are summarized in Table 1.2 (10).

KEY CONCEPTS
- Soft tissue tumors are classified histologically on the basis of the adult tissues that they resemble.
- Poorly differentiated tumors may lack the microscopic features required for histological classification.
- Immunohistochemistry and genetic analysis may aid in further classification.

TABLE 1.1
WORLD HEALTH ORGANIZATION CLASSIFICATION OF SOFT TISSUE TUMORS

Adipocytic Tumors

Benign
Lipoma
Lipomatosis
Lipomatosis of nerve
Lipoblastoma/lipoblastomatosis
Angiolipoma
Myolipoma of soft tissue
Chondroid lipoma
Spindle cell lipoma/pleomorphic lipoma
Hibernoma

Intermediate (Locally Aggressive)
Atypical lipomatous tumor/well-
     differentiated liposarcoma

Malignant
Dedifferentiated liposarcoma
Myxoid liposarcoma
Round cell liposarcoma
Pleomorphic liposarcoma
Mixed-type liposarcoma
Liposarcoma, not otherwise specified

Fibroblastic/Myofibroblastic Tumors

Benign
Nodular fasciitis
Proliferative fasciitis
Proliferative myositis
Myositis ossificans and fibroosseous
     pseudotumor of digits
Ischemic fasciitis
Elastofibroma
Fibrous hamartoma of infancy
Myofibroma/myofibromatosis
Fibromatosis coli
Juvenile hyaline fibromatosis
Inclusion body fibromatosis
Fibroma of tendon sheath
Desmoplastic fibroblastoma
Mammary-type myofibroblastoma
Calcifying aponeurotic fibroma
Angiomyofibroblastoma
Cellular angiofibroma
Nuchal-type fibroma
Gardner fibroma
Calcifying fibrous tumor
Giant cell angiofibroma

Intermediate (Locally Aggressive)
Superficial fibromatosis
Desmoid-type fibromatosis
Lipofibromatosis

Intermediate (Rarely Metastasizing)
Solitary fibrous tumor and
     hemangiopericytoma
Inflammatory myofibroblastic tumor
Low-grade myofibroblastic sarcoma
Myxoinflammatory fibroblastic sarcoma
Infantile fibrosarcoma

Malignant
Adult fibrosarcoma
Myxofibrosarcoma
Low-grade fibromyxoid sarcoma
Sclerosing epithelioid fibrosarcoma

So-called Fibrohistiocytic Tumors

Benign
Giant cell tumor of tendon sheath
Diffuse-type giant cell tumor
Deep benign fibrous histiocytoma

Intermediate (Rarely Metastasizing)
Plexiform fibrohistiocytic tumor
Giant cell tumor of soft tissue

Malignant
Pleomorphic MFH/undifferentiated
     pleomorphic sarcoma
Giant cell MFH/undifferentiated
     pleumorphic sarcoma with giant cells
Inflammatory MFH/undifferentiated
     pleomorphic sarcoma with prominent
     inflammation

Smooth Muscle Tumors

Benign
Angioleiomyoma
Deep leiomyoma
Genital leiomyoma

Malignant
Leiomyosarcoma

Pericytic (Perivascular) Tumors
Glomus tumor
Myopericytoma

Skeletal Muscle Tumors

Benign
Rhabdomyoma

Malignant
Embryonal rhabdomyosarcoma
Alveolar rhabdomyosarcoma
Pleomorphic rhabdomyosarcoma

Vascular Tumors
Hemangiomas
Epithelioid hemangioma
Angiomatosis
Lymphangioma

Intermediate (Locally Aggressive)
Kaposiform hemangioendothelioma

Intermediate (Rarely Metastasizing)
Retiform hemangioendothelioma
Papillary intralymphatic
     angioendothelioma
Composite hemangioendothelioma
Kaposi sarcoma

Malignant
Epithelioid hemangioendothelioma
Angiosarcoma of soft tissue

Chondro-Osseous Tumors
Soft tissue chondroma
Mesenchymal chondrosarcoma
Extraskeletal osteosarcoma

Tumors of Uncertain Differentiation

Benign
Intramuscular myxoma
Juxta-articular myxoma
Deep "aggressive" angiomyxoma
Pleomorphic hyalinizing angiectatic
     tumor of soft parts
Ectopic hamartomatous thymoma

Intermediate (Rarely Metastasizing)
Angiomatoid fibrous histiocytoma
Ossifying fibromyxoid tumor
Mixed tumor/myoepithelioma/
     parachordoma

Malignant
Synovial sarcoma
Epithelioid sarcoma
Alveolar soft part sarcoma
Clear cell sarcoma of soft tissue
Extraskeletal myxoid chondrosarcoma
PNET/extraskeletal Ewing tumor
Desmoplastic small round cell tumor
Extrarenal rhabdoid tumor
Malignant mesenchymoma
Neoplasms with perivascular epithelioid
     cell differentiation (PEComa)
Intimal sarcoma

PNET, primitive neuroectodermal tumor.

Immunohistochemistry

Although the diagnosis of soft tissue tumors can frequently be made on the basis of light microscopic features, as many as 20% of cases cannot be definitively classified, even by experienced pathologists (12). Many soft tissue tumors have features that overlap. This includes various spindle cell tumors as well as other nonsarcomatous lesions such as carcinoma, melanoma, and lymphoma; therefore, additional methods may be required to further classify these lesions (12–14).

In addition to standard hematoxylin-eosin–stained slides, additional staining referred to as *histochemical techniques* may be used (12–14). For example, trichrome stain may be used to distinguish fibrous tissue from muscle tissue (13). Intracytoplasmic glycogen usually seen in lesions such as Ewing sarcoma may be identified with periodic acid–Schiff (PAS) stain (13). More recently, immunohistochemical techniques have been applied to the diagnosis of soft tissue tumors.

Immunohistochemistry is the process of detecting the presence of specific proteins in a cell or tissue with the use of antibodies. In soft tissue pathology, the main application of immunohistochemistry is in the detection of differentiation markers specifically related to certain mesenchymal phenotypes (15). Immunohistochemistry is also useful in the detection of various cell proliferation markers, oncoproteins, and tumor suppressor proteins (15). Although immunohistochemistry is not totally specific, it is currently the best way to further characterize soft tissue sarcomas for which light microscopy is not diagnostic (13,16).

For those not directly involved with immunology, the nomenclature is difficult, confusing, and at times overwhelming. Historically, immunohistochemistry was initially developed to distinguish among classes of lymphocytes on the basis of their cell surface antigens by producing antibodies that would selectively recognize different cell subpopulations (17). Surface antigens (markers) were initially named according to the antibodies that reacted with them, and in an attempt to eliminate confusion with their designation, a uniform nomenclature system was adopted. According to this system, surface markers were given a "CD" (cluster of differentiation) designation (17). This system was initially used for human leukocyte antigens and has since been more widely applied to other cells. The most important markers used in the diagnosis of soft tissue tumors and their diagnostic targets are listed in Table 1.3.

Cytogenetics

Advances in molecular biology have added a new dimension to the diagnosis of soft tissue tumors. The ability to detect specific genetic abnormalities, in the form of chromosomal translocations and the resulting translocation fusion products, can be used as a disease-specific marker in diagnosis (18). A review of medical genetics is beyond the scope of this text; however, some basic definitions may be useful.

A translocation is the interchange of genetic material between nonhomologous chromosomes—the movement of a DNA fragment from one chromosomal location to another. The result is an abnormal chromosome that contains genetic material from two or more chromosomes (18). A fusion gene is the joining of heterologous gene fragments that occurs as a result of a translocation.

Translocations are generally specific for particular types of tumors and as such are useful diagnostic markers. They are detected by cytogenetics or gene fusion assay. A list of the lesions detectable by specific chromosome translocations and other gene fusions is shown in Table 1.4.

TEXT ORGANIZATION

This text is broadly organized by tissue type. Whereas many chapters, such as the chapter on lipomatous tumors, will closely follow the classification system used by the WHO, other chapters will not. We have retained the broad tissue-type organization because it is more functional and useful for radiologists in establishing radiologic differential diagnoses.

TABLE 1.2

CLASSIFICATION OF PERIPHERAL NERVE SHEATH TUMORS[a]

Nonneoplastic Lesions
Morton neuroma
Traumatic neuroma

Neurofibroma
Cutaneous
Cellular
Diffuse
Epithelioid

Schwannoma
Conventional
Cellular
Plexiform
Epithelioid

Nerve Sheath Myxoma

Perineurioma
Intraneural perineurioma
Soft tissue perineurioma

Granular Cell Tumor
Granular cell tumor
Malignant granular cell tumor

Malignant Peripheral Nerve Sheath Tumor (MPNST)
Malignant peripheral nerve sheath tumor
MPNST with rhabdomyoblastic differentiation

---

[a]Adapted from Refs. 10 and 11.

TABLE 1.3

IMMUNOHISTOCHEMICAL MARKERS USED IN THE DIAGNOSIS OF SOFT TISSUE TUMORS[a]

Marker	Useful In Diagnosis/Positive In
Endothelial Markers	
CD31	Angiosarcoma, Kaposi sarcoma
CD34	Kaposi sarcoma, many vascular fibroblastic and other tumors
CD141	Variable in angiosarcoma, positive in mesothelioma, squamous carcinoma
Fli-1	Angiosarcoma, Ewing sarcoma
Muscle Cell Markers	
Actin, common muscle	Smooth and skeletal muscle tumors, myofibroblastic tumors
Actin, smooth muscle	Smooth muscle and myofibroblastic tumors
Actin, sarcomeric	Skeletal muscle and rhabdomyosarcoma
Desmin	Smooth and skeletal muscle tumors, some other tumors
HCD	Smooth muscle and its tumors, myoepithelia, GI stromal tumors
Calponin	Smooth muscle, myofibroblasts, myoepithelia, synovial sarcoma (often)
MyoD1, myogenin	Rhabdomyosarcoma (reactive skeletal muscle)
Myoglobin	Rhabdomyosarcoma (differentiated)
Myosins	Isoforms for smooth and skeletal muscle tumors
Neural and Neuroendocrine-Specific Markers	
Synaptophysin	Neuroblastoma, paraganglioma, neuroendocrine carcinoma
Chromogranin	Paraganglioma, neuroendocrine carcinoma (especially low-grade)
NSE	General neuroendocrine marker (poor specificity)
NF proteins	Neuroblastoma, paraganglioma, Merkel cell carcinoma
S-100 Protein and Other Multispecific Neural Markers	
S-100 protein	Melanocytic, schwannian, chondroid, Langerhans cell
Nerve growth factor receptor p75	Dermatofibrosarcoma protuberans and other nerve sheath tumors
CD56 (NCAM)	Neuroendocrine carcinoma, rhabdomyosarcoma, many other sarcomas
CD57	Nerve sheath tumor, synovial sarcoma, leiomyosarcoma (relatively nonspecific)
Melanoma Markers Other Than S-100 Protein	
HMB45	Melanoma, clear cell sarcoma, angiomyolipoma
Tyrosinase	Nevi, melanoma
Melinoma	Nevi, melanoma, angiomyolipoma
Microphthalmia	Melanoma, osteoclastic giant cells
CD63	Melanoma, some carcinomas, alveolar soft parts sarcoma
Histiocytic Markers	
Lysozyme	Histiocytes, myelomonocytic cells
Factor Xiia	Histiocytes, especially dendritic ones
CD68	Histiocytes, melanoma, paraganglioma, schwannoma, granular cell tumor
CD163	Histiocytes
Keratin	
Keratin	Carcinoma, synovial and epithelioid sarcoma, chordoma
Other Markers	
EMA	Epithelial tumors, perineural tumors
CEA	Many adenocarcinomas, biphasic synovial sarcoma
Desmoplakin	Epithelial tumors in general, meningioma, Ewing sarcoma
HBME-1	Mesothelioma, some adenocarcinoma, synovial sarcoma, chondroma
CD99	Ewing sarcoma, widespread in different tumors
CD117	GI stromal tumor, angiosarcoma, Ewing sarcoma, and others
GFAP	Glial tumors, schwannomas, myoepithelial tumors
Osteocalin	Osteosarcoma, osteoid material
Vimentin	Mesenchymal tumors, many poorly differentiated carcinomas

[a]Adapted from Table 3-1, Ref. 16.

TABLE 1.4
USEFUL DIAGNOSTIC GENETIC TUMOR MARKERS[a]

Tumor	Aberration
Aggressive angiomyxoma	t(8;12)(p12;q15)
Alveolar soft parts sarcoma	t(X;17)(p;11;q25)
Angiomatoid fibrous histiocytoma	t(12;16)(q13;p11)
Clear cell sarcoma	t(12;22)(q13;q12)
Desmoplastic small round cell tumor	t(11;22)(p13;q12)
Dermatofibrosarcoma protuberans	t(17;22)(q21;q13)
Ewing sarcoma (PNET)	t(11;22)(q24;q12), t(21;22)(q22;q12), t(7;22)(p22;q12), and others
Extraskeletal chondrosarcoma	t(9;22)(q22;q12), t(9;17)(q22;q11), and others
Fibrosarcoma, infantile	t(12;15)(p12;q25)
Hemangioendothelioma, epithelioid	t(1;3)(p36.3;q25)
Hemangiopericytoma	t(12;19)(q13;q13)
Leiomyoma, uterine	t(12;14)(q15;q24)
Lipoblastoma	8q12 rearrangement
Lipoma	t(3;12)(q27;q14-q15), t(12;13)(q13-q15; q12-q14), and others
Liposarcoma, myxoid	t(12;16)(q13;p11), t(12;22)(q13;q12)
Rhabdomyosarcoma, alveolar	t(2;13)(q35;q14), t(1;13)(p36;q14)
Synovial sarcoma	t(X;18)(p11;q11)

[a]Adapted from Table 4-1, Ref. 18.

For example, a radiologist may recognize a mass as originating from a joint or synovial-lined structure and direct the differential accordingly. The WHO classification system does not include a category of synovial lesions. Lesions that typically occur in the juxta-articular region are classified by the WHO on their histogenesis and may be included in the chapters on tumors of uncertain differentiation or on so-called fibrohistiocytic tumors (19). The former group includes synovial sarcoma, whereas the latter includes the spectrum of benign proliferative disorders of the synovium (giant cell tumor of tendon sheath and pigmented villonodular synovitis). Whereas the histiogenic approach is best for the pathologist, the adherence to a broad tissue typing remains more useful for the radiologist. Using the previous example, it gives us greater freedom to include relevant tumor-like lesions and allows us to include synovial cysts and ganglions in the chapter on synovial lesions.

REFERENCES

1. Jemal A, Murray T, Ward E, et al. Cancer statistics, 2005. *CA Cancer J Clin.* 2005;55:16–30.
2. Du Boulay CEH. Immunohistochemistry of soft tissue tumors: a review. *J Pathol.* 1985;146:77–94.
3. Greelee RT, Hill-Harmon MB, Murray T, et al. Cancer statistics 2001. *CA Cancer J Clin.* 2001;51:15–36.
4. Baldursson G, Agnarsson BA, Benediktsdottir KR, et al. Soft tissue sarcomas in Iceland 1955–1988. *Acta Oncol.* 1991;30:563–568.
5. Rydholm A. Management of patients with soft-tissue tumors. Strategy developed at a regional oncology center. *Acta Orthopaed.* 1983;54(suppl 203):1–77.
6. Weiss SW, Goldblum JR. General considerations. In: Weiss SW, Goldblum JR, eds. *Enzinger and Weiss's Soft Tissue Tumors*. St. Louis: Mosby, 2001:1–19.
7. Angervall L, Kindblom LG. Principles for pathologic-anatomic diagnosis and classification of soft-tissue sarcomas. *Clin Orthop.* 1993;289:9–18.
8. Mettlin C, Priore R, Rao U, et al. Results of the national soft-tissue sarcoma registry. *J Surg Oncol.* 1982;19:224–227.
9. Christopher DM, Unni KK, Mertens F. WHO classification of soft tissue tumors. *Pathology and Genetics: Tumors of Soft Tissue and Bone.* Lyon, France: IARC Press, 2002.
10. Kleihues P, Cavenee WK. WHO classification of soft tissue tumors. *Pathology and Genetics of Tumors of the Nervous System.* Lyon, France: IARC Press, 2000:63–222.
11. Miettinen M. Nerve sheath tumors. In: Miettinen M, ed. *Diagnostic Soft Tissue Pathology.* New York: Churchill Livingstone, 2003:343–378.
12. Ordonez NG. Application of immunocytochemistry in the diagnosis of soft tissue sarcomas: a review and update. *Adv Anat Pathol.* 1998;5:67–85.
13. Angervall L, Kindblom LG. Principles for pathologic-anatomic diagnosis and classification of soft-tissue sarcomas. *Clin Orthop.* 1993;289:9–18.
14. Carbone A, Gloghini A, Volpe R. The value of immunohistochemistry in the diagnosis of soft tissue sarcomas. *Ann Oncol.* 1992;3:S51–S54.
15. Zhang P, Brooks JS. Modern pathological evaluation of soft tissue sarcoma specimens and its potential role in soft tissue sarcoma research. *Curr Treat Options Oncol.* 2004;5:441–450.
16. Miettinen M. Immunohistochemistry of soft tissue tumors. *Diagnostic Soft Tissue Pathology.* New York: Churchill Livingstone, 2003:41–98.
17. Abbas AK, Lichtman AH, Pober JS. *Cellular and Molecular Immunology.* Philadelphia: WB Saunders, 1997:15–33.
18. Lasota J. Genetics of soft tissue tumors. In: Miettinen M, ed. *Diagnostic Soft Tissue Pathology.* New York: Churchill Livingstone, 2003:99–142.
19. Christopher DM, Unni KK, Mertens F. WHO classification of tumors. *Pathology and Genetics: Tumors of Soft Tissue and Bone.* Lyon, France: IARC Press, 2002:185.

Soft Tissue Tumors in a Large Referral Population: Prevalence and Distribution of Diagnoses by Age, Sex, and Location

The evaluation of soft tissue tumors has undergone a dramatic change with the advent of computed tomography (CT) and magnetic resonance (MR) imaging. Despite these sophisticated techniques and the increasing number of lesions that may have a characteristic imaging appearance (e.g., lipoma, hemangioma, subacute hematoma, pigmented villonodular synovitis), the majority of lesions remain nonspecific; consequently, a correct histologic diagnosis on the basis of *imaging studies alone* is reached in only approximately one-quarter to one-third of cases (1–4).

It is often not possible to establish a meaningful differential diagnosis for nonspecific soft tissue lesions or to determine reliably whether they are benign or malignant. Unlike their intraosseous counterparts, soft tissue lesions cannot be assessed by evaluation of their growth rate or physical parameters. In these cases, knowledge of the tumor's prevalence, along with the patient's age and the lesion's location, allows one to develop a suitably ordered differential diagnosis.

This chapter presents the results of a retrospective analysis of 31,047 soft tissue tumors seen in consultation by the Department of Soft Tissue Pathology, Armed Forces Institute of Pathology, during the 10-year period beginning January 1, 1980 (5,6). The purpose of this analysis was (i) to determine the relative prevalence, age at presentation, sex distribution, and skeletal distribution of soft tissue tumors and (ii) to ascertain the relative frequency of these tumors in specific anatomic locations and age groups among a population of patients in a large pathologic consultation service.

Only mesenchymal lesions originating in soft tissue were included in the study. Intra-abdominal and retroperitoneal lesions were also included when the lesions were not thought to originate in bowel or abdominal viscera. Hence, leiomyosarcoma of the vena cava was included, whereas an angiosarcoma of the spleen was not. Lesions arising in the chest and abdominal walls and the paraspinal region were also included, as they are frequently within the purview of the musculoskeletal radiologist.

All soft tissue tumors and tumor-like lesions were placed in one of 121 major diagnostic categories. For purposes of analysis, all lesions were placed in one of 10 locations: hand and wrist, upper extremity, proximal limb girdle (axilla and shoulder), foot and ankle, lower extremity, hip and buttocks region, head and neck, trunk, retroperitoneum, and other lesions. This last category included lesions coded as abdomen, pelvis, mediastinum, or location unknown.

In total, the records of 42,490 lesions occurring in 38,484 patients were reviewed. Multiple lesions were seen in

(*Text continues on p. 36*)

TABLE 2.1
MALIGNANT SOFT TISSUE TUMORS[a]

Diagnosis	Total No.	%
Malignant fibrous histiocytoma	2,978	24.1
Liposarcoma	1,755	14.2
Sarcoma, not further classified	1,457	11.8
Leiomyosarcoma	1,039	8.4
Malignant schwannoma	775	6.3
Dermatofibrosarcoma protuberans	771	6.2
Synovial sarcoma	672	5.4
Fibrosarcoma, adult	553	4.5
Extraskeletal chondrosarcoma	263	2.1
Angiosarcoma	251	2.0
Rhabdomyosarcoma	239	1.9
Angiomatoid malignant fibrous histiocytoma	199	1.6
Epithelioid sarcoma	170	1.4
Kaposi sarcoma	152	1.2
Malignant hemangiopericytoma	141	1.1
Extraskeletal Ewing sarcoma	131	1.1
Clear cell sarcoma	130	1.1
Atypical fibroxanthoma	121	1.0
Hemangioendothelioma	109	0.9
Infantile fibrosarcoma	97	0.8
Extraskeletal osteosarcoma	79	0.6
Alveolar soft part sarcoma	65	0.5
Malignant mesothelioma	46	0.4
Neuroblastoma	35	0.3
Giant cell fibroblastoma	31	0.3
Malignant mesenchymoma	24	0.2
Malignant granular cell tumor	23	0.2
Peripheral neuroepithelioma	19	0.2
Ganglioneuroblastoma	18	0.2
Malignant giant cell tumor of tendon sheath	10	0.1
Primative neuroectodermal tumor	9	0.1
Malignant paraganglioma	8	0.1

[a]Based on an analysis of 12,370 cases seen in consultation over 10 years.

TABLE 2.2
BENIGN SOFT TISSUE TUMORS[a]

Diagnosis	Total No.	%
Lipoma and lipoma variants	2,999	16.1
Fibrous histiocytoma	2,385	12.8
Nodular fasciitis	2,116	11.3
Hemangioma (all)	1,418	7.6
Fibromatosis (all)	1,297	6.9
Neurofibroma	973	5.2
Schwannoma	895	4.8
Giant cell tumor of tendon sheath	731	3.9
Myxoma (all)	597	3.2
Granuloma annulare/necrobiotic nodule	408	2.2
Hemangiopericytoma	384	2.1
Granular cell tumor	348	1.9
Leiomyoma (including angiomyoma)	311	1.7
Chondroma (all)	277	1.5
Fibroma of tendon sheath	272	1.5
Fibroma (all)	217	1.2
Myofibromatosis	178	1.0
Glomus tumor	164	0.9
Pigmented villonodular synovitis	161	0.9
Lymphangioma (all)	160	0.9
Ganglion	159	0.9
Proliferative fasciitis	144	0.8
Myositis ossificans (all)	139	0.7
Papillary endothelial hyperplasia	136	0.7
Infantile fibromatosis	116	0.6
Lipoblastoma	114	0.6
Neurothekeoma	92	0.5
Fibrous hamartoma of infancy	84	0.5
Neuroma	76	0.4
Calcifying aponeurotic fibroma	75	0.4
Mesothelioma	72	0.4
Juvenile xanthogranuloma	71	0.4
Proliferative myositis	57	0.3
Paraganglioma	56	0.3
Tumoral calcinosis	55	0.3
Elastofibroma	51	0.3
(Teno)synovial chondromatosis	46	0.3
Sclerosing retroperitonitis	44	0.2
Hibernoma	41	0.2
Ganglioneuroma	37	0.2
Other	144	0.8
Mesenchymal lesion, not further classified	577	3.1

[a]Based on an analysis of 18,677 cases seen in consultation over 10 years.

TABLE 2.3
LESIONS OF BLOOD AND LYMPH VESSELS

A. Age Distribution of Lesions of Blood and Lymph Vessels

Diagnosis	<1	1–5	6–10	11–15	16–20	21–25	26–30	31–35	36–40	41–45	46–50	51–55	56–60	61–65	66–70	71–75	76–80	81–85	>85	Unknown Age
Benign Lesions of Blood Vessels																				
Capillary hemangioma[a]	32	17	12	20	24	18	23	27	28	21	23	16	13	20	10	10	3	6	2	16
Cavernous hemangioma	21	15	12	10	12	7	7	9	9	5	4	4	5	7	3	3	2			3
Arteriovenous hemangioma	1	13	4	8	4	11	5	5	5	1	3			2	4					
Epithelioid hemangioma			1	1	10	12	16	23	18	11	8	6	4	4	4	1	1		1	10
Intramuscular hemangioma	3	15	23	24	29	46	44	31	20	13	18	8	9	1	8	2	3	1		3
Hemangioma, not further classified	8	26	18	39	35	46	36	29	31	16	18	19	22	8	18	8	1	2	4	12
Angiomatosis	3	6	6	5	6	2		2		3	4	1	1							
Glomus[b]			2	6	9	13	7	7	15	13	13	12	8	12	14	10	6	3	2	12
Hemangiopericytoma	9	1	3	7	11	22	42	34	41	39	40	24	25	21	24	19	9	6	1	6
Papillary endothelial hyperplasia	2		1	5	13	16	9	11	12	16	7	8	9	6	6	7	4		2	2
Benign Lesions of Lymph Vessels																				
Lymphangioma	10	45	11	20	11	12	7	5	3	6	5	2	4	4	1	1	1	2		1
Lymphangiomatosis		3			1	2						1		1				1		
Lymphangiomyoma/ lymphangiomyomatosis					1	1	1	1	1	1	1									
Malignant Tumors																				
Hemangioendothelioma			3	5	7	13	12	5	14	7	9	6	8	4	6	3	1	2		4
Angiosarcoma	3	3	8	8	11	16	18	12	14	10	9	23	23	22	21	11	14	9	9	7
Kaposi sarcoma					2		7	10	5	5	3	3	9	18	20	16	29	9	11	5
Malignant hemangiopericytoma	5		2	2	3	12	10	10	10	9	12	18	7	9	8	10	7	2	2	3

[a]Includes juvenile hemangioma.
[b]Includes glomangioma and glomangiomyoma.

B. Mean Age, Sex, and Skeletal Distribution of Lesions of Blood and Lymph Vessels

Diagnosis	Total No.	Mean Age	Std Dev	Sex			Hand Wrist	Upper Ext	Prox Limb	Foot Ankle	Lower Ext	Hip Butt	Head Neck	Trunk	Retro	Other
				M	F	Unknown										
Benign Lesions of Blood Vessels	**2,102**															
Capillary hemangioma	347	33.9	23.0	164	173	4	121	28	10	20	22	4	103	31	2	6
Cavernous hemangioma	138	25.3	22.6	66	70	2	21	14	9	8	24	3	22	33	2	2
Arteriovenous hemangioma	66	23.6	18.8	37	29		14	8	1	6	13	2	9	7	5	1
Epithelioid hemangioma	131	37.7	15.0	83	45	3	16	12	3	5	2	5	71	11	2	4
Intramuscular hemangioma	301	28.8	16.9	161	140		10	44	21	9	76	9	30	88	6	8
Hemangioma, not further classified	396	32.1	20.6	183	211	2	81	42	12	40	59	21	59	65	6	11
Angiomatosis	39	20.2	17.6	16	22	1	3	2		12	13	1	1	6	1	
Glomus tumor	164	47.1	19.9	107	55	2	52	38	3	12	38	7	4	7	1	2
Hemangiopericytoma	384	44.0	18.5	159	225		11	24	19	10	59	57	73	59	69	3
Papillary endothelial hyperplasia	136	40.9	19.5	70	64	2	42	12	12	12	8	2	29	15	2	2
Benign Lesions of Lymph Vessels	**167**															
Lymphangioma	151	19.1	20.3	67	84		12	14	15	5	21	9	21	19	32	3
Lymphangiomatosis	9	28.3	27.0	3	6			2	1	1	2		1	1		1
Lymphangiomyoma/lymphangiomatosis	7	32.1	10.7	1	6									1	6	
Malignant Lesions	**653**															
Hemangioendothelioma	109	40.1	18.5	45	63	1	18	21	2	27	15	5	9	9		3
Angiosarcoma	251	48.7	23.1	129	117	5	13	18	4	13	39	25	62	47	12	18
Kaposi sarcoma	152	64.4	17.9	105	44	3	12	16	3	73	16	10	11	4		7
Malignant hemangiopericytoma	141	46.4	20.7	71	69	1	2	8	6		27	13	19	23	23	20
	2,922															

TABLE 2.4
LESIONS OF CARTILAGE AND BONE-FORMING TISSUE

A. Age Distribution of Lesions of Cartilage and Bone-Forming Tissue

Diagnosis	<1	1–5	6–10	11–15	16–20	21–25	26–30	31–35	36–40	41–45	46–50	51–55	56–60	61–65	66–70	71–75	76–80	81–85	>85	Unknown Age
Benign Lesions																				
Panniculitis ossificans				5	7	7	3	7	2	6	2	1	2	2		1				1
Myositis ossificans	1	5	7	10	8	6	9	7	3	4	5	3	1	2	3	2	2			
Fibro-osseous pseudotumor	1	1				3	1	2	1		1			2						
Fibrodysplasia ossificans progessiva	2	1																		
Chondroma/osteochondroma/osteoma[a]	1	1	7	17	13	18	22	20	20	14	22	21	28	19	17	15	7	3	1	11
Malignant Lesions																				
Extraskeletal chondrosarcoma	2	5	5	9	16	7	23	16	18	22	23	25	30	26	17	7	4	1		7
Extraskeletal osteosarcoma		3		1	1	3	2	3	3	6	9	9	13	7	8	9			2	

[a]Includes a single osteoma.

B. Mean Age, Sex, and Skeletal Distribution of Lesions of Cartilage and Bone-Forming Tissue

Diagnosis	Total No.	Mean Age	Std Dev	Sex M	Sex F	Sex Unknown	Hand Wrist	Upper Ext	Prox Limb	Foot Ankle	Lower Ext	Hip Butt	Head Neck	Trunk	Retro	Other
Benign Lesions	**416**															
Panniculitis ossificans	46	32.3	15.4	21	25		9			1	19	3	2	11		1
Myositis ossificans	78	35.1	20.3	42	36		8	9	10		27	8	3	12	1	
Fibro-osseous pseudotumor	12	31.9	18.7	4	8		12									
Fibrodysplasia ossificans progressiva	3	5.7	4.0	2	1				1				1	1		
Chondroma/osteochondroma/osteoma	277	43.8	20.2	149	125	3	150	8	2	76	17	3	6	11	1	3
Malignant Lesions	**342**															
Extraskeletal chondrosarcoma	263	49.1	18.7	154	108	1	10	18	15	23	92	30	13	37	8	17
Extraskeletal osteosarcoma	79	56.9	18.0	49	29	1	3	5	2	4	20	10	3	16	10	6
	758															

TABLE 2.5
FIBROHISTIOCYTIC LESIONS

A. Age Distribution of Fibrohistiocytic Lesions

Diagnosis	<1	1–5	6–10	11–15	16–20	21–25	26–30	31–35	36–40	41–45	46–50	51–55	56–60	61–65	66–70	71–75	76–80	81–85	>85	Unknown Age
Benign Lesions																				
Fibrous histiocytoma[a]	8	59	85	148	185	305	312	268	241	192	106	103	82	72	50	26	13	8	6	116
Juvenile xanthogranuloma	40	16	6	3	3	1		1				1								
Reticulohistiocytoma			3	2	2	1	3	5	4		1	2	1	1						1
Malignant Lesions																				
Dermatofibrosarcoma protuberans	2	14	13	25	34	77	110	100	98	72	56	49	32	28	23	12	4	4	3	15
Giant cell fibroblastoma	2	18	7		2	1		1												
Atypical fibroxanthoma			2	2	6	6	7	7	7	4	8	6	8	5	11	19	8	8	6	1
Angiomatoid MFH	1	13	41	55	31	19	12	6	6	6	2	1	2		2					2
Malignant fibrous histiocytoma (MFH)	1	5	14	34	45	78	83	115	129	134	182	203	330	343	346	338	255	170	118	55

[a]Includes dermatofibroma.

B. Mean Age, Sex, and Skeletal Distribution of Fibrohistiocytic Lesions

Diagnosis	Total No.	Mean Age	Std Dev	Sex			Hand Wrist	Upper Ext	Prox Limb	Foot Ankle	Lower Ext	Hip Butt	Head Neck	Trunk	Retro	Other
				M	F	Unknown										
Benign Lesions	**2,482**															
Fibrous histiocytoma	2,385	33.3	16.6	1,283	1,078	24	354	340	234	178	561	88	300	283		47
Juvenile xanthogranuloma	71	4.3	8.6	43	27	1		7	3	2	11	2	16	25	1	4
Reticulohistiocytoma	26	26.7	15.8	15	11		2		4		5	2	4	6		3
Malignant Lesions	**4,100**															
Dermatofibrosarcoma protuberans	771	37.6	16.1	398	366	7	19	35	99	39	96	78	111	268		26
Giant cell fibroblastoma	31	5.9	6.7	22	9			4	11		7	5	3	11		
Atypical fibroblastoma	121	54.8	22.4	83	37	1	5	17	7	3	16	2	58	11		2
Angiomatoid MFH	199	17.9	12.2	93	105	1	17	54	15	3	49	14	13	32		2
Malignant fibrous histiocytoma (MFH)	2,978	59.3	18.2	1,683	1,271	24	90	416	176	103	1,072	235	174	377	230	105
	6,582															

TABLE 2.6

FIBROUS LESIONS

A. Age Distribution of Fibrous Lesions

Diagnosis	<1	1–5	6–10	11–15	16–20	21–25	26–30	31–35	36–40	41–45	46–50	51–55	56–60	61–65	66–70	71–75	76–80	81–85	>85	Unknown Age
Benign Fibrous Lesions																				
Fibroma	2	8	7	12	11	12	12	20	13	15	19	9	14	12	9	6	3	3	2	2
Nodular fasciitis	14	77	100	137	197	247	273	262	235	166	122	78	62	28	34	16	5	3	1	59
Proliferative fasciitis			5	3			3	9	8	11	12	10	20	24	16	8	7	3	1	4
Proliferative myositis	1			2				1		3	7	6	11	8	6	3	3	4	1	1
Fibroma of tendon sheath		3	11	14	15	30	33	31	37	24	10	16	18	5	8	1	1	1		14
Elastofibroma									1	2	8	5	7	9	8	4	4	1		2
Nuchal fibroma					1	3		1	2	2	6	2	3	3		1				
Nasopharyngeal angiofibroma					1			1												
Keloid			1	1	2	1		1		1	1			2						
Fibrous Tumors of Infancy/Childhood																				
Fibrous hamartoma of infancy	45	37			2															
Myofibromatosis	71	21	22	8	7	4	6	1	5	6	1	7	2	4	2	1	1	1		8
Fibromatosis coli	2																			
Infantile digital fibromatosis	5	10	3	1																
Infantile fibromatosis (desmoid type)	35	45	9	2	1	1				1										1
Calcifying aponeurotic fibroma		8	22	18	9	6	4	2	2		2			1						
Fibromatosis																				
Superficial fibromatosis		3	12	9	12	29	22	30	21	26	18	26	22	24	15	8	3	1		14
Deep fibromatosis	19	28	28	50	79	129	141	103	95	68	44	48	54	34	23	20	17	3		19
Malignant Fibrous Lesions																				
Fibrosarcoma	6	10	24	29	46	48	48	38	44	36	27	24	45	29	25	30	21	9	6	8
Fibrosarcoma, infantile type	55	35	2	2																3

B. Mean Age, Sex, and Skeletal Distribution of Fibrous Lesions

Diagnosis	Total No.	Mean Age	Std Dev	Sex			Hand Wrist	Upper Ext	Prox Limb	Foot Ankle	Lower Ext	Hip Butt	Head Neck	Trunk	Retro	Other
				M	F	Unknown										
Benign Fibrous Lesions	**2,857**															
Fibroma	193	39.7	21.1	113	78	2	39	12	11	22	32	17	30	25		5
Nodular fasciitis	2,116	31.1	15.5	1,136	967	13	152	612	130	13	288	80	418	391		32
Proliferative fasciitis	144	54.2	17.4	82	62		3	39	9	5	53	3	5	27		
Proliferative myositis	57	58.3	17.2	26	31			9	7		11	1	12	16		1
Fibroma of tendon sheath	272	35.1	15.8	174	97	1	228	5		22	9		1	1		6
Elastofibroma	51	60.6	10.7	27	24						1	1		49		
Nuchal fibroma	24	46.0	14.9	18	6								15	9		
Fibrous Tumors of Infancy and Childhood	**453**															
Fibrous hamartoma of infancy	84	1.4	2.8	52	29	3	1	15	23		9	14	5	15	1	1
Myofibromatosis	178	14.0	20.4	106	68	4	18	13	13		27	9	63	30	1	4
Infantile digital fibromatosis	19	3.2	3.4	10	9		11			8						
Infantile fibromatosis (desmoid type)	97	3.0	5.8	59	35	3	14	14	4	13	10	6	19	17		
Calcifying aponeurotic fibroma	75	15.8	11.7	48	27		43	3	1	12	7		1	8		
Fibromatoses	**1,297**															
Superficial fibromatosis	295	41.1	18.3	199	94	2	76			218				1		
Deep fibromatosis	1,002	34.3	18.0	412	585	5	70	69	69	82	103	70	72	327	76	64
Malignant Fibrous Tumors	**650**															
Fibrosarcoma	553	40.7	21.9	285	267	1	35	72	34	37	113	45	62	102	28	25
Fibrosarcoma, infantile type	97	1.5	2.4	49	46	2	3	11	9	6	25	6	20	12	2	3
	5,257															

TABLE 2.7
LESIONS OF ADIPOSE TISSUE

A. Age Distribution of Lesions of Adipose Tissue

Diagnosis	<1	1–5	6–10	11–15	16–20	21–25	26–30	31–35	36–40	41–45	46–50	51–55	56–60	61–65	66–70	71–75	76–80	81–85	>85	Unknown Age
Benign Lesions																				
Lipoma	2	11	17	30	31	46	76	114	124	115	147	125	186	166	87	59	31	14	7	61
Perineural fibrolipoma		2	2	5	2	2	4	3	1	1		1	1							1
Lipomatosis	1	2			1		1		1		1	3								
Angiolipoma				4	11	26	19	39	20	16	16	15	10	12	11	4	2		2	28
Spindle cell lipoma		1			2	9	16	34	65	60	79	96	92	118	85	67	49	11	2	30
Pleomorphic lipoma							7	10	14	10	17	21	31	31	27	15	11	3	2	8
Angiomyolipoma						1	1	1	2	6	1	3	4	4	2	1	3			1
Myelolipoma									1				4		1	1	2	1		
Intramuscular lipoma	1	1	1	9	5	7	7	11	15	23	26	32	26	25	22	20	11	6	1	4
Hibernoma				2	2	14	6	6	2	3	2	1	1		1	1				
Lipoblastoma	18	46	15	7	2															
Lipoblastomatosis	5	18	2		1															
Liposarcoma																				
Well-differentiated			1		6	10	15	23	43	58	69	74	101	121	101	99	60	24	16	13
Myxoid		1	5	12	26	22	38	42	38	37	29	21	19	22	20	14	4	2	2	6
Round cell				1	3	2	4	17	13	11	8	6	7	3	6	1				2
Pleomorphic				1		1	4	2	3	10	11	8	11	9	19	8	10	9	1	2
Dedifferentiated						1	2	2	7	6	11	10	22	23	22	21	14	6	5	4
Not further classified			3		3	5	8	8	17	14	10	21	25	26	26	18	14	7	1	6

B. Mean Age, Sex, and Skeletal Distribution of Lesions of Adipose Tissue

Diagnosis	Total No.	Mean Age	Std Dev	Sex			Hand Wrist	Upper Ext	Prox Limb	Foot Ankle	Lower Ext	Hip Butt	Head Neck	Trunk	Retro	Other
				M	F	Unknown										
Benign Lesions	**3,194**															
Lipoma	1,453	48.4	17.1	960	484	9	89	102	189	62	233	132	252	332	19	43
Perineural fibrolipoma	25	23.9	14.9	14	11		14	4		4	3					
Lipomatosis	10	30.3	22.7	3	7				1	3	2		2	2		
Angiolipoma	235	40.6	16.1	180	50	5	4	104	4	3	28	2	4	76	1	9
Spindle cell lipoma	816	56.3	14.1	714	98	4	24	17	150	7	21	32	331	223	1	10
Pleomorphic lipoma	207	57.3	13.8	143	61	3	9	25	36	4	7	1	83	40		2
Angiomyolipoma	30	53.8	14.8	3	26	1								1	29	
Myelolipoma	10	65.0	12.3	7	3									2	7	1
Intramuscular lipoma	253	52.0	17.7	143	108	2	1	26	31	2	113	8	22	44	2	4
Hibernoma	41	32.2	13.7	20	21			2	4		9	4	5	15	2	
Lipoblastoma	88	4.0	4.3	52	33	3	3	5	8	10	11	13	10	17	5	6
Lipoblastomatosis	26	3.1	3.9	11	14	1			5		4	5	2	7	3	
Liposarcoma	**1,755**															
Well-differentiated	834	50.1	14.7	480	349	5	14	49	58	10	287	83	43	103	178	9
Myxoid	360	41.5	17.6	203	155	2	3	5	13	13	220	42	8	25	29	2
Round cell	84	43.3	13.4	52	32			2	2	3	58	10		3	4	2
Pleomorphic	109	59.9	15.8	66	43		1	15	6	1	41	11	8	9	16	1
Dedifferentiated	156	62.9	13.4	80	75	1		3	4	1	21	14	1	8	103	1
Not further classified	212	55.7	17.0	125	86	1	3	13	17	3	48	19	6	21	77	5
	4,949															

TABLE 2.8
LESIONS OF MESOTHELIAL TISSUE

A. Age Distribution of Lesions of Mesothelial Tissue

Diagnosis	<1	1–5	6–10	11–15	16–20	21–25	26–30	31–35	36–40	41–45	46–50	51–55	56–60	61–65	66–70	71–75	76–80	81–85	>85	Unknown Age
Mesothelioma			2	1		3	6	7	4	10	5	4	6	5	7	5	5	2		
Malignant mesothelioma		2				1		1	3	1	4	3	5	7	8	6	5			

B. Mean Age, Sex, and Skeletal Distribution of Lesions of Mesothelial Tissue

Diagnosis	Total No.	Mean Age	Std Dev	Sex M	Sex F	Sex Unknown	Hand Wrist	Upper Ext	Prox Limb	Foot Ankle	Lower Ext	Hip Butt	Head Neck	Trunk	Retro	Other
Mesothelioma	**72**	49.9	18.3	32	40								1	11	18	42
Malignant mesothelioma	**46**	58.5	16.9	24	21	1		1	1			1		18	6	19
	118															

LESIONS OF PLURIPOTENTIAL MESENCHYME AND TUMOR-LIKE LESIONS

A. Age Distribution of Lesions of Pluripotential Mesenchyme and Tumor-Like Lesions

Diagnosis	<1	1–5	6–10	11–15	16–20	21–25	26–30	31–35	36–40	41–45	46–50	51–55	56–60	61–65	66–70	71–75	76–80	81–85	>85	Unknown Age
Tumor-Like Lesions																				
Ganglion				6	11	17	19	20	12	14	7	6	14	10	5	4	4	2		8
Inflammatory pseudotumor	1	1	3	1	1		2	1		5	4		1	5	1	1				
Granuloma annulare[a]	2	111	35	32	42	36	28	17	16	7	9	13	14	14	9	7	1	1		14
Sclerosing retroperitonitis[b]					2	1	1	2	3	3	3	9	6	7	2		3			2
Synovial cyst			1		2		2			2	1	3	2	3			1	1		2
Malignant Mesenchymoma								1	1			1	4	7	5	3		1		

[a]Includes necrobiotic nodule.
[b]Includes sclerosing mediastinitis.

B. Mean Age, Sex, and Skeletal Distribution of Lesions of Pluripotential Mesenchyme and Tumor-Like Lesions

Diagnosis	Total No.	Mean Age	Std Dev	Sex M	Sex F	Sex Unknown	Hand Wrist	Upper Ext	Prox Limb	Foot Ankle	Lower Ext	Hip Butt	Head Neck	Trunk	Retro	Other
Tumor-Like Lesions	**658**															
Ganglion	159	40.4	17.9	88	70	1	84	6	3	17	36	7	2	1		3
Inflammatory pseudotumor	27	39.3	22.2	13	14		1	2			3	1	5	1	11	3
Granuloma annulare	408	22.7	20.6	186	218	4	79	89		110	79	9	31	2		9
Sclerosing retroperitonitis	44	51.7	14.6	30	13	1									41	3
Synovial cyst	20	48.4	20.5	11	7	2	6	1	1	6	6					
Malignant Mesenchymoma	24	61.8	10.7	15	9		1				1	2	1		16	3
	682															

TABLE 2.10
MUSCLE TUMORS

A. Age Distribution of Muscle Tumors

Diagnosis	<1	1–5	6–10	11–15	16–20	21–25	26–30	31–35	36–40	41–45	46–50	51–55	56–60	61–65	66–70	71–75	76–80	81–85	>85	Unknown Age
Benign Lesions																				
Leiomyoma	1	6	3	4	5	11	11	8	8	16	15	6	7	5	6	4	1	1	1	7
Angiomyoma (vascular angiomyoma)	1	1	3		3	4	10	7	16	19	12	23	24	19	11	11	7	3	1	10
Rhabdomyoma	5	1					1	1		2		1	2	1			1			1
Myofibroblastoma									1			1	1	2	1	1		1		
Malignant Lesions																				
Leiomyosarcoma	1	6	3	3	15	17	22	40	53	65	77	91	115	129	119	115	90	41	19	18
Rhabdomyosarcoma	10	53	32	37	26	26	9	8	9	2	2	4	6	4	1	1	3			6

B. Mean Age, Sex, and Skeletal Distribution of Muscle Tumors

Diagnosis	Total No.	Mean Age	Std Dev	M	F	Unknown	Hand Wrist	Upper Ext	Prox Limb	Foot Ankle	Lower Ext	Hip Butt	Head Neck	Trunk	Retro	Other
Benign Lesions	**335**															
Leiomyoma	126	39.5	19.6	41	85		3	9	3	19	17	27	8	9	13	18
Angiomyoma (vascular leiomyoma)	185	51.0	17.0	125	60		32	24	2	58	55	3	7	1		3
Rhabdomyoma	16	31.2	28.2	14	2				1			1	10	3		1
Myofibroblastoma	8	62.4	13.9	7	1		1					3	4			
Malignant Lesions	**1,278**															
Leiomyosarcoma	1,039	58.2	16.9	501	525	13	16	56	26	46	187	96	35	70	338	169
Rhabdomyosarcoma	239	18.1	17.3	123	109	7	16	22	13	12	37	21	55	25	22	16
	1,613															

TABLE 2.11
PARAGANGLIONIC TUMORS

A. Age Distribution of Paraganglionic Tumors

Diagnosis	<1	1–5	6–10	11–15	16–20	21–25	26–30	31–35	36–40	41–45	46–50	51–55	56–60	61–65	66–70	71–75	76–80	81–85	>85	Unknown Age
Paraganglioma			1		4	3		5	8	2	3	1	4	6	7	5	5		1	1
Malignant paraganglioma									1	3				2	2					

B. Mean Age, Sex, and Skeletal Distribution of Paraganglionic Tumors

Diagnosis	Total No.	Mean Age	Std Dev	Sex			Hand Wrist	Upper Ext	Prox Limb	Foot Ankle	Lower Ext	Hip Butt	Head Neck	Trunk	Retro	Other
				M	F	Unknown										
Paraganglioma	56	47.4	18.9	24	31	1					1	2	24		22	7
Malignant paraganglioma	8	48.9	14.2	2	6								4		4	
	64															

TABLE 2.12
LESIONS OF PERIPHERAL NERVES

A. Age Distribution of Lesions of Peripheral Nerves

Diagnosis	<1	1–5	6–10	11–15	16–20	21–25	26–30	31–35	36–40	41–45	46–50	51–55	56–60	61–65	66–70	71–75	76–80	81–85	>85	Unknown Age
Benign Lesions																				
Neuroma		3	3	1	3	9	6	7	9	5	6	4	2	1	6	2	1			8
Schwannoma		4	7	19	34	76	79	92	90	63	53	54	59	75	57	58	29	13	7	26
Neurothekeoma	1	4	8	15	11	11	9	8	8	4	2	5	1	1	2					2
Neurofibroma	5	18	26	36	95	130	110	104	84	58	42	30	46	50	43	29	20	6	3	38
Granular cell tumor	1	4	14	18	28	42	36	38	30	21	28	33	19	9	5	3	2			17
Ganglioneuroma		6	4	4	4	7	2	3	1	1	1	2	1							1
Malignant Lesions																				
Malignant schwannoma	5	11	17	29	56	85	65	73	54	55	62	43	37	49	50	28	23	18	6	9
Malignant granular cell tumor			2	1	3	1	2	2	2	2	2		1	1	2		1	1		
Clear cell sarcoma			4	10	12	16	10	19	13	6	5	10	7	5	1	3	2	3		4
Ganglioneuroblastoma	2	5	1		2	3	1		3									1		
Primitive neuroectodermal tumor	1			2	1	1	1						1				2			
Peripheral neuroepithelioma			1	2	2	5	3	1	3	1					1					
Neuroblastoma	7	6		7	5	2		2			1	1	1	1			1		1	

B. Mean Age, Sex, and Skeletal Distribution of Lesions of Peripheral Nerves

Diagnosis	Total No.	Mean Age	Std Dev	Sex M	Sex F	Sex Unknown	Hand Wrist	Upper Ext	Prox Limb	Foot Ankle	Lower Ext	Hip Butt	Head Neck	Trunk	Retro	Other
Benign Lesions	2,421															
Neuroma	76	37.9	18.8	43	32	1	16	5		31	6	1	13	1		3
Schwannoma	895	45.7	19.0	504	387	4	77	107	39	81	157	52	97	120	102	63
Neurothekeoma	92	26.0	15.7	33	59		10	15	6	6	22	2	16	12		3
Neurofibroma	973	36.8	19.1	529	439	5	92	106	37	58	176	86	178	171	30	39
Granular cell tumor	348	35.1	16.2	143	204	1	37	47	29	12	51	31	34	97	2	8
Ganglioneuroma	37	21.7	15.4	17	20				1			2	4	7	18	5
Malignant Lesions	1,009															
Malignant schwannoma	775	41.7	20.6	391	376	8	20	92	70	29	183	58	82	132	62	47
Malignant granular cell tumor	23	39.3	22.5	7	16		4	3	4		4			5	1	2
Clear cell sarcoma	130	36.5	18.3	67	61	2	23	9	4	49	26	9	2	8		
Ganglioneuroblastoma	18	19.5	22.1	6	12				1			1	1	1	10	4
Primitive neuroectodermal tumor	9	35.0	25.3	2	7				1		2		1	2	2	1
Neuroepithelioma	19	28.1	13.4	12	7				1	1	7	2		5	3	
Neuroblastoma	35	19.2	21.4	15	20				4		3			3	16	6
	3,430															

TABLE 2.13
LESIONS OF SYNOVIAL TISSUE

A. Age Distribution of Lesions of Synovial Tissue

Diagnosis	<1	1–5	6–10	11–15	16–20	21–25	26–30	31–35	36–40	41–45	46–50	51–55	56–60	61–65	66–70	71–75	76–80	81–85	>85	Unknown Age
Benign Lesions																				
Giant cell tumor of tendon sheath (GCTTS)	5	13	26	43	101	75	68		59	50	62	47	43	37	31	12	12	7	1	39
Pigmented villonodular synovitis[a]		1	11	11	19	23	16		13	13	10	15	12	1	4	1	4	2		5
(Teno)synovial (osteo)chondromatosis			2	1	3	5	2		7	6	4	5		5	2	2		1		1
Malignant Lesions																				
Synovial sarcoma	3	19	61	93	102	91	80		30	31	43	33	31	17	15	11	5	1		6
Malignant GCTTS[b]	1	1	2					1				1	1	1		1		1		

[a]Includes diffuse giant cell tumor of tendon sheath.
[b]Malignant giant cell tumor of tendon sheath.

B. Mean Age, Sex, and Skeletal Distribution of Lesions of Synovial Tissue

Diagnosis	Total No.	Mean Age	Std Dev	M	F	Unknown	Hand Wrist	Upper Ext	Prox Limb	Foot Ankle	Lower Ext	Hip Butt	Head Neck	Trunk	Retro	Other
Benign Lesions	938															
Giant cell tumor of tendon sheath	731	39.2	17.6	384	339	8	474	23	1	113	90	4		4		22
Pigmented villonodular synovitis	161	37.7	17.0	93	67	1	22	1	1	52	72	5	1	2		5
Tenosynovial (osteo)chondromatosis	46	43.9	17.0	29	17		23	1	2	7	11		1	1		
Malignant Lesions	682															
Synovial sarcoma	672	32.2	16.7	331	339	2	51	91	28	120	234	53	32	44	2	17
Malignant GCTTS	10	39.4	30.2	4	6		4	1		1	3					1
	1,620															

TABLE 2.14
LESIONS OF UNCERTAIN HISTOGENESIS

A. Age Distribution of Lesions of Uncertain Histogenesis

Diagnosis	<1	1–5	6–10	11–15	16–20	21–25	26–30	31–35	36–40	41–45	46–50	51–55	56–60	61–65	66–70	71–75	76–80	81–85	>85	Unknown Age
Benign Lesions																				
Tumoral calcinosis	1	2	1	3	2	1	2	6	2	3	3	3	5	5	4	7		1	2	2
Myxoma		3	1	6	15	10	21	23	24	20	30	30	26	27	15	17	17	4	2	8
Intramuscular myxoma					1	4	11	23	24	25	33	32	38	31	10	16	5	2		7
Juxta-articular myxoma						4	2		3	2	4	3	2	5	4	3	3	1		
Malignant Lesions																				
Alveolar soft part sarcoma		3	2	7	17	13	10	8	2		1				1					1
Epithelioid sarcoma		1	6	13	15	33	35	18	15	4	4	4	5	6	4	1	1			5
Extraskeletal Ewing sarcoma	1	4	8	22	31	17	12	14	7	5		1	4			3	2			

B. Mean Age, Sex, and Skeletal Distribution of Lesions of Unknown Histogenesis

Diagnosis	Total No.	Mean Age	Std Dev	Sex M	Sex F	Sex Unknown	Hand Wrist	Upper Ext	Prox Limb	Foot Ankle	Lower Ext	Hip Butt	Head Neck	Trunk	Retro	Other
Benign Lesions	652															
Tumoral calcinosis	55	47.7	23.5	18	35	2	17	9	4	3	6	9	1	3	1	2
Myxoma	299	48.3	18.5	164	131	4	37	34	20	21	55	46	39	40	1	6
Intramuscular myxoma	262	56.0	13.3	99	162	1	2	39	20	1	139	36	9	13		3
Juxta-articular myxoma	36	53.9	17.9	23	13			1	5	2	25	2	1			
Intramuscular myxoma																
Malignant Lesions	366															
Alveolar soft part sarcoma	65	22.7	10.2	27	37	1		6	6		26	4	7	11	2	3
Epithelioid sarcoma	170	30.7	14.9	116	50	4	69	33	3	15	26	15	2	5		2
Extraskeletal Ewing sarcoma	131	24.5	14.9	75	56		2	8	10	4	24	11	8	39	13	12
	1,018															

TABLE 2.15

AGE 0–5 YEARS: COMMON LESIONS BY LOCATION

Location		Malignant Diagnoses	No. (%)	Benign Diagnoses	No. (%)
Hand and Wrist		Fibrosarcoma	5 (45)	Fibromatosis	21 (22)
Total This Location	108	Angiosarcoma	1 (9)	Hemangioma	15 (15)
Malignant	11	Epithelioid sarcoma	1 (9)	Granuloma annulare	14 (14)
Benign	97	Malignant GCTTS	1 (9)	Infantile digital fibromatosis	8 (8)
		DFSP	1 (9)	Aponeurotic fibroma	7 (7)
		Malignant schwannoma	1 (9)	Fibrous histiocytoma	5 (5)
		Rhabdomyosarcoma	1 (9)	Nodular fasciitis	5 (5)
				Other	22 (23)
Upper Extremity		Fibrosarcoma	9 (29)	Fibrous hamartoma infancy	15 (16)
Total This Location	125	Rhabdomyosarcoma	7 (23)	Granuloma annulare	15 (16)
Malignant	31	Angiomatoid MFH	3 (10)	Hemangioma	14 (15)
Benign	94	DFSP	2 (6)	Fibromatosis	13 (14)
		Giant cell fibroblastoma	2 (6)	Fibrous histiocytoma	6 (6)
		Malignant schwannoma	2 (6)	Juvenile xanthogranuloma	6 (6)
		MFH	2 (6)	Myofibromatosis	6 (6)
		Other	4 (13)	Other	19 (20)
Axilla and Shoulder		Fibrosarcoma	9 (56)	Fibrous hamartoma infancy	23 (29)
Total This Location	96	Rhabdomyosarcoma	4 (25)	Hemangioma	12 (15)
Malignant	16	Angiomatoid MFH	1 (6)	Lipoblastoma	11 (14)
Benign	80	Chondrosarcoma	1 (6)	Fibrous histiocytoma	7 (9)
		Malignant schwannoma	1 (6)	Myofibromatosis	6 (8)
				Lymphangioma	5 (6)
				Nodular fasciitis	4 (5)
				Other	12 (15)
Foot and Ankle		Fibrosarcoma	5 (45)	Granuloma annulare	23 (30)
Total This Location	87	DFSP	2 (18)	Fibromatosis	19 (25)
Malignant	11	Malignant schwannoma	2 (18)	Hemangioma	8 (11)
Benign	76	Rhabdomyosarcoma	2 (18)	Infantile digital fibromatosis	7 (9)
		Infantile digital fibromatosis	7 (9)	Lipoblastoma	6 (8)
				Lipoma	4 (5)
				Neurofibroma	3 (4)
				Other	6 (8)
Lower Extremity		Fibrosarcoma	24 (45)	Granuloma annulare	42 (23)
Total This Location	233	Rhabdomyosarcoma	8 (15)	Hemangioma	26 (14)
Malignant	53	Giant cell fibroblastoma	5 (9)	Myofibromatosis	16 (9)
Benign	180	Malignant schwannoma	5 (9)	Fibrous histiocytoma	15 (8)
		Angiomatoid MFH	3 (6)	Lipoblastoma	13 (7)
		DFSP	3 (6)	Lymphangioma	10 (6)
		Angiosarcoma	2 (4)	Juvenile xanthogranuloma	10 (6)
		Other	3 (6)	Other	48 (27)
Hip, Groin, and Buttocks		Fibrosarcoma	7 (32)	Fibrous hamartoma infancy	14 (20)
Total This Location	92	Giant cell fibroblastoma	3 (14)	Lipoblastoma	14 (20)
Malignant	22	Rhabdomyosarcoma	3 (14)	Myofibromatosis	8 (11)
Benign	70	DFSP	2 (9)	Lymphangioma	7 (10)
		MFH	2 (9)	Fibromatosis histiocytoma	5 (7)
		Leiomyosarcoma	1 (5)	Nodular fasciitis	4 (6)
		Synovial sarcoma	1 (5)	Fibromatosis	4 (6)
		Other	3 (14)	Other	14 (20)
Head and Neck		Fibrosarcoma	22 (37)	Nodular fasciitis	47 (20)
Total This Location	297	Rhabdomyosarcoma	20 (33)	Hemangioma	43 (18)
Malignant	60	Malignant hemangiopericytoma	3 (5)	Fibromatosis	30 (13)
Benign	237	Alveolar soft part sarcoma	2 (3)	Myofibromatosis	27 (11)
		DFSP	2 (3)	Granuloma annulare	14 (6)
		Malignant schwannoma	2 (3)	Fibrous histiocytoma	13 (5)
		Giant cell fibroblastoma	2 (3)	Lipoblastoma	11 (5)
		Other	7 (12)	Other	52 (22)

continued

TABLE 2.15
(continued)

Location		Malignant Diagnoses	No. (%)	Benign Diagnoses	No. (%)
Trunk		Fibrosarcoma	13 (26)	Hemangioma	36 (18)
Total This Location	253	Giant cell fibroblastoma	8 (16)	Juvenile xanthogranuloma	24 (12)
Malignant	50	Rhabdomyosarcoma	8 (16)	Myofibromatosis	24 (12)
Benign	203	Angiomatoid MFH	6 (12)	Fibromatosis	23 (11)
		DFSP	4 (8)	Lipoblastoma	17 (8)
		Ewing sarcoma	3 (6)	Nodular fasciitis	17 (8)
		Neuroblastoma	3 (6)	Fibrous hamartoma infancy	15 (7)
		Other	5 (10)	Other	47 (23)
Retroperitoneum		Fibrosarcoma	4 (20)	Lipoblastoma	7 (37)
Total This Location	39	Neuroblastoma	4 (20)	Lymphangioma	5 (26)
Malignant	20	Rhabdomyosarcoma	4 (20)	Hemangioma	4 (21)
Benign	19	Ganglioneuroblastoma	3 (15)	Ganglioneuroma	2 (11)
		Angiosarcoma	2 (10)	Fibrous hamartoma infancy	1 (5)
		Leiomyosarcoma	2 (10)		
		Alveolar soft part sarcoma	1 (5)		

DFSP, dermatofibrosarcoma protuberans; GCTTS, giant cell tumor of tendon sheath; MFH, malignant fibrous histiocytoma.

TABLE 2.16
AGE 6–15 YEARS: COMMON LESIONS BY LOCATION

Location		Malignant Diagnoses	No. (%)	Benign Diagnoses	No. (%)
Hand and wrist		Epithelioid sarcoma	9 (21)	Fibrous histiocytoma	32 (14)
Total This Location	278	Angiomatoid MFH	7 (16)	Hemangioma	31 (13)
Malignant	43	Synovial sarcoma	5 (12)	Aponeurotic fibroma	25 (11)
Benign	235	MFH	4 (9)	Fibroma of tendon sheath	22 (9)
		Angiosarcoma	3 (7)	GCTTS	17 (7)
		Rhabdomyosarcoma	3 (7)	Fibromatosis	13 (6)
		Clear cell sarcoma	2 (5)	Lipoma	9 (4)
		Other	10 (23)	Other	86 (37)
Upper Extremity		Angiomatoid MFH	30 (33)	Fibrous histiocytoma	41 (23)
Total This Location	274	Synovial sarcoma	14 (15)	Nodular fasciitis	39 (21)
Malignant	92	Fibrosarcoma	8 (9)	Hemangioma	24 (13)
Benign	182	Malignant schwannoma	7 (7)	Granuloma annulare	12 (7)
		MFH	7 (7)	Fibromatosis	11 (6)
		Rhabdomyosarcoma	7 (7)	Neurofibroma	7 (4)
		Epithelioid sarcoma	4 (4)	Neurothekeoma	6 (3)
		Other	15 (16)	Other	42 (23)
Axilla and Shoulder		Angiomatoid MFH	8 (21)	Fibrous histiocytoma	25 (34)
Total This Location	112	MFH	5 (13)	Nodular fasciitis	18 (25)
Malignant	39	Ewing sarcoma	4 (10)	Hemangioma	7 (10)
Benign	73	Malignant schwannoma	4 (10)	Granular cell tumor	4 (5)
		Rhabdomyosarcoma	4 (10)	Neurofibroma	3 (4)
		Fibrosarcoma	3 (8)	Lymphangioma	2 (3)
		Synovial sarcoma	3 (8)	Myofibromatosis	2 (3)
		Other	8 (21)	Other	12 (16)
Foot and Ankle		Synovial sarcoma	11 (21)	Fibromatosis	35 (22)
Total This Location	214	DFSP	9 (17)	Granuloma annulare	21 (13)
Malignant	53	Rhabdomyosarcoma	5 (9)	Hemangioma	21 (13)
Benign	161	Angiosarcoma	4 (8)	Fibrous histiocytoma	14 (9)
		Clear cell sarcoma	4 (8)	GCTTS	13 (8)
		Fibrosarcoma	4 (8)	Chondroma	11 (7)
		Chondrosarcoma	3 (6)	Lipoma	9 (6)
		Other	13 (25)	Other	37 (23)

continued

TABLE 2.16
(continued)

Location		Malignant Diagnoses	No. (%)	Benign Diagnoses	No. (%)
Lower Extremity		Synovial sarcoma	28 (22)	Hemangioma	47 (22)
Total This Location	344	Angiomatoid MFH	22 (17)	Fibrous histiocytoma	34 (16)
Malignant	128	MFH	13 (10)	Nodular fasciitis	22 (10)
Benign	216	Liposarcoma	11 (9)	Granuloma annulare	20 (9)
		Malignant schwannoma	9 (7)	Fibromatosis	14 (6)
		DFSP	8 (6)	Lipoma	13 (6)
		Rhabdomyosarcoma	6 (5)	Neurofibroma	8 (4)
		Other	31 (24)	Other	58 (27)
Hip, Groin, and Buttocks		Angiomatoid MFH	8 (21)	Nodular fasciitis	15 (27)
Total This Location	93	Synovial sarcoma	7 (19)	Fibroma	7 (13)
Malignant	38	Rhabdomyosarcoma	6 (16)	Fibrous histiocytoma	6 (11)
Benign	55	MFH	4 (11)	Fibromatosis	5 (9)
		Epithelioid sarcoma	2 (5)	Lipoma	5 (9)
		Fibrosarcoma	2 (5)	Lipoblastoma	3 (5)
		Malignant schwannoma	2 (5)	Neurofibroma	3 (5)
		Other	7 (18)	Other	11 (20)
Head and Neck		Rhabdomyosarcoma	17 (26)	Nodular fasciitis	75 (33)
Total This Location	293	Fibrosarcoma	13 (20)	Fibrous histiocytoma	34 (15)
Malignant	65	Synovial sarcoma	7 (11)	Neurofibroma	23 (10)
Benign	228	Malignant schwannoma	6 (9)	Hemangioma	21 (9)
		MFH	6 (9)	Myofibromatosis	14 (6)
		Angiomatoid MFH	4 (6)	Fibromatosis	12 (5)
		DFSP	2 (3)	Lipoma	6 (3)
		Other	10 (15)	Other	43 (19)
Trunk		Angiomatoid MFH	14 (15)	Nodular fasciitis	54 (28)
Total This Location	286	Fibrosarcoma	13 (14)	Fibrous histiocytoma	43 (22)
Malignant	91	Ewing sarcoma	12 (13)	Hemangioma	25 (13)
Benign	195	DFSP	12 (13)	Lipoma	9 (5)
		Malignant schwannoma	9 (10)	Neurofibroma	7 (4)
		Rhabdomyosarcoma	8 (9)	Fibromatosis	6 (3)
		MFH	3 (3)	Granular cell tumor	6 (3)
		Other	20 (22)	Other	45 (23)
Retroperitoneum		Rhabdomyosarcoma	9 (31)	Lymphangioma	7 (37)
Total This Location	48	Malignant schwannoma	5 (17)	Ganglioneuroma	4 (21)
Malignant	29	Neuroblastoma	4 (14)	Schwannoma	2 (11)
Benign	19	Ewing sarcoma	2 (7)	Fibromatosis	2 (11)
		Fibrosarcoma	2 (7)	Paraganglioma	1 (5)
		MFH	2 (7)	Hemangioma	1 (5)
		Malignant hemangiopericytoma	2 (7)	Inflammatory pseudotumor	1 (5)
		Other	3 (10)	Other	1 (5)

DFSP, dermatofibrosarcoma protuberans; GCTTS, giant cell tumor of tendon sheath; MFH, malignant fibrous histiocytoma.

TABLE 2.17

AGE 16–25 YEARS: COMMON LESIONS BY LOCATION

Location		Malignant Diagnoses	No. (%)	Benign Diagnoses	No. (%)
Hand and Wrist		Epithelioid sarcoma	25 (29)	GCTTS	84 (20)
Total This Location	506	MFH	11 (13)	Fibrous histiocytoma	57 (14)
Malignant	86	DFSP	7 (8)	Hemangioma	40 (10)
Benign	420	Synovial sarcoma	7 (8)	Fibroma of tendon sheath	40 (10)
		Rhabdomyosarcoma	7 (8)	Nodular fasciitis	26 (6)
		Angiomatoid MFH	5 (6)	Granuloma annulare	21 (5)
		Hemangioendothelioma	5 (6)	Ganglion	20 (5)
		Other	19 (22)	Other	132 (31)
Upper Extremity		Synovial sarcoma	32 (23)	Nodular fasciitis	130 (35)
Total This Location	514	MFH	19 (14)	Fibrous histiocytoma	87 (23)
Malignant	138	Malignant schwannoma	16 (12)	Hemangioma	36 (10)
Benign	376	Fibrosarcoma	12 (9)	Neurofibroma	24 (6)
		Angiomatoid MFH	10 (7)	Granuloma annulare	20 (5)
		Epithelioid sarcoma	9 (7)	Granular cell tumor	17 (5)
		Hemangioendothelioma	6 (4)	Schwannoma	11 (3)
		Other	34 (25)	Other	51 (14)
Axilla and Shoulder		Synovial sarcoma	13 (18)	Fibrous histiocytoma	62 (36)
Total This Location	246	DFSP	12 (16)	Nodular fasciitis	35 (20)
Malignant	74	Malignant schwannoma	11 (15)	Fibromatosis	16 (9)
Benign	172	Fibrosarcoma	8 (11)	Lipoma	14 (8)
		MFH	8 (11)	Neurofibroma	12 (7)
		Rhabdomyosarcoma	4 (5)	Hemangioma	4 (2)
		Angiomatoid MFH	3 (4)	Schwannoma	4 (2)
		Other	15 (20)	Other	25 (15)
Foot and Ankle		Synovial sarcoma	27 (30)	Fibromatosis	46 (22)
Total This Location	295	Clear cell sarcoma	10 (11)	GCTTS	29 (14)
Malignant	90	Fibrosarcoma	7 (8)	Granuloma annulare	25 (12)
Benign	205	DFSP	7 (8)	Fibrous histiocytoma	24 (12)
		MFH	6 (7)	Hemangioma	13 (6)
		Hemangioendothelioma	6 (7)	PVNS	12 (6)
		Malignant schwannoma	5 (6)	Neurofibroma	11 (5)
		Other	22 (24)	Other	45 (22)
Lower Extremity		Synovial sarcoma	76 (25)	Fibrous histiocytoma	118 (24)
Total This Location	822	Liposarcoma	45 (13)	Nodular fasciitis	61 (13)
Malignant	338	Malignant schwannoma	44 (13)	Hemangioma	55 (11)
Benign	484	MFH	36 (11)	Neurofibroma	48 (10)
		Fibrosarcoma	24 (7)	Fibromatosis	38 (8)
		DFSP	18 (5)	Lipoma	22 (5)
		Angiomatoid MFH	15 (4)	Schwannoma	20 (4)
		Other	80 (24)	Other	122 (25)
Hip, Groin, and Buttocks		Synovial sarcoma	15 (18)	Neurofibroma	20 (16)
Total this location	205	Malignant schwannoma	13 (16)	Fibromatosis	18 (15)
Malignant	83	Liposarcoma	8 (10)	Fibrous histiocytoma	18 (15)
Benign	122	DFSP	6 (7)	Nodular fasciitis	12 (10)
		MFH	6 (7)	Hemangioma	9 (7)
		Rhabdomyosarcoma	5 (6)	Lipoma	8 (7)
		Leiomyosarcoma	4 (5)	Hemangiopericytoma	8 (7)
		Other	26 (31)	Other	29 (24)
Head and Neck		MFH	17 (17)	Nodular fasciitis	61 (21)
Total This Location	376	DFSP	14 (16)	Hemangioma	48 (17)
Malignant	89	Malignant schwannoma	8 (9)	Fibrous histiocytoma	45 (16)
Benign	287	Synovial sarcoma	8 (9)	Neurofibroma	37 (13)
		Rhabdomyosarcoma	8 (9)	Schwannoma	19 (7)
		MFH	7 (8)	Fibromatosis	11 (4)
		Angiomatoid MFH	6 (7)	Lipoma	10 (4)
		Other	21 (24)	Other	56 (20)

continued

TABLE 2.17
(continued)

Location		Malignant Diagnoses	No. (%)	Benign Diagnoses	No. (%)
Trunk		DFSP	37 (23)	Nodular fasciitis	112 (24)
Total This Location	623	MFH	21 (13)	Fibromatosis	72 (16)
Malignant	161	Malignant schwannoma	19 (12)	Fibrous histiocytoma	71 (15)
Benign	462	Fibrosarcoma	15 (9)	Hemangioma	52 (11)
		Synovial sarcoma	13 (8)	Neurofibroma	38 (8)
		Ewing sarcoma	12 (7)	Lipoma	21 (5)
		Angiomatoid MFH	6 (4)	Schwannoma	17 (4)
		Other	38 (24)	Other	79 (17)
Retroperitoneum		Malignant schwannoma	9 (20)	Fibromatosis	14 (20)
Total This Location	115	Ewing sarcoma	8 (18)	Schwannoma	10 (14)
Malignant	44	Leiomyosarcoma	6 (14)	Neurofibroma	9 (13)
Benign	71	Ganglioneuroblastoma	4 (9)	Hemangiopericytoma	8 (11)
		Neuroblastoma	4 (9)	Lymphangioma	8 (11)
		Rhabdomyosarcoma	3 (7)	Ganglioneuroma	6 (8)
		Malignant hemangiopericytoma	2 (7)	Hemangioma	4 (6)
		Other	8 (18)	Other	12 (17)

DFSP, dermatofibrosarcoma protuberans; GCTTS, giant cell tumor of tendon sheath; MFH, malignant fibrous histiocytoma; PVNS, pigmented villonodular synovitis.

TABLE 2.18
AGE 26–35 YEARS: COMMON LESIONS BY LOCATION

Location		Malignant Diagnoses	No. (%)	Benign Diagnoses	No. (%)
Hand and Wrist		Epithelioid sarcoma	19 (23)	GCTTS	78 (16)
Total this Location	576	Synovial sarcoma	14 (17)	Fibrous histiocytoma	78 (16)
Malignant	83	Fibrosarcoma	11 (13)	Fibroma of tendon sheath	55 (11)
Benign	493	MFH	11 (13)	Hemangioma	46 (9)
		Clear cell sarcoma	7 (8)	Nodular fasciitis	43 (9)
		Liposarcoma	5 (6)	Chondroma	21 (4)
		Malignant schwannoma	3 (4)	Neurofibroma	20 (4)
		Other	13 (16)	Other	152 (31)
Upper Extremity		MFH	38 (29)	Nodular fasciitis	178 (40)
Total This Location	575	Fibrosarcoma	16 (12)	Fibrous histiocytoma	90 (20)
Malignant	133	Synovial sarcoma	15 (11)	Angiolipoma	30 (7)
Benign	442	Malignant schwannoma	14 (11)	Hemangioma	23 (5)
		DFSP	13 (10)	Schwannoma	20 (5)
		Liposarcoma	8 (6)	Neurofibroma	20 (5)
		Angiomatoid MFH	6 (5)	Fibromatosis	15 (3)
		Other	23 (17)	Other	66 (15)
Axilla and shoulder		DFSP	25 (33)	Fibrous histiocytoma	65 (33)
Total This Location	271	Malignant schwannoma	11 (15)	Lipoma	34 (17)
Malignant	75	MFH	9 (12)	Nodular fasciitis	31 (16)
Benign	196	Fibrosarcoma	5 (7)	Fibromatosis	12 (6)
		Synovial sarcoma	5 (7)	Hemangioma	11 (6)
		Ewing sarcoma	4 (5)	Schwannoma	9 (5)
		Leiomyosarcoma	3 (4)	Neurofibroma	7 (4)
		Other	13 (17)	Other	27 (14)
Foot and Ankle		Synovial sarcoma	35 (33)	Fibromatosis	57 (22)
Total This Location	369	Clear cell sarcoma	14 (13)	Fibrous histiocytoma	38 (14)
Malignant	106	MFH	11 (10)	GCTTS	32 (12)
Benign	263	Malignant schwannoma	7 (8)	Hemangioma	22 (8)
		Liposarcoma	7 (8)	Schwannoma	17 (6)
		DFSP	6 (6)	Granuloma annulare	15 (6)
		Hemangioendothelioma	6 (6)	Neurofibroma	15 (6)
		Other	20 (19)	Other	67 (25)

continued

TABLE 2.18
(continued)

Location		Malignant Diagnoses	No. (%)	Benign Diagnoses	No. (%)
Lower Extremity		Liposarcoma	79 (22)	Fibrous histiocytoma	131 (25)
Total This Location	891	MFH	63 (18)	Nodular fasciitis	85 (16)
Malignant	357	Synovial sarcoma	57 (16)	Lipoma	45 (8)
Benign	534	Malignant schwannoma	39 (11)	Neurofibroma	44 (8)
		DFSP	26 (7)	Hemangioma	32 (6)
		Fibrosarcoma	17 (5)	Schwannoma	32 (6)
		Leiomyosarcoma	12 (3)	Fibromatosis	23 (4)
		Other	64 (18)	Other	142 (27)
Hip, Groin, and Buttocks		Liposarcoma	22 (18)	Lipoma	27 (15)
Total This Location	304	DFSP	20 (17)	Fibromatosis	25 (14)
Malignant	119	Synovial sarcoma	12 (10)	Neurofibroma	23 (12)
Benign	185	MFH	12 (10)	Fibrous histiocytoma	21 (11)
		Malignant schwannoma	10 (8)	Nodular fasciitis	17 (9)
		Leiomyosarcoma	9 (8)	Schwannoma	13 (7)
		Epithelioid sarcoma	8 (7)	Myxoma	13 (7)
		Other	26 (22)	Other	46 (25)
Head and Neck		DFSP	35 (36)	Nodular fasciitis	80 (20)
Total This Location	498	Malignant schwannoma	13 (13)	Fibrous histiocytoma	78 (19)
Malignant	97	Synovial sarcoma	8 (8)	Lipoma	65 (16)
Benign	401	Liposarcoma	7 (7)	Hemangioma	57 (14)
		Angiosarcoma	5 (5)	Neurofibroma	35 (9)
		Fibrosarcoma	4 (4)	Hemangiopericytoma	22 (5)
		Angiomatoid MFH	6 (7)	Schwannoma	12 (3)
		Other	19 (20)	Other	52 (13)
Trunk		DFSP	76 (31)	Fibromatosis	96 (18)
Total This Location	778	MFH	32 (13)	Nodular fasciitis	89 (17)
Malignant	245	Malignant schwannoma	26 (11)	Fibrous histiocytoma	69 (13)
Benign	533	Fibrosarcoma	23 (9)	Lipoma	67 (13)
		Liposarcoma	18 (7)	Hemangioma	50 (9)
		Synovial sarcoma	17 (7)	Neurofibroma	39 (7)
		Angiosarcoma	8 (3)	Schwannoma	29 (5)
		Other	45 (18)	Other	94 (18)
Retroperitoneum		Leiomyosarcoma	20 (29)	Schwannoma	19 (24)
Total This Location	147	Liposarcoma	15 (22)	Fibromatosis	13 (16)
Malignant	68	Malignant schwannoma	8 (12)	Hemangiopericytoma	10 (13)
Benign	79	MFH	7 (10)	Neurofibroma	9 (11)
		Malignant hemangiopericytoma	4 (6)	Hemangioma	7 (9)
		Fibrosarcoma	2 (3)	Paraganglioma	5 (6)
		Ewing sarcoma	2 (3)	Lymphangioma	3 (4)
		Other	10 (15)	Other	13 (16)

DFSP, dermatofibrosarcoma protuberans; GCTTS, giant cell tumor of tendon sheath; MFH, malignant fibrous histiocytoma.

TABLE 2.19

AGE 36–45 YEARS: COMMON LESIONS BY LOCATION

Location		Malignant Diagnoses	No. (%)	Benign Diagnoses	No. (%)
Hand and Wrist		MFH	18 (29)	Fibrous histiocytoma	89 (20)
Total This Location	513	Synovial sarcoma	7 (11)	GCTTS	70 (16)
Malignant	63	Fibrosarcoma	6 (10)	Fibroma of tendon sheath	51 (11)
Benign	450	Epithelioid sarcoma	5 (8)	Hemangioma	40 (9)
		Liposarcoma	4 (6)	Nodular fasciitis	36 (8)
		Malignant schwannoma	4 (6)	Fibromatosis	26 (5)
		Hemangioendothelioma	4 (4)	Chondroma	21 (5)
		Other	15 (24)	Other	117 (26)
Upper Extremity		MFH	27 (26)	Nodular fasciitis	131 (36)
Total This Location	471	Malignant schwannoma	15 (15)	Fibrous histiocytoma	55 (15)
Malignant	103	Liposarcoma	12 (12)	Schwannoma	23 (6)
Benign	368	Fibrosarcoma	9 (9)	Lipoma	22 (6)
		Synovial sarcoma	8 (8)	Hemangioma	20 (5)
		Epithelioid sarcoma	7 (7)	Angiolipoma	18 (5)
		Leiomyosarcoma	5 (5)	Neurofibroma	17 (5)
		Other	20 (19)	Other	82 (22)
Axilla and Shoulder		DFSP	30 (32)	Lipoma	71 (39)
Total This Location	278	MFH	21 (22)	Fibrous histiocytoma	27 (15)
Malignant	94	Liposarcoma	19 (20)	Nodular fasciitis	24 (13)
Benign	184	Malignant schwannoma	10 (11)	Fibromatosis	17 (9)
		Fibrosarcoma	5 (5)	Hemangioma	6 (3)
		Chondrosarcoma	3 (3)	Neurofibroma	6 (3)
		Synovial sarcoma	2 (2)	Myxoma	6 (3)
		Other	4 (4)	Other	27 (15)
Foot and Ankle		Synovial sarcoma	15 (18)	Fibromatosis	42 (21)
Total This Location	282	MFH	14 (17)	Fibrous histiocytoma	36 (18)
Malignant	83	Clear cell sarcoma	11 (13)	Hemangioma	14 (7)
Benign	199	Hemangioendothelioma	8 (10)	Schwannoma	13 (7)
		DFSP	7 (8)	Chondroma	10 (5)
		Liposarcoma	6 (7)	Lipoma	10 (5)
		Fibrosarcoma	5 (6)	GCTTS	9 (5)
		Other	17 (20)	Other	65 (33)
Lower Extremity		Liposarcoma	117 (33)	Fibrous histiocytoma	114 (25)
Total This Location	812	MFH	88 (25)	Nodular fasciitis	59 (13)
Malignant	351	Malignant schwannoma	31 (9)	Lipoma	56 (12)
Benign	461	Synovial sarcoma	21 (6)	Myxoma	38 (8)
		DFSP	21 (6)	Schwannoma	27 (6)
		Leiomyosarcoma	18 (5)	Neurofibroma	27 (6)
		Fibrosarcoma	16 (5)	Hemangioma	20 (4)
		Other	39 (11)	Other	120 (26)
Hip, Groin, and Buttocks		MFH	26 (21)	Lipoma	30 (21)
Total This Location	268	Liposarcoma	23 (18)	Fibrous histiocytoma	16 (11)
Malignant	125	DFSP	22 (18)	Neurofibroma	15 (10)
Benign	143	Leiomyosarcoma	17 (14)	Nodular fasciitis	14 (10)
		Fibrosarcoma	10 (8)	Hemangiopericytoma	12 (8)
		Malignant schwannoma	5 (4)	Fibromatosis	11 (8)
		Malignant hemangiopericytoma	4 (3)	Myxoma	9 (6)
		Other	18 (14)	Other	36 (25)
Head and Neck		DFSP	24 (25)	Lipoma	103 (29)
Total This Location	455	Malignant schwannoma	14 (14)	Nodular fasciitis	65 (18)
Malignant	97	MFH	13 (13)	Fibrous histiocytoma	59 (16)
Benign	358	Liposarcoma	11 (11)	Hemangioma	40 (11)
		Fibrosarcoma	10 (10)	Neurofibroma	22 (6)
		Leiomyosarcoma	4 (4)	Hemangiopericytoma	15 (4)
		Rhabdomyosarcoma	3 (3)	Schwannoma	15 (4)
		Other	18 (19)	Other	39 (11)

continued

TABLE 2.19
(continued)

Location		Malignant Diagnoses	No. (%)	Benign Diagnoses	No. (%)
Trunk		DFSP	53 (28)	Lipoma	111 (27)
Total This Location	603	MFH	45 (24)	Nodular fasciitis	61 (15)
Malignant	188	Liposarcoma	23 (12)	Fibromatosis	52 (13)
Benign	415	Malignant schwannoma	19 (10)	Fibrous histiocytoma	29 (7)
		Fibrosarcoma	13 (7)	Hemangioma	28 (7)
		Angiosarcoma	7 (4)	Neurofibroma	26 (6)
		Leiomyosarcoma	7 (4)	Schwannoma	22 (5)
		Other	21 (11)	Other	86 (21)
Retroperitoneum		Leiomyosarcoma	37 (33)	Schwannoma	19 (22)
Total This Location	198	Liposarcoma	37 (33)	Fibromatosis	17 (20)
Malignant	111	MFH	15 (14)	Hemangiopericytoma	15 (17)
Benign	87	Fibrosarcoma	5 (5)	Angiomyolipoma	8 (9)
		Malignant schwannoma	3 (3)	Sclerosing retroperitonitis	5 (6)
		Malignant hemangiopericytoma	3 (3)	Neurofibroma	4 (5)
		Neuroblastoma	2 (2)	Mesothelioma	4 (5)
		Other	9 (8)	Other	15 (17)

DFSP, dermatofibrosarcoma protuberans; GCTTS, giant cell tumor of tendon sheath; MFH, malignant fibrous histiocytoma.

TABLE 2.20
AGE 46–55 YEARS: COMMON LESIONS BY LOCATION

Location		Malignant Diagnoses	No. (%)	Benign Diagnoses	No. (%)
Hand and Wrist		MFH	5 (13)	GCTTS	79 (23)
Total This Location	383	Synovial sarcoma	5 (13)	Hemangioma	35 (10)
Malignant	40	Liposarcoma	4 (10)	Fibrous histiocytoma	35 (10)
Benign	343	Epithelioid sarcoma	4 (10)	Lipoma	32 (9)
		Leiomyosarcoma	4 (10)	Fibromatosis	31 (9)
		Clear cell sarcoma	3 (8)	Fibroma of tendon sheath	21 (6)
		Chondrosarcoma	3 (8)	Chondroma	21 (6)
		Other	12 (30)	Other	89 (26)
Upper Extremity		MFH	39 (37)	Nodular fasciitis	63 (26)
Total This Location	349	Synovial sarcoma	11 (10)	Lipoma	38 (16)
Malignant	106	Liposarcoma	9 (8)	Fibrous histiocytoma	28 (12)
Benign	243	Fibrosarcoma	8 (8)	Myxoma	13 (5)
		Leiomyosarcoma	8 (8)	Schwannoma	12 (5)
		Malignant schwannoma	8 (8)	Hemangioma	10 (4)
		Hemangioendothelioma	5 (5)	Neurofibroma	10 (4)
		Other	18 (17)	Other	69 (28)
Axilla and Shoulder		MFH	25 (26)	Lipoma	84 (52)
Total This Location	260	Liposarcoma	20 (20)	Fibrous histiocytoma	17 (10)
Malignant	98	DFSP	15 (15)	Nodular fasciitis	10 (6)
Benign	162	Malignant schwannoma	14 (14)	Fibromatosis	7 (4)
		Leiomyosarcoma	7 (7)	Schwannoma	7 (4)
		Fibrosarcoma	6 (6)	Granular cell tumor	7 (4)
		Synovial sarcoma	3 (3)	Myxoma	7 (4)
		Other	8 (8)	Other	23 (14)
Foot and Ankle		MFH	19 (29)	Fibromatosis	35 (20)
Total This Location	239	Synovial sarcoma	14 (22)	Fibrous histiocytoma	21 (12)
Malignant	65	Liposarcoma	6 (9)	Lipoma	17 (10)
Benign	174	Clear cell sarcoma	4 (6)	GCTTS	14 (8)
		Fibrosarcoma	4 (6)	Chondroma	12 (7)
		Leiomyosarcoma	4 (6)	Schwannoma	11 (6)
		Malignant schwannoma	3 (5)	Hemangioma	9 (5)
		Other	11 (17)	Other	55 (32)

continued

TABLE 2.20
(continued)

Location		Malignant Diagnoses	No. (%)	Benign Diagnoses	No. (%)
Lower Extremity		MFH	145 (38)	Lipoma	72 (20)
Total This Location	741	Liposarcoma	103 (27)	Fibrous histiocytoma	59 (16)
Malignant	383	Synovial sarcoma	27 (7)	Myxoma	48 (13)
Benign	358	Malignant schwannoma	21 (5)	Nodular fasciitis	27 (8)
		Leiomyosarcoma	21 (5)	Schwannoma	18 (5)
		Chondrosarcoma	20 (5)	Hemangiopericytoma	14 (4)
		DFSP	12 (3)	Hemangioma	12 (3)
		Other	34 (9)	Other	108 (30)
Hip, Groin, and Buttocks		Liposarcoma	31 (24)	Lipoma	34 (30)
Total This Location	243	MFH	24 (19)	Myxoma	17 (15)
Malignant	128	Leiomyosarcoma	15 (12)	Fibrous histiocytoma	13 (11)
Benign	115	DFSP	12 (9)	Nodular fasciitis	9 (8)
		Synovial sarcoma	10 (8)	Hemangioma	8 (7)
		Fibrosarcoma	9 (7)	Hemangiopericytoma	7 (6)
		Chondrosarcoma	8 (6)	Neurofibroma	5 (4)
		Other	19 (15)	Other	22 (19)
Head and Neck		MFH	20 (23)	Lipoma	150 (43)
Total This Location	431	Malignant schwannoma	15 (17)	Nodular fasciitis	43 (12)
Malignant	86	DFSP	15 (17)	Hemangioma	32 (9)
Benign	345	Liposarcoma	11 (13)	Fibrous histiocytoma	20 (6)
		Leiomyosarcoma	7 (8)	Neurofibroma	13 (4)
		Angiosarcoma	5 (6)	Myxoma	12 (4)
		Fibrosarcoma	3 (3)	Schwannoma	11 (3)
		Other	10 (12)	Other	64 (19)
Trunk		MFH	46 (24)	Lipoma	110 (37)
Total This Location	494	DFSP	43 (22)	Nodular fasciitis	30 (10)
Malignant	194	Liposarcoma	35 (18)	Fibromatosis	27 (9)
Benign	300	Malignant schwannoma	18 (9)	Hemangioma	19 (6)
		Angiosarcoma	10 (5)	Hemangiopericytoma	13 (4)
		Leiomyosarcoma	9 (5)	Fibrous histiocytoma	13 (4)
		Malignant hemangiopericytoma	9 (5)	Schwannoma	13 (4)
		Other	24 (12)	Other	75 (25)
Retroperitoneum		Leiomyosarcoma	69 (34)	Schwannoma	14 (18)
Total This Location	280	Liposarcoma	56 (27)	Sclerosing retroperitonitis	12 (16)
Malignant	204	MFH	47 (23)	Hemangiopericytoma	11 (14)
Benign	76	Malignant schwannoma	12 (6)	Fibromatosis	10 (13)
		Malignant hemangiopericytoma	5 (2)	Angiomyolipoma	4 (5)
		Angiosarcoma	3 (1)	Paraganglioma	4 (5)
		Neuroblastoma	2 (1)	Neurofibroma	4 (5)
		Other	10 (5)	Other	17 (22)

DFSP, dermatofibrosarcoma protuberans; GCTTS, giant cell tumor of tendon sheath; MFH, malignant fibrous histiocytoma.

TABLE 2.21
AGE 56–65 YEARS: COMMON LESIONS BY LOCATION

Location		Malignant Diagnoses	No. (%)	Benign Diagnoses	No. (%)
Hand and Wrist		MFH	11 (25)	GCTTS	64 (22)
Total This Location	331	Synovial sarcoma	7 (16)	Chondroma	31 (11)
Malignant	44	Fibrosarcoma	6 (14)	Fibrous histiocytoma	28 (10)
Benign	287	Chondrosarcoma	4 (9)	Lipoma	27 (9)
		Kaposi sarcoma	4 (9)	Hemangioma	26 (9)
		Epithelioid sarcoma	3 (7)	Fibroma of tendon sheath	16 (6)
		Liposarcoma	3 (7)	Fibromatosis	12 (4)
		Other	6 (14)	Other	83 (29)
Upper Extremity		MFH	94 (51)	Lipoma	42 (22)
Total This Location	372	Liposarcoma	25 (13)	Nodular fasciitis	23 (12)
Malignant	186	Leiomyosarcoma	14 (8)	Schwannoma	18 (10)
Benign	189	Fibrosarcoma	10 (5)	Fibrous histiocytoma	16 (8)
		Malignant schwannoma	9 (5)	Neurofibroma	14 (7)
		DFSP	5 (3)	Myxoma	11 (6)
		Synovial sarcoma	5 (3)	Hemangioma	9 (5)
		Other	24 (13)	Other	56 (30)
Axilla and Shoulder		MFH	41 (46)	Lipoma	105 (63)
Total This Location	256	Liposarcoma	19 (21)	Fibrous histiocytoma	11 (7)
Malignant	90	DFSP	7 (8)	Myxoma	9 (5)
Benign	166	Leiomyosarcoma	7 (8)	Fibromatosis	7 (4)
		Malignant schwannoma	6 (7)	Schwannoma	5 (3)
		Fibrosarcoma	2 (2)	Granular cell tumor	5 (3)
		Granular cell tumor	2 (2)	Proliferative myositis	4 (2)
		Other	6 (7)	Other	20 (12)
Foot and Ankle		MFH	20 (22)	Fibromatosis	48 (30)
Total This Location	249	Leiomyosarcoma	15 (17)	Fibrous histiocytoma	22 (14)
Malignant	90	Synovial sarcoma	13 (14)	Lipoma	18 (11)
Benign	159	Kaposi sarcoma	12 (13)	Schwannoma	14 (9)
		Chondrosarcoma	6 (7)	Chondroma	9 (6)
		Fibrosarcoma	4 (6)	GCTTS	7 (4)
		Liposarcoma	3 (3)	Hemangioma	7 (4)
		Other	17 (19)	Other	34 (21)
Lower Extremity		MFH	254 (47)	Lipoma	85 (26)
Total This Location	862	Liposarcoma	129 (24)	Myxoma	61 (19)
Malignant	537	Leiomyosarcoma	42 (8)	Fibrous histiocytoma	34 (10)
Benign	325	Malignant schwannoma	17 (3)	Schwannoma	21 (6)
		Chondrosarcoma	17 (3)	Neurofibroma	20 (6)
		Fibrosarcoma	15 (3)	Proliferative fasciitis	19 (6)
		Synovial sarcoma	13 (2)	Nodular fasciitis	13 (4)
		Other	50 (9)	Other	71 (22)
Hip, Groin, and buttocks		MFH	42 (27)	Lipoma	42 (41)
Total This Location	257	Liposarcoma	36 (23)	Myxoma	19 (19)
Malignant	155	Leiomyosarcoma	25 (16)	Schwannoma	12 (12)
Benign	102	Malignant schwannoma	9 (6)	Fibromatosis	4 (4)
		DFSP	8 (5)	Hemangiopericytoma	4 (4)
		Fibrosarcoma	7 (5)	Fibrous histiocytoma	4 (4)
		Chondrosarcoma	6 (4)	Neurofibroma	4 (4)
		Other	22 (14)	Other	13 (13)
Head and Neck		MFH	34 (33)	Lipoma	156 (48)
Total This Location	426	DFSP	13 (13)	Nodular fasciitis	23 (7)
Malignant	104	Liposarcoma	11 (11)	Hemangioma	23 (7)
Benign	322	Angiosarcoma	11 (11)	Fibrous histiocytoma	22 (7)
		Atypical fibroxanthoma	9 (9)	Neurofibroma	17 (5)
		Malignant schwannoma	8 (8)	Schwannoma	14 (4)
		Leiomyosarcoma	4 (4)	Myxoma	11 (3)
		Other	14 (13)	Other	56 (17)

continued

TABLE 2.21
(continued)

Location		Malignant Diagnoses	No. (%)	Benign Diagnoses	No. (%)
Trunk		MFH	85 (37)	Lipoma	180 (49)
Total This Location	592	Liposarcoma	45 (20)	Fibromatosis	36 (10)
Malignant	228	Leiomyosarcoma	18 (8)	Neurofibroma	19 (5)
Benign	364	Malignant schwannoma	17 (7)	Fibrous histiocytoma	16 (4)
		DFSP	17 (7)	Schwannoma	15 (4)
		Fibrosarcoma	16 (7)	Nodular fasciitis	14 (4)
		Chondrosarcoma	10 (4)	Hemangioma	12 (3)
		Other	20 (9)	Other	72 (20)
Retroperitoneum		Liposarcoma	114 (37)	Schwannoma	19 (19)
Total This Location	406	Leiomyosarcoma	85 (28)	Fibromatosis	15 (15)
Malignant	307	MFH	64 (21)	Sclerosing retroperitonitis	13 (13)
Benign	99	Malignant schwannoma	11 (4)	Hemangiopericytoma	10 (10)
		Fibrosarcoma	8 (3)	Angiomyolipoma	8 (8)
		Malignant mesenchymoma	8 (3)	Lipoma	7 (7)
		Rhabdomyosarcoma	3 (1)	Paraganglioma	5 (5)
		Other	14 (5)	Other	22 (22)

DFSP, dermatofibrosarcoma protuberans; GCTTS, giant cell tumor of tendon sheath; MFH, malignant fibrous histiocytoma.

TABLE 2.22
AGE 66–75 YEARS: COMMON LESIONS BY LOCATION

Location		Malignant Diagnoses	No. (%)	Benign Diagnoses	No. (%)
Hand and Wrist		MFH	12 (27)	GCTTS	33 (19)
Total This Location	219	Leiomyosarcoma	6 (13)	Schwannoma	21 (12)
Malignant	45	Synovial sarcoma	5 (11)	Hemangioma	18 (10)
Benign	174	Kaposi sarcoma	3 (7)	Chondroma	18 (10)
		Malignant schwannoma	3 (7)	Fibromatosis	13 (7)
		DFSP	2 (4)	Neurofibroma	12 (7)
		Liposarcoma	2 (4)	Lipoma	9 (5)
		Other	12 (27)	Other	50 (29)
Upper Extremity		MFH	91 (55)	Lipoma	31 (23)
Total This Location	300	Liposarcoma	19 (12)	Nodular fasciitis	15 (11)
Malignant	165	Leiomyosarcoma	13 (8)	Schwannoma	12 (9)
Benign	135	Malignant schwannoma	12 (7)	Myxoma	10 (7)
		Fibrosarcoma	5 (3)	Neurofibroma	9 (7)
		Chondrosarcoma	5 (3)	Angiolipoma	8 (6)
		Kaposi sarcoma	5 (3)	Fibromatosis	7 (5)
		Other	15 (9)	Other	43 (32)
Axilla and Shoulder		MFH	43 (48)	Lipoma	62 (64)
Total This Location	187	Liposarcoma	21 (23)	Myxoma	7 (7)
Malignant	90	Malignant schwannoma	8 (9)	Fibromatosis	4 (5)
Benign	97	DFSP	5 (6)	Hemangioma	3 (3)
		Fibrosarcoma	3 (3)	Fibrous histiocytoma	3 (3)
		Leiomyosarcoma	2 (2)	Proliferative fasciitis	3 (3)
		Chondrosarcoma	2 (2)	Schwannoma	2 (2)
		Other	6 (7)	Other	13 (13)
Foot and Ankle		Kaposi sarcoma	19 (27)	Fibromatosis	13 (14)
Total This Location	163	MFH	15 (21)	Fibrous histiocytoma	11 (12)
Malignant	70	Leiomyosarcoma	14 (20)	Chondroma	9 (10)
Benign	93	Fibrosarcoma	5 (7)	Schwannoma	9 (10)
		Chondrosarcoma	4 (6)	Lipoma	7 (7)
		Malignant schwannoma	3 (4)	GCTTS	6 (6)
		Synovial sarcoma	2 (3)	Granuloma annulare	6 (6)
		Other	8 (11)	Other	32 (34)

continued

TABLE 2.22
(continued)

Location		Malignant Diagnoses	No. (%)		Benign Diagnoses	No. (%)	
Lower Extremity		MFH	242	(50)	Lipoma	46	(26)
Total This Location	660	Liposarcoma	126	(26)	Myxoma	30	(17)
Malignant	481	Leiomyosarcoma	47	(10)	Fibrous histiocytoma	25	(14)
Benign	179	Chondrosarcoma	13	(3)	Schwannoma	17	(9)
		Synovial sarcoma	9	(2)	Hemangioma	7	(4)
		Malignant schwannoma	9	(2)	Proliferative fasciitis	7	(4)
		Fibrosarcoma	8	(2)	Hemangiopericytoma	7	(4)
		Other	27	(6)	Other	40	(22)
Hip, Groin, and Buttocks		MFH	67	(44)	Lipoma	13	(17)
Total This Location	227	Liposarcoma	31	(20)	Neurofibroma	12	(16)
Malignant	152	Leiomyosarcoma	14	(9)	Myxoma	9	(12)
Benign	75	Fibrosarcoma	10	(7)	Schwannoma	8	(11)
		Malignant schwannoma	7	(5)	Hemangiopericytoma	7	(9)
		DFSP	4	(3)	Hemangioma	4	(5)
		Chondrosarcoma	4	(3)	Nodular fasciitis	4	(5)
		Other	15	(10)	Other	18	(24)
Head and Neck		MFH	37	(27)	Lipoma	108	(51)
Total This Location	348	Atypical fibroxanthoma	23	(17)	Hemangioma	14	(7)
Malignant	138	Liposarcoma	17	(12)	Schwannoma	13	(6)
Benign	210	Angiosarcoma	14	(10)	Fibrous histiocytoma	11	(5)
		Malignant schwannoma	9	(7)	Neurofibroma	11	(5)
		Fibrosarcoma	7	(5)	Nodular fasciitis	11	(5)
		Leiomyosarcoma	7	(5)	Hemangiopericytoma	9	(4)
		Other	24	(17)	Other	33	(16)
Trunk		MFH	86	(43)	Lipoma	99	(45)
Total This Location	420	Liposarcoma	32	(16)	Fibromatosis	17	(8)
Malignant	200	Leiomyosarcoma	15	(8)	Neurofibroma	13	(6)
Benign	220	DFSP	15	(8)	Schwannoma	13	(6)
		Malignant schwannoma	12	(6)	Fibrous histiocytoma	12	(5)
		Chondrosarcoma	8	(4)	Myxoma	12	(5)
		Fibrosarcoma	8	(4)	Hemangioma	11	(5)
		Other	24	(12)	Other	43	(20)
Retroperitoneum		Liposarcoma	104	(40)	Hemangiopericytoma	11	(25)
Total This Location	307	Leiomyosarcoma	71	(27)	Schwannoma	9	(20)
Malignant	263	MFH	60	(23)	Paraganglioma	4	(9)
Benign	44	Malignant schwannoma	11	(4)	Mesothelioma	4	(9)
		Fibrosarcoma	5	(2)	Lipoma	3	(7)
		Malignant mesenchymoma	5	(2)	Hemangioma	2	(5)
		Malignant hemangiopericytoma	3	(1)	Sclerosing retroperitonitis	2	(5)
		Other	4	(2)	Other	9	(20)

DFSP, dermatofibrosarcoma protuberans; GCTTS, giant cell tumor of tendon sheath; MFH, malignant fibrous histiocytoma.

TABLE 2.23
AGE 76 AND OLDER: COMMON LESIONS BY LOCATION

Location		Malignant Diagnoses	No. (%)	Benign Diagnoses	No. (%)
Hand and Wrist		MFH	16 (47)	GCTTS	18 (26)
Total This Location	102	Kaposi sarcoma	2 (6)	Neurofibroma	9 (13)
Malignant	34	Leiomyosarcoma	2 (6)	Hemangioma	6 (9)
Benign	68	Clear cell sarcoma	2 (6)	Chondroma	6 (9)
		Fibrosarcoma	2 (6)	Fibrous histiocytoma	6 (9)
		DFSP	2 (6)	Lipoma	4 (6)
		Liposarcoma	1 (3)	Schwannoma	3 (4)
		Other	7 (21)	Other	16 (24)
Upper Extremity		MFH	92 (66)	Myxoma	9 (20)
Total This Location	184	Leiomyosarcoma	10 (7)	Lipoma	8 (18)
Malignant	139	Malignant schwannoma	8 (6)	Glomus tumor	6 (13)
Benign	45	Liposarcoma	6 (4)	Schwannoma	5 (11)
		Kaposi sarcoma	5 (4)	Nodular fasciitis	3 (7)
		DFSP	3 (2)	Hemangioma	2 (4)
		Fibrosarcoma	3 (2)	Angiolipoma	2 (4)
		Other	12 (9)	Other	10 (22)
Axilla and Shoulder		MFH	24 (56)	Lipoma	21 (45)
Total This Location	90	Liposarcoma	9 (21)	Myxoma	7 (15)
Malignant	43	Malignant schwannoma	4 (9)	Schwannoma	4 (9)
Benign	47	Kaposi sarcoma	2 (5)	Fibroma	2 (4)
		Fibrosarcoma	1 (2)	Fibrous histiocytoma	2 (4)
		Leiomyosarcoma	1 (2)	Proliferative fasciitis	2 (4)
		DFSP	1 (2)	Lymphangioma	2 (4)
		Other	1 (2)	Other	7 (15)
Foot and Ankle		Kaposi sarcoma	30 (47)	Schwannoma	6 (24)
Total This Location	89	MFH	11 (17)	Fibromatosis	3 (12)
Malignant	64	Leiomyosarcoma	6 (9)	Lipoma	3 (12)
Benign	25	Fibrosarcoma	4 (6)	PVNS	3 (12)
		Malignant schwannoma	2 (3)	Chondroma	2 (8)
		Liposarcoma	2 (3)	Fibrous histiocytoma	2 (8)
		Chondrosarcoma	2 (3)	Granuloma annulare	2 (8)
		Other	7 (11)	Other	4 (16)
Lower Extremity		MFH	213 (62)	Lipoma	22 (28)
Total This Location	425	Liposarcoma	52 (15)	Myxoma	14 (18)
Malignant	345	Leiomyosarcoma	39 (11)	Schwannoma	12 (15)
Benign	80	Fibrosarcoma	14 (4)	Fibrous histiocytoma	8 (10)
		Malignant schwannoma	6 (2)	Neurofibroma	4 (5)
		Kaposi sarcoma	5 (1)	Hemangiopericytoma	3 (4)
		Chondrosarcoma	3 (1)	Nodular fasciitis	3 (4)
		Other	13 (4)	Other	14 (18)
Hip, Groin, and Buttocks		MFH	44 (48)	Lipoma	9 (29)
Total This Location	122	Liposarcoma	18 (20)	Myxoma	7 (23)
Malignant	91	Leiomyosarcoma	10 (11)	Hemangioma	4 (13)
Benign	31	Angiosarcoma	7 (8)	Hemangiopericytoma	3 (10)
		Malignant schwannoma	4 (4)	Schwannoma	2 (6)
		Malignant hemangiopericytoma	3 (3)	Neurofibroma	1 (3)
		Chondrosarcoma	3 (3)	Fibromatosis	1 (3)
		Other	2 (2)	Other	4 (13)
Head and Neck		MFH	45 (44)	Lipoma	50 (48)
Total This Location	206	Atypical fibroxanthoma	18 (18)	Hemangioma	8 (8)
Malignant	102	Angiosarcoma	13 (13)	Fibrous histiocytoma	6 (6)
Benign	104	Malignant schwannoma	7 (7)	Schwannoma	5 (5)
		Leiomyosarcoma	6 (6)	Neurofibroma	5 (5)
		Liposarcoma	3 (3)	Myxoma	5 (5)
		Fibrosarcoma	3 (3)	Fibromatosis	4 (4)
		Other	7 (7)	Other	21 (20)

continued

TABLE 2.23

(continued)

Location		Malignant Diagnoses	No. (%)	Benign Diagnoses	No. (%)
Trunk		MFH	51 (46)	Lipoma	25 (33)
Total This Location	187	Liposarcoma	24 (22)	Fibromatosis	9 (12)
Malignant	111	Leiomyosarcoma	8 (7)	Neurofibroma	7 (9)
Benign	76	Malignant schwannoma	8 (7)	Elastofibroma	5 (7)
		Angiosarcoma	5 (5)	Myxoma	4 (5)
		Fibrosarcoma	4 (4)	Hemangioma	3 (4)
		Chondrosarcoma	3 (3)	Hemangiopericytoma	3 (4)
		Other	8 (7)	Other	20 (26)
Retroperitoneum		Liposarcoma	60 (39)	Schwannoma	10 (36)
Total This Location	181	Leiomyosarcoma	47 (31)	Angiomyolipoma	3 (11)
Malignant	153	MFH	33 (22)	Fibromatosis	3 (11)
Benign	28	Osteosarcoma	5 (3)	Hemangiopericytoma	3 (11)
		Fibrosarcoma	3 (2)	Lipoma	3 (11)
		Malignant schwannoma	2 (1)	Sclerosing retroperitonitis	3 (11)
		Malignant hemangiopericytoma	1 (1)	Mesothelioma	2 (7)
		Other	2 (1)	Other	1 (4)

DFSP, dermatofibrosarcoma protuberans; GCTTS, giant cell tumor of tendon sheath; MFH, malignant fibrous histiocytoma; PVNS, pigmented villonodular synovitis.

639 patients (1.7%), including 592 patients with 2 lesions, 39 patients with 3 lesions, 7 patients with 4 lesions, and 1 patient with 5 lesions. Sequential biopsy specimens were found in 3,311 cases. A total of 39,179 soft tissue tumors (and tumor-like masses) were available for detailed analysis. From this group, 8,132 nonmesenchymal lesions were excluded.

There were 12,370 malignant mesenchymal lesions. More than 80% were classified into seven pathologic diagnoses: malignant fibrous histiocytoma (24%), liposarcoma (14%), leiomyosarcoma (8%), malignant peripheral nerve sheath tumor (6%), dermatofibrosarcoma protuberans (6%), synovial sarcoma (5%), and fibrosarcoma (5%); 12% could not be further classified. There were 18,677 benign mesenchymal lesions. Approximately 70% of benign lesions were classified into 8 pathologic diagnostic categories: lipoma and lipoma variants (16%), fibrous histiocytoma (13%), nodular fasciitis (11%), hemangioma (8%), fibromatosis (7%), neurofibroma (5%), schwannoma (5%), and giant cell tumor of tendon sheath (4%).

A summary of the malignant and benign lesions is presented in Tables 2.1 and 2.2. A summary of the age, sex, and distribution of lesions for all histologic diagnoses is shown in Tables 2.3 to 2.14.

The patient age and lesion location were known in 26,854 patients. For this group, the number and percentage of the seven most common malignant and benign lesions for each age and location are shown in Tables 2.15 to 2.23. All liposarcomas and fibrosarcomas have been grouped together for this analysis, as have all hemangiomas, lym-

phangiomas, and superficial and deep fibromatoses. Lipoma, lipomatosis, spindle cell lipoma, pleomorphic lipoma, and intramuscular lipoma have been combined and classified as lipoma. In total, 31 malignant and 52 benign diagnostic categories were used for this analysis.

The referral nature of the cases may introduce a bias for difficult case material and may be responsible for the relatively high percentage of malignancies (approximately 40%). This is greater than the 16% noted by Lattes (7) in citing the records of Columbia University during the 45.5 years from February 1, 1906, to September 1, 1951 (1,349 malignant and 7,337 benign lesions) and considerably greater than the 5% reported by Myhre-Jensen (8) during the 7-year period from April 1970 to April 1977 (72 malignant and 1,331 benign lesions) at the University Institute of Pathology, Aarhus, Denmark. Because of the increased number of malignancies, benign and malignant lesions have been considered separately in order to reflect accurately their relative prevalence.

In 2002, the World Health Organization (WHO) revised its classification of soft tissue tumors, incorporating new cytogenetic and molecular genetic information (9). The major changes in the WHO classification are highlighted in Chapter 1 and are not repeated here. For this analysis, we have retained the original tumor nomenclature and doubt this will cause any difficulty. Sufficient time has not elapsed since the publication of the 2002 WHO classification of bone and soft tissue tumors (9) to assess the effect of the classification changes on tumor prevalence and distribution.

REFERENCES

1. Crim JR, Seeger LL, Yao L, et al. Diagnosis of soft-tissue masses with MR imaging: can benign masses be differentiated from malignant ones? *Radiology.* 1992;185:581–586.
2. Kransdorf MJ, Jelinek JS, Moser RP, et al. Soft-tissue masses: diagnosis using MR imaging. *AJR Am J Roentgenol.* 1989;153: 541–547.
3. Berquist TH, Ehman RL, King BF, et al. Value of MR imaging in differentiating benign from malignant soft-tissue masses: study of 95 lesions. *AJR Am J Roentgenol.* 1990;155:1251–1255.
4. Sundaram M, McLeod RA. MR imaging of tumor and tumorlike lesions of bone and soft tissue. *AJR Am J Roentgenol.* 1990;155: 817–824.
5. Kransdorf MJ. Malignant soft-tissue tumors in a large referral population: distribution of diagnoses by age, sex and location. *AJR Am J Roentgenol.* 1995;164:129–134.
6. Kransdorf MJ. Benign soft-tissue tumors in a large referral population: distribution of diagnoses by age, sex and location. *AJR Am J Roentgenol.* 1995;164:395–402.
7. Lattes R. *Tumors of the Soft Tissue.* Second series. Washington, DC: Armed Forces Institute of Pathology, 1982.
8. Myhre-Jensen O. A consecutive 7-year series of 1331 benign soft tissue tumors. Clinicopathologic data. Comparison with sarcomas. *Acta Orthop Scand.* 1981;52:287–293.
9. Fletcher CDM, Unni KK, Mertens F. WHO classification of soft tissue tumors. *Pathology and Genetics: Tumors of Soft Tissue and Bone.* Lyon, France: IARC Press, 2002.

Imaging of Soft Tissue Tumors

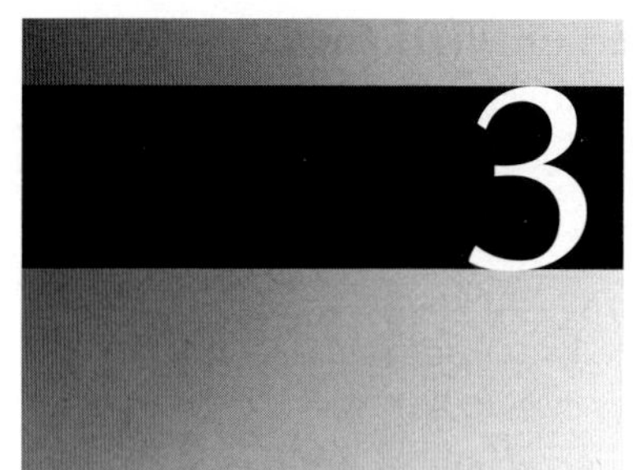

The radiologic evaluation of soft tissue masses has changed dramatically within the last two decades. Prior to the advent of computer-assisted imaging, assessment of clinically suspicious soft tissue masses was usually limited to radiographs. Although radiographs were sensitive to the identification of adipose tissue and soft tissue mineralization, they provided little other diagnostic information. When lesions were small, radiologists of those dark days were happy just to confirm the presence of a mass, much less give a confident diagnosis. The emergence of CT improved this situation dramatically. Masses could be delineated with great confidence and generally well-staged with excellent depiction of anatomic detail. Diagnosis, however, remained problematic, with images sufficiently characteristic to suggest the correct histology in only a minority of cases, typically lipomas and hemangiomas (1). The introduction of MR imaging was met with great enthusiasm because of the markedly improved soft tissue contrast and multiplanar image acquisition capabilities. The imaging of soft tissue masses was now on a par with that of other imaging-intense radiologic subspecialties, with exquisite depiction of anatomic detail. This ability to accurately characterize masses anatomically spurred new interest in the evaluation of soft tissue tumors. Attempts were made to develop rules, analogous to those for bone tumors, for differentiating benign from malignant processes based on lesion morphology and signal intensity; however, with few exceptions, these proved unreliable (2–7).

What has emerged is an approach to evaluation that is a combination of science and gestalt: a few well-tested general principles, as well as a number of lesions with a characteristic imaging appearance. Despite the initial fervor for the superiority of MR imaging in assessing soft tissue tumors, it remains relatively limited in its ability to characterize them precisely, with a correct histological diagnosis reached solely on the basis of imaging studies in only approximately one-quarter to one-third of cases (5–7). More recently, the superiority of MR imaging in the staging of musculoskeletal tumors has also come into question. In a multi-institutional study of 133 patients with primary soft tissue malignancies, the Radiology Diagnostic Oncology Group found no statistically significant difference between CT and MR imaging in determining tumor involvement of muscle, bone, joint, or neurovascular structures (8).

Despite these limitations, most radiologists are comfortable with the use of MR in the evaluation of soft tissue lesions. We strongly believe it is the modality of choice. When used in conjunction with a systematic approach, the majority of masses can be diagnosed correctly. Accordingly, this chapter presents a systematic approach to the evaluation of soft tissue tumors, highlighting the use of MR imaging in diagnosing and in differentiating benign from malignant soft tissue lesions. In addition, an approach is provided for establishing a differential diagnosis for those lesions with a nonspecific imaging appearance, as well as indications for contrast-enhanced imaging.

We also briefly review the use of other imaging modalities in the evaluation of soft tissue tumors, emphasizing their applications and limitations. Finally, information required for staging is presented, as well as a review of the imaging appearance of patients following treatment.

IMAGING EVALUATION

The initial evaluation of a patient with a soft tissue mass begins with a thorough clinical history and radiologic evaluation.

Clinical History

The clinical history is an important factor in establishing an accurate diagnosis. In many circumstances it provides key information that allows a specific diagnosis when imaging is nonspecific. Is there a history of a previous

KEY CONCEPTS
- Clinical history is essential in establishing an accurate diagnosis.
- Important information includes answering these questions:
  - Is there a history of a previous lesion or underlying malignancy?
  - Is the lesion painful, or did the patient note a painless mass?
  - Is there a history of notable trauma or anticoagulants?
  - Has the lesion remained stable over a long period of time, varied in size, or is it growing?
  - Is there more than one lesion?

lesion or underlying malignancy? Has there been previous surgery or radiation? It is essential to know how the patient presented: Is the lesion painful or did the patient note a painless mass? A painful mass always requires including an inflammatory process in the differential diagnosis. Is there a history of notable trauma or anticoagulants? Has the lesion remained stable over a long period of time, varied in size, or is it growing? A history of continued growth is always suspicious for malignancy. Unlike bone tumors, however, a slowly growing soft tissue mass is not invariably indicative of a benign process. Variation in lesion size with time or activity is exceedingly unusual for a malignancy and suggests a process such as a ganglion or hemangioma.

Is there more than one lesion? Soft tissue tumors are typically solitary; therefore, the identification of multiple lesions markedly limits the differential diagnosis. Multiple lipomas are seen in 5% to 15% of patients presenting with a soft tissue mass (9–11). The diagnosis in these cases can be made confidently on the basis of MR signal intensity. Aggressive fibromatosis is multifocal in 10% to 15% of patients (12,13). A second soft tissue mass in a patient with a previously confirmed desmoid tumor should be regarded as a second desmoid tumor until proven otherwise (14). Patients with neurofibromatosis have multiple lesions, and although the diagnosis is often known or suspected, such is not always the case (Fig. 3.1). The diagnosis may be suggested on the basis of imaging findings by the identification of multiple lesions in a major nerve distribution.

Angiomatous lesions are quite common, and they are multiple in as many as 20% of patients (15). In such cases, superficial and deep lesions may coexist. Multiple lesions may also be seen with metastatic disease. The soft tissue is relatively resistant to metastasis, and although it comprises about 40% of total body weight, soft tissue metastases are quite rare. The skin and subcutaneous tissue are also a frequent site of extraosseous involvement in patients with multiple myeloma, with involvement typically seen as multiple subcutaneous nodules (16). Extraosseous manifestations are found in less than 5% of patients with multiple

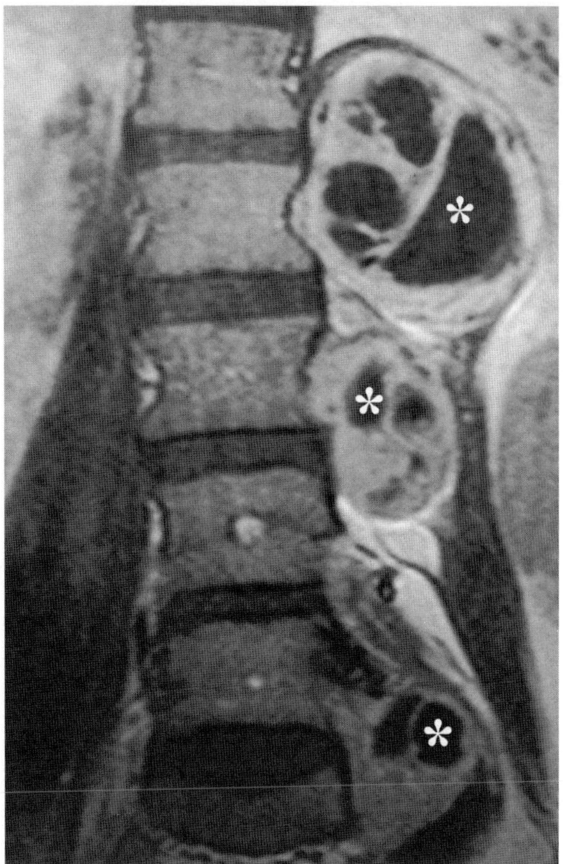

Figure 3.1 Neurofibromatosis: Woman 36 years of age presenting with multiple soft tissue masses. Coronal contrast-enhanced T1-weighted (TR/TE; 500/15) spin-echo MR image shows multiple left paraspinal masses with cystic change (*asterisks*).

myeloma and are associated with a more aggressive clinical course (16). Metastatic melanoma may display a similar pattern of multiple nodular subcutaneous metastases (17). These are seen in more than 30% of patients with melanoma metastatic disease, usually in patients with Clark level IV or V disease (depth on tumor invasion into the deep dermis or through the dermis into the subcutaneous fat), and may be the only radiologic manifestation of metastases (17). Finally, multiple myxomas may be seen in association with fibrous dysplasia of bone (Mazabraud syndrome) (18). These myxomas are usually intramuscular and the association is most frequent with polyostotic disease (18,19).

Radiographic Evaluation

KEY CONCEPTS
- Evaluation must begin with radiographs.
- Radiographs may be diagnostic of a palpable lesion caused by a skeletal deformity or exostosis.
- Radiographs may reveal soft tissue calcifications that can suggest a specific diagnosis.

Despite dramatic technological advances in our ability to image soft tissue tumors, the radiologic evaluation of a suspected soft tissue mass must begin with the radiograph. Although frequently unrewarding, it is impossible to predetermine those cases in which radiographs will be critical for diagnosis. Radiographs may be diagnostic of a palpable lesion caused by an underlying skeletal deformity (such as exuberant callus related to prior trauma) or exostosis, which may masquerade as a soft tissue mass. Radiographs may also reveal soft tissue calcifications, which can be suggestive and, at times, very characteristic of a specific diagnosis. For example, they may reveal the phleboliths within a hemangioma (Fig. 3.2), the juxta-articular osteocartilaginous masses of synovial chondromatosis, the peripherally more mature ossification of myositis ossificans, or the characteristic bone changes of other processes with associated soft tissue involvement. When not characteristic of a specific process, soft tissue calcification can suggest certain diagnoses. For example, nonspecific dystrophic calcifications within a slowly growing lower extremity mass in an adolescent or young adult should suggest a synovial sarcoma as the diagnosis of exclusion (Fig. 3.3).

In addition, radiographs are the best initial method of assessing coexistent osseous involvement, such as remodeling, periosteal reaction, or overt osseous invasion and

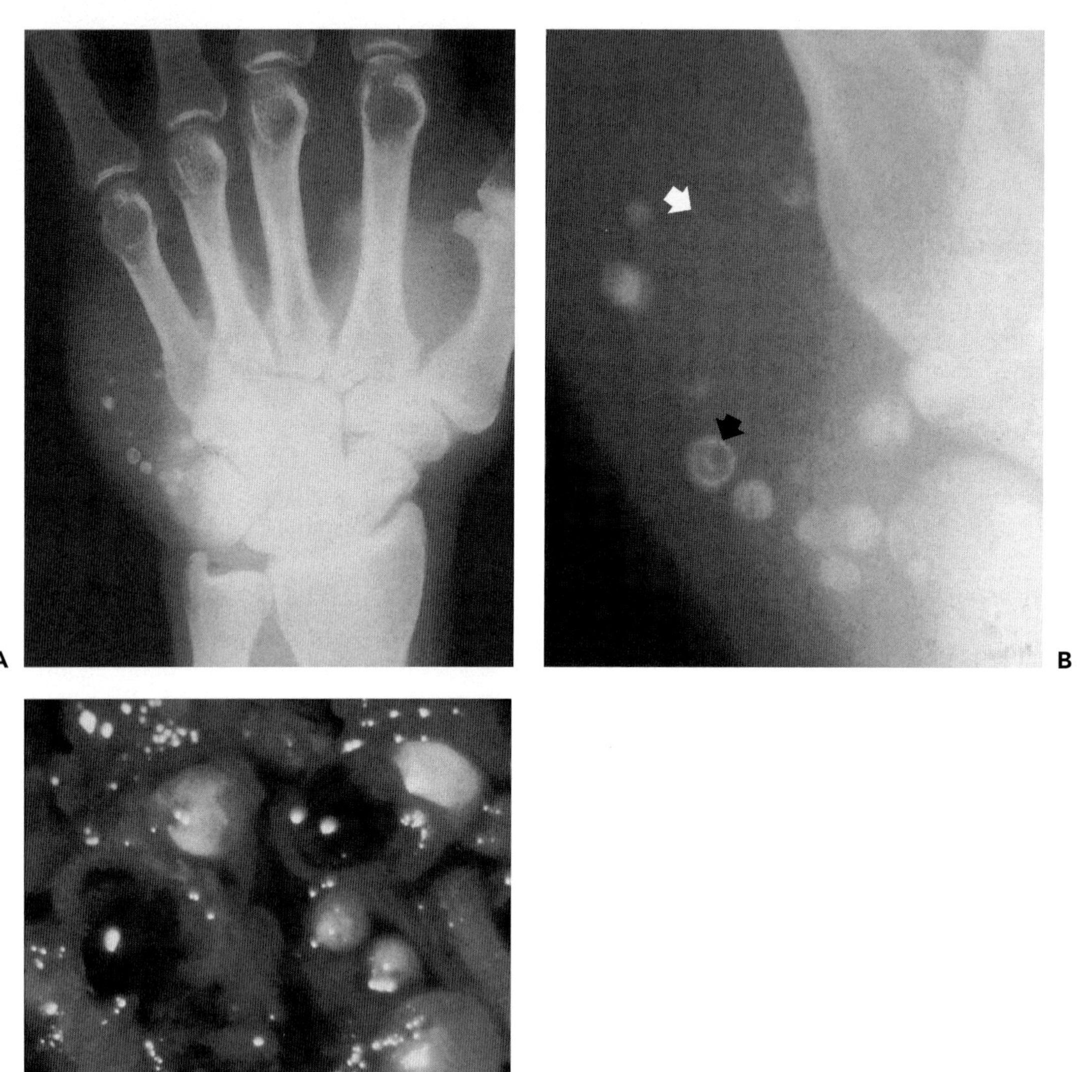

Figure 3.2 Phleboliths: Hemangioma in the hypothenar eminence of hand of a man 52 years of age. **A:** Radiograph shows hypothenar mass with multiple calcifications. **B:** Columnated radiograph shows multiple, small, smooth, rounded calcifications (*black arrow*), more opaque peripherally, characteristic of phleboliths. Note small, nonspecific calcifications (*white arrow*). **C:** Corresponding intraoperative photograph shows multiple phleboliths within interstices of hemangioma.

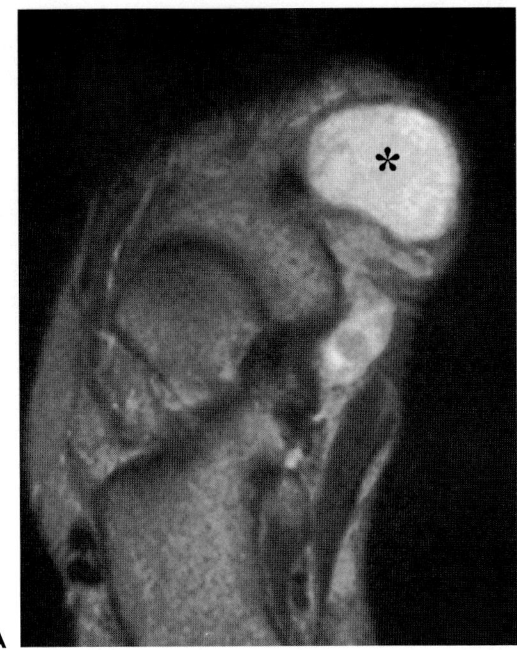
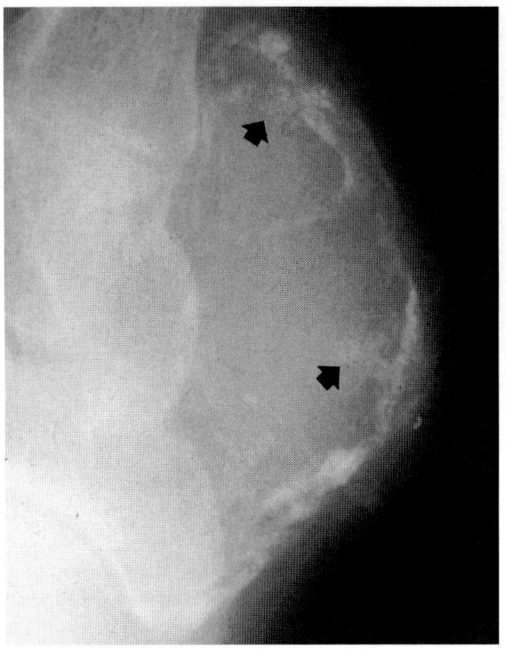

Figure 3.3 Synovial sarcoma: Mass in the foot of a girl 17 years of age presenting with slowly growing painless mass. **A:** Axial conventional T2-weighted (TR/TE; 1800/80) spin-echo MR image shows well-defined, nonspecific, soft tissue mass (*asterisk*). **B:** Corresponding radiograph shows peripheral and central calcification. The peripheral mineralization (*arrows*) does not show the ossification required to suggest myositis ossificans. This radiographic appearance (calcified soft tissue mass), in context of slowly growing juxta-articular mass in a young adult, strongly suggests the appropriate diagnosis.

destruction (20). However, unlike bone tumors, the biologic activity of a soft tissue mass cannot be reliably assessed by its growth rate. A slowly growing soft tissue mass that remodels adjacent bone (causing a scalloped area with well-defined sclerotic margins) may still be highly malignant on histologic examination (20).

A soft tissue mass may also be the initial presentation of a primary bone tumor or inflammatory process. In such cases, the radiograph can also be useful in identifying the osseous origin of the lesion. The diagnosis of a malignant bone tumor, such as Ewing sarcoma or primary lymphoma of bone, should be considered when a large circumferential soft tissue mass is associated with an underlying destructive bone lesion. A subtle radiologic feature, which may help separate inflammatory and neoplastic processes, is that an inflammatory process typically obliterates fascial planes, rather than displaces them.

Magnetic Resonance Imaging

MR imaging is the preferred modality for evaluating soft tissue lesions (2–4,21–28). It provides superior soft tissue contrast, allows multiplanar image acquisition, obviates the need for iodinated contrast agents or for ionizing radiation, and is devoid of streak artifact commonly encountered with CT imaging (2,21–23). When clinical findings are equivocal, MR imaging evaluation can confirm the presence of a soft tissue lesion or reassuringly identify a suspected "bump" or "mass" as normal tissue (Fig. 3.4).

Technique

> ### KEY CONCEPTS
> - Lesions should be imaged in at least two orthogonal planes.
> - Standard spin-echo images are most useful in establishing a specific diagnosis.
> - Fast scanning techniques shorten imaging times and decrease motion artifacts.
> - Gradient-echo imaging may be a useful supplement in demonstrating hemosiderin.
> - Gradient-echo imaging accentuates susceptibility artifacts caused by metal, hemorrhage, and air.
> - Short-tau inversion recovery (STIR) imaging enhances the identification of abnormal tissue.
> - STIR and fat-suppressed imaging reduces variations in signal intensities that are helpful in tissue characterization.
> - Field of view is dictated by the size and location of the lesion.
> - Small field of view is preferred.

Lesions should be imaged in at least two orthogonal planes, using T1-weighted and T2-weighted spin-echo MR pulse sequences in at least one of these. When possible, standard spin-echo images are most useful in establishing a specific diagnosis. It is the most reproducible technique and the one most often referenced in the tumor-imaging literature. It is the most familiar imaging technique for

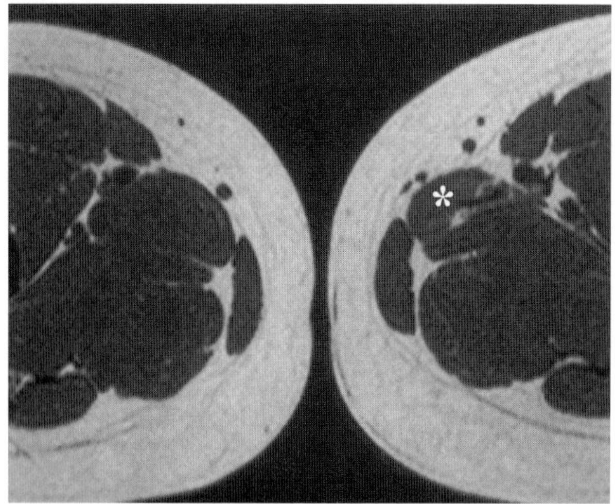

Figure 3.4   Atrophied muscle: Masslike soft tissue asymmetry in the right thigh suggesting a mass in a woman 24 years of age. Axial T1-weighted (TR/TE; 600/16) spin-echo MR image shows the marked atrophy to the left adductor longus muscle (*asterisk*). Atrophy was secondary to a previous muscle injury.

(29). Radiologists are most familiar with conventional axial anatomy, and axial T1- and T2-weighted spin-echo images should be obtained in almost all cases. The choice of additional imaging plane or planes varies with the involved body part, the lesion location, and its relationship to crucial structures. In general, the additional plane is *sagittal* with anterior or posterior masses, and *coronal* with medial or lateral lesions. Oblique planes may also be a useful adjunct. In these additional planes, it is valuable to use a combination of conventional T1- and T2-weighted spin-echo images, turbo (fast) spin-echo images, gradient images, and short-tau inversion recovery (STIR) images, as the case requires.

Fast scanning techniques may be helpful in the evaluation of soft tissue masses. They allow for shorter imaging times, decreased motion artifact, and increased patient tolerance, as well as patient throughput (29,30). They may add additional information and be helpful in specific instances, although fast scanning techniques have not replaced standard spin-echo imaging. Gradient-echo imaging may be a useful supplement in demonstrating hemosiderin because of its greater magnetic susceptibility. Also, in general, susceptibility artifacts related to metallic material, hemorrhage, and air are accentuated on gradient-echo images (38) (Fig. 3.5). Gradient-echo images may also be

tumor evaluation and the standard by which other imaging techniques must be judged (29). The main disadvantage of spin-echo imaging remains the relatively long acquisition times, particularly for double-echo T2-weighted sequences

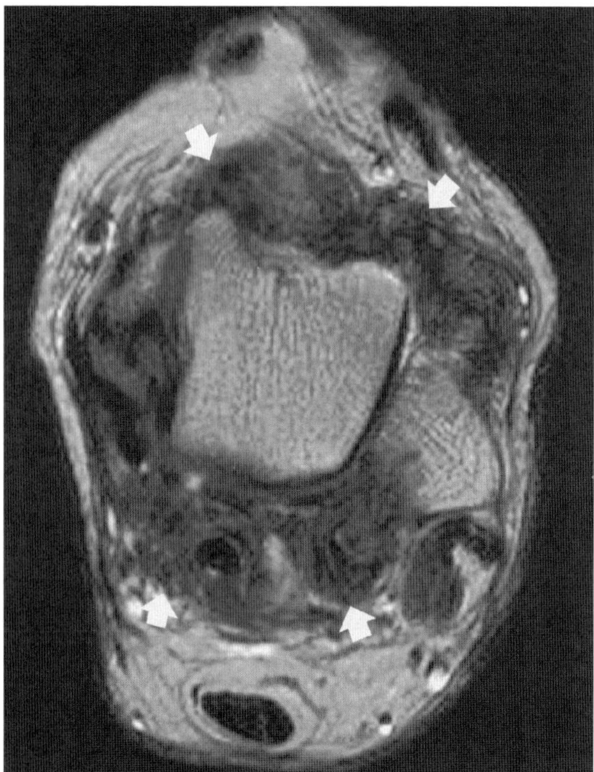

A

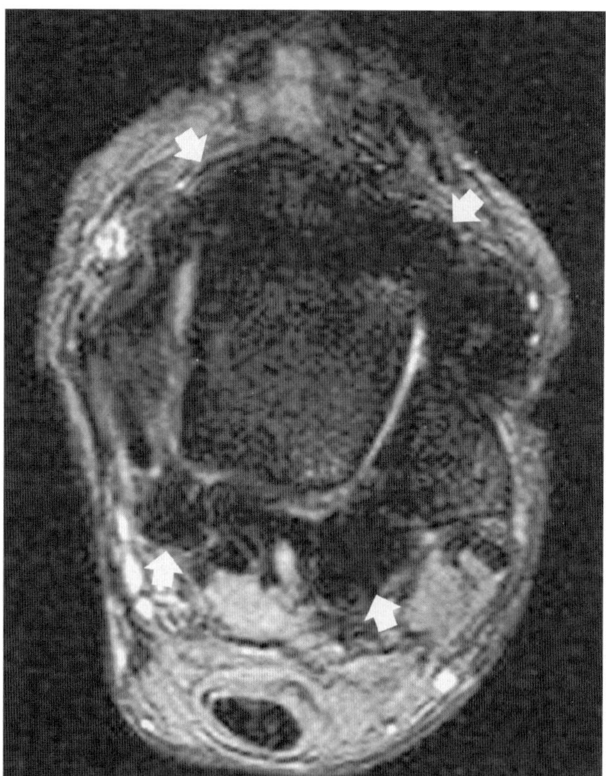

B

Figure 3.5   Hemosiderin identification with gradient-echo imaging: Pigmented villonodular synovitis (PVNS) in the ankle of a woman 23 years of age. **A:** Axial fast spin-echo T2-weighted (TR/TE; 4570/80) MR image shows a mass surrounding the ankle (*arrows*) with intermediate-to-decreased signal intensity. **B:** Corresponding axial gradient-echo (TR/TE; 785/20) MR image shows marked decreased signal from the mass (*arrows*) caused by the greater magnetic susceptibility of the hemosiderin-laden tissue, characteristic of PVNS.

better in some instances to demonstrate the lesion-to-fat interfaces and to depict small surrounding vessels (31).

STIR imaging can be an adjunct in selective cases. STIR imaging produces fat suppression and enhances the identification of abnormal tissue with increased water content, and, as such, is useful in confirming subtle areas of soft tissue abnormality (32). This technique increases lesion conspicuity (32,33) but typically has lower signal-to-noise than does spin-echo imaging, and it is also more susceptible to degradation by motion (29,32). Lesions are generally well-seen on standard imaging, and, in our opinion, STIR imaging tends to reduce the variations in signal intensities identified on conventional spin-echo MR imaging, signal intensities which are most helpful in tissue characterization.

Fat suppression on T2-weighted images is useful in increasing lesion-to-background signal intensity differences for high signal intensity lesions within the marrow or fatty soft tissue (37). Fat-suppression imaging is also useful in decreasing or eliminating the MR signal from fat, allowing increased conspicuity of lesions containing paramagnetic substances (such as methemoglobin) on T1-weighted images, and in identifying contrast enhancement. As with STIR techniques, fat-suppressed T2-weighted imaging decreases variations in tumor signal intensities, and we do not use this in place of T2-weighted images.

Field of view is dictated by the size and location of the lesion. In general, a small field of view is preferred; however, the field of view must be large enough to evaluate the lesion and allow appropriate staging (Fig. 3.6). When an extremity is being evaluated, it is not usually necessary to obtain the contralateral extremity for comparison, unless no lesion is detected on initial sequences (Fig. 3.7). It is useful to place a marker over the area of clinical concern, to ensure it is appropriately imaged. This becomes important in evaluating lesions such as subcutaneous lipoma or lipomatosis, in which the lesion may not be appreciated as being distinct from the adjacent adipose tissue. When small superficial lesions are being evaluated, care should be taken to ensure that the marker or patient position does not compress the mass.

Magnetic Resonance Imaging Contrast Enhancement

> **KEY CONCEPTS**
> - Magnetic resonance contrast agents:
>   - Enhance the signal intensity on T1-weighted spin-echo MR images of many tumors.
>   - Enhance the demarcation between tumor and muscle and tumor and edema.
>   - Enhance tissue vascularity and tissue perfusion.
> - Malignant lesions generally show greater enhancement and greater rate of enhancement than benign lesions.
> - Overlap in enhancement patterns and rates between benign and malignant lesions are sufficiently great that they are of limited practical value in any specific case.
> - Gadolinium-enhanced imaging is useful in:
>   - Evaluating hematomas.
>   - Differentiating solid from cystic (or necrotic) lesions.
>   - Identifying cystic or necrotic areas within solid tumors.

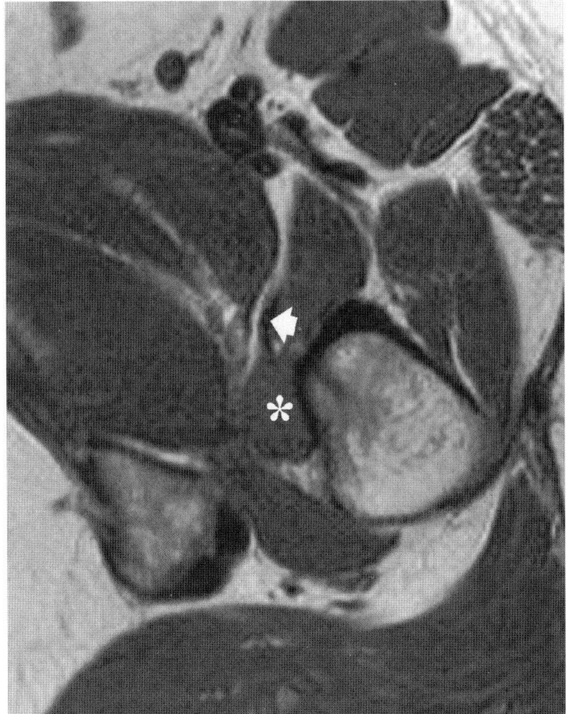

Figure 3.6 Field of view: Giant cell tumor of tendon sheath arising from the iliopsoas tendon in a woman 50 years of age presenting with hip pain. Columnated T1-weighted (TR/TE; 683/17) spin-echo MR image obtained with a 20-cm field of view shows the mass (*asterisk*) to be intimately associated with the iliopsoas tendon (*arrow*). This relationship was essential in suggesting the diagnosis preoperatively.

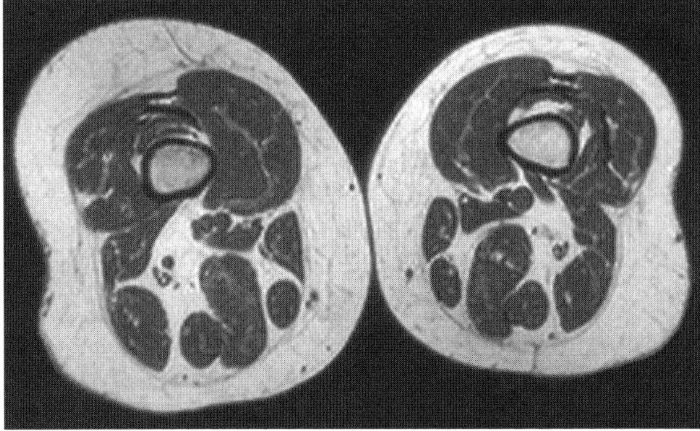

Figure 3.7 Contralateral extremity: Mild lipomatosis of the right lower extremity in a woman 54 years of age who presented with "fullness" around knee. Axial T1-weighted (TR/TE; 700/16) spin-echo MR image of both distal thighs shows increased adipose tissue on right as compared to contralateral side. Images of both distal thighs were obtained after no cause for clinical findings was found on axial images of right knee.

Although there is general agreement on the value of MR in the detection, diagnosis, and staging of soft tissue tumors and tumorlike lesions, the use of intravenous contrast in their evaluation remains controversial. In general, MR contrast agents enhance the signal intensity on T1-weighted spin-echo MR images of many tumors, in some cases enhancing the demarcation between tumor and muscle and tumor and edema, as well as providing information on tumor vascularity (34,35). In actuality, differentiation between tumor and muscle is usually quite well-delineated without enhanced imaging on T2-weighted images, and the accurate distinction between tumor and edema is probably of little practical value. Edema, which is infrequent without superimposed trauma or hemorrhage, is considered part of the reactive zone around the neoplasm and, as such, is removed en bloc with the tumor (36).

Other investigators have evaluated whether the rate of enhancement of soft tissue masses with gadolinium may help differentiate benign from malignant lesions (37–43). Enhancement reflects tissue vascularity and tissue perfusion, and, in general, malignant lesions show a greater enhancement, as well as a greater rate of enhancement. Van Rijswijk et al. (44) prospectively evaluated the use of static and dynamic gadopentetate dimeglumine–enhanced MR imaging relative to that of nonenhanced MR imaging in differentiating benign from malignant soft tissue lesions to evaluate which MR imaging parameters are most predictive of malignancy. In a study of 140 patients, they found that diagnostic accuracy was significantly improved for combined nonenhanced and contrast-enhanced MR imaging compared to nonenhanced MR imaging alone. They also noted that dynamic contrast-enhanced MR imaging parameters were significantly superior to nonenhanced MR imaging parameters in predicting malignancy.

Although dynamic contrast-enhanced imaging is promising, the overlap between benign and malignant lesions is sufficiently great that it is of limited practical value in any specific case (38,45). Consequently, we do not use it routinely.

Information on tumor enhancement is not without a price. The use of intravenous contrast increases the length and cost of the examination. Although contrast-enhanced MR imaging may provide some additional information, it does not increase lesion conspicuity or replace the diagnostic value of T2-weighted imaging (46). Moreover, although the incidence of untoward reaction as a result of contrast administration is small, it is real. Severe reactions are reported with both gadopentetate dimeglumine (Magnevist; Berlex Laboratories, Wayne, NJ) and gadoteridol (ProHance; Squibb Diagnostics, Princeton, NJ), including hypotension, laryngospasm, bronchospasm, anaphylactoid reaction, and anaphylactic shock (47–51), as well as a full spectrum of less serious reactions. Jordan and Mintz (52) described a fatal reaction to gadopentetate dimeglumine that was presumed to be caused by an anaphylactic reaction with associated bronchospasm. Consequently, gadolinium-enhanced

imaging should be reserved for those cases in which the results influence patient management.

There are several circumstances in which gadolinium-enhanced imaging is useful. We find it particularly valuable in the evaluation of hematomas. In such cases, contrast-enhanced imaging may reveal a small tumor nodule that may not be apparent within hemorrhage on conventional MR imaging (Fig. 3.8) (53,54). Caution is required, however, in that the fibrovascular tissue in organizing hematomas may show enhancement (55). Gadolinium-enhanced imaging is also used to differentiate solid from cystic (or necrotic) lesions or to identify cystic or necrotic areas within solid tumors, with these necrotic or cystic areas showing no enhancement (34). This distinction may be difficult or impossible to detect on conventional T2-weighted images when both tumor and fluid show high signal intensity, well-defined margins, and homogeneous signal intensity, and it is especially important to guide biopsy. Care is needed, however, because myxoid lesions, such as intramuscular myxoma or myxoid liposarcoma, and hyaline cartilage lesions, such as synovial chondromatosis, may demonstrate little or mild enhancement and may mimic cysts or lesions with cystic components (Fig. 3.9). In general, ultrasound is fast and inexpensive and an ideal method for differentiating solid from cystic lesions when the lesion is in an anatomic location accessible to sonographic evaluation.

Magnetic Resonance Imaging Diagnosis

KEY CONCEPTS

- A correct diagnosis is reached on the basis of imaging studies alone in 25% to 35% of cases.
- MR diagnosis is usually made on lesion signal intensity, pattern of growth, location, and associated "signs" and findings.
- When a lesion has a nonspecific MR imaging appearance, it is useful to formulate a suitably ordered differential diagnosis on tumor prevalence, patient age, and lesion anatomic location.
- Differential can be refined by considering clinical history and diagnostic radiologic features, such as pattern of growth, signal intensity, and localization (subcutaneous, intramuscular, intermuscular, etc.).
- A systematic approach markedly improves diagnostic results.

Despite the superiority of MR imaging in delineating soft tissue tumors, it remains limited in its ability to characterize them precisely, with most lesions demonstrating prolonged T1- and T2-relaxation times. The majority of lesions remain nonspecific, with a correct histologic diagnosis reached on the basis of imaging studies alone in only approximately 25% to 35% of cases (5–7). There are instances, however, in which a specific diagnosis may be

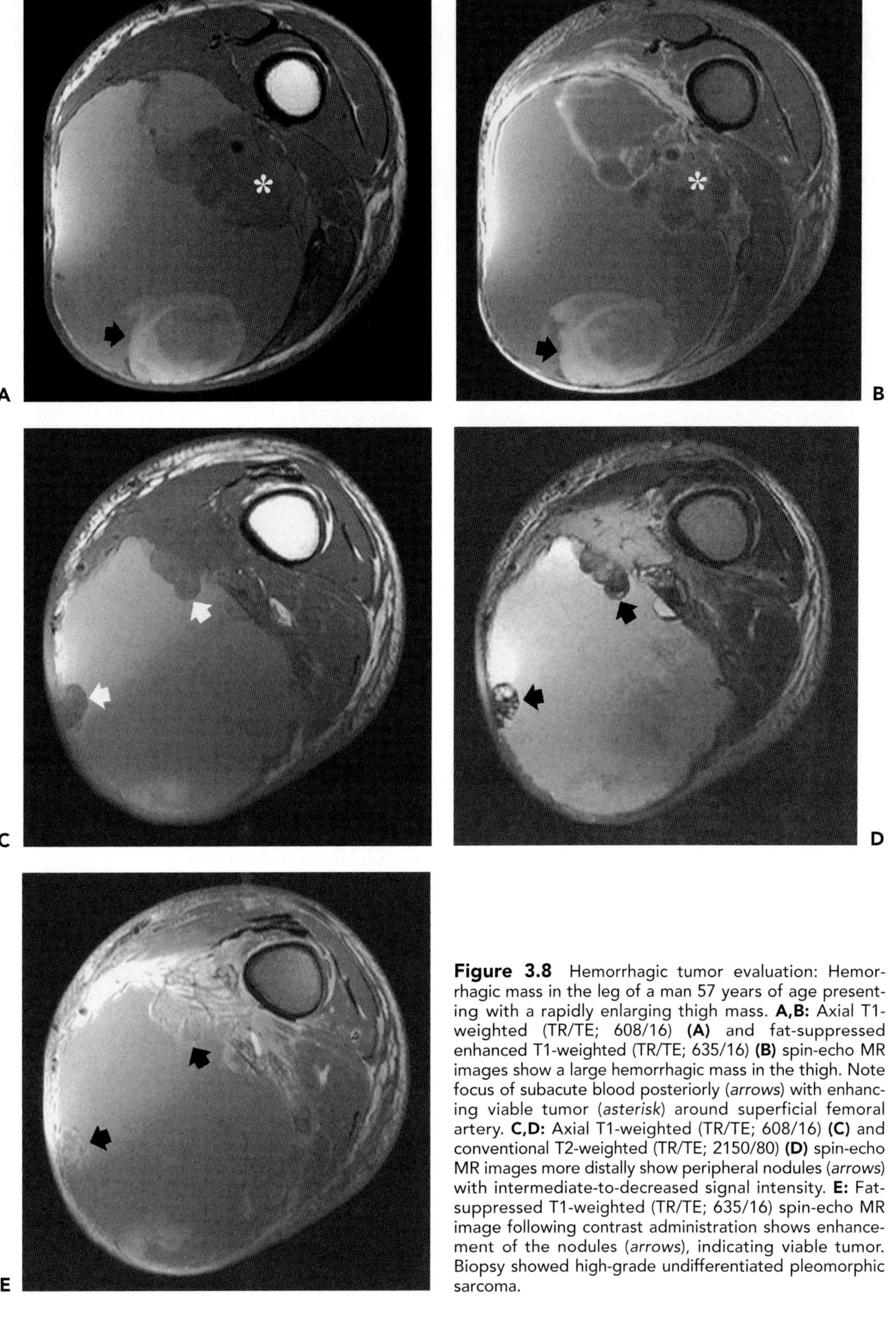

Figure 3.8 Hemorrhagic tumor evaluation: Hemorrhagic mass in the leg of a man 57 years of age presenting with a rapidly enlarging thigh mass. **A,B:** Axial T1-weighted (TR/TE; 608/16) **(A)** and fat-suppressed enhanced T1-weighted (TR/TE; 635/16) **(B)** spin-echo MR images show a large hemorrhagic mass in the thigh. Note focus of subacute blood posteriorly (*arrows*) with enhancing viable tumor (*asterisk*) around superficial femoral artery. **C,D:** Axial T1-weighted (TR/TE; 608/16) **(C)** and conventional T2-weighted (TR/TE; 2150/80) **(D)** spin-echo MR images more distally show peripheral nodules (*arrows*) with intermediate-to-decreased signal intensity. **E:** Fat-suppressed T1-weighted (TR/TE; 635/16) spin-echo MR image following contrast administration shows enhancement of the nodules (*arrows*), indicating viable tumor. Biopsy showed high-grade undifferentiated pleomorphic sarcoma.

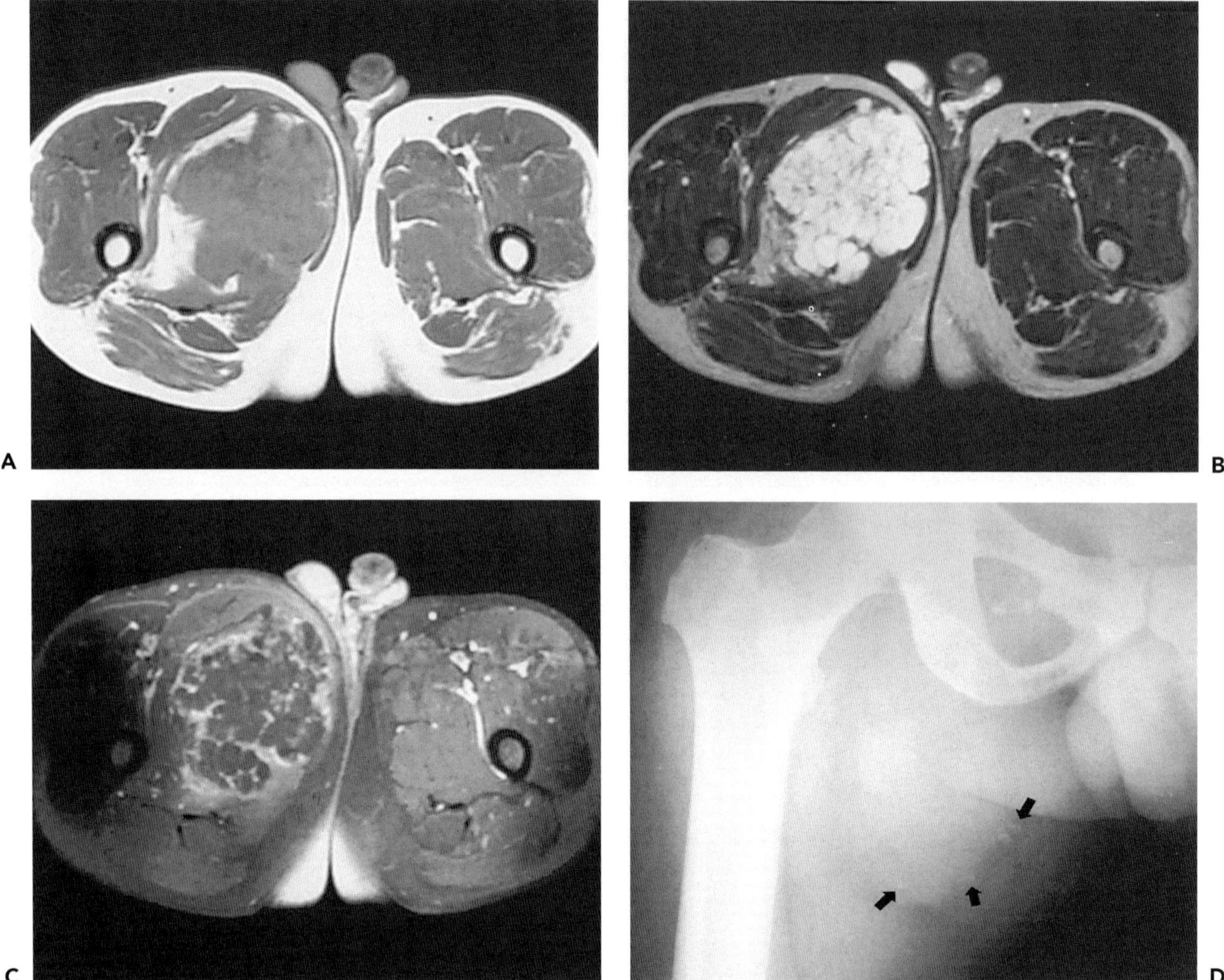

Figure 3.9 Cyst mimic: Extra-articular synovial chondromatosis in the thigh of a man 35 years of age mimicking loculated fluid. **A:** Axial T1-weighted (TR/TE; 763/18) spin-echo MR image shows large lobulated mass, with signal intensity similar to that of skeletal muscle, in adductor compartment. **B:** Corresponding conventional T2-weighted (2912/80, TR/TE) spin-echo MR image shows lesion to have signal intensity greater than that of fat. **C:** Fat-suppressed axial T1-weighted (475/18, TR/TE) spin-echo MR image following contrast administration shows peripheral and septal enhancement, suggesting loculated fluid. **D:** Radiograph shows nonspecific calcifications (*arrows*) within mass.

made or strongly suspected on an analysis of the MR imaging features. This is usually done on the basis of lesion signal intensity, pattern of growth, location, and associated "signs" and findings. The MR imaging appearance of these lesions is discussed throughout this volume and not reviewed here. They are listed in Table 3.1.

More commonly, MR imaging may reveal a nonspecific appearance. In such cases, it is often not possible to establish a meaningful differential diagnosis or to determine reliably whether a lesion is benign or malignant. In such situations, it is useful to formulate a suitably ordered differential diagnosis on the basis of a knowledge of tumor prevalence, patient age, and lesion anatomic location. This differential diagnosis can be further refined by considering clinical history and radiologic features, such as pattern of growth, signal intensity, and localization (subcutaneous, intramuscular, intermuscular, etc.). Table 3.2 lists the most common lesions in each compartment. The most common malignant and benign lesions, by tumor location and patient age, are reviewed in Chapter 2. The use of this prevalence data is demonstrated by the diagnostic examples at the end of this chapter.

Benign versus Malignant

Although there is general agreement on the diagnostic value of MR in many cases, the issue of whether MR can reliably distinguish benign from malignant is much less clear. One study suggested that MR can differentiate benign from malignant masses in greater than 90% of cases based on the morphology of the lesion (6). Criteria

TABLE 3.1
SPECIFIC DIAGNOSES MADE OR SUSPECTED ON THE BASIS OF MR IMAGING

Vascular lesions:
  Aneurysm and pseudoaneurysm
  Hemangioma
  Hemangiomatosis (angiomatosis)
  Arteriovenous hemangioma (arteriovenous malformation)
  Lymphangioma
  Lymphangiomatosis

Bone- and cartilage-forming lesions:
  Extraskeletal chondroma
  Myositis ossificans
  Panniculitis ossificans

Fibrous lesions:
  Elastofibroma
  Musculoaponeurotic fibromatosis
  Superficial fibromatosis
  Fibroma of tendon sheath

Lipomatous lesions:
  Lipoma
  Lipomatosis
  Intramuscular lipoma
  Lipomatosis of nerve
  Lipoblastoma
  Lipoblastomatosis
  Liposarcoma
  Periosteal lipoma

Tumorlike lesions:
  Calcific myonecrosis
  Cystic adventitial disease
  Ganglion
  Granuloma annulare
  Hematoma
  Intramuscular myxoma
  Popliteal (synovial) cyst
  Tumoral calcinosis

Peripheral nerve lesions:
  Malignant peripheal nerve sheath tumor
  Neurofibroma
  Schwannoma

Synovial lesions:
  Giant cell tumor of tendon sheath
  Lipoma arborescens
  Nodular synovitis
  Pigmented villonodular synovitis
  Synovial chondromatosis
  Synovial lipoma
  Synovial sarcoma

KEY CONCEPTS
- Malignancies generally are deep and large.
- Only 5% of benign soft tissue tumors exceed 5 cm in diameter.
- When sarcomas are superficial, they generally have a less aggressive biologic behavior.
- Malignancies usually grow as deep space-occupying lesions, enlarging in a centripetal fashion.
- As malignancies enlarge, a pseudocapsule of compressed fibrous connective tissue is formed.
- Malignancy is predicted with the highest sensitivity when lesions:
  - Have a high signal intensity on T2-weighted images.
  - Are larger than 33 mm in diameter.
  - Have a heterogeneous signal intensity on T1-weighted images.
- Malignancy is predicted with the highest specificity when lesions show:
  - Tumor necrosis.
  - Bone or neurovascular involvement.
  - Mean diameter of more than 66 mm.

used for predicting benign lesions included smooth, well-defined margins, small size, and homogeneous signal intensity, especially on T2-weighted images. Other studies, however, note that malignant lesions may appear as smoothly marginated, homogeneous masses, and MR cannot reliably distinguish benign from malignant processes (2–5,7,34). This discrepancy likely reflects differences within the studied populations.

When the MR images of a lesion are not sufficiently characteristic to suggest a specific diagnosis, a conservative approach is warranted. Malignancies, by virtue of their very nature and potential for autonomous growth, are generally larger and more likely to outgrow their vascular supply with subsequent infarction and necrosis and heterogeneous signal intensity on T2-weighted spin-echo MR images. Consequently, the larger the mass and the greater its heterogeneity, the greater is the concern for malignancy. Only 5% of benign soft tissue tumors exceed 5 cm in diameter (56,57). In addition, most malignancies are deep lesions, whereas only about 1% of all benign soft tissue tumors are deep (56,57). Although these figures are based on surgical and not imaging series, these trends are likely still valid for radiologists. Also, an increasing percentage of malignant lesions are found with increasing age. Location is also important in predicting benign and malignant lesions (58,59). In the Armed Forces Institute of Pathology (AFIP) series, for example, 70% of retroperitoneal lesions (for all age groups) were malignant, whereas only 15% of hand and wrist lesions were malignant (Table 3.3) (58,59).

TABLE 3.2
MOST COMMON LESIONS BY COMPARTMENT

Lesion Localization

Intermuscular	Extraskeletal myxoid chondrosarcoma		Synovial hemangioma
	Fibromatosis		Synovial sarcoma
	Ganglion		Tumoral calcinosis
	Leiomyosarcoma	Subcutaneous	Angiomatous lesions
	Nodular fasciitis		Benign fibrous histiocytoma
	Neurogenic tumors		DFSP (dermatofibrosarcoma protuberans)
	Synovial cyst		Granuloma annulare
Intra-articular	Lipoma arborescens		Leiomyosarcoma
	Nodular synovitis		Lipoma
	Pigmented villonodular synovitis		Lymphoma
	Synovial chondromatosis		MFH (malignant fibrous histiocytoma)
	Synovial hemangioma		Metastasis (especially melanoma)
			Myxoma
Intramuscular	Angiomatous lesions		Nodular fasciitis
	Lipoma		Skin appendage tumor
	MFH (malignant fibrous histiocytoma)		
	Myxoma	Tendinous/	Clear cell sarcoma
	Sarcoma (not specific)	Musculoaponeurotic	Giant cell tumor of tendon sheath (nodular tenosynovitis)
Juxta-articular	Ganglion		Fibroma of tendon sheath
	Giant cell tumor of tendon sheath		Fibromatosis
	Myxoma		
	Synovial cyst		

When sarcomas are superficial, they generally have a less aggressive biologic behavior than deep lesions (60). As a rule, most malignancies grow as deep space-occupying lesions, enlarging in a centripetal fashion (60), pushing, rather than infiltrating adjacent structures (although clearly there are exceptions to this general rule). As they enlarge, a pseudocapsule of fibrous connective tissue is formed around them by compression and layering of normal tissue, associated inflammatory reaction, and vascularization (Fig. 3.10) (60). They generally respect fascial borders and remain within anatomic compartments until late in their course (60). It is this pattern of growth that gives most sarcomas relatively well-defined margins, in contradistinction to the general concepts of margin definition used in the evaluation of osseous tumors (Fig. 3.11).

Although well-defined margins surrounding sarcomas are common, a rind of increased signal intensity may be seen surrounding tumors on fluid-sensitive sequences. This rind is often termed *peritumoral edema* or *reactive change* and is composed of inflammatory cell infiltration, vascular congestion, muscle atrophy, as well as edema (61,62). These areas may also contain tumors cells, either singly or in clusters, and are identified in as many as 67% of patients with high-grade sarcomas (61). Malignant cells are usually located within 1 cm of the tumor margin but can be found at a distance of up to 4 cm (Fig. 3.12).

Although our experience with metastatic carcinoma to soft tissue is limited, we have generally found these lesions to be more infiltrative, with ill-defined margins, often violating fascial planes and anatomic compartments. This pattern of growth is quite different from that seen in most primary soft tissue tumors (Fig. 3.13).

Increased signal intensity in the skeletal muscle surrounding a musculoskeletal mass on T2-weighted spin-echo MR images or other fluid-sensitive sequences (i.e., STIR) is also suggested as a reliable indicator of malignancy (63,64). These results are based on studies in which both bone and soft tissue lesions were evaluated. Although this increased signal intensity may be seen with malignancy, in our experience this finding is quite nonspecific. In fact, prominent high signal intensity surrounding a soft tissue mass more commonly suggests an inflammatory process, abscess, myositis ossificans, local trauma, hemorrhage, biopsy, or radiation therapy rather than a primary soft tissue neoplasm (Fig. 3.14).

Gadolinium imaging is also proposed as useful in differentiating benign from malignant soft tissue lesions, with malignant lesions showing a greater enhancement as well as a greater rate of enhancement (35,46,48,65). Enhancement reflects tissue vascularity and tissue perfusion, and, in general, the rate of enhancement of malignant lesions is greater than that seen in benign lesions. However, the overlap between benign and malignant is so great, in our opinion, that this is of little practical value in any specific case (65). When a lesion has a nonspecific MR appearance, one is ill-advised to suggest that a lesion is benign or malignant based solely on its MR imaging characteristics and rate or degree of enhancement.

TABLE 3.3
BENIGN AND MALIGNANT TUMOR DISTRIBUTION BY LOCATION AND AGE

Age	Number	Malignant Benign	% Malignant % Benign	Hand Wrist	Upper Extremity	Prox Limb	Foot Ankle	Lower Extremity	Hip Buttocks	Head Neck	Trunk	Retro
0–5	1330	274	20.6	11 (10%)*	31 (25%)	16 (17%)	11 (13%)	53 (23%)	22 (24%)	60 (20%)	50 (20%)	20 (51%)
		1056	79.4	97 (90%)	94 (75%)	80 (83%)	76 (87%)	180 (77%)	70 (76%)	237 (80%)	203 (80%)	19 (49%)
6–15	1942	578	29.8	43 (15%)	92 (34%)	39 (35%)	53 (25%)	128 (37%)	38 (41%)	65 (22%)	91 (32%)	29 (60%)
		1364	20.2	235 (85%)	182 (66%)	73 (65%)	161 (75%)	216 (63%)	55 (59%)	228 (78%)	195 (68%)	19 (40%)
16–25	3702	1103	29.8	86 (17%)	138 (27%)	74 (30%)	90 (31%)	338 (39%)	83 (40%)	89 (24%)	161 (26%)	44 (38%)
		2599	70.2	420 (83%)	376 (73%)	172 (70%)	205 (69%)	484 (61%)	122 (60%)	287 (76%)	462 (74%)	71 (62%)
26–35	4409	1283	29.1	83 (14%)	133 (23%)	75 (28%)	106 (29%)	357 (42%)	119 (39%)	97 (19%)	245 (46%)	68 (46%)
		3126	70.9	493 (86%)	442 (77%)	196 (72%)	263 (71%)	534 (58%)	185 (61%)	401 (81%)	533 (54%)	79 (54%)
36–45	3880	1215	31.3	63 (12%)	103 (22%)	94 (34%)	83 (29%)	351 (43%)	125 (47%)	97 (21%)	188 (31%)	111 (56%)
		2665	68.7	450 (88%)	368 (78%)	184 (66%)	199 (71%)	461 (57%)	143 (53%)	358 (79%)	415 (69%)	87 (44%)
46–55	3420	1304	38.1	40 (10%)	106 (30%)	98 (38%)	65 (27%)	383 (52%)	128 (53%)	86 (20%)	194 (39%)	204 (73%)
		2116	61.9	343 (90%)	243 (70%)	162 (62%)	174 (73%)	358 (48%)	115 (47%)	345 (80%)	300 (61%)	76 (27%)
56–65	3754	1741	46.4	44 (13%)	186 (50%)	90 (35%)	90 (36%)	537 (62%)	155 (60%)	104 (24%)	228 (39%)	307 (76%)
		2013	53.6	287 (87%)	189 (50%)	166 (65%)	159 (64%)	325 (38%)	102 (40%)	322 (76%)	364 (61%)	99 (24%)
66–75	2831	1604	56.7	45 (21%)	165 (55%)	90 (48%)	70 (43%)	481 (73%)	152 (67%)	138 (40%)	200 (48%)	263 (86%)
		1227	43.3	174 (79%)	135 (45%)	97 (52%)	93 (57%)	179 (27%)	75 (33%)	210 (60%)	220 (52%)	44 (14%)
>76	1586	1082	68.2	34 (33%)	139 (76%)	43 (48%)	64 (72%)	345 (81%)	91 (75%)	102 (50%)	111 (59%)	153 (85%)
		504	31.8	68 (67%)	45 (24%)	47 (52%)	25 (28%)	80 (19%)	31 (25%)	104 (50%)	76 (41%)	28 (15%)
Total	26854	10184	37.9	449 (15%)*	1093 (35%)	619 (34%)	632 (32%)	2973 (51%)	913 (50%)	838 (25%)	1468 (35%)	1199 (70%)
		16670	62.1	2567 (85%)*	2974 (65%)	1177 (66%)	1355 (68%)	2817 (49%)	898 (50%)	2492 (75%)	2768 (65%)	522 (30%)
% of all lesions				11.2	11.8	6.7	7.4	21.5	6.7	12.5	15.8	6.4

*11 (10%): Indicates 11 malignant and 97 benign hand and wrist lesions for ages 0–5 years and that 10% of the lesions are malignant and 90% are benign.
97 (90%)

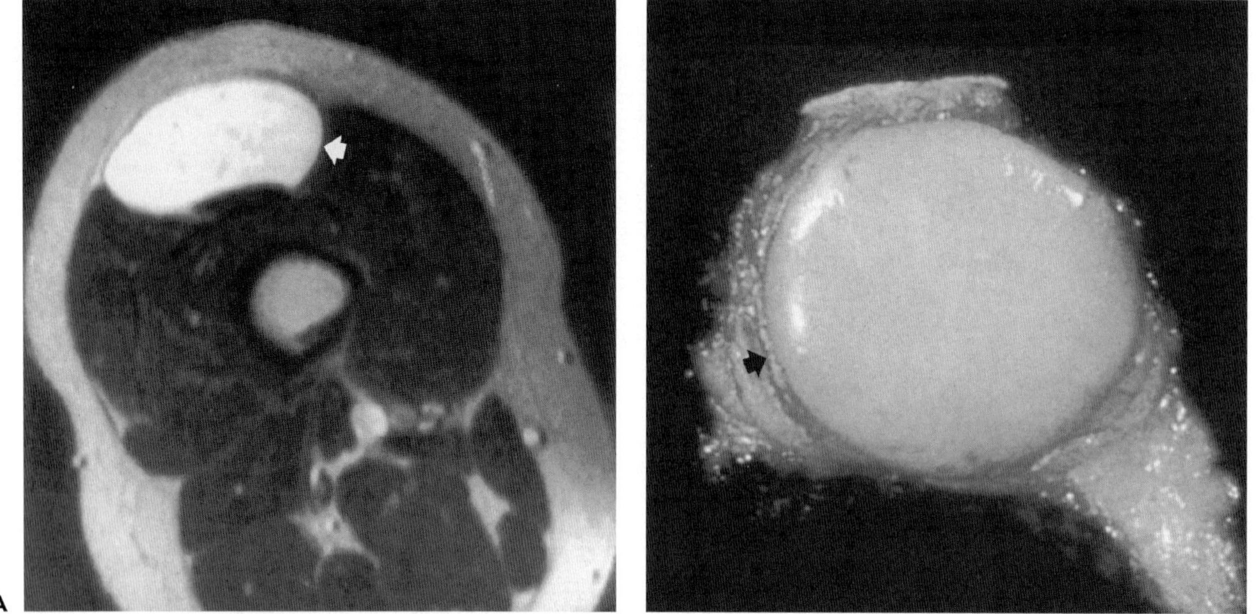

Figure 3.10 Pseudocapsule: Myxoid liposarcoma in the thigh of a man 26 years of age. **A:** Axial T2-weighted (TR/TE; 2000/80) spin-echo MR image shows a homogeneous well-defined mass with an internal cystlike appearance (*arrow*). **B:** Gross photograph from a different patient with a high-grade sarcoma shows the thin pseudocapsule (*arrow*) at the periphery of the mass.

DeSchepper et al. (66) performed a multivariate statistical analysis of ten imaging parameters, individually and in combination. These researchers found that malignancy was predicted with the highest sensitivity when lesions had a high signal intensity on T2-weighted images, were larger than 33 mm in diameter, and had heterogeneous signal intensity on T1-weighted images. Signs that had the greatest specificity for malignancy included tumor necrosis, bone or neurovascular involvement, and mean diameter of more than 66 mm (Fig. 3.15).

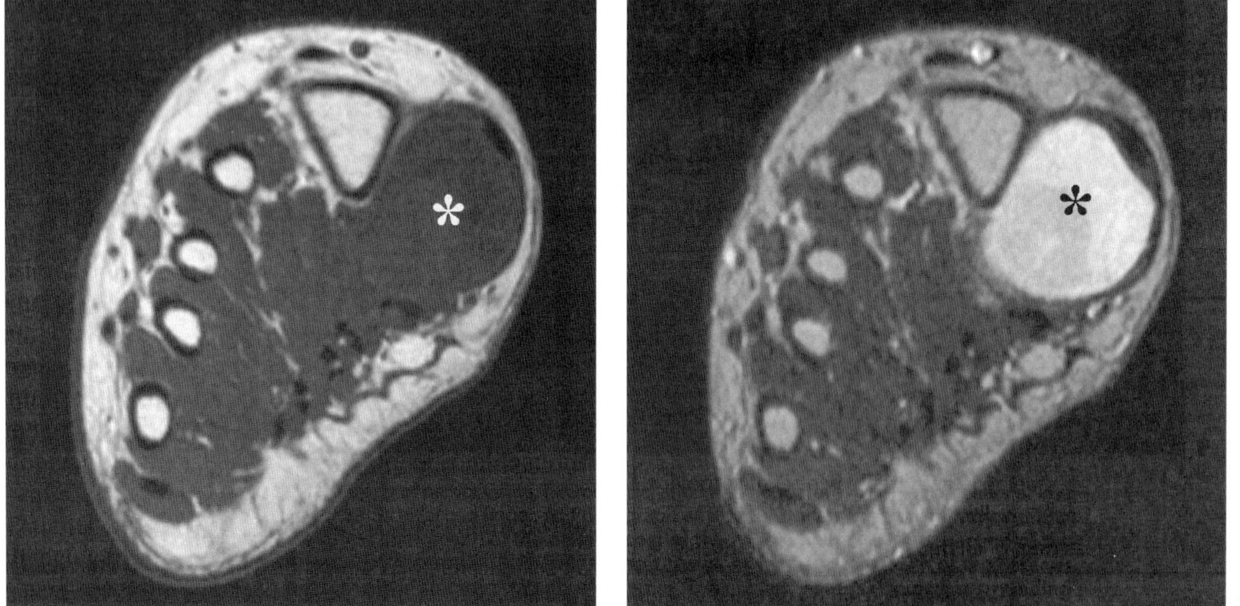

Figure 3.11 Well-defined high grade malignancy with pseudocapsule: Synovial sarcoma in the foot of a girl 10 years of age. **A,B:** Coronal T1-weighted (TR/TE; 450/12) **(A)** and T2-weighted (TR/TE; 2000/80) **(B)** spin-echo MR images shows a well-defined mass (*asterisk*) within the flexor hallucis brevis muscle. (*continued*)

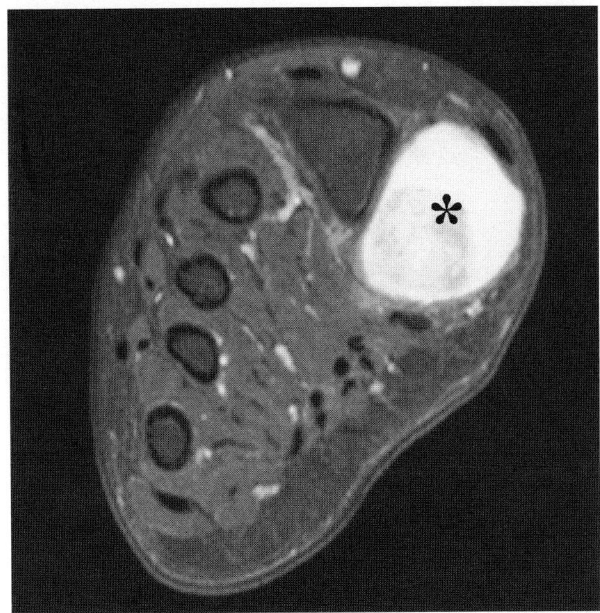

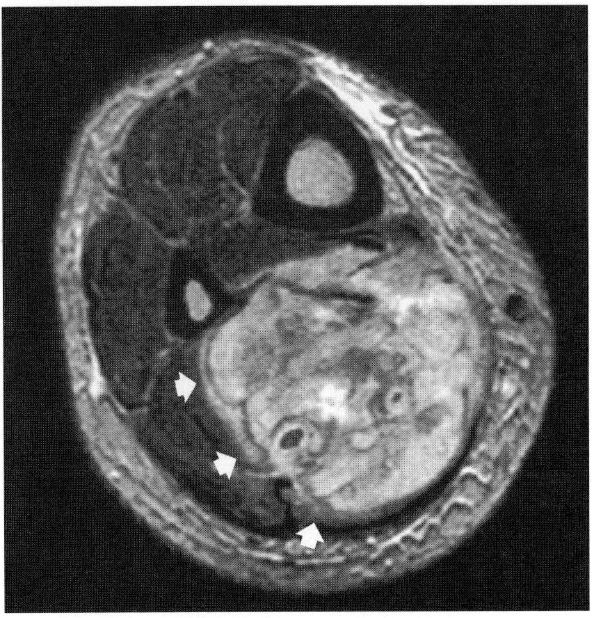

Figure 3.11 *(continued)* **C:** Fat-suppressed axial T1-weighted (TR/TE; 850/12) spin-echo MR image following contrast administration shows intense diffuse enhancement.

Figure 3.12 Peritumoral reactive change: High-grade undifferentiated pleomorphic sarcoma in a woman 41 years of age. Axial T2-weighted (TR/TE; 2500/80) spin-echo MR image shows rind of increased signal surrounding the tumor (*arrows*).

Other Imaging Modalities

Although MR imaging is the preferred modality for evaluating soft tissue lesions, a number of additional modalities may be useful. These modalities, along with their primary uses and limitations, are discussed later.

Spectroscopy

Phosphorus-31 (P-31) nuclear MR spectroscopy detects phosphorus-containing metabolites in intact living tissue (67). Shinkwin et al. (67) evaluated 18 patients with

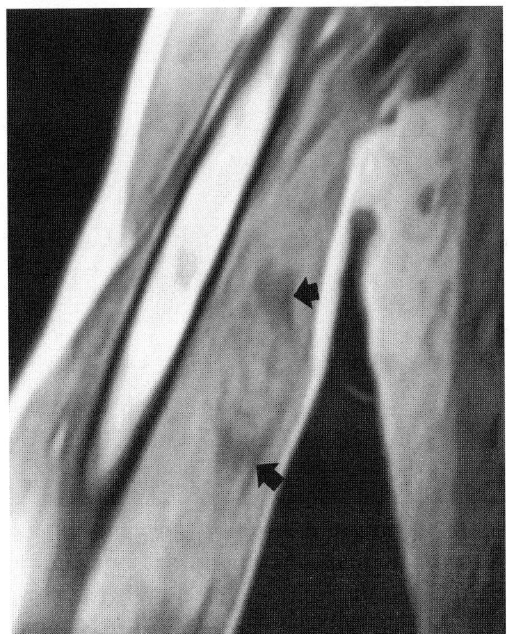

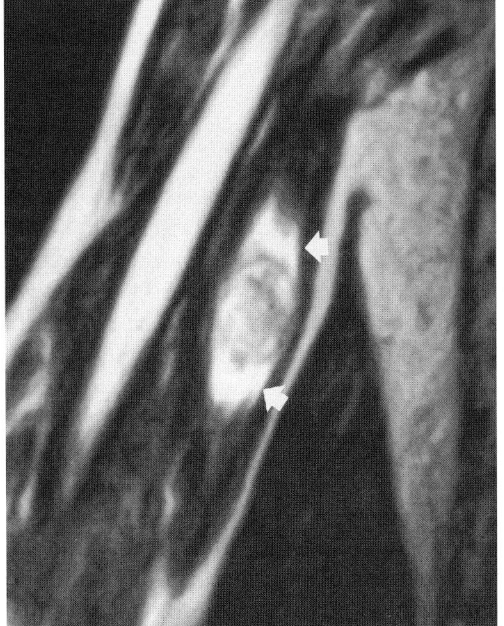

Figure 3.13 Peritumoral reactive change: Metastatic carcinoma (poorly differentiated) in the upper arm of a man 66 years of age with head and neck cancer. **A,B:** Coronal gradient-echo (TR/TE/FA; 69/24/60) image and T2-weighted (TR/TE; 1800/105) spin-echo MR image show a heterogeneous mass in the upper arm with peritumoral reactive changes (*arrows*).

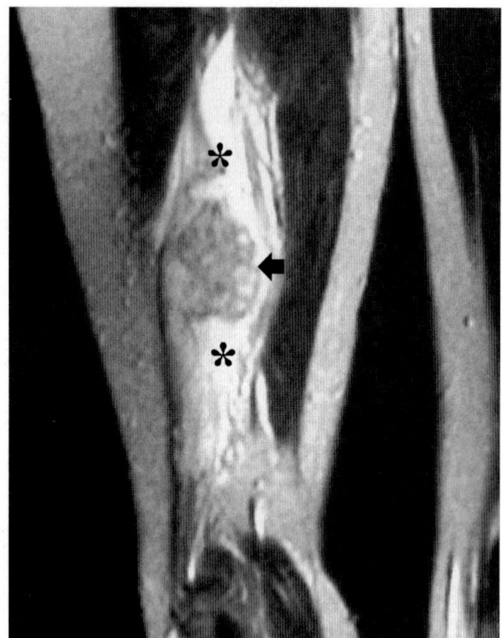

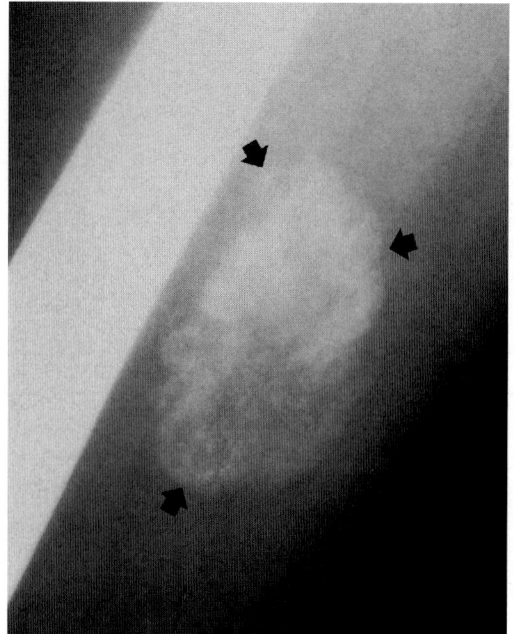

Figure 3.14 Inflammatory change: Myositis ossificans in the thigh of a woman 24 years of age. **A:** Coronal conventional T2-weighted (TR/TE; 2200/80) spin-echo MR image shows large edemalike signal (*asterisks*) around myositis ossificans (*arrow*). **B:** Corresponding lateral radiograph shows the peripherally mature ossification (*arrows*) of myositis ossificans.

> **KEY CONCEPTS**
> - Spectroscopy is still not ready for prime time.
> - ^{31}P MR spectroscopy detects phosphorus-containing metabolites in intact living tissue.
> - Proton magnetic resonance spectroscopy (^{1}HMRS), used routinely in neuroradiology but only recently applied to musculoskeletal imaging, detects choline.
> - The great variability in tumor size and necrosis, as well as muscle contamination, limits the usefulness of MR spectroscopy in differentiating benign from malignant tumors.

soft tissue masses and found that soft tissue tumors had a significantly higher proportion of phosphate in the low-energy portion of the P-31 spectrum, with a concomitant decrease in phosphocreatine as compared with that in normal muscle, and a greater relative amount of phospho-monoesters, inorganic phosphate, and phosphodiesters. The great variability in tumor size, necrosis, and muscle contamination makes spectroscopy of limited value in separating benign from malignant lesions. Sostman et al. (68) found that spectroscopy could be useful in evaluating tumor necrosis; consequently, it could be useful in establishing the prognosis of patients with soft tissue sarcomas.

^{1}H MR spectroscopy is used routinely in neuroradiology but only recently was applied to musculoskeletal imaging. Wang and colleagues (69) reported the use of ^{1}H MR spectroscopy in the evaluation of 36 musculoskeletal tumors. They noted that they could differentiate accurately between benign and malignant tumors by detection of choline.

They reported a sensitivity of 95%, specificity of 89%, and an accuracy of 89%. Although this technique is promising, it is not applicable to tumors smaller than 1.5 cm and is subject to sampling limitations.

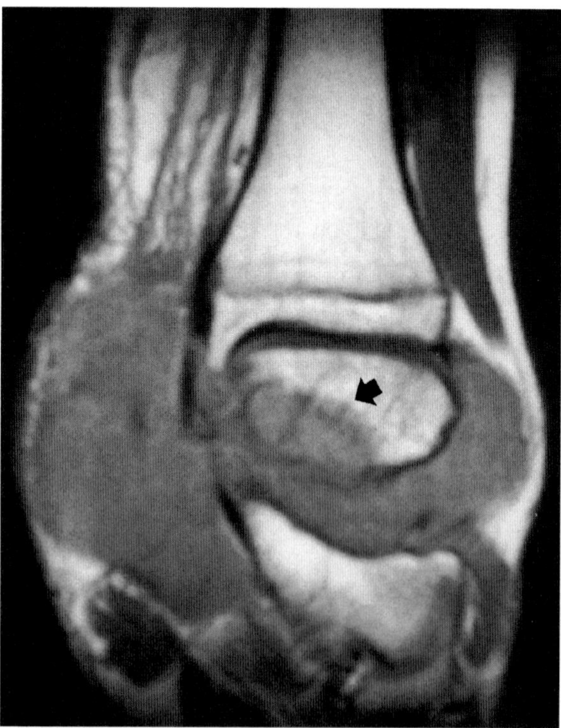

Figure 3.15 Bone invasion: Synovial sarcoma in the ankle of a boy 16 years of age. Coronal T1-weighted spin-echo image shows osseous invasion (*arrow*), a specific sign of malignancy.

Computed Tomography

In general, MR has replaced CT in the evaluation of patients with soft tissue masses, and CT is redundant rather than complementary in the majority of cases (23). Although initial investigations maintained that CT was superior to MR imaging in detecting destruction of cortical bone (22,23,28), newer studies suggest these two modalities are comparable in this regard (21,71). We still find CT scanning superior for the delineation of fine osseous detail (Fig. 3.16).

The identification of adipose tissue within a mass may be accomplished equally well with either CT or MR imaging; however, further characterization of fat-containing masses (other than simple lipomas) is better accomplished with MR imaging. CT scanning is unequivocally superior in detecting and characterizing calcification or ossification within a soft tissue mass (findings that may be sufficiently subtle to be undetectable on radiographs) and therefore may be complementary to MR in such specific cases. The zonal pattern of mineralization essential to the radiologic diagnosis of early myositis ossificans may be seen on CT while radiographs remain nonspecific (72).

In selected instances, CT may also be a useful adjunct when subtle bone abnormalities are suspected and radiographs do not evaluate a lesion adequately. This may occur in skeletal locations in which the osseous anatomy is complex, such as in the shoulder girdle, pelvis, or paraspinal region. Such cases are uncommon, however, and CT scanning is only required infrequently. CT remains the modality of choice for the evaluation of the chest in order to exclude pulmonary metastases.

Sonography

> **KEY CONCEPTS**
> - Sonography is readily available, noninvasive, and relatively inexpensive.
> - Sonography is useful for:
>   - Confirming the presence of a suspected lesion.
>   - Differentiating a localized mass from diffuse edema.
>   - Differentiating solid from cystic lesions.
> - Unfortunately, sonographic characteristics are typically nonspecific.
> - Sonography is ideal in directing percutaneous biopsy.

Sonography is a readily available, noninvasive, and relatively inexpensive method of detecting and determining the size and consistency of a soft tissue mass. In addition, sonography may be helpful in differentiating a localized mass from diffuse edema and differentiating solid from cystic lesions (73,74). Ultrasound is also useful for confirming the cystic nature of a suspected ganglion (in the appropriate clinical setting), identifying fluid surrounding a tendon affected by acute tenosynovitis, and showing the relationship between a mass and the adjacent neurovascular structures (Fig. 3.17) (73). Because the sonographic characteristics of soft tissue masses are more often nonspecific, the role of ultrasound is in confirming the presence of a suspected lesion, identifying its size, determining its internal characteristics, guiding percutaneous biopsy, and monitoring response

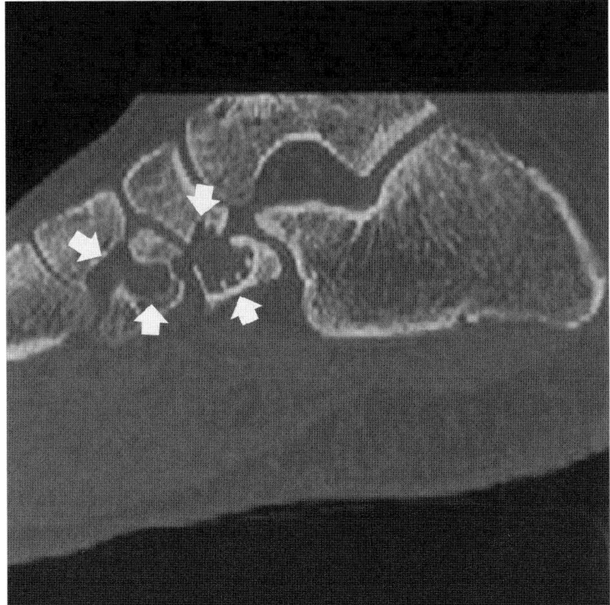
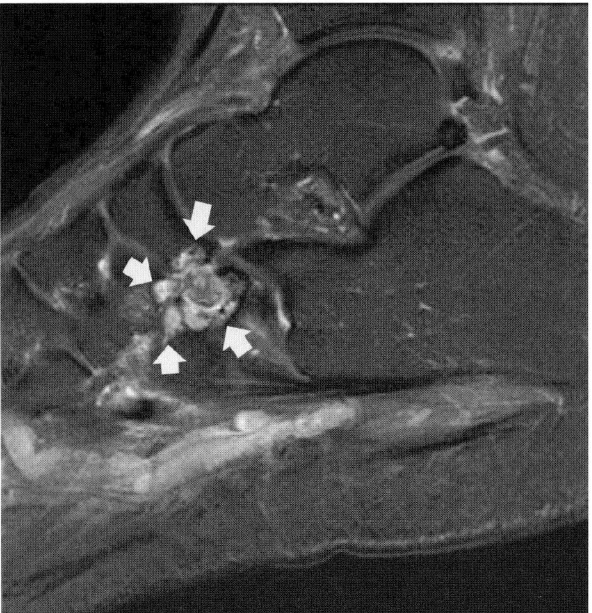

Figure 3.16   CT and MR comparison: Pigmented villonodular synovitis (PVNS) in the foot of a 51-year-old woman. **A:** Reformatted sagittal CT image shows osseous erosions (*arrows*) in multiple tarsal bones. **B:** Sagittal fat-suppressed, enhanced, T1-weighted (TR/TE; 766/17) spin-echo MR image shows the osseous erosions (*arrows*), although the fine sclerotic margins are appreciated to better advantage in **A**.

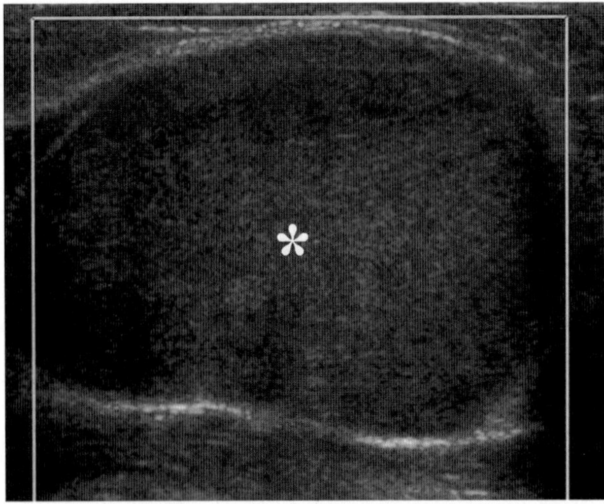

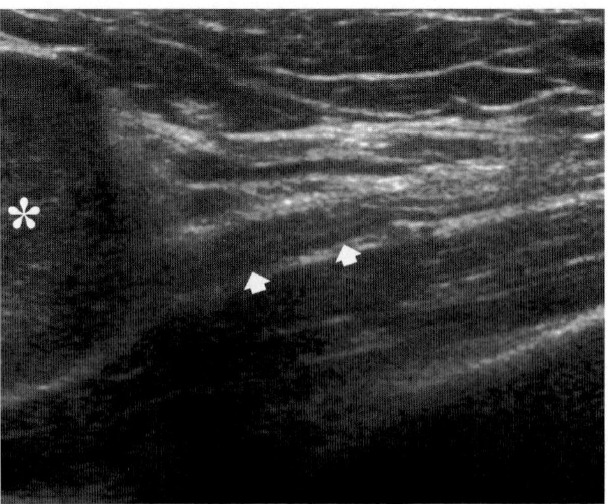

Figure 3.17 Sonography: Schwannoma in the forearm of a man 52 years of age. **A:** Sonogram shows a nonspecific, solid, soft tissue mass (*asterisk*). **B:** Imaging more proximally shows the mass (*asterisk*) to be intimately associated with the median nerve (*arrows*). The eccentric relation of the mass to the nerve suggests a schwannoma.

to therapy (Fig. 3.18) (74), rather than in establishing a precise diagnosis.

Color Doppler is useful in assessing the degree of intratumoral blood flow in solid lesions as well as in indicating the origin and pattern of vascular supply (75). Although color Doppler is typically not useful for establishing a specific diagnosis (76), establishing a vascular supply to a lesion should exclude the diagnosis of an abscess (75). Power Doppler sonography is also useful in establishing the hyperemia associated with inflammatory processes (77). In patients with vascular anomalies, ultrasound can detect arterial flow and distinguish arterial venous hemangiomas (vascular malformations) from other hemangiomas (78).

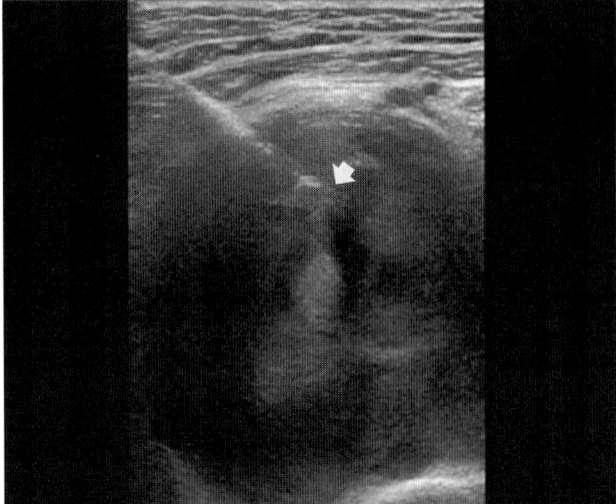

Figure 3.18 Sonography: Biopsy guidance in a man 56 years of age with a groin mass. Sonogram shows the tip of the needle (*arrow*) within the mass. Biopsy with a coaxial needle revealed a schwannoma with central hemorrhage.

Scintigraphy

> ### KEY CONCEPTS
> - Bone metastases are unusual as an isolated manifestation of metastatic disease, and routine scintigraphy in patients with no other evidence of metastatic disease is probably unnecessary.
> - Dynamic scintigraphy (including both flow and blood-pool studies) is generally useful in identifying the vascular nature of a musculoskeletal mass.

The natural history of a soft tissue sarcoma varies with histologic subtype, but is one of local recurrence, usually at the primary site, or of pulmonary metastases (79). Bone metastases are unusual as an isolated manifestation of metastatic disease and routine 99m-technetium–labeled diphosphonate scintigraphy in patients with no other evidence of metastatic disease is probably unnecessary. Dynamic scintigraphy (including both flow and blood-pool studies) is generally useful, however, in identifying the vascular nature of a musculoskeletal mass (Fig. 3.19).

Although 99m-technetium–labeled diphosphonate scintigraphy is used most frequently, more specific agents are available. Gallium-67 may be useful in distinguishing benign from malignant nerve sheath tumors (80,81). Thallium has also been reported to be useful in predicting response to radiation (82).

Positron Emission Tomography

Positron emission tomography (PET) is the proven gold standard in metabolic imaging. PET uses radioisotopes that undergo positron emission decay. A sophisticated ring detector surrounding the patient then detects the coincident photons and registers the interaction in the

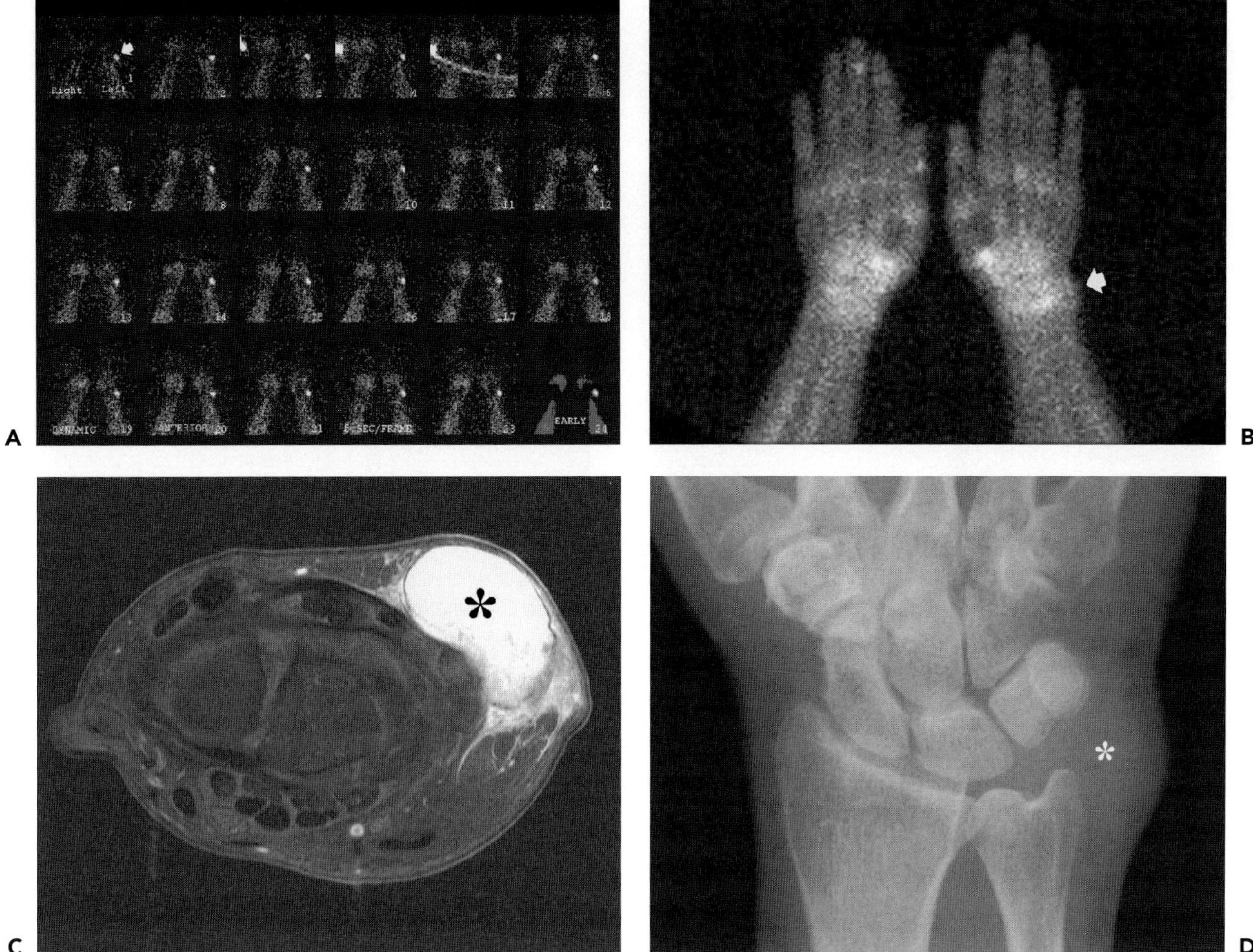

Figure 3.19 99m-Tc–labeled diphosphonate scintigraphy: High-grade undifferentiated sarcoma in the wrist of a woman 56 years of age. **A:** Flow study shows increased flow to the left wrist (*arrow*). **B:** Delayed static images show relatively symmetric distribution with very slight increased tracer accumulation to the area of the tumor (*arrow*). **C:** Corresponding enhanced, fat-suppressed, axial T1-weighted (TR/TE; 750/15) spin-echo MR image shows intense enhancement of the mass. **D:** Anteroposterior radiograph of the wrist shows the mass (*asterisk*) with no adjacent osseous abnormality.

KEY CONCEPTS

- Positron emission tomography (PET) is the gold standard in metabolic imaging.
- It uses radioisotopes that undergo positron emission decay.
- Fluorodeoxyglucose (FDG) behaves like glucose and provides a means of quantifying glucose metabolism.
- High-grade malignancies tend to have higher rates of glycolysis and FDG uptake.
- Studies show FDG-PET to be 95% sensitive and 75% specific in the diagnosis of soft tissue sarcomas.
- FDG-PET is useful in directing biopsy to the most metabolically active area.

---

ing glucose metabolism. Unlike glucose, the metabolite of FDG is not a substrate for glycolytic enzymes. Therefore, the radioactive tracer is trapped in the cell, allowing subsequent imaging. The amount of tracer accumulation reflects the tissue's glucose metabolism. Many types of tumors have higher rates of glycolysis than uninvolved normal tissue (83). High-grade malignancies tend to have higher rates of glycolysis and FDG uptake than those of low-grade malignancies and benign lesions. There are multiple reports in the literature of significantly greater standardized uptake value (SUV) in malignant tumors compared to that of benign tumors. However, there can be a higher accumulation of FDG in some benign tumors, especially histiocytic or giant cell–containing lesions.

In general, sarcomas tend to be FDG avid (Fig. 3.20) (84,85), although there is significant variability. Studies show FDG-PET to be 95% sensitive and 75% specific in the

form of an image. The radionuclide most commonly used for PET is fluorodeoxyglucose (FDG). In vivo, FDG behaves like glucose and provides a means of quantify-

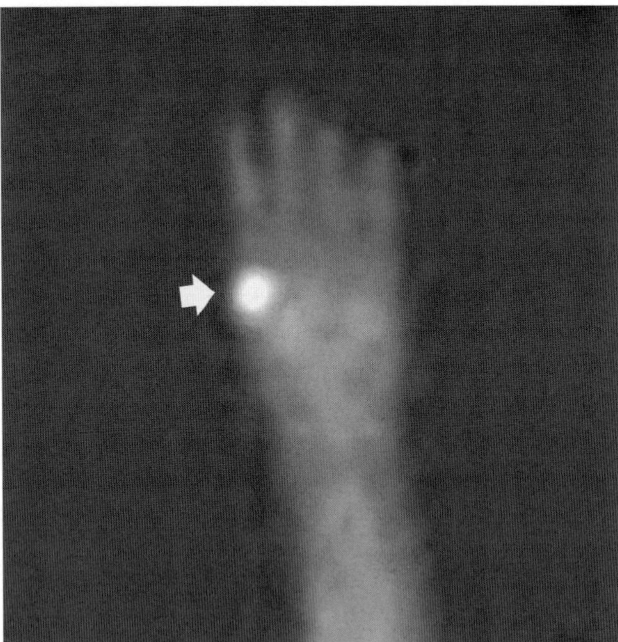

A

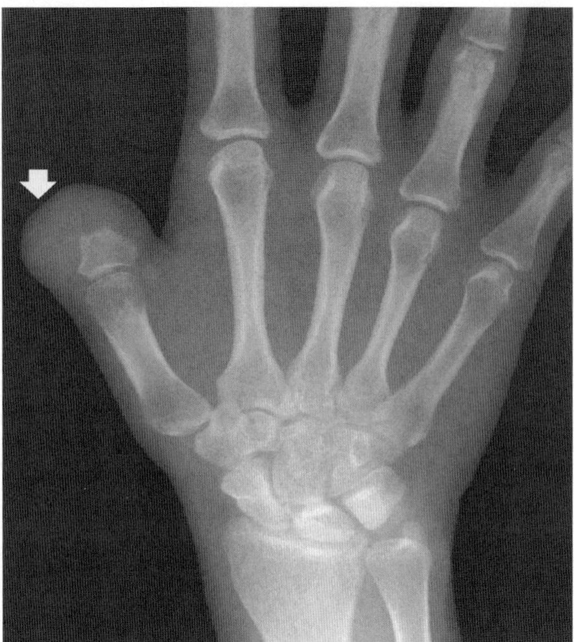

B

Figure 3.20   Positron emission tomography (PET): Recurrent epithelioid sarcoma in a woman 35 years of age with prior amputation of the right first digit at the level of the first proximal phalanx. **A:** FDG-PET demonstrates marked increased metabolic activity (*arrow*) corresponding to the nodular focus at the prior amputation site indicating the presence of recurrent tumor. **B:** Anteroposterior radiograph shows the prior amputation and recurrent tumor (*arrow*).

diagnosis of soft tissue sarcomas (86,87). A systematic review and meta-analysis of the value of FDG-PET in the detection, grading, and therapy response of musculoskeletal sarcomas was completed by Bastiannet et al. (88) in 2003. A review of 29 clinical studies revealed a pooled sensitivity, specificity, and accuracy of 91%, 85%, and 88%, respectively. FDG-PET is useful in directing biopsy to the most metabolically active area of a tumor to improve diagnostic yield (Fig. 3.21) (89).

Arteriography

> **KEY CONCEPTS**
> - MR angiography depicts major tumor vessels.
> - Angiographic findings of soft tissue tumors are nonspecific.
> - CT and MR imaging are more accurate in compartmental localization.

With the advent of computerized imaging, especially MR and now magnetic resonance angiography (MRA), the role of conventional arteriography in evaluating soft tissue tumors has decreased markedly. MR angiography is capable of depicting the major vessels in a tumor bed and detecting most of those seen by conventional angiographic techniques, except for those that are quite small, such as sural or geniculate arteries (Figs. 3.22 and 3.23) (90). These small vessels are of little importance in planning

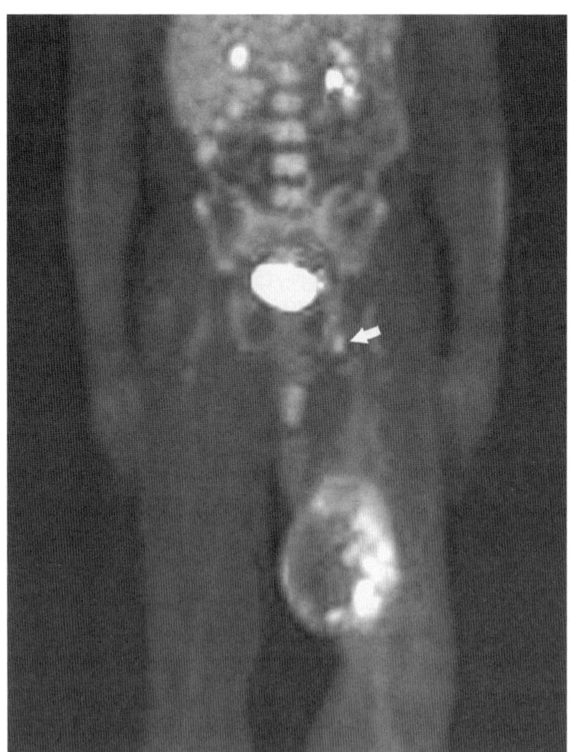

Figure 3.21   Positron emission tomography (PET): Directing biopsy to the most metabolically active areas in a hemorrhagic, high-grade, undifferentiated pleomorphic sarcoma (same patient; see Fig. 3.8). PET shows hypermetabolic activity at the periphery of the mass compatible with viable tumor, as well as absent activity centrally caused by hemorrhage and necrosis. Note small hypermetabolic focus in the left groin corresponding to lymphadenopathy (*arrow*).

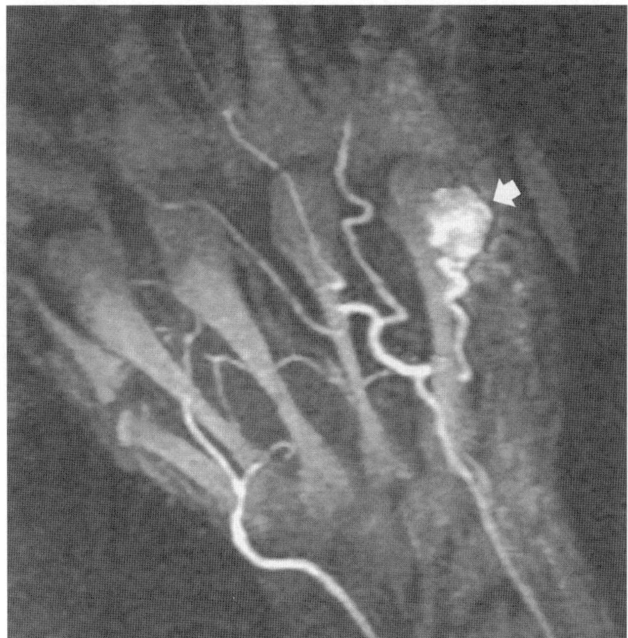

Figure 3.22 Magnetic resonance angiography (MRA): Spindle cell hemangioma in the hand of a man 60 years of age. MRA shows the mass (*arrow*) and its vascular supply. The ulnar artery is intact.

limb-salvage surgery (90). Computed imaging is more accurate in compartmental localization of lesions, as well as in determining the relationship of the lesion to the vascular structures (91). Moreover, the angiographic findings of soft tissue tumors are nonspecific; therefore, they cannot be used to reliably distinguish benign from malignant lesions (92–97). Arteriography (either conventional or intra-arterial digital subtraction) remains useful for providing an operative road map, identifying normal anatomic variants prior to surgery and establishing access for intra-arterial chemotherapy.

Arteriography is also helpful in evaluating patients with arteriovenous malformations (arteriovenous hemangiomas) and occasionally for preoperative or therapeutic embolization. Preoperative embolization of hypervascular tumors may dramatically reduce intraoperative bleeding. Therapeutic embolization, accomplished intra-arterially (transcatheter) or percutaneously, is used in the treatment of vascular malformations (98,99). These techniques are highly effective in palliating symptomatic vascular malformations. Embolic materials used include polyvinyl alcohol foam particles (Ivalon; Unipont Laboratories, High Point, NC), Gelfoam (Upjohn, Kalamazoo, MI), absolute ethanol, sodium tetradecyl sodium (Sotradecol; Elkins-Sinn, Cherry Hill, NJ), and isobutyl cyanoacrylate (glue) (98,99).

IMAGING FOLLOWING TREATMENT

Overall, approximately half of patients with soft tissue sarcomas have local recurrence (79,100). Consequently, routine follow-up is essential. As with patients presenting for the initial evaluation of a mass, the evaluation of a patient following treatment begins with a thorough clinical history

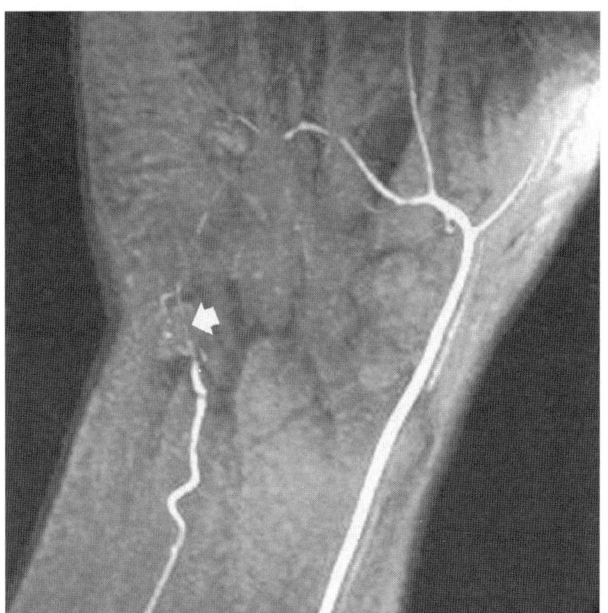

A

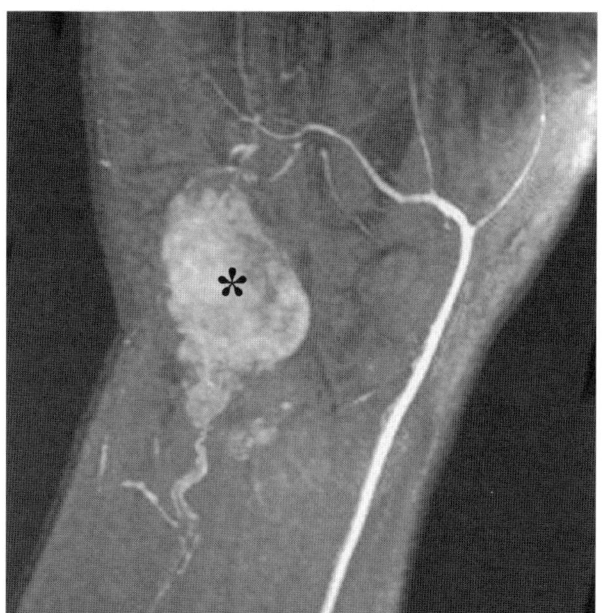

B

Figure 3.23 Magnetic resonance angiography (MRA): Recurrent ulnar nerve schwannoma in a 28-year-old woman. **A:** First-pass image from enhanced MRA of the hand shows the mass to be occluding the ulnar artery (*arrow*). **B:** Second-pass image shows intense enhancement of the mass (*asterisk*) with draining veins.

and radiologic evaluation. Examination of the operative site may also provide considerable additional information.

Clinical History

KEY CONCEPTS
- Clinical history is critically important in evaluating patients following treatment.
- Important information includes addressing these questions:
  - What was the original tumor diagnosis?
  - What was the tumor grade and location?
  - What type of surgical resection was done?
  - What type of reconstructive surgery was done?
  - Was there a history of radiation surgery?
  - Any new lumps or bumps?
  - Any evidence or history of metastatic disease?

The clinical history is critically important in evaluating patients following treatment and may be the key factor in establishing an accurate diagnosis. In many circumstances it may provide information that allows a specific diagnosis when imaging is nonspecific. Important information includes identification of the original tumor diagnosis. Certain tumors show much greater predilection for local recurrence. Fibromatosis, for example, is reported to recur locally in as many as three-quarters of patients (101,102). What was the tumor grade? High-grade tumors are at much greater risk for local recurrence. Tumor grade and type influence recurrence risk as does location. Deep tumors, and those in which wide margins cannot be obtained, are at greater risk for local recurrence than are superficial lesions. A well-differentiated liposarcoma of the extremity may be "cured" by wide local excision, whereas the same tumor in the retroperitoneum has virtually a 100% local recurrence rate (103).

An appropriate clinical history should include the details of surgery. What type of surgical resection was done? The type of surgical resection has significant implications on the risk of local recurrence; ranging from exceedingly low risk with radical resection (amputation) to exceedingly high risk with marginal excision. Surgical data should include the details of the surgical margins. Patients with positive surgical margins may show no mass or discrete lesion on imaging while having histologic evidence of residual tumor.

It is also essential to identify whether there was radiation therapy or reconstructive surgery, and, if so, their time course in relation to the current study. Both radiation and reconstructive surgery influence the postoperative imaging appearance, and both demonstrate time-dependent changes (104–106).

Other important information includes any change in the areas of previous surgery and any new lumps or bumps. A new mass in the face of anticoagulation may suggest the possibility of a hematoma; however, in our experience such lesions are highly suspect for hemorrhagic tumor. Finally, is there any evidence or history of metastatic disease? Documented metastases indicate a more aggressive biological potential and serve to raise the index of suspicion for local recurrence.

Imaging Evaluation

KEY CONCEPTS
- The radiologic evaluation for the postoperative patient begins with the radiograph.
- Radiographs can show:
  - Postoperative skeletal deformity or heterotopic ossification.
  - Soft tissue calcifications that may not be appreciated on MR imaging.
- Review should include previous MR imaging studies:
  - Although not all change is indicative of recurrence, no change is reassuring in excluding recurrence.
  - Recurrent tumor frequently exhibits an imaging appearance similar to that of the primary tumor.
- MR imaging of patients following treatment mirror those for initial tumor evaluation:
  - Markers noting the margins of the surgical scar can be helpful to ensure complete coverage.
  - Contrast is especially important in the evaluation of post-treatment hemorrhage.

Similar to the evaluation of a primary mass, the radiologic evaluation for the postoperative patient begins with the radiograph. Radiographs can show postoperative skeletal deformity or heterotopic ossification, which may be difficult to appreciate on MR imaging and may masquerade as recurrent tumor. This is especially helpful in cases in which the normal marrow signal has altered. Radiographs can also reveal soft tissue calcifications that may not be appreciated on MR imaging. CT is a useful adjunct in specific circumstances. We generally reserve CT for those patients in whom radiographs do not adequately depict the lesion, its pattern of mineralization, or its relationship to the host. This is typically in areas in which the osseous anatomy is complex, such as in the pelvis, shoulder, and paraspinal regions.

In the postoperative patient, preliminary radiologic evaluation should include a review of the previous MR imaging studies, as well as the presenting and pretreatment studies when available. Although not all change is indicative of tumor recurrence, no change is very reassuring in excluding recurrence. Additionally, it has been our experience that recurrent tumor frequently exhibits an imaging appearance similar to that of the primary tumor, information that can be useful in distinguishing tumor recurrence from postoperative change.

Although the technical considerations for MR imaging of the patient following treatment mirror those for initial tumor evaluation, there are some additional considerations. It is essential to evaluate the entire operative or treated area. Markers noting the margins of the surgical scar can be helpful to ensure complete coverage. Contrast may also be a useful adjunct. Although in general we find that in most cases recurrent tumor is usually well-seen without contrast, in specific instances contrast is especially useful; these include the distinction of postoperative hematoma from recurrent tumor and the evaluation of recurrent fibromatosis. In the evaluation of lesions with increased signal intensity on T1-weighted images, comparison of precontrast fat-suppressed T1-weighted images with postcontrast fat-suppressed T1-weighted images is preferred. Hemorrhage shows increased signal on enhanced fat-suppressed imaging and may be mistaken for enhancement without careful comparison to precontrast imaging. If precontrast fat-suppressed imaging is not done, comparison with non–fat-suppressed enhanced imaging is useful.

Clinical Examination

> ### KEY CONCEPTS
> - Clinical examination allows confirmation of a clinically suspected palpable abnormality.
> - It allows inspection of the operative bed to identify:
>   - The scope of the surgical change.
>   - The presence of reconstructive procedures.
>   - The presence of associated conditions.

Examination of the operative site may provide considerable additional information. It allows confirmation of a clinically suspected palpable abnormality. It also allows inspection of the operative bed to identify the scope of the surgical change, the presence of reconstructive procedures, as well as any associated conditions such as radiation dermatitis, cellulitis, or cutaneous ulcers (Fig. 3.24).

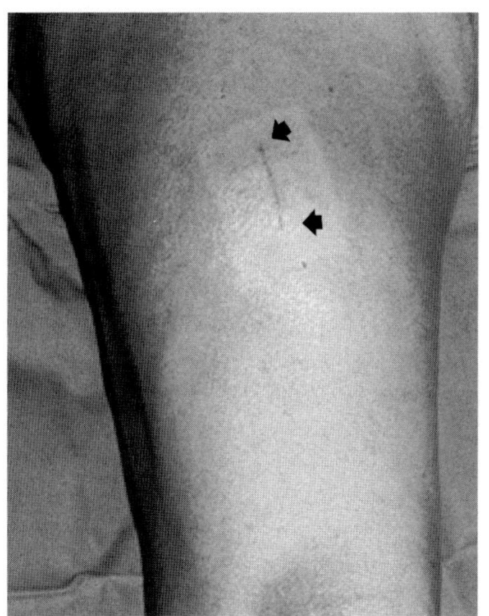

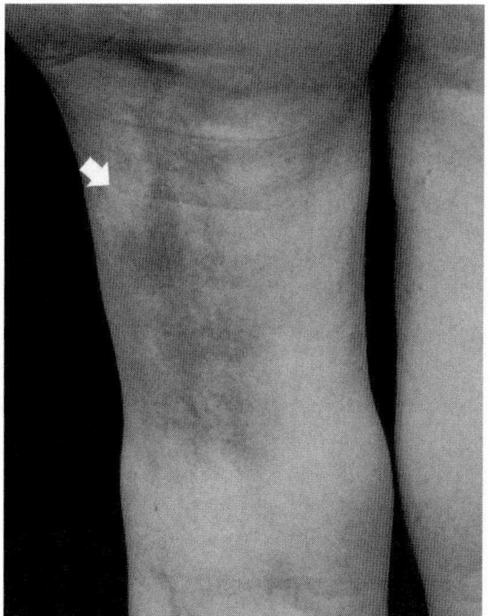

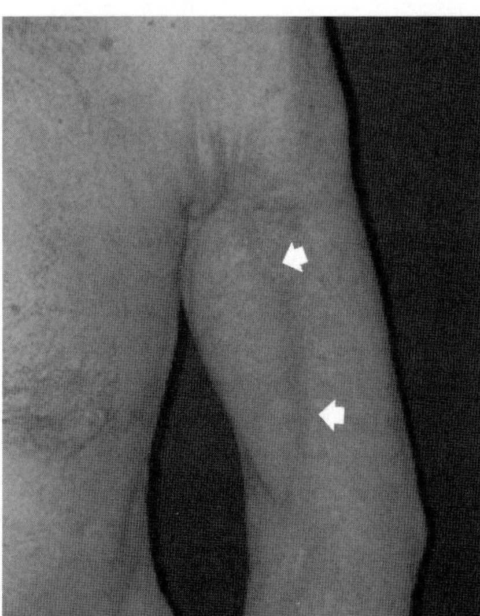

Figure 3.24 Clinical examination: Clinical photographs of postoperative site. **A:** Photograph shows scar (*arrows*) following surgical excision. **B:** Photograph shows scar and hyperpigmentation (*arrow*) from radiation dermatitis in patient treated with excision and radiation therapy. **C:** Photograph shows a rotational myocutaneous flap (*arrows*) providing coverage and function following excision of upper arm sarcoma.

Local Recurrence

> ## KEY CONCEPTS
> - Recurrent tumor is characterized by the presence of a discrete nodule or mass.
> - When a masslike area is found, it must be distinguished from postoperative change.

MR imaging and ultrasonography are both useful in detecting local recurrence (100). Recurrent tumor is characterized by the presence of a discrete nodule or mass. On MR imaging recurrent tumor typically shows prolonged T1- and T2-relaxation times, usually demonstrating prominent contrast enhancement (Figs. 3.25 and 3.26). Tumor recurrence, however, is usually well-seen without enhanced imaging. When identification of a discrete high-signal-intensity nodule on fluid-sensitive images is used as criterion for local recurrence, MR imaging is quite accurate (107).

Postsurgical changes are more variable and usually show areas of low or intermediate signal intensity or fluid collections, without a discrete nodule (100,107). The spectrum of post-treatment changes is described more fully later. When a mass with high signal intensity on T2-weighted images is found, tumor must be differentiated from postoperative hygroma. In most cases, this differentiation is straightforward, with fluid characterized by a homogeneous, well-defined mass with prolonged T1- and T2-weighted spin-echo MR images.

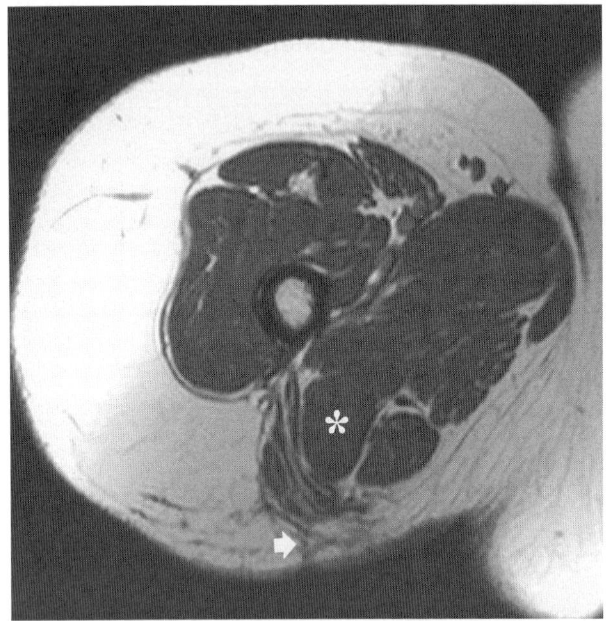

A

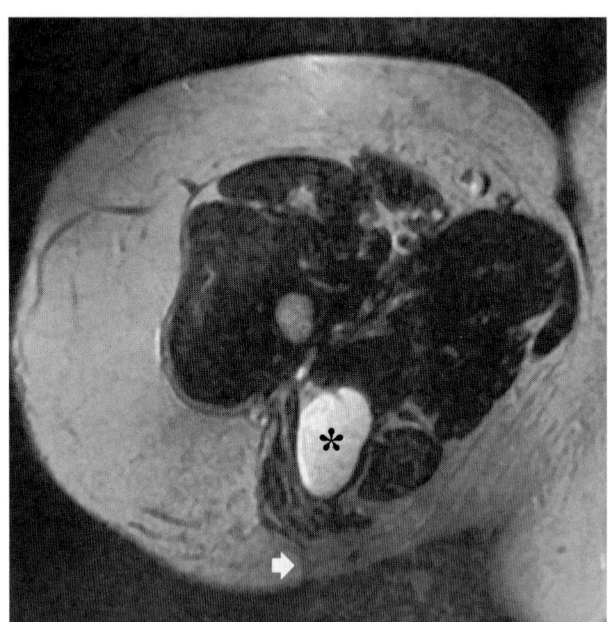

B

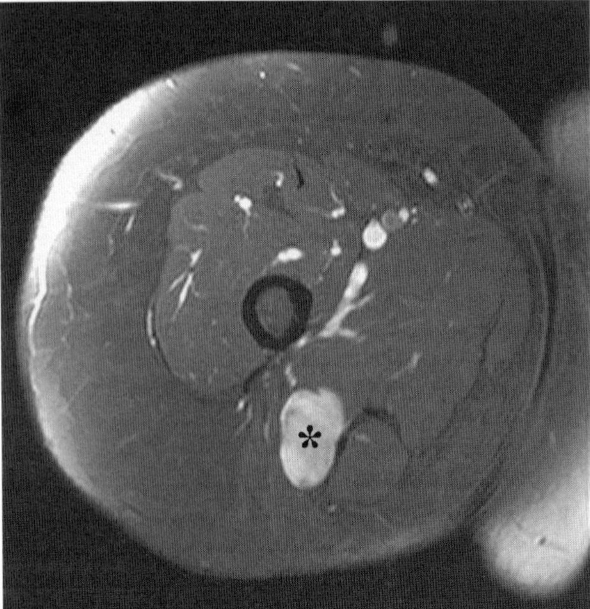

C

Figure 3.25 Local recurrence: Recurrent myxoid liposarcoma in the thigh of a woman 57 years of age. **A,B:** Axial T1-weighted (TR/TE; 400/16) **(A)** and T2-weighted (TR/TE; 2060/80) **(B)** spin-echo MR images show focal intermuscular mass (*asterisk*) with a fluidlike signal intensity. Note posterior surgical scar (*arrow*). **C:** Axial fat-suppressed T1-weighted (TR/TE; 438/18) spin-echo MR image following intravenous contrast shows intense enhancement (*asterisk*).

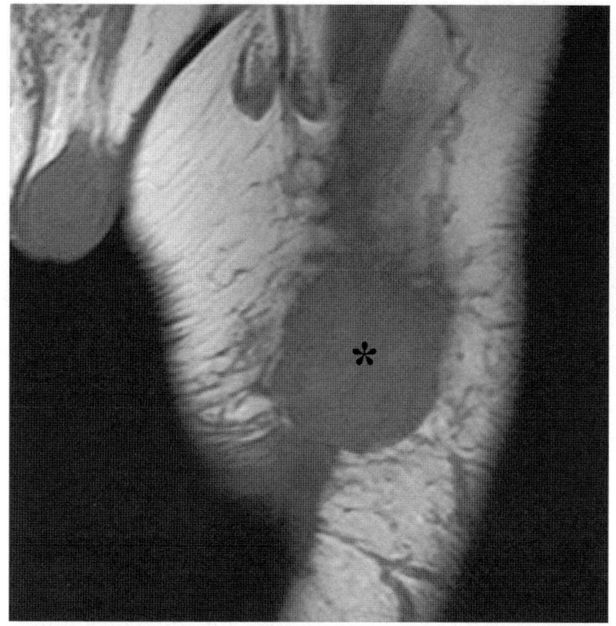

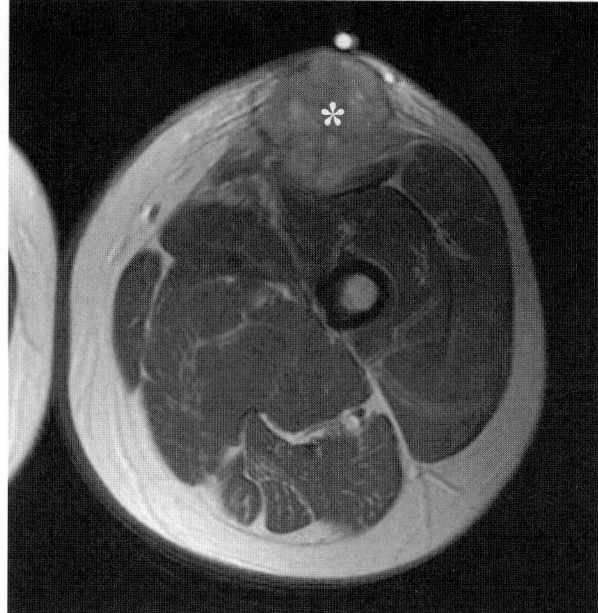

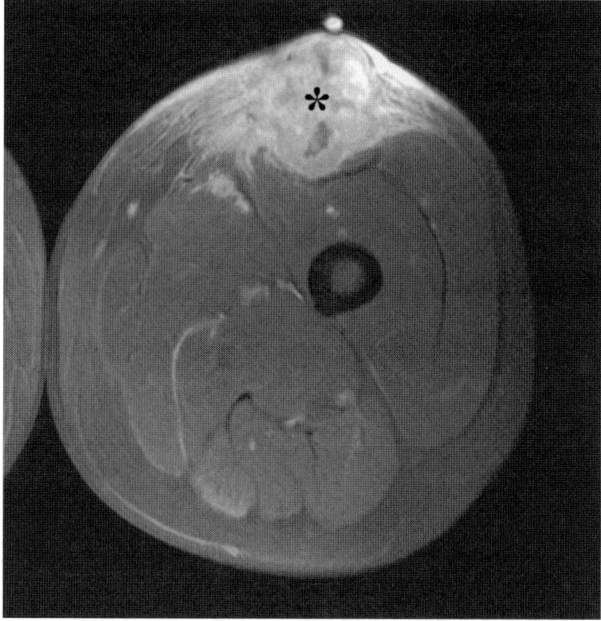

Figure 3.26 Local recurrence: Recurrent high-grade, undifferentiated pleomorphic sarcoma (malignant fibrous histiocytoma) in the thigh of a man 39 years of age. The patient received 5000 cGy postoperative radiation therapy to the surgical site. **A,B:** Coronal T1-weighted (TR/TE; 300/17) **(A)** spin-echo and axial fast spin-echo T2-weighted (TR/TE; 2060/80) **(B)** MR images show a focal mass (*asterisk*) with an intermediate signal intensity. Note surrounding peritumoral reactive change. **C:** Axial fat-suppressed T1-weighted (TR/TE; 654/16) spin-echo MR image following intravenous contrast shows intense enhancement (*asterisk*).

As noted previously, comparison with pretreatment images is essential. For example, myxoid tumors may mimic cysts on MR imaging, and differentiation between a postoperative fluid collection and recurrent tumor would be considerably more difficult if the patient's original tumor were a myxoid liposarcoma. When there is a question of whether an area of high signal intensity on T2-weighted images represents fluid, ultrasound examination is an ideal method for further evaluation. It is easy, inexpensive, and highly accurate. Alternatively, gadolinium-enhanced MRI may be used.

Ultrasound may be used as the primary modality to follow patients for recurrence, with a discrete hypoechoic mass considered to be recurrent tumor (100). Ultrasound is still very operator dependent and of limited value in cases where the osseous anatomy is complex, such as in the shoulder girdle or pelvis. Consequently, we prefer MR imaging for identification of recurrent tumor.

Post-Treatment Changes

A number of imaging features are commonly seen following treatment for a soft tissue sarcoma. Knowledge of these imaging features minimizes the likelihood they will be misconstrued for recurrent tumor. Post-treatment changes include the effects of chemotherapy, pre- or postoperative radiation on bone and soft tissue, postsurgical fluid collections, hemorrhage, and reconstructive myocutaneous flaps.

Chemotherapy

> ### KEY CONCEPTS
> - Effects of chemotherapy are variable.
> - Chemotherapy may result in an increase in tumor size as a result of intralesional hemorrhage.
> - Chemotherapy may decrease tumor size significantly.

The effects of chemotherapy are often thought to be inconsequential; however, significant increase in tumor size secondary to chemotherapy-induced hemorrhage has been reported (108). In other cases, chemotherapy may significantly reduce tumor size, with only degenerated and reactive tissue identified at subsequent surgery (109). We have found contrast-enhanced imaging useful in determining the degree of intralesional necrosis, a feature that may be useful in establishing the effectiveness of chemotherapy and tumor biological potential.

Radiation Therapy

It has been long recognized that resection of high-grade sarcomas without adjuvant therapy results in unacceptably high rates of local recurrence (110). This led oncologists in the 1970s to evaluate the use of adjuvant radiation therapy and chemotherapy in improving functional outcome of limb-sparing surgery (110). In current practice, radiation may be administered prior to, during, or following tumor surgical resection (111).

Administering radiation following tumor resection avoids the increased risk of wound complications associated

> ### KEY CONCEPTS
> - MR imaging can detect radiation marrow changes as early as 8 days following onset of therapy.
> - Complete fatty replacement usually occurs within 6 to 8 weeks.
> - Irradiated bone is at increased risk for fracture.
> - Irradiated soft tissue shows abnormal edemalike signal intensity.
> - Soft tissue MR imaging signal abnormalities are greater and persist longer in the intermuscular septa than in the fat or muscle.

with operating on compromised tissue. It also eliminates the potential difficulty of determining the histologic diagnosis from radiated tissue. Finally, it allows surgery to be performed without delay (110,111). Although preoperative radiation is associated with increased wound complication, it reduces tumor volume and therefore improves tumor resectability (110,111).

Radiation changes are readily identified in both bone and soft tissue. Osseous changes following radiation are well documented; however, for the current discussion we focus on those changes primarily identified on MR imaging. MR imaging can detect radiation-induced marrow changes as early as 8 days following onset of therapy (112). Between 3 and 6 weeks post-radiation the marrow shows increasingly heterogeneous signal intensity with increasing fat signal. In the vast majority of patients, complete fatty replacement usually occurs within 6 to 8 weeks (Figs. 3.27

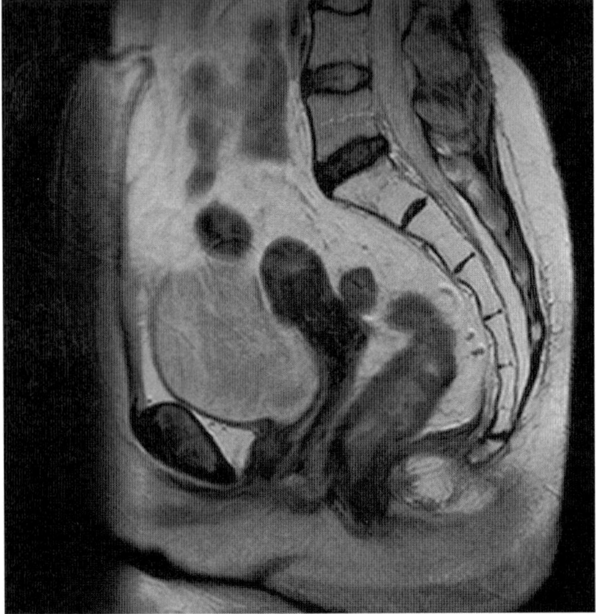

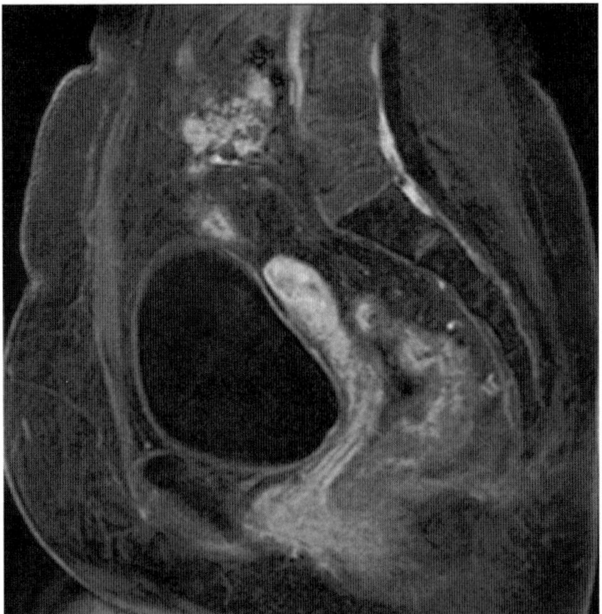

Figure 3.27 Radiation therapy changes: Osseous radiation change in the sacrum of a woman 46 years of age following radiation for anal carcinoma. **A,B:** Sagittal fast spin-echo T2-weighted **(A)** and enhanced fat-suppressed T1-weighted **(B)** MR images show increased fat within the sacrum caused by previous radiation therapy.

and 3.28) (112,113). Uncommonly, a band of peripheral intermediate signal surrounding central fat may be seen (113). About half of those patients receiving radiation show marrow changes immediately adjacent to the radiated field. These changes are milder and are more common in patients with highly cellular pretreatment marrow (112,114).

As a result of the cellular damage caused by radiation, irradiated bone is at increased risk for fracture (115). The pelvis is the most likely area to be involved, although the incidence of pelvic-associated injury is small (0.1% to 0.3%) (116). This is considerably less than the 1.8% estimated incidence of sacral insufficiency fractures in women 55 years of age and older (61).

We also occasionally note the appearance of somewhat poorly defined areas of nonspecific nonadipose tissue within the marrow of radiated extremities. This is usually several months following the completion of radiation; moreover, these changes may become more prominent during the succeeding months before stabilizing (Fig. 3.29).

Soft tissue changes are more variable and differ with the type of radiotherapy. Richardson et al. (118) characterized the soft tissue changes following radiation and noted that irradiated soft tissue showed abnormal edemalike signal intensity. The signal intensity showed great variability but was generally greater on STIR images than on T2-weighted spin-echo images. Signal alterations increase with time and are greatest in photon-treated patients at 12 to 18 months post-treatment and return to normal in about half of these in 2 to 3 years. The edema signal in the subcutaneous tissue appears as a trabecular or latticelike pattern of low-to-inter-

mediate signal intensity on T1-weighted spin-echo images and high signal intensity on fluid-sensitive sequences (108). Radiation-induced changes in muscle are more diffuse with minimal enhancement following contrast administration and preservation of muscle shape and texture (107,108,119).

MR imaging signal abnormalities are greater and persist longer in the intermuscular septa than in the subcutaneous fat or muscle. The size of the fat and intramuscular septa increase mildly; muscle shows a decrease in size following treatment (Figs. 3.29 and 3.30) (118).

Following radiation therapy, patients may also develop inflammatory pseudotumors (Fig. 3.31). Scant documentation exists for this phenomenon in the imaging literature, but Vanel et al. (107) noted two such cases in a review of follow-up imaging of 182 patients with aggressive soft tissue tumors. Both lesions presented as high signal intensity masses, 1 year following and the other 12 years following radiation and surgery. Both of these lesions were investigated with dynamic contrast enhancement and showed delayed enhancement (4 to 7 minutes) as compared to tumor recurrence (1 to 3 minutes).

Postoperative Fluid and Hemorrhage

> **KEY CONCEPTS**
> - Postoperative fluid collections and hemorrhage show a similar appearance to that seen following nononcology procedures.
> - The distinction of postoperative hematoma from postoperative recurrence or residual tumor may be especially difficult, and post contrast imaging is helpful in this distinction.

Postoperative fluid collections and hemorrhage following sarcoma surgery show a similar appearance to that seen following nononcology procedures (Fig. 3.32). In the oncology patient, however, the masslike appearance of these complications may mimic that of local tumor recurrence, and the distinction may be especially difficult in selected cases. In these instances, post contrast imaging is especially helpful (Fig. 3.33).

Uncomplicated postoperative fluid collections are more readily distinguished from tumor recurrence. Recurrent tumor is usually more heterogeneous and the margins are usually more irregular than those seen in simple postoperative hygroma. Contrast-enhanced imaging may prove helpful in cases in which seromas demonstrate increased (intermediate) signal intensity on T1-weighted images (Fig. 3.34) (107). Most seromas appear to resolve in 3 to 18 months (109), although this is variable, and they may persist for an extended period of time.

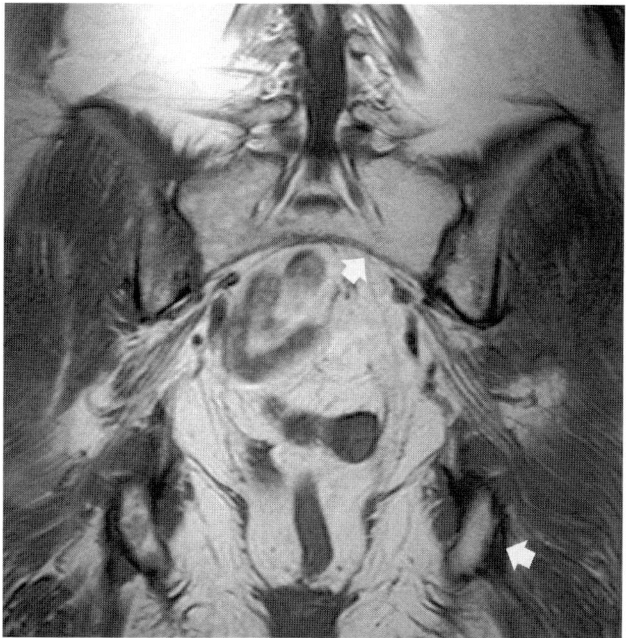

Figure 3.28 Radiation therapy changes: Osseous radiation change in the pelvis and sacrum of a woman 59 years of age following radiation for lymphoma. The patient received 4500 cGy to the left hemipelvis. Coronal T1-weighted spin-echo MR image of the pelvis. Note increased fatty marrow in ischium and sacrum (*arrows*).

Reconstructive Surgery

The extensive tissue resection required to achieve adequate surgical margins in oncologic surgery often require soft tissue

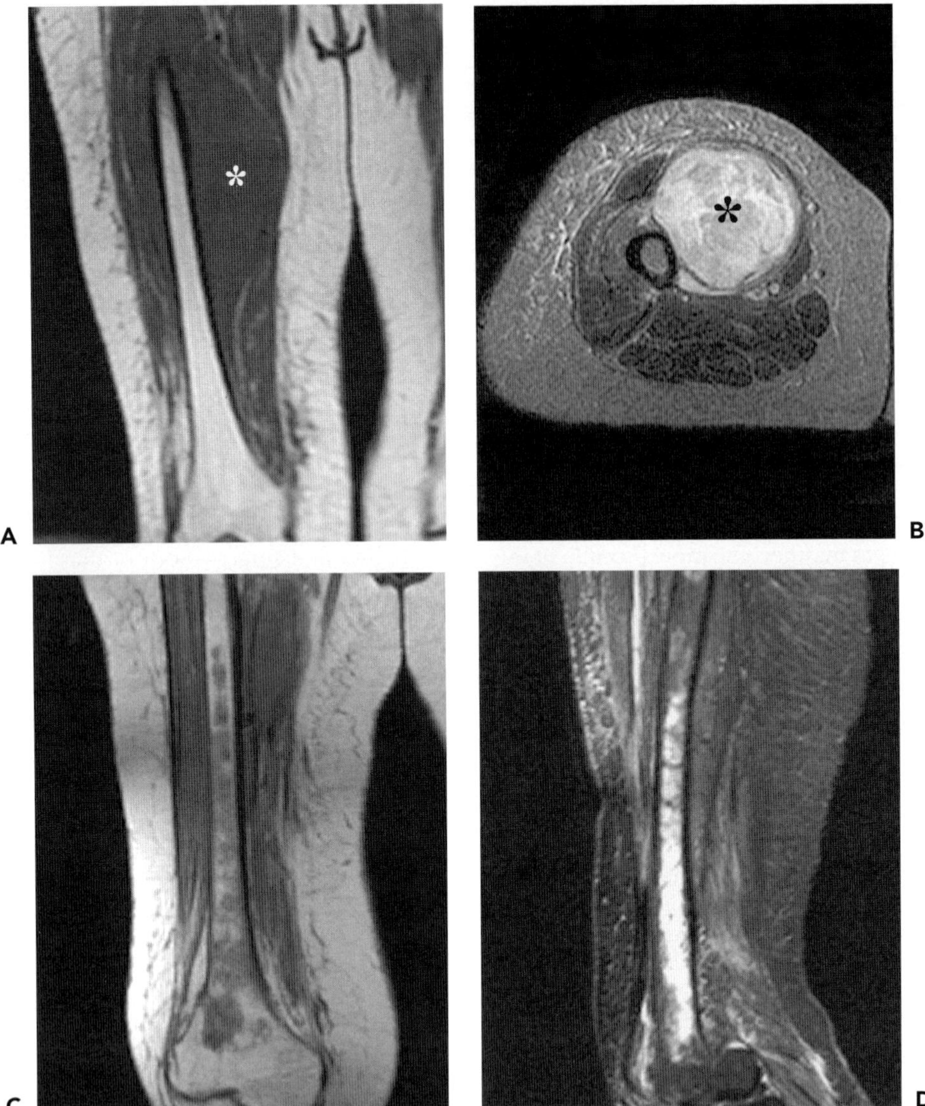

Figure 3.29 Radiation therapy marrow changes: High-grade undifferentiated pleomorphic sarcoma (malignant fibrous histiocytoma) in the thigh of a woman 89 years of age treated with 5040 cGy preoperative radiation. **A,B:** Coronal T1-weighted **(A)** and axial T2-weighted **(B)** spin-echo MR images obtained 1 month following start of radiation therapy show edema of the soft tissues surrounding the mass (*asterisk*). **C,D:** Coronal T1-weighted **(C)** and axial T2-weighted **(D)** spin-echo MR images obtained 41 months following start of radiation therapy show nonspecific abnormal signal within the femoral marrow. Note postoperative and postradiation changes.

KEY CONCEPTS
- Myocutaneous flaps contain both muscle and overlying skin.
- Rotational flaps are rotated into position, preserving native neurovascular supply via a pedicle.
- Free flaps are completely detached and the vascular pedicle is reanastomosed.
- Time-dependent changes in musculoskeletal flaps on MR imaging include:
  - Initial increased signal intensity on T2-weighted images that returns to normal in approximately one-third of cases.
  - Contrast enhancement in about three-quarters that returns to normal in approximately one-third.
  - Atrophy, which is variable, but can be marked.

reconstructive surgery. Myocutaneous flaps are employed in more than two-thirds of extremity sarcoma surgeries (106).

Myocutaneous flaps contain both muscle and overlying skin. *Rotational flaps* are rotated into position, covering the soft tissue defect while preserving the native neurovascular supply via a pedicle (Fig. 3.35). *Free flaps* are completely detached, placed into the soft tissue defect, and the vascular pedicle is reanastomosed using a microvascular technique (Fig. 3.36). Although most flaps are used for coverage only, rotational flaps using muscles such as the latissimus dorsi may provide both coverage and function when they are used for the upper arm.

As the MR imaging appearance of radiated tissue changes with time, so does the appearance of myocutaneous flaps.

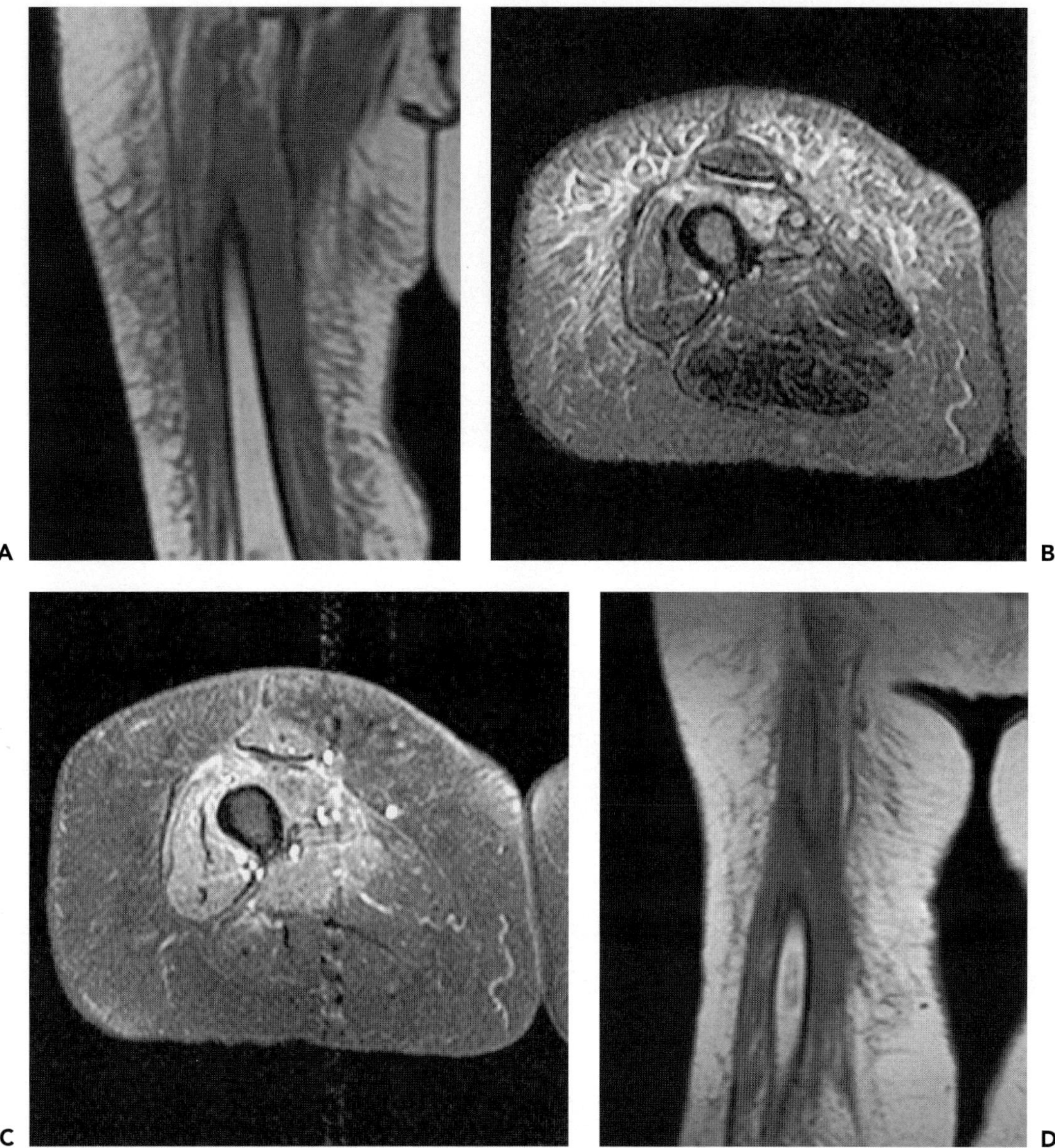

Figure 3.30 Radiation therapy soft tissue changes: Same patient as in Figure 3.29. **A,B:** Coronal T1-weighted (TR/TE; 633/16) **(A)** and axial T2-weighted (TR/TE; 2800/80) **(B)** spin-echo MR images obtained 6.5 months following radiation therapy show extensive edema in the muscle and subcutaneous soft tissues. **C:** Corresponding axial fat-suppressed T1-weighted (TR/TE; 450/10) spin-echo MR image following contrast shows enhancement of the muscle but little enhancement of the subcutaneous edema. **D,E:** Coronal T1-weighted (TR/TE; 829/15) **(D)** and axial T2-weighted (TR/TE; 3262/80) **(E)** spin-echo MR images obtained 16 months following radiation therapy show interval improvement. *(continued)*

A recent report by Fox et al. (106) reviewed the MR imaging findings in 30 myocutaneous flaps. They noted that all flaps demonstrate time-dependent changes in size, signal intensity, and enhancement. All flaps atrophy with time, demonstrating decreased muscle mass and progressive fatty replacement. The amount of atrophy was variable, however, ranging from mild to marked, but was less in flaps providing coverage and function (Fig. 3.37). In addition, all flaps initially demonstrate increased signal intensity on T2-weighted images, which return to baseline (similar to the signal intensity of the surrounding muscle) in one-third of cases

between 5 and 21 months (Fig. 3.38). Finally, enhancement was seen in about three-quarters of cases, returning to baseline in about one-third, in 18 months. Postoperative radiation therapy increased the likelihood a flap will exhibit increased T-2 weighted signal and enhancement.

STAGING

The radiologic staging of soft tissue tumors is an essential part of a patient's evaluation. Simply stated, the purpose of

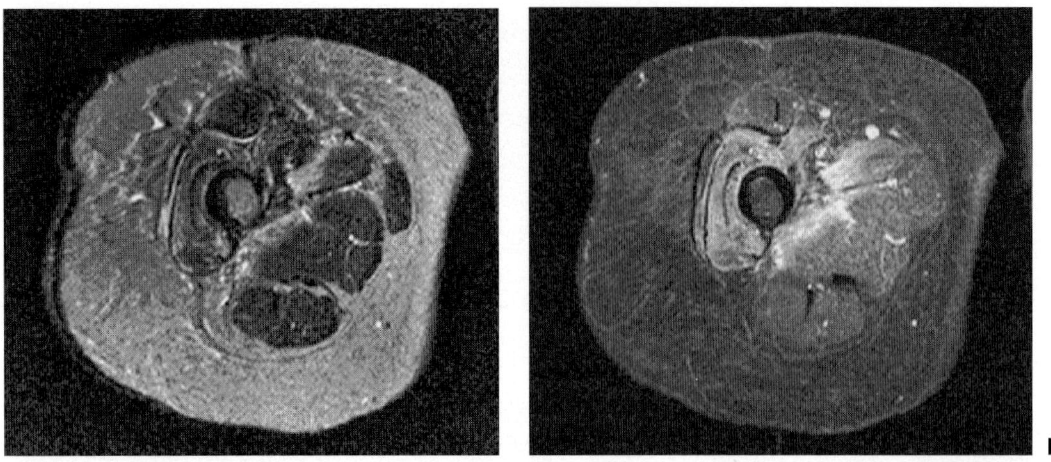

Figure 3.30 *(continued)* **D,E:** Coronal T1-weighted (TR/TE; 829/15) **(D)** and axial T2-weighted (TR/TE; 3262/80) **(E)** spin-echo MR images obtained 16 months following radiation therapy show interval improvement. **F:** Corresponding axial fat-suppressed T1-weighted (TR/TE; 644/15) spin-echo MR image following contrast shows persistent abnormal muscle enhancement.

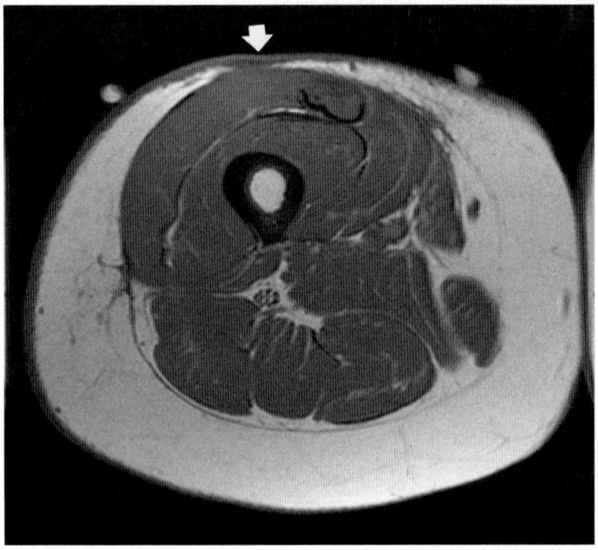

Figure 3.31 Radiation pseudotumor: Woman 61 years of age with a history of a dedifferentiated liposarcoma treated with surgery, chemotherapy, and 4500 cGy radiation therapy. **A,B:** Axial T1-weighted **(A)** and T2-weighted **(B)** spin-echo MR images obtained 3 years following surgery and radiation show a somewhat ill-defined area of abnormal signal in the surgical bed, but no discrete mass is identified. **C:** Axial fat-suppressed T1-weighted (TR/TE; 450/10) spin-echo MR image following contrast shows intense enhancement. Surgical biopsy showed atrophic skeletal muscle and fibrosis.

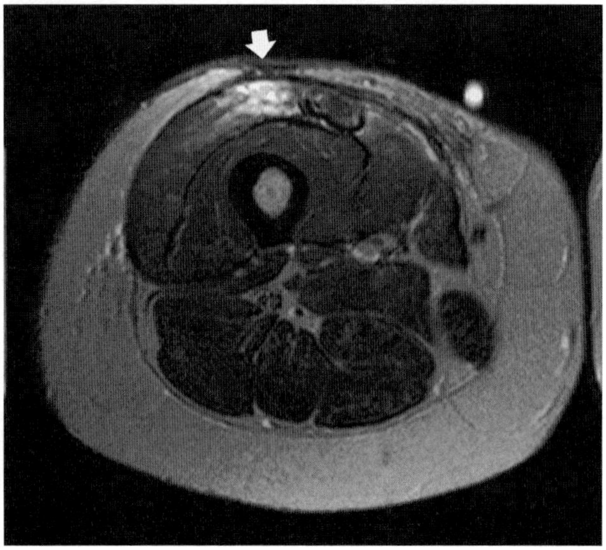

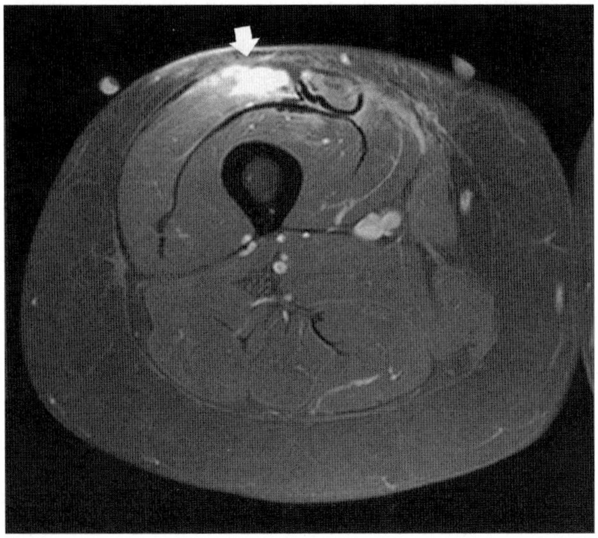

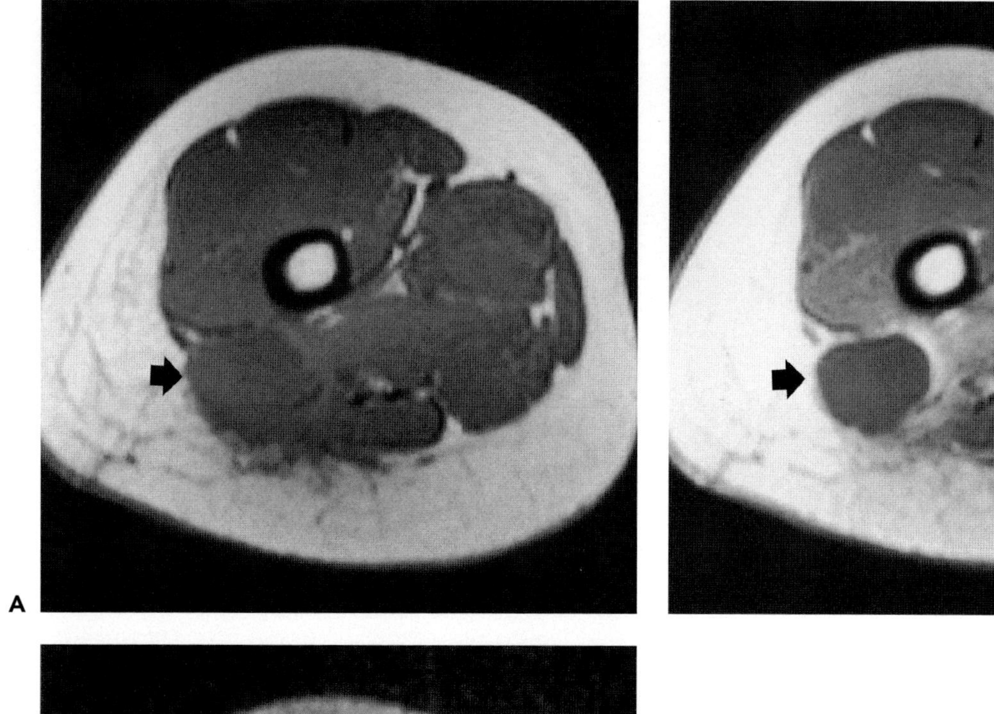

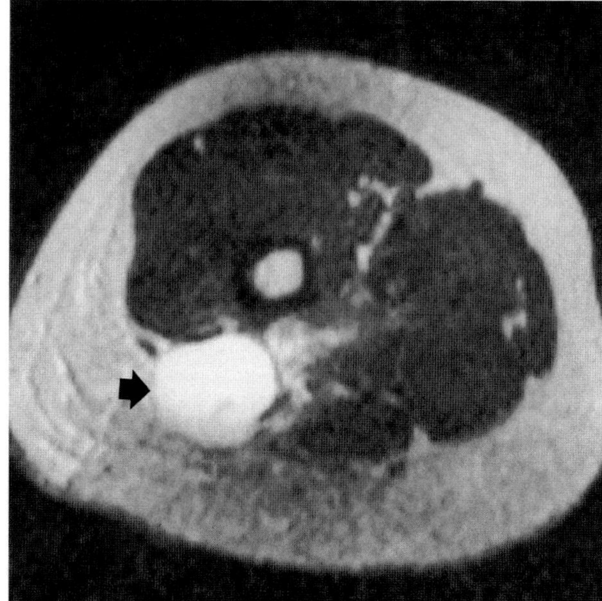

Figure 3.32 Postoperative hygroma: Follow-up examination in a girl 15 years of age following resection of a clear cell sarcoma. **A,B:** Axial T1-weighted (TR/TE; 720/15) spin-echo MR images preceding **(A)** and following **(B)** intravenous contrast administration show a nonenhancing masslike area (*arrow*) in the posterior thigh. Lesion has a cystlike margin and shows peripherally ill-defined enhancement. **C:** Axial T2-weighted (TR/TE; 2180/80) spin-echo MR image shows the lesion to have a "fluid" signal intensity.

a staging system is to provide a standard manner in which to readily communicate the state of a malignancy. Accurate staging is essential to (a) incorporate the most significant prognostic factors into a system that describes progressive degrees of risk to which a patient is subject, (b) delineate progressive stages of disease that have specific implications for surgical management, and (c) provide guidelines to the use of adjunctive therapies (120). The staging systems most commonly used are the Enneking system and the staging system of the American Joint Committee.

Enneking Staging System

The surgical staging system most commonly used in the evaluation of musculoskeletal tumors is that of Enneking (120). The Enneking staging system addresses the surgical grade of a tumor (G), its local extent (T), and the presence or absence of regional or distant metastases (M) (120). The Enneking staging system was designed for the evaluation of musculoskeletal mesenchymal tumors and not intended for use with lesions derived from marrow or reticuloendothelial system because of their different natural history, surgical management, and response to treatment (120). The Enneking staging system is also not applicable to rhabdomyosarcoma (121).

Lesions are divided into two grades: low (G1) and high (G2), on the basis of histologic appearance. In general, low-grade lesions are well-differentiated and have a low potential for the development of metastatic disease. Lesions in this category include myxoid liposarcoma, and

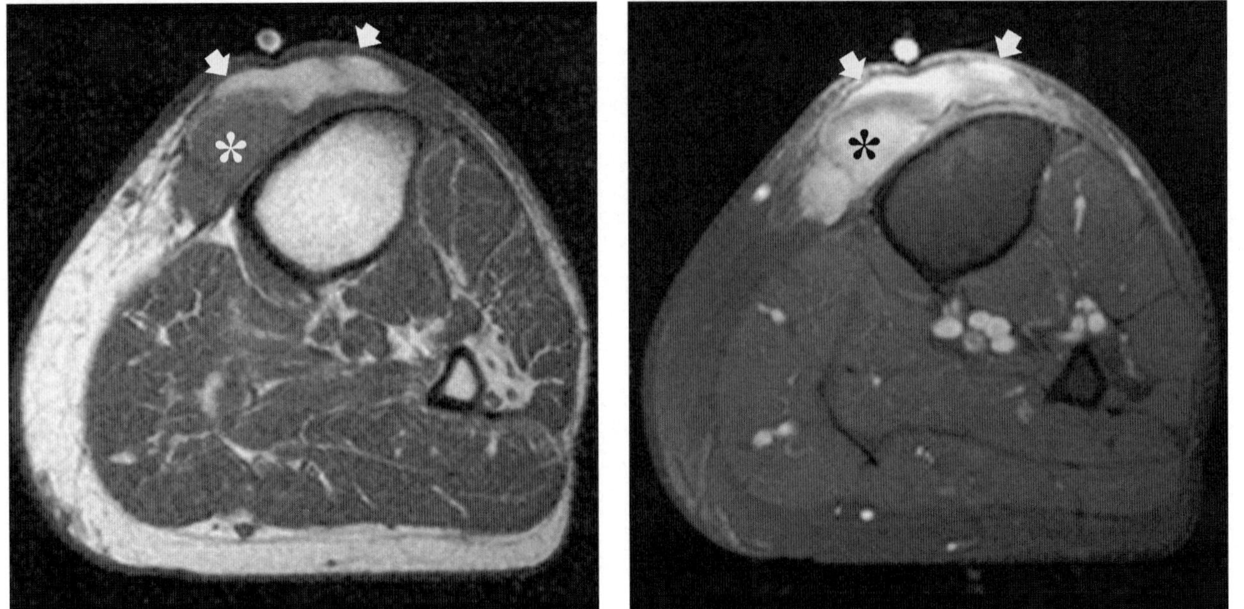

Figure 3.33 Postoperative hematoma and tumor recurrence: Recurrent leiomyosarcoma in a man 66 years of age following surgical excision complicated by a large hematoma. **A:** Axial T1-weighted (TR/TE; 740/15) spin-echo image shows a small residual hematoma (*arrows*) with an adjacent mass (*asterisk*). **B:** Axial fat-suppressed T1-weighted (TR/TE; 475/15) spin-echo MR image following intravenous contrast shows marked enhancement to the recurrent tumor. Note high signal intensity of subacute blood on fat-suppressed image (*arrows*).

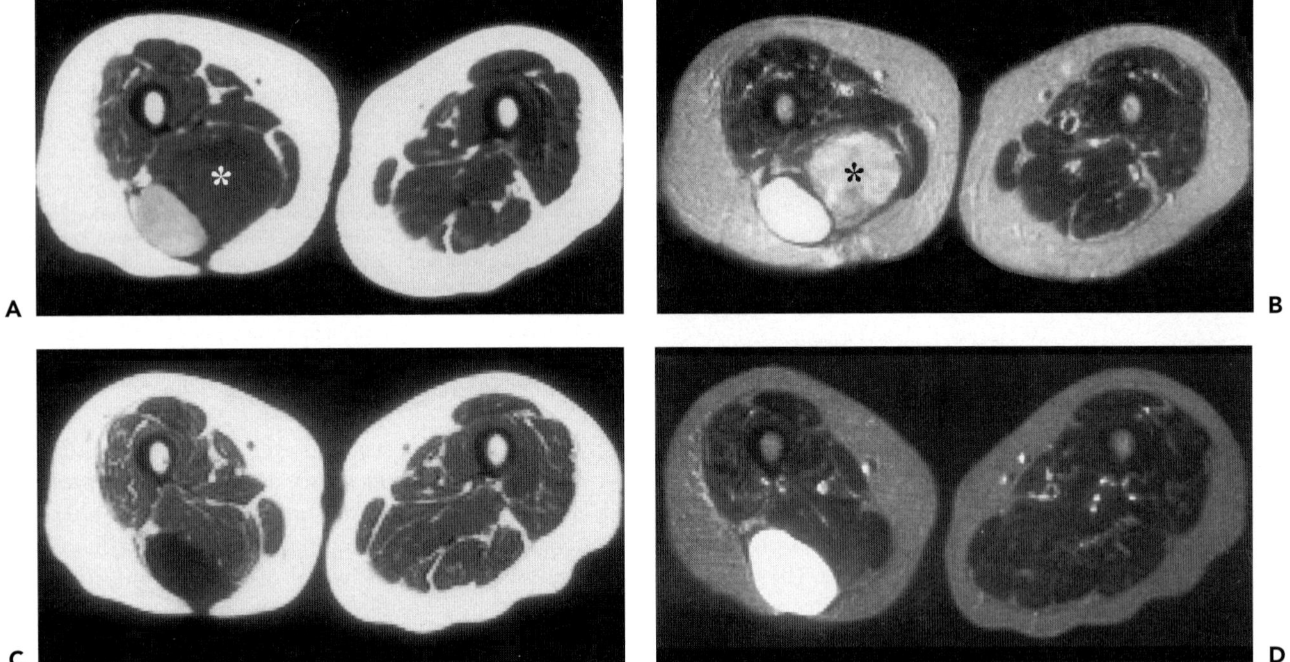

Figure 3.34 Postoperative seroma and tumor recurrence: Recurrent high-grade undifferentiated pleomorphic sarcoma (malignant fibrous histiocytoma) in a woman 70 years of age presenting with a painless mass in the posterior thigh. She had a malignant fibrous histiocytoma resected approximately 2 years earlier and received radiation therapy and chemotherapy. **A,B:** Axial T1-weighted (TR/TE; 500/17) **(A)** and T2-weighted (TR/TE; 2100/90) **(B)** spin-echo MR images of the right thigh show a discrete mass (*asterisk*) as well as a well-defined homogeneous fluid collection. **C,D:** Axial T1-weighted (TR/TE; 500/17) **(C)** and T2-weighted (TR/TE; 2100/90) **(D)** spin-echo MR images 18 months earlier, also show the postoperative fluid collection (seroma). Note that the signal intensity of the fluid has increased significantly over time on T1-weighted images, likely reflecting increased protein content.

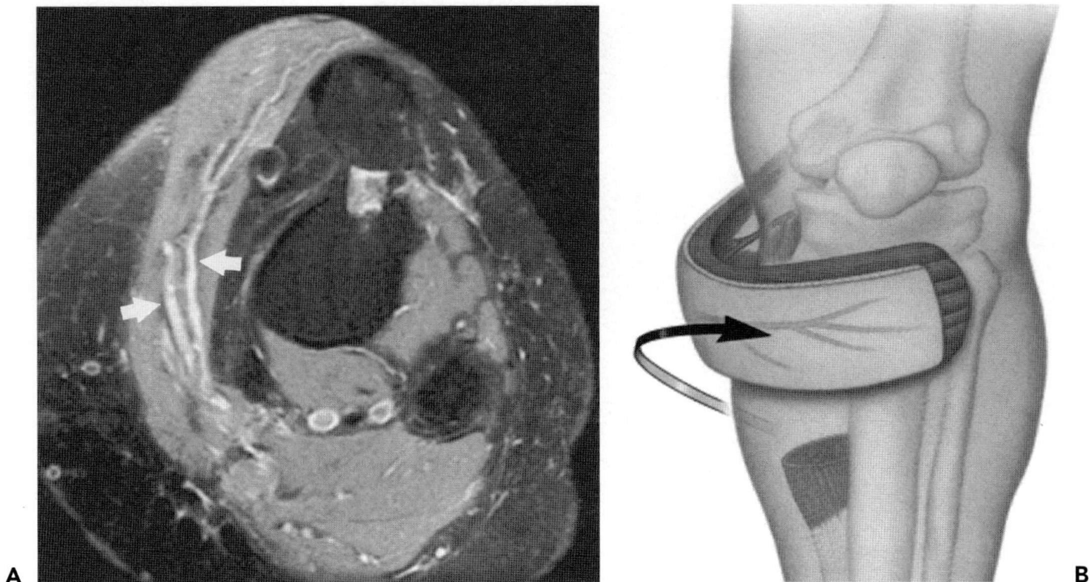

Figure 3.35 Rotational flap: Woman 41 years of age with rotational medial gastrocnemius flap used for coverage after debridement for osteomyelitis. **A:** Axial fat-suppressed proton-density (TR/TE; 4000/15) image obtained 35 months after surgery demonstrates preserved vascular pedicle (*arrows*) and flap signal characteristics similar to that of background muscle. **B:** Diagram of rotational gastrocnemius flap.

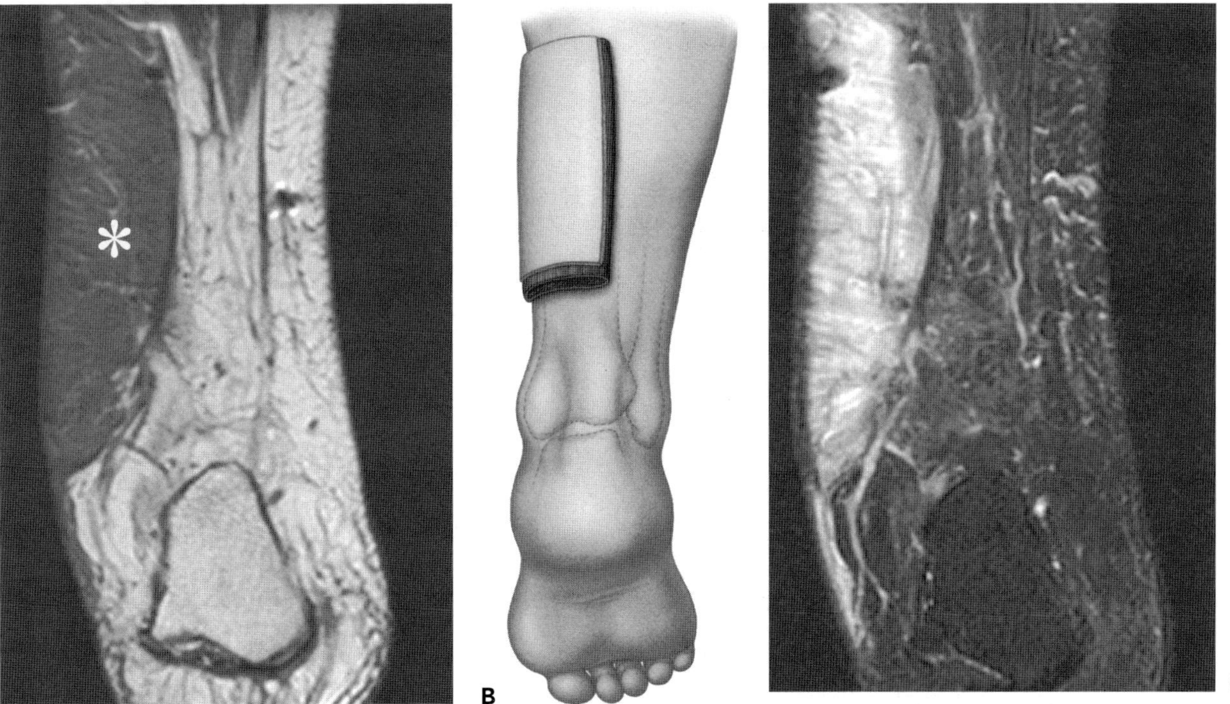

Figure 3.36 Free flap: Woman 39 years of age with a rectus abdominus free flap to ankle following resection of dermatofibrosarcoma protuberans. **A:** Coronal T1-weighted (TR 683/TE 17) spin-echo MR image at 4 months after placement of free flap (*asterisk*). **B:** Diagram of free flap. **C:** Coronal fast spin-echo T2-weighted (TR/TE; 3000/95) MR image demonstrates markedly increased T2-weighted signal at 4 months after flap placement. Signal intensity returns to that of adjacent muscle in approximately one-third of patients.

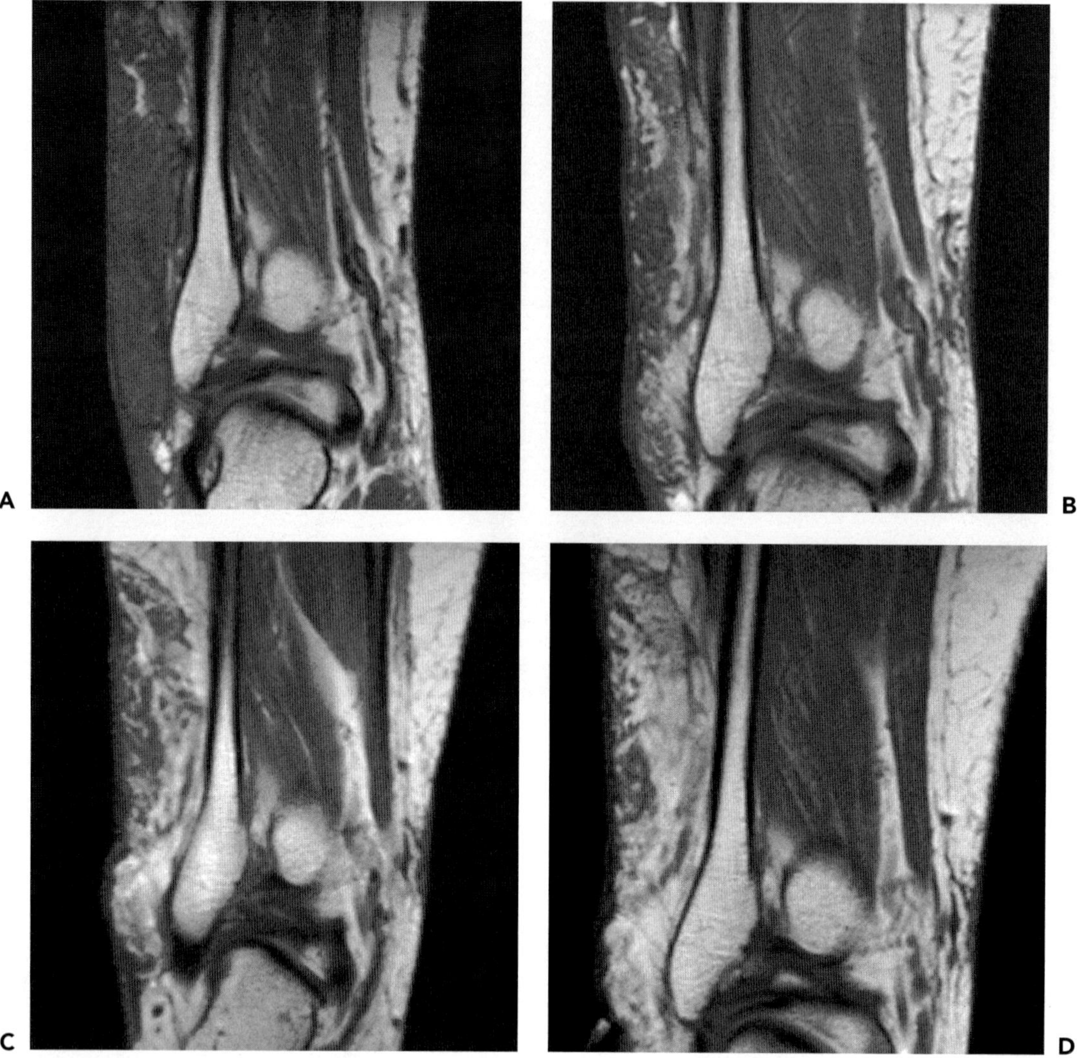

Figure 3.37   Time-dependent changes: Progressive fatty atrophy of rectus abdominus free flap to ankle (same patient as Fig. 3.36). Patient did not receive any radiation therapy. **A–D:** Coronal T1-weighted images obtained at 5 months (**A**), 15 months (**B**), 28 months (**C**), and 41 months (**D**).

hemangiopericytoma. In contrast, high-grade lesions are in general poorly differentiated, with a high mitotic rate and aggressive clinical course. Synovial sarcoma and pleomorphic liposarcoma are considered to be high-grade lesions.

Local extent is divided into lesions that are intracompartmental (T1) and extracompartmental (T2). The designation of intracompartmental indicates the lesion remains confined to the compartment of origin and has not crossed a major fascial septae dividing anatomic compartments. Typical anatomic compartments include the anterior thigh, medial thigh, posterior thigh, volar forearm, dorsal forearm, and so on. Compartmental anatomy is reviewed in Chapter 14.

The presence (M1) or absence (M0) of regional or distant metastases is the third and final component of staging. On the basis of these considerations, lesions are staged as shown in Table 3.4.

American Joint Committee Staging System

The Enneking system is well-suited for the evaluation of extremity lesions because of its emphasis on compartmentalization. It does not, however, consider tumor size, type, or depth. In addition, the division of all lesions into either high- or low-grade may not be sufficient to be applicable to the wide range of all soft tissue sarcomas. An alternative staging system is that of the American Joint Committee (AJC), which is based on the tumor, node, metastasis (TNM) classification (122). This system is more complex, with four stages and several subclassifications. It is applicable to all soft tissue sarcomas, except Kaposi sarcoma, dermatofibrosarcoma protuberans, desmoid tumor, and rhabdomyosarcoma.

The AJC staging system addresses the surgical grade of a tumor (G), its size and local extent (T), the presence or

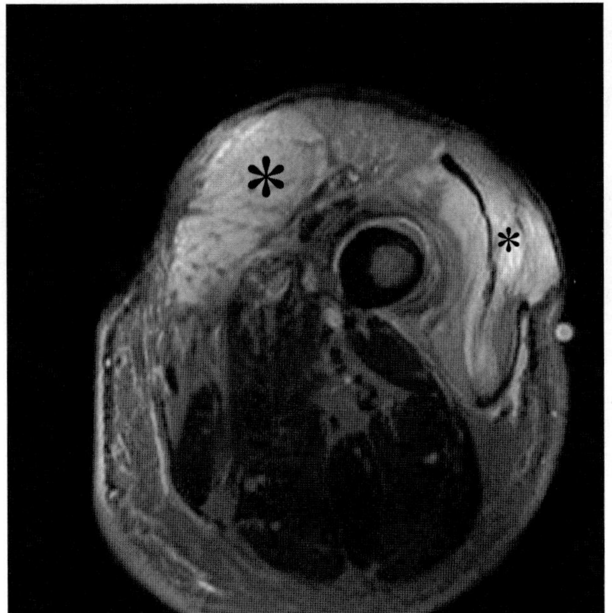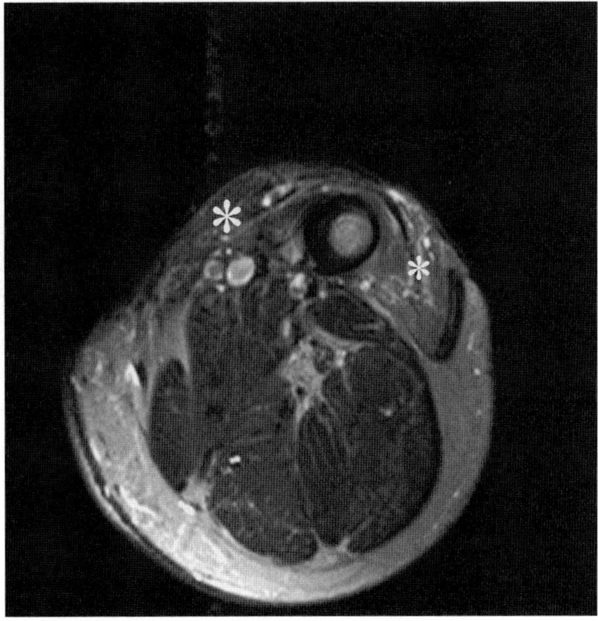

Figure 3.38 Time-dependent changes: Resolution of hyperintense T2-weighted flap signal in a man 42 years of age with a latissimus free flap to the upper thigh for high-grade malignant fibrous histiocytoma. **A:** Axial conventional T2-weighted (TR/TE; 2930/80) spin-echo MR image obtained 2 months postoperatively displays hyperintense signal in flap (*large asterisk*) relative to background musculature. Patient had received postoperative radiation, and increased signal is also seen in the native muscle of the anterior compartment (*small asterisk*). **B:** Axial conventional T2-weighted (TR/TE; 2250/80) spin-echo MR image obtained during follow-up at 27 months shows marked atrophy of the flap (*large asterisk*) with near reversion of flap signal to that of adjacent muscles. Slight increased signal is seen within the flap caused by fatty infiltration. Note slight residual increased signal in radiated muscle (*small asterisk*).

absence of nodal involvement (N), and the presence or absence of distal metastasis (M) (122). Tables 3.5 and 3.6 list the classification criteria and subsequent surgical staging. Unfortunately, the AJC gives no detailed guidelines for the standardization of grading (121).

Rhabdomyosarcoma Staging

Although there is no universal agreement, the most widely used staging system for rhabdomyosarcoma is that proposed by the Intergroup Rhabdomyosarcoma Study (IRS) (123,124). This system is based on the clinical trials of the IRS, which divides patients into four clinical groups. Table 3.7 presents the classification criteria.

TABLE 3.5

AMERICAN JOINT COMMITTEE STAGING OF SOFT TISSUE SARCOMAS[a]

Histologic Grade (G)

G_1	Well-differentiated
G_2	Moderately well-differentiated
G_3	Poorly differentiated
G_4	Undifferentiated

Primary Site (T*)

T_{1a}	Superficial tumor 5 cm or less in diameter
T_{1b}	Deep tumor more than 5 cm in diameter
T_{2a}	Superficial tumor 5 cm or less in diameter
T_{2b}	Deep tumor more than 5 cm in diameter

Nodal Involvement (N)

N_0	No histologically verified metastases to lymph nodes
N_1	Histologically verified regional lymph nodal metastases

Distant Metastasis (M)

M_0	No distant metastasis
M_1	Distant metastasis present

---

[a]Adapted from Ref. 122.
*Tumors deep to the fascia or in the retroperitoneum or mediastinum are designated "b."

TABLE 3.4

ENNEKING SURGICAL STAGING OF SOFT TISSUE SARCOMAS[a]

Stage	Grade	Site
IA	Low (G_1)	Intracompartmental (T_1)
IB	Low (G_1)	Extracompartmental (T_2)
IIA	High (G_2)	Intracompartmental (T_1)
IIB	High (G_2)	Extracompartmental (T_2)
III	Any (G)	Any (T) with Metastases

[a]Adapted from Ref. 120.

TABLE 3.6

AMERICAN JOINT COMMITTEE STAGING OF SOFT TISSUE SARCOMAS[a]

Stage	Classification	Description
I	$G_{1,2}T_{any}N_0M_0$	Tumor grade 1 or 2, any size, superficial or deep, no regional lymph nodes or distant metastases
II	$G_{3,4}T_{1a,1b,2a}N_0M_0$	Tumor grade 3 or 4, any superficial tumor or deep tumor 5 cm or less in diameter, no regional lymph nodes or distant metastases
III	$G_{3,4}T_{2b}N_0M_0$	Tumor grade 3 or 4, deep tumor more than 5 cm in diameter, no regional lymph nodes or distant metastases
IV	$G_{any}T_{any}N_1M_0$ $G_{any}T_{any}N_0M_1$	Any tumor grade, any size, superficial or deep, positive regional lymph nodes or distant metastases

[a]Adapted from Ref. 122.

SURGICAL CONSIDERATIONS

With increasing frequency, radiologists are asked to perform percutaneous biopsy of soft tissue masses. It must be emphasized that coordination with the orthopedic surgeon who does the definitive surgery is essential prior to biopsy.

Gadopentetate-enhanced MR imaging can be used to direct the biopsy to a vascular, and therefore presumed viable portion of the tumor, avoiding necrotic and/or cystic areas. The biopsy tract is excised with the specimen at the time of surgery and an approach that facilitates this is desirable. An approach that violates anatomic compartments, contaminates vital structures such as major nerves, vessels or tendons; or results in a hematoma or infection adversely impacts patient care (125).

Patient imaging for diagnosis and staging should be done prior to biopsy. When associated edema, characterized by poorly defined high signal intensity, is present around a lesion on T2-weighted images, a rigid distinction between tumor and edema should not be made. Edema, when present, is considered to be part of the reactive zone around the neoplasm, and as such, it is removed en bloc with the tumor (125).

ALGORITHM FOR THE IMAGING EVALUATION OF SOFT TISSUE MASSES

Figure 3.39 presents an algorithm for the evaluation of a patient with a soft tissue mass. Imaging and staging of lesions should be done prior to biopsy.

TABLE 3.7

INTERGROUP RHABDOMYOSARCOMA STUDY STAGING OF RHABDOMYOSARCOMA[a]

Clinical Group	Description
I	Localized disease, completely resected, no lymph node involvement (A) Tumor confined to muscle or organ of origin (B) Tumor infiltration outside muscle or organ of origin
II	Localized or regional disease with total gross resection (A) Primary tumor grossly resected with "microscopic residual" disease at margin of resection, negative nodes (B) Primary tumor grossly resected with "no microscopic residual" disease, positive regional nodes (C) Primary tumor resected with "microscopic residual" disease, positive regional nodes
III	Incomplete resection, with residual unresected disease (A) Biopsy of resection of <50% of gross tumor (B) Resection of ≥50% of gross tumor
IV	Distant metastatic disease present at diagnosis

[a]Adapted from Ref. 123.

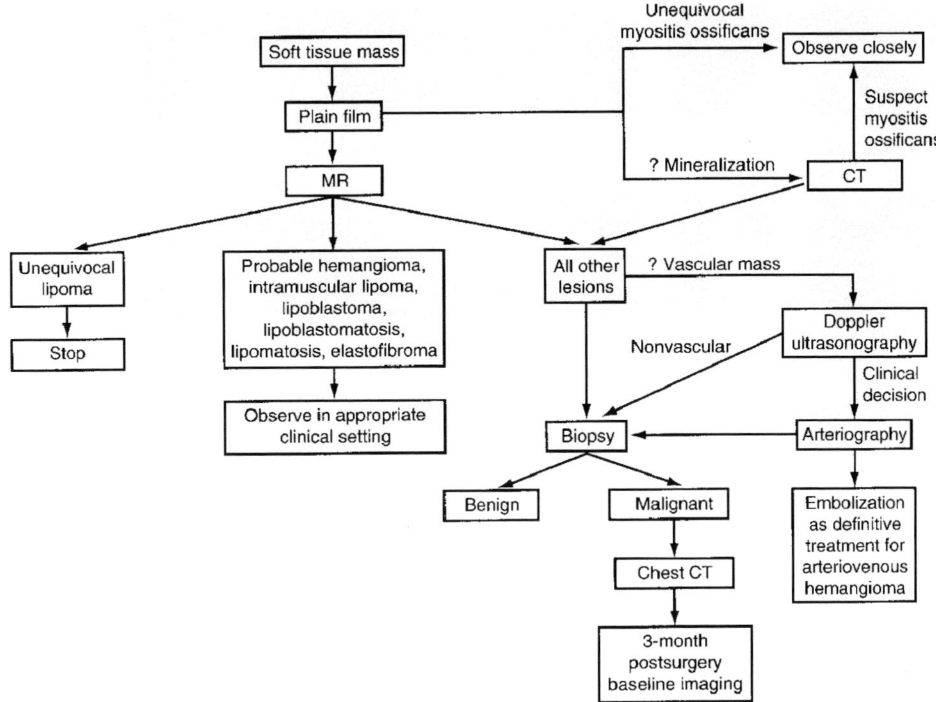

Figure 3.39 Algorithm for the workup of soft tissue tumors.

The question of whether all clinically apparent lesions need to be biopsied is not easily answered, nor is it a question on which there is uniform agreement. As a general rule, we do not recommend biopsy for an unequivocal superficial lipoma. Our referring orthopedic surgeons follow selected patients with presumed diagnoses, such as hemangioma, intramuscular lipoma, lipomatosis, myositis ossificans, and so on, in the appropriate clinical setting. When imaging characteristics are nonspecific, however, a malignancy must be considered.

SAMPLE CASES

When evaluating a soft tissue mass, all of the information available must be used. The following examples use a systematic approach. Although there are no absolutes, a systematic approach to diagnosis can make evaluation easier.

CASE 1

HISTORY

The patient is a woman 56 years of age who noted a mass in her left thigh. The mass has grown slowly over the previous 6 months with no associated pain or discomfort. The patient has no history of previous malignancy or systemic disease.

Analysis

The clinical history of a slowly growing mass is always suspicious for a neoplasm, and a malignancy needs to be excluded. The absence of pain, inflammation, or systemic symptoms make an infectious cause less likely.

MULTIPLICITY

Only one lesion was noted by the patient.

Analysis

A history of additional lesions would help limit our differential diagnosis. The lack of additional lesions is most frequently the case.

RADIOGRAPHS

Radiographs (not shown) were unremarkable.

Analysis

Although radiographs are often unremarkable, this step should *never* be omitted.

MAGNETIC RESONANCE IMAGING

Figures 3.40A and 3.40B show typical T1-weighted and T2-weighted spin-echo MR images.

Analysis

Review of the MR images shows the lesion to be located within the vastus medialis muscle. The lesion has a smooth, well-defined margin, with no associated edema or hemorrhage. It is homogeneous with a signal intensity less than that of muscle on T1-weighted spin-echo images and greater than that of fat on corresponding T2-weighted images. This appearance is not characteristic of a specific diagnosis. Although it is tempting to say the lesion is cystic on the basis of its MR appearance, this can be misleading and one can only say it is homogeneous with signal characteristics similar to those of fluid. A distinction between solid and cystic is made with much greater accuracy on ultrasound. Absence of contrast

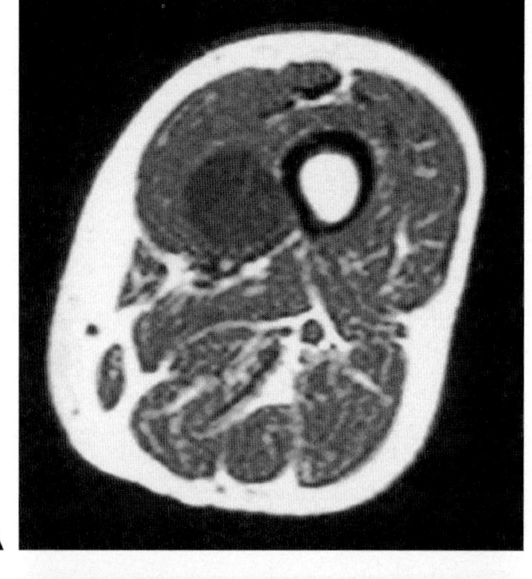

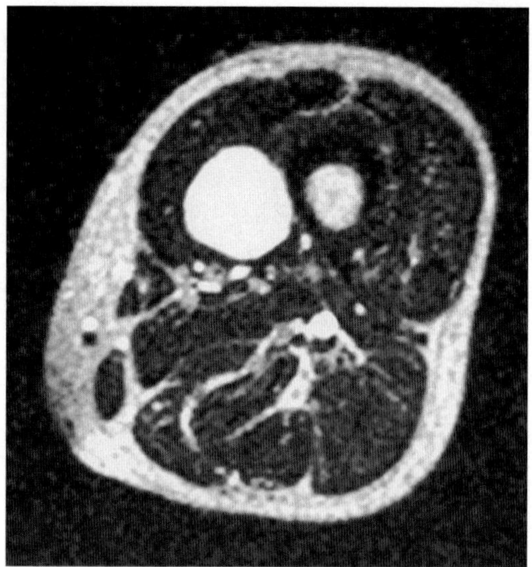

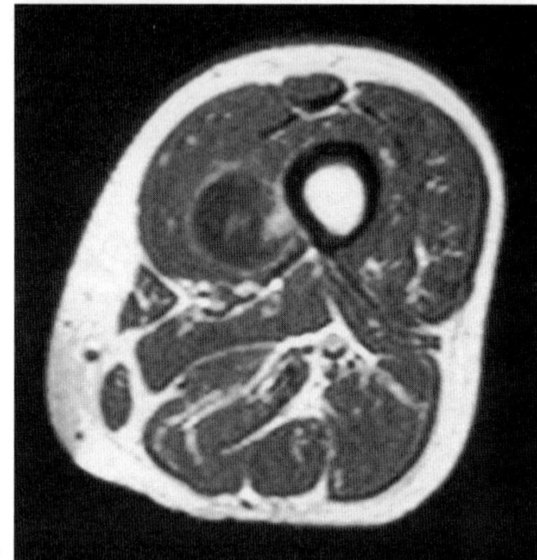

Figure 3.40 Example 1: Mass in the thigh of a woman 56 years of age that has been slowly growing over the previous 6 months. **A,B:** Axial T1-weighted (TR/TE; 650/20) **(A)** and T2-weighted (TR/TE; 2000/80) **(B)** spin-echo MR images show a well-defined homogeneous mass in the anterior compartment of the left thigh. **C:** Axial T1-weighted (TR/TE; 650/20) spin-echo MR image, following intravenous contrast administration, shows mild heterogeneous peripheral enhancement. Biopsy demonstrated myxoid liposarcoma.

enhancement on MR imaging suggests a cystic lesion, but caution is required. Necrosis does not enhance, and the enhancement in myxoid tumors is variable. Hyaline cartilage may also simulate a multiloculated fluid collection on enhanced MR imaging. Should a malignant or a benign lesion be favored? The relatively small size, homogeneous signal, and well-defined margins favor a benign process, whereas the deep intramuscular location and older age of the patient favor a malignancy. Clearly, the lesion must be considered to be nonspecific.

GADOLINIUM-ENHANCED IMAGING

Figure 3.40C shows a typical gadolinium-enhanced T1-weighted spin-echo MR image.

Analysis

Gadolinium-enhanced images add little, but the pattern of enhancement suggests this is not a cystic lesion. The homogeneity and smooth margin also suggest the lesion is not necrotic, favoring a myxoid lesion.

DIFFERENTIAL

Based on the patient's age and the lesion's location, the following lesions would be most likely (see Chapter 2):

Benign		Malignant	
Lipoma	26%	Malignant fibrous histiocytoma	47%
Myxoma	19%	Liposarcoma	24%
Fibrous histiocytoma	10%	Leiomyosarcoma	8%
Schwannoma	6%	Malignant schwannoma	3%
Neurofibroma	6%	Extraskeletal chondrosarcoma	3%
Proliferative fasciitis	6%		
Nodular fasciitis	4%	Fibrosarcoma	3%
Other	22%	Synovial sarcoma	2%
		Other	9%

Analysis

This type of analysis is based on the concept that "common things are common." We can exclude a lipoma on the basis of signal intensity. Proliferative fasciitis is subcutaneous by definition and can also be excluded. Similarly, fibrous histiocytoma and nodular fasciitis are usually subcutaneous. Although they can be deep, such lesions are unusual. Moreover, both of these lesions are typically solid. Extensive diffuse enhancement is typically seen with nodular fasciitis, and the pattern demonstrated in the current case would be quite atypical. The pattern of enhancement would also be unusual for a peripheral nerve sheath tumor, as would the conventional imaging appearance. Thus, the most likely benign lesion would be an intramuscular myxoma. Of the malignant lesions, a malignant fibrous histiocytoma (MFH) would be statistically most likely. These lesions tend to be large and heterogeneous and often have central necrosis. A similar case could be made for leiomyosarcoma, malignant peripheral nerve sheath tumor (MPNST, previously termed malignant schwannoma), fibrosarcoma, and synovial sarcoma. Extraskeletal chondrosarcoma is most often a slowly growing myxoid lesion. An extraskeletal myxoid chondrosarcoma and a myxoid liposarcoma may both show a cystlike appearance on conventional spin-echo MR imaging. Of these two lesions, the liposarcoma is far more common. No fat is seen within the lesion; however, this is of no concern in that fat is seen in only about 50% to 80% of liposarcomas (not including the well-differentiated type). Approximately 20% of myxoid liposarcomas have an imaging appearance similar to that of a cyst on conventional spin-echo MR imaging. Thus, the most likely malignant lesion is a myxoid liposarcoma. The distinction between intramuscular myxoma and myxoid liposarcoma can be difficult. The well-defined margin, absence of associated muscle atrophy and fatty replacement, and absence of surrounding peritumoral increased signal, however, all mitigate against the diagnosis of an intramuscular myxoma.

DIAGNOSIS

On the basis of all radiologic and clinical information available, we would favor a myxoid liposarcoma as the diagnosis of exclusion. The relatively short history of a growing mass is of concern and a malignancy must be excluded. The final diagnosis was a myxoid liposarcoma.

CASE 2

HISTORY

The patient is a man 30 years of age who has a mass in the thigh that has been rapidly growing over the previous 3 weeks. There is no significant pain, although the mass is tender to deep palpation.

Analysis

The clinical history of a rapidly growing mass is always suspicious for an infection, although a neoplasm with hemorrhage may also present as a rapidly growing mass. Repeat physical examination confirmed only mild tenderness to deep palpation, as well as the absence of erythema or associated adenopathy.

MULTIPLICITY

Only one lesion was present.

RADIOGRAPHS

Radiographs (not shown) were unremarkable.

MAGNETIC RESONANCE IMAGING

Figures 3.41A and 3.41B show typical T1-weighted and T2-weighted spin-echo MR images.

Analysis

Review of the MR images shows the lesion to be located within the vastus lateralis muscle. It has a relatively smooth, well-defined margin, with increased signal intensity in the entire anterior compartment of the thigh, compatible with diffuse muscle edema. There is no evidence of subacute or chronic hemorrhage. The lesion is mildly heterogeneous with a signal intensity very slightly less than that of skeletal muscle on T1-weighted images and greater than that of fat on corresponding T2-weighted images. The presumed edema is very helpful. Our experience is that this is most frequently seen in inflammatory processes. It may be found in association with malignancies, but this is usually in the absence of hemorrhage, biopsy, or previous radiation. There is no MR evidence of subacute hemorrhage, nor is there a history of biopsy or radiation therapy. The radiologic picture is not specific, but the mass has features that strongly suggest an inflammatory process. Thus, despite the absence of associated clinical evidence of an abscess, we would favor this diagnosis. Could the patient be immunocompromised, accounting for a lack of adenopathy?

GADOLINIUM-ENHANCED IMAGING

Figure 3.41C shows a typical gadolinium-enhanced T1-weighted spin-echo MR image.

Analysis

In this situation, gadolinium-enhanced imaging is quite helpful. Imaging following intravenous contrast administration shows diffuse uniform peripheral enhancement. There are no focal enhancing nodules or evidence of an underlying tumor. Based on the MR imaging features, a soft tissue abscess would be strongly favored.

DIAGNOSIS

The final diagnosis was a *Staphylococcus aureus* abscess. The lack of associated adenopathy may have been caused by an immunocompromised state; however, the patient refused HIV testing.

In summary, MR is the preferred modality for the evaluation of a soft tissue mass following radiography. The radiologic appearance of certain soft tissue tumors or tumorlike processes may be sufficiently unique to allow a

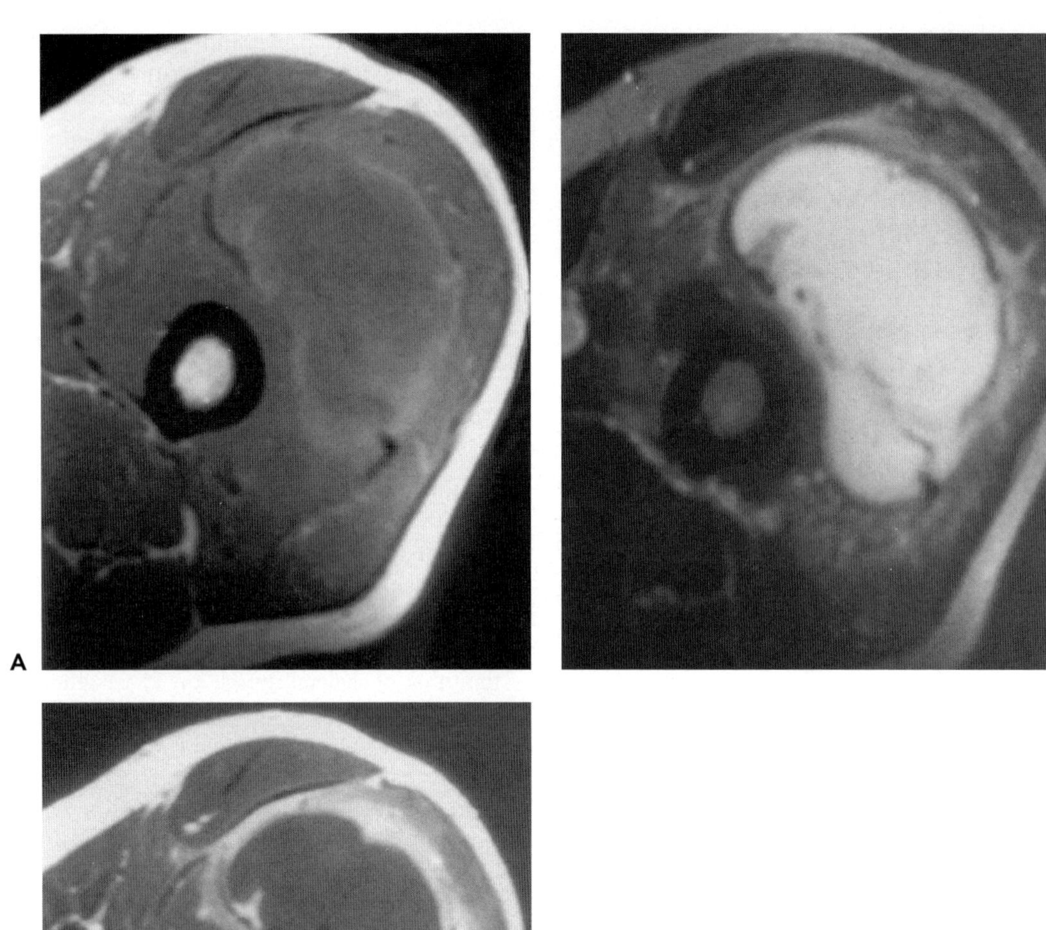

Figure 3.41 Case 2: Mass in the thigh of a man 39 years of age that had been rapidly growing over the previous 3 weeks. **A,B:** Axial T1-weighted (TR/TE; 522/25) **(A)** and T2-weighted (TR/TE; 2303/90) **(B)** spin-echo MR images show a well-defined relatively homogeneous mass in the anterior compartment of the left thigh. The mass shows a signal intensity very slightly less than that of the surrounding muscle on T1-weighted images and greater than that of fat on corresponding T2-weighted images. Some heterogeneity, as well as diffuse increased signal intensity, is seen in the entire anterior compartment, suggesting diffuse muscle edema. Also note rind of slight increased signal intensity surrounding the lesion in **A. C:** Axial T1-weighted (TR/TE; 522/25) MR image, following intravenous contrast administration, shows diffuse, uniform, peripheral enhancement. Biopsy demonstrated *Staphylococcus aureus* abscess.

strong presumptive radiologic diagnosis. It must be emphasized that MR cannot *reliably* distinguish between benign and malignant lesions, and when radiologic evaluation is nonspecific, clinicians are ill-advised to suggest a lesion is benign or malignant solely on its MR appearance.

REFERENCES

1. Weekes RG, McLeod RA, Reiman HM, et al. CT of soft-tissue neoplasms. *AJR Am J Roentgenol.* 1985;144:355–360.
2. Sundaram M, McGuire MH, Herbold DR. Magnetic resonance imaging of soft tissue masses: an evaluation of fifty-three histologically proven tumors. *Magn Reson Imaging.* 1988;6:237–248.
3. Petasnick JP, Turner DA, Charters JR, et al. Soft-tissue masses of the locomotor system: comparison of MR imaging with CT. *Radiology.* 1986;160:125–133.
4. Totty WG, Murphy WA, Lee JKT. Soft-tissue tumors: MR imaging. *Radiology.* 1986;160:135–141.
5. Kransdorf MJ, Jelinek JS, Moser, et al. Soft-tissue masses: diagnosis using MR imaging. *AJR Am J Roentgenol.* 1989;153:541–547.
6. Berquist TH, Ehman RL, King BF, et al. Value of MR imaging in differentiating benign from malignant soft tissue masses: study of 95 lesions. *AJR Am J Roentgenol.* 1990;155:1251–1255.
7. Crim JR, Seeger LL, Yao L, et al. Diagnosis of soft-tissue masses with MR imaging: can benign masses be differentiated from malignant ones? *Radiology.* 1992;185:581–586.
8. Panicek DM, Gatsonis C, Rosenthal DI, et al. CT and MR imaging in the local staging of primary malignant musculoskeletal

neoplasms: report of the Radiology Diagnostic Oncology Group. *Radiology.* 1997;202:237–246.

9. Osment LS. Cutaneous lipomas and lipomatosis. *Surg Gynecol Obstet.* 1968;127:129–132.

10. Leffert RD. Lipomas of the upper extremity. *J Bone Joint Surg Am.* 1972;54-A:1262–1266.

11. Rydholm A, Berg NO. Size, site and clinical incidence of lipoma. Factors in the differential diagnosis of lipoma and sarcoma. *Acta Orthop Scand.* 1983;54:929–934.

12. Disler DG, Alexander AA, Mankin HJ, et al. Multicentric fibromatosis with metaphyseal dysplasia. *Radiology.* 1993;187:489–492.

13. Rock MG, Pritchard DJ, Reiman HM, et al. Extra-abdominal desmoid tumors. *J Bone Joint Surg Am.* 1984;66-A:1369–1374.

14. Sundaram M, Duffrin H, McGuire MH, et al. Synchronous multicentric desmoid tumors (aggressive fibromatosis) of the extremities. *Skeletal Radiol.* 1988;17:16–19.

15. Murphey MD, Fairbairn KJ, Parman LM, et al. Musculoskeletal angiomatous lesions: radiologic-pathologic correlation. *Radiographics.* 1995;15:893–917.

16. Moulopoulos LA, Granfield CAJ, Dimopoulos MA, et al. Extraosseous multiple myeloma: imaging features. *AJR Am J Roentgenol.* 1993;161:1083–1087.

17. Patten RM, Shuman WP, Teefey S. Subcutaneous metastases from malignant melanoma: prevalence and findings on CT. *AJR Am J Roentgenol.* 1989;152:1009–1012.

18. Sundaram M, McDonald DJ, Merenda G. Intramuscular myxoma: a rare but important association with fibrous dysplasia of bone. *AJR Am J Roentgenol.* 1989;153:107–108.

19. Wirth WA, Leavitt D, Enzinger FM. Multiple intramuscular myxomas: another extraskeletal manifestation of fibrous dysplasia. *Cancer.* 1971;27:321–340.

20. Kransdorf MJ, Murphey MD. *Imaging of Soft Tissue Tumors.* Philadelphia: WB Saunders; 1997:37–56.

21. Dalinka MK, Zlatkin MD, Chao P, et al. The use of magnetic resonance imaging in the evaluation of bone and soft tissue tumors. *Radiol Clin North Am.* 1990;28:461–470.

22. Pettersson H, Gillespy T, Hamlin DJ, et al. Primary musculoskeletal tumors: examination with MR imaging compared with conventional modalities. *Radiology.* 1987;164:237–241.

23. Tehranzadeh J, Mnaymneh W, Ghavam C, et al. Comparison of CT and MR imaging in musculoskeletal neoplasms. *J Comput Assist Tomogr.* 1989;13:466–472.

24. Aisen AM, Martel W, Braunstein EM, et al. MRI and CT evaluation of primary bone and soft-tissue tumors. *AJR Am J Roentgenol.* 1984;146:749–756.

25. Chang AE, Matory YL, Dwyer AJ, et al. Magnetic resonance imaging versus computed tomography in the evaluation of soft tissue tumors of the extremities. *Ann Surg.* 1987;205:340–348.

26. Demas BE, Heelan RT, Lane J, et al. Soft-tissue sarcomas of the extremities: comparison of MR and CT in determining the extent of disease. *AJR Am J Roentgenol.* 1988;150:615–620.

27. Hudson TM, Hamlin DJ, Enneking MD, et al. Magnetic resonance imaging of bone and soft-tissue tumors: early experience in 31 patients compared with computed tomography. *Skeletal Radiol.* 1985;13:134–146.

28. Weekes RG, Berquist TH, McLeod RA, et al. Magnetic resonance imaging of soft-tissue tumors: comparison with computed tomography. *Magn Reson Imaging.* 1985;3:345–352.

29. Rubin DA, Kneeland JB. MR imaging of the musculoskeletal system: technical considerations for enhancing image quality and diagnostic yield. *AJR Am J Roentgenol.* 1994;163:1155–1163.

30. Mirowitz SA. Fast scanning and fat-suppression MR imaging of musculoskeletal disorders. *AJR Am J Roentgenol.* 1993;161:1147–1157.

31. Fujimoto H, Murakami K, Ichikawa T, et al. MRI of soft-tissue lesions: opposed-phase T2*-weighted gradient-echo images. *J Comput Assist Tomogr.* 1993;17:418–424.

32. Shuman WP, Baron RL, Peters MJ, et al. Comparison of STIR and spin-echo MR imaging at 1.5T in 90 lesions of the chest, liver and pelvis. *AJR Am J Roentgenol.* 1989;152:853–859.

33. Dwyer AJ, Frank JA, Sank VJ, et al. Short-Ti inversion-recovery pulse sequence: analysis and initial experience in cancer imaging. *Radiology.* 1988;168:827–836.

34. Beltran J, Chandnani V, McGhee RA, et al. Gadopentetate dimeglumine-enhanced MR imaging of the musculoskeletal system. *AJR Am J Roentgenol.* 1991;156:457–466.

35. Verstraete KL, De Deene Y, Roels H, et al. Benign and malignant musculoskeletal lesions: dynamic contrast-enhanced MR imaging-parametric "first pass" images depict tissue vascularization and perfusion. *Radiology.* 1994;192:835–843.

36. McDonald DJ. Limb-salvage surgery for treatment of sarcomas of the extremities. *AJR Am J Roentgenol.* 1994;163:509–513.

37. Erlemann R, Reiser MF, Peters PE, et al. Musculoskeletal neoplasms: static and dynamic Gd-DTPA-enhanced MR imaging. *Radiology.* 1989;171:767–773.

38. Fletcher BD, Hanna SL. Musculoskeletal neoplasms: dynamic Gd-DTPA-enhanced imaging [Letter]. *Radiology.* 1990;177:287–288.

39. Pettersson H, Eliasson J, Egund N, et al. Gadolinium-DTPA enhancement of soft-tissue tumors in magnetic resonance imaging—preliminary clinical experience in five patients. *Skeletal Radiol.* 1988;17:319–323.

40. Benedikt RA, Jelinek JS, Kransdorf MJ, et al. MR imaging of soft-tissue masses: role of gadopentetate dimeglumine. *J Magn Reson Imaging.* 1994;4:485–490.

41. Beltran J, Chandnani V, McGhee RA, et al. Gadopentetate dimeglumine-enhanced MR imaging of the musculoskeletal system. *AJR Am J Roentgenol.* 1991;156:457–466.

42. Erlemann R, Vassallo P, Bongartz G, et al. Musculoskeletal neoplasms: fast low-angle shot imaging with and without Gd-DTPA. *Radiology.* 1990;176:489–495.

43. Verstraete KL, De Deene Y, Roels H, et al. Benign and malignant musculoskeletal lesions: dynamic contrast-enhanced MR imaging-parametric "first pass" images depict tissue vascularization and perfusion. *Radiology.* 1994;192:835–843.

44. van Rijswijk CS, Geirnaerdt MJ, Hogendoorn PC, et al. Soft-tissue tumors: value of static and dynamic gadopentetate dimeglumine–enhanced MR imaging in prediction of malignancy. *Radiology.* 2004;233:493–502.

45. Mirowitz SA, Totty WG, Lee JKT. Characterization of musculoskeletal masses using dynamic Gd-DTPA enhanced spin-echo MRI. *J Comput Assist Tomogr.* 1992;16:120–125.

46. Benedikt RA, Jelinek JS, Kransdorf MJ, et al. MR imaging of soft-tissue masses: role of gadopentetate dimeglumine. *J Magn Reson Imaging.* 1994;4:485–490.

47. Takebayashi S, Sugiyama M, Nagase M, et al. Severe adverse reaction to IV gadopentetate dimeglumine. *AJR Am J Roentgenol.* 1993;160:659.

48. Tardy B, Guy C, Barral G, et al. Anaphylactic shock induced by intravenous gadopentetate dimeglumine. *Lancet.* 1992;339:494.

49. Tisher S, Hoffman JC. Anaphylactoid reaction to IV gadopentetate dimeglumine. *AJNR Am J Neuroradiol.* 1990;174:17–23.

50. Omohundro JE, Elderbrook MK, Ringer TV. Laryngospasm after administration of gadopentetate dimeglumine. *J Magn Reson Imaging.* 1992;2:729–730.

51. Shellock FG, Hahn HP, Mink JH, et al. Adverse reaction to intravenous gadoteridol. *Radiology.* 1993;189:151–152.

52. Jordan RM, Mintz RD. Fatal reaction to gadopentetate dimeglumine. *AJR Am J Roentgenol.* 1995;164:743–744.

53. Harkens KL, Moore TE, Yuh WTC, et al. Gadolinium-enhanced MRI of soft tissue masses. *Australas Radiol.* 1993;37:30–34.

54. Seeger LL, Widoff BE, Bassett LW, et al. Preoperative evaluation of osteosarcoma: value of gadopentetate dimeglumine-enhanced MR imaging. *AJR Am J Roentgenol.* 1991;157:347–351.

55. Kransdorf MJ, Murphey MD. The use of gadolinium in the MR evaluation of soft tissue tumors. *Semin Ultrasound CT MR.* 1997;18:251–268.

56. Myhre-Jensen O. A consecutive 7-year series of 1331 benign soft tissue tumors. Clinicopathologic data. Comparison with sarcomas. *Acta Orthop Scand.* 1981;52:287–293.

57. Rydholm A. Management of patients with soft-tissue tumors. Strategy developed at a regional oncology center. *Acta Orthop Scand Suppl.* 1983;203:13–77.

58. Kransdorf MJ. Malignant soft-tissue tumors in a large referral population: distribution of diagnoses by age, sex and location. *AJR Am J Roentgenol.* 1995;164:129–134.

59. Kransdorf MJ. Benign soft-tissue tumors in a large referral population: distribution of diagnoses by age, sex and location. *AJR Am J Roentgenol.* 1995;164:395–402.

60. Peabody TD, Simon MA. Principles of staging of soft-tissue sarcomas. *Clin Orthop.* 1993;289:19–31.

61. White LM, Wunder JS, Bell RS, et al. Histologic assessment of peritumoral edema in soft tissue sarcoma. *Int J Radiat Oncol Biol Phys.* 2005;61:1439–1445.

62. Hanna SL, Fletcher BD, Parham DM, et al. Muscle edema in musculoskeletal tumors: MR imaging characteristics and clinical significance. *J Magn Reson Imaging.* 1991;1:441–449.

63. Beltran J, Simon DC, Katz W, et al. Increased MR signal intensity in skeletal muscle adjacent to malignant tumors: pathologic correlation and clinical relevance. *Radiology.* 1987;162: 251–255.

64. Hanna SL, Fletcher BD, Parham DM, et al. Muscle edema in musculoskeletal tumors: MR imaging characteristics and clinical significance. *J Magn Reson Imaging.* 1991;1:441–449.

65. Mirowitz SA, Totty WG, Lee JKT. Characterization of musculoskeletal masses using dynamic Gd-DTPA enhanced spin-echo MRI. *J Comput Assist Tomogr.* 1992;16:120–125.

66. De Schepper A, Ramon F, Degryse H. Statistical analysis of MRI parameters predicting malignancy in 141 soft tissue masses. *Rofo Fortschr Geb Rontgenstr Neuen Bildgeb Verfahr.* 1992;156: 587–591.

67. Shinkwin MA, Lenkinski RE, Daly JM, et al. Integrated magnetic resonance imaging and phosphorus spectroscopy of soft tissue tumors. *Cancer.* 1991;67:1849–1858.

68. Sostman HD, Prescott DM, Dewhirst MW, et al. MR imaging and spectroscopy for prognostic evaluation in soft-tissue sarcomas. *Radiology.* 1994;190:269–275.

69. Wang CK, Li CW, Hsieh TJ, et al. Characterization of bone and soft-tissue tumors with in vivo 1H MR spectroscopy: initial results. *Radiology.* 2004;232:599–605.

70. Tehranzadeh J, Manymneh W, Ghavam C, et al. Comparison of CT and MR imaging in musculoskeletal neoplasms. *J Comput Assist Tomogr.* 1989;13:466–472.

71. Bloem JL, Taminiau AHM, Eulderink F, et al. Radiologic staging of primary bone sarcoma: MR imaging, scintigraphy, angiography, and CT correlated with pathologic examination. *Radiology.* 1988;169:805–810.

72. Kransdorf MJ, Meis JM, Jelinek JS. Myositis ossificans: MR appearance with radiologic-pathologic correlation. *AJR Am J Roentgenol.* 1991;157:1243–1248.

73. Fornage BD, Rifkin MD. Ultrasound examination of the hand and foot. *Radiol Clin North Am.* 1988;26:109–129.

74. Pathria MN, Zlatkin M, Sartoris DJ, et al. Ultrasonography of the popliteal fossa and lower extremities. *Radiol Clin North Am.* 1988;26:77–85.

75. Taylor GA, Perlman EJ, Scherer LR, et al. Vascularity of tumors in children: evaluation with color Doppler imaging. *AJR Am J Roentgenol.* 1991;157:1267–1271.

76. Inampudi P, Jacobson JA, Fessell DP. Soft-tissue lipomas: accuracy of sonography in diagnosis with pathologic correlation. *Radiology.* 2204;233:763–767.

77. Newman JS, Adler RS, Bude RO, et al. Detection of soft-tissue hyperemia: value of power Doppler sonography. *AJR Am J Roentgenol.* 1994;163:385–389.

78. Paltiel HJ, Burrows PE, Kozakewich HP, et al. Soft tissue vascular anomalies: utility of US for diagnosis. *Radiology.* 2000;214: 747–754.

79. Vezeridis MP, Moore R, Karakousis CP. Metastatic patterns in soft-tissue sarcomas. *Arch Surg.* 1983;118:915–918.

80. Hodler J, Yu JS, Steinert HC, et al. MR imaging versus alternative imaging techniques. *Magn Reson Imaging Clin North Am.* 1995;3: 591–608.

81. Schwartz HS, Jones CK. The efficacy of gallium scintigraphy in detecting malignant soft tissue neoplasms. *Ann Surg.* 1992;215: 78–82.

82. Levine E, Huntrakoon M, Wetzel LH. Malignant nerve-sheath neoplasms in neurofibromatosis: distinction from benign tumors by using imaging techniques. *AJR Am J Roentgenol.* 1987;149:1059–1064.

83. Aoki J, Watanabe H, Shinozaki T, et al. FDG PET of primary benign and malignant bone tumors: standardized uptake value in 52 Lesions. *Radiology.* 2001;219:774–777.

84. Jadvar H, Gamie S, Ramanna L, et al. Musculoskeletal system. *Semin Nucl Med.* 2004;34:254–261.

85. Israel-Mardirosian N, Adler LP. Positron emission tomography of soft tissue sarcomas. *Curr Opin Oncol.* 2003;15:327–330.

86. Lucas JD, O'Doherty MJ, Wong JC, et al. Evaluation of fluorodeoxyglucose positron emission tomography in the management of soft-tissue sarcomas. *J Bone Joint Surg Br.* 1998;80: 441–447.

87. Lucas JD, O'Doherty MJ, Cronin BF, et al. Prospective evaluation of soft tissue masses and sarcomas using fluorodeoxyglucose positron emission tomography. *Br J Surg.* 1999;86:550–556.

88. Bastiaannet E, Groen H, Jager PL, et al. The value of FDG-PET in the detection, grading and response to therapy of soft tissue and bone sarcomas; a systematic review and meta-analysis. *Cancer Treat Rev.* 2004;30:83–101.

89. Hain SF, O'Doherty MJ, Cronin BF, et al. Can FDG-PET be used to successfully direct preoperative biopsy of soft tissue tumors? *Nucl Med Commun.* 2003;24:1139–1143.

90. Swan JS, Grist TM, Sproat IA, et al. Musculoskeletal neoplasms: preoperative evaluation with MR angiography. *Radiology.* 1995; 194:519–524.

91. Ekelund L, Herrlin K, Rydholm A. Comparison of computed tomography and angiography in the evaluation of soft tissue tumors of the extremities. *Acta Radiol Diagn (Stockh).* 1982;23: 15–28 (Fasc 1).

92. Levine E, Lee KRL, Neff JR, et al. Comparison of computed tomography and other imaging modalities in the evaluation of musculoskeletal tumors. *Radiology.* 1979; 131:431–437.

93. Martell W, Abell MR. Radiologic evaluation of soft tissue tumors. *Cancer.* 1973;32:352–366.

94. Viamonte MM, Roen S, LePage J. Nonspecificity of abnormal vascularity in the angiographic diagnosis of malignant neoplasms. *Radiology.* 1973;106:59–63.

95. Lois JF, Fischer HJ, Deutsch LS, et al. Angiography in soft tissue sarcomas. *Cardiovasc Intervent Radiol.* 1984;7:309–316.

96. Herzberg DL, Schreiber MH. Angiography in mass lesions of the extremities. *AJR Am J Roentgenol.* 1971;111:541–546.

97. Halpern M, Freiberger RH. Arteriography in orthopedics. *AJR Am J Roentgenol.* 1965;94:194–206.

98. Widlus DM, Murray RR, White RI, et al. Congenital arteriovenous malformations: tailored embolotherapy. *Radiology.* 1988;169:511–516.

99. Yakes WF, Pevsner R, Reed M, et al. Serial embolizations of an extremity arteriovenous malformation with alcoholin via direct percutaneous puncture. *AJR Am J Roentgenol.* 1986;146: 1038–1040.

100. Choi H, Varma DGK, Fornage BD, et al. Soft-tissue sarcoma: MR imaging vs sonography for the detection of local recurrence after surgery. *AJR Am J Roentgenol.* 1991;157:353–358.

101. Rock MG, Pritchard DJ, Reiman HM, et al. Extra-abdominal desmoid tumors. *J Bone Joint Surg Am.* 1984;66A:1369–1374.

102. Griffiths HJ, Robinson K, Bonfiglo TA. Agressive fibromatosis. *Skeletal Radiol.* 1983;9:179–182.

103. Peterson JJ, Kransdorf MJ, Bancroft LW, et al. Malignant fatty tumors: classification, clinical course, imaging appearance and treatment. *Skeletal Radiol.* 2003;32:493–503.

104. Som P, Urken M, Biller H, et al. Imaging of the postoperative neck. *Radiology.* 1993;187:593–603.

105. Wester D, Whiteman M, Singer S, et al. Imaging of the postoperative neck with emphasis on surgical flaps and their complications. *AJR Am J Roentgenol.* 1995;164:989–993.

106. Fox MG, Bancroft LW, Peterson JJ, et al. MR imaging appearance of myocutaneous flaps commonly used in orthopedic reconstructive surgery. *AJR Am J Roentgenol.* In press.

107. Vanel D, Shapeero LG, De Baere T, et al. MR imaging in the follow-up of malignant and aggressive soft-tissue tumors: results of 511 examinations. *Radiology.* 1994;190:263–268.

108. Varma DGK, Jackson EF, Pollock RE, et al. Soft-tissue sarcoma of the extremities. MR appearance of post-treatment changes and local recurrence. *MRI Clin North Am.* 1995;3:695–710.

109. Pezzi CM, Pollock RE, Evans HL, et al. Preoperative chemotherapy for soft-tissue sarcomas of the extremities. *Ann Surg.* 1990;476:476–481.

110. Fuller BG. The role of radiation therapy in the treatment of bone and soft-tissue sarcomas. In: Malawer M, Suarbaker PH, eds. *Musculoskeletal Cancer Surgery. Treatment of Sarcomas and Allied Diseases.* Dordrecht: Kluwer Academic Publishers; 2001: 85–133.

111. Khatri VP, Goodnight JE Jr. Extremity soft tissue sarcoma: controversial management issues. *Surg Oncol.* 2005;14:1–9.
112. Blomlie V, Rofstad EK, Skjonsberg A, et al. Female pelvic bone marrow: serial MR imaging before, during, and after radiation therapy. *Radiology.* 1995;194:537–543.
113. Stevens SK, Moore SG, Kaplan ID. Early and late bone-marrow changes after irradiation: MR evaluation. *AJR Am J Roentgenol.* 1990;154:745–750.
114. Kauczor HU, Dieti B, Brix G, et al. Fatty replacement of bone marrow after radiation therapy for Hodgkin disease: quantification with chemical shift imaging. *J Magn Reson Imaging.* 1993; 3:575–580.
115. Mumber MP, Greven KM, Haygood TM. Pelvic insufficiency fractures associated with radiation atrophy: clinical recognition and diagnostic evaluation. *Skeletal Radiol.* 1997;26: 94–99.
116. Fu AL, Greven KM, Maruyama Y. Radiation osteitis and insufficiency fractures after pelvic irradiation for gynecologic malignancies. *Am J Clin Oncol.* 1994;17:248–254.
117. Weber M, Hasler P, Gerber H. Insufficiency fractures of the sacrum. Twenty cases and review of the literature. *Spine.* 1993; 18:2507–2512.
118. Richardson ML, Zink-Brody GC, Patten RM, et al. MR characterization of post-irradiation soft tissue edema. *Skeletal Radiol.* 1996;25:537–543.
119. Biondetti PR, Ehman RL. Soft-tissue sarcomas: use of textural patterns in skeletal muscle as a diagnostic feature in postoperative MR imaging. *Radiology.* 1992;183:845–848.
120. Enneking WF, Spanier SS, Goodman MA. A system for the surgical staging of musculoskeletal sarcoma. *Clin Orthop.* 1980;153: 106–120.
121. Peabody TD, Simon MA. Principles of staging of soft-tissue sarcomas. *Clin Orthop.* 1993;289:19–31.
122. Greene FL, Page DL, Fleming FD, et al. (eds). American Joint Committee on Cancer: Cancer Staging Manual, 6th ed. New York, NY: Springer; 2002:221–226.
123. Hays DM, Soule EH, Lawrence W, et al. Extremity lesions in the Intergroup Rhabdomyosarcoma Study (IRS-I): a preliminary report. *Cancer.* 1982;48:1–8.
124. Shimada H, Newton WA, Soule EH, et al. Pathology of fatal rhabdomyosarcoma. Report from Intergroup Rhabdomyosarcoma Study (IRS-I and IRS-II). *Cancer.* 1987;59:459–465.
125. McDonald DJ. Limb-salvage surgery for treatment of sarcomas of the extremities. *AJR Am J Roentgenol.* 1994;163:509–513.

Lipomatous Tumors

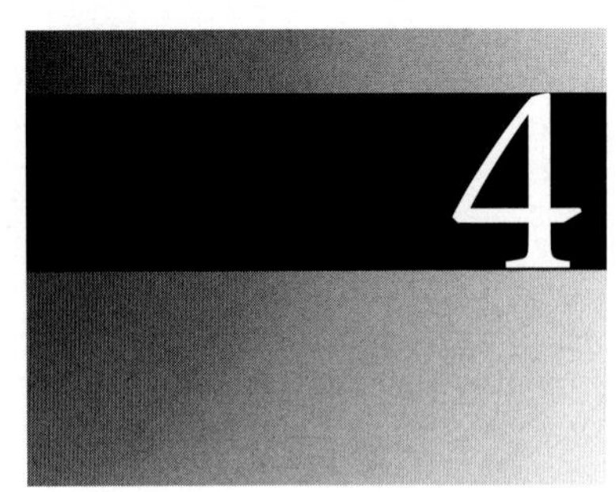

Lipomatous lesions are quite common and represent the largest single group of mesenchymal tumors (1). It is impossible to estimate their incidence accurately because they are often diagnosed clinically and untreated; however, nearly half of all surgically excised benign mesenchymal tumors are lipomas (2).

Current imaging techniques have markedly improved our ability to detect and diagnose soft tissue tumors. Computed tomography (CT) and magnetic resonance (MR) images of fatty masses are frequently sufficiently characteristic to suggest a specific diagnosis. This is typically the case with lipoma. However, when a mass does not meet the diagnostic criteria for a lipoma, a presumptive diagnosis of liposarcoma may be suggested. Although liposarcoma is often the diagnosis of exclusion, there are frequently other differential considerations.

BENIGN FATTY TUMORS

Classification

KEY CONCEPTS

Benign fatty tumors are classified into five groups:

- Lipoma
- Variants of lipoma: angiolipoma, myolipoma, chondroid lipoma, lipoblastoma, and spindle cell lipoma
- Lipomatous tumors: intramuscular lipoma, intermuscular lipoma, lipomatosis of nerve, and lipoma of tendon sheath and joint
- Infiltrating lipoma: lipomatosis, symmetric lipomatosis, and adiposis dolorosa
- Hibernoma

At present, the World Health Organization (WHO) Committee for the Classification of Soft Tissue Tumors divides benign lipomatous tumors into nine distinct diagnoses:

1. Lipoma
2. Lipomatosis
3. Lipomatosis of nerve
4. Lipoblastoma/lipoblastomatosis
5. Angiolipoma
6. Myolipoma of soft tissue
7. Chondroid lipoma
8. Spindle cell lipoma/pleomorphic lipoma
9. Hibernoma

This system of classification recognizes two newly characterized entities: myolipoma and chondroid lipoma, and it acknowledges the renaming of fibrolipomatous hamartoma of nerve to lipomatosis of nerve (1).

Although the new (2002) WHO classification system provides an excellent basis for diagnosis, we find greater clinical usefulness for radiologic diagnosis in the classification used by Weiss and Goldblum, in which benign lipomatous lesions are grouped into five major categories, some of which are subsequently further divided (2). This categorization includes the following:

1. *Lipoma:* A tumor composed of mature fat and further classified as superficial or deep, single or multiple.
2. *Variants of lipoma:* Fatty lesions with a characteristic histologic picture and specific clinical setting. Entities in this group include angiolipoma, myolipoma, chondroid lipoma, lipoblastoma, and spindle cell/pleomorphic lipoma.
3. *Lipomatous tumors:* Lesions in this group are intimately associated with specific nonadipose tissue. Included in this category are intramuscular lipoma, intermuscular lipoma, lipomatosis of nerve, and lipoma of tendon sheath and joint.
4. *Infiltrating lipomas:* Proliferative fatty lesions that compress adjacent structures, including diffuse lipomatosis, symmetric lipomatosis, and adiposis dolorosa.
5. *Hibernoma:* A benign tumor of brown fat.

This classification system recognizes the radiologic similarities between the members of each group and helps in the formulation of a differential diagnosis. These major groups are discussed in greater detail here, emphasizing the typical features of lesions as encountered in the musculoskeletal system.

Lipoma

> **KEY CONCEPTS**
>
> Lipoma is the most common soft tissue tumor, representing approximately half of all soft tissue tumors:
> - Characterized by anatomic location as superficial or deep; usually, but not invariably, encapsulated.
> - Typically occurs in adults in the fifth to sixth decade.
> - An estimated 80% are smaller than 5 cm; deep lesions tend to be larger.
> - Superficial lesions are much more common than deep lesions.

The lipoma is the most common soft tissue tumor and comprises nearly half of all benign mesenchymal tumors in surgical series, with an incidence as high as 2.1 per 100 people (3,4). A benign lesion composed of mature adipose tissue, it is not distinguishable histologically from normal fat (3). Despite the microscopic similarities to normal adipose tissue, studies identify cytogenetic abnormalities in approximately 50% to 60% of typical cutaneous lipomas (5,6).

The majority of lipomas are discrete masses, categorized by anatomic location as either superficial (subcutaneous) or deep. The superficial lipoma alone accounts for 16% to 50% of all soft tissue tumors in some large series (3,7,8). Superficial lipoma is far more common, with deep lipoma accounting for only approximately 1% of cases (3,9,10).

Grossly, a lipoma is a soft, well-circumscribed mass, usually encapsulated, with a distinct lobular pattern. The shape of a deep-seated lipoma is more variable than that of a superficial lipoma. On cross-section, a lipoma is pale yellow to tan in color, with a lobular to smooth and variably greasy to myxoid cut surface. Microscopically, the mass is composed of mature fat cells (adipocytes) that are uniform in size and shape. Lipomas are well-vascularized, but the vascular network is not readily discernible microscopically because of compression of the blood vessels by plump adipocytes (2). Interestingly, the fat within the lipoma is unavailable for systemic metabolism, and, paradoxically, a lipoma may actually increase in size during starvation (11). A few cases of malignant transformation of lipoma are reported, but these probably represent cases in which the subtle histologic features of malignancy were initially overlooked (2). The concept of malignant transformation is addressed more fully in the section on liposarcoma.

Superficial Lipoma

Patients with a superficial soft tissue lipoma typically present in middle age (fifth and sixth decades), although there is a wide spectrum, with 80% of lesions presenting in patients between 26 and 65 years of age (12). Both men and women are reported as being more commonly affected, depending on the series (7,13–15). Patients usu-

ally present with a slowly growing soft tissue mass (15). After an initial period of discernible growth, lesions typically stabilize in size (2). Lipomas usually do not produce symptoms, although local pain, tenderness, or compression of peripheral nerves is present in up to approximately one-quarter of patients (15,16). Most lipomas are small; 80% are less than 5 cm and the remainder are typically less than 10 cm (7). Rydholm and Berg (7) noted that only 4 (1%) of 338 superficial lipomas were larger than 10 cm. Lesions are most commonly located on the trunk, shoulder, upper arm, and neck. They are unusual in the hand and foot (7). Diagnosis on the basis of clinical findings is accurate in approximately 85% of cases (17). Recurrence following surgery is seen in approximately 4% of patients (15).

The pathogenesis of lipoma is unknown, although it is thought to represent a true mesenchymal neoplasm. Lipoma is usually a solitary lesion, although patients may demonstrate multiple tumors that can vary in number from very few to numerous (10,13–15). The incidence of multiple lipomas varies from 5% to 15% (3,7,10,15). Rydholm and Berg (7) noted a striking male predilection of 6.6:1 in 61 patients with multiple lipomas, in contrast to 1.2:1 in 338 patients with solitary lesions.

Deep Lipoma

The deep-seated lipoma (as distinguished from other deep fatty lesions, such as intramuscular lipoma) occurs most commonly in the chest wall and deep soft tissue of the hands and feet. It may rarely occur in the retroperitoneum, although most fatty retroperitoneal tumors are well-differentiated or dedifferentiated liposarcomas (12,17). Deep-seated lipomas are less well-defined and typically considerably larger in size than their superficial counterparts. Myhre-Jensen (3) noted that deep-seated lipomas accounted for less than 1% of 707 lipomas seen by the surgical pathology department over a 7-year period. Our experience indicates that these lesions are considerably more common. We suspect that this is the result of a bias for imaging of deep lesions and the fact that many small superficial lipomas are excised without imaging.

Weiss and Goldblum (2) separate deep lipomas from lesions in an intramuscular or intermuscular location. This division is confusing, and in clinical practice, all lipomas deep to the superficial fascia are considered to be deep-seated lesions.

Imaging of Lipoma

> **KEY CONCEPTS**
> - Lipoma typically images identical to fat on CT scanning and MR imaging.
> - Thin fibrous septa are occasionally seen.
> - Calcification is uncommon, and osseous erosions are rare.

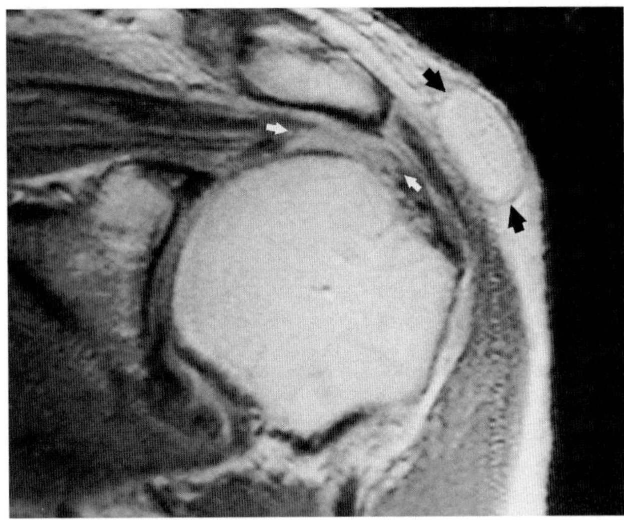

Figure 4.1 Encapsulated superficial (subcutaneous) lipoma: MR imaging in man 74 years of age. Oblique coronal proton (TR/TE; 2000/20) spin-echo MR image of the shoulder shows a well-defined lipomatous mass (*black arrows*) in the subcutaneous fat. The lesion images identical to fat on all pulse sequences. There is a thin surrounding fibrous capsule of low signal intensity. Note full-thickness tear of the supraspinatus tendon (*white arrows*).

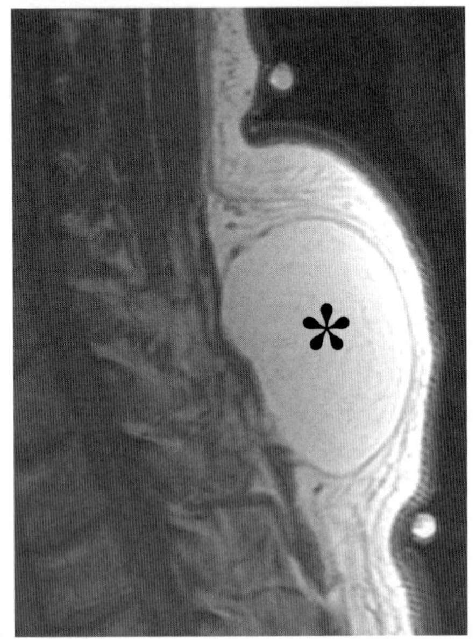

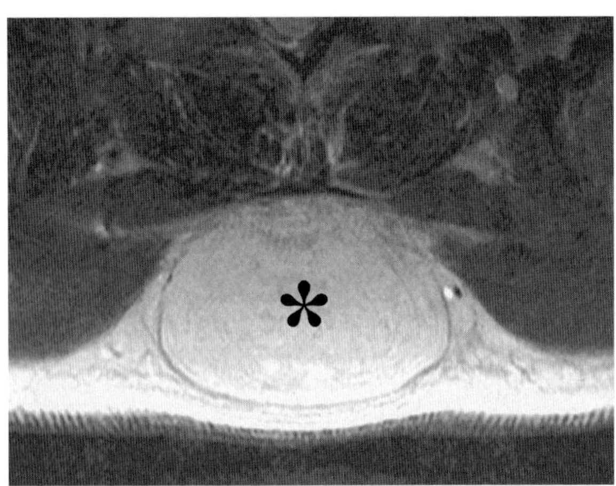

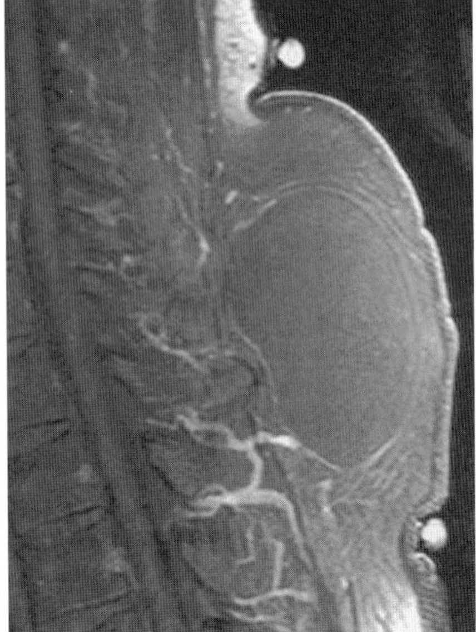

Figure 4.2 Encapsulated superficial (subcutaneous) lipoma: MR imaging in a man 51 years of age presenting with an enlarging posterior neck mass. **A,B:** Sagittal T1-weighted (620/17) **(A)** and axial turbo T2-weighted (TE/TE; 4000/87) **(B)** spin-echo MR images show a well-encapsulated lipomatous mass (*asterisk*) in the subcutaneous fat. The signal intensity of the lesion is identical to that of fat on all pulse sequences. **C:** Sagittal enhanced fat-suppressed T1-weighted (TR/TE; 579/17) spin-echo image shows no enhancement. Note thin surrounding fibrous capsule of low signal intensity that enhances following contrast administration.

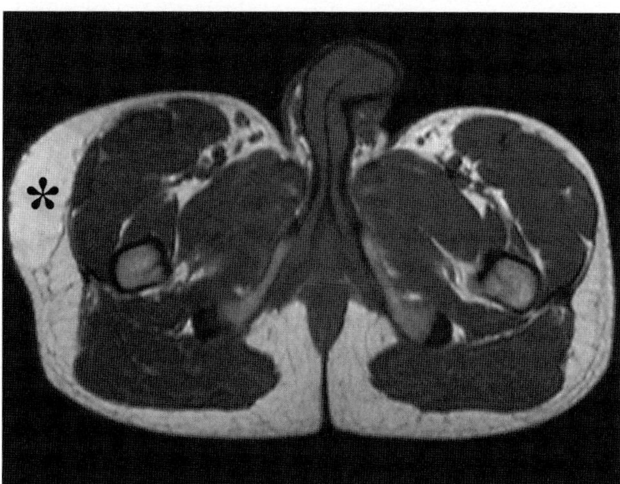

Figure 4.3 Partially encapsulated superficial (subcutaneous) lipoma: MR imaging in a man 35 years of age presenting with an enlarging hip mass. Axial T1-weighted (TR/TE; 728/16) spin-echo MR image shows a subcutaneous lipoma (*asterisk*). The signal intensity of the lesion is identical to that of fat on all pulse sequences. Although there is a well-defined capsule along the deep margin of the mass, it is less defined posteriorly and anteriorly.

Depending on the size and location of the lesion, radiographs may be unremarkable or demonstrate a mass of fat density. Superficial lipomas may be difficult to distinguish from the adjacent adipose tissue. Although reported, bone erosion is extremely unusual (15). Calcification is uncommon but reported in up to 11% of benign fatty tumors (18). Calcification is more common in malignant fatty tumors (18). Soft tissue lipoma may occasionally be associated with changes in the skeleton. Cortical thickening may be seen in association with adjacent parosteal lipoma, and congenital osseous anomalies are described adjacent to deep lipomas (19).

The lipoma is well-characterized on CT and MR, with the lesion having an appearance identical to that of subcutaneous fat (20–26). The MR signal intensity of a lipoma should be identical to that of the subcutaneous adipose tissue on all pulse sequences (20,25). If the lesion is minimally heterogeneous, we have found it useful to compare the appearance of the lesion to that of the surrounding fat. When imaging is done with a surface coil, comparison of lesional tissue should be made to the adipose tissue at a similar distance from the coil. A lipoma should not have discernible enhancement following the administration of intravenous gadopentetate dimeglumine (27). When a lipoma is encapsulated, a surrounding fibrous capsule of low signal intensity on MR may be delineated (Figs. 4.1 and 4.2). Such capsules may be incompletely visualized (Fig. 4.3). Alternatively, a superficial lipoma may blend imperceptibly with the surrounding subcutaneous fat on MR and may not be recognizable as a distinct encapsulated mass. In such cases, the capsule may not be present or may be too thin to resolve on imaging studies. These lesions may be referred to as *nonencapsulated lipomas* (Fig. 4.4) (27). A marker placed over the area of clinical concern aids in identifying the lesion. Comparison with the contralateral side or extremity can also be useful to identify subtle focal asymmetry.

On CT scanning, a lipoma demonstrates a homogeneous low attenuation (approximately −65 to −120 HU), without enhancement following administration of intravenous contrast (20,22,26,28). Comparison of the tissue attenuation of tumor to that of surrounding normal fat, either visually or numerically, is more reliable for diagnosis than an absolute

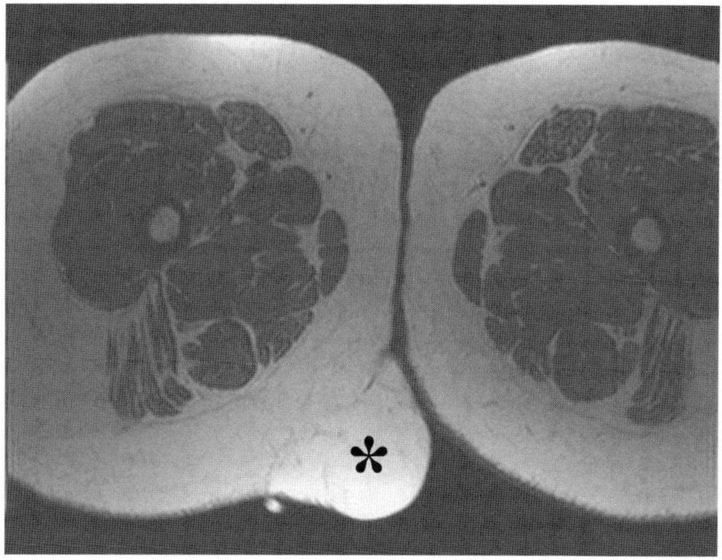

A

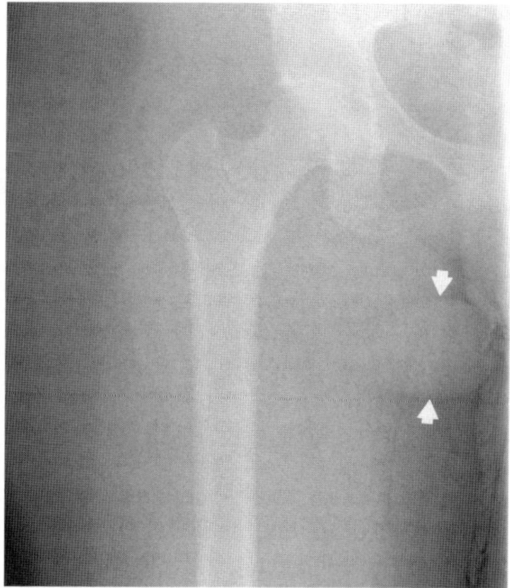

B

Figure 4.4 Nonencapsulated superficial (subcutaneous) lipoma: MR imaging in a woman 29 years of age. **A:** Axial T1-weighted (TR/TE; 584/16) spin-echo MR image shows an unencapsulated, pedunculated fatty mass (*asterisk*) in the posterior thigh. **B:** Anteroposterior radiograph shows the pedunculated character of the mass (*arrows*).

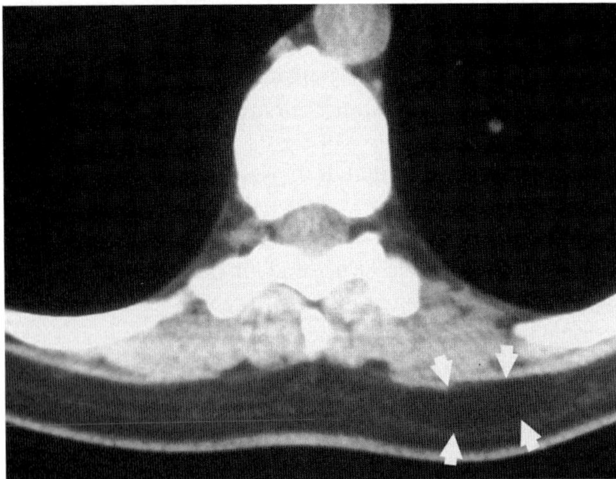

Figure 4.5   Encapsulated superficial (subcutaneous) lipoma: CT imaging in a woman 44 years old presenting with a paraspinal mass. Axial unenhanced CT scan shows a subtle mass (*arrows*) with attenuation identical to that of the subcutaneous adipose tissue.

CT number (Fig. 4.5) (22). Moreover, in any one individual, fat densities vary among different locations within the body (29). When present, a fibrous capsule shows an attenuation similar to that of muscle on CT scan.

The sonographic appearance of superficial lipoma is typically an elliptical mass parallel to the skin surface that is hyperechoic relative to the adjacent muscle and contains linear echogenic lines at right angles to the ultrasound beam (30,31). Superficial lipomas show no increased through transmission and compress with moderate transducer pressure (Fig. 4.6) (30). Although these features are relatively constant on superficial lesions evaluated with high-frequency high-resolution transducers, there is variability. In the evaluation of 25 patients with head and neck lipoma, Ahuja et al. (30) found 76% to be hyperechoic, 8% to be isoechoic, and 16% to be hypoechoic to

adjacent muscle. These authors also noted that whereas 88% of lesions were well-defined, 12% had an incomplete capsule.

In general, we are more confident with the CT and MR imaging appearance of lipoma. MR imaging is also far better suited to assess the internal architecture of lesions when lesions do not meet the imaging requirements for a lipoma. Sonography can be useful for follow-up in patients with established diagnoses.

Imaging Variations

> **KEY CONCEPTS**
> - Imaging variations are more common in large or long-standing lesions.
> - Fat necrosis is suggested by identification of a globular or laminated lesion with fatty signal centrally and surrounding hypointense rim without a discrete mass.
> - The term *fibrolipoma* is used when significant fibrous tissue is present.
> - *Benign mesenchymoma* is the term previously used when metaplastic cartilage or bone forms within a lipoma.

Although the imaging diagnosis of lipoma is usually not difficult, complicating features may alter the typical imaging picture. These changes may be on a microscopic level as a result of a vascular or traumatic injury with infarction, hemorrhage, and calcification, or they may be macroscopic with fat necrosis and liquefaction (2). Additionally, lipomas may be associated with other mesenchymal elements, including fibrous tissue, cartilage, and bone. These imaging variations may be seen in superficial or deep lesions, but generally in our experience they are more commonly encountered on imaging examinations in deep fatty lesions.

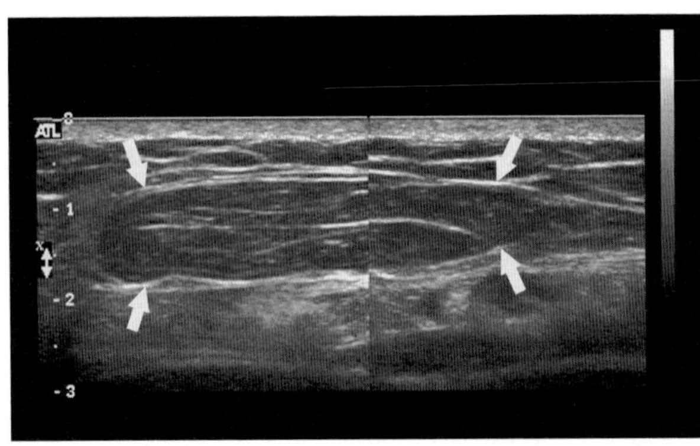

A

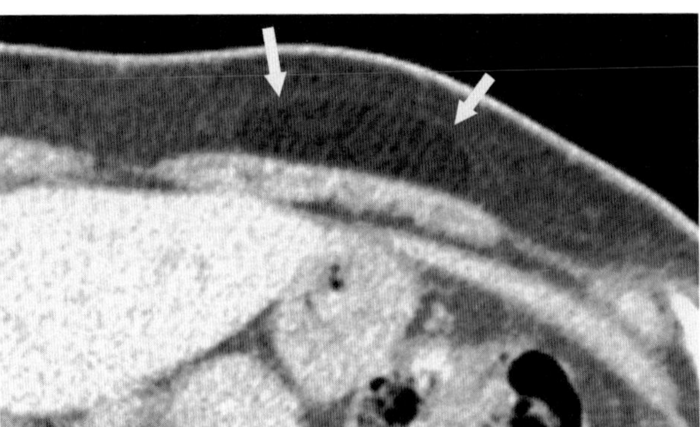

B

Figure 4.6   Superficial (subcutaneous) lipoma: Imaging in a woman 73 years of age with an abdominal wall mass. **A:** Ultrasound reveals an elliptical mass (*arrows*) parallel to the skin surface that is hypoechoic relative to the adjacent muscle of the abdominal wall and contains linear echogenic lines. The lesion is well-defined and compressible with transducer pressure. **B:** Corresponding axial noncontrast CT scan shows the lesion (*arrows*) as a well-defined homogeneous fatty mass. Note slight difference in texture and attenuation of the lesion and the surrounding adipose tissue.

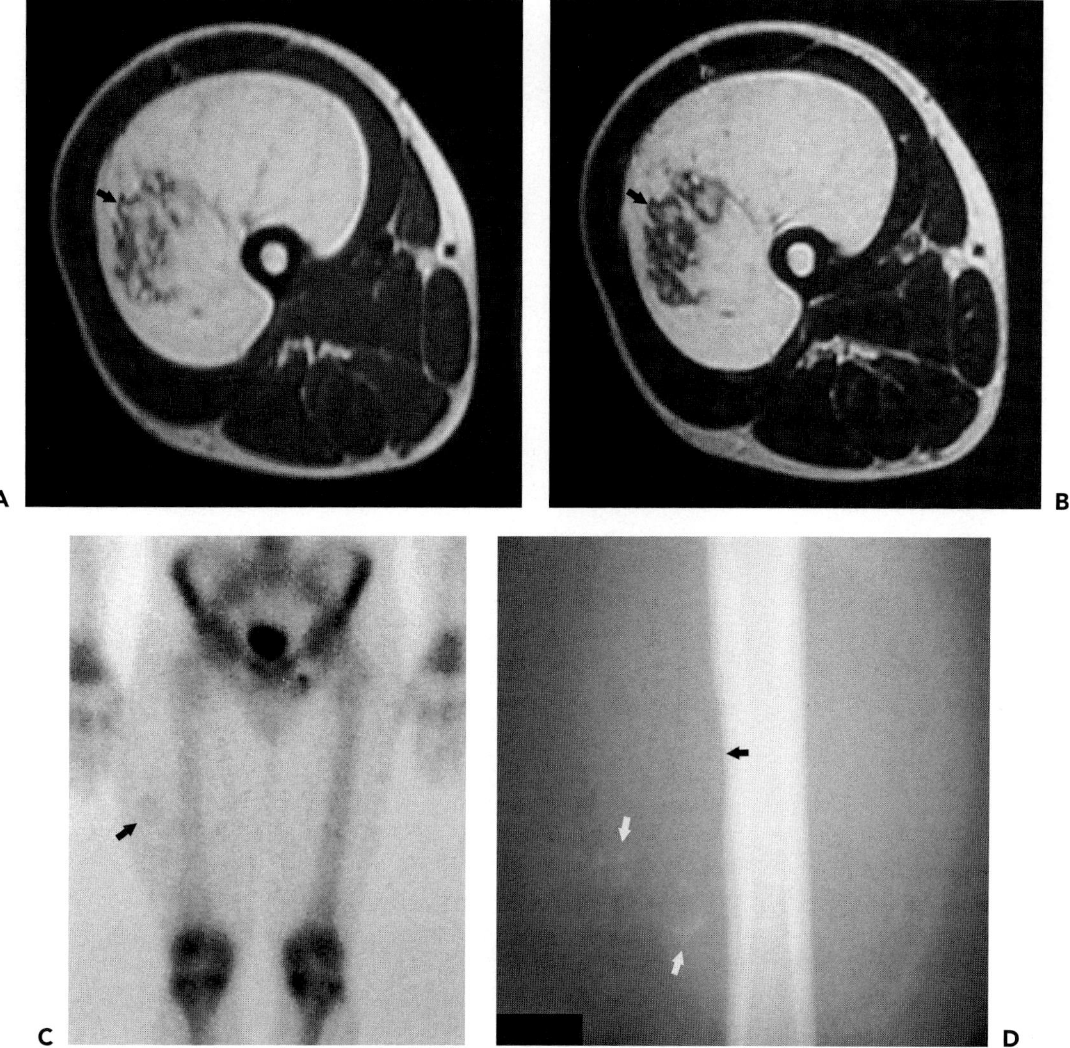

Figure 4.7.   Fat necrosis within a lipoma: Typical MR imaging features in a man 30 years of age with a large lipoma. **A,B:** Corresponding axial T1-weighted (TR/TE; 730/11) **(A)** and turbo T2-weighted (TR/TE; 3133/91) **(B)** spin-echo MR images show a multilobulated masslike area within the lipoma with fatty signal intensity centrally and surrounding irregular-curvilinear hypointense rim (*arrow*). **C:** Anteroposterior image from MDP scintigram shows slight increased tracer accumulation within the area of fat necrosis (*arrow*). **D:** Anteroposterior radiograph shows globular, amorphous calcifications (*white arrows*). The lipoma has remodeled the adjacent femoral cortex (*black arrow*).

Fat Necrosis

Although the cause of fat necrosis is frequently unknown, it is often attributed to nonpenetrating trauma because fat necrosis is most frequently seen in the superficial adipose tissue and often found overlying osseous protuberances. Fat necrosis is also not uncommon in large deep fatty masses (18,32). When trauma is the initiating cause, the time interval between the initial injury and the observation of a palpable lump may be prolonged (32). Fat necrosis is also reported in the newborn, usually becoming apparent clinically within the first month of life (33). Lesions are usually superficial, firm, well-defined, and mobile (33).

There are few reports detailing the appearance of fat necrosis, and in some of these reports, histologic confirma-tion of the diagnosis is limited. The diagnosis of fat necrosis can be made, however, when imaging shows a globular or laminated lesion with fatty signal intensity centrally and a surrounding irregular hypointense rim (Fig. 4.7) without a discrete mass (32,34).

Gadolinium enhancement is variable and may be absent or irregular at the periphery of the lesion (32). The adipose tissue within the lesion may show increased signal on fluid-sensitive sequences (32). Calcification may also be seen, and it is likely that the microscopic or macroscopic calcification causes the increased tracer accumulation seen on scintigra-phy (Fig. 4.7). The spectrum of imaging appearances of fat necrosis is varied and may demonstrate amorphous and cloudlike stranding, inflammation, cyst formation, and a masslike appearance (Fig. 4.8). When these involutional

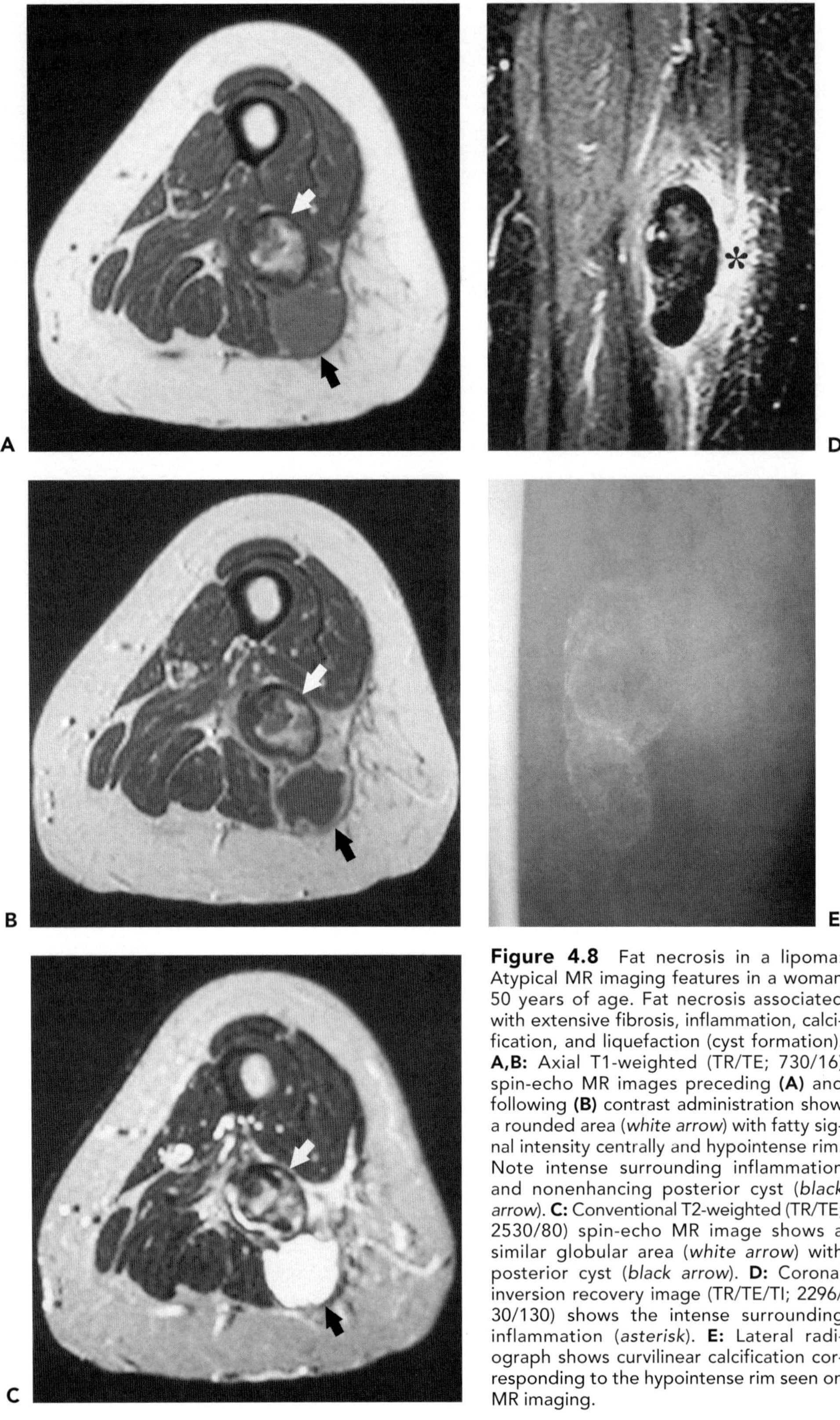

Figure 4.8 Fat necrosis in a lipoma: Atypical MR imaging features in a woman 50 years of age. Fat necrosis associated with extensive fibrosis, inflammation, calcification, and liquefaction (cyst formation). **A,B:** Axial T1-weighted (TR/TE; 730/16) spin-echo MR images preceding **(A)** and following **(B)** contrast administration show a rounded area (*white arrow*) with fatty signal intensity centrally and hypointense rim. Note intense surrounding inflammation and nonenhancing posterior cyst (*black arrow*). **C:** Conventional T2-weighted (TR/TE; 2530/80) spin-echo MR image shows a similar globular area (*white arrow*) with posterior cyst (*black arrow*). **D:** Coronal inversion recovery image (TR/TE/TI; 2296/30/130) shows the intense surrounding inflammation (*asterisk*). **E:** Lateral radiograph shows curvilinear calcification corresponding to the hypointense rim seen on MR imaging.

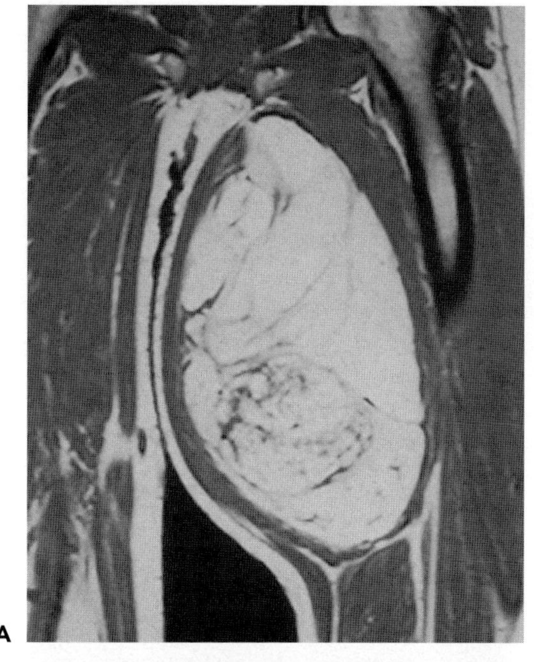

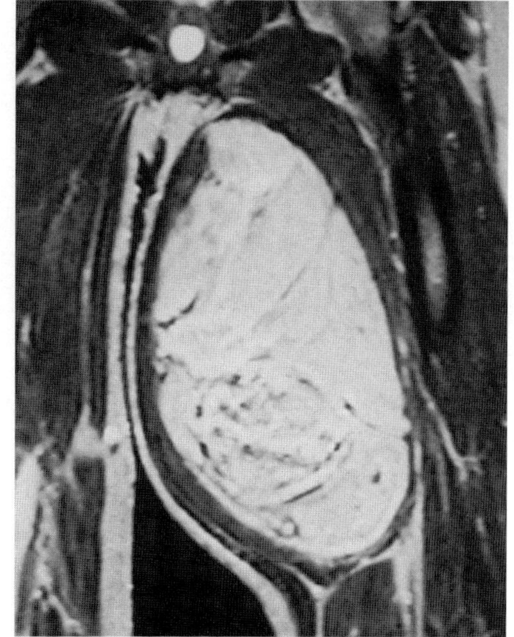

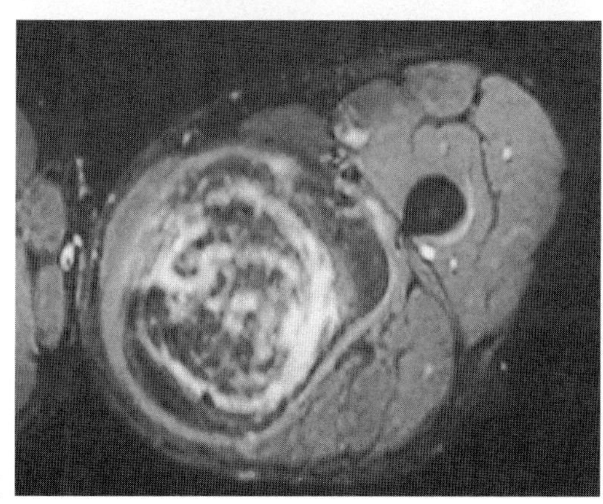

Figure 4.9 Involutional changes: MR imaging features of a long-standing lipoma simulating a liposarcoma in a man 48 years of age. **A,B:** Coronal T1-weighted (TE/TE; 633/16) **(A)** and T2-weighted (TR/TE; 2080/80) **(B)** spin-echo MR images show a large fatty mass with thickened nodular septations. **C:** Axial STIR (TR/TE/TI; 2183/40/150) MR image shows thickened linear, nodular, and globular areas of increased signal intensity. Similar findings are commonly seen in a liposarcoma.

changes occur within a lipoma, they may simulate the MR appearance of a liposarcoma (Fig. 4.9) (18,35). Fat necrosis may be seen in association with panniculitis.

Fibrolipoma

Lipomas occasionally contain other mesenchymal elements. The most common of these is fibrous connective tissue, which may demonstrate a septal configuration, appearing as linear densities on CT (21,23) or as linear areas of decreased signal on MR imaging, regardless of pulse sequence (Figs. 4.10 and 4.11) (36). When significant fibrous tissue is present, these lesions may be termed *fibrolipoma,* although this term is not a recognized WHO diagnosis.

Benign Mesenchymoma

Cartilage and bone formation may occasionally be seen within a lipoma, particularly if the lesion is long-standing (2,36,38). Plaut et al. (38) noted that calcified areas were reported in lipomata in the early literature, and they were termed *lipoma petrificum ossificans* by Virchow in 1864,

attributing the ossification to "previous mucoid and calcareous degeneration, presumably a result of mechanical pressure." This cartilage and bone formation is now regarded as metaplastic (2,36,38), and the term *benign mesenchymoma* was previously employed to describe this type of lesion. When mature ossification dominates, radiographs may suggest myositis ossificans. CT and MR are especially useful in revealing the fatty nature of the mass (Fig. 4.12). On occasion, extensive bone and cartilage within the mass make identification of the lipoma difficult (Fig. 4.13). Benign mesenchymoma is *not* related to malignant mesenchymoma (39), the latter term being used to describe a malignant mesenchymal tumor displaying features of at least two unrelated distinct sarcomas. (Malignant mesenchymoma is discussed further in Chapter 12.) A lipoma with metaplastic cartilage may occasionally be termed a *chondrolipoma* and should not be called a *chondroid lipoma,* which refers to a specific lesion recognized by the WHO and discussed later (9). Similarly, a lipoma with metaplastic bone may occasionally be called an *osteolipoma* (9).

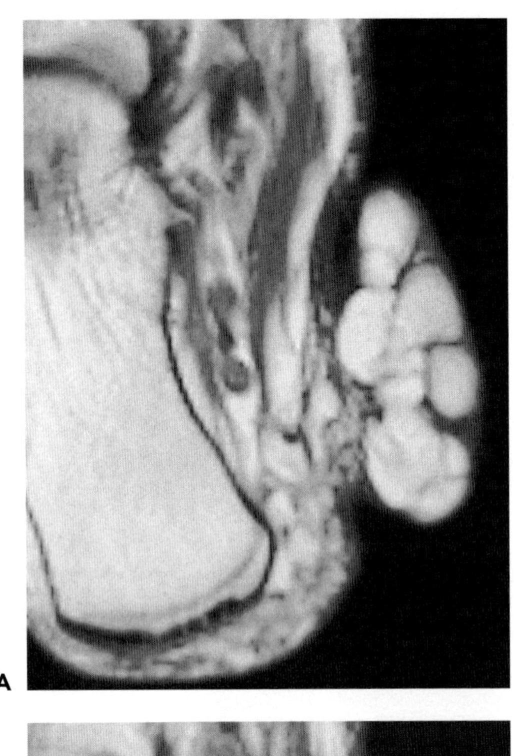

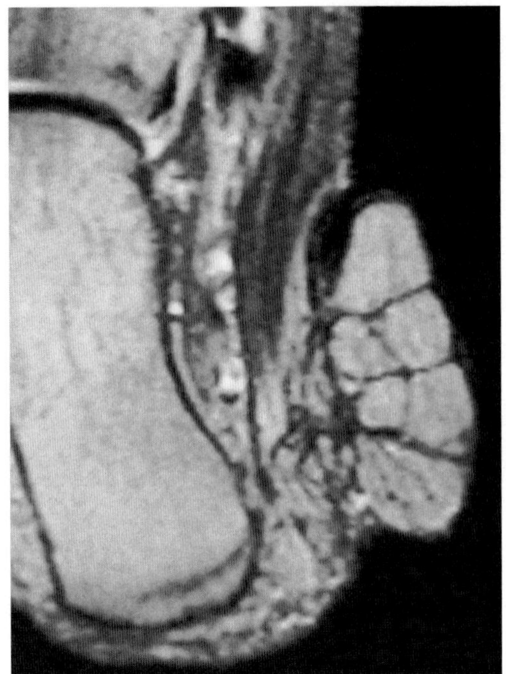

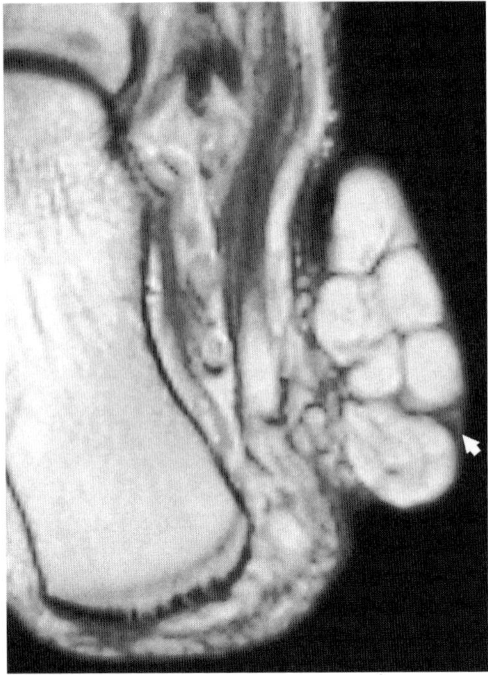

Figure 4.10 Superficial fibrolipoma: MR imaging in a woman 69 years of age with a recurrent mass. **A,B:** Axial T1-weighted (600/15) **(A)** and T2-weighted (2500/80) **(B)** spin-echo MR images show the mass to have a lobulated contour with a signal intensity identical to that of subcutaneous fat. The lesion has multiple linear septations of decreased signal intensity coursing through its substance on all pulse sequences. **C:** Corresponding axial T1-weighted (600/15) spin-echo MR image following gadopentetate dimeglumine injection shows minimal enhancement within the fibrovascular septae (*arrow*).

Multiple Lipomas

KEY CONCEPTS
- Familial lipomatosis (multiple lipomas) is usually autosomal dominant, with a strong male predominance.
- Lesions are superficial and most common in the forearm, trunk, thighs, and arms.
- Encephalocraniocutaneous lipomatosis is a rare congenital disorder characterized by mental retardation, seizures, cerebral malformations, and cutaneous lipomas of the scalp.

As noted earlier, lipoma is usually a solitary lesion; however, multiple lesions are not uncommon and are seen in 5% to 15% of patients (7,8,13,15). Lipomatosis syndromes, in contrast, are quite rare; two such syndromes are discussed here.

Familial Multiple Lipomas

Familial lipomatosis (multiple lipomas) is a rare disorder characterized by the development of multiple encapsulated, subcutaneous lipomas (14,40). Lipomas are quite common, as are patients with multiple lipomas; however,

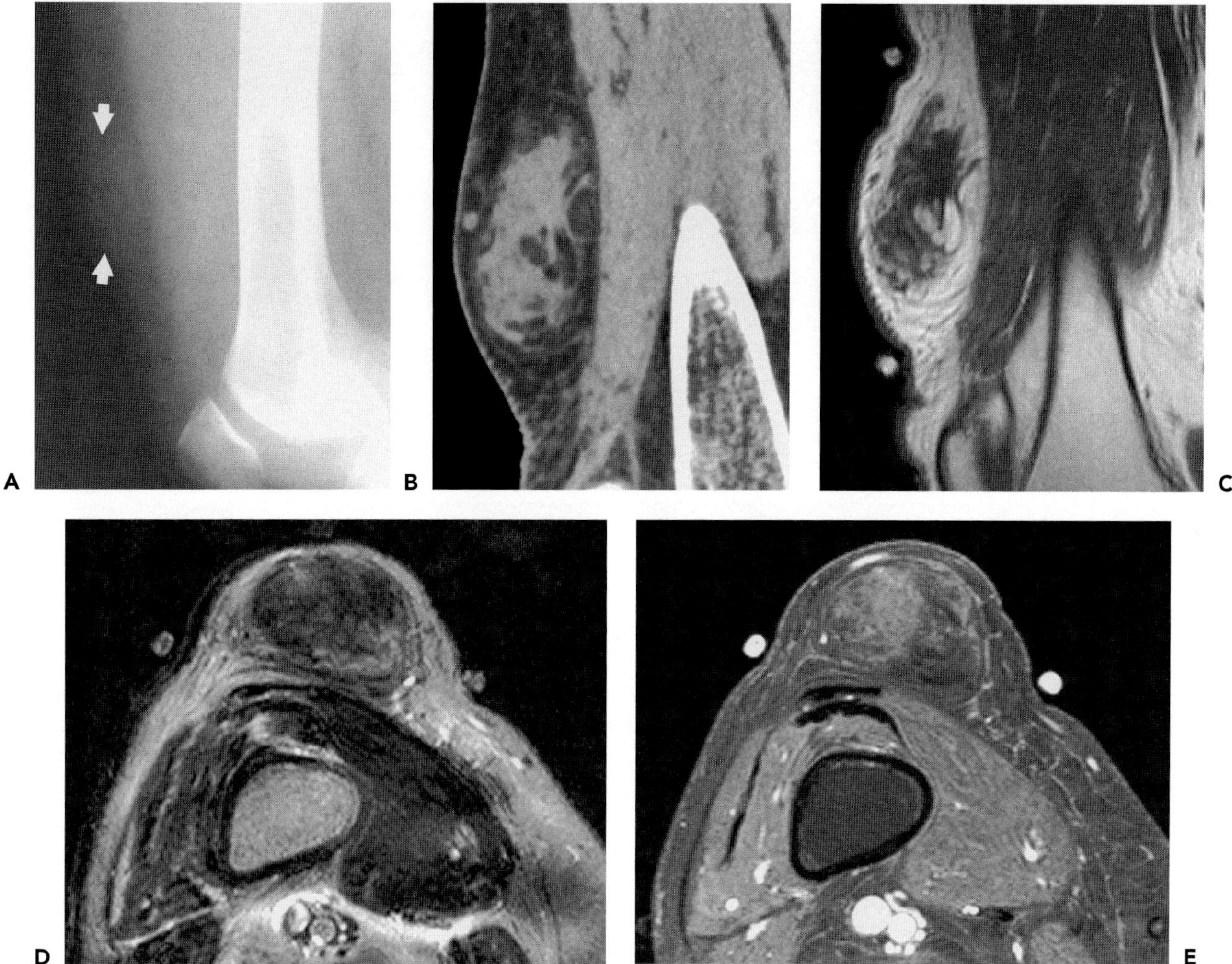

Figure 4.11. Fibrolipoma: MR and CT imaging in a woman 72 years of age. **A:** Lateral radiograph shows a soft tissue mass (*arrows*) in the anterior subcutaneous adipose tissue. **B,C:** Sagittal reformatted CT scan **(B)** and corresponding T1-weighted (589/12) spin-echo MR image **(C)** show a mass in the subcutaneous adipose tissue with a significant nonadipose component. **D:** Axial T2-weighted (2610/80) spin-echo MR image shows the nonadipose component to have a decreased signal intensity, similar to that of muscle. Note adipose tissue in the interstices of the mass. **E:** Axial fat-suppressed, enhanced, T1-weighted (519/12) spin-echo MR image shows no significant enhancement.

only a small number of familial cases have been reported. The pattern of inheritance in familial multiple lipomas is variable and probably polygenic (40). Although usually autosomal dominant, an autosomal recessive inheritance pattern is also reported (41). Patients in affected families show the same male predominance seen in patients with multiple lipomas, and they present at a similar age (14,40,42,43). Patients have no detectable metabolic or lipid metabolism abnormalities, and subcutaneous lipomatosis has no clinical significance except for the cosmetic disability, which can be significant and lead to grotesque deformity (40,42). Research identifies the genetic abnormality in this disorder to chromosome 12q15, resulting from a translocation involving the high-mobility-group protein isoform I-C (HMGIC) on chromosome 12 and

the lipoma preferred partner gene (LLP) on chromosome 3 (44).

In familial multiple lipomas, lesions are superficial and composed of mature adipocytes. They are identical to ordinary lipomas, although larger in size (Fig. 4.14) (42). Clinically, patients typically present in the third or fourth decade with multiple smooth, round to oval, nontender, subcutaneous nodules on the forearms, trunk, thighs, and arms (40,41,43). The neck and shoulders are usually spared (40,43). The number of lesions varies from a few to greater than 100 (45). Although the lesions are painless and benign, surgical removal is usually sought for cosmesis or relief from discomfort and disfigurement because of size or location (4). Treatment can include simple excision, endoscopic removal, or liposuction (44).

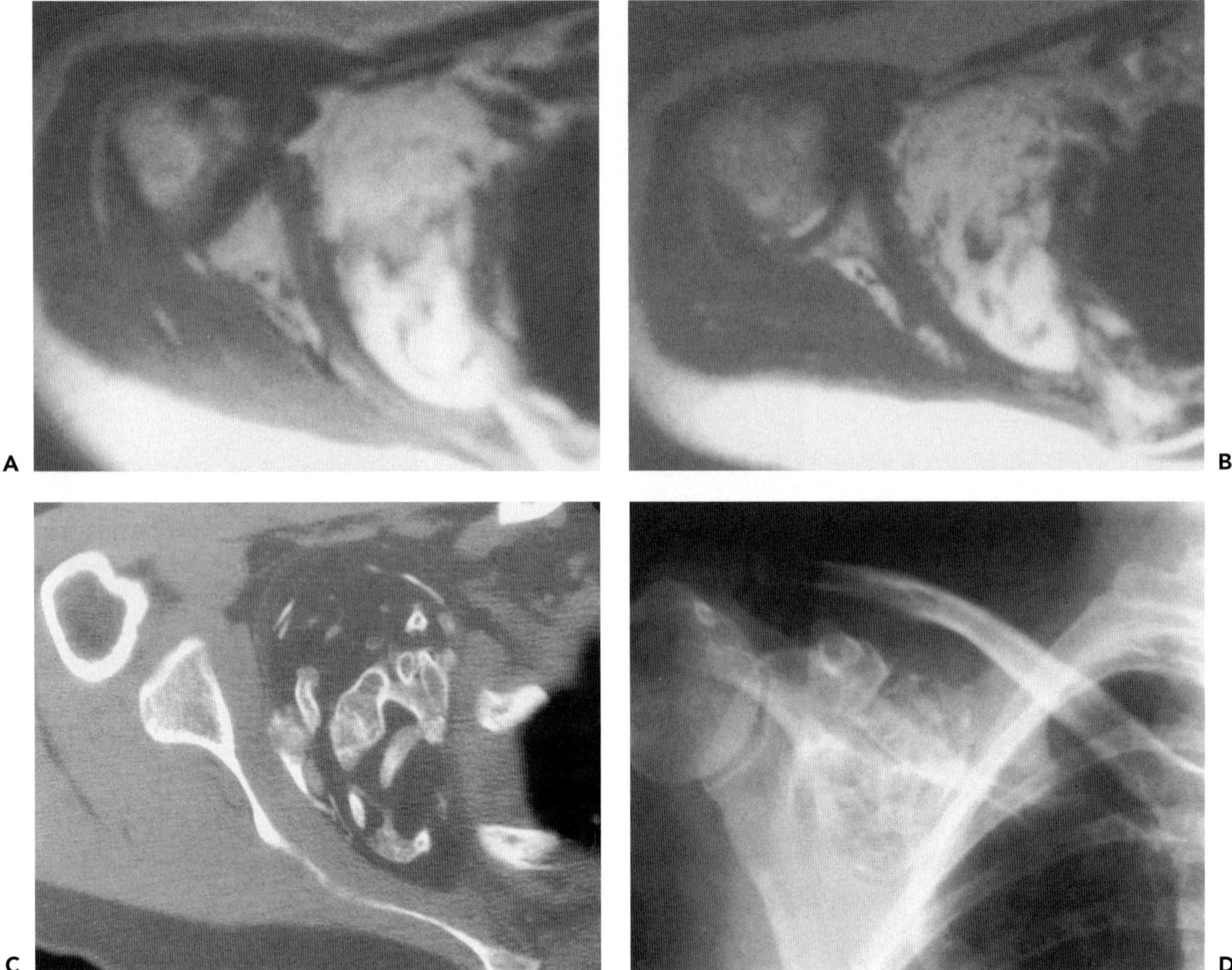

Figure 4.12   Lipoma with metaplastic bone (benign mesenchymoma): MR and CT imaging in the shoulder of a woman 60 years of age. **A,B:** Axial T1-weighted (TR/TE; 700/16) **(A)** and turbo T2-weighted (TR/TE; 3000/85) **(B)** MR images show a lipomatous mass in the right axilla with multiple central well-defined areas of decreased signal intensity. These areas of decreased signal intensity represent mature cortical bone surrounding areas of fatty marrow, with signal intensity similar to that of subcutaneous fat (and the surrounding lipoma). **C:** Corresponding axial CT scan at bone window shows the fatty nature of the mass as well as the mature ossification. **D:** Anteroposterior radiograph of the shoulder shows the well-formed bone. The fatty nature of the mass is difficult to appreciate.

The asymmetric distribution of multiple familial lipomas helps separate this entity from the rare multiple symmetric lipomatosis (see subsequent discussion). Rubinstein et al. (42) reported a family who had lipomatosis with hyperlipidemia and associated elevated serum total cholesterol, low-density lipoprotein (LDL), and high-density lipoprotein (HDL). There was also a correlation between the degree of hyperlipidemia and the number of subcutaneous lipomas. Familial multiple lipomatosis is also reported in association with peripheral neuropathy (41).

Encephalocraniocutaneous Lipomatosis

Encephalocraniocutaneous lipomatosis, first described in 1970 by Haberland and Perou (46), is a rare congenital disorder characterized by profound mental retardation, early onset of seizures, unilateral temporofrontal lipomatosis, ipsilateral cerebral and leptomeningeal lipomatosis, cerebral malformation and calcification, and cutaneous lipomas (47–50). In these rare cases, the cutaneous lipomas are mainly confined to the scalp, but they may be seen in the lower limbs and back (48). Encephalocraniocutaneous lipomatosis is classified as a congenital neurocutaneous syndrome and may be a localized form of Proteus syndrome because both syndromes have some overlapping manifestations (49,51).

Central nervous system abnormalities predominate and ocular abnormalities are invariably present, typically presenting as small skin tags around the eyelids (49,52). Neurocutaneous findings are ipsilateral in almost three-quarters of patients and include intracranial calcifications,

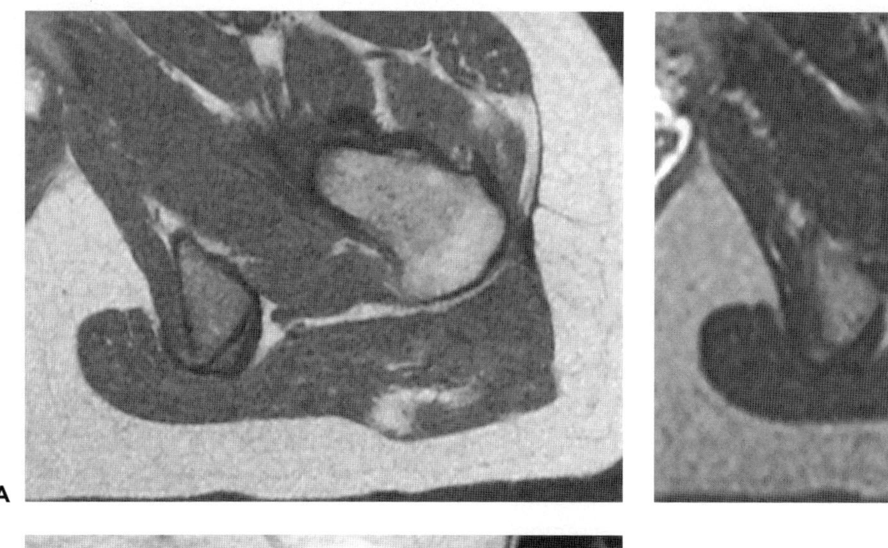

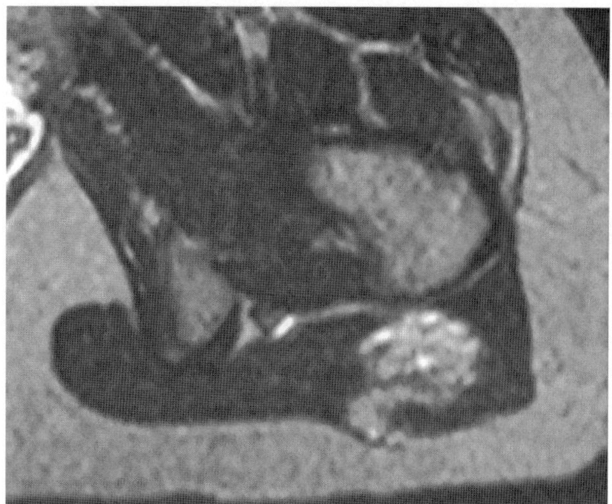

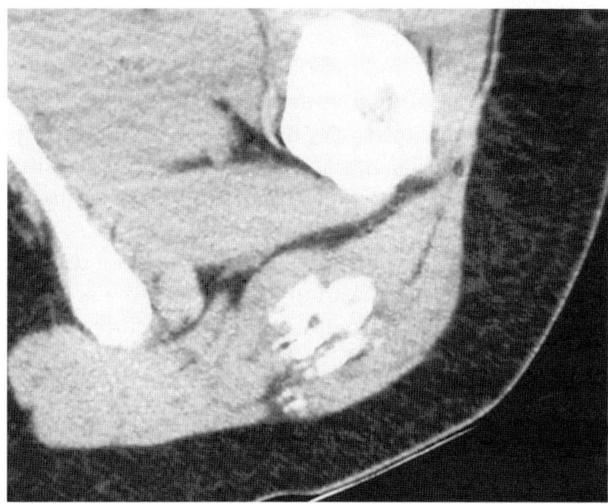

Figure 4.13 Lipoma with extensive metaplastic cartilage and bone (benign mesenchymoma): MR and CT imaging in the buttocks of a woman 27 years of age. **A,B:** Axial T1-weighted (TR/TE; 700/16) **(A)** and conventional T2-weighted (TR/TE; 2000/85) **(B)** MR images show a lipomatous mass with extensive metaplastic cartilage and bone. **C:** Corresponding axial CT scan at soft tissue window shows the extensive mineralization in the mass. The decreased attenuation adjacent to the mineralization represents the fatty component, which was seen to better advantage on MR imaging.

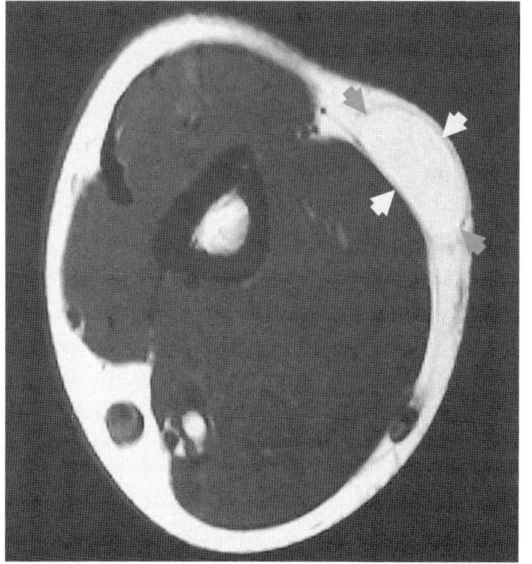

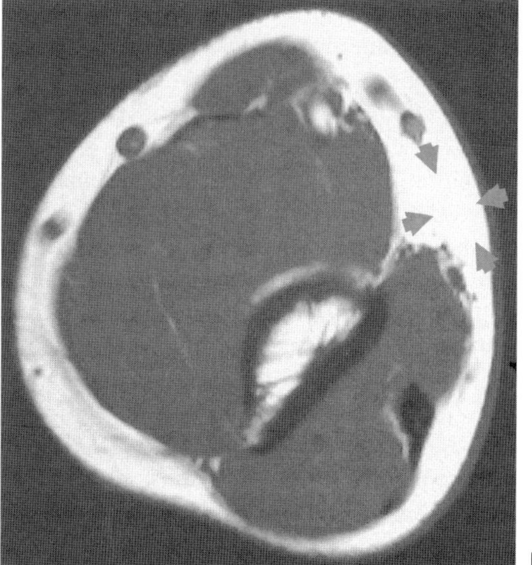

Figure 4.14 Familial multiple lipomas: MR imaging features in a man 45 years of age. **A:** Axial T1-weighted (TR/TE; 600/15) spin-echo MR image through the distal arm shows one of innumerable subcutaneous (superficial) lipomas (*arrows*). **B:** Axial T1-weighted just distal to **(A)** shows an additional smaller lesion (*arrows*).

porencephalic cysts, and enlargement of the lateral ventricles (49,52). Seizures and mental retardation are frequent (52). The most commonly reported intracranial lesion is epibulbar choristoma, occurring in almost three-quarters of cases (52).

Lipoma Variants

Although the so-called ordinary lipoma is overwhelmingly the most frequently encountered fatty soft tissue tumor, there are numerous lipoma variants. These are well-described in the pathology literature; however, they have received relatively little attention in the radiology literature. These lipoma variants differ from the classic soft tissue lipoma with regard to both clinical presentation and microscopic appearance. The following entities are considered lipoma variants: lipoblastoma, angiolipoma, spindle cell lipoma/pleomorphic lipoma, myolipoma, and chondroid lipoma.

Lipoblastoma

KEY CONCEPTS

- Lipoblastoma is a relatively rare cellularly immature lipoma.
- It appears almost exclusively in infants, usually presents by 3 years of age, and males are affected two to three times more frequently than females.
- Two-thirds to three-quarters are discrete; when diffuse, they are termed *lipoblastomatosis*.
- Radiologically, lipoblastomas may be indistinguishable from liposarcoma, although the latter is exceedingly rare in children.

Established as a distinct clinical entity in 1958 by Vellios et al. (53), who presented a girl 8 months of age with an infiltrating lesion in the anterior chest wall, lipoblastoma is a relatively immature lipoma that occurs almost exclusively in infancy and early childhood (54). Vellios chose the name *lipoblastomatosis* because the lesion resembles the histologic appearance of fetal fat (53). In 1973, Chung and Enzinger suggested the term *benign lipoblastoma* be used for well-encapsulated lesions and *lipoblastomatosis* be used to describe unencapsulated, infiltrating tumors (54). The natural history of the lesion is one of maturation to a lipoma. This progression was demonstrated in 1943 by Van Meurs (55), who reported a case in a girl 5 years of age with an axillary mass in which five resections over 20 months showed this progressive transformation. Ha et al. (56) showed similar results over a 5-year period of progression to an infiltrating lipoma. As with other lipomatous tumors, lipoblastomas have pseudodiploid karyotypes with structural chromosome aberrations, with a characteristic rearrangement of 8q11–13 in the vast majority of cases (1).

O'Donnell et al. suggest the term *infantile lipoma* to describe lipoblastoma and the designation *infiltrating*

infantile lipoma to replace lipomatosis (57). They note that these terms reflect more accurately the lesions' characteristic early occurrence, benign course, and documented ability to transform into mature adipose tissue.

Lipoblastoma is typically encountered in infants. More than 90% of cases occur in patients younger than 3 years; it is rarely seen in adults (2,58,59). The vast majority of lipoblastomas are situated in the superficial soft tissue or subcutis of the extremities, but they can occur in the neck, trunk, perineum, and retroperitoneum (59).

Patients frequently present with a progressive, painless soft tissue mass. As with other benign fatty tumors, symptoms are usually a function of the size and position of the mass (56,59–68). Lesions may reach considerable size but lack the ability to metastasize. Lipoblastomas are typically nontender, but symptoms may occur related to mass effect. Symptoms associated with these lesions are directly related to the location and the size of the mass. Upper respiratory symptoms, fever, and intermittent airway obstruction are described in patients with pleural-based mediastinal, pulmonary, and lower neck lipoblastomas (70,71). Emesis, diarrhea, anorexia, and abdominal pain are described in patients with mesenteric or retroperitoneal lipoblastomas (65).

Complete local excision without radical resection is the treatment of choice. Although these tumors are benign, without potential for metastatic spread, recurrence is common and seen in 14% to 25% of patients (53,54,69). Recurrence rates are greater in cases of lipoblastomatosis because the margins of the tumor are often less defined than in cases of lipoblastoma. A report of a newborn with biopsy-confirmed lipoblastomatosis of the thigh and hip showed spontaneous regression of the lesion. Regression was documented by serial imaging examinations, suggesting that a wait-and-see approach may be a reasonable alternative in infants with extensive lesions in which corrective surgery may be mutilating (70).

Previous reports show that males are affected two to three times more frequently than females (54,59). Two-thirds to three-quarters of these masses are well-circumscribed, comprising the classic lipoblastoma. The remaining cases are diffuse, meeting the definition of lipoblastomatosis and infiltrating both the musculature and the subcutis (12,71). In the Armed Forces Institute of Pathology (AFIP) experience, the mean age at presentation of patients with lipoblastoma was approximately 4 years (range: newborn to 10 years). The male predilection in the AFIP experience is approximately 1.3:1; with the male-to-female ratios for discrete and infiltrating forms of lipoblastoma at 1.6:1 and 0.8:1, respectively (12).

The circumscribed or focal lipoblastoma is well-encapsulated and composed of immature adipose tissue arranged in multiple lobules, which are delineated by fibrous septa (59). The diffuse form is unencapsulated and infiltrates subcutaneous fat as well as muscle (2,56,72). Microscopy reveals a signet-ring appearance, as well as multivacuolated lipoblasts interspersed between spindle or stellate mesenchymal cells, suspended in a myxoid stroma. (The histologic similarity of lipoblastoma, spindle cell lipoma, and myxoid liposarcoma is sometimes striking.) Ultrastructural studies (i.e., electron microscopy) suggest that lipoblastoma is a postnatal proliferation of mesenchymal cells with a spectrum of differentiation ranging from prelipoblasts (spindle cells) to mature adipocytes (13,71,73). Lipoblastomas have chromosomal aberrations with pseudodiploid karyotypes. The characteristic cytogenetic abnormalities of deletions and rearrangement of 8q11–13 are seen in the vast majority of patients (74–76). Lipoblastomas lack the t(12;16) translocation seen in myxoid liposarcomas (1).

The imaging appearance of lipoblastoma or lipoblastomatosis reflects its pathology. Although lipoblastoma is usually well-defined, the margins in lipoblastomatosis are infiltrating and difficult to identify. CT and MR show a predominantly fatty mass, with the nonlipomatous (cellularly immature) areas of the mass showing a nonspecific imaging appearance (Figs. 4.15–4.17) (13,56,72). Fat is the predominant feature in many patients, particularly in older children. However, in very young patients (infants), the nonlipomatous myxoid component may predominate, with only small elements of fat (13,56,63). These myxoid areas enhance following contrast administration because of the rich capillary network. Consequently, lipoblastoma and liposarcoma may be indistinguishable. Although the radiologic differential diagnosis is that of liposarcoma, this entity is exceedingly rare in children. In a review of more than 2,500 cases of liposarcoma at the AFIP, only 2 (0.08%) occurred in children younger than 10 years. Fifteen additional cases were identified in children between 11 and 15 years of age (77).

Angiolipoma

KEY CONCEPTS

- Angiolipoma is a lipoma variant with two forms: encapsulated (superficial) and unencapsulated (deep).
- The deep infiltrating form is better classified as an intramuscular hemangioma.
- Most lesions image as a predominantly fatty mass with associated nonspecific areas showing hemangioma-like imaging characteristics as well as postcontrast enhancement.

Howard and Helwig first described angiolipoma in 1960 as a lipoma variant containing varying proportions of mature fat cells and thin-walled blood vessels (1,78,79). Other terms used to describe this lesion include *vascular lipoma, hemangiolipoma,* and *fibromyxolipoma* (80). Angiolipoma is subdivided into noninfiltrative (encapsulated) and infiltrative (nonencapsulated) types.

The encapsulated form of angiolipoma is a cutaneous lesion that typically occurs on the trunk and extremities of adults in the third through fifth decades, with the forearm being the most common location (Fig. 4.18). Histologically, these lesions are composed of adipose tissue, small vessels, and capillaries. The latter elements characteristically contain fibrin thrombi (2). As cutaneous lesions, they are typically not subject to radiologic examination, and the diagnosis is usually established clinically. Lesions that involve the subcutaneous tissues of the trunk and extremities are commonly multiple, firm, and often painful to palpation. Superficial angiolipomas are easily cured with surgical resection. Rare familial cases (demonstrating an autosomal dominant

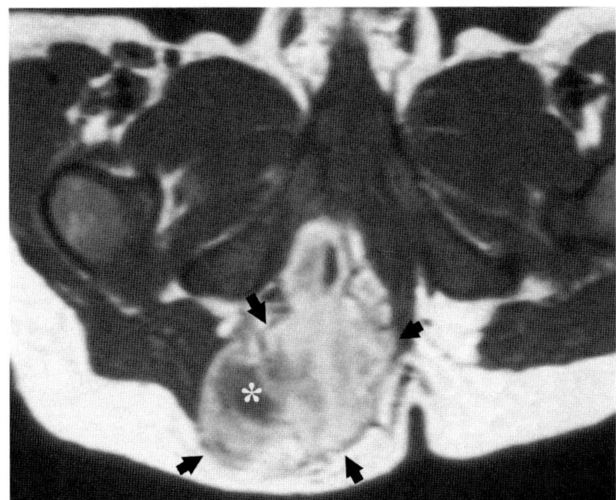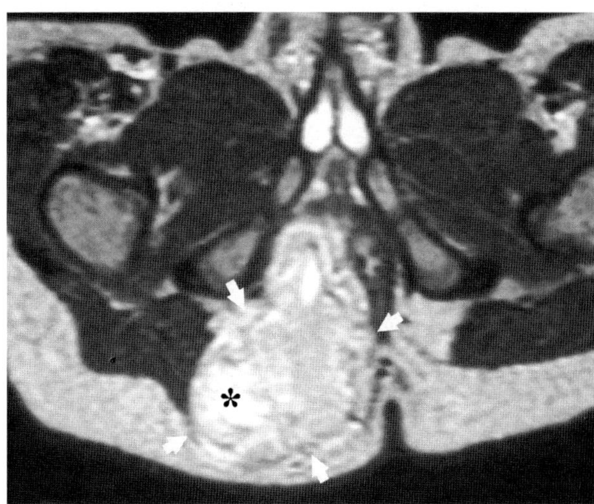

Figure 4.15 Lipoblastoma: MR imaging features in a boy 11 months of age with a perineal mass. **A,B:** Axial T1-weighted (TR/TE; 500/20) **(A)** and T2-weighted (TR/TE; 2000/70) **(B)** spin-echo MR images show the fatty nature of the mass (*arrows*) as well as nonspecific areas within the tumor (*asterisk*) with decreased signal intensity on T1-weighted and increased signal intensity on T2-weighted images.

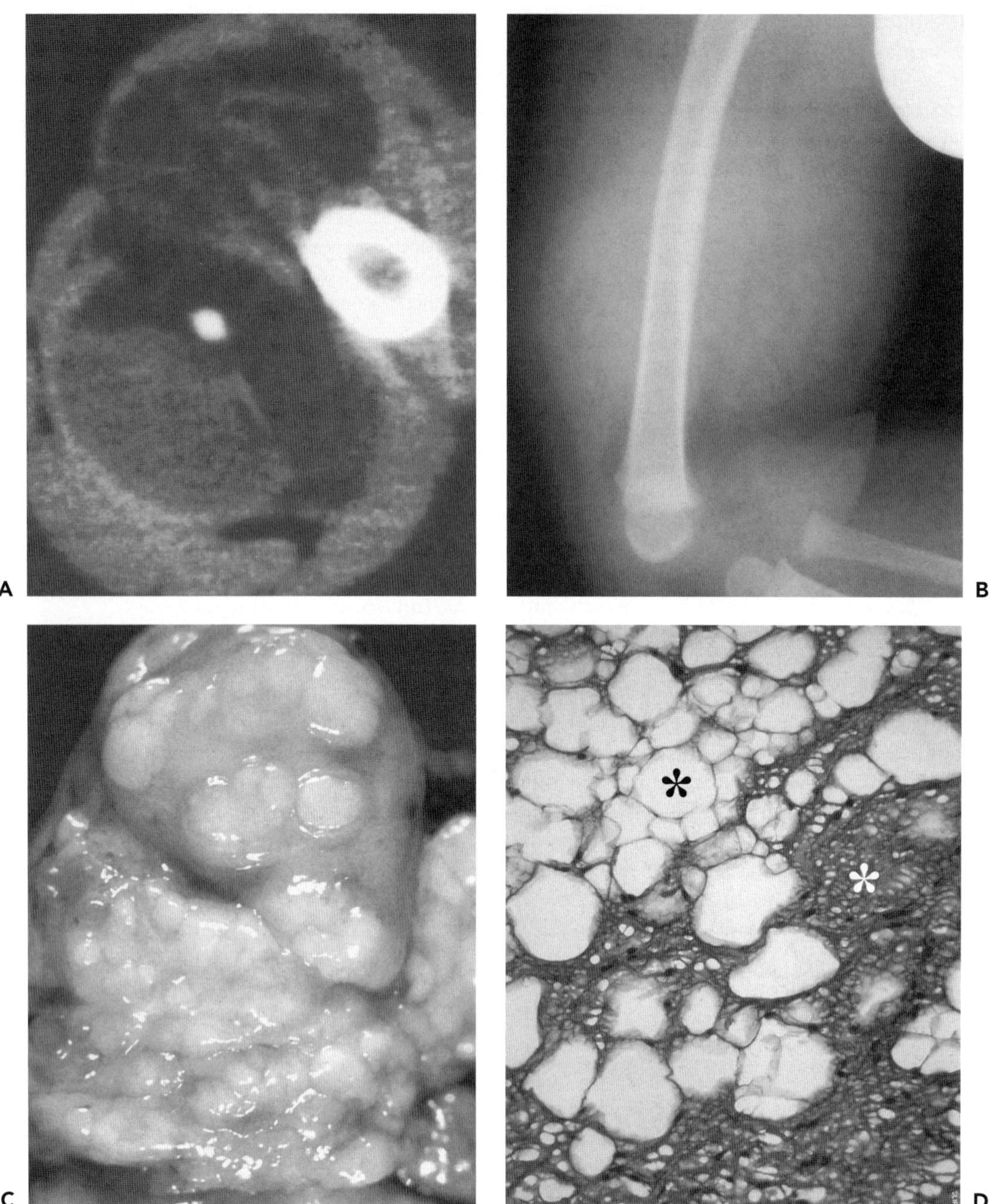

Figure 4.16 Lipoblastoma: CT imaging features in a boy 18 months of age with a thigh mass. **A:** Axial CT scan displayed at soft tissue window shows a well-defined predominantly fatty mass with large nonadipose areas. **B:** Lateral radiograph of the thigh shows a nonspecific mass. The fatty nature of the mass is not appreciated. **C:** Photograph of the gross specimen shows the glistening cut surface of the multilobular mass, with the tumor lobules separated by fibrous septa. **D:** Microscopy reveals typical adipocytes (*black asterisk*) and immature fat composed of stellate and primitive spindle cells (*white asterisk*).

inheritance) are described (2,81–83). Clinically, familial cases may mimic familial multiple lipomatosis (81). The standard treatment of angiolipoma is surgical resection.

As with most small superficial lesions, angiolipomas are often excised without imaging. Our experience with this lesion is similar to that reported, imaging as a well-defined encapsulated, predominantly fatty mass, with nonadipose areas demonstrating a nonspecific signal intensity (89). The nonadipose areas show low signal intensity on T1-weighted images, high signal intensity on T2-weighted and other fluid-sensitive sequences, enhanced following intravenous contrast administration, and they may demonstrate a serpentine character (Fig. 4.19). Calcification representing phleboliths may also be seen.

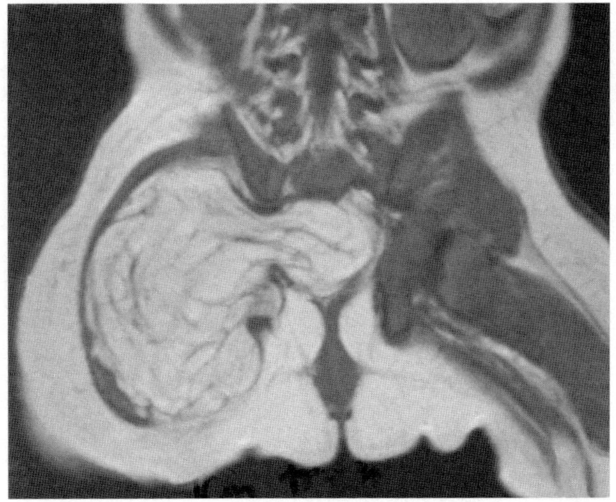
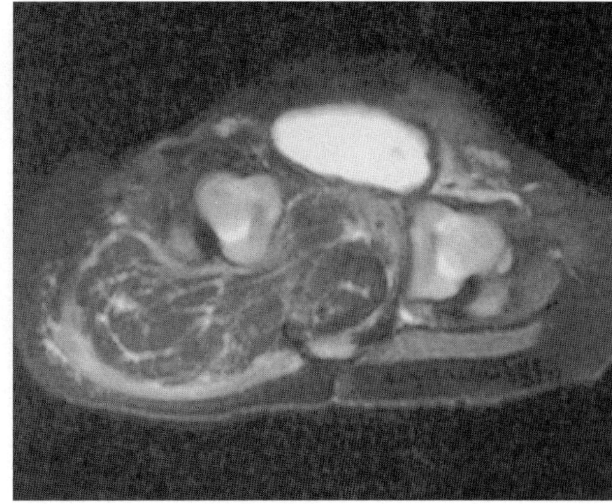

A

B

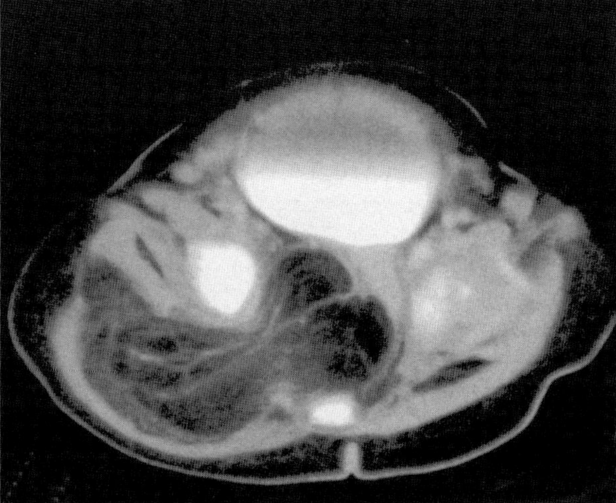

C

Figure 4.17 Lipoblastoma: MR and CT imaging features in a boy 4 months of age presenting with partial paralysis of the right leg. **A:** Coronal T1-weighted (TR/TE; 640/20) spin-echo MR image shows a large bilobed fatty mass with thickened irregular septa. **B,C:** Axial fast spin-echo T2-weighted (TR/TE; 5000/96) MR image **(B)** and enhanced CT **(C)** show the thickened septa as well as increased signal on T2-weighted image **B.**

The rare infiltrating angiolipoma sometimes grows as a deep infiltrating mass and may be the subject of radiologic evaluation. The infiltrating angiolipoma is described as a nonencapsulated infiltrating lesion composed of mature adipose tissue and benign vascular elements. It is distin-guished from the cutaneous (encapsulated) form because of its growth pattern and tendency to recur locally (84–88). This infiltrative lesion is best classified as an intramuscular hemangioma and is recognized as such by the WHO Classification of Soft Tissue Tumors (1,2). As expected, the deep infiltrating angiolipomas demonstrate serpentine densities intermixed with fat and an imaging appearance identical to that of an intramuscular hemangioma, with associated fatty overgrowth (Fig. 4.20) (90–92). Intramuscular hemangioma is discussed in Chapter 5.

Spindle Cell Lipoma/Pleomorphic Lipoma

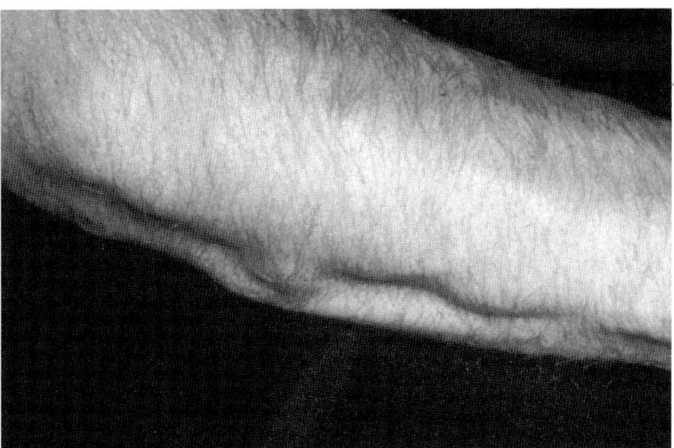

Figure 4.18 Angiolipoma: Clinical presentation in a young man with a superficial forearm mass.

> **KEY CONCEPTS**
> - Spindle cell lipoma/pleomorphic lipoma is typically seen in men (>90%) from 45 to 65 years of age.
> - It is most commonly located in the subcutaneous tissues of the posterior neck, back, or shoulder.
> - This complex fatty mass is usually composed of 25% to 75% fat with the remainder of the lesion nonspecific.
> - The nonspecific component enhances extensively.

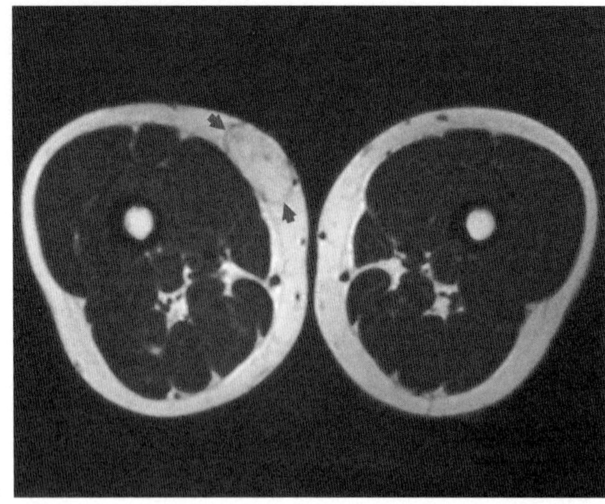 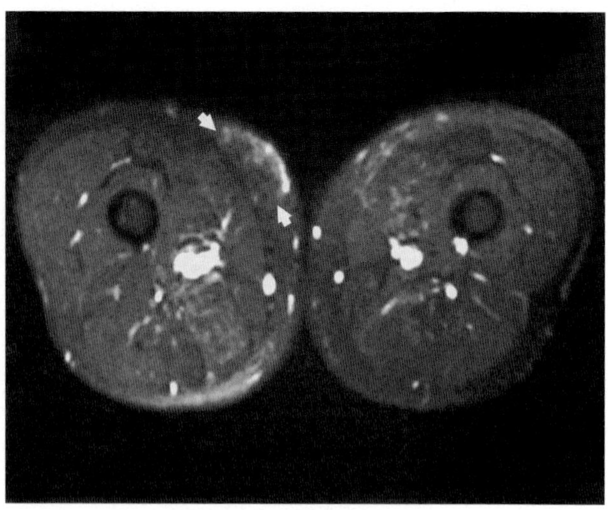

Figure 4.19 Angiolipoma: MR imaging in a man 21 years of age with a thigh mass. **A,B:** Corresponding axial T1-weighted (TR/TE; 500/14) **(A)** and fat-suppressed fast T2-weighted (TR/TE; 2000/60) **(B)** spin-echo MR images show an encapsulated, well-defined fatty mass (*arrows*) in the anterior medial thigh. The mass is predominantly fatty with a small amount of nonadipose tissue that shows high signal intensity on fat-suppressed fluid-sensitive image **(B).**

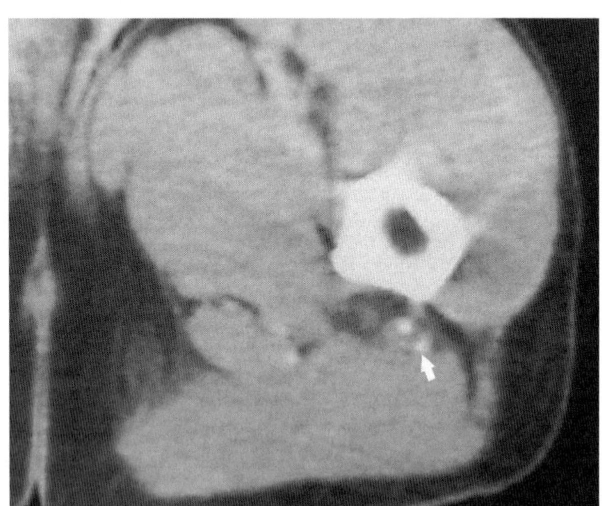 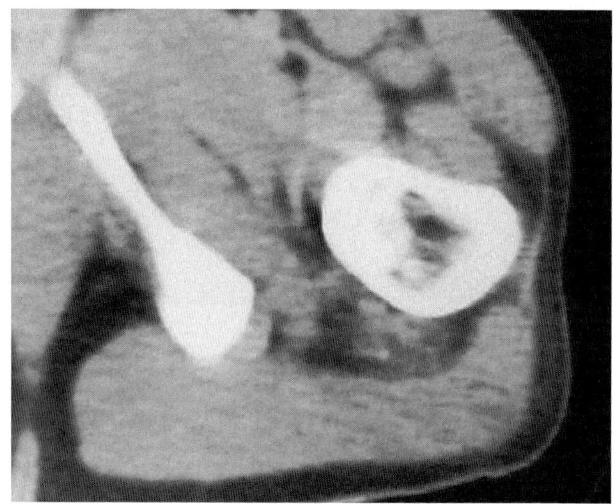

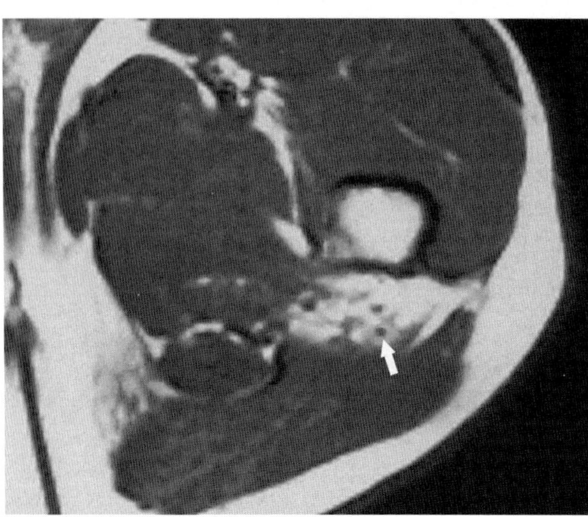

Figure 4.20 Intramuscular hemangioma with increased adipose tissue (deep infiltrating angiolipoma): CT and MR imaging features in a man 24 years of age. **A:** Axial contrast-enhanced CT scan of the hip shows a fatty mass just posterior to the left hip. Within the mass are small calcifications compatible with phleboliths (*arrow*), as well as soft tissue compatible with the vascular elements of the hemangioma. **B:** Axial CT image just cranial to **A** shows a greater amount of associated adipose tissue. **C:** Axial T1-weighted (TR/TE; 700/32) spin-echo MR image shows the fatty nature of the mass as well as the vascular component. Phleboliths image as signal voids (*arrow*).

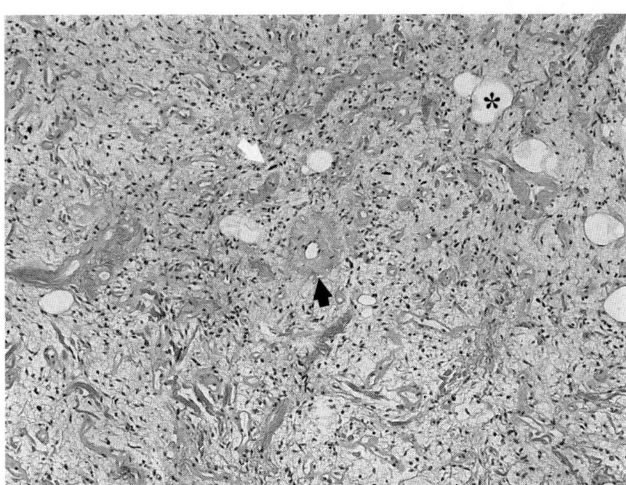

Figure 4.21 Spindle cell lipoma: Histology. Photomicrograph of a spindle cell lipoma demonstrates spindle cells (*white arrow*) throughout the specimen, scattered vascular channels (*black arrow*), and lipocytes (*asterisk*) in a background of mucoid matrix (hematoxylin and eosin ×100).

Enzinger and Harvey first described spindle cell lipoma in 1975 as a benign lesion in which mature fat is replaced by collagen-forming spindle cells (93). In their original description, these authors described spindle cell lipomas as being "relatively common," yet these tumors are perceived as rare by radiologists because they are typically small, superficial, and often excised without imaging. Spindle cell and pleomorphic lipoma represent ends of a histologic spectrum, with the latter representing an extremely pleomorphic variant of the spindle cell lipoma (2). Both spindle cell lipoma and pleomorphic lipoma show similar cytogenetic aberrations, although the karyotypes are more complex than those seen with conventional lipoma (1).

Spindle cell lipoma is a benign, slow-growing, usually solitary, painless lipomatous variant. It typically presents in men between 45 and 65 years of age (2,93,94). The lesion is cured by local excision and has never been reported to metastasize (2,93,94). In their original report, Enzinger and Harvey noted a striking proclivity for men, accounting for 91% (104 of 114) of their patients, a trend substantiated in subsequent reports (12). The lesion also has a significant tendency to occur in the subcutaneous tissues of the posterior neck, shoulder, and back (2,12,93,94). Approximately two-thirds of lesions occur in these regions, although they may occur elsewhere in the body. Intramuscular and extremity lesions are occasionally seen; rare locations include oral cavity, larynx, bronchus, scalp, and perianal region (94–98).

Prior to its designation as a separate entity, spindle cell lipoma was frequently misdiagnosed pathologically as liposarcoma (99,100). Microscopically, the spindle cell lipoma is comprised of mature fat with areas replaced by fibroblast-like spindle cells within a matrix of mucin and collagen fibrils (101). Although most cases have a relatively equal ratio of fat and spindle cells, either component may predominate. The vascular pattern of spindle cell lipoma is usually inconspicuous, although some tumors have a prominent plexiform vascular pattern similar to that of myxoid liposarcoma (102); a hemangiopericytomalike vascular pattern or a pseudoangiomatous variant is also described (103). This prominent vascularity likely accounts for the intense enhancement seen in the nonadipose components of the tumor following contrast administration (Fig. 4.21).

The variation in the ratio of fat to spindle cells causes a wide spectrum of imaging features. Imaging reveals a lesion with between 25% and 75% fat in approximately 80% of cases (Figs. 4.22 and 4.23). Uncommonly, lesions are principally soft tissue or fat. The imaging appearance of the nonadipose component is nonspecific and enhances intensely following contrast administration (94). Osseous erosions are reported, but they are rare (104). Primarily soft tissue lesions are nonspecific, whereas predominantly fatty lesions may mimic an angiolipoma (Fig. 4.24).

Although the imaging appearance of spindle cell lipoma is not pathognomonic and may overlap with that of liposarcoma, angiolipoma, or possibly hibernoma, the diagnosis of spindle cell lipoma should be suggested when a well-defined complex fatty mass is encountered in the subcutis of a middle-aged man, especially when the mass is localized to the posterior neck. Intense enhancement of the nonadipose component further supports this diagnosis.

Myolipoma

> **KEY CONCEPTS**
> - Myolipoma is a rare lesion composed of smooth muscle and fat; most commonly found in women.
> - The smooth muscle component usually dominates.
> - Imaging shows a fatty mass with a prominent nonadipose component.
> - Imaging appearance suggests a well-differentiated liposarcoma.

Meis and Enzinger described myolipoma of soft tissue as a distinctive tumor in 1991 with a report of nine cases (105). They noted the lesion is composed of varying amounts of smooth muscle and mature adipose tissue. Myolipoma of soft tissue should not be confused with uterine leiomyoma with fatty degeneration, termed *lipoleiomyoma,* which is exceedingly rare in soft tissues (106).

Patients with myolipoma are typically adults, although rare cases are reported in children (105–108). A female predilection was noted in the original report. Lesions are most frequently found in the retroperitoneum and

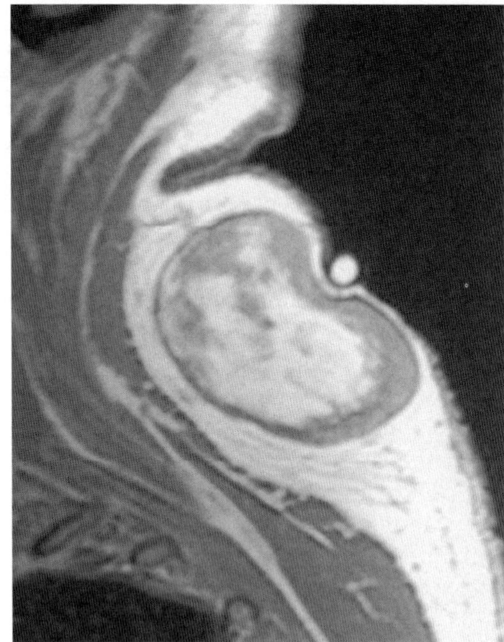
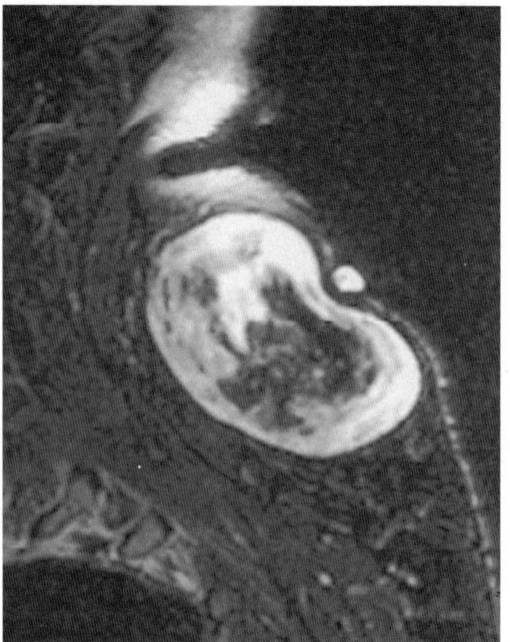

Figure 4.22   Spindle cell lipoma: Typical MR imaging features in a man 53 years of age with a mass in the posterior neck. **A:** Sagittal fast spin-echo (FSE) T1-weighted (TR/TE; 550/13) MR image shows an ovoid, well-circumscribed tumor with a fairly equal ratio of adipose and nonadipose tissue. **B:** Corresponding sagittal FSE T2-weighted (TR/TE; 4000/104) fat-suppressed image depicts hyperintense nonadipose soft tissue nodules, thick septae, and fat-suppressed low-signal adipose tissue.

abdomen, including the inguinal region and abdominal wall. Less common locations include the subcutaneous tissues, mediastinum, and orbit (105–108). Patients may present with evidence of a soft tissue mass; however, large retroperitoneal lesions may be identified as an incidental finding (1,105,107). Local recurrence and metastatic disease are not reported (106,107).

Histologically, the lesion is composed of both smooth muscle and adipose tissue, with the smooth muscle component predominating in seven of nine cases reported by Meis and Enzinger (105). The smooth muscle component is interspersed with adipose tissue, giving the lesion a sievelike appearance (105).

There is a paucity of literature describing the radiologic appearance of myolipoma. The imaging appearance reflects the histologic composition of the lesion with variable amounts of adipose and nonadipose tissue. The smooth muscle component typically dominates the microscopic picture, which is reflected in the radiologic imaging, with an appearance suggesting a well-differentiated liposarcoma: a fatty mass with poorly defined internal areas of nonadipose tissue (Fig. 4.25). Coarse calcification is reported in large lesions (107).

Chondroid Lipoma

Chondroid lipoma is a rare, newly recognized, benign fatty tumor that bears a strikingly close resemblance to myxoid liposarcoma and extraskeletal myxoid chondrosarcoma (1). The first probable case of chondroid lipoma was

> **KEY CONCEPTS**
> - Chondroid lipoma is a variant that resembles myxoid liposarcoma and extraskeletal myxoid chondrosarcoma.
> - It is more common in women (approximately 80%).
> - Limited reports are available; imaging reflects myxoid character with heterogeneous fluid-like signal.
> - Chondroid lipoma may show calcification on radiographs and imaging studies.

described in 1986 by Chan et al., although the lesion was identified as a distinct entity by Meis and Enzinger in 1993, who coined the term *chondroid lipoma* (2,109,110).

Most patients present with a slowly growing, painless mass. The lesion is typically located in the subcutaneous or deeper soft tissues of the limbs and limb girdles. Women are affected far more commonly than men, with women comprising 16 (80%) of the 20 patients in the original report, which is still the largest series to date (110). Reported patients range from 14 to 70 years of age (110–112). Conservative surgical excision is the treatment of choice, with no cases of local recurrence or metastasis reported.

At gross pathologic examination, chondroid lipoma is an encapsulated, often multilobular, yellow to white mass with a size range of 1 to 11 cm (mean: 4 cm). Microscopically, the characteristic appearance is nests and cords of lipoblasts in an admixed bed of prominent myxoid or hyalinized chondroid matrix and a variable amount of mature adult fat (112). These features may closely resemble myxoid

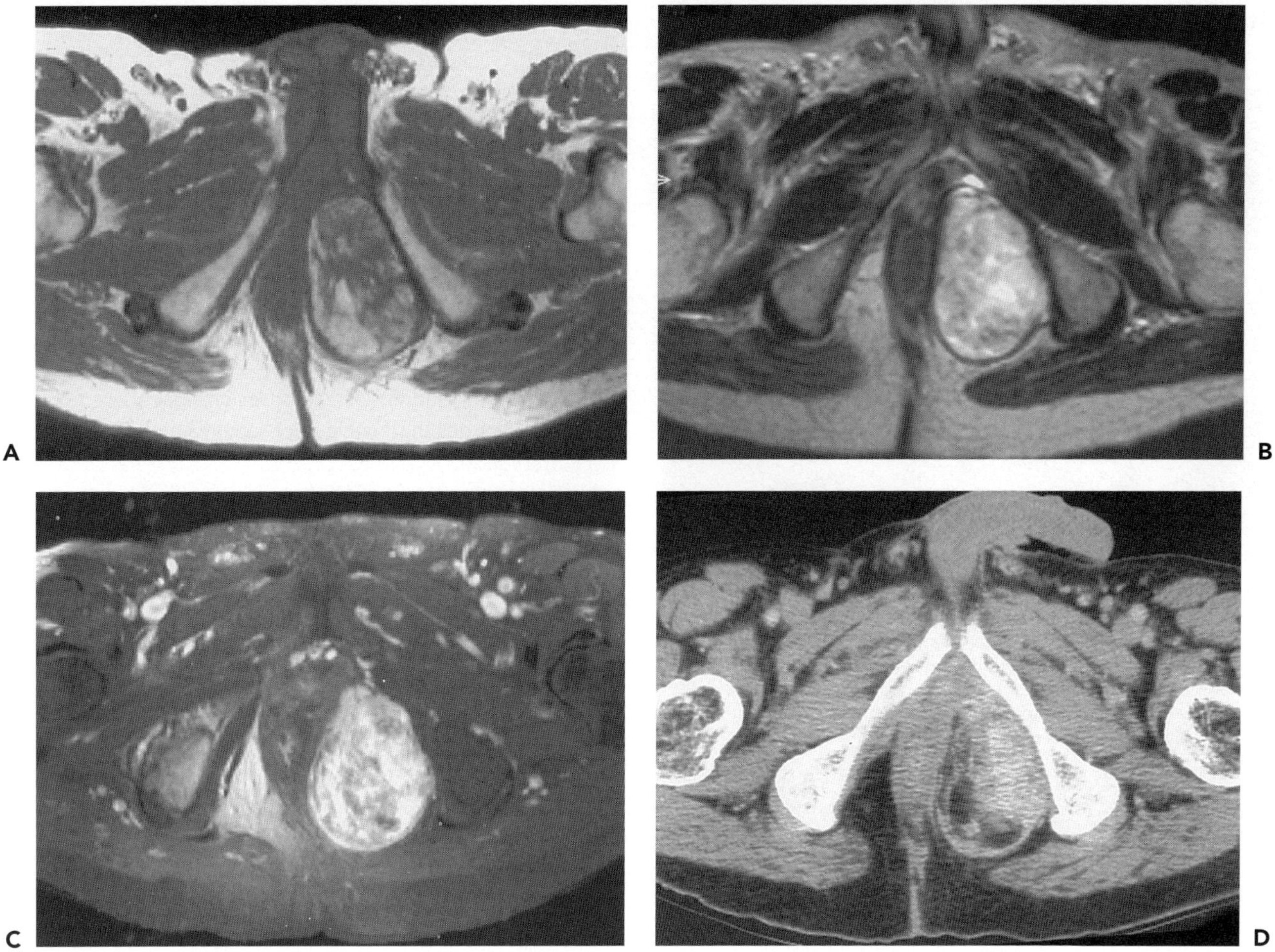

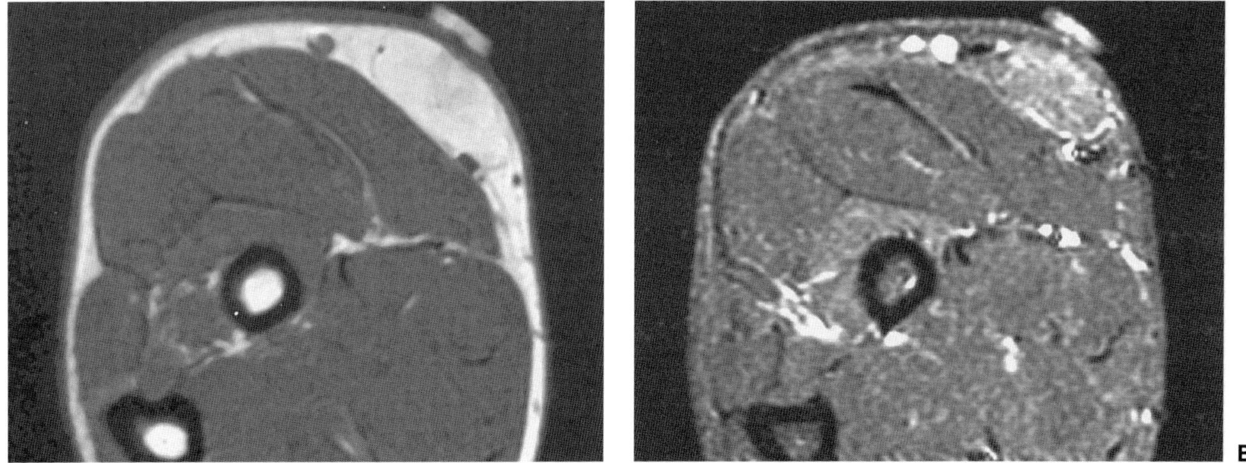

Figure 4.23 Spindle cell lipoma: Typical MR and CT findings in ischiorectal fossa of man 69 years of age. **A,B:** Corresponding axial T1-weighted (TR/TE; 690/15) **(A)** and fast spin-echo T2-weighted (TR/TE; 6498/130) **(B)** images through mass show a relatively equal distribution of adipose and nonadipose tissue characteristic of a spindle cell lipoma. **C:** Axial T1-weighted (TR/TE; 450/15) enhanced fat-suppressed image demonstrates intense enhancement of the nonadipose components of the tumor. **D:** Contrast-enhanced axial CT image through lower pelvis demonstrates a well-circumscribed ovoid mass that contains both adipose and markedly enhancing, nonadipose tissue nodules. Thin septae are also identified in the medial portion of the mass.

Figure 4.24 Spindle cell lipoma: Predominantly fatty lesion in the subcutaneous tissue of the forearm in a man 43 years of age. **A,B:** Corresponding axial T1-weighted (TR/TE; 400/14) **(A)** and fat-suppressed T2-weighted (TR/TE; 2300/60) **(B)** axial images demonstrate a 3-cm fatty mass in the subcutaneous fat, with scattered, thin septae and vascular elements. The subcutaneous location, predominantly fatty nature, and vascularity mimic an angiolipoma.

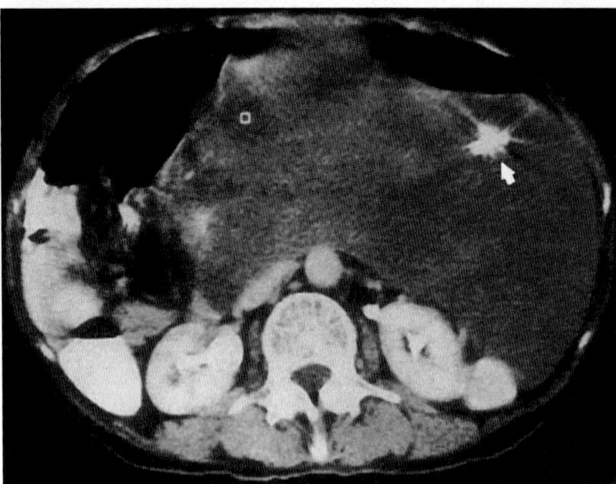

Figure 4.25 Myolipoma: CT findings in a woman 79 years of age presenting with fever and right lower quadrant abdominal pain. Contrast-enhanced CT scan displayed at soft tissue window shows a sharply circumscribed, heterogeneous mass, with attenuation varying between that of fat and soft tissue. Note coarse calcification (*arrow*). The radiologic features suggest a liposarcoma. (From reference 107 with permission.)

liposarcoma or extraskeletal myxoid chondrosarcoma, leading to pseudosarcomatous misdiagnosis. Cytogenetic aberrations with t(11;16) translocations are reported with chondroid lipoma similar to hibernomas, suggesting a histogenetic link between these lesions (1).

Imaging data on this unusual tumor is scant. Reported cases reflect the predominantly myxoid nature of the lesion, showing a well-defined mass with fluidlike signal intensity. A small amount of fatty signal is also noted, both peripherally as well as centrally, demonstrating fine lacy strands (111,112). Calcification may be seen on radiographs as well as on CT and MR imaging studies (Fig. 4.26).

Lipomatous Tumors

Intramuscular and intermuscular lipoma are relatively common benign lipomatous lesions that arise, respectively, either within or between skeletal muscles. They are members of a subgroup of fatty lesions referred to as *lipomatous tumors,* which arise in intimate association with nonadipose tissue. Previously, this group of lesions was referred to as *heterotopic lipomas.* Other entities in this category include lipomatosis of nerve and lipoma of tendon sheath and joint.

Intramuscular and Intermuscular Lipoma

Arising within the muscle, intramuscular lipoma may actually involve both muscular and intermuscular tissue; however, involvement isolated to the intermuscular region (intermuscular lipoma) is less common. Intramuscular lipoma occurs in patients of all ages, although principally in adults. There is a slight male predominance. Patients typically present with a mass in the large muscles of the extremities, especially the thigh, shoulder, and upper arm.

The fat within an intramuscular lipoma may infiltrate the adjacent skeletal muscle. The amount of marginal infiltration is variable, but may be extensive. Rarely, it may completely infiltrate the muscle, giving it a striated appearance on gross inspection. In such cases the lesion is referred to as an infiltrating lipoma (16).

Intramuscular lipomas are rare in comparison to superficial lipomas. Myhre-Jensen (8) noted only 3 (0.4%) intramuscular lipomas in a review of 707 lipomas seen over 7 years. In the AFIP experience, intramuscular lipoma represents approximately 8% of all benign fatty lesions seen in consultation (12). The mean age at patient presentation was 52 years of age, with 80% of patients between 26 and 73 years of age. There was a slight male predilection (1.3:1). Our anecdotal experience is that in a clinical radiology practice, these lipomas are not uncommon. Their deep intramuscular location often precludes a definitive clinical diagnosis, and they are imaged in the evaluation of patients presenting with a soft tissue mass.

Intramuscular lipoma is found most commonly in the lower extremity, with approximately 45% of lesions occurring in this location. The trunk is the next most common location, followed by the shoulder girdle and upper extremity, accounting for 17%, 12%, and 10%, respectively.

Radiographs may reveal an intramuscular mass of fat density (Fig. 4.27). When adjacent to bone, lesions may be associated with cortical thickening (19). On CT and MR imaging, the lesion is a predominantly fatty mass, which is usually well-defined and sharply circumscribed (Figs. 4.28 and 4.29). As a rule, intramuscular lipomas tend to be uninodular masses or, less commonly, multinodular masses (113). In spite of the well-defined margins on radiographs and imaging studies, intramuscular lipomas are frequently infiltrating at microscopy (Fig. 4.30). Although well-defined margins are usually the case, partially infiltrating margins are noted but less common (Fig. 4.31) (113). Uncommonly, intramuscular lipomas demonstrate completely irregular margins on radiologic examination with fatty tissue interdigitating with skeletal muscle (113); such lesions are termed *infiltrating lipomas* (Fig. 4.32). Infiltrating lipomas may affect multiple muscles and simulate lipomatosis (114). Completely irregular margins are not noted in liposarcoma (113).

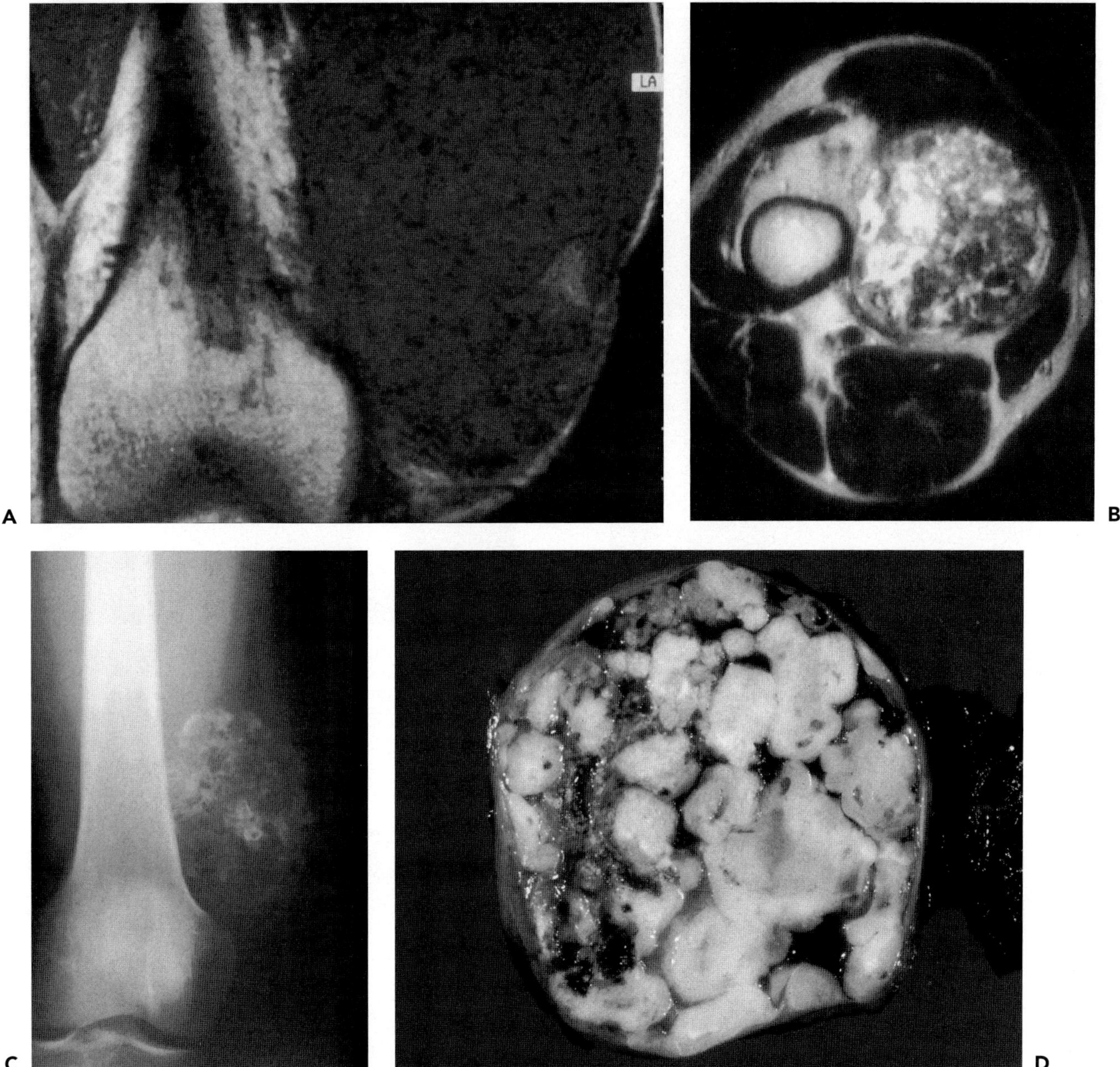

Figure 4.26 Chondroid lipoma in the vastus medialis muscle. **A,B:** Coronal T1-weighted **(A)** and axial fast T2-weighted **(B)** spin-echo MR images of the knee show a mass with heterogeneous high signal intensity in **B**, reflecting its myxoid nature. The heterogeneity in this case is caused by the prominent calcification. **C:** Anteroposterior radiograph shows the extensive mineralization within the mass. **D:** Photograph of the bisected mass shows its heterogeneous character and myxoid nature.

Intramuscular lipoma shows an imaging appearance similar to that of a lipoma, with a signal intensity or tissue attenuation identical to that of subcutaneous fat. The diagnosis is made with confidence when lesions are entirely composed of adipose tissue and without a nonadipose component (18,113). Frequently, thin septa of nonadipose tissue 2 mm or less in thickness may be present (18,113). These septa showed no enhancement on MR imaging relative to muscle in 11 of 19 benign lipomas reported by Ohguri et al., whereas septa in 8 well-differentiated liposarcomas in the same study showed moderate or marked enhancement (113). Thick septa or the presence of nodular and globular or nonadipose masslike areas also suggest a well-differentiated liposarcoma (see following discussion). The MR imaging criteria pertaining to the presence and character of septa are well-applied to CT scanning, although enhancement characteristics are not yet adequately studied. In the diagnosis of intramuscular lipoma, we have found it useful to compare the signal intensity of the lesion to that of the adjacent subcutaneous fat. This is especially useful when the lesion is somewhat heterogeneous. When lesions are imaged with a surface coil, the fat within the lesion should be compared to that of the subcutaneous fat at a similar distance from the coil to compensate for depth-related signal loss (Fig. 4.33).

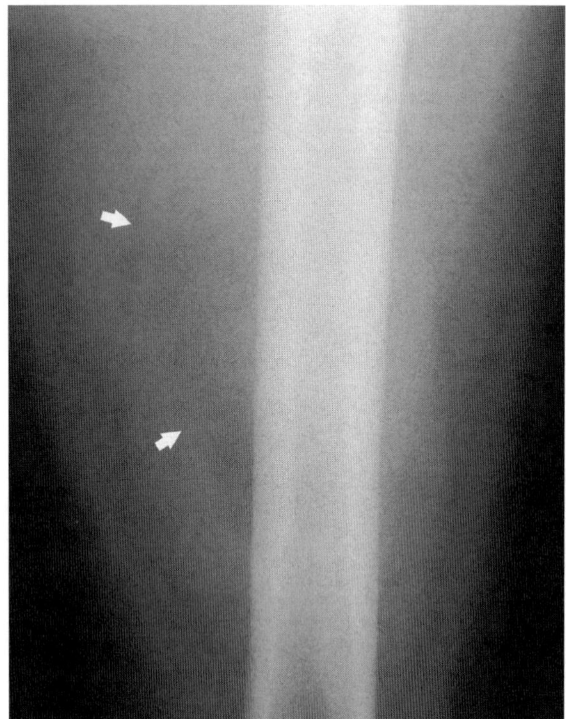

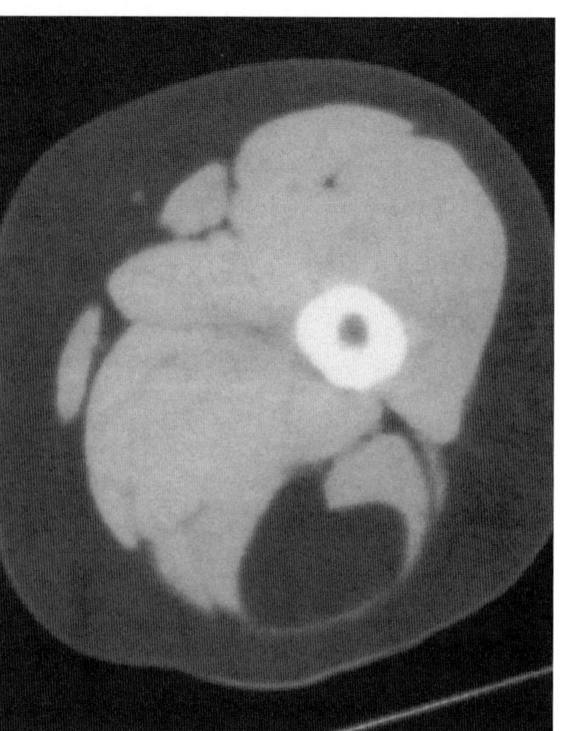

Figure 4.27 Intramuscular lipoma: Radiographic features. Radiograph shows a well-defined radiolucent area within the thigh (*arrows*). The left margin of the lesion is obscured by overlying bone.

Figure 4.28 Intramuscular lipoma: CT scanning features. Noncontrast axial CT scan of the thigh shows a well-defined intramuscular mass with an attenuation identical to that of the subcutaneous fat. The lesion is homogeneous with no nonadipose component.

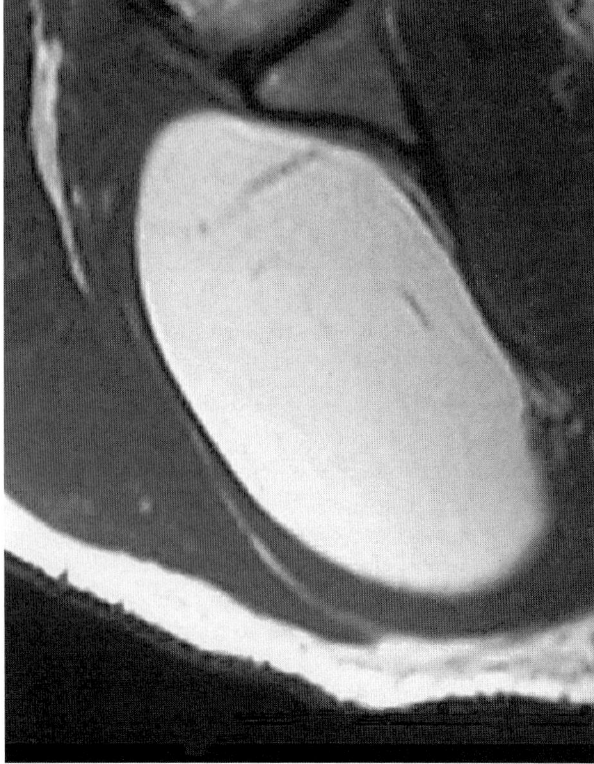

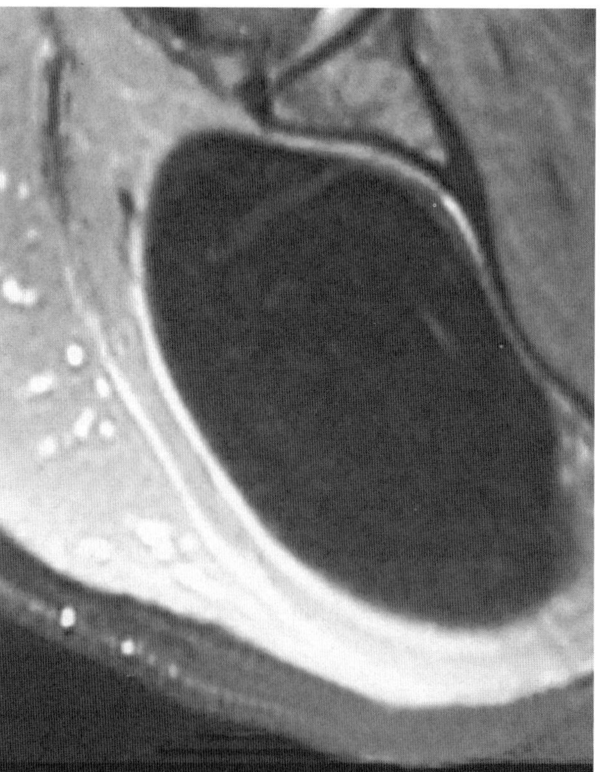

Figure 4.29 Intramuscular lipoma: MR imaging features. **A,B:** Corresponding axial T1-weighted **(A)** and STIR **(B)** images demonstrate a well-defined fatty intramuscular mass without nodularity or associated mass.

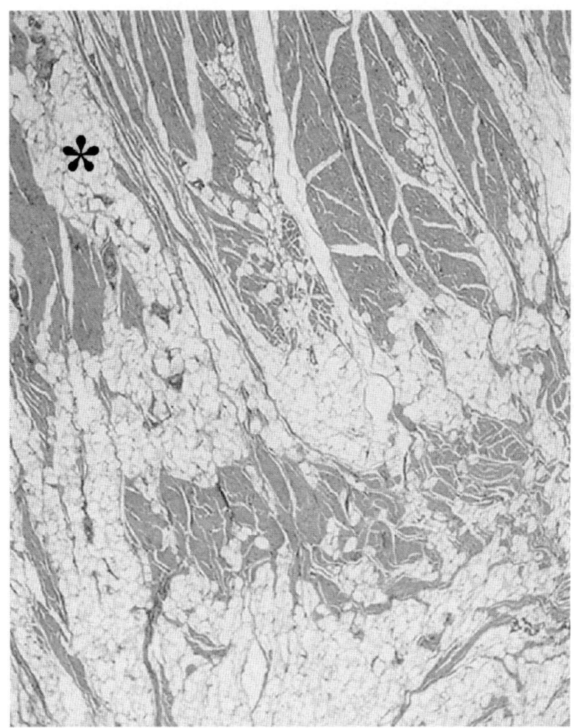

Figure 4.30 Intramuscular lipoma: Histologic features. Microscopy of the margin of an intramuscular lipoma show fat (*asterisk*) infiltrating between skeletal muscle fibers (hematoxylin and eosin).

Mature fat is subject to a variety of superimposed secondary inflammatory processes, and these findings are not uncommon. As in superficial lipoma, these secondary features may be seen in intramuscular lipoma and may complicate its imaging appearance. In a report of 35 intramuscular lipomas, 11 (31%) showed significant nonadipose areas (18). Although nonadipose areas in this study were not mapped and correlated with images, histologic analysis of the nonadipose areas demonstrated fat necrosis and associated calcification, fibrosis, inflammation, and myxoid change (Fig. 4.9). In this same report, masslike areas were present in two lipomas and suggested dedifferentiation (see following discussion on dedifferentiated liposarcoma). Similarly, intramuscular lipomas may be associated with other mesenchymal elements, including fibrous tissue, cartilage, and bone. Although these imaging variations are also seen in superficial lesions (and were described earlier), in our experience they are more prevalent in larger deep lesions. In general, MR imaging is highly specific for the diagnosis of a superficial or intramuscular lipoma. When a lesion does not meet the imaging criteria for a lipoma, it is more likely a lipoma variant or a lipoma with involution change rather than a liposarcoma (115).

Lipomatosis of Nerve

Fibrofatty enlargement of the median nerve was initially described in the English literature in 1952, with the presentation of two cases at the American Society for Surgery of the Hand (116). This lesion is reported under a variety of names, including *neural fibrolipoma, fibrolipomatous hamar-*

KEY CONCEPTS

- Lipomatosis of nerve is a fibrofatty infiltration of the nerve.
- It is most common in an upper extremity; 80% in median nerve distribution.
- MR imaging shows 3 mm longitudinally oriented cylindrical low signal areas on a fatty background.
- Macrodactyly, termed *macrodystrophia lipomatosa* or *nerve territory–oriented macrodactyly*, occurs in 27% to 67% of affected patients.
- Macrodactyly shows overgrowth of both bone and soft tissue.

toma of nerve, perineural lipoma, fatty infiltration of the nerve, and *intraneural lipoma* (116,117); however, the term *lipomatosis of nerve* is the new designation adopted by the 2002 WHO Classification of Soft Tissue Tumors (1).

The cause of this disorder remains unclear, but it may be related to hypertrophy of mature fat and fibroblasts in the epineurium (117). There is no known associated syndrome or hereditary predisposition (1).

Patients typically present during early adulthood with a soft, slowly enlarging mass occurring in the volar aspect of the hand, wrist, or forearm. Lesions may be noted in early childhood or even at birth (1,117–121). Most patients are adolescents or young adults in the second through fourth decades (1), and males and females are equally affected. There is a striking predilection for the upper extremity, with 78% to 96% of lesions occurring in this location (117,120). Approximately 80% of upper extremity lesions originate in the median nerve (117–121); the lower extremity is involved much less frequently (4% to 22%) (117–120).

Amadio et al. (120) reviewed the Mayo Clinic institutional experience with macrodactyly from 1950 to 1985. Neural fibrolipoma was the most common condition associated with macrodactyly of the upper extremity, seen in 10 of 22 cases. Other lesions include five each of vascular and idiopathic cases and two cases of neurofibromatosis. In contradistinction, these researchers noted that lipomatosis of nerve was the least common cause associated with macrodactyly of the lower extremity, identified in 1 of 43 cases. Other lower extremity lesions included 31 idiopathic, 10 vascular, and 1 neurofibromatosis. In this study, idiopathic causes were defined as lesions in patients with no stigmata of neurofibromatosis or congenital malformation. The authors also noted nine cases of hemihypertrophy. The differential diagnosis of localized gigantism also includes Proteus syndrome (122).

Accompanying symptoms include pain, tenderness, decreased sensation, or paresthesia. Carpal tunnel syndrome may be a late sequela (123). Patients may demonstrate macrodactyly (117,121), referred to as *macrodystrophia lipomatosa,* which may involve multiple digits. Macrodactyly usually involves the second and third digits of the hand or foot. It is seen in 27% to 67% of cases, more

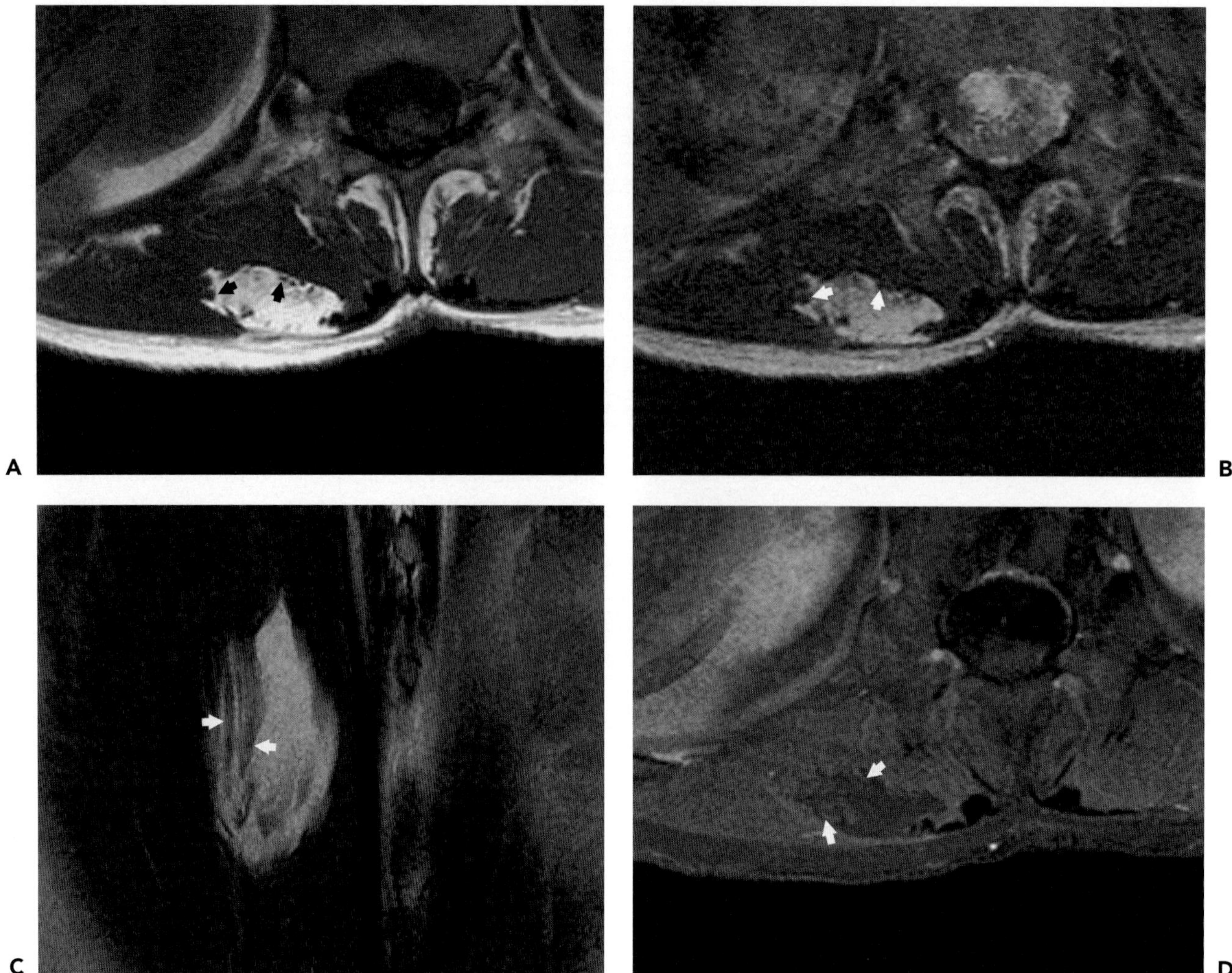

Figure 4.31   Intramuscular lipoma with partially irregular margins: MR imaging features in a woman 58 years of age with a paraspinal mass. **A,B:** Axial T1-weighted (TR/TE; 625/12) **(A)** and conventional T2-weighted (TR/TE; 2419/80) **(B)** spin-echo MR images demonstrate a fatty intramuscular mass with a partially irregular margin. Tissue with signal intensity identical to that of skeletal muscle (*arrows*) is seen within the lesion. **C:** Coronal T1-weighted spin-echo MR image (TR/TE; 490/12) shows the grossly interdigitating margin to better advantage. **D:** Axial enhanced fat-saturated T1-weighted spin-echo MR image (TR/TE; 522/12) shows no enhancement of the adipose tissue of the lesion; the skeletal muscle within and surrounding the lesion show an identical appearance.

commonly in females (117,120). Surgical excision is not without risk, and motor and sensory deficits are reported following resection (121,123). The infiltrative growth pattern of the lesion makes complete resection with a residual intact nerve virtually impossible (116).

Grossly, the lesion is described as a fusiform, sausagelike enlargement of the nerve by fibrofatty tissue (117), appearing as a tannish yellow mass within the nerve sheath (121). Microscopy demonstrates infiltration of the epineurium and perineurium by varying amounts of fibroadipose tissue (Fig. 4.34) (116–119). The nerve fascicle typically appears normal, although atrophy is reported as a late finding (121). Lipomatosis of nerve in which nerve bundles are infiltrated with varying amounts of fibrofatty tissue (120), must be distinguished from a nerve sheath lipoma in which the individual nerve bundles are

not involved (117). Cases in which there is macrodactyly are indistinguishable histologically from those in which there is no macrodactyly (117). The macrodactyly associated with lipomatosis of nerve is sometimes referred to as *nerve territory–oriented macrodactyly* (124).

The MR imaging appearance of lipomatosis of nerve is characteristic, reflecting the morphology of the lesion. MR imaging demonstrates small, approximately 3 mm in diameter, longitudinally oriented cylindrical decreased signal intensity on a background of increased signal intensity (121). This is thought to represent the nerve fascicles with epineural and perineural fibrosis on a background of fatty tissue (Figs. 4.34 and 4.35) (121,125). The MR imaging findings are quite constant, even when the lesion is in unusual locations (Fig. 4.36); however, it has been our experience that lesions in the carpal tunnel often show less

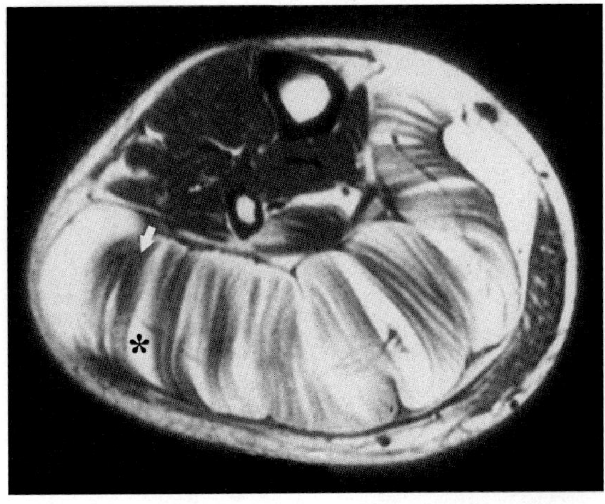 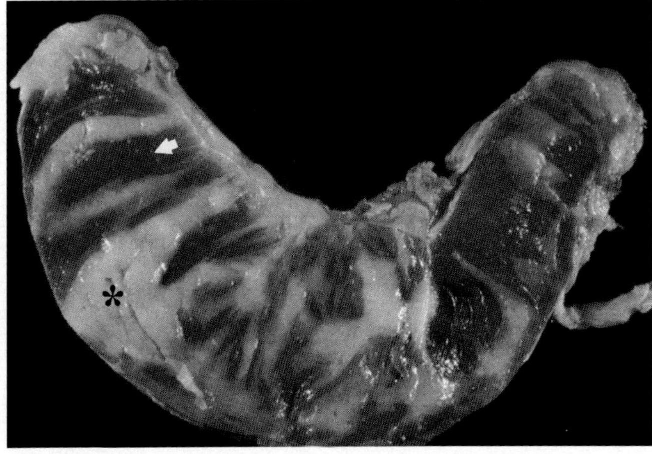

Figure 4.32 Infiltrating lipoma: MR imaging features in calf. **A,B:** Axial T1-weighted **(A)** spin-echo MR image and correlating photograph **(B)** demonstrate an infiltrating lipoma of the gastrocnemius muscle, showing the adipose tissue (*asterisk*) infiltrating skeletal muscle (*arrow*).

adipose tissue. Ultrasound imaging of lipomatosis of nerve may demonstrate alternating hyperechoic and hypoechoic bands (cablelike appearance) (Fig. 4.35) (125).

Radiographs of patients with lipomatosis of nerve may show a soft tissue mass. When there is associated macrodystrophia lipomatosa, it demonstrates both bone and soft tissue abnormalities. The phalanges are long, broad, and often splayed at their distal ends. The osseous overgrowth may be marked and disproportionately large, with extensive secondary degenerative change (Fig. 4.34) (13,125).

Lipoma of Tendon Sheath and Joint

> ## KEY CONCEPTS
> - Lipomas of tendon sheath and joint are rare and image as discrete lipomatous masses.
> - Lipoma arborescens is a diffuse lipoma of the joint; it is rare but more common than the discrete form.
> - Lipoma arborescens is most common in the knee.
> - MR imaging of lipoma arborescens shows a large, villous, frondlike mass with joint effusion.

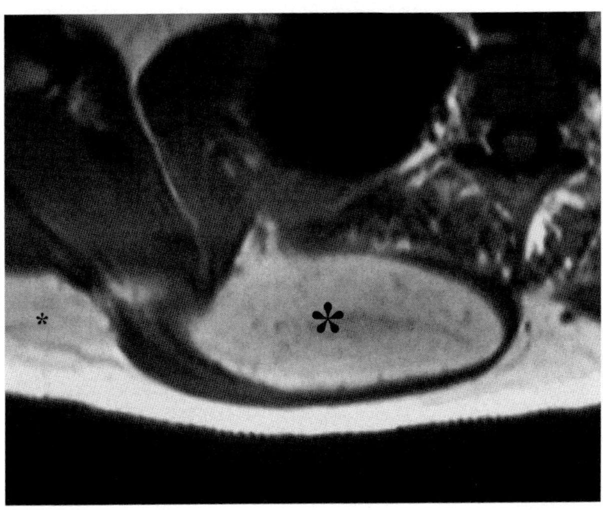 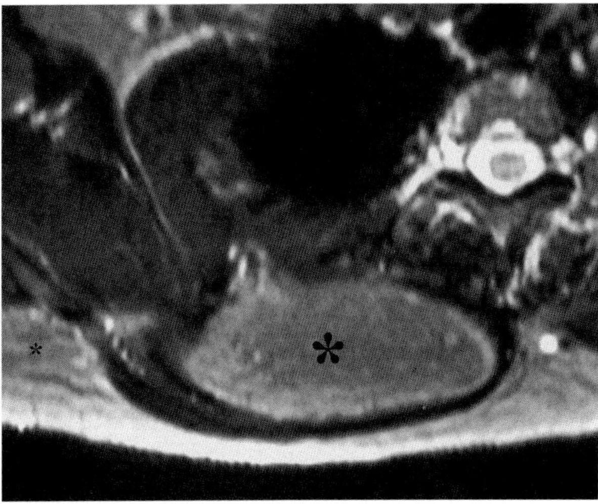

Figure 4.33 Intramuscular lipoma: MR imaging features of a heterogeneous lesion in a woman presenting with a shoulder mass. **A,B:** Corresponding axial T1-weighted (TR/TE; 600/16) **(A)** and conventional T2-weighted (TR/TE; 2300/80) **(B)** spin-echo MR images show a somewhat heterogeneous intramuscular fatty mass (*large asterisk*). The heterogeneity is not appreciated in the subcutaneous fat superficial to the lesion because of coil burnout. Note that the signal intensity of the lesion is identical to that of the subcutaneous fat lateral to the lesion (*small asterisk*), at the same distance from the coil.

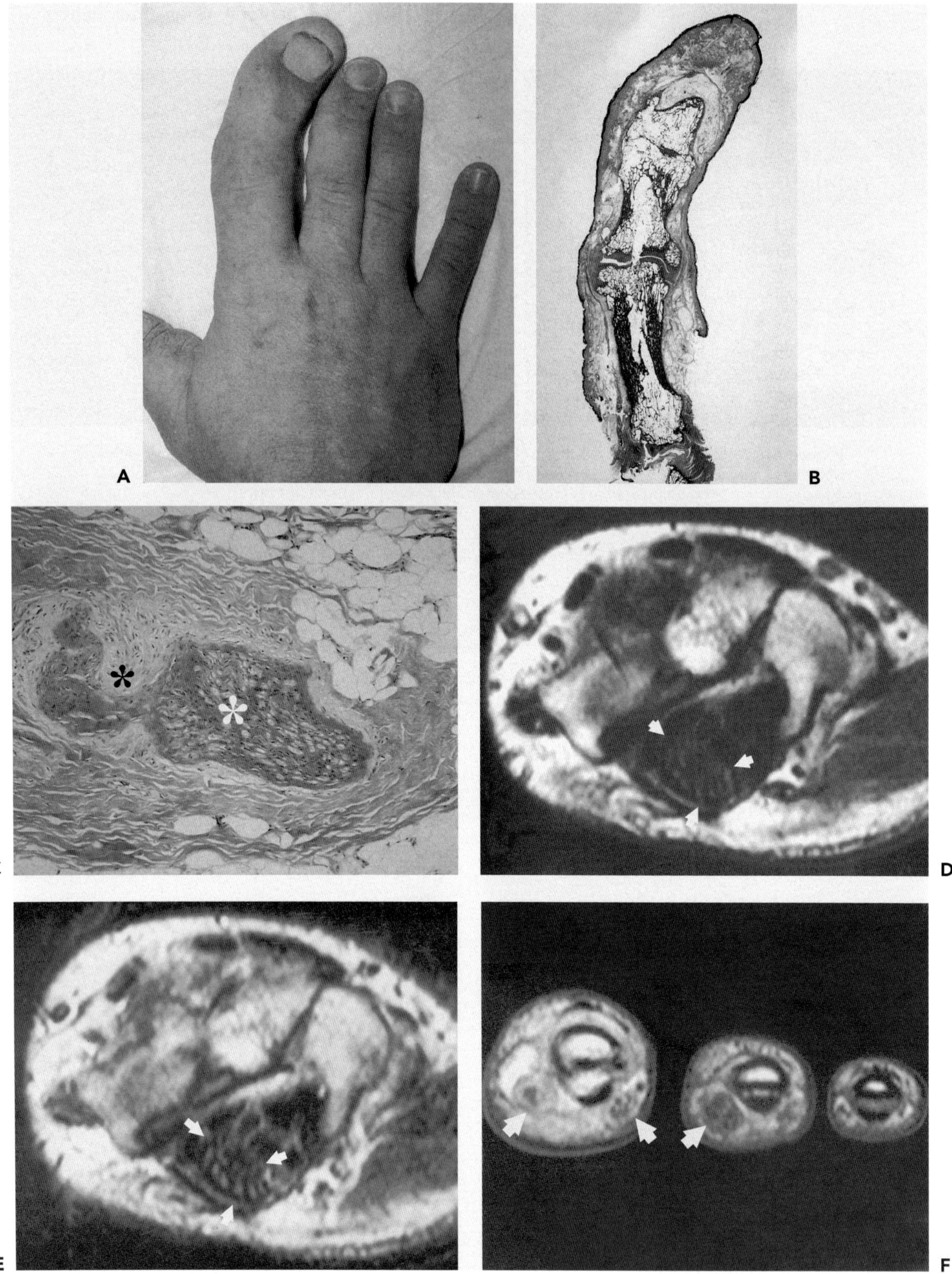

Figure 4.34 Lipomatosis of nerve: Gross, microscopic, and imaging features in a man 34 years of age with a lifelong history of an enlarged finger. **A:** Photograph of hand shows marked enlargement of the index finger. Note subtle overgrowth of the radial aspect of the middle finger. **B:** Macrosection of the resected index finger shows increased fat within the soft tissue, as well as overgrowth of the osseous structures. **C:** High-power photomicrograph of a nerve fiber (*white asterisk*) shows surrounding dense fibrous tissue (*black asterisk*) and fat. **D,E:** Axial T1-weighted (TR/TE; 800/18) **(D)** and turbo T2-weighted axial (TR/TE; 6000/88) **(E)** spin-echo MR images of the wrist at the level of the carpal tunnel show marked enlargement of the medial nerve (*arrows*). Note small, rounded nerve fascicles surrounded by fibrous tissue. No significant macroscopic fat is seen at this level. **F,G:** Axial **(F)** and coronal **(G)** T1-weighted (TR/TE; 500/16) spin-echo MR images through the fingers show marked fat overgrowth and enlargement of the digital nerves (*arrows*) in the affected areas. (*continued*)

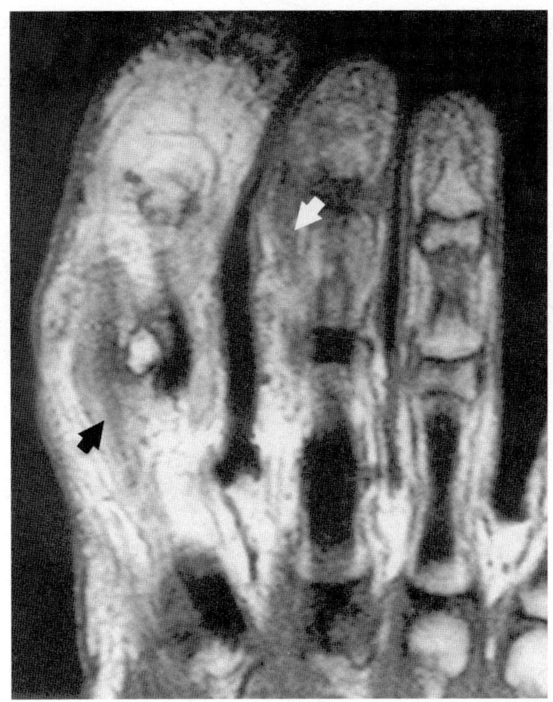

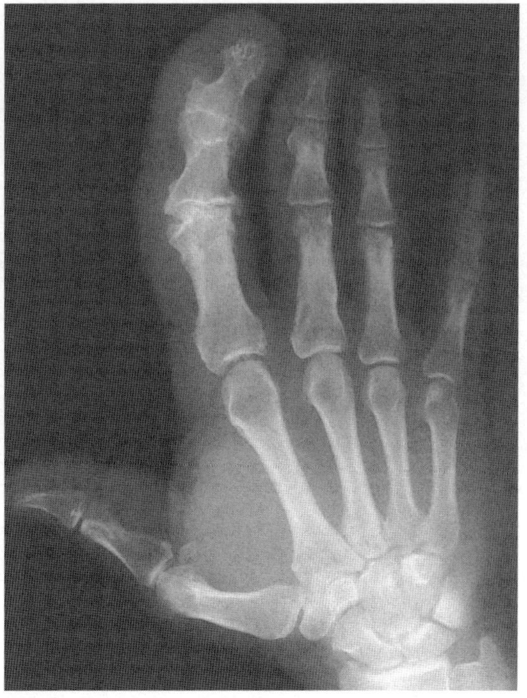

Figure 4.34 *(continued)* **F,G:** Axial **(F)** and coronal **(G)** T1-weighted (TR/TE; 500/16) spin-echo MR images through the fingers show marked fat overgrowth and enlargement of the digital nerves *(arrows)* in the affected areas. **H:** Anteroposterior radiograph of the hand shows marked overgrowth of the bones and soft tissues of the index finger, most marked distally. There is milder involvement of the radial aspect of the middle finger.

There are two variants of these rare tumors: a discrete, solid fatty mass that extends along the affected tendon or within the affected joint and a lipomalike lesion composed of hypertrophic synovial villi distended with fat, typically seen in the knee and termed *lipoma arborescens* (2).

Discrete Lipoma of Tendon Sheath

The discrete lipoma of tendon sheath most commonly arises in the hand and wrist and less commonly in the ankle and foot. These lesions are most frequent in young adults in the second through fourth decades and have no gender predilection (2). Bilateral symmetric lesions are not uncommon (2). Despite the fact that lipomas are the most common soft tissue tumor, discrete lesions associated with the tendon sheath or joint are quite rare. Fatty tumors of the hand and wrist rarely produce neurologic symptoms and are more typically associated with nonspecific findings (126). When a peripheral nerve is secondarily affected by a lipomatous lesion, sensory rather than motor symptoms are exhibited, and tendon sheath lipoma of the wrist is reported as a rare cause of carpal tunnel syndrome (126).

A lipoma of tendon sheath is evident radiographically as a focal lipomatous mass, imaging similar to that of a superficial or deep lipoma. Consequently, the lesion shows attenuation and signal intensity identical to that of fat (Fig. 4.37). Osseous erosion may be seen rarely.

Discrete Lipoma of Joint

True intra-articular lipoma is quite rare and must be distinguished from the diffuse synovial lipoma, which is considerably more common. Marui et al. reported a case in the knee and reviewed the literature in 2002, noting seven previously reported cases (127). The knee accounted for 75% of reported cases, with additional cases occurring in the hip and lumbar facet joint.

Radiologically, a discrete synovial lipoma has an imaging appearance similar to that of a discrete lipoma of tendon sheath. The imaging appearance mirrors that of a focal superficial or deep lipoma (Fig. 4.38). Although quite rare, a focal intra-articular lipoma may show a nonspecific appearance with more fluidlike signal intensity, which is attributed to mucoid degeneration within the tumor (127).

Lipoma Arborescens (Diffuse Lipoma of Joint)

Lipoma arborescens is a lipomalike lesion in which the subsynovial connective tissue is infiltrated by mature adipocytes, often associated with scattered inflammatory cells (1). Also referred to as *diffuse synovial lipoma*, lipoma arborescens is now thought to be a reactive

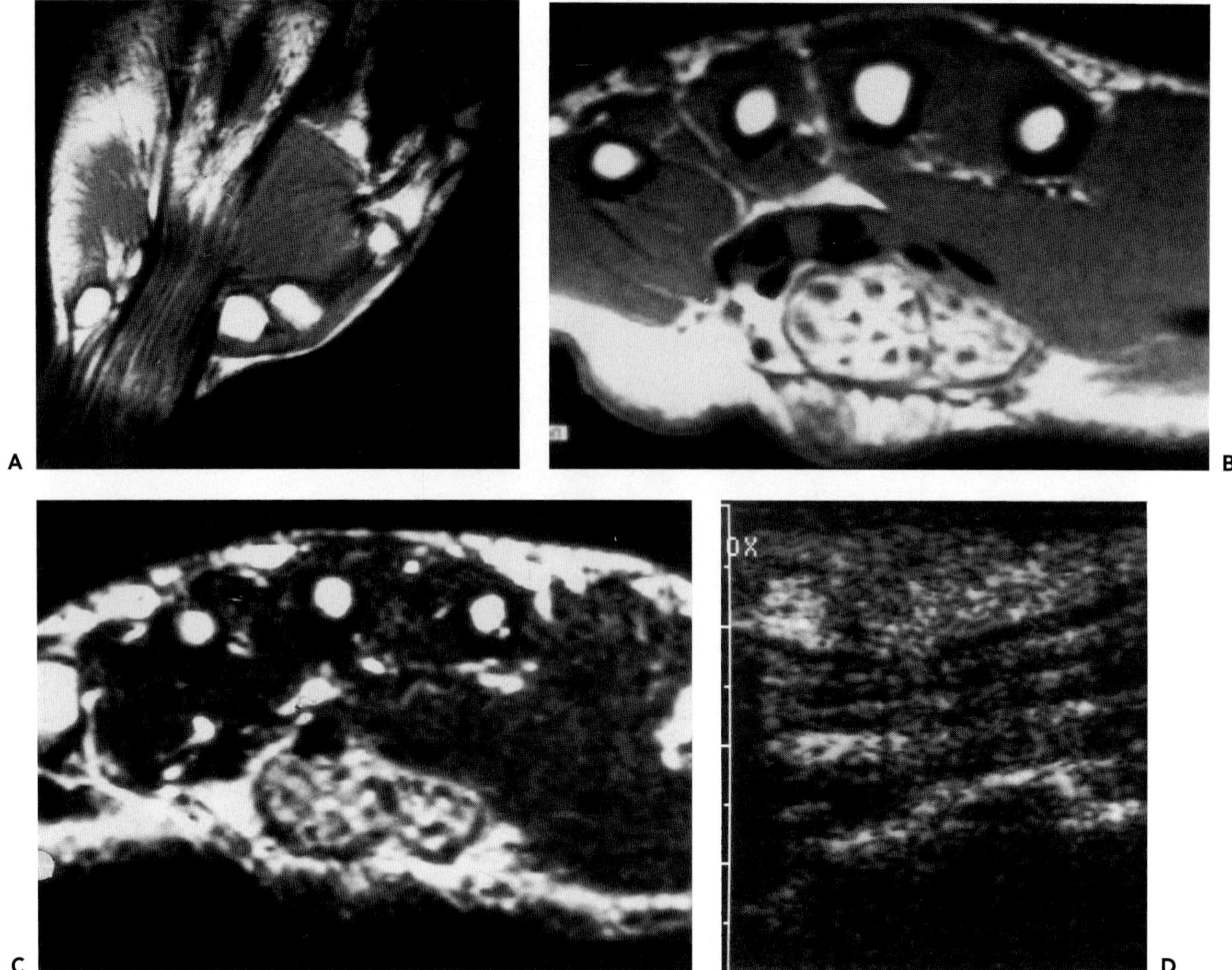

Figure 4.35 Lipomatosis of nerve: MR and ultrasound features in the median nerve of a man 22 years of age. **A,B:** Coronal **(A)** and axial **(B)** T1-weighted (TR/TE; 500/15) spin-echo MR images show small diameter, longitudinally oriented cylindrical areas of decreased signal on a background of increased signal intensity, identical to that of subcutaneous fat, in the distribution of the median nerve. **C:** Corresponding T2-weighted MR image shows a similar appearance. **D:** Longitudinally oriented sonogram shows linear areas of increased and decreased echogenicity corresponding to the findings in **A.** This appearance represents the nerve fascicles with epineural and perineural fibrosis on a background of fatty tissue.

process and is frequently associated with degenerative joint disease, chronic rheumatoid arthritis, or prior trauma involving the affected joint (2). All synovial lipomas are rare; lipoma arborescens, however, is encountered more frequently than the discrete form of synovial lipoma. In a review of 707 lipomas, Myhre-Jensen found 2 (0.3%) intra-articular cases of lipoma arborescens (3). Hallel et al. (128) suggested that the lesion be termed *villous lipomatous proliferation of the synovial membrane* because the designation *lipoma arborescens* implies a tumor.

Patients present with symptoms that progress over several years and include painless synovial thickening and intermittent effusions (128–134). Although few cases with long-term follow-up are available, Hallel et al. (128) reported detailed histories on five patients and noted

duration of symptoms present from 5 to 30 years prior to presentation. The clinical course is typically marked by intermittent exacerbations (128). Patients range from 9 to 66 years of age, with males affected much more commonly than females (128–131). Most reported cases occur in the knee. In reviewing the literature in 1989, Armstrong and Watt (130) noted nine cases in the knee: six unilateral and three bilateral. They also noted one patient with bilateral wrist involvement and one final case involving the hip unilaterally. Although lipoma arborescens is typically observed as an intra-articular lesion involving the synovial lining of the joint, bursal involvement as well as bilateral bursal involvement are described (135,136). The suggested treatment remains synovectomy, which alleviates the synovial thickening and effusions but not the associated

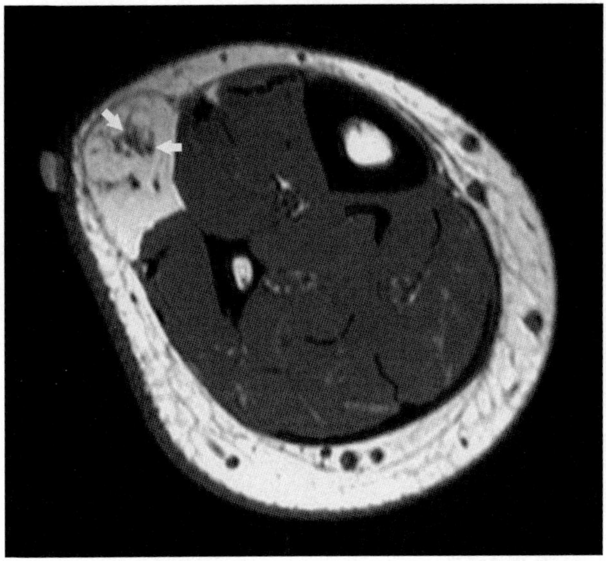
A

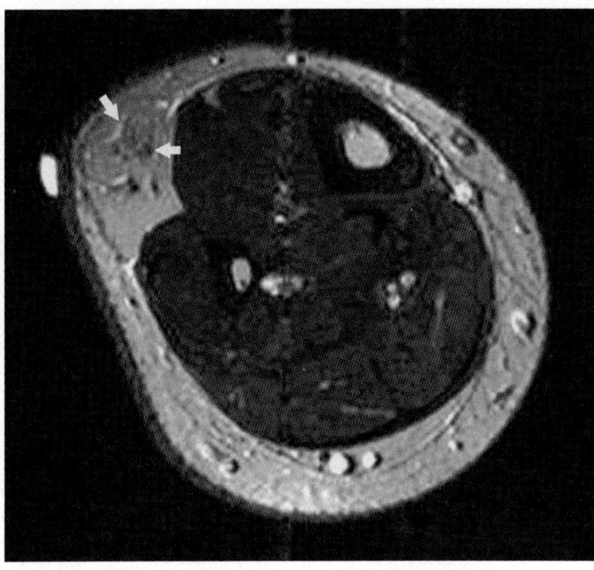
B

Figure 4.36 Lipomatosis of the superficial peroneal nerve: MR imaging features of an unusual location in a boy 15 years of age. **A,B:** Corresponding axial T1-weighted (TR/TE; 589/16) **(A)** and conventional T2-weighted (TR/TE; 2068/80) **(B)** MR images of the lower leg show a fatty mass with multiple small diameter regions of decreased signal (*arrows*). Serial imaging showed these cablelike regions to be oriented longitudinally, extending through the associated fatty mass.

osteoarthritis (128). Recurrence following synovectomy is reported (129).

Laboratory tests, including erythrocyte sedimentation rate and serologic tests for rheumatoid arthritis, are generally negative, as are cultures (128,130). Grossly, the lesion has a frondlike contour, and joint fluid is negative for crystals and cells (128,130,132). Microscopically, there is replacement of the subsynovial tissue by mature adipose tissue with the formation of proliferative villous projections, most prominently in the suprapatellar pouch with associated chronic inflammation (Fig. 4.39) (128,132). Extension into an associated popliteal cyst is reported (131).

MR imaging shows a large villous, frondlike mass, mainly within the suprapatellar bursa, with an associated joint effusion. The signal intensity of the lesion mirrors that of fat on all pulse sequences (Fig. 4.40) (131–136). Enhancement may be seen within the inflamed synovium. Lesions may be mistaken for liposarcoma, and the key to diagnosis is recognition of the synovial (joint or bursal) origin, as well as the multilobulated frondlike contour (135). CT also shows a frondlike mass of fat attenuation (130,132,133), although the frondlike nature may be more difficult to recognize on CT imaging.

Radiographs in patients afflicted with the lipoma arborescens form of synovial lipoma show soft tissue swelling around the joint that may or may not be radiolucent. Sonography is useful to document the joint effusion as well as the villous nature of the mass (Fig. 4.40) (131,133,135). Associated imaging findings include degenerative changes, meniscal tear, synovial cysts, and bone

erosions (134). Arthrography shows multiple and/or lobulated intra-articular filling defects (132,137).

Infiltrating Lipomas

Infiltrating lipoma and *lipomatosis* are terms used to describe a diffuse overgrowth of mature adipose tissue (1).

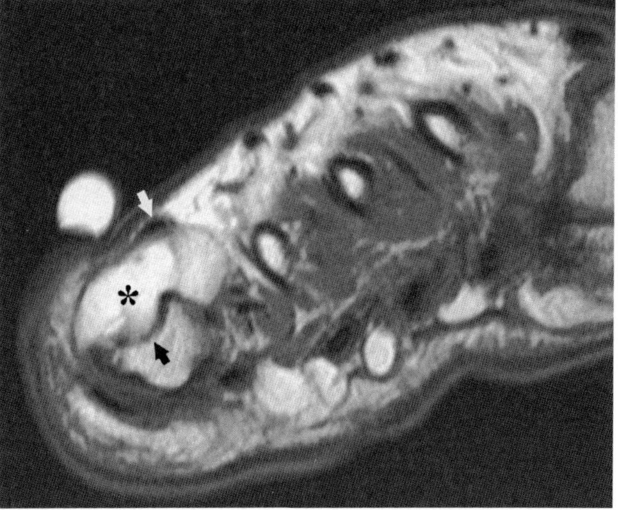

Figure 4.37 Lipoma of tendon sheath: Imaging features in a woman 57 years of age presenting with a soft tissue mass. Axial T1-weighted (TR/TE; 621/17) spin-echo MR image shows a discrete lipoma (*asterisk*) of the extensor tendon of the small toe (*white arrow*). The lesion demonstrated a signal intensity identical to that of fat on all pulse sequences. Note focal osseous erosion (*black arrow*).

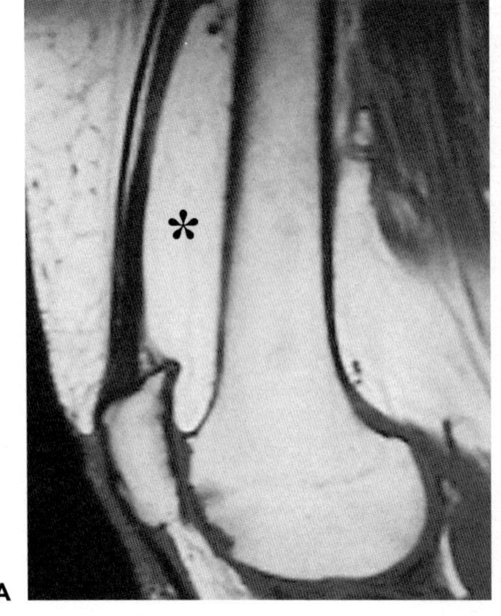

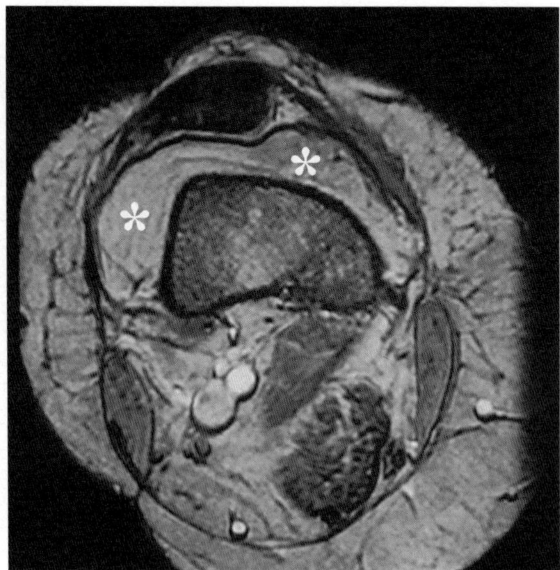

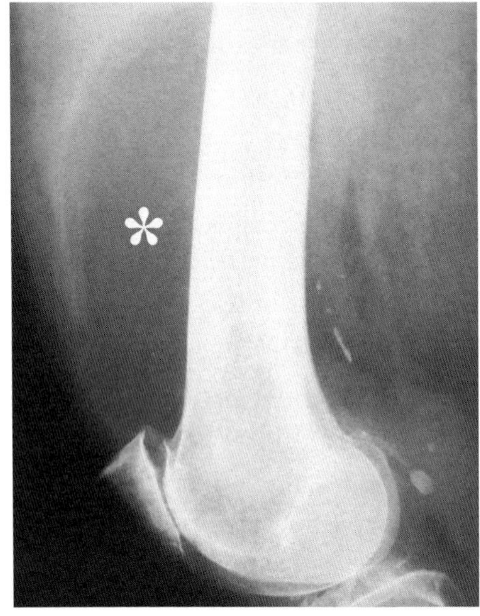

Figure 4.38   Discrete synovial lipoma: MR imaging features in a woman 73 years of age. **A,B:** Sagittal T1-weighted (TR/TE; 462/15) spin-echo **(A)** and axial gradient-echo (TR/TE; 40/13) **(B)** MR images show a discrete fatty mass (*asterisks*) filling the suprapatellar bursa. **C:** Lateral radiograph shows the fatty mass (*asterisk*) filling the suprapatella bursa.

This fatty overgrowth occurs in a variety of clinical settings that affect various anatomic areas. These lesions compress adjacent structures, and the members of this group of fatty lesions are histologically indistinguishable, divided clinically by location and distribution.

Several different types of lipomatosis are described (138). These include diffuse lipomatosis, infiltrating congenital lipomatosis of the face, multiple symmetric lipomatosis, shoulder girdle lipomatosis, adiposis dolorosa, mediastinal lipomatosis, pelvic lipomatosis, and renal sinus lipomatosis. Those lesions typically associated with evaluation of the soft tissues are further characterized in the following sections.

Diffuse Lipomatosis

Diffuse lipomatosis is an entity characterized by diffuse overgrowth of mature adipose tissue infiltrating through the soft tissues of the affected extremity or even the trunk

> **KEY CONCEPTS**
> - Diffuse lipomatosis is microscopically indistinguishable from lipoma or intramuscular lipoma.
> - Usually present by 2 years of age, it typically affects an extremity or trunk; nerve is not affected.
> - Imaging shows diffuse overgrowth and infiltration of adipose tissue.
> - Osseous overgrowth and deformity may be observed.

of the body (Fig. 4.41). Microscopically, this lesion is indistinguishable from lipoma or intramuscular lipoma, and the distinction between infiltrating lipoma and diffuse lipomatosis may be blurred at times (56).

Patients affected with diffuse lipomatosis usually present during the early years of life, usually by 2 years of age, although there are scattered reports of presentation in

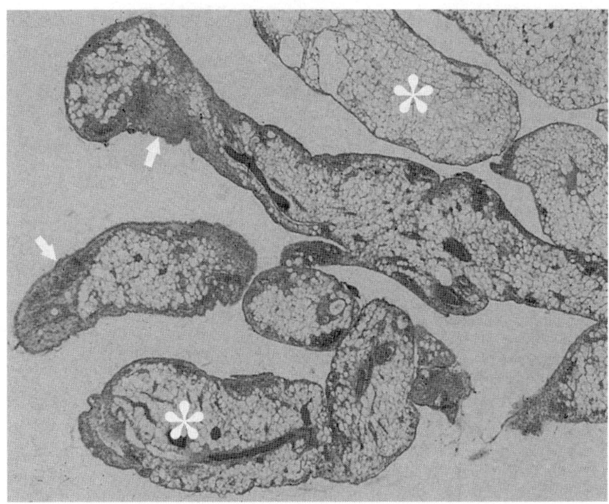
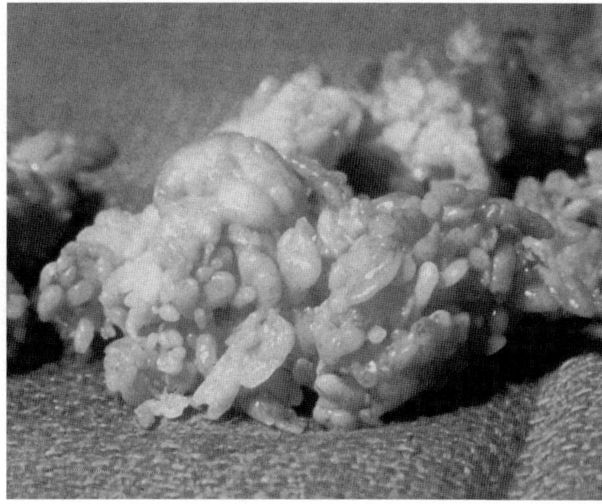

Figure 4.39 Lipoma arborescens: Microscopic and gross features. **A:** Low-power photomicrograph shows synovial villi distended with fat (*asterisk*) and associated subsynovial inflammation (*arrows*). Villous configuration is well-appreciated on the microscopic section. **B:** Gross photograph of resected specimen shows the villous growth pattern to better advantage.

adulthood (2,139). Coode et al. (139) note that the designation of *diffuse congenital lipomatosis* is suggested on the assumption that adult cases represent delayed presentation. Diffuse lipomatosis may be associated with coexistent osseous hypertrophy and gigantism, but unlike macrodystrophia lipomatosa, the nerve is unaffected and the disease is not confined to an extremity. Diffuse lipomatosis should be distinguished from diffuse infiltrating intramuscular lipoma, in which the subcutaneous tissues are spared (114).

Radiologic evaluation reflects the underlying pathologic process, showing diffuse overgrowth and infiltration of adipose tissue (Figs. 4.42 and 4.43). Mild cases of diffuse extremity lipomatosis may go unrecognized and may only be identified as an incidental finding in adults (Fig. 4.44). The adipose tissue in diffuse lipomatosis is neither well-circumscribed nor homogeneous. Diffuse swelling of the soft tissues and osseous overgrowth and deformity may be observed (13). Radiographs may demonstrate nonspecific soft tissue swelling or mottled lucent areas.

Infiltrating Congenital Lipomatosis of the Face

KEY CONCEPTS

- Infiltrating congenital lipomatosis of the face is a rare congenital disorder characterized by subcutaneous lipomatous masses of the face and cheek.
- Fatty lesions infiltrate adjacent muscle and soft tissue; they may have osseous hypertrophy.
- Associated anomalies include macroglossia, cutaneous capillary blush, and mucosal neuromas.

Infiltrating congenital lipomatosis of the face is a rare, but distinct clinical entity, described in 1983 by Slavin et al. (140). Patients present with a congenital subcutaneous mass, usually limited to the face and cheek (141,142). Lesions may increase in size causing facial asymmetry, which may be considerable (141,142). Osseous hypertrophy is also reported (143). Although infiltrating congenital lipomatosis of the face is benign, complete excision is surgically difficult and local recurrence is common, occurring in more than 60% of patients (141–143). The lesion infiltrates the adjacent muscles, fibrous tissue, and parotid gland (142).

The optimal timing and extent of surgical excision is unclear. Although early intervention prevents extensive infiltration, delayed resection lessens the chance of damaging the facial nerve at surgery, as well as decreasing the ultimate number of surgeries required (143). Liposuction is also advocated as the best method of achieving facial symmetry (143); alternatively, intervention may be postponed until the end of facial growth (144,145).

Slavin et al. noted that all of their cases shared the following morphologic criteria: (a) nonencapsulated tumors containing mature fat cells, (b) infiltration of adjacent muscle and soft tissue, (c) absence of malignant characteristics, (d) absence of lipoblasts, (e) presence of fibrous elements in conjunction with increased numbers of nerve bundles and vessels, and (f) hypertrophy of subjacent bone (140). Reported associated anomalies include ipsilateral macroglossia, cutaneous capillary blush, and mucosal neuromas (143,144). The clinical differential diagnosis for infiltrating lipomatosis of the face includes Proteus syndrome, encephalocraniocutaneous lipomatosis, and facial hemangioma.

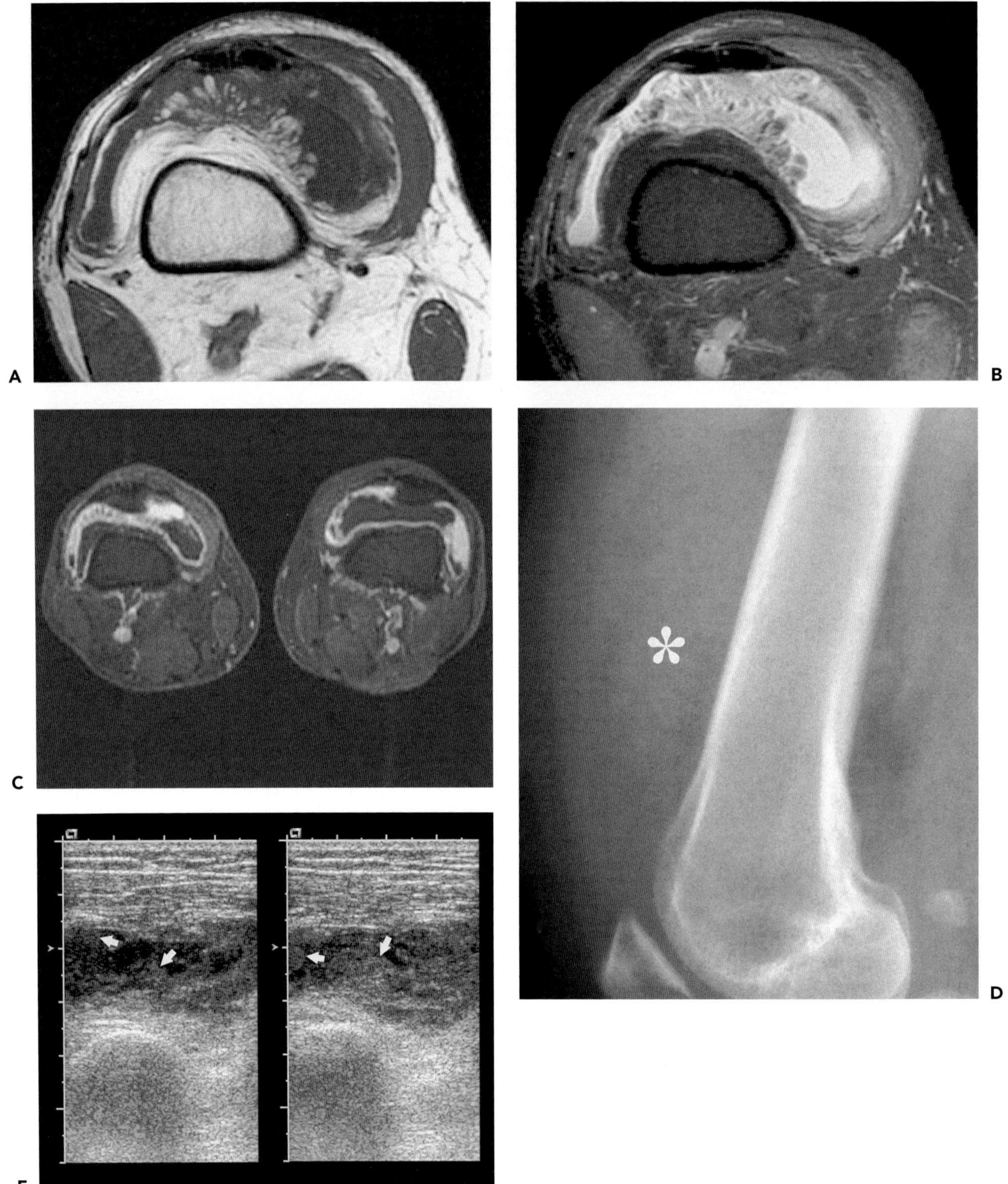

Figure 4.40   Lipoma arborescens: Imaging features in a man 60 years of age with chronic bilateral knee pain and swelling. **A,B:** Corresponding axial T1-weighted (TR/TE; 550/16) **(A)** and fat-suppressed fast proton density (TR/TE; 5016/16) **(B)** spin-echo MR images show a large joint effusion with fatty frondlike excrescences extending from the synovial surface. Similar findings were seen in the left knee. **C:** Enhanced fat-suppressed axial T1-weighted (TR/TE; 733/16) MR image shows intense synovial enhancement caused by the associated inflammation. **D:** Lateral radiograph shows a mass (*asterisk*) within the suprapatella bursa with a slightly heterogeneous appearance and areas of slight radiolucency. **E:** Sonography shows a joint effusion with a diffuse villous synovial-based mass. The villous nature of the mass (*arrows*) is well seen.

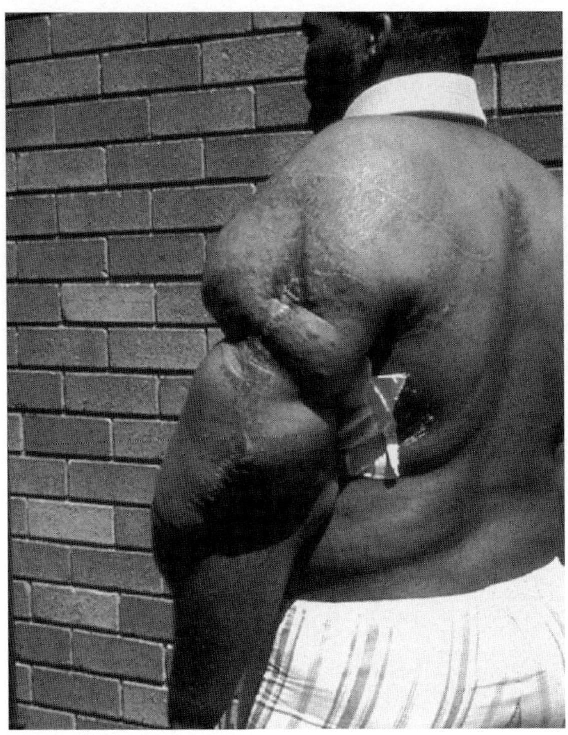

Figure 4.41 Diffuse lipomatosis: Clinical appearance of lipomatosis of the upper extremity. Clinical photograph shows marked residual overgrowth of the left upper extremity despite extensive prior surgery. (Courtesy of Sharon W. Weiss, M.D., Atlanta, GA.)

Lipomatous infiltration may involve the parotid gland, and typical cytomegalovirus (CMV) inclusions are noted within the secretory cells of the parotid gland. This finding suggests the possibility of a causal relationship between the two conditions (141,142).

Multiple Symmetric Lipomatosis

> **KEY CONCEPTS**
>
> Multiple symmetric lipomatosis has the following characteristics:
>
> - Symmetric deposition of adipose tissue in the head, neck, and trunk.
> - Strong male prevalence; 50% of patients have history of excessive alcohol intake.
> - Commonly associated with peripheral motor and sensory neuropathy.
> - Diagnosis based on clinical and radiologic features.

Multiple symmetric lipomatosis is a rare form of lipomatosis, characterized by symmetric deposits of adipose tissue in the head, neck, and trunk. Initially reported by Brodie in 1846 (146–149), Madelung established it as a distinct entity in 1888, and it is sometimes referred to as *Madelung disease*. Launois and Bensaude reviewed the literature in 1898, presenting 65 cases, and this entity is also referred to

as *Launois-Bensaude syndrome* (147,149,150). To date, more than 270 cases are reported (151).

Multiple symmetric lipomatosis is typically seen in middle-aged men. In their 2003 review of the literature, Chong et al. noted that 84% of affected individuals were males, with an average age of 45 years (151). Interestingly, the male-to-female ratio in a report of 32 Korean patients was 31:1 (152). A history of excessive alcohol intake was reported in approximately half the cases; however, in some reports this figure is much higher (151). Multiple symmetric lipomatosis is rare in nondrinkers (153). Other associations include liver disease and glucose intolerance (146,154–156). Most cases are solitary, although a familial history was noted in 23% of reported cases (151). An autosomal dominant mode of inheritance is postulated (146,147,150,157), and an increased frequency is noted in the Mediterranean regions (150). A mitochondrial gene mutation is found in approximately 28% of patients with symmetric lipomatosis and may be the cause of clinical and pathologic features (151). Mitochondria are important for alcohol metabolism; consequently, alcohol abuse may lead to the production of factors promoting lipogenesis (158).

The fatty deposits tend to be lobular and symmetric, occurring most commonly in the cervical regions and upper trunk (146,155). In the neck, the fatty masses are usually deep to the sternocleidomastoid and trapezius muscles, in the supraclavicular fossa, or between the paraspinal muscles (159). Rarer locations include the anterior neck, superior mediastinum, and pretracheal and prevertebral spaces (159). The fatty deposits may extend into the back, producing a hump, or into the upper neck and parotid region, giving a so-called chipmunk appearance to the face (146,155). Less commonly, the axilla and groin are involved (146,157).

The etiology is unclear. A "hyperplastic mechanism for fatty tumor formation and growth" was postulated by Enzi (157), who identified two types of benign symmetric lipomatosis: one in which the fatty lesions present as discrete masses, with pronounced atrophy of the uninvolved adipose tissue (type I) and one in which the lipomatous tissue diffuses into the subcutaneous fat, giving the outward appearance of obesity (type II). In the first type, patients are underweight and the uninvolved subcutaneous fat is reduced or atrophic. In the second group, Enzi was able to identify the nodular configuration of the fatty masses early in the course of the disease, prior to the development of the generalized appearance of obesity. In women, the morphologic pattern of involvement is type II, with lipomatous masses most frequently in the proximal arms (91%) and legs (55%) (153). Men also demonstrate type II involvement, although in only approximately 64% of cases (153). The submental deposition of fat seen in both types of symmetric lipomatosis is usually not seen in women; mediastinal involvement is more common in men (153).

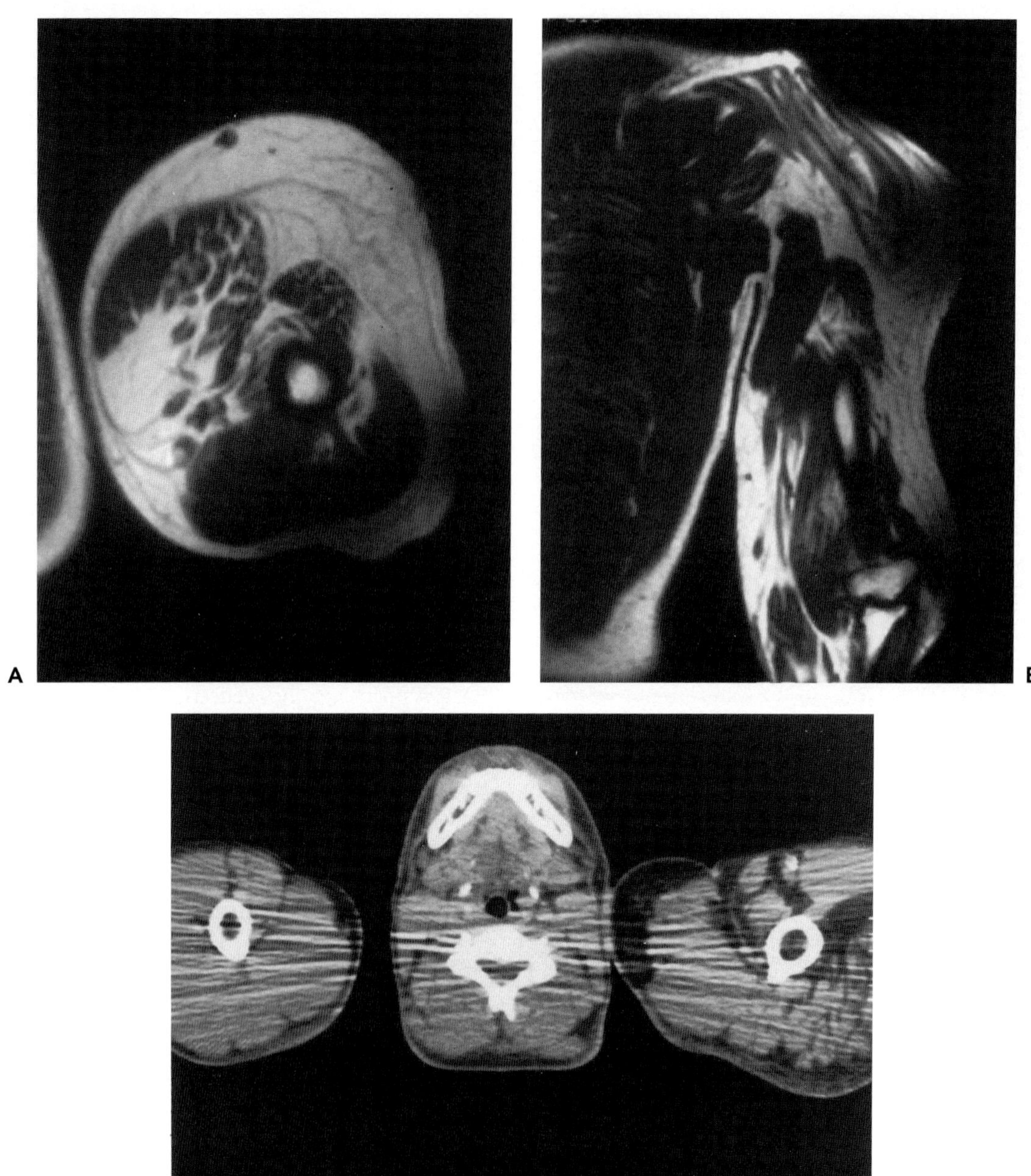

Figure 4.42 Diffuse lipomatosis of the upper extremity: MR and CT imaging features in a man 23 years of age. **A,B:** Axial **(A)** and coronal **(B)** T1-weighted (TR/TE; 400/20) spin-echo MR images of the left upper extremity show diffuse overgrowth of adipose tissue. **C:** Corresponding axial CT shows overgrowth of fat in the left upper extremity. Comparison of osseous structures shows slight overgrowth of left humerus.

Patients' symptoms are related to the size and location of the lesions, and significant associated deformity is possible (146). Masses may appear suddenly and grow rapidly (155,157). The growth rate is irregular, and the lesion may cease to grow spontaneously or become intermittently quiescent (155,157). Mediastinal involvement may be associated with tracheal compression (157). Pericardial and abdominal fatty masses have not been reported (157).

Signs and symptoms of peripheral motor and sensory neuropathy are commonly present and were seen in the vast majority of 19 patients presented by Enzi, and some evidence of neuropathy is seen in approximately 59% to 84% of patients with multiple symmetric lipomatosis (151,153, 157,160). These neuropathies were most typically in the lower extremities and varied from minor loss of vibratory sensation to severe or incapacitating neuroarthropathy. Multiple symmetric lipomatosis is also associated with hypertriglyceridemia, hyperuricemia, impaired glucose tolerance, and elevated HDL cholesterol (41,157). Lesions are treated by surgical excision, which is

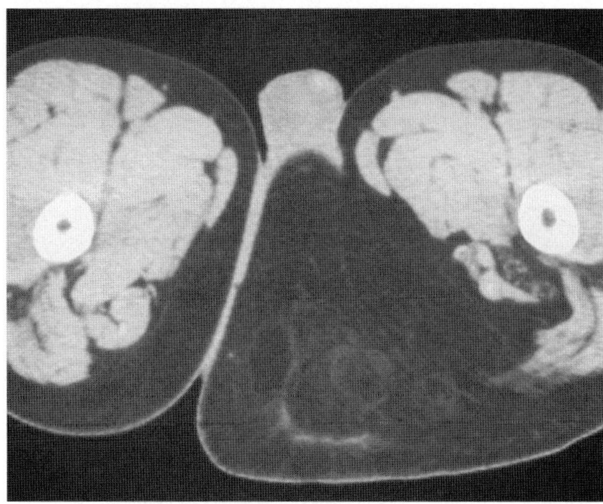
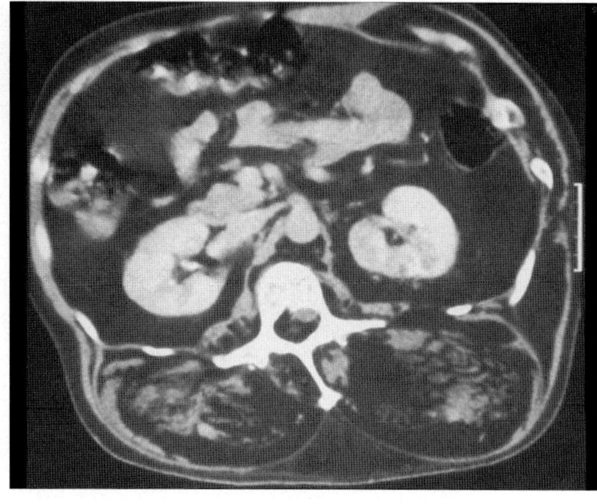

Figure 4.43 Diffuse lipomatosis of the trunk: CT imaging features in a man 29 years of age. **A:** Axial CT scan of the buttocks shows a large fatty mass infiltrating the left buttocks. **B:** Axial image at the level of the kidneys shows diffuse infiltration of the paraspinal muscles and left abdominal wall. Note epidural involvement.

usually done for cosmetic reasons (146). Abstinence from alcohol may arrest further progression but does not lead to regression of the disease (152).

Microscopically, the lesions are unencapsulated and infiltrate the adjacent tissue (150). They are identical to the adipose tissue in other lipomatous tumors, except for some increase in fibrous and vascular elements (146). CT and MR imaging are well-suited to identify the fatty nature of the masses as well as to establish their extent (Fig. 4.45) (161,162). Sonography is also used but is less effective (163). Enzi et al. (150) evaluated 15 patients using CT scanning and found narrowing of the tracheal lumen in three (75%) of four patients with involvement of the thoracic inlet. Two of these patients were asymptomatic. Calcification within the fatty masses is also reported (150,157).

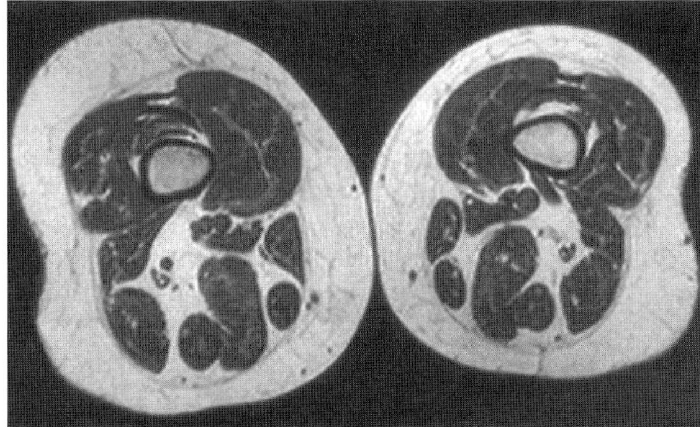

Figure 4.44 Diffuse lipomatosis of the lower extremity: Subtle MR features in a woman 42 years of age with diffuse leg swelling. Axial T1-weighted (TR/TE; 700/16) spin-echo MR image of the lower extremities at the level of the knees shows mild diffuse increased adipose tissue in the right leg as compared to the left.

Shoulder Girdle Lipomatosis

> **KEY CONCEPTS**
> - Shoulder girdle lipomatosis is a rare form of lipomatosis reported most frequently in women.
> - It is characterized by a unilateral accumulation of fat between the chest wall and overlying muscle.
> - This lipomatosis is commonly associated with airway compression and neuromyopathy.

Shoulder girdle lipomatosis was described in 1992 by Enzi et al. (121) as a lipomatosis characterized by a unilateral accumulation of adipose tissue between the bands of muscle that connect the upper limb to the thoracic wall. They reported six cases, all in women, between 38 and 72 years of age. Three (50%) of these six patients had compression of the upper airway or infiltration of the laryngeal wall. Patients with shoulder girdle lipomatosis present with gradual enlargement and deformity of the shoulder and proximal arm (146). Signs and symptoms of neuromyopathy are present in most patients, likely caused by mechanical compression or possibly by neural fatty degeneration. An association between lipomatosis and neuropathy is also seen in multiple symmetric lipomatosis.

Imaging of shoulder girdle lipomatosis shows increased accumulations of fat between the chest wall and the overlying muscle, the latter of which may appear wasted (121). The increased fat images identically to normal subcutaneous fat, with no areas of increased signal intensity on T2-weighted images or short-tau inversion recovery (STIR) images (Fig. 4.46) (164).

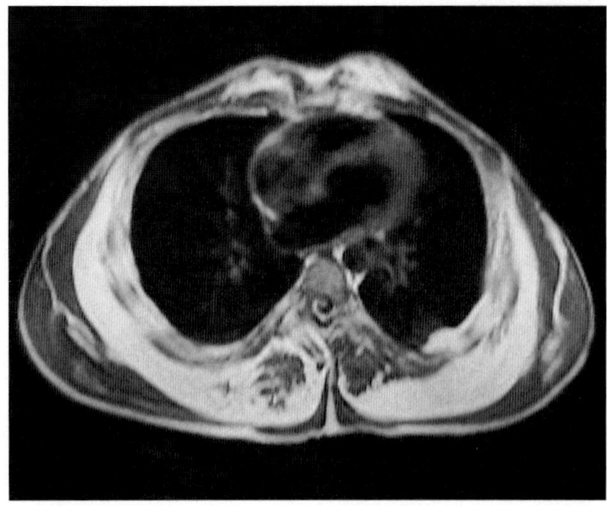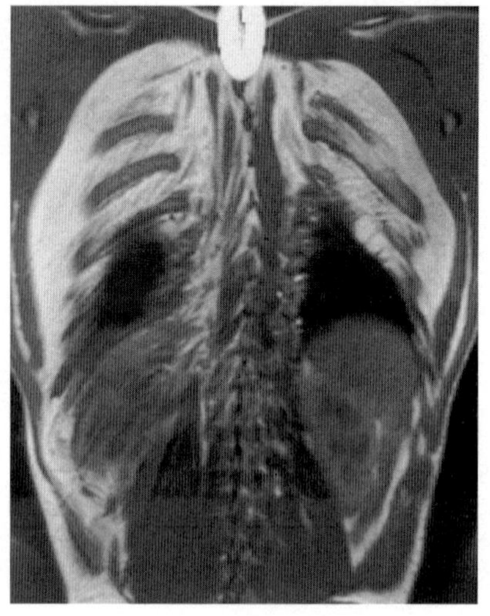

Figure 4.45 Multiple symmetric lipomatosis (Madelung disease): MR imaging features in a man 28 years of age. **A,B:** Axial T1-weighted (TR/TE; 775/20) **(A)** and coronal T1-weighted (TR/TE; 700/15) **(B)** spin-echo MR images show extensive, but symmetric, involvement of the chest wall. Note relative paucity of subcutaneous fat and other uninvolved adipose tissue.

Adiposis Dolorosa

KEY CONCEPTS

- Adiposis dolorosa is a rare form of lipomatosis most common in postmenopausal obese women.
- Characteristics are: (1) multiple painful fatty masses, (2) generalized obesity, (3) weakness and fatigability, and (4) psychiatric disturbances.
- Adiposis dolorosa cannot be distinguished histologically from other forms of lipomatosis.

Adiposis dolorosa was originally described by Dercum at the American Neurological Association in 1888 and reported in the literature later that same year by the title "A Subcutaneous Connective-tissue Dystrophy of the Arms and Back Associated with Symptoms Resembling Myxoedema" (165). Dercum subsequently collected and published three cases in 1892, separating them from lipomatosis by the associated "nervous symptoms." Adiposis dolorosa is characterized by the accumulation of multiple subcutaneous lipomatous masses, which may become quite extensive, with associated pain, tenderness, motor weakness, and esthesia (loss of strength and fatigue with minimal

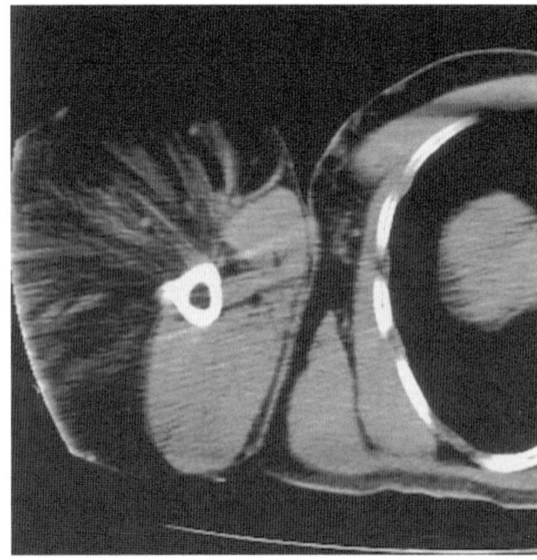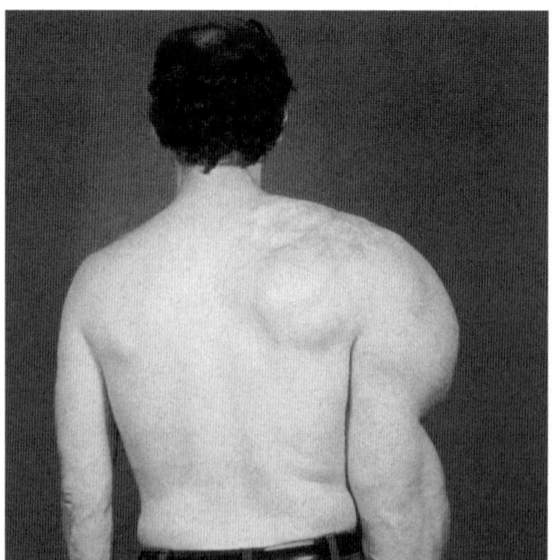

Figure 4.46 Shoulder girdle lipomatosis: CT imaging features in a man 40 years of age. **A:** Axial CT scan reveals extensive lipomatous infiltration of the shoulder girdle, largely affecting the subcutaneous adipose tissue. **B:** Clinical photograph shows marked fatty overgrowth and clinical disfigurement.

effort) (2). Dercum chose the term *adiposis dolorosa* to describe this disease because of the multiple painful lipomas (166). The prevalence of adiposis dolorosa is unknown, but it may be more common than previously recognized (167).

Because there are no unique pathognomonic features, the term *Dercum syndrome* is suggested. This syndrome has four cardinal symptoms: multiple painful fatty masses; generalized obesity, usually in women of menopausal age; asthenia, weakness, and fatigability; and mental disturbances (166).

Adiposis dolorosa is most common in postmenopausal obese females, with the female-to-male ratio greater than 30:1 (167). The etiology is unknown, but some evidence indicates it is hereditary, with an autosomal dominant transmission and variable penetrance (167,168). Adiposis dolorosa is also associated with endocrine and lipid metabolic dysfunction (168). The fatty masses are usually found in the extremities, especially near the joints, and less commonly in the trunk, with sparing of the hands and face (167). In addition to the multiple fatty masses, the disease is characterized by pain, asthenia, and psychiatric disturbances (169). The latter includes emotional instability, depression, epilepsy, and true dementia (168). Onset of pain is often spontaneous, or it may follow minor trauma (149). The cause of the pain is unclear; however, it is sometimes attributed to pressure on adjacent peripheral nerves by the fatty masses (2,167). The asthenia is noted to be out of proportion to all physical activity and may be physically debilitating (169).

The fatty masses of adiposis dolorosa cannot be distinguished from other forms of lipomatosis histologically (167). It may be distinguished from multiple symmetric lipomatosis in that the fatty masses associated with multiple symmetric lipomatosis are not associated with pain or tenderness.

The treatment of adiposis dolorosa is directed to symptomatic control. Medical treatment includes lidocaine infusion and steroids; surgical options range from liposuction to surgical resection of fatty masses (166,168). At present, no treatment is known to alter the progressive course of the disease (166).

Hibernoma

KEY CONCEPTS

- Hibernoma is a rare tumor of brown fat, named for its similarity to brown adipose tissue found in hibernating animals.
- It usually presents as a slowly growing mass located in the thigh, shoulder, back, or neck.
- Four variants: typical (most common), myxoid (<10%), lipomalike (<10%), and spindle cell (rare).
- Imaging shows fatty nature with prominent septations and serpentine/branching vessels.
- Less often, imaging shows appearance similar, but not identical, to fat, suggesting liposarcoma.

Hibernoma is a rare benign soft tissue tumor consisting of brown fat. The original description was by Merkel in 1906, who named it a "pseudolipoma." Gery coined the term *hibernoma* in 1914 because of the tumor's resemblance to the brown fat in hibernating animals, and approximately 100 cases have been reported to date (170,171,172). Brown fat, once thought to represent a stage in the development of "white" adipose tissue, is now considered distinct, with specific functions in nonshivering thermogenesis in hibernating animals and in the newborn (173). In the human fetus and newborn, brown fat is found in the subpleural and axillary regions (174); consequently, hibernomas are often (but not invariably) found in the periscapular or interscapular regions, as well as in the soft tissues of the axilla, chest wall, and neck. Ahn and Harvey (172) note that brown fat was first described by Welch in 1670, when he noted a glandlike structure in the mediastinum of a woodchuck. This was initially thought to be associated with the thymus but was later recognized to be separate from it.

Clinical presentation of hibernoma is typically that of a slowly growing, painless mass (173,175,176), with patients usually in the third and fourth decades of life. In a recent report of 170 cases, the average patient age was 38 years (range: 2 to 72 years of age) (177). In this study, only nine patients (5%) were younger than 18 years. There is a slight female predominance in the literature (173,178), although in the AFIP series, 58% of patients were male. Interestingly, seven (78%) of the nine patients younger than 18 years were female. Hibernoma was always thought to arise in the neck, axilla, back, and mediastinum, which are areas of residual brown fat. Newer evidence, however, suggests that lesions are most common in the thigh, with this location accounting for 30% of lesions (177). Less common locations include the shoulder, back, and neck, in descending order of frequency (177). Symptoms depend on the size and location of the lesion, and the duration of symptoms may vary from days to 10 years (174,177). Malignant transformation has not been reported (2).

The gross appearance of hibernoma is that of a well-demarcated, encapsulated, soft, lobulated mass. Lesions usually measure 5 to 10 cm in diameter, although there are reports of hibernomas reaching 20 cm (1,2,9). Hibernoma varies in color from brown to yellow, depending on the relative lipid content of the tumor. On microscopy, univacuolar or multivacuolar adipocytes are commonly interspersed among the granular to eosinophilic cells of hibernoma, which result in a lipoma with hibernomalike areas. Such intermediate forms or mixtures are more frequent than pure hibernomas, which are exceedingly rare. In the AFIP series, approximately 2% of lipomas were coded as having focal areas of hibernomatous change (12). The point at which a mixed lesion changes from a lipoma with hibernomatous change to a hibernoma is not clearly defined.

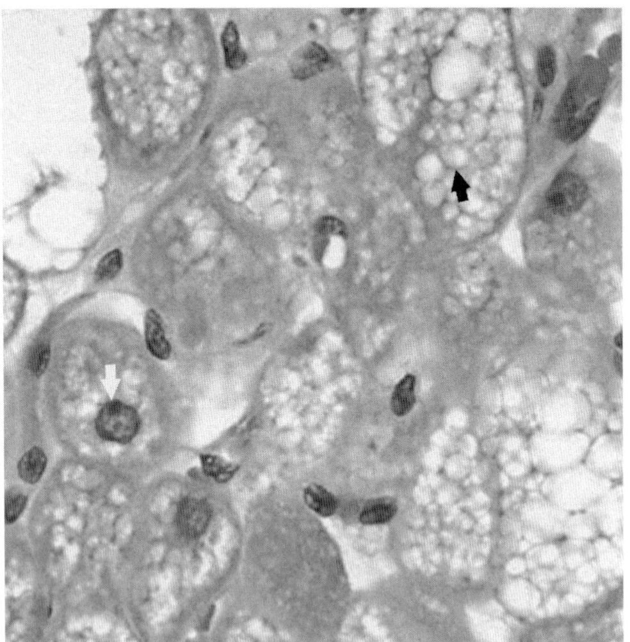

Figure 4.47 Typical hibernoma: Histology. Low-power photomicrograph shows the characteristic microscopic features of a hibernoma with finely granular round to oval cells with central nuclei (*white arrow*) and multivacuolated cytoplasm (*black arrow*). Scattered mature adipocytes are interspersed (hematoxylin and eosin).

Four histologic variants of hibernoma are identified: typical, myxoid, lipomalike, and spindle cell (177). The typical variant is most common, comprising 82% of lesions. Intramuscular lesions are usually the typical variant. The myxoid variant represents 8% of lesions and occurs predominantly in men. The lipomalike variant, which accounts for 7% of hibernomas, is most commonly located in the thigh. The spindle cell variant makes up 2% of lesions and has features of hibernoma as well as of spindle cell lipoma. As would be expected, the spindle cell variant is found in the superficial adipose tissue of the posterior neck (177).

Hibernoma is composed of multivacuolated fat cells with small central nuclei and no atypia (Fig. 4.47). The marked hypervascularity of hibernoma, both microscopically and angiographically, is typically in sharp contrast to that of mature adult fat (175–180). The lesion shows an intense, homogeneous blush, with arteriovenous shunting that may resemble a soft tissue sarcoma (Fig. 4.48) (173,174). Hibernoma is often arranged in lobules, which are separated by fibrous septae (178). It is typically encapsulated but may infiltrate muscle or skin (172,173). The specific cytogenetic abnormality for hibernoma has been isolated to the long arm of chromosome 11 (11q13-21) and 10q22 (2;177).

There is limited experience with hibernoma on MR imaging. The MR appearance reflects the underlying pathology (171,173,181–184). Three distinct patterns are identified on CT and MR imaging (184). The typical hibernoma images similar, but not identical, to mature adult fat. These lesions also show prominent septations, with some lobular growth and serpentine/branching vessels (Fig. 4.49). In such cases, imaging may suggest a liposarcoma, but hibernoma can be distinguished by the vascular pattern. Diffuse hyperintensity is reported throughout the lesion on STIR imaging (185). Somewhat less commonly, the lipomalike hibernoma presents as a

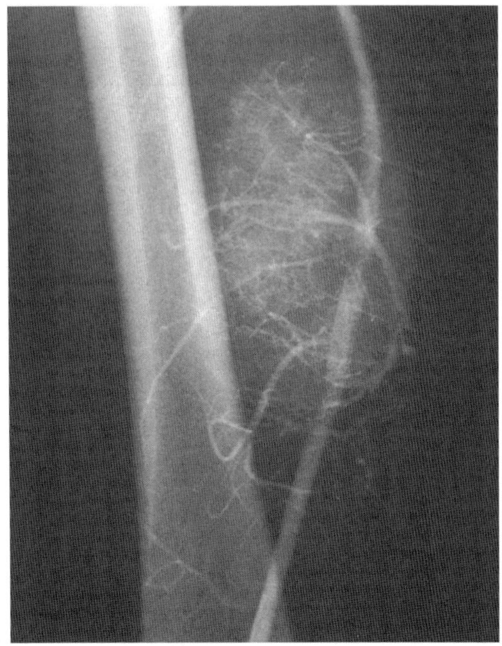

A

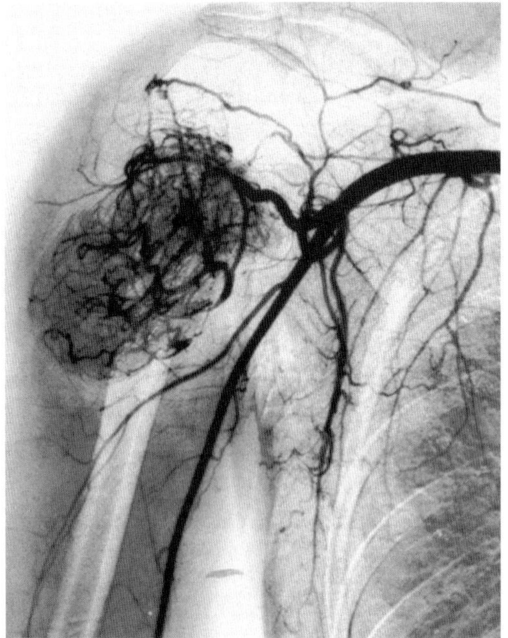

B

Figure 4.48 Hibernoma: Spectrum of angiographic findings. **A:** Midarterial phase film from conventional arteriogram in a man 27 years of age shows draping of vessels caused by mass, as well as areas of neovascularity. **B:** Early arterial phase subtraction film from conventional arteriogram in a woman 23 years of age shows a markedly hypervascular axillary mass with an intense blush and neovascularity. Early draining veins were identified on late arterial film.

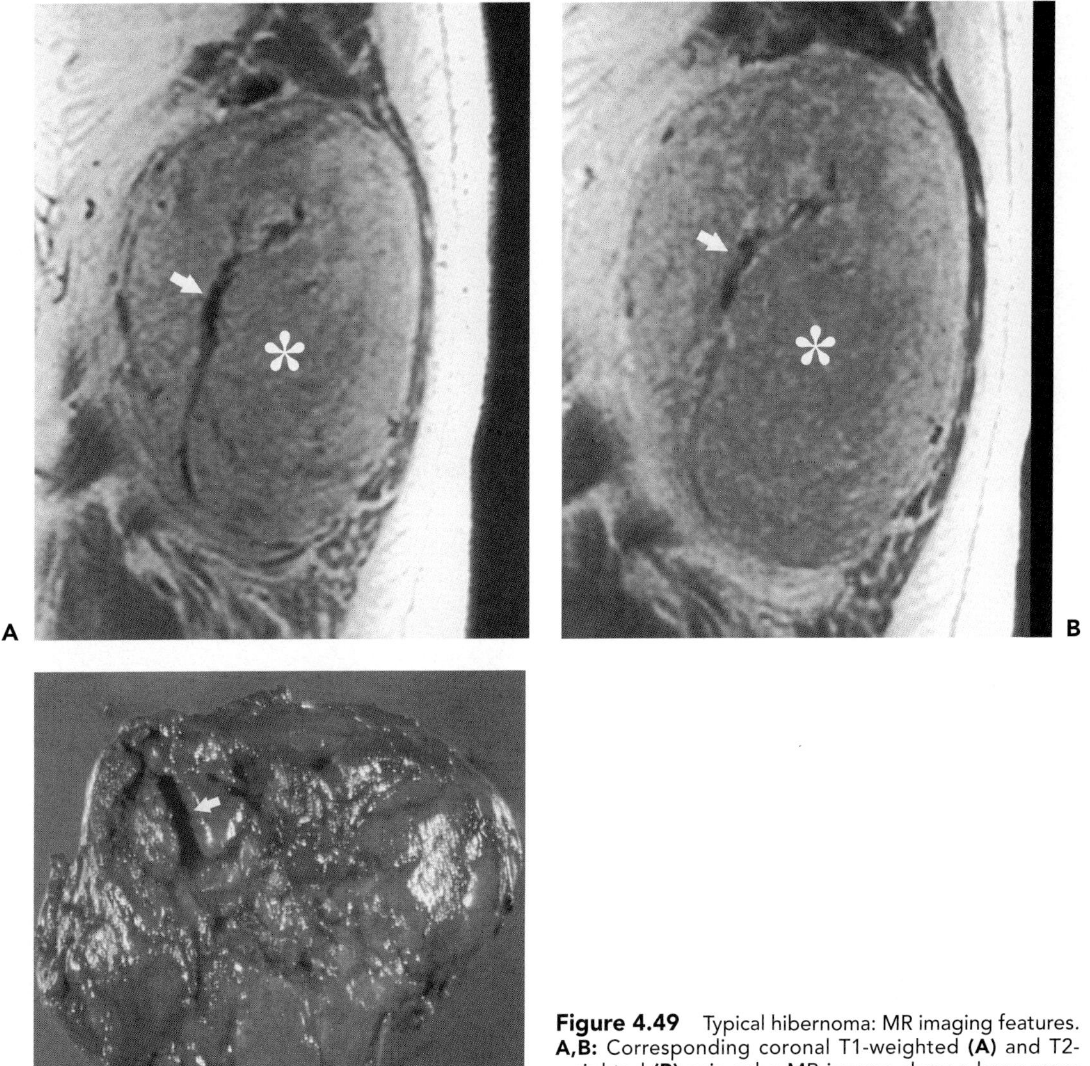

Figure 4.49 Typical hibernoma: MR imaging features. **A,B:** Corresponding coronal T1-weighted **(A)** and T2-weighted **(B)** spin-echo MR images show a large mass (*asterisk*) with a signal intensity similar to, but not identical to mature adult fat. Note prominent vascularity (*arrow*). **C:** Gross specimen shows lobulated mass with large branching vessels (*arrow*).

lesion largely composed of fat, with prominent septations and serpentine/branching vessels, with the vascularity demonstrating areas of both high and low flow (Fig. 4.50). The rare myxoid variant may show a nonspecific appearance with fluidlike signal intensity, reflecting its gross character (Fig. 4.51). Lesions enhance following gadolinium administration.

When imaged on CT, hibernoma is usually a well-defined lesion with tissue attenuation intermediate between that of fat and skeletal muscle, depending on the lipid content of the tumor (Fig. 4.50) (175,181,183). Lateur et al. (173), reported a case in which the margins were ill-defined on both CT and MR imaging, likely reflecting infiltration into adjacent muscle. On CT scanning, variable and heterogeneous enhancement may be seen following the administration of intravenous contrast material (171,173,175,179,181,183).

Sonography is nonspecific, showing the lesion to be well-circumscribed and hyperechoic (171,173,183). Doppler vascular ultrasound can demonstrate the increased tumor vascularity as well as large feeding vessels (183) (Fig. 4.52). Bone scintigraphy may demonstrate moderate uptake on blood-pool imaging and mild uptake on static imaging (186,187). Intense uptake is reported on Tc-99m Tetrofosmin and FDG positron emission tomographic (PET) scanning (186,187). These scintigraphic features are not typically seen with lipoma or well-differentiated liposarcoma and are a reflection of the hypervascularity and increased cellular activity and glucose turnover.

Treatment is complete surgical resection, and local recurrence does not occur with complete excision. There are no reports of metastases or malignant transformation.

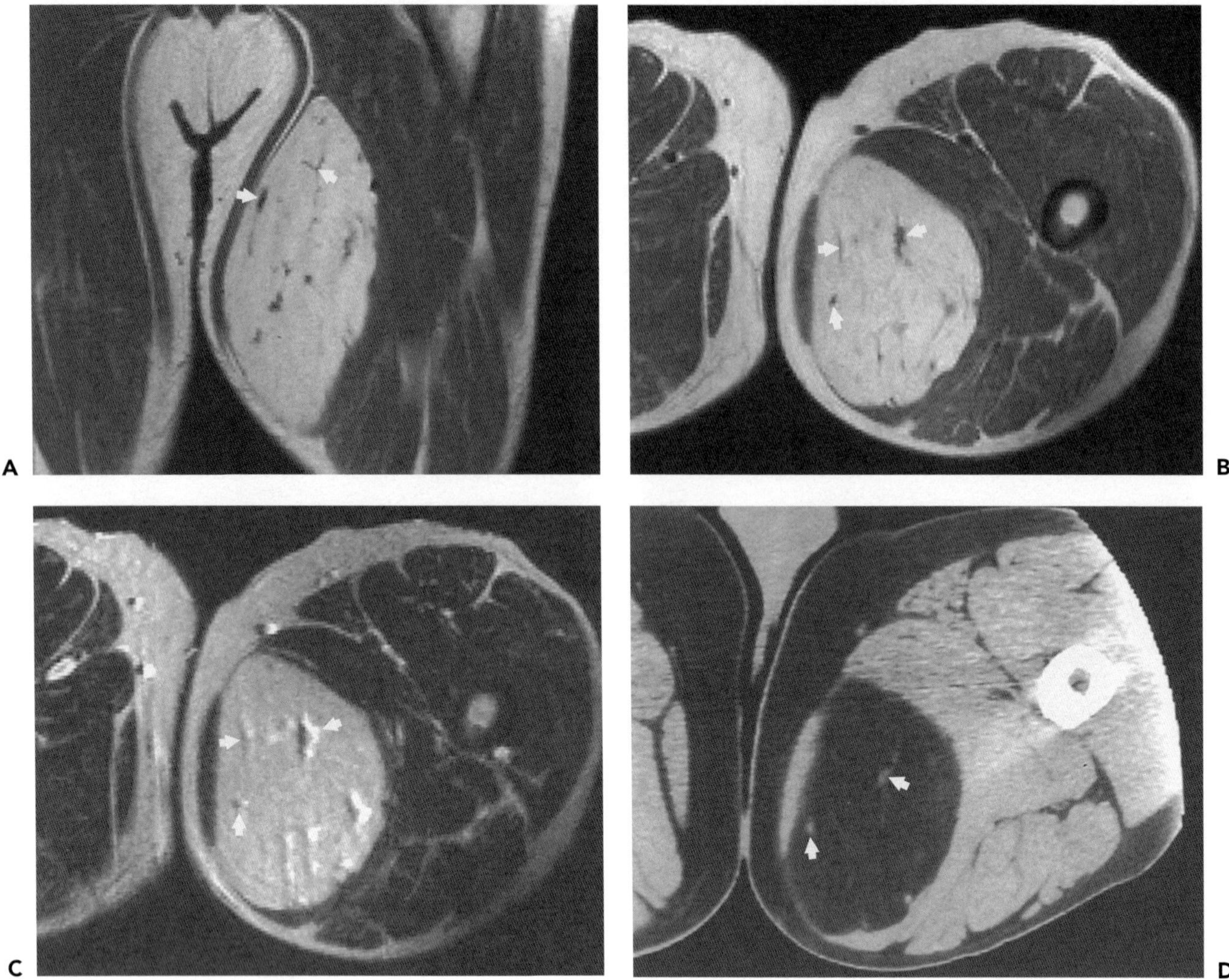

Figure 4.50 Lipomalike hibernoma: MR and CT imaging features. **A,B:** Coronal **(A)** and axial **(B)** T1-weighted spin-echo MR images of the thigh show a fatty mass with signal intensity identical to that of the adjacent fat. Note prominent vascularity within mass (*arrows*). **C:** Axial T2-weighted spin-echo MR image shows a similar signal intensity with prominent vessels (*arrows*). **D:** Axial noncontrast CT scan also shows the fatty nature of the mass and prominent vessels (*arrows*).

Parosteal Lipoma

KEY CONCEPTS
- Parosteal lipoma is a rare, fatty lesion arising from the surface of bone.
- It may be associated with compressive neuropathy, most commonly in the upper extremity.
- An osseous excrescence or cortical thickening is seen in most cases (67% to 100%).
- Surrounding fatty mass may show fibrovascular septations that may enhance.

Parosteal lipoma is an unusual lesion that represents approximately 0.3% of all lipomas (188). The lesion was originally described as a *periosteal lipoma* by Seering in 1836 (189), with the term *parosteal lipoma* subsequently suggested by Power (190), to indicate that the lesion does not arise within the periosteum. The term *parosteal lipoma* is generally accepted over *periosteal lipoma* because it indicates the juxtaposition of the lesion to the surface of the bone, without identifying the tissue of origin (188).

Patients are usually adults, averaging approximately 50 years of age (range: 4 to 64 years of age). There is a male predilection; lesions are most commonly in the thigh, forearm, calf, and arm, adjacent to the diaphysis or meta-diaphysis of bone (188,191–203). Approximately one-third of cases are adjacent to the femur (192). Virtually all lesions are solitary, with the exception of a single case reported by Goldman et al. (188), in which there was a coincident intramuscular lipoma. Patients typically present with a painless soft tissue mass; muscle atrophy is not uncommon (191). Parosteal lipoma occurring in the proximal radius has been associated with posterior interosseous nerve palsy (204,205). This complication is reported in

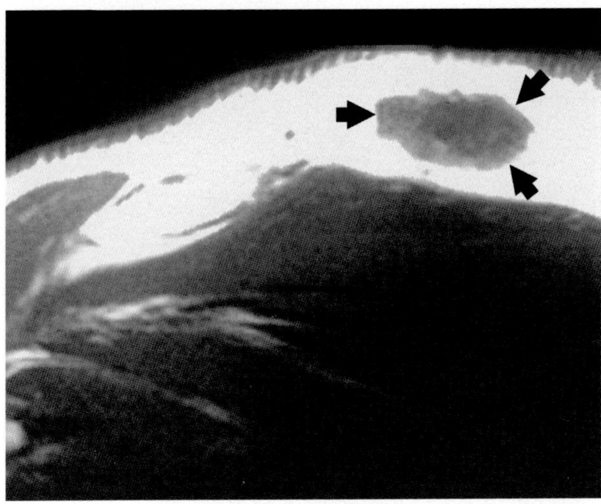
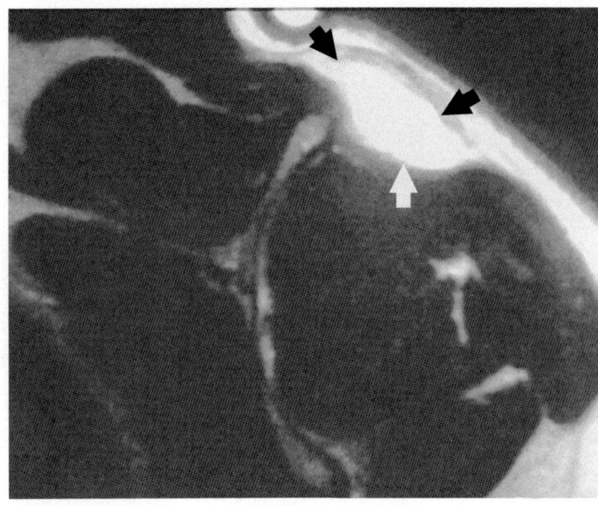

Figure 4.51   Myxoid hibernoma: MR imaging features. **A,B:** Oblique coronal T1-weighted (TR/TE; 583/16) **(A)** and oblique sagittal fast T2-weighted (TR/TE; 5833/114) **(B)** spin-echo MR images of the shoulder show a nonspecific mass with fluidlike signal intensity (*arrows*).

approximately a third of parosteal lipomas occurring in this location in patients who presented with weakness of the extensor muscles of the fingers, (without sensory loss) and the gradual onset of pain (204). In one study by Moon and Marmor, 11 of 20 cases (55%) showed nerve palsy that most commonly affected the posterior interosseus nerve (194). Involvement of the radial, sciatic, ulnar, and median nerves (in descending order) have also been reported (204–206).

Lesions are encapsulated and adherent to the underlying periosteum (191,207). Histologically, a parosteal lipoma is identical to a superficial or deep lipoma (188). Genetic analysis suggests a common histopathogenesis

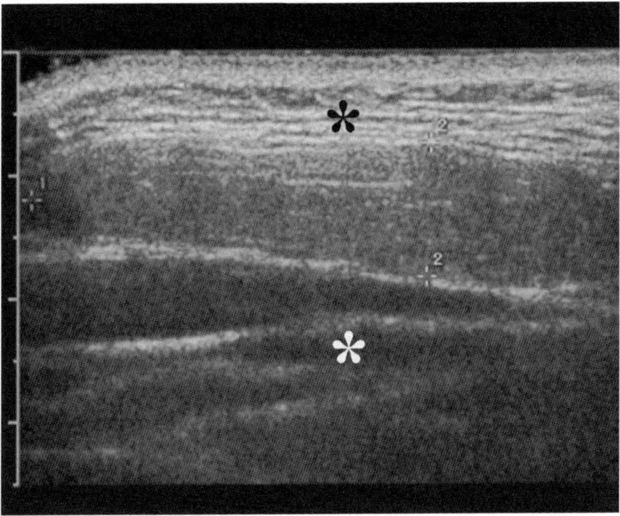

Figure 4.52   Typical hibernoma: Ultrasound imaging. Long axis imaging shows a well-defined mass that is slightly less echogenic than the adjacent subcutaneous fat (*black asterisk*) and more echogenic than the adjacent muscle (*white asterisk*). This appearance is similar to that of a lipoma.

between parosteal and soft tissue lipoma, in that both lesions demonstrate a 3;12 translocation (208); the diagnosis of a parosteal lipoma is made on the basis of the relationship of the lesion to the adjacent bone (207). Cases with malignant transformation have not been reported. Cartilage and bone metaplasia may be present. Cartilage is typically hyaline, but small foci of fibrocartilage may be seen at the periphery of large osseous excrescences (191). Depending on the degree of chondroid modulation and enchondral ossification, a parosteal lipoma may abut the cortex or have an osseous excrescence extending into a surrounding lipomatous mass (209). An osseous excrescence or cortical thickening is seen in most cases and may be because of tugging on the periosteum by the lipoma. Bone formation and mature hyaline cartilage is uncommonly seen within the body of the tumor (210). As with other lipomatous lesions, internal fibrovascular tissue septa may be present (191).

Radiographs reveal a well-defined radiolucent mass (162,188,191), and variable septa may be present within the mass (191). The adjacent bone may demonstrate solid periosteal reaction, cortical thickening, saucerization, or osseous excrescences (162,188,191). Osseous changes are seen in 67% to 100% of cases (188,191,207), although these changes may be subtle. The periosteal reaction in 2 of the 8 cases reported by Murphey et al. (191) was minimal, identified only on magnification radiography. The osseous excrescences associated with parosteal lipoma do not demonstrate cortical and medullary continuity as seen with a true osteochondroma (Fig. 4.53) (188). Bone scintigraphy typically shows increased tracer accumulation in areas of new bone production (191) (Fig. 4.53).

CT scanning demonstrates an osseous excrescence, as well as areas of cortical thickening and periosteal new bone.

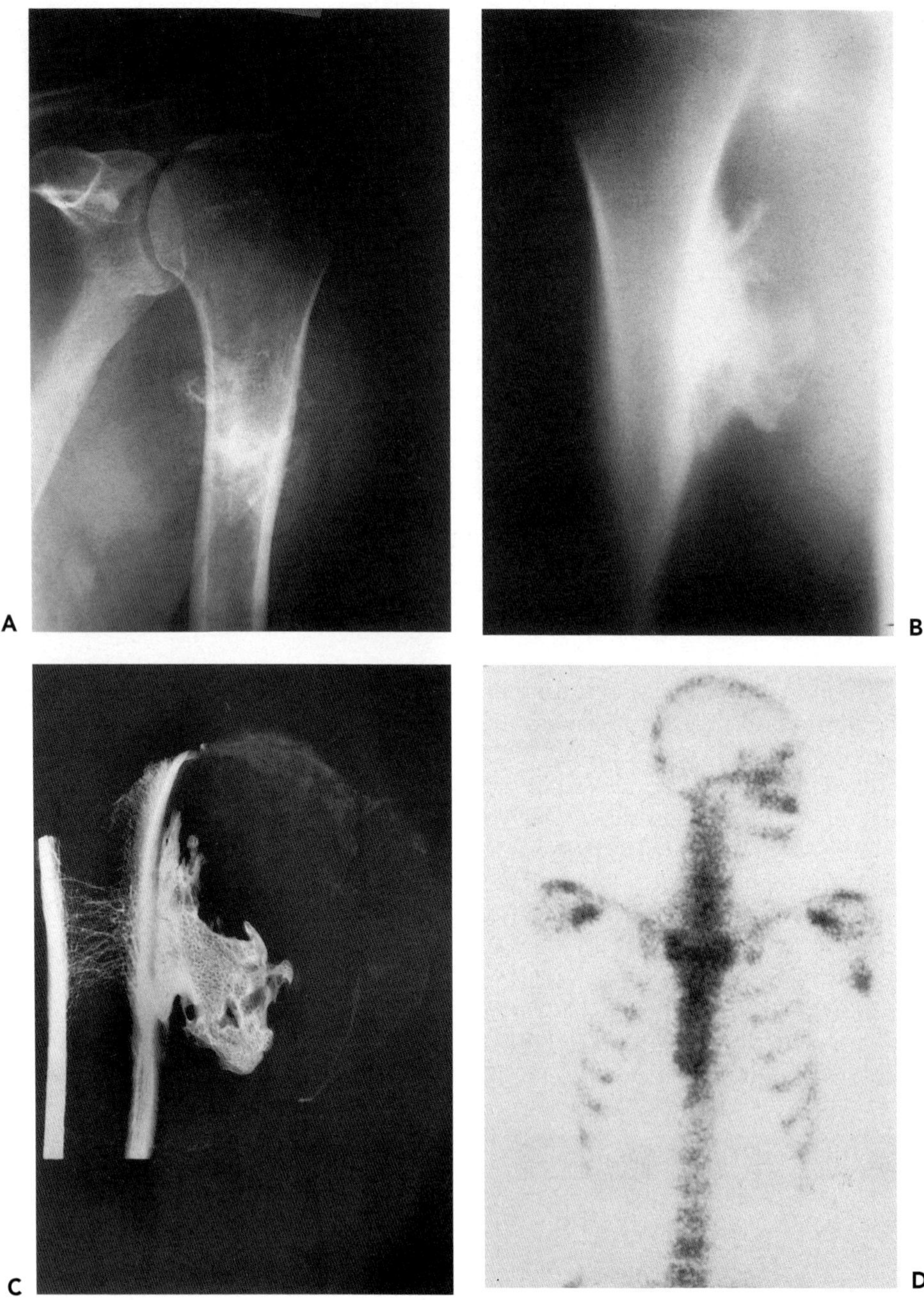

Figure 4.53 Parosteal lipoma: Radiographic and scintigraphic features in a woman 32 years of age with an upper extremity mass. **A:** Anteroposterior radiograph shows an osseous excrescence adjacent to the proximal humerus. **B,C:** Conventional tomogram **(B)** and specimen radiograph **(C)** nicely show the cortical thickening and mature bone formation, without the cortical and medullary continuity, as seen with a true osteochondroma. **D:** Delayed static image from bone scintigram shows focal increased tracer accumulation in the proximal left arm corresponding to uptake in the osseous excrescence.

CT also shows the lipomatous nature of the mass and septations that may be present within the mass (Fig. 4.54) (191). MR imaging demonstrates the fatty nature of the mass with a signal intensity identical to that of the subcutaneous fat on all pulse sequences (191,204,209). Fibrovascular tissue septa may demonstrate an increased signal intensity on long TR images, as may hyaline cartilage, which can also be found within lesions (191). MR imaging may also identify muscle atrophy as increased striations of fat within skeletal muscle resulting from compressive neuropathy, particularly in forearm lesions (Fig. 4.55). Following administration of intravenous gadolinium, the fibrous portions of the lesion may show mild enhancement (162).

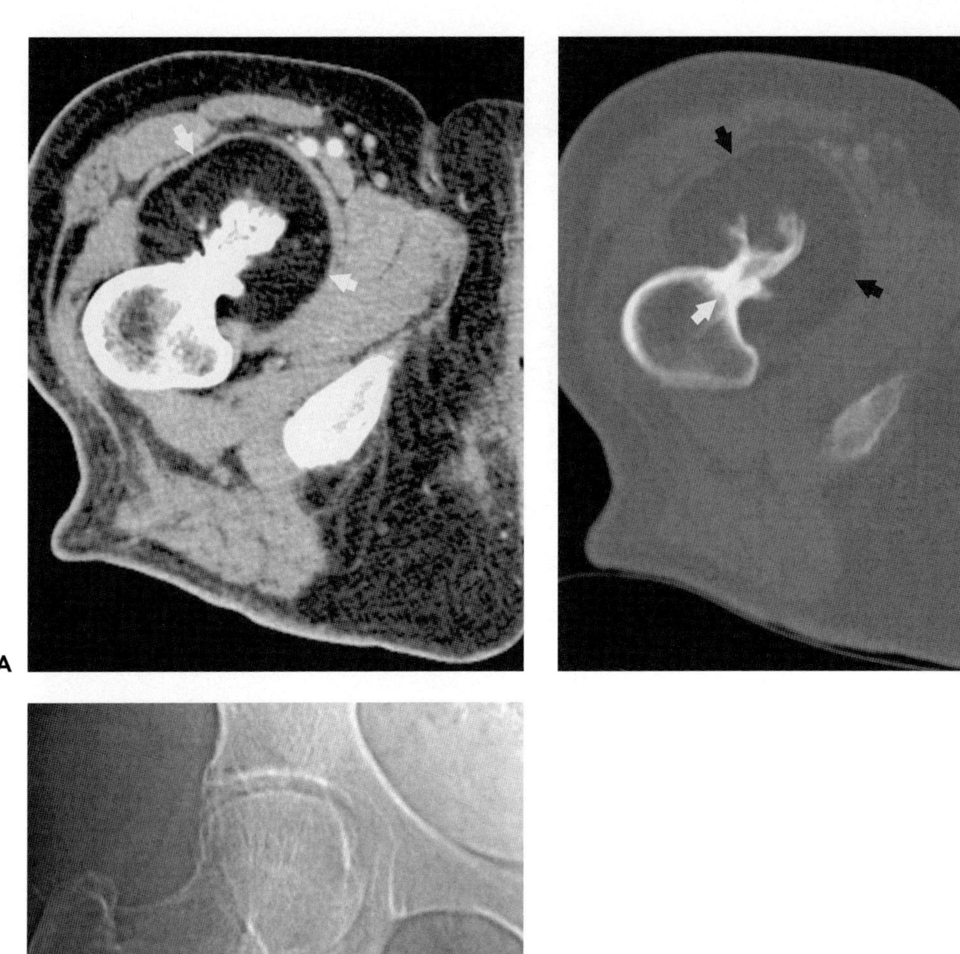

Figure 4.54 Parosteal lipoma: CT scanning features in a woman 68 years of age. **A:** Axial unenhanced CT scan displayed at soft tissue window shows a well-defined fatty mass (*arrows*) with an osseous excrescence arising from the surface of the femur. **B:** The same image displayed at bone window shows the osseous excrescence (*white arrow*) to better advantage. Note osseous character of excrescence and absence of cortical and medullary continuity. The fatty nature of the mass (*black arrows*) is readily appreciated. **C:** Scout image shows the osseous nature of the lesion. The surrounding fatty mass (*arrows*) is difficult to appreciate.

Treatment of parosteal lipoma is complete surgical resection. In cases with nerve entrapment, removal prior to irreversible muscle atrophy is important to maintain function (191, 204–206). The nerve must also be separated from the parosteal lipoma and spared during surgical excision. At surgery, parosteal lipomas are characteristically encapsulated and strongly adherent to the underlying periosteum. The site of the strongest attachment to the underlying bone is at the areas of most prominent osseous proliferation. This is important for surgical removal, in that resection requires either subperiosteal dissection or segmental resection for adequate removal, unlike a soft tissue lipoma, which simply lies adjacent to bone. Local recurrence is unusual but is reported. There are no reports of malignant transformation.

Treatment of Benign Fatty Tumors

> KEY CONCEPTS
> - Small asymptomatic lesions do not require excision.
> - When surgery is required, the goal is to remove the lesion completely, to minimize risk of local recurrence while avoiding significant functional impairment.

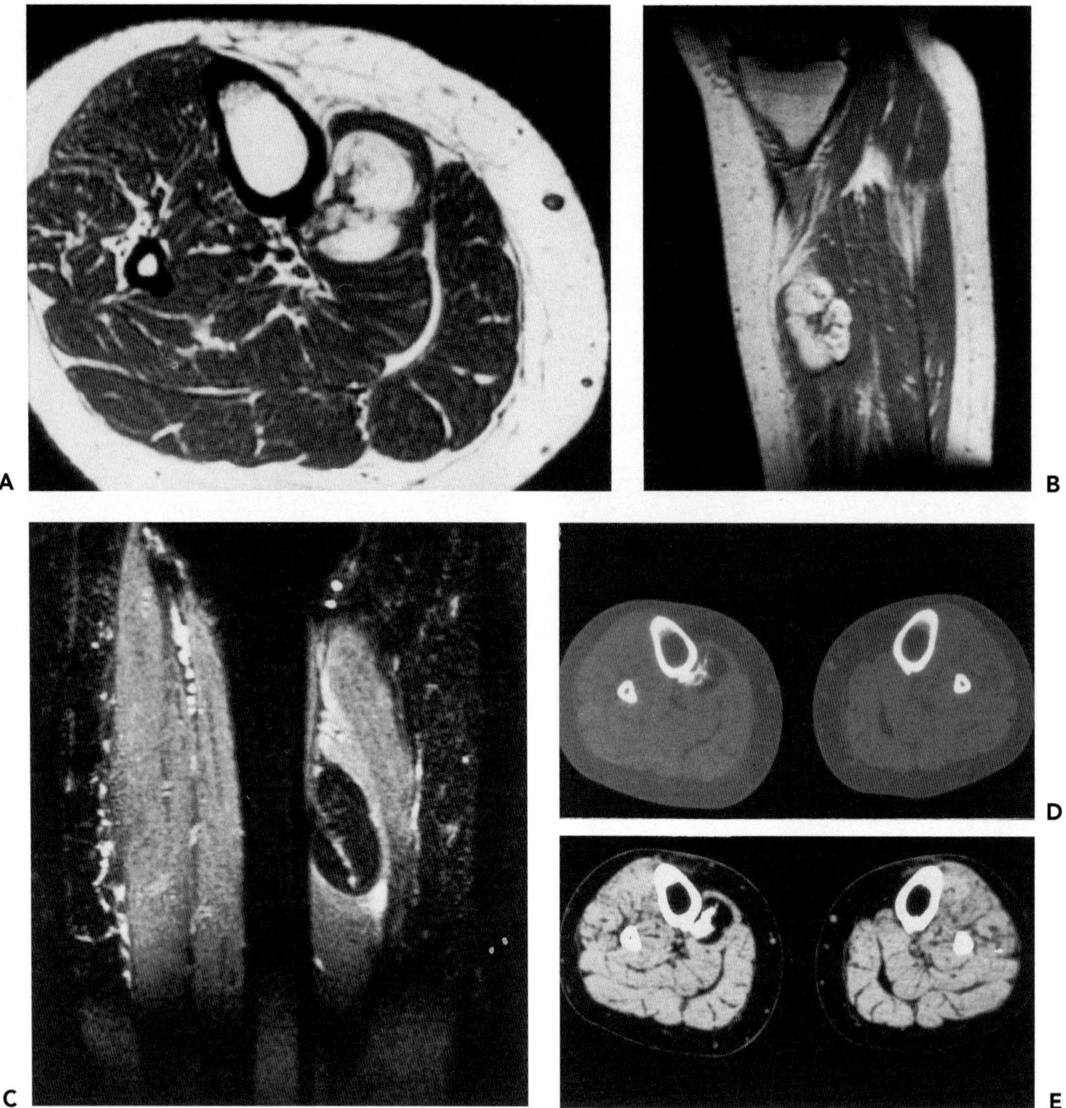

Figure 4.55 Parosteal lipoma: MR and CT imaging features in a woman 40 years of age with lesion in the lower leg. **A,B:** Axial T1-weighted (TR/TE; 500/20) **(A)** and sagittal T2-weighted (TR/TE; 2500/100) **(B)** MR images show the fatty nature of the mass with a signal intensity identical to that of subcutaneous fat on all pulse sequences. The osseous excrescence appears as an irregular linear region of decreased signal intensity. **C:** Coronal STIR (TR/TE/TI; 2000/43/160) image shows some increased signal within the lesion, which is likely caused by fibrovascular tissue and hyaline cartilage. **D,E:** Axial CT scans at bone **(D)** and soft tissue **(E)** windows demonstrate the osseous excrescence as well as the lipomatous nature of the mass. Areas of cortical thickening and periosteal new bone may be better seen on CT. *(continued)*

Treatment of benign fatty tumors depends on the degree of clinical symptoms related to the lesion, the location and growth pattern of the tumor, and concern regarding a potential malignant histology. From a surgical treatment standpoint, fatty tumors can be categorized as superficial versus deep and well-defined versus infiltrative. In general, small subcutaneous lipomas (either encapsulated or not) that are asymptomatic do not require surgical excision; however, observation of such lesions is still appropriate. If the patient notes growth of the mass or the development of symptoms, reevaluation by the physician is appropriate. Excision of a subcutaneous fatty tumor should be approached with the goal of complete removal of the lesion while not performing an overly aggressive procedure. This may be achieved with a so-called shelling-out procedure if the lesion is encapsulated. For nonencapsulated superficial fatty tumors, the margins of surgical resection are defined by the clinical and radiographic extent of the lesion.

Deep-seated lipomas are typically treated with surgical excision. The goal is to remove the lesion completely and minimize the risk of recurrence while sparing the normal surrounding tissue to avoid functional impairment. For a

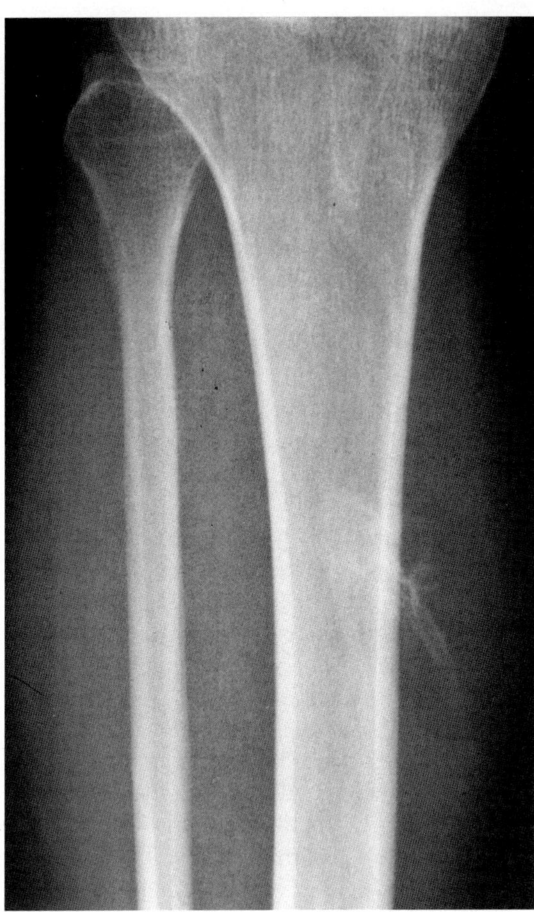

F

Figure 4.55 *(continued)*   **F:** Anteroposterior radiograph shows a well-defined radiolucent mass with associated osseous excrescence.

typical well-defined intramuscular lipoma, the mass can be excised with a thin cuff of surrounding muscle, without functional compromise. Infiltrative deep lipomas can be challenging resections with residual microscopic disease. This is typically the case when the lesion is adjacent to or encircles vital neurovascular structures. Such residual microscopic disease portends a high risk of local recurrence. Although local failure can be minimized with a more aggressive surgical resection, the potential for permanent functional loss tempers this approach. Such patients are appropriately followed with serial MR imaging to monitor for local disease relapse.

In unusual cases in which there is extensive infiltrative growth, function-sparing surgery may not permit even gross tumor removal. Surgery may be considered if symptoms related to the mass justify intervention. A debulking procedure can then be performed with the expectation by the patient that tumor regrowth is possible and even likely.

LIPOSARCOMA

Liposarcoma is a relatively common, yet diverse, soft tissue malignancy with a variety of clinical presentations. It is the second most common soft tissue sarcoma following malignant fibrous histiocytoma, accounting for approximately 16% to 18% of all soft tissue tumors (17) and having an estimated annual incidence of 2.5 per million (211). It remains the most variable and diverse mesenchymal tumor, with a wide spectrum of imaging appearances that reflect this histologic heterogeneity (212). Several subtypes are described, ranging from lesions nearly entirely composed of mature adipose tissue to tumors with very sparse fatty elements. The imaging appearance of these fatty masses is frequently sufficiently characteristic to allow a specific diagnosis. In other cases, although a specific diagnosis is not achievable, a meaningful limited differential diagnosis can be established. Unfortunately, there are those lesions in which imaging remains completely nonspecific.

Classification

KEY CONCEPTS

Malignant fatty tumors are classified into four main groups:
- Well-differentiated liposarcoma; low-grade tumor that recurs locally but does not metastasize; termed *atypical lipomatous tumor* when superficial.
- Dedifferentiated liposarcoma; bimorphic lesion with high-grade pleomorphic sarcoma (of nonadipose cell line) intimately associated with low-grade well-differentiated liposarcoma.
- Myxoid liposarcoma; intermediate-grade tumor, hypercellular form is a high-grade tumor (hypercellular form formerly designated as *round cell liposarcoma*).
- Pleomorphic liposarcoma; high-grade, least common form.

The current system used for the classification of liposarcoma stems from the landmark work by Enzinger and Winslow in 1962 (213). In a review of 103 cases, they recognized the diversity of liposarcoma and proposed the division of tumors into subtypes. At present, the WHO Committee for the Classification of Soft Tissue Tumors uses an extension of this division and identifies four distinct subtypes of liposarcoma: well-differentiated, dedifferentiated, myxoid, and pleomorphic (1). These subtypes recognize the great variation in clinical behavior and histologic appearance of liposarcoma. Additionally, a *mixed-type* liposarcoma, showing combinations of the previously noted subtypes, is defined (1).

For radiologic diagnosis, we find it useful to group together well-differentiated and dedifferentiated liposarcoma, as described by Weiss and Goldblum (213). This grouping recognizes the radiologic similarities between the well-differentiated and dedifferentiated subtypes because the former may give rise to the latter. Well-differentiated liposarcoma is the most common subtype of liposarcoma,

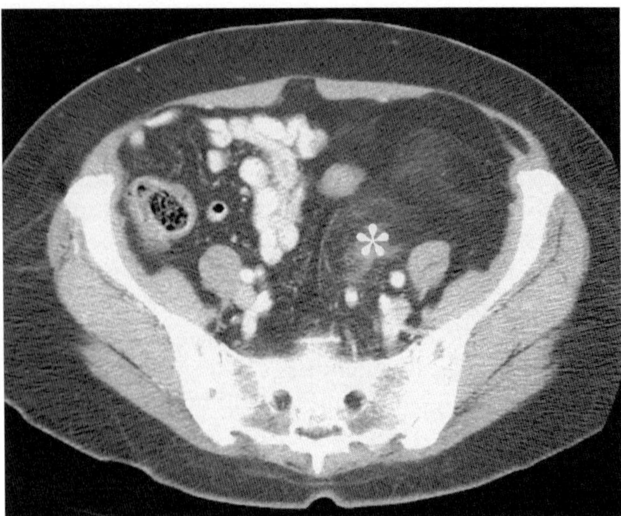

Figure 4.56 Liposarcoma: Infiltrating margin of retroperitoneal tumor in a 60-year-old woman. Axial enhanced CT scan shows a retroperitoneal well-differentiated liposarcoma (*asterisk*). The margins of the lesion are quite poorly defined, making complete excision virtually impossible.

representing approximately half of all liposarcomas (211,214). Grossly, and it may resemble a lipoma (212). Well-differentiated liposarcoma is a low-grade tumor with no propensity to metastasize, and is also designated *atypical lipomatous tumor* by the WHO. Other names for well-differentiated liposarcoma/atypical lipomatous tumor include *atypical lipoma-like liposarcoma* and *adipcytic liposarcoma*.

The terms *atypical lipoma* and *atypical intramuscular lipoma* were introduced into the medical literature by Evans et al. in 1979 (100). They argued that subcutaneous and intramuscular tumors having the histologic appearance of well-differentiated liposarcoma should be designated as atypical lipoma and atypical intramuscular lipoma, respectively, "because they do not constitute a sufficient danger to life to be considered sarcoma" (100). In 1988, Evans grouped these lesions with well-differentiated liposarcoma under the designation of atypical lipomatous tumor, concluding that differences in behavior are related to tumor location rather than to histologic appearance (215). Accordingly, the new WHO Classification of Soft Tissue Tumors notes that atypical lipomatous tumor and well-differentiated liposarcoma are identical morphologically and karyotypically; consequently, it recommends that the term *well-differentiated liposarcoma* be retained for lesions located at sites at which a wide surgical margin cannot be obtained (1). Such sites include the retroperitoneum and mediastinum (1). Although there is no agreement on the terminology for lesions in the deep somatic soft tissues, we agree with Weiss and Goldblum and their use of the term *atypical lipoma* only for subcutaneous extremity lesions, reserving the term *well-differentiated liposarcoma* for lesions with similar histologies in all remaining sites (5,212).

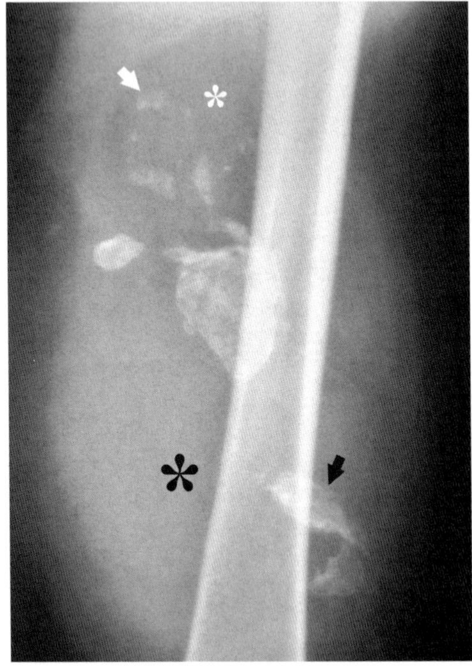

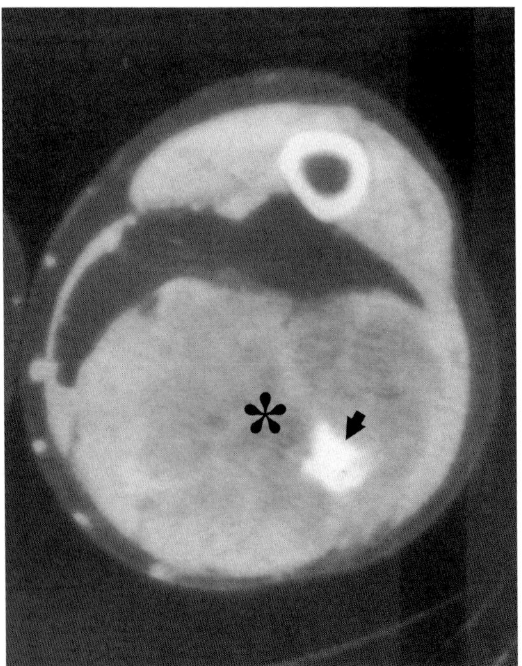

A   **B**

Figure 4.57 Liposarcoma: Radiographic features. **A:** Anteroposterior radiograph of the thigh shows a large mass. The fatty nature of the proximal aspect of the mass (*white asterisk*) is well-seen, whereas the distal portion of the mass (*black asterisk*) is not specific. Note metaplastic bone (*white arrow*) and nonspecific calcifications proximally as well as distally (*black arrow*). **B:** Axial CT scan through the lower portion of this dedifferentiated liposarcoma shows a large nonadipose component to the mass (*black asterisk*) with focal mineralization (*arrow*).

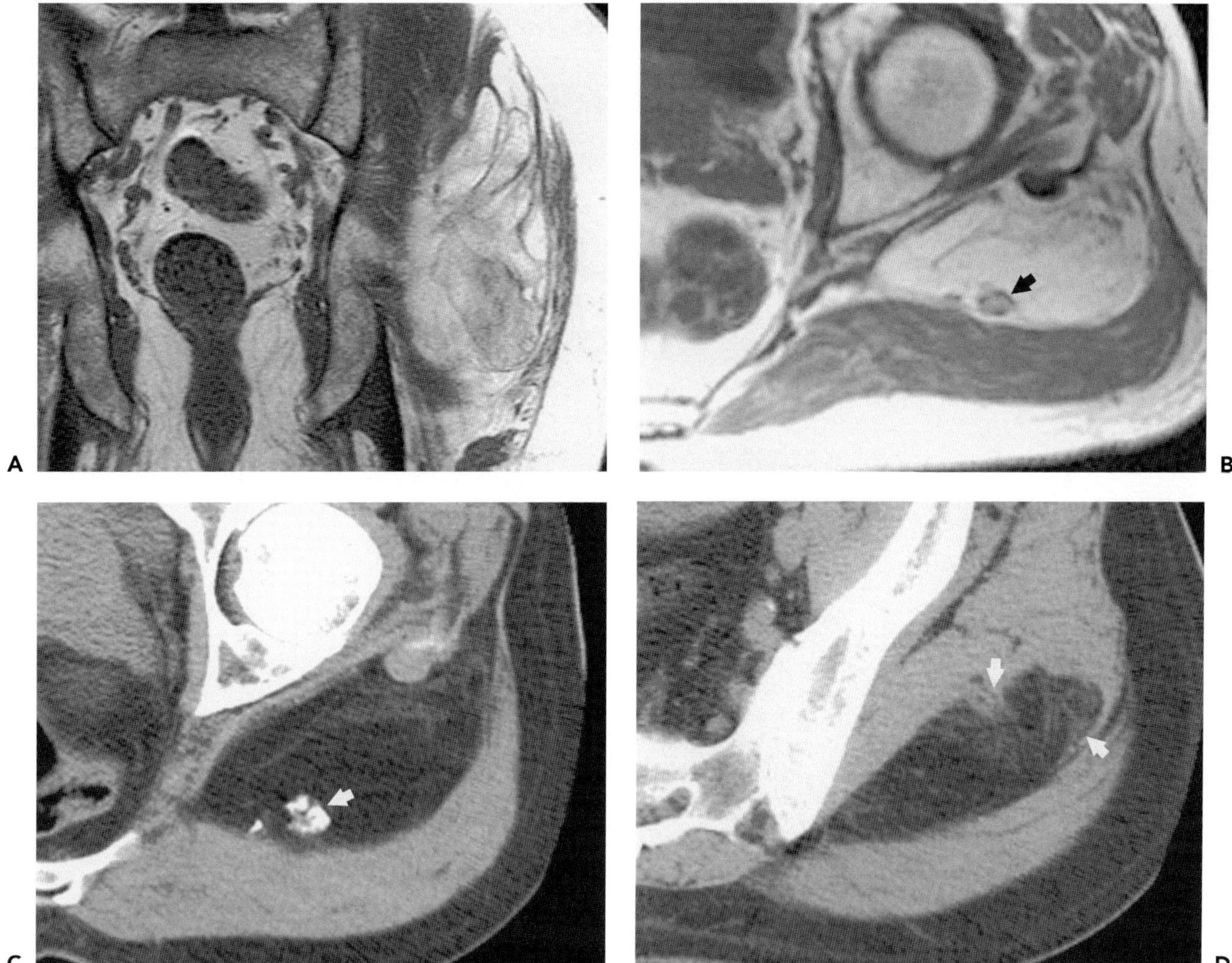

Figure 4.58 Well-differentiated liposarcoma: Typical MR and CT imaging features in a woman 76 years of age with a mass in the buttocks. **A:** Coronal T1-weighted (TR/TE; 400/12) spin-echo MR image shows a predominantly fatty mass with multiple thickened septa, as well as poorly defined areas of nonadipose tissue infiltrating the fat. **B:** Axial T1-weighted (TR/TE; 683/16) spin-echo MR image also demonstrates prominent nonadipose areas laterally, as well as a rounded soft tissue density posteriorly (*arrow*), representing a calcification. **C:** Corresponding axial noncontrast CT shows the calcification to better advantage. **D:** Axial CT cranial to C shows a greater amount of nonadipose tissue within the lesion laterally (*arrows*). (*continued*)

The dedifferentiated liposarcoma is a distinct subtype of liposarcoma, although it is closely related to the well-differentiated liposarcoma pathogenetically (212). The dedifferentiated liposarcoma is a bimorphic neoplasm in which a histologically different high-grade sarcoma, typically a malignant fibrous histiocytoma or fibrosarcoma, arises in intimate association with a well-differentiated liposarcoma (99,214,216). Dedifferentiated liposarcoma is uncommon outside the retroperitoneum but is being reported with increasing frequency (217,218). The risk of dedifferentiation is estimated at 15% for retroperitoneal lesions and approximately 5% for extremity tumors (212,217). Dedifferentiation may be, at least in part, time-related, and when present, dedifferentiation occurs approximately 7 to 8 years following presentation, although there is a wide spectrum (217).

Although previously identified as distinct subtypes by the WHO Classification of Soft Tissue Tumors, the myxoid and round cell liposarcoma are now combined under the designation of *myxoid liposarcoma* (1). These lesions are known to form a histologic continuum and represent the ends of a common spectrum (5). Now under a single diagnosis, the pure myxoid lesion is considered an intermediate-grade tumor at the low-grade end of this spectrum, whereas the hypercellular (round cell) morphology represents the histologically similar high-grade counterpart. The presence of the hypercellular (round cell) component is associated with a more aggressive clinical course and a significantly worse prognosis (214). The radiologic images of these lesions also form an overlapping spectrum, which further supports this classification.

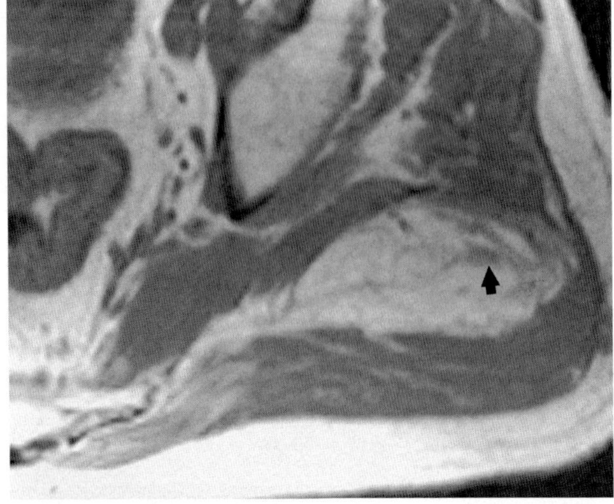

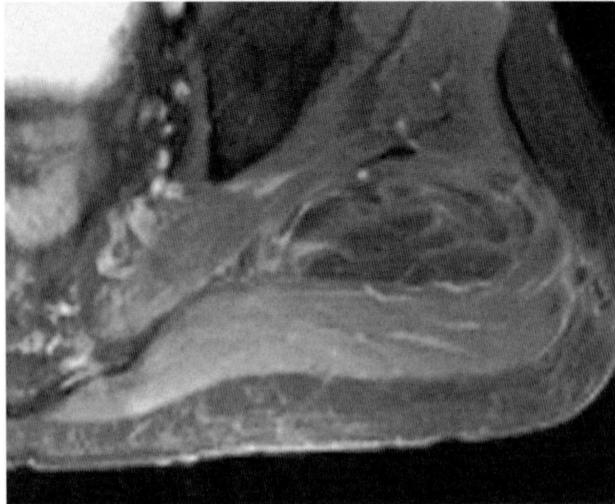

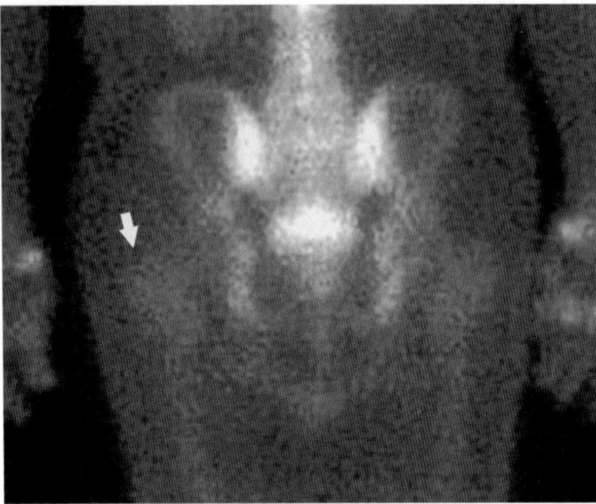

Figure 4.58 *(continued)*   **E:** Axial T1-weighted (TR/TE; 638/16) spin-echo MR image cranial to the calcification shows irregularly thickened septa (*arrow*) with poorly defined nonadipose signal laterally. **F:** Corresponding axial fat-suppressed T1-weighted (TR/TE; 650/15) spin-echo MR image following gadolinium administration shows significant enhancement of the nonadipose components. **G:** Delayed posterior image from bone scintigram shows minimal increased tracer accumulation in the mass (*arrow*).

Pleomorphic is the rarest subtype of liposarcoma, accounting for 5% to 10% of all liposarcomas (17,212, 214). Pleomorphic liposarcoma is a high-grade lesion, typically occurring in the extremities. Pleomophic liposarcoma has two distinct, but related forms: that resembling a malignant fibrous histiocytoma (MFH) and the less common cellular pleomorphic/mononuclear cell form. On occasion, the latter mimics carcinoma or melanoma (212,214). Approximately 5% to 12% of liposarcomas cannot be readily subclassified (17,212).

Clinical Presentation

Most patients with liposarcoma, as with other soft tissue sarcomas, present with a painless soft tissue mass. Pain and tenderness, however, is reported in approximately 10% to 15% of patients. Liposarcoma has a predilection for the extremities, with this location accounting for approximately 66% to 75% of lesions (17,212,217,219). The lower extremity is involved approximately four times more commonly than the upper extremity, although distal extremity

> ### KEY CONCEPTS
> - Liposarcoma is relatively common, representing 16% to 18% of all soft tissue sarcomas.
> - Most patients present with a painless mass; pain and tenderness is seen in 10% to 15%.
> - Lesions are most common in extremities (66% to 75%); lower extremity involvement is four times more common than upper extremity.
> - Liposarcomas are very rare in children; most pediatric fatty masses are lipoblastoma.

lesions (wrist/hand and ankle/foot) are quite rare and account for only 1% to 2% of all lesions (17). Approximately 20% to 33% of lesions originate in the retroperitoneum (212,217,219).

It is difficult to determine the true prevalence and distribution of the liposarcoma subtypes in that extremity and retroperitoneal tumors are often reported separately. Moreover, such data must be acquired from a referral

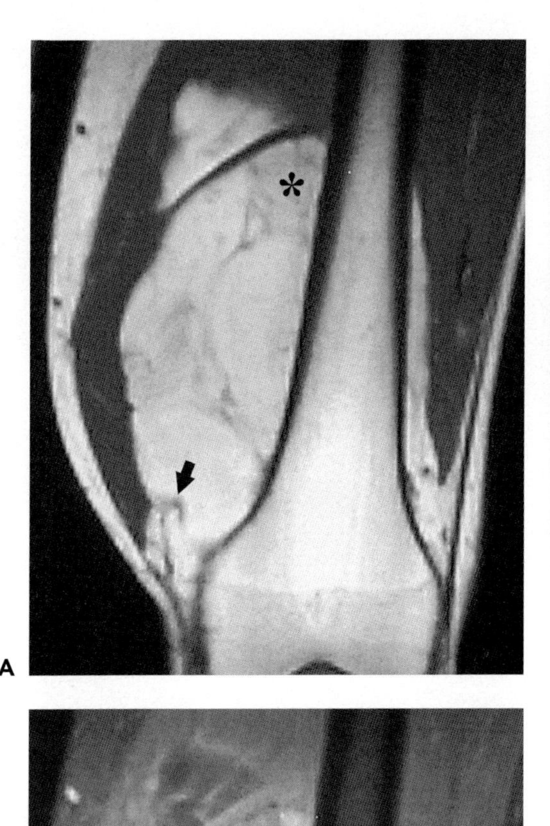

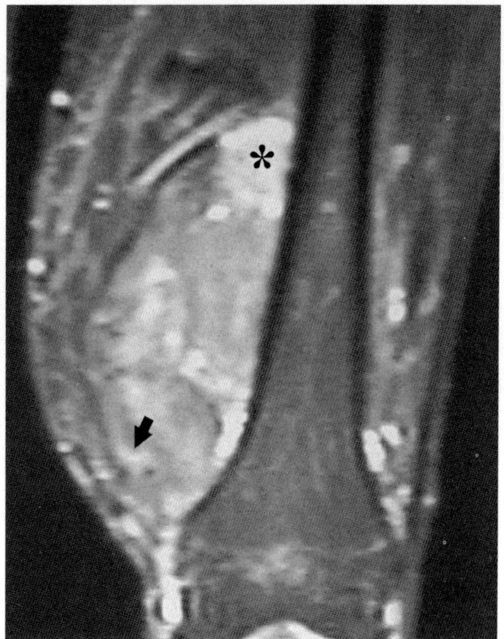

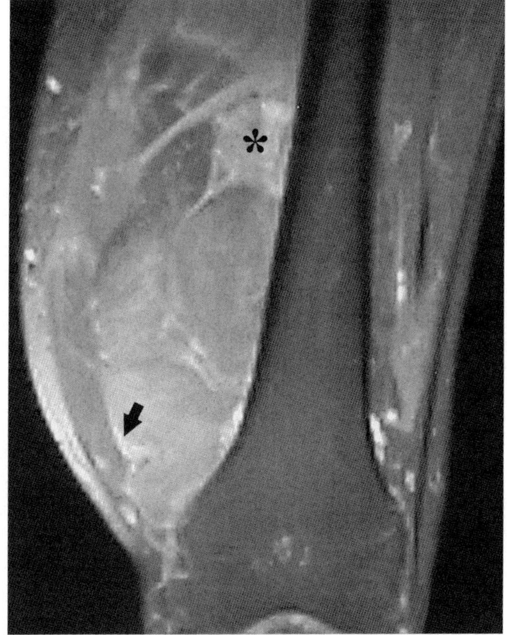

Figure 4.59 Well-differentiated liposarcoma: Typical MR imaging features in a man 74 years of age with a mass in the thigh. **A:** Coronal T1-weighted (TR/TE; 493/14) spin-echo MR image shows irregular septa (*arrow*) with a large amount of "altered" fat, most prominent in the proximal aspect of the mass (*asterisk*). **B:** Corresponding STIR (TR/TE/TI; 5542/60/150) MR image shows the nonadipose areas to have an increased signal intensity relative to that of fat. **C:** Fat-saturated T1-weighted (TR/TE; 782/14) spin-echo MR image following administration of contrast shows moderate heterogeneous enhancement of the nonadipose areas.

population and, as such, surely incorporate a referral bias. These caveats must be kept in mind in reviewing the AFIP data presented here (12,17).

Patients with extremity lesions present 5 to 10 years prior to patients with retroperitoneal tumors, presumably because the former are more readily detected (212). The age range of patients with liposarcomas parallels that of benign lipomas, with a majority occurring in the fifth and sixth decades. Liposarcomas are exceedingly rare in infants and children. Most lipomatous lesions in children that do not meet the requirements for lipoma are lipoblastoma (13). In a review of more than 2,500 cases of liposarcoma at the AFIP, only 2 (0.08%) occurred in children younger

than 10 years. Fifteen additional cases were identified in children between 11 and 15 years of age (77). Childhood liposarcoma is typically myxoid (76%), located in the extremities (51%), and has a lower recurrence rate than its adult counterpart (37% versus 72%) (185,186).

Natural History and Prognosis

The clinical course and prognosis of liposarcoma vary according to subtype, as does propensity for local recurrence and distant metastases. In general terms, local recurrence is more common and seen in approximately 25% to 43% of extremity lesions, whereas it is found in 90% to 100% of

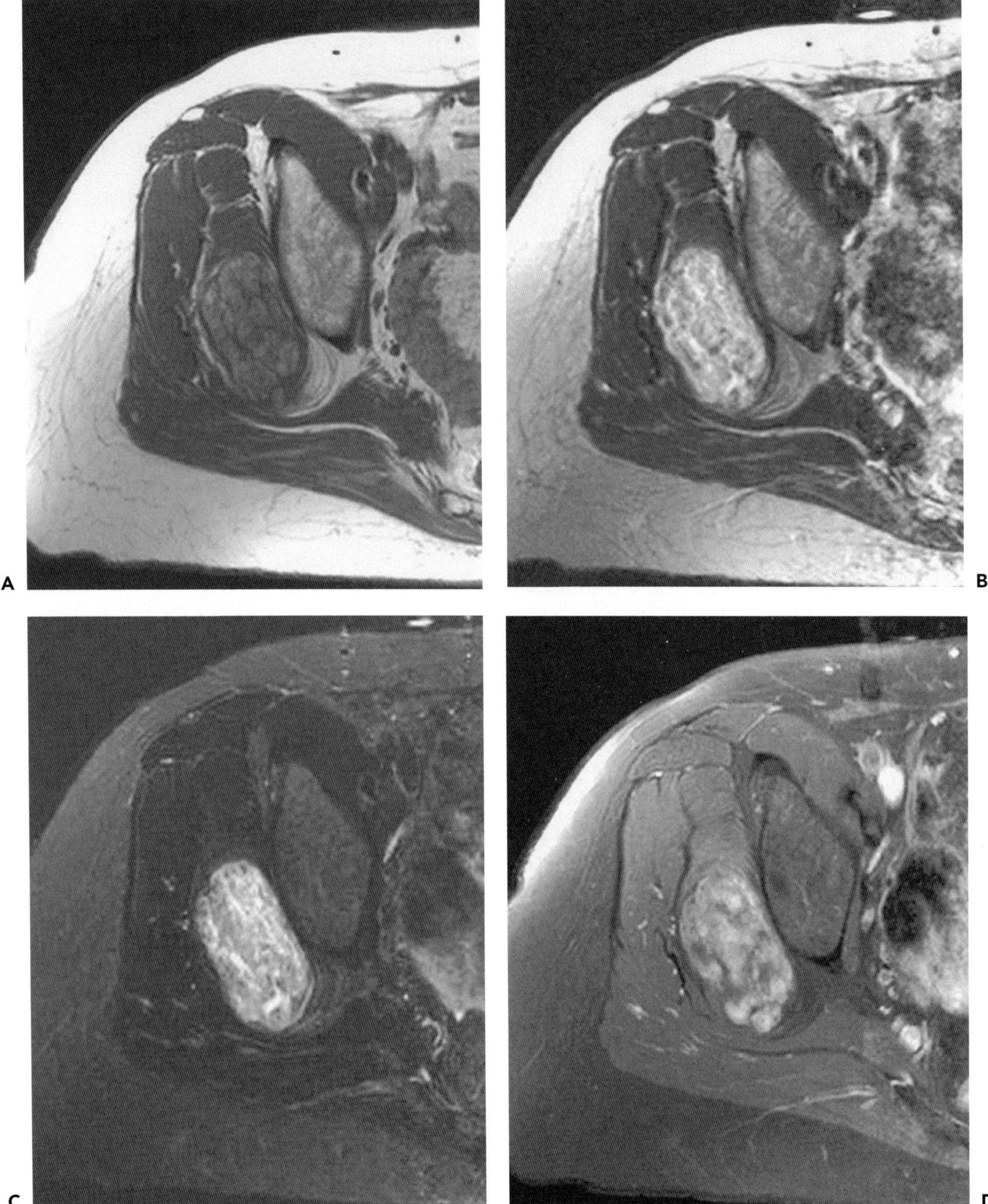

Figure 4.60 Well-differentiated liposarcoma: Atypical MR and CT imaging features in a woman 79 years of age with a mass in the buttocks. **A,B:** Axial T1-weighted (TR/TE; 400/12) **(A)** and T2-weighted (TR/TE; 2000/80) **(B)** spin-echo MR images show a heterogeneous mass with extensive "dirty" fat and nonspecific nonadipose tissue. **C:** Axial STIR (TR/TE/TI; 6270/80/150) image shows a greater signal intensity to the nonadipose areas. **D:** Axial enhanced fat-suppressed T1-weighted (TR/TE; 594/16) spin-echo MR image shows extensive enhancement. (*continued*)

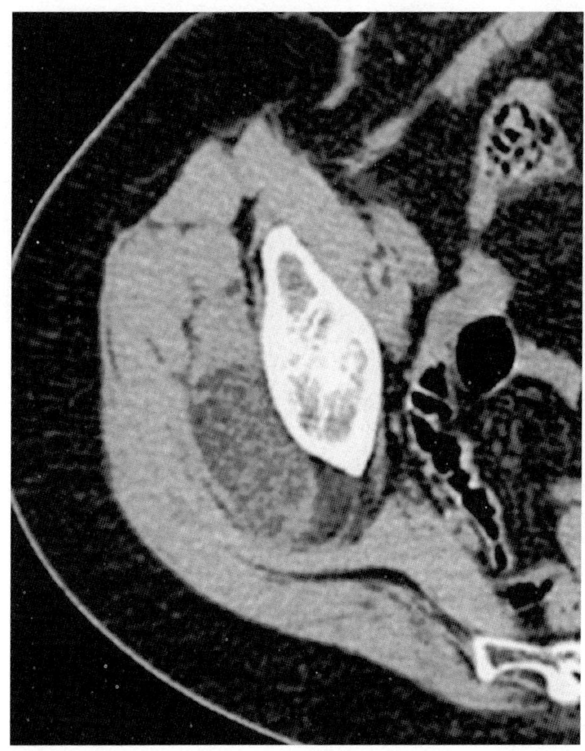

E

Figure 4.60 *(continued)*   **E:** Corresponding noncontrast axial CT shows the heterogeneous character of the mass with prominent nonadipose tissue.

KEY CONCEPTS

- Clinical course varies with subtype; overall recurrence in 67%, metastases in 50%; local recurrence approaches 100% for retroperitoneal tumors.
- Well-differentiated lesions are considered to be non-metastasizing.
- Myxoid lesions show a variable natural history depending on the hypercellular (round cell) component; 10-year survival is 70%, but falls to 40% if there is a dominant round cell component.
- Pleomorphic subtype is a high-grade sarcoma with a 40% 5-year survival.
- Dedifferentiation occurs in 10% to 15% of retroperitoneal tumors; uncommon in extremity lesions; guarded prognosis.

---

retroperitoneal tumors (212,217). Overall, local recurrence is seen in approximately two-thirds of patients, whereas metastases are seen in approximately half of patients (222–224). Metastases are most common to the lungs, and patients with pulmonary metastases have a 5-year survival rate approaching 60% (212,224). These figures vary with subtype, tumor location, and size.

Patients with well-differentiated liposarcoma have a relatively good prognosis compared to that for the other subtypes. In clinical practice, a well-differentiated liposarcoma is considered to be a nonmetastasizing lesion, although it demonstrates a significant propensity for local recurrence

when in the retroperitoneum because of the difficulty in obtaining adequate surgical margins.

The natural history of myxoid liposarcoma is difficult to define accurately in that the lesion may coexist with the hypercellular, higher grade (round cell) component. Failure to separate these lesions likely accounts for the wide spectrum of reported survival rates (5). Evans (215) correlated survival rate with the round cell component, dividing tumors into those with less than 5% round cell; those with 5% to 25% round cell; and those having more than 25% round cell. The 10-year survival rate for patients with these lesions ranges from approximately 70% for lesions that were myxoid (<5% round cell) to 40% for lesions with a dominant hypercellular (round cell) component (215).

The myxoid subtype also has a striking predilection for extrapulmonary metastases. In a 13-year study of 102 patients with extremity myxoid liposarcoma, Pearlstone et al. (225) found a 5-year disease-free survival rate of 73%. Of the 33 (32%) patients who developed metastatic disease, 31 (94%) had metastases to the extrapulmonary soft tissue (retroperitoneum, chest wall, pleura, pericardium, pelvic sidewall, and soft tissue), whereas only 2 (6%) had metastases to the lung. This was in sharp contrast to the 18 patients with the pleomorphic subtype, 10 (56%) of whom developed metastatic disease, 7 (70%) of which were to the lungs and only 3 (30%) to extrapulmonary sites. The pleomorphic liposarcoma is an aggressive, high-grade sarcoma with a high propensity for metastases and local recurrence, and it has a 5-year survival rate of only 40% (226). In a long-term study of 66 patients who were followed at least 10 years, Evans noted metastases and recurrence in all of 3 pleomorphic liposarcomas, and metastases in 16 (48%) and recurrence in 23 (70%) of 33 patients with myxoid liposarcoma (215). In that study, myxoid liposarcoma metastasized almost as frequently in cases without local recurrence as in those with recurrence. Tateishi et al. (227), in a multivariate analysis of 36 patients with myxoid liposarcoma, noted that pronounced enhancement on MR imaging is the most significant factor in predicting an adverse prognosis.

Local recurrence rates for retroperitoneal tumors approach 100%, and accordingly, retroperitoneal liposarcoma may be considered to be incurable (Fig. 4.56) (5). The frequency of dedifferentiation of retroperitoneal tumors is unknown but estimated at approximately 10% to 15% (212,217). Dedifferentiated liposarcoma occurring outside of the mediastinum, retroperitoneum, or inguinal regions (the inguinal regions can be considered an extension of the retroperitoneum) is uncommon; however, it is reported with increasing frequency (215,217,219,228). Brooks and Connor (229) reported two extremity dedifferentiated liposarcomas, both occurring in patients with previous radiation therapy. Dedifferentiation is well-documented in the absence of radiation, and radiation's role in the development of dedifferentiation is unclear. Dedifferentiated liposarcoma may also occur de novo (228).

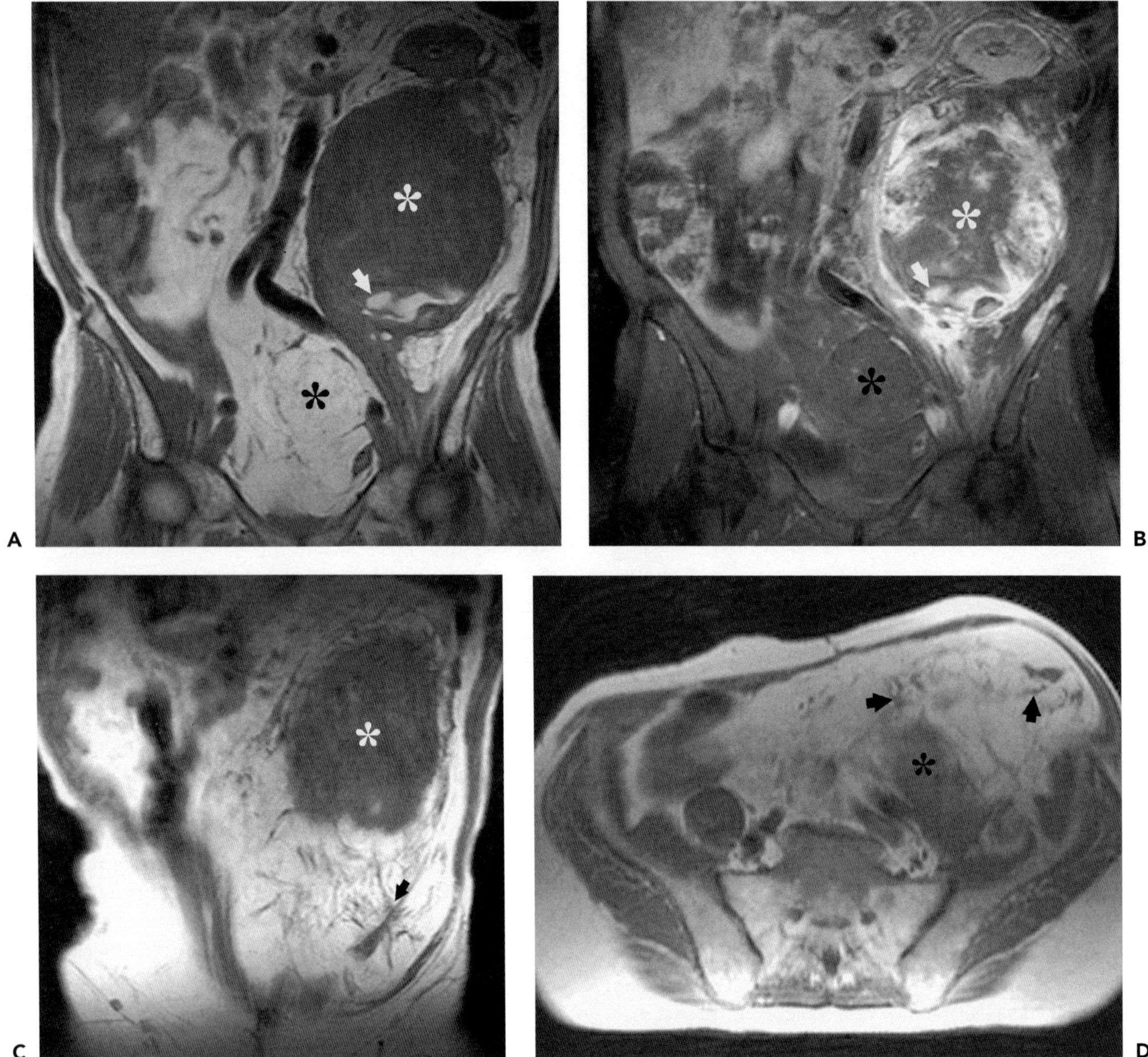

Figure 4.61   Dedifferentiated liposarcoma: Typical MR and CT features in the retroperitoneum of a man 74 years of age. **A,B:** Coronal T1-weighted (TR/TE; 549/12) **(A)** and fat-suppressed enhanced T1-weighted (TR/TE; 757/12) **(B)** spin-echo MR images show a large mass (*white asterisk*) with a juxtaposed poorly marginated, well-defined liposarcoma (*black asterisk*). The high-grade component shows evidence of internal hemorrhage (*arrow*) and displaces the kidney superiorly. **C:** Coronal T1-weighted image more anteriorly shows to better advantage the thickened irregular septa (*arrow*) in the well-differentiated liposarcoma, as well as the juxtaposed high-grade sarcoma (*asterisk*). **D:** Axial T1-weighted (TR/TE; 634/16) spin-echo image at lower aspect of dedifferentiated component (*asterisk*), shows infiltrating nature of well-differentiated portion of tumor (*arrows*). (*continued*)

Malignant Transformation

Although there are scattered, well-documented reports of patients having both liposarcoma and lipoma (or lipomatosis) (230–232), the concept of liposarcoma arising from lipoma is generally not accepted. Although a few possible cases of malignant transformation of lipoma are reported in the literature (233–236), the cases have not clearly established this phenomenon, and the most likely explanations relate to the great histologic variability of liposarcoma, lesion heterogeneity, and possibility of diagnostic sampling error (212).

Radiologic Appearance

Radiographs of patients with liposarcoma may depict the presence of a soft tissue mass but are rarely specific. Calcification is uncommon but reported in up to 10% to 15% of patients (18,222,237). Calcification may be seen in both benign and malignant fatty tumors, and reports vary whether calcification is more common in benign or in malignant disease; however, in our experience, it is more common in liposarcoma. Although the fatty nature of the lesion may sometimes be appreciated on radiographs, radiographs rarely allow a specific diagnosis, and they serve

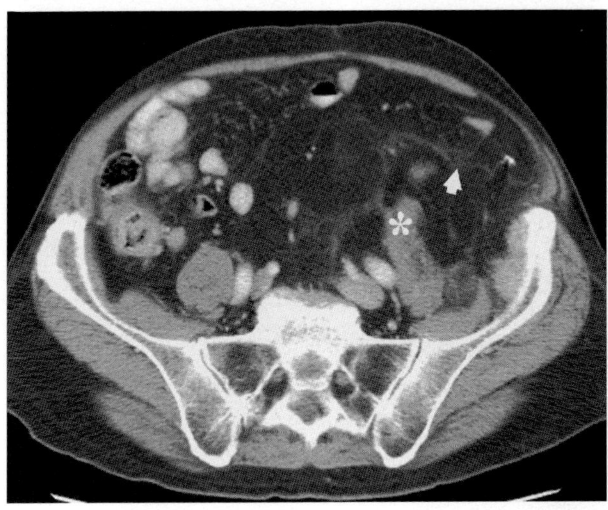

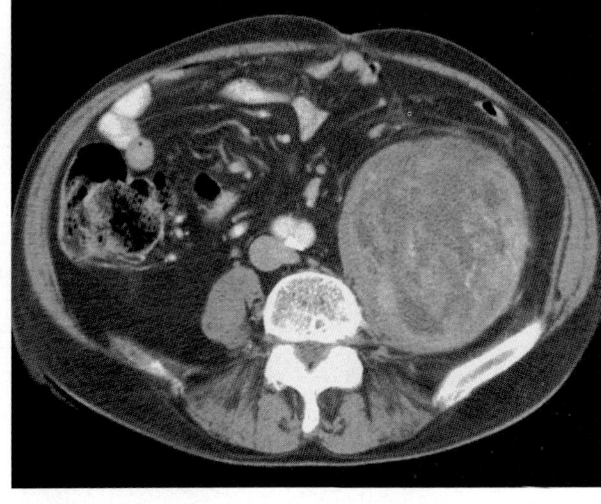

Figure 4.61 *(continued)*   **E:** Corresponding axial enhanced CT scan at the level of the inferior margin of the dedifferentiated component (*asterisk*), show the well-differentiated portion (*arrow*) infiltrating the adjacent retroperitoneal fat, highlighting the difficulty of obtaining appropriate surgical margins. **F:** Axial contrast-enhanced CT through the dedifferentiated component highlights the contrasting appearance of the difficult-to-define well-differentiated liposarcoma component and focal masslike appearance of the dedifferentiated component.

KEY CONCEPTS

- Radiographic calcification is uncommon (10% to 15%); more common in liposarcoma than in lipoma.
- Well-differentiated liposarcoma images as a predominantly fatty mass (>75% fat), with irregular, thickened, linear, swirled, and/or nodular septa; nodular and globular areas may be seen.
- Myxoid and pleomorphic lesions usually show less than 25% fat; pleomorphic and hypercellular myxoid (round cell) lesions are more heterogeneous.
- About 20% of myxoid lesions have a cystlike appearance.
- Dedifferentiated liposarcoma has features of a well-differentiated liposarcoma with a juxtaposed, focal, nonadipose mass.

---

primarily to identify calcification and osseous involvement (Fig. 4.57).

Imaging Appearance

The appearance of liposarcoma on CT and MR imaging reflects the degree of tumor differentiation. The more differentiated the tumor, the more its imaging appearance approaches that of adipose tissue. On MR imaging and CT scanning, a well-differentiated liposarcoma typically images as a predominantly fatty mass having irregularly thickened, linear, swirled, and/or nodular septa (Figs. 4.58 and 4.59). These nonadipose areas demonstrate a nonspecific decreased signal on T1-weighted and variably increased signal on T2-weighted or fluid-sensitive images and increased attenuation on CT (18,238–244). The amount of radiologically identifiable fat is variable: A well-differentiated liposarcoma generally demonstrates at least 75% adipose tissue, although uncommonly this is as little as 25% of the lesion volume (Fig. 4.60) (18). Thin septa, uniform in thickness and no more than 2 mm thick, may be seen in both benign and malignant lesions; however, thick septa or nodular areas are significant predictors of malignancy (18). It has been our experience that the characterization of the nonadipose portion of the lesion is best made on high-quality T1-weighted spin-echo MR images. In a study of 60 fatty tumors, 24 of 25 (96%) fatty lesions with thick septa, as well as 10 of 12 (83%) lesions with nodular/globular areas, proved to be malignant (18).

Gadolinium contrast enhancement of the nonadipose areas is variable and described as faint to significant (18,242,243). Our experience mirrors that of Hosono et al. (242), who noted that the septal structures in liposarcoma were thick, had irregular width, and enhanced significantly on fat-suppressed T1-weighted images following gadolinium-diethylenetriamine pentaacetic acid (Gd-DTPA) administration (Figs. 4.58–4.60). In contradistinction, these investigators found that the septa in lipoma were thin, with faint enhancement, suggesting this pattern might be useful in distinguishing liposarcoma from lipoma.

The diagnosis of a dedifferentiated liposarcoma is suggested when a lesion shows the imaging characteristics of a well-differentiated liposarcoma with an associated or juxtaposed focal, nonlipomatous mass. The associated mass typically shows a nonspecific MR appearance with prolonged T1- and T2-relaxation times or a tissue attenuation approximating that of skeletal muscle on CT scanning. Hemorrhage and necrosis may be seen within the high-grade dedifferentiated component (Figs. 4.61 and 4.62) (228).

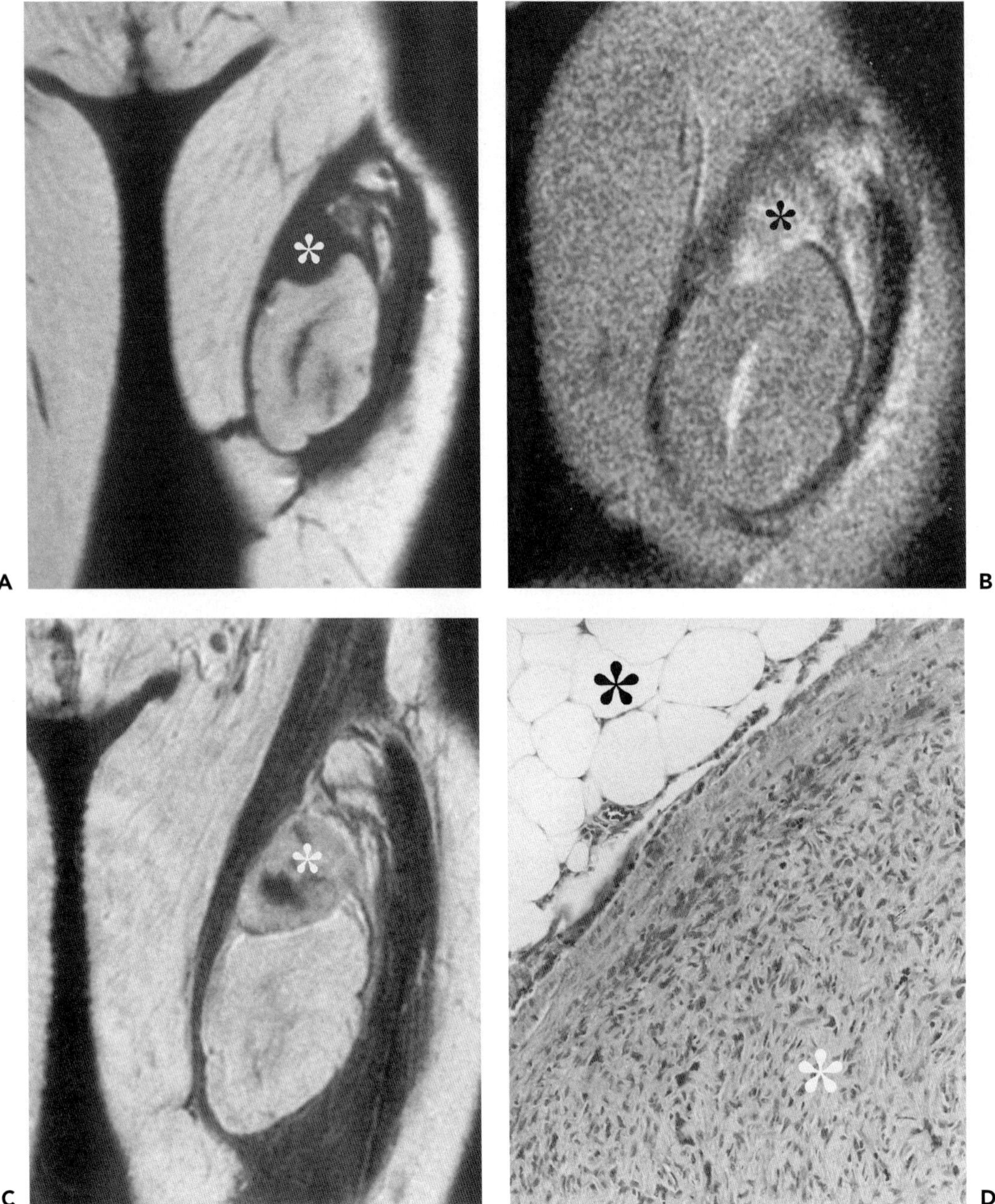

Figure 4.62   Dedifferentiated liposarcoma: Typical extremity imaging appearance in a woman 33 years of age with a recurrent thigh mass. **A,B:** Coronal T1-weighted (TR/TE; 650/20) **(A)** and conventional T2-weighted (TR/TE; 1800/80) **(B)** spin-echo MR images show a mass in anterior aspect of the left thigh. Well-differentiated portion of the mass shows signal intensity similar to that of subcutaneous fat, whereas the high-grade component (*asterisk*) in its superior aspect does not. Note thickened septa in the well-differentiated component. **C:** Corresponding enhanced coronal T1-weighted (TR/TE; 650/20) spin-echo MR image shows significant enhancement of nonfatty component (*asterisk*), as well as enhancement of nonfatty areas within the well-differentiated portion of tumor. Note central nonenhancing area in the high-grade components compatible with central necrosis. **D:** Low-power photomicrograph of recurrent tumor shows juxtaposed, well-differentiated lipomatous (*black asterisk*) and higher grade nonlipogenic spindle cell components (*white asterisk*) (hematoxylin and eosin). (*continued*)

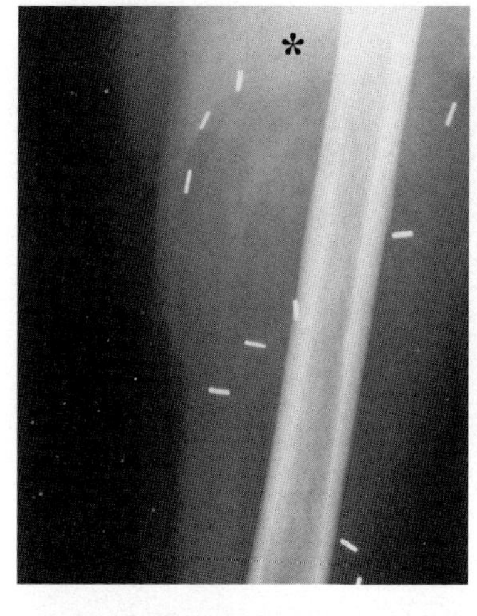
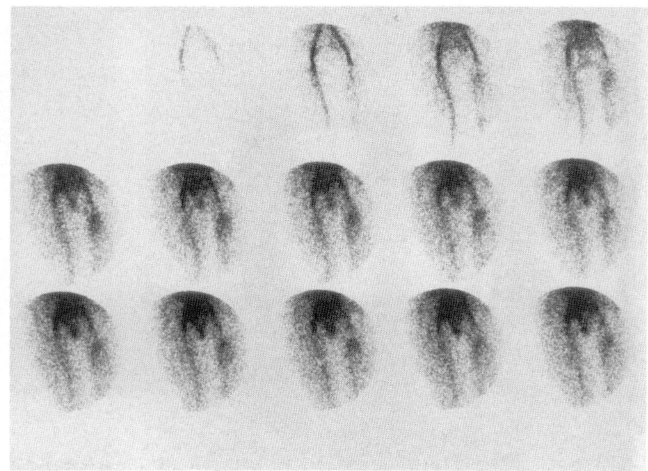
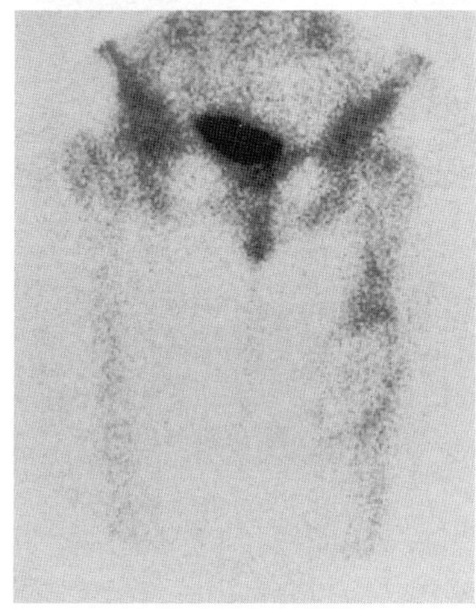

Figure 4.62 *(continued)* **E:** Anteroposterior radiograph of the thigh shows a fatty mass. The high-grade component (*asterisk*) cannot be differentiated from adjacent muscle. **F,G:** Flow **(F)** and delayed static **(G)** images from technetium bone scan show markedly increased tracer accumulation in the high-grade portion of the lesion.

Usually only the well-differentiated liposarcoma is predominantly fatty on radiologic evaluation. The other histologic subtypes of liposarcoma typically contain less fat radiologically: usually less than 25% of tumor volume (Fig. 4.63). Approximately half of the higher grade liposarcomas are reported to show no fat at imaging (13,240). This figure of 50% is based on small early studies, and newer investigations identified fat on T1-weighted MR images in 78% of cases (244), which is in keeping with our clinical experience. The appearance of these fatty areas within the tumor is described as lacy, linear, and amorphous (240,244). Myxoid liposarcoma may also demonstrate an imaging appearance that may simulate a cyst in 21% to 22% of patients (Fig. 4.64) (240,244). A cyst and cystlike myxoid liposarcoma can usually be readily separated clinically; however, they may be distinguished radiologically by either ultrasound or contrast-enhanced MR imaging (Fig. 4.64). Ultrasound of a myxoid mass reveals a complex hypoechoic lesion, in sharp contrast to the findings in a simple cyst (Fig. 4.65). Similarly, Sung et al. (244) reported enhanced MR imaging of myxoid liposarcoma to show complete or heterogeneous (partial) contrast enhancement in more than 96% of cases.

As would be expected by the histological similarities between pure myxoid and myxoid lesions with hypercellular areas (round cell components), the imaging features show similarities. Lesions with hypercellular components are considerably less common, comprising only approximately 5% of all liposarcomas. There are only anecdotal reports of the imaging features of these lesions; however, in our experience, they are generally more heterogeneous but may demonstrate an appearance similar to that of the pure myxoid liposarcoma, including its cystlike appearance (Figs. 4.66 and 4.67). The pleomorphic subtype tends to be more heterogeneous, often with areas of necrosis and hemorrhage (Figs. 4.68 and 4.69) (243).

Differentiating Features

The distinction of lipoma from well-differentiated liposarcoma is simple when the former is homogeneous with an imaging appearance identical to that of the subcutaneous adipose tissue. When nonadipose elements are present, however, this distinction may be quite problematic. Newer literature documents a wider spectrum for the imaging features of lipoma than was appreciated previously, with a small but significant number of lipomas demonstrating

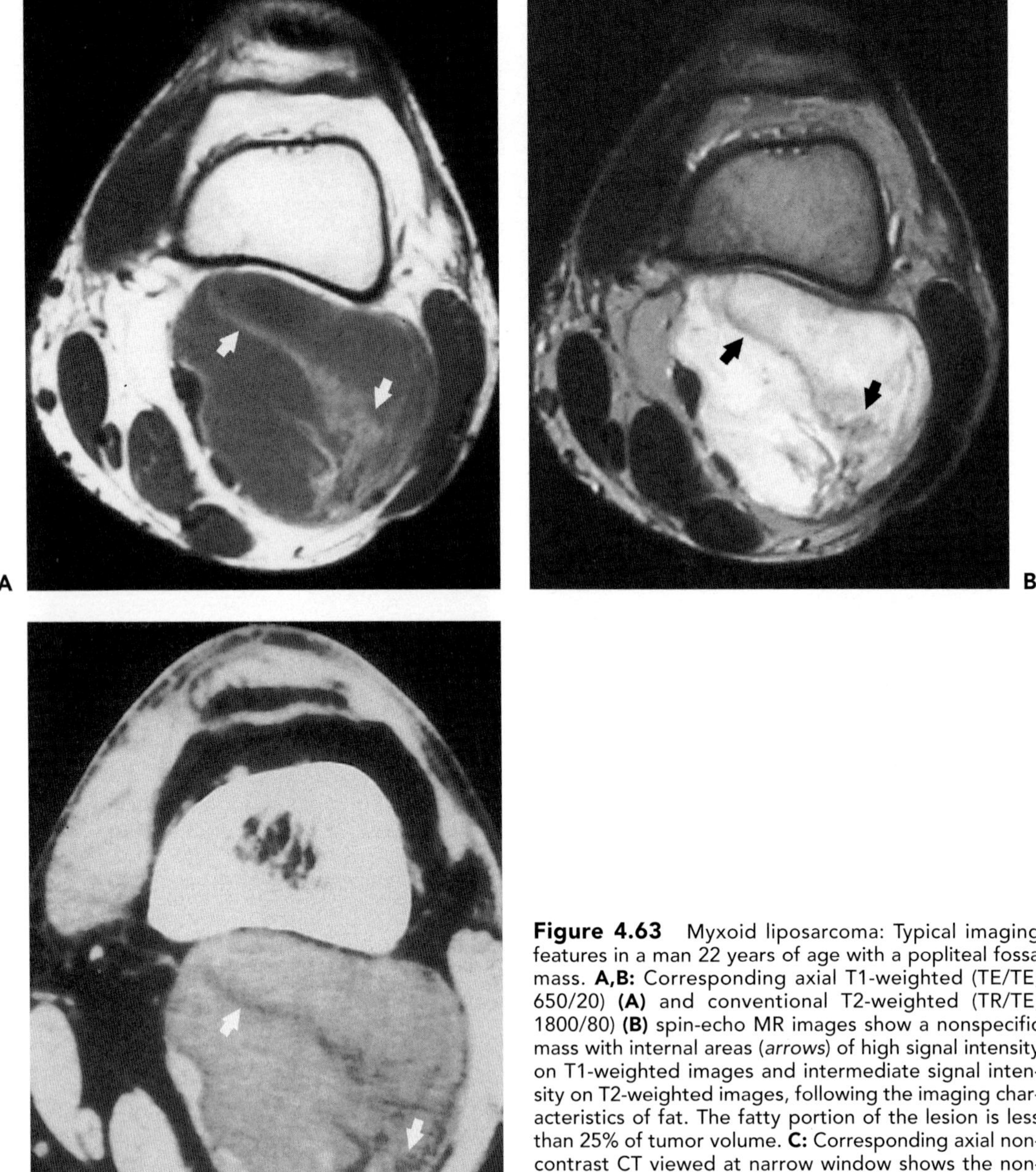

Figure 4.63 Myxoid liposarcoma: Typical imaging features in a man 22 years of age with a popliteal fossa mass. **A,B:** Corresponding axial T1-weighted (TE/TE; 650/20) **(A)** and conventional T2-weighted (TR/TE; 1800/80) **(B)** spin-echo MR images show a nonspecific mass with internal areas (*arrows*) of high signal intensity on T1-weighted images and intermediate signal intensity on T2-weighted images, following the imaging characteristics of fat. The fatty portion of the lesion is less than 25% of tumor volume. **C:** Corresponding axial noncontrast CT viewed at narrow window shows the nonspecific mass with central area of decreased attenuation (*arrows*), corresponding to the area of fatty differentiation seen on MR imaging.

prominent nonadipose areas and an imaging appearance that may mimic what was traditionally ascribed to well-differentiated liposarcoma (18). In these cases, the nonadipose areas represent fat necrosis and associated calcification, fibrosis, inflammation, and myxoid change. As a generalization, lesion size may also be useful, in that well-differentiated liposarcoma tends to be significantly larger than lipoma. In a review of 60 well-differentiated fatty tumors, the average largest dimension of malignant lesions was nearly twice that of benign lipomas (24 cm versus 13 cm) (18). Similarly, patients with liposarcoma were older than those with lipoma (65 versus 52 years).

Although many lesions can mimic a liposarcoma, the lesion that is perhaps the most problematic to radiologists is the intramuscular myxoma. The intramuscular myxoma may have a striking similarity to the cystlike form of myxoid liposarcoma, both radiologically and histologically. Although there is an overlap, intramuscular myxoma can be differentiated from myxoid liposarcoma on MR most confidently when there is a rind of perilesional fat (rather than intralesional fat), a globular heterogeneous peripheral and central enhancement pattern, and increased signal in the adjacent muscle on T2-weighted/fluid-sensitive sequences. These features are all statistically significant,

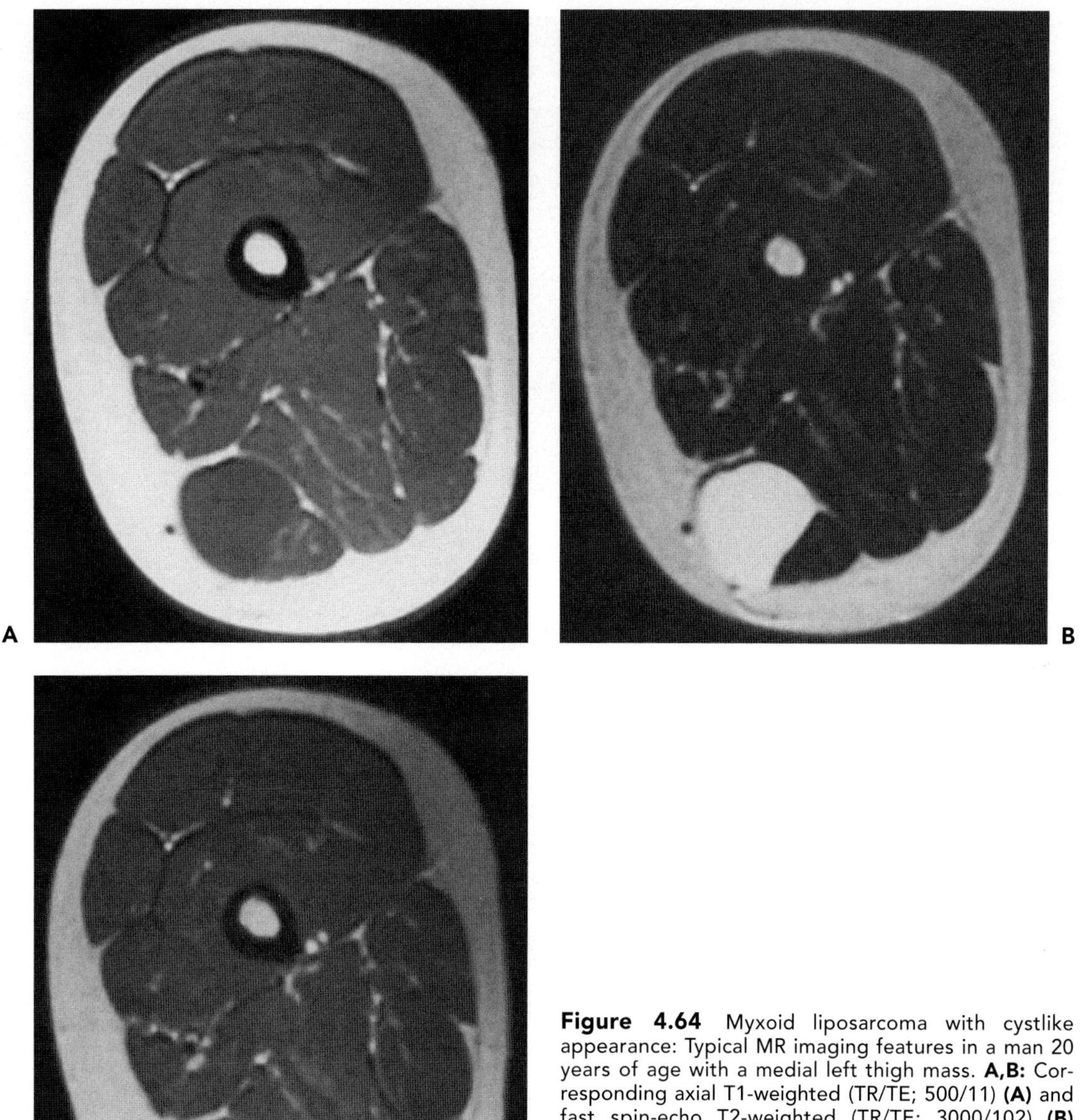

Figure 4.64 Myxoid liposarcoma with cystlike appearance: Typical MR imaging features in a man 20 years of age with a medial left thigh mass. **A,B:** Corresponding axial T1-weighted (TR/TE; 500/11) **(A)** and fast spin-echo T2-weighted (TR/TE; 3000/102) **(B)** images of the left thigh demonstrate a well-defined lesion closely applied to the gracilis muscle. Homogeneous low signal intensity on T1-weighted images and high signal intensity on T2-weighted images simulate the appearance of a cyst. **C:** Immediate postcontrast axial T1-weighted (TR/TE; 500/11) spin-echo MR image demonstrates diffuse enhancement, excluding the diagnosis of a cyst.

and their presence markedly increases the likelihood that a lesion is a myxoma rather than a myxoid liposarcoma by 13- to 20-fold (245).

Treatment

> **KEY CONCEPTS**
> - Treatment is based on lesion grade, location, and extent.
> - Surgery is the mainstay of treatment.
> - Adjuvant radiotherapy is frequently used when wide excision is not possible.

Treatment of liposarcoma is based on the histologic aggressiveness of the lesion, its anatomic location and extent, as well as various patient factors. Surgery is the mainstay of treatment for liposarcoma. Limb-sparing resections are appropriate if a satisfactory surgical margin can be achieved and resultant function would surpass that of amputation and prosthetic usage. Fortunately, most patients with liposarcoma are candidates for limb salvage surgery.

Although surgery is a critical treatment modality, adjuvant therapies may also be appropriate for some patients. Wide surgical excision (excision of the sarcoma with a

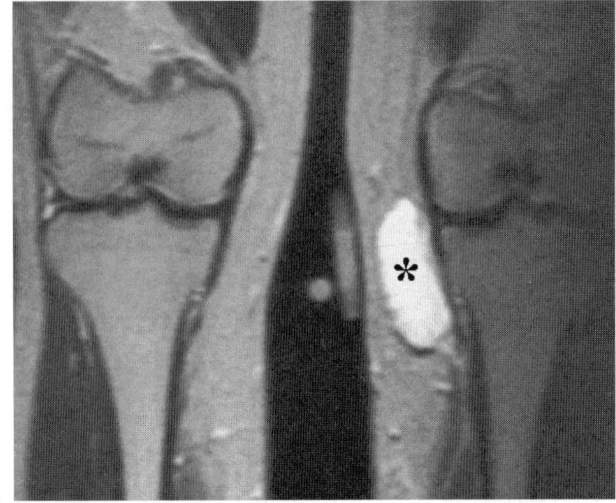

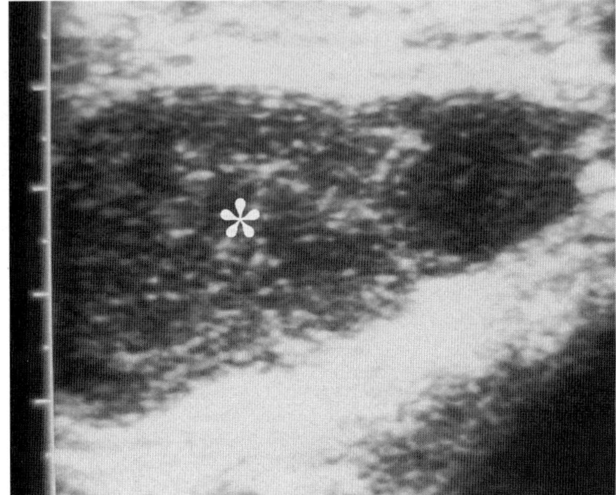

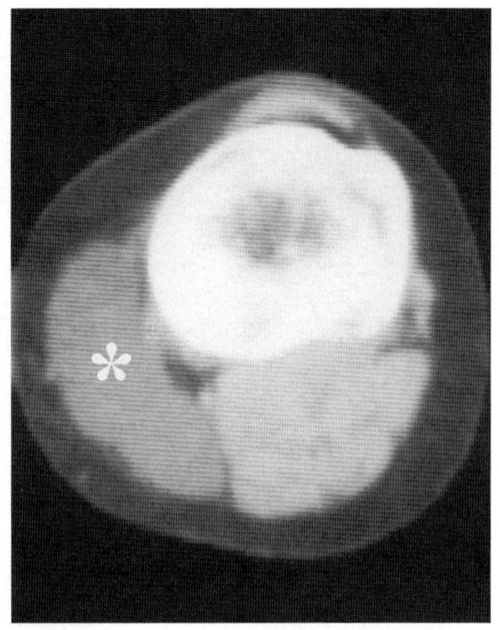

Figure 4.65 Myxoid liposarcoma with cystlike appearance: Distinction from cyst in a woman 28 years of age with a mass adjacent to the medial aspect of the knee. **A:** Coronal conventional T2-weighted (TR/TE; 2000/80) spin-echo MR image shows a well-defined, homogeneous, cystlike mass (*asterisk*) adjacent to the knee. **B:** Axial noncontrast CT shows well-defined mass (*asterisk*) with decreased attenuation. **C:** Sonogram shows the mass (*asterisk*) to be hypoechoic and clearly not a simple cyst.

cuff of surrounding normal tissue) alone is appropriate for most low-grade subcutaneous liposarcomas (246). However, deep-seated low-grade liposarcomas may be managed with wide resection alone or surgery combined with adjuvant radiotherapy, depending on the anatomic location and extent of the tumor (247). Because wide excision may not be possible in sarcomas adjacent to critical neurovascular structures, adjuvant radiotherapy is frequently employed in these patients in an attempt to decrease the risk of local recurrence. Radiation may be administered as preoperative external beam irradiation, intraoperative radiotherapy, postoperative brachytherapy, postoperative external beam irradiation, or combinations thereof.

Patients with high-grade liposarcoma remain a very challenging treatment subgroup. Although advances over the past several decades have resulted in greater frequency and effectiveness of limb salvage surgeries, little impact has been made on the incidence of metastatic disease, prompting introduction of adjuvant chemotherapy.

Experience with combined chemotherapy, radiation therapy, and surgical excision of high-grade liposarcomas is favorable (248).

LESIONS MIMICKING FATTY TUMORS

> ### KEY CONCEPTS
> Lesions that mimic fatty tumors include:
> - Myxoid tumors: myxoma, extraskeletal myxoid chondrosarcoma, myxofibrosarcoma.
> - Lesions with associated subacute hematoma.
> - Normal muscle with fatty replacement.
> - Tumors that invade or engulf adjacent fat.
> - Mesenteric or other fat-containing hernias.

Myxoid tumors may mimic lipomatous neoplasms both histologically and radiographically. Included in this group are intramuscular myxoma, extraskeletal myxoid

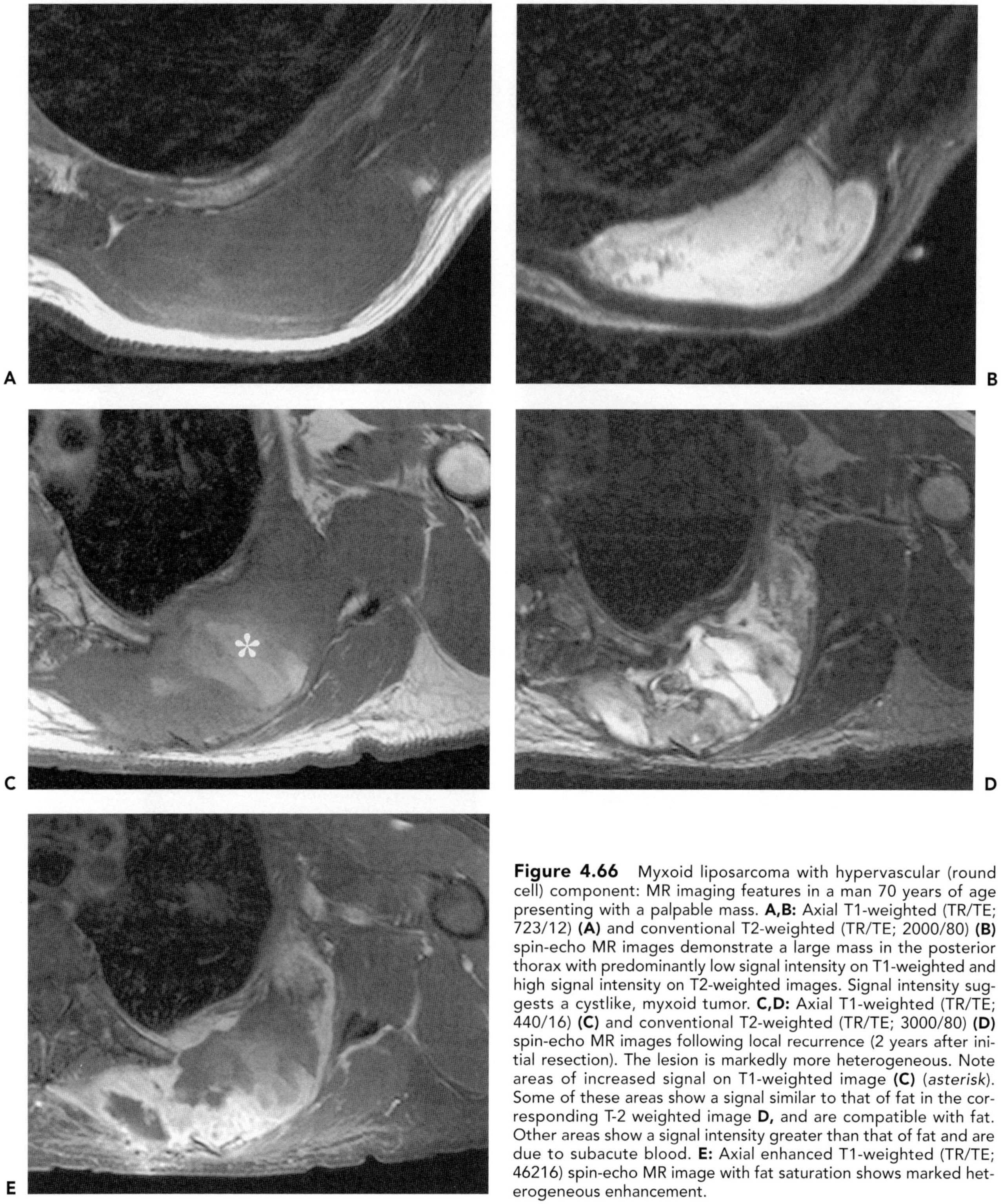

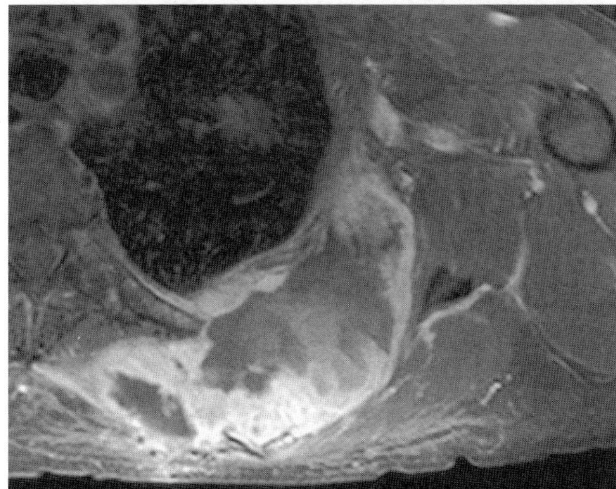

Figure 4.66 Myxoid liposarcoma with hypervascular (round cell) component: MR imaging features in a man 70 years of age presenting with a palpable mass. **A,B:** Axial T1-weighted (TR/TE; 723/12) **(A)** and conventional T2-weighted (TR/TE; 2000/80) **(B)** spin-echo MR images demonstrate a large mass in the posterior thorax with predominantly low signal intensity on T1-weighted and high signal intensity on T2-weighted images. Signal intensity suggests a cystlike, myxoid tumor. **C,D:** Axial T1-weighted (TR/TE; 440/16) **(C)** and conventional T2-weighted (TR/TE; 3000/80) **(D)** spin-echo MR images following local recurrence (2 years after initial resection). The lesion is markedly more heterogeneous. Note areas of increased signal on T1-weighted image **(C)** (*asterisk*). Some of these areas show a signal similar to that of fat in the corresponding T-2 weighted image **D,** and are compatible with fat. Other areas show a signal intensity greater than that of fat and are due to subacute blood. **E:** Axial enhanced T1-weighted (TR/TE; 46216) spin-echo MR image with fat saturation shows marked heterogeneous enhancement.

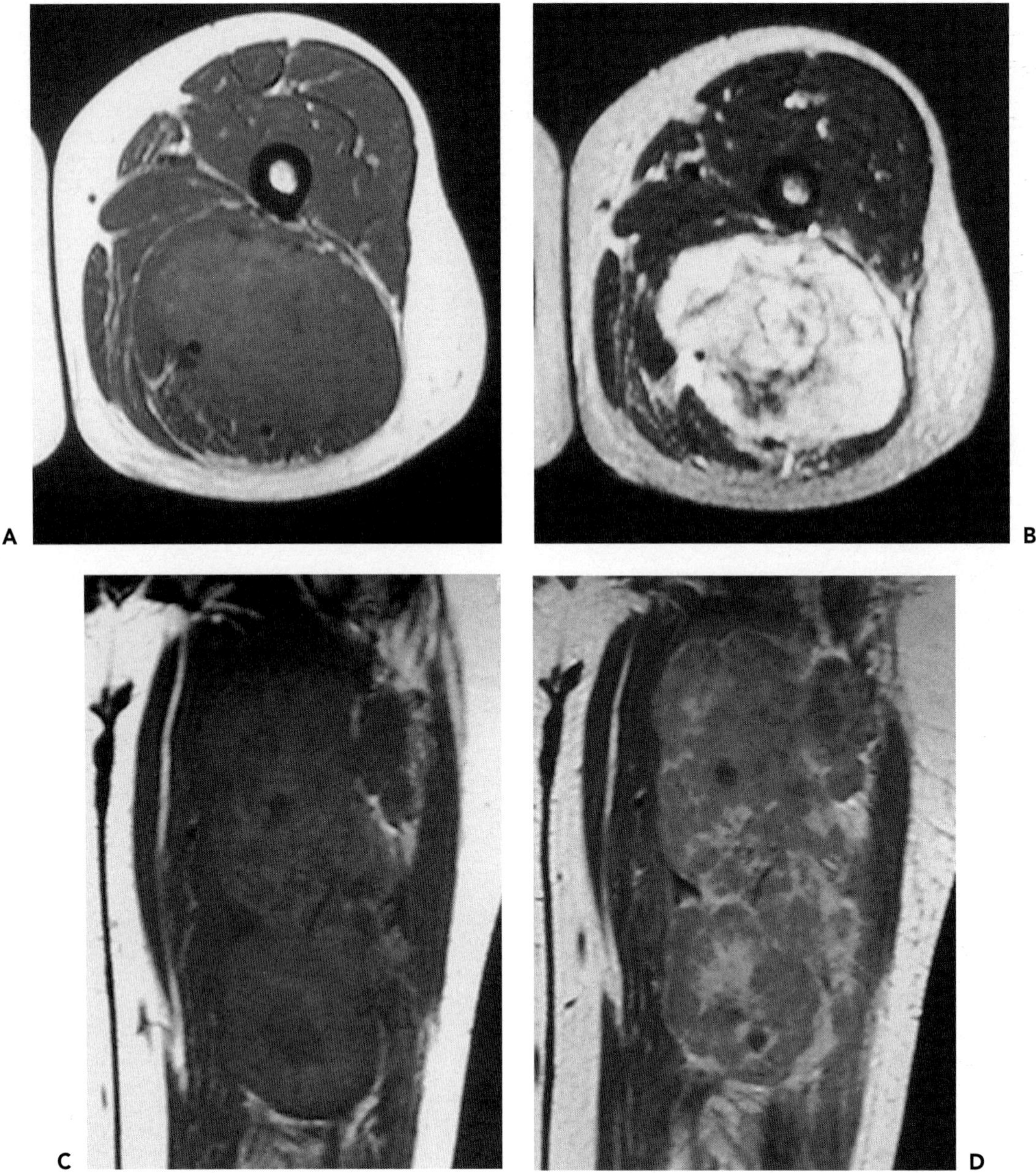

Figure 4.67 Myxoid liposarcoma with prominent hypervascular (round cell) component: MR imaging features in a man 43 years of age demonstrating no appreciable fatty component. **A,B:** Axial T1-weighted (TR/TE; 700/16) **(A)** and conventional T2-weighted (TR/TE; 2500/80) **(B)** spin-echo MR images demonstrate a nonspecific heterogeneous mass. **C,D:** Corresponding coronal T1-weighted (TR/TE; 600/16) spin-echo MR pre- **(C)** and post-contrast **(D)** images depict the heterogeneous enhancement pattern with small foci of central necrosis.

chondrosarcoma, and myxoid malignant fibrous histiocytoma.

On MR imaging, subacute hematoma demonstrates increased signal on both T1- and T2-weighted images (249). Consequently, differentiation between lipoma and hematoma can be difficult; however, T1- and T2-relaxation times of hematoma are usually longer than those of fat (signal intensity less than fat on T1-weighted

and greater than fat on T2-weighted images) (20). Fat suppression may be useful to separate the two on MR imaging.

Fatty replacement secondary to muscle atrophy may also be seen and may mimic a fatty lesion. Care must be taken to ensure the fat identified on imaging studies is within the lesion and not surrounding it. Tumors may invade adjacent adipose tissue and engulf a portion of it,

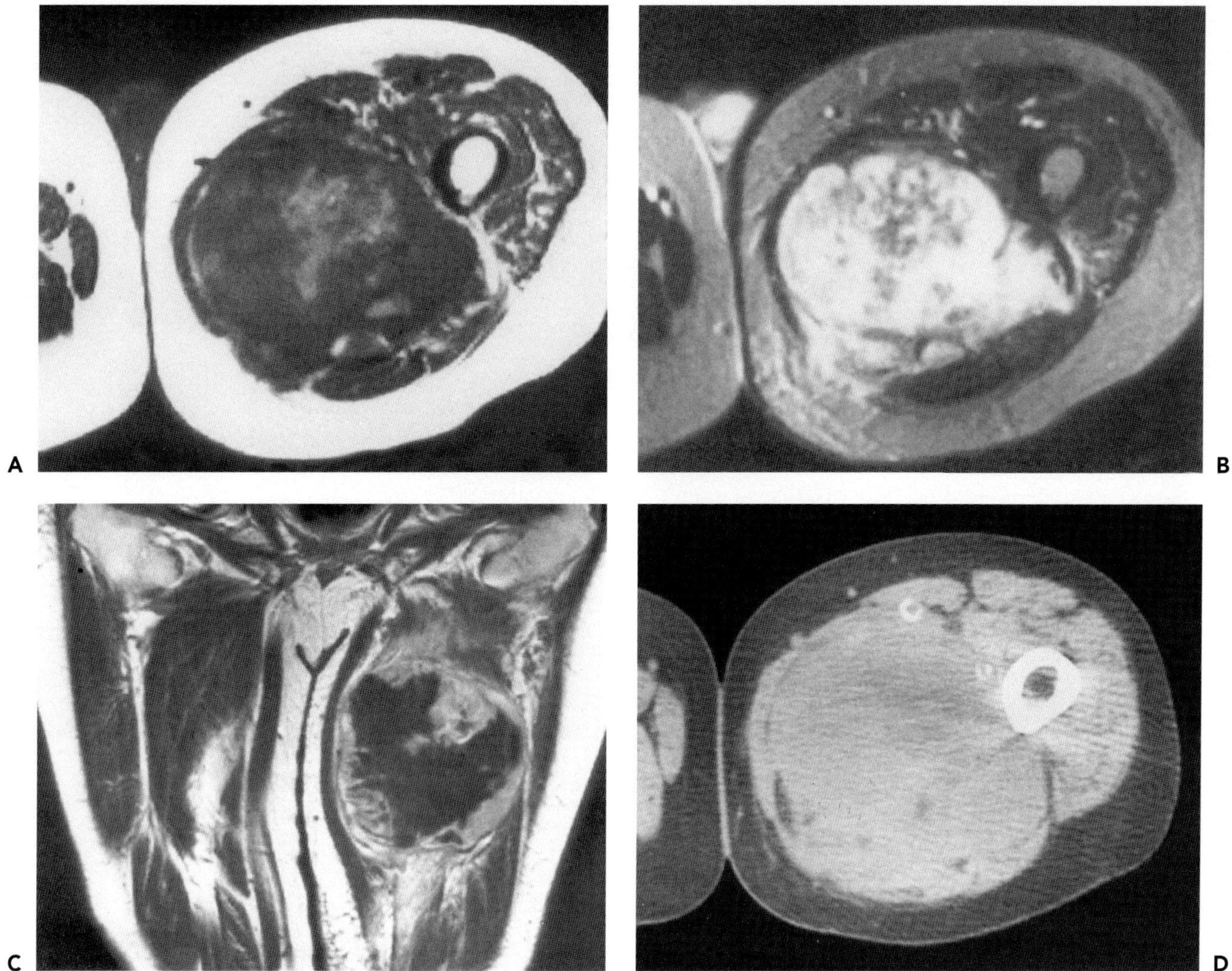

Figure 4.68 Pleomorphic liposarcoma: MR and CT imaging features in a man 85 years of age with a thigh mass. **A,B:** Axial T1-weighted (TR/TE; 600/15) **(A)** and conventional T2-weighted (TR/TE; 2500/90) **(B)** spin-echo MR images show a large mass in the adductor compartment. Scattered areas within the mass show increased signal intensity in **A** and intermediate signal in **B,** representing areas of mature fat within the mass. **C:** Enhanced coronal T1-weighted (TR/TE; 600/16) spin-echo MR image shows marked inhomogeneous contrast enhancement, reflecting underlying necrosis. **D:** Axial enhanced CT scan at level similar to **A** shows a nonspecific appearance. *(continued)*

simulating a fatty lesion (Fig. 4.70) (250). Engulfment of adjacent fat is suggested as the cause of the fat found in elastofibroma.

On CT scanning, nerve sheath tumors show a tissue attenuation value significantly less than that of muscle in almost 75% of cases and may mimic the tissue attenuation of fatty lesions (251,252). The histologic basis for this is postulated to include a population of lipid-rich Schwann cells, the presence of adipocytes intimately intermingled with neurofibromas, and entrapment of perineural adipose tissue by plexiform neurofibromas (252). Conceivably, hemorrhage or cystic degeneration, as well as

clusters of xanthomatous change (foamy macrophages) and predominance of Antoni B areas (less compact myxoid foci) in schwannomas, could contribute to the low attenuation values.

Hernias occasionally may mimic a fatty tumor. Our anecdotal experience is that this is most common in the anterior abdominal wall (Fig. 4.71). Finally, muscular dystrophy may show marked atrophy and fatty replacement of muscle simulating lipomatosis, although these diagnoses are usually easily distinguished by the distribution of the affected muscles and clinical presentation (Fig. 4.72).

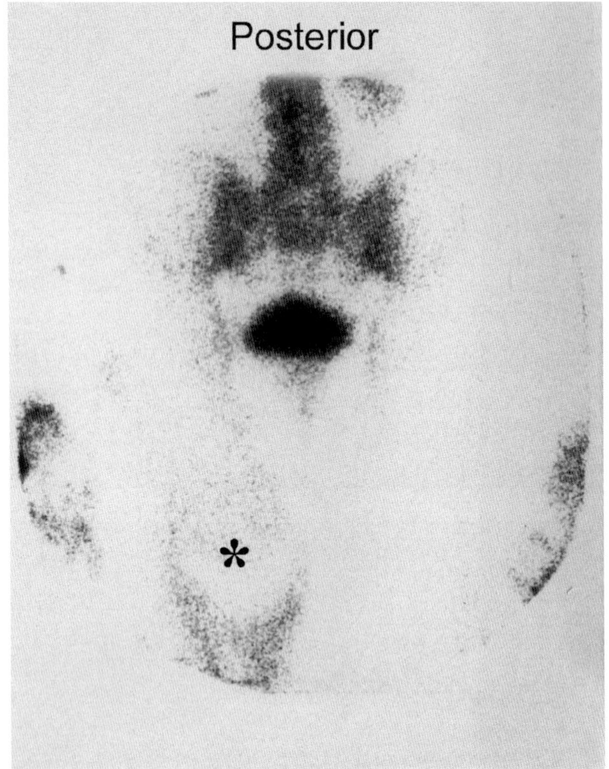

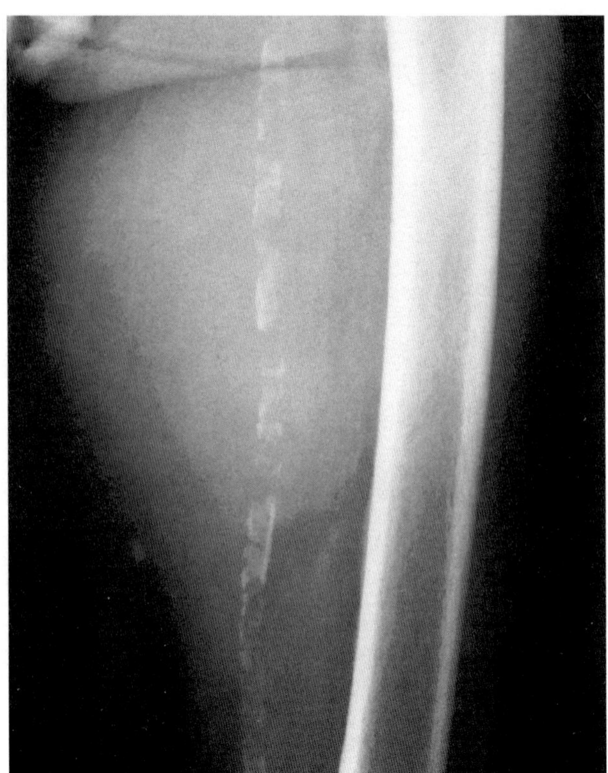

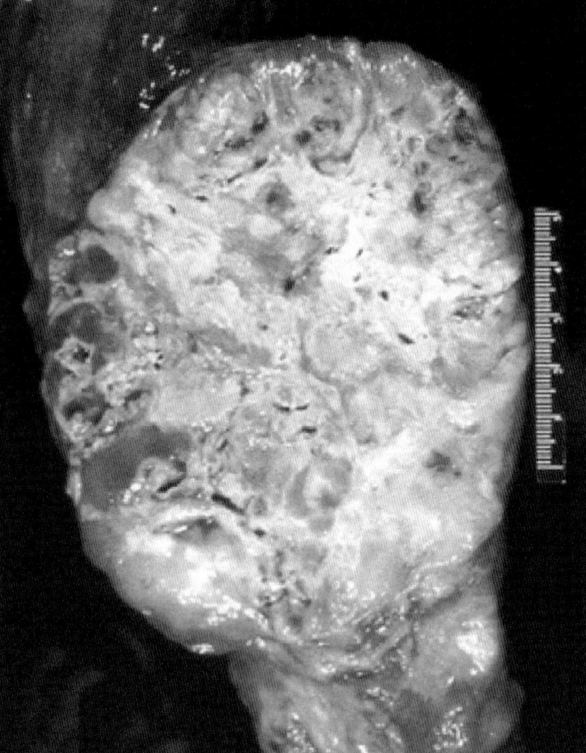

Figure 4.68 *(continued)*   **E:** Bone scintigram shows focal tracer accumulation within the mass *(asterisk)*, with relative central photopenia, compatible with central necrosis. **F:** Radiograph shows nonspecific mass in the medial aspect of the left thigh. **G:** Photograph of the resected mass shows the marked heterogeneity of the mass.

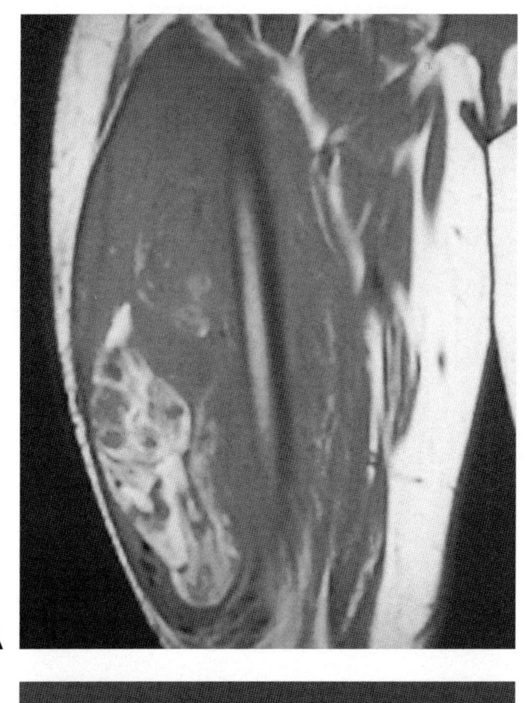
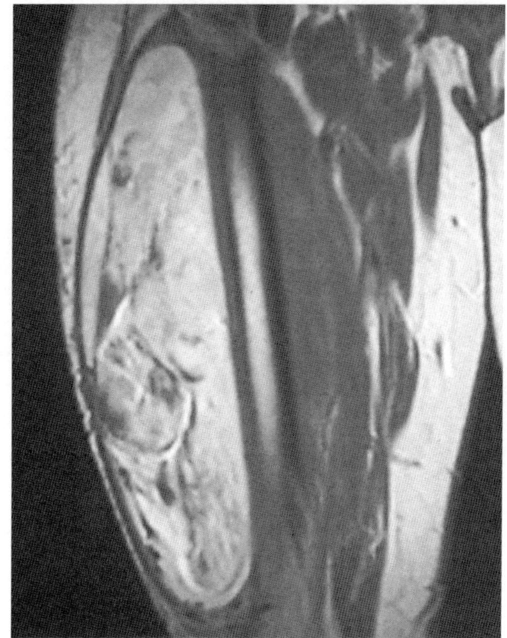
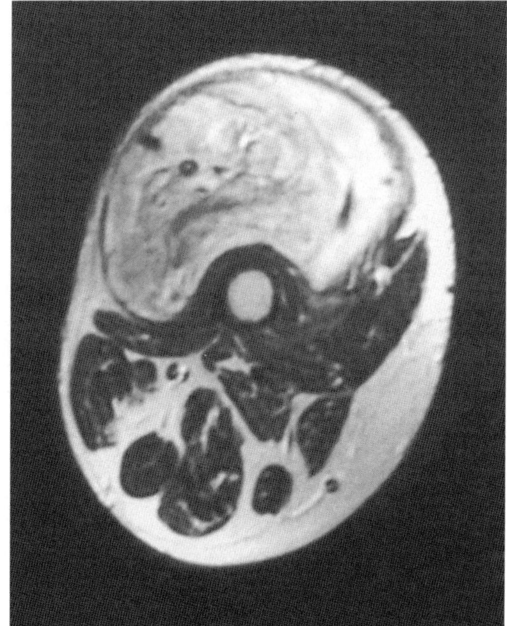

Figure 4.69 Pleomorphic liposarcoma: MR imaging features in a woman 57 years of age. **A:** Coronal T1-weighted (TR/TE; 600/16) spin-echo MR image demonstrates a large heterogeneous soft tissue mass in the right thigh that contains fatty elements. **B:** Enhanced coronal T1-weighted (TR/TE; 600/16) spin-echo MR image of the thigh demonstrates enhancement of a majority of the lesion. **C:** Axial fast spin-echo T2-weighted (TR/TE; 3200/102) MR image shows predominantly high signal intensity, with thick nodular septations traversing the lesion.

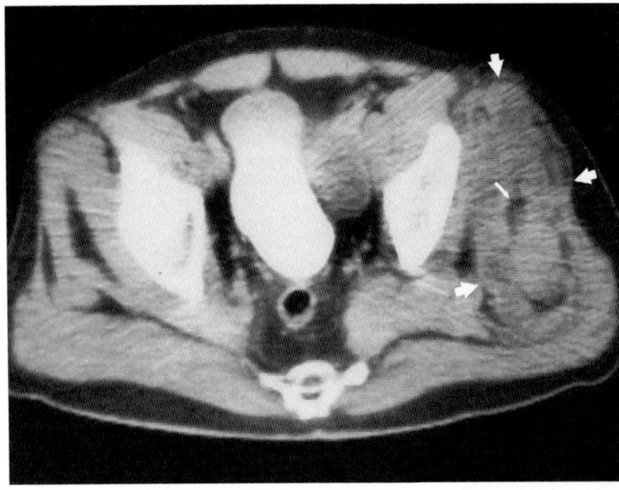

Figure 4.70   Liposarcoma mimic: Mass engulfing adjacent fat. CT imaging features in a man 56 years of age with an extraskeletal myxoid chondrosarcoma of the buttocks. Axial CT image shows a large mass in the left hip (*arrows*). Small amount of fat within the mass (*small arrow*) represented fat between the gluteal muscle that was engulfed as the lesion grew. Note metastatic node in pelvis.

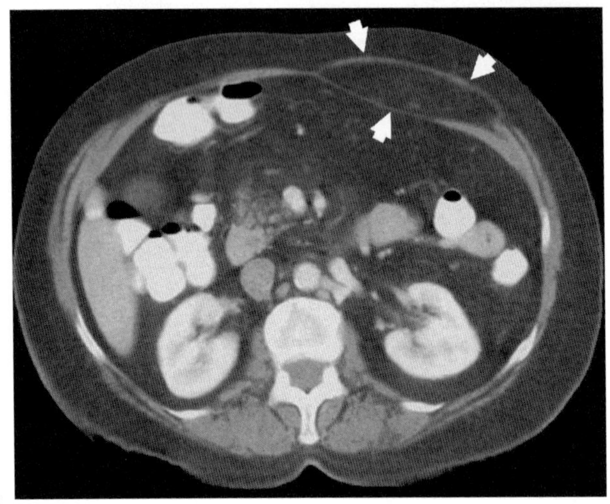

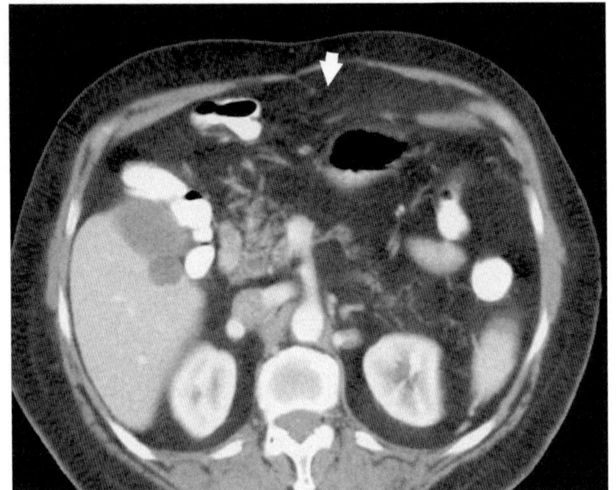

Figure 4.71   Liposarcoma mimic: Abdominal wall hernia in a woman. **A:** CT shows a fatty mass (*arrows*) within the anterior abdominal wall. The initial diagnosis was a well-differentiated liposarcoma. **B:** Image cranial to **A** shows the fascial defect (*arrow*) allowing herniation of mesenteric fat and vessels into the anterior abdominal wall.

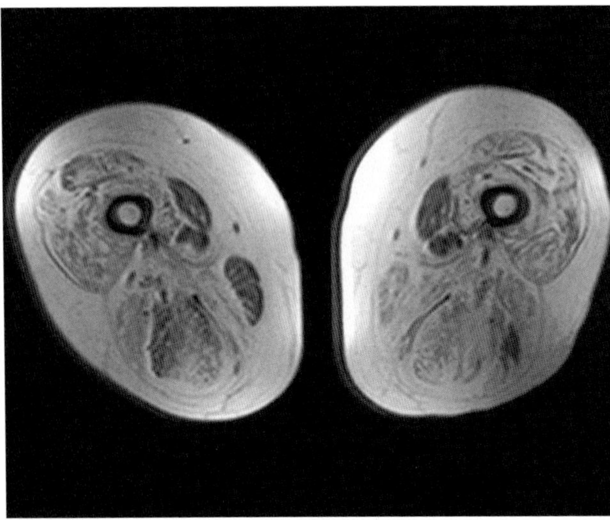

Figure 4.72   Liposarcoma mimic: Muscular dystrophy in a man 50 years of age presenting with proximal muscle weakness. Axial T1-weighted (TR/TE; 748/17) spin-echo MR image demonstrates extensive symmetric fatty replacement of skeletal muscle.

REFERENCES

1. Fletcher DM, Unni KK, Mertens F. Adipocytic tumors. In: *WHO Classification of Soft Tissue Tumors. Pathology and Genetics: Tumors of Soft Tissue and Bone*. Lyon, France: IARC Press; 2002:19.
2. Weiss SW, Goldblum JR. Benign lipomatous tumors. In: *Enzinger and Weiss's Soft Tissue Tumors*. 4th ed. St. Louis: Mosby; 2001: 571–639.
3. Myhre-Jensen O. A consecutive 7-year series of 1331 benign soft tissue tumors. Clinicopathologic data. Comparison with sarcomas. *Acta Orthop Scand*. 1981;52:287–293.
4. Ronan SJ, Broderick. Minimally invasive approach to familial multiple lipomatosis. *Plastic Reconstr Surg*. 2000;106:878–880.
5. Weiss SW. Lipomatous tumors. In: Weiss SW, Brooks JSJ, eds. *Soft Tissue Tumors*. Baltimore: Williams & Wilkins; 1996:207–251.
6. Dei Tos AP, Cin PD. The role of cytogenetics in the classification of soft tissue tumors. *Virchows Arch*. 1997;431:83–94.
7. Rydholm A, Berg NO. Size, site and clinical incidence of lipoma. Factors in the differential diagnosis of lipoma and sarcoma. *Acta Orthop Scand*. 1983;54:929–934.
8. Meis-Kindblom JM, Enzinger FM. Lipomatous tumors. In: *Color Atlas of Soft Tissue Tumors*. St. Louis: Mosby-Wolfe; 1996:74–105.
9. Miettinen M. Benign fatty tumors. In: *Diagnostic Soft Tissue Pathology*. New York: Churchill Livingstone; 2003:207–225.
10. Osment LS. Cutaneous lipomas and lipomatosis. *Surg Gynecol Obstet*. 1968;127:129–132.
11. Lattes R. *Tumors of the Soft Tissue*. Fascicle 1. Second Series. Washington, DC: Armed Forces Institute of Pathology; 1982: 53–59.
12. Kransdorf MJ. Benign soft-tissue tumors in a large referral population: distribution of diagnoses by age, sex and location. *AJR Am J Roentgenol*. 1995;164:395–402.
13. Kransdorf MJ, Moser RP, Meis JM, et al. Fat containing soft tissue masses of the extremities. *Radiographics*. 1991;11:81–106.
14. Humphrey AA, Kingsley PC. Familial multiple lipomas. Report on a family. *Arch Dermatol Syphil*. 1938;37:30–34.
15. Leffert RD. Lipomas of the upper extremity. *J Bone Joint Surg*. 1972;54A:1262–1266.
16. Regan JM, Bickel WH, Broders AC. Infiltrating benign lipomas of the extremities. *West J Surg Obstet Gynecol*. 1946;54:87–93.
17. Kransdorf MJ. Malignant soft-tissue tumors in a large referral population: distribution of diagnoses by age, sex and location. *AJR Am J Roentgenol*. 1995;164:129–134.
18. Kransdorf MJ, Bancroft LW, Peterson JJ, et al. Well-differentiated fatty tumors: distinction of lipoma from well-differentiated liposarcoma. *Radiology*. 2002;224:99–104.
19. Sauer JM, Ozonoff MD. Congenital bone anomalies associated with lipomas. *Skeletal Radiol*. 1985;13:276–279.
20. Dooms GC, Hricak H, Sollitto RA, et al. Lipomatous tumors and tumors with fatty component: MR imaging potential and comparison of MR and CT results. *Radiology*. 1985;157:479–483.
21. Waligore MP, Stephens DH, Soule EH, et al. Lipomatous tumors of the abdominal cavity: CT appearance and pathologic correlation. *AJR Am J Roentgenol*. 1981;137:539–545.
22. Friedman AC, Hartman DS, Sherman J, et al. Computed tomography of abdominal fatty masses. *Radiology*. 1981;139:415–429.
23. Weekes RG, McLeod RA, Reiman HM, et al. CT of soft-tissue neoplasms. *AJR Am J Roentgenol*. 1985;144:355–360.
24. Egund N, Ekelund L, Sako M, et al. CT of soft-tissue tumors. *AJR Am J Roentgenol*. 1981;137:725–729.
25. Sundaram M, McGuire MH, Herbold DR. Magnetic resonance imaging of soft tissue masses: an evaluation of fifty-three histologically proven tumors. *Magnetic Reson Imaging*. 1988;6:237–248.
26. Genant HK, Helms CA. Computed tomography of the appendicular musculoskeletal system. In: Moss AA, Gamsu G, Genant HK, eds. *Computed Tomography of the Body*. Philadelphia: WB Saunders; 1983:475–534.
27. Roberts CC, Liu PT, Colby TV. Encapsulated versus nonencapsulated superficial fatty masses: a proposed MR imaging classification. *AJR Am J Roentgenol*. 2003;180:1419–1422.
28. Hunter JC, Johnston WH, Genant HK. Computed tomography evaluation of fatty tumors of the somatic soft tissues, clinical utility and radiographic-pathologic correlation. *Skeletal Radiol*. 1979;4:79–91.
29. Tyrrel TM, Montemayor KA, Bernardino ME. CT density of mesenteric, retroperitoneal and subcutaneous fat in cirrhotic patients: comparison with control subjects. *AJR Am J Roentgenol*. 1990;155:73–75.
30. Ahuja AT, King AD, Kew J, et al. Head and neck lipomas: sonographic appearance. *AJNR Am J Neuroradiol*. 1998;19:505–508.
31. Gitzman N, Schratter M, Traxler M, et al. Sonographic and computer tomography in deep cervical lipomas and lipomatosis of the neck. *J Ultrasound Med*. 1988;7:451–456.
32. Tsai TS, Evans HA, Donnelly LF, et al. Fat necrosis after trauma: a benign cause of palpable lumps in children. *AJR Am J Roentgenol*. 1997;169:1623–1626.
33. Anderson DR, Narla LD, Dunn NL. Subcutaneous fat necrosis of the newborn. *Pediatr Radiol*. 1999;29:794–796.
34. Lopez JA, Saez F, Alejandro Larena J, et al. MRI diagnosis and follow-up of subcutaneous fat necrosis. *J Magn Reson Imaging*. 1997;7:929–932.
35. Chan LP, Gee R, Keogh C, et al. Imaging features of fat necrosis. *AJR Am J Roentgenol*. 2003;181:955–959.
36. Kransdorf MJ, Jelinek JS, Moser RP, et al. Soft-tissue masses: diagnosis using MR imaging. *AJR Am J Roentgenol*. 1989;153: 541–547.
37. Murphy NB. Ossifying lipoma. *Br J Radiol*. 1974;47:97–98.
38. Plaut GS, Salm R, Truscott DE. Three cases of ossifying lipoma. *J Pathol Bacteriol*. 1959;78:292–295.
39. Le Ber MS, Stout AP. Benign mesenchymomas in children. *Cancer*. 1962;15:598–605.
40. Dolph JL, Demuth RJ, Miller SH. Familial multiple lipomatosis. *Plast Reconst Surg*. 1980;66:620–622.
41. Keskin D, Ezirmik N, Celik H. Familial multiple lipomatosis. *Isr Med Assoc J*. 2002;4:1121–1123.
42. Rubinstein A, Goor Y, Gazit E, et al. Non-symmetric subcutaneous lipomatosis associated with familial combined hyperlipidaemia. *Br J Dermatol*. 1989;120:689–694.
43. Leffell DJ, Braverman IM. Familial multiple lipomatosis. Report of a case and a review of the literature. *J Am Acad Dermatol*. 1986;15:275–279.
44. Troy BR. Familial multiple lipomatosis. *Dermatology Online J*. 2003;9:9.
45. Shanks JA, Paranchych W, Tuba J. Familial multiple lipomatosis. *Can Med Assoc J*. 1957;77:881–884.
46. Haberland C, Perou M. Encephalocraniocutaneous lipomatosis. A new example of ectomesodermal dysgenesis. *Arch Neurol*. 1970;22:144–155.
47. Grimalt R, Ermacora E, Mistura L, et al. Encephalocraniocutaneous lipomatosis: case report and review of the literature. *Pediatric Dermatol*. 1993;10:164–168.
48. McCall S, Ramzy MI, Curé JK, et al. Encephalocraniocutaneous lipomatosis and the Proteus syndrome: distinct entities with overlapping manifestations. *Am J Med Genet*. 1992;43:662–668.
49. Almer Z, Vishnevskia-Dai V, Zadok D. Encephalocraniocutaneous lipomatosis: case report and review of the literature. *Cornea*. 2003;22:389–390.
50. Rubegni P, Risulo M, Sbano P, et al. Encephalocraniocutaneous lipomatosis (Haberland syndrome) with bilateral cutaneous and visceral involvement. *Clin Exp Dermatol*. 2003;28:387–390.
51. Legius E, Wu R, Eyssen M, et al. Encephalocraniocutaneous lipomatosis with a mutation in the NF1 gene. *J Med Genet*. 1995;32:316–319.
52. Cruz A, Schirmbeck T, Pina-Neto JM, et al. Cicatricial upper eyelid retraction in encephalocraniocutaneous lipomatosis: a report of two cases and review of the literature. *Opthal Plast Reconst Surg* 2002;18:151–155.
53. Vellios F, Baez J, Shumacker HB. Lipoblastomatosis: a tumor of fetal fat different from hibernoma. Report of a case, with observations on the embryogenesis of human adipose tissue. *Am J Pathol*. 1958;34:1149–1159.
54. Chung EB, Enzinger FM. Benign lipoblastomatosis: an analysis of 35 cases. *Cancer*. 1973;32:482–492.
55. Van Meurs DP. The transformation of an embryonic lipoma to a common lipoma. *Br J Surg*. 1947;34:282–284.

56. Ha TV, Kleinman PK, Fraire A, et al. MR imaging of benign fatty tumors in children: report of four cases and review of the literature. *Skeletal Radiol.* 1994;23:361–367.

57. O'Donnell KA, Caty MG, Allen JE, et al. Lipoblastoma: better termed infantile lipoma? *Pediatr Surg Int.* 2000;16:458–461.

58. Carcassonne F, Bonneau H, Peschard JJ, et al. Le lipoblastome. *J Int Coll Surg.* 1964;42:311–331.

59. Jimenez JF. Lipoblastoma in infancy and childhood. *J Surg Oncol.* 1986;32:238–244.

60. Sciot R, De Wever I, Debiec-Rychter M. Lipoblastoma in a 23-year-old male: distinction from atypical lipomatous tumor using cytogenetic and fluorescence in-situ hybridization analysis. *Virchows Arch.* 2003;442:468–471.

61. Kwak JY, Ha DH, Kim YA, et al. Lipoblastoma of the parietal pleura in a 7-month-old infant. *J Compute Assist Tomogr.* 1999;23:952–954.

62. Stringel G, Shandling B, Mancer K, et al. Lipoblastoma in infants and children. *J Pediatr Surg.* 1982;17:277–280.

63. Seidel FG, Magill HL, Burton EM, et al. Cases of the day. Pediatric. Lipoblastoma. *Radiographics.* 1990;10:728–731.

64. Rasmussen IS, Kirkegaard J, Kaasbol M. Intermittent airway obstruction in a child caused by a cervical lipoblastoma. *Acta Anaesthesiol Scand.* 1997;41:945–946.

65. Fisher MF, Fletcher BD, Dahms BB, et al. Abdominal lipoblastomatosis: radiographic, echographic, and computed tomographic findings. *Radiology.* 1981;138:593–596.

66. Beebe MM, Smith MD. Omental lipoblastoma. *J Pediatr Surg.* 1993;28:1626–1627.

67. Collins MH, Chatten J. Lipoblastoma/lipoblastomatosis: a clinicopathologic study of 25 tumors. *Am J Surg Pathol.* 1997;21:1131–1137.

68. Coffin CM. Lipoblastoma: an embryonal tumor of soft tissue related to organogenesis. *Semin Diagn Pathol.* 1994;11:98–103.

69. Ko SF, Shieh CS, Shih TY, et al. Mediastinal lipoblastoma with intraspinal extension: MRI demonstration. *Magn Reson Imaging.* 1998;16:445–448.

70. Mognato G, Cecchetto G, Carli M, et al. Is surgical treatment of lipoblastoma always necessary? *J Pediatr Surg.* 2000;35:1511–1513.

71. Black WC, Burke JW, Feldman PS, et al. CT appearance of cervical lipoblastoma. *J Comput Assist Tomogr.* 1986;10:696–698.

72. Reiseter T, Nordshus T, Borthne A, et al. Lipoblastoma: MRI appearances of a rare paediatric soft tissue tumor. *Pediatr Radiol.* 1999;29:543–545.

73. Bolen JW, Thorning D. Benign lipoblastoma and myxoid liposarcoma. A comparative light- and electron-microscopic study. *Am J Surg Pathol.* 1980;4:163–174.

74. Hibbard MK, Kozakewich HP, Dal Cin P, et al. PLAG1 fusion oncogenes in lipoblastoma. *Cancer Res.* 2000;60:4869–4872.

75. Fletcher JA, Kozakewich HP, Schoenberg ML, et al. Cytogenetic findings in pediatric adipose tumors: consistent rearrangement of chromosome 8 in lipoblastoma. *Genes Chromosomes Cancer.* 1993;6:24–29.

76. Gisselsson D, Hibbard MK, Dal Cin P, et al. PLAG1 alterations in lipoblastoma: involvement in varied mesenchymal cell types and evidence for alternative oncogenic mechanisms. *Am J Pathol.* 2001;159:955–962.

77. Shmookler BM, Enzinger FM. Liposarcoma occurring in children. *Cancer.* 1983;52:567–574.

78. Howard WR, Helwig EB. Angiolipoma. *Arch Dermatol.* 1960;82:924–931.

79. Provenzale JM, McLendon RE. Spinal angiolipomas: MR features. *AJNR Am J Neuroradiol.* 1996;17:713–719.

80. Leu NH, Chen CY, Shy CG, et al. MR imaging of an infiltrating spinal epidural angiolipoma. *AJNR Am J Neuroradiol.* 2003;24:1008–1011.

81. Kanter WR, Wolfort FG. Multiple familial angiolipomatosis: treatment of liposuction. *Ann Plast Surg.* 1988;20:277–279.

82. Kumar R, Pereira BJG, Sakhuja V, et al. Autosomal dominant inheritance in familial angiolipomatosis. *Clin Genet.* 1989;35:202–204.

83. Hapnes SA, Boman H, Skeie SO. Familial angiolipomatosis. *Clin Genet.* 1980;17:202–208.

84. Lin JJ, Lin F. Two entities in angiolipoma: a study of 459 cases of lipoma with review of literature on infiltrating angiolipoma. *Cancer.* 1974;34:720–727.

85. Chew FS, Hudson TM, Hawkins IF. Radiology of infiltrating angiolipoma. *AJR Am J Roentgenol.* 1980;135:781–787.

86. Gonzalez-Crussi F, Enneking WF, Arean VM. Infiltrating angiolipoma. *J Bone Joint Surg Am.* 1966;48A:1111–1124.

87. DeOrchis DD, Ozonoff MB. Infiltrating angiolipoma with phlebolith formation. *Skeletal Radiol.* 1986;15:464–467.

88. Pribyl C, Burke SW, Roberts JM, et al. Infiltrating angiolipoma or intramuscular hemangioma? A report of five cases. *J Pediatr Orthop.* 1986;6:172–176.

89. Kim JY, Park JM, Lim GY, et al. Atypical benign lipomatous tumors in soft tissue: radiographic and pathologic correlation. *J Comput Assist Tomogr.* 2002;26:1063–1068.

90. Chew FS, Hudson TM. Hawkins IF. Radiology of infiltrating angiolipoma. *AJR Am J Roentgenol.* 1980;135:781–787.

91. De Orchis D, Ozonoff MB. Infiltrating angiolipoma with phlebolith formation. *Skeletal Radiol.* 1986;15:464–467.

92. Murphey MD, Fairbairn KJ, Parman LM, et al. Musculoskeletal angiomatous lesions: radiologic-pathologic correlation. *Radiographics.* 1995;15:893–917.

93. Enzinger FM, Harvey DA. Spindle cell lipoma. *Cancer.* 1975;36:1852–1859.

94. Bancroft LW, Kransdorf MJ, Peterson JJ, et al. Imaging characteristics of spindle cell lipoma. *AJR Am J Roentgenol.* 2003;181:1251–1254.

95. Sund S, Hordvik M, Maehle B, et al. Large intramuscular spindle-cell lipoma. A case report. *APMIS.* 1988;96:347–351.

96. Braunschweig IJ, Stein IH, Dodwad MIM, et al. Case Report 751. Spindle cell lipoma causing marked bone erosion. *Skeletal Radiol.* 1992;21:414–417.

97. Christopoulos P, Nicolatou O, Patrikiou A. Oral spindle cell lipoma: report of a case. *Int J Oral Maxillofac Surg.* 1989;18:208–209.

98. Nonaka S, Enomoto K, Kawabori S, et al. Spindle cell lipoma within the larynx: a case report with correlated light and electron microscopy. *Orl J Otorhinolaryngol Relat Spec.* 1993;55:147–149.

99. Evans HL. Liposarcoma: a study of 55 cases with a reassessment of its classification. *Am J Surg Pathol.* 1979;3:507–523.

100. Evans HL, Soule EH, Winkelmann RK. Atypical lipoma, atypical intramuscular lipoma, and well differentiated retroperitoneal liposarcoma. A reappraisal of 30 cases formerly classified as well differentiated liposarcoma. *Cancer.* 1979;43:574–584.

101. Bolen JW, Thorning D. Spindle-cell lipoma: a clinical, light- and electron-microscopical study. *Am J Surg Pathol.* 1981;5:435–541.

102. Fletcher CDM, Martin-Bates E. Spindle cell lipoma: a clinicopathological study with some original observations. *Histopathology.* 1987;11:803–817.

103. Hawley IC, Krausz T, Evans DJ, et al. Spindle cell lipoma—a pseudoangiomatous variant. *Histopathology.* 1994;24:565–569.

104. Math KR, Pavlov H, DiCarlo E, et al. Spindle cell lipoma of the foot: a case report and literature review. *Foot Ankle Int.* 1995;16:220–226.

105. Meis JM, Enzinger FM. Myolipoma of soft tissue. *Am J Surg Pathol.* 1991;15:121–125.

106. Guillou L, Coindre J. Newly described adipocytic lesions. *Semin Diagn Pathol.* 2001;18:238–249.

107. Liang EY, Cooper JE, Lam WWM, et al. Case report: Myolipoma or liposarcoma—a mistaken identity in the retroperitoneum. *Clin Radiol.* 1996;51:295–297.

108. Brown PG, Shaver EG. Myolipoma in a tethered cord. Case report and review of the literature. *J Neurosurg.* 2000;92:214–216.

109. Chan JKC, Lee KC, Saw D. Extraskeletal chondroma with lipoblast-like cells. *Hum Pathol.* 1986;17:1285–1287.

110. Meis JM, Enzinger FM. Chondroid lipoma: a unique tumor simulating liposarcoma and myxoid chondrosarcoma. *Am J Surg Pathol.* 1993;17:1103–1112.

111. Logan PM, Janzen DL, O'Connell JX, et al. Chondroid lipoma: MRI appearances with clinical and histologic correlation. *Skeletal Radiol.* 1996;25:592–595.

112. Yang YJ, Damron TA, Ambrose JL. Diagnosis of chondroid lipoma by fine-needle aspiration biopsy. *Arch Pathol Lab Med.* 2001;125:1224–1226.

113. Ohguri T, Aoki T, Hisaoka M, et al. Differential diagnosis of benign peripheral lipoma from well-differentiated liposarcoma on MR imaging: is comparison of margins and internal characteristics useful? *AJR Am J Roentgenol.* 2003;180:1689–1694.

114. Morris AD, Jane MJ, Ritchie D, et al. Diffuse intramuscular lipomatosis of a lower limb. *Sarcoma.* 1998;2:53–56.

115. Gaskin CM, Helms CA. Lipomas, lipoma variants, and well-differentiated liposarcomas (atypical lipomas): results of MRI evaluations of 126 consecutive fatty masses. *AJR Am J Roentgenol.* 2004;182:733–739.

116. Mason ML. Presentation of cases. In: Proceedings of the American Society for Surgery of the Hand. *J Bone Joint Surg Am.* 1953;35A:273–275.

117. Silverman TA, Enzinger FM. Fibrolipomatous hamartoma of nerve. A clinicopathologic analysis of 26 cases. *Am J Surg Pathol.* 1985;9:7–14.

118. Blacksin M, Barnes FJ, Lyons MM. MR diagnosis of macrodystrophia lipomatosa. *AJR Am J Roentgenol.* 1992;158:1295–1297.

119. Jain R, Sawhney S, Berry M. CT diagnosis of macrodystrophia lipomatosa: a case report. *Acta Radiol.* 1992;33:554–555.

120. Amadio PC, Reiman HM, Dobyns JH. Lipofibromatous hamartoma of nerve. *J Hand Surg.* 1988;13A:67–75.

121. Cavallaro MC, Taylor JAM, Gorman JD, et al. Imaging findings in a patient with fibrolipomatous hamartoma of the median nerve. *AJR Am J Roentgenol.* 1993;161:837–838.

122. Samlaska CP, Levin SW, James WD, et al. Proteus syndrome. *Arch Dermatol.* 1989;125:1109–1114.

123. Langa V, Posner MA, Steiner GE. Lipofibroma of the median nerve: a report of two cases. *J Hand Surg.* 1987;12B:221–223.

124. Weissman BN, Wong M, Smith D. Image interpretation session: 1996. *Radiographics.* 1997;17:243–267.

125. Murphey MD, Smith WS, Smith SE, et al. Imaging of musculoskeletal neurogenic tumors: radiologic-pathologic correlation. *Radiographics.* 1999;19:1253–1280.

126. Kremchek TE, Kremchek EJ. Carpal tunnel syndrome caused by flexor tendon sheath lipoma. *Orthop Rev.* 1988;17:1083–1085.

127. Marui T, Yamamoto T, Kimura T, et al. A true intra-articular lipoma of the knee in a girl. *Arthroscopy.* 2002;18:E24.

128. Hallel T, Lew S, Bansal M. Villous lipomatous proliferation of the synovial membrane (lipoma arborescens). *J Bone Joint Surg Am.* 1988;70A:264–270.

129. Coventry MB, Harrison EG, Martin JF. Benign synovial tumors of the knee: a diagnostic problem. *J Bone Joint Surg Am.* 1966;48A:1350–1358.

130. Armstrong SJ, Watt I. Lipoma arborescens of the knee. *Br J Radiol.* 1989;62:178–180.

131. Grieten M, Buckwalter KA, Cardinal E, et al. Case report 873. Lipoma arborescens (villous lipomatous proliferation of the synovial membrane). *Skeletal Radiol.* 1994;23:652–655.

132. Martinez D, Millner PA, Coral A, et al. Case report 745. Synovial lipoma arborescens. *Skeletal Radiol.* 1992;21:393–395.

133. Feller JF, Rishi M, Hughes EC. Lipoma arborescens of the knee: MR demonstration. *AJR Am J Roentgenol.* 1994;163:162–164.

134. Vilanova JC, Barcelo J, Villalon M, et al. MT imaging of lipoma arborescens and associated lesions. *Skeletal Radiol.* 2003;32:504–509.

135. Doyle AJ, Miller MV, French JG. Lipoma arborescens in the bicipital bursa of the elbow: MRI findings in two cases. *Skeletal Radiol.* 2002;31:656–660.

136. Dinauer P, Bojescul JA, Kaplan KJ, et al. Bilateral lipoma arborescens of the bicipitoradial bursa. *Skeletal Radiol.* 2002;31:661–665.

137. Burgan DW. Lipoma arborescens of the knee: another cause of filling defects on a knee arthrogram. *Radiology.* 1971;101:583–584.

138. Enzi G, Carraro R, Alfieri P, et al. Shoulder girdle lipomatosis. *Ann Int Med.* 1992;117:749–750.

139. Coode PE, McGuinness FE, Rawas MM, et al. Diffuse lipomatosis involving the thoracic and abdominal wall: CT features. *J Comput Assist Tomogr.* 1991;15:341–343.

140. Slavin SA, Baker DC, McCarthy JG, et al. Congenital infiltrating lipomatosis of the face: clinicopathologic evaluation and treatment. *Plast Reconst Surg.* 1983;72:158–164.

141. Donati L, Candiani P, Grappolini S, et al. Congenital infiltrating lipomatosis of the face related to cytomegalovirus infection. *Br J Plast Surg.* 1990;43:124–126.

142. Patel RV, Gondalia JS. Congenital infiltrating lipomatosis of the face [letter]. *Br J Plast Surg.* 1991;44:157–158.

143. Ünal S, Demirkan F, Arslan E, et al. Infiltrating lipomatosis of the face: a case report and review of the literature. *J Oral Maxillofac Surg.* 2003;61:1098–1101.

144. Padwa BL, Mulliken JB. Facial infiltrating lipomatosis. *Plast Reconstr Surg.* 2001;108:1544–1554.

145. Bouletreau P, Breton P, Freidel M. Congenital infiltrating lipomatosis of the face. Case report. *J Oral Maxillofac Surg.* 2000;58:807–810.

146. Shugar MA, Gavron JP. Benign symmetrical lipomatosis (Madelung's disease). *Otolaryngol Head Neck Surg.* 1985;93:109–112.

147. Chalk CH, Mills KR, Jacobs JM, et al. Familial multiple symmetric lipomatosis with peripheral neuropathy. *Neurology.* 1990;40:1246–1250.

148. Brodie DC. *Lectures Illustrative of Various Subjects in Pathology and Surgery.* London: Longman; 1846:275–276.

149. Lee MS, Lee MH, Hur KB. Multiple symmetric lipomatosis. *J Korean Med Sci.* 1988;3:163–167.

150. Enzi G, Biondetti PR, Fiore D, et al. Computed tomography of deep fat masses in multiple symmetrical lipomatosis. *Radiology.* 1982;144:121–124.

151. Chong PST, Vucic S, Hedley-Whyte ET, et al. Multiple symmetric lipomatosis (Madelung's disease) caused by the MERRF (A8344G) mutation. *J Clin Neuromusc Dis.* 2003;5:1–7.

152. Lee HW, Kim TH, Cho JW, et al. Multiple symmetric lipomatosis: Korean experience. *Dermatol Surg.* 2003;29:235–240.

153. Busetto L, Strater D, Enzi G, et al. Differential clinical expression of multiple symmetric lipomatosis in men and women. *Int J Obes Relat Metab Disord.* 2003;27:1419–1422.

154. Gabriel YA, Chew DKW, Wedderburn RV. Multiple symmetrical lipomatosis (Madelung's disease). *Surgery.* 2001;129:117–118.

155. Comings DE, Glenchur H. Benign symmetric lipomatosis [letter]. *JAMA.* 1968;203:305.

156. Martin DS, Sharafuddin M, Boozan J, et al. Multiple symmetric lipomatosis (Madelung's disease). *Skeletal Radiol.* 1995;24:72–73.

157. Enzi G. Multiple symmetric lipomatosis: an updated clinical report. *Medicine.* 1984;63:56–64.

158. Morelli F, Feliciani C, De Benedetto A, et al. Alcoholism as a trigger of multiple symmetric lipomatosis [letter]. *J Eur Acad Dermatol Venerol.* 2003;17:367–368.

159. Salgado R, Bernaerts A, de Beeck BO, et al. Madelung's neck: cross-sectional imaging observations. *AJR Am J Roentgenol.* 2004;182:1344–1345.

160. Enzi G, Angelini C, Negrin P, et al. Sensory, motor and autonomic neuropathy in patients with multiple symmetric lipomatosis. *Medicine.* 1986;64:388–393.

161. Watt AJB, McMillan N. Multiple symmetric lipomatosis—MR appearances. *Clin Radiol.* 1999;54:778–780.

162. Yu JS, Weis L, Becker W. MR imaging of a parosteal lipoma. *Clin Imaging.* 2000;24:15–18.

163. Ahuja AT, King AD, Chan ESY, et al. Madelung disease: distribution of cervical fat and preoperative findings at sonography, MR and CT. *AJNR Am J Neuroradiol.* 1998;19:707–710.

164. McEachern A, Janzen DL, O'Connell JX. Shoulder girdle lipomatosis. *Skeletal Radiol.* 1995;24:471–473.

165. Dercum FX. Three cases of a hitherto unclassified affection resembling in its grosser aspects obesity, but associated with special nervous symptoms-adiposis dolorosa. *Am J Med Sci.* 1892;104:521–535.

166. Brodovsky S, Westreich M, Leibowitz A, et al. Adiposis dolorosa (Dercum's disease): 10-year follow-up. *Ann Plast Surg.* 1994;33:664–668.

167. Bonatus TJ, Alexander AH. Dercum's disease (adiposis dolorosa). A case report and review of the literature. *Clin Orthop.* 1986;205:251–253.

168. Reece PH, Wyatt M, O'Flynn P. Dercum's disease (adiposis dolorosa). *J Laryngol Otol.* 1999;113:174–176.

169. Wohl MG, Pastor N. Adiposis dolorosa (Dercum's disease). *JAMA.* 1938;110:1261–1264.

170. Gery L. Discussions. *Bull Mem Soc Anat Paris.* 1914;89:111.

171. Kallas KM, Vaughan L, Haghighi P, et al. Hibernoma of the left axilla; a case report and review of the literature. *Skeletal Radiol.* 2003;32:290–294.

172. Ahn C, Harvey JC. Mediastinal hibernoma, a rare tumor. *Ann Thorac Surg.* 1990;50:828–830.

173. Lateur L, Van Ongeval C, Samson I, et al. Case report 842. Benign hibernoma. *Skeletal Radiol.* 1994;23:306–309.

174. Shaw HB. Contribution to the study of the morphology of adipose tissue. *J Anat Physiol.* 1902;36:1–13.

175. Nigrisoli M, Ruggieri P, Picci P, et al. Case report 489. *Skeletal Radiol.* 1988;17:432–435.

176. Alvine G, Rosenthal H, Murphey H, et al. Hibernoma. *Skeletal Radiol.* 1996;25:493–496.

177. Furlong MA, Fanburg-Smith JC, Miettinen M. The morphologic spectrum of hibernoma. A clinicopathologic study of 170 cases. *Am J Surg Pathol.* 2001;25:809–816.

178. McLane RC, Meyer LC. Axillary hibernoma: review of the literature with report of a case examined angiographically. *Radiology.* 1978;127:673–674.

179. Rigor VU, Goldstone SE, Jones J, Bernstein R, Gold MS, Weiner S. Hibernoma: a case report and discussion of a rare tumor. *Cancer.* 1986;57:2207–2211.

180. Angervall L, Nilsson L, Stener B. Microangiographic and histologic studies in 2 cases of hibernoma. *Cancer.* 1964;17:685–692.

181. Deseran MW, Seeger LL, Doberneck SA, et al. Case report 840. Hibernoma of the right gracilis muscle. *Skeletal Radiol.* 1994;23:301–302.

182. Seynaeve P, Mortelmans L, Knockx M, et al. Case report 813. Hibernoma of the left thigh. *Skeletal Radiol.* 1994;23:137–138.

183. Anderson SE, Schwab C, Stauffer E, et al. Hibernoma: imaging characteristics of a rare benign soft tissue tumor. *Skeletal Radiol.* 2001;30:590–595.

184. Murphey MD, Kransdorf MJ, Choi JJ, et al. Imaging of hibernoma. *Radiology.* 2000;217(P):573.

185. Atilla S, Eilenberg SS, Brown JJ. Hibernoma: MRI appearance of a rare tumor. *Magn Reson Imaging.* 1995;13:335–337.

186. Chatterton BE, Mensforth D, Coventry BJ, et al. Hibernoma: intense uptake seen on Tc-99m tetrofosmin and FDG positron emission tomographic scanning. *Clin Nucl Med.* 2002;27:369–370.

187. Oller JD, Gomez JD, Kortazar JF, et al. Scapular hibernoma fortuitously discovered on myocardial perfusion imaging through Tc-99m tetrofosmin. *Clin Nucl Med.* 2001;26:69–70.

188. Goldman AB, DiCarlo EF, Marcove RC. Case report 774. Coincidental lipoma with osseous excrescence and intramuscular lipoma. *Skeletal Radiol.* 1993;22:138–145.

189. Seering G. Geschicte eines sehr grossen steatoms im hinterhaupte eines 2 und 1/2 jährigen kindes. *Mag Ges Heil.* 1836;511–514.

190. Power D. Parosteal lipoma, or congenital fatty tumor, connected with periosteum of femur. *Trans Pathol Soc London.* 1888;39:270–272.

191. Murphey MD, Johnson DL, Bhatia PS, et al. Parosteal lipoma: MR imaging characteristics. *AJR Am J Roentgenol.* 1994;162:105–110.

192. Imbriaco M, Ignarra R, De Rosa N, et al. Parosteal lipoma of the rib. CT findings and pathologic correlation. *Clin Imaging.* 2003;27:435–437.

193. Jacobs P. Parosteal lipoma with hyperostosis. *Clin Radiol.* 1972;23:196–198.

194. Moon N, Marmor L. Parostel lipoma of the proximal part of the radius. A clinical entity with frequent radial-nerve injury. *J Bone Joint Surg Am.* 1964;46A:608–614.

195. Khan AA, Mathew B. Parosteal lipoma. *J Indian Med Assoc.* 1974;63:285–286.

196. Steiner M, Gould AR, Rasmussen J, et al. Parosteal lipoma of the mandible. *Oral Surg Oral Med Oral Pathol.* 1981;52:61–65.

197. Krajewska I, Vernon-Roberts B, Sorby-Adams G. Parosteal (periosteal) lipoma. *Pathology.* 1988;20:179–183.

198. Rosen H. Parosteal lipoma. *Bull Hosp Joint Dis.* 1959;20:96–102.

199. Jones JG, Habermann ET, Dorfman HD. Case report 553. Parosteal ossifying lipoma of femur. *Skeletal Radiol.* 1989;18:537–540.

200. Berry JB, Moiel RH. Parosteal lipoma producing paralysis of the deep radial nerve. *South Med J.* 1973;66:1298–1300.

201. Brooks ML, Mayer DP, Grannick MS, et al. Parosteal lipoma of the finger: preoperative evaluation with computed tomography. *Comput Med Imaging Graph.* 1989;13:481–485.

202. Demos TC, Bruno E, Armin A, et al. Parosteal lipoma with enlarging osteochondroma. *AJR Am J Roentgenol.* 1984;143:365–366.

203. Kurland KZ, Kennard JW. Parosteal lipoma arising from the proximal radius: a case report. *Clin Orthop.* 1965;41:140–144.

204. Nishida J, Shimamura T, Ehara S, et al. Posterior interosseous nerve palsy caused by parosteal lipoma of proximal radius. *Skeletal Radiol.* 1998;27:375–379.

205. Fitzgerald A, Anderson W, Hooper G. Posterior interosseous nerve palsy due to parosteal lipoma. *J Hand Surg [Br].* 2002;27:535–537.

206. Henrique A. A high radial neuropathy by parosteal lipoma compression. *J Shoulder Elbow Surg.* 2002;11:386–388.

207. Fleming RJ, Alpert M, Garcia A. Parosteal lipoma. *AJR Am J Roentgenol.* 1962;87:1075–1084.

208. Petit MM, Swarts S, Bridge JA, et al. Expression of reciprocal fusion transcripts of the HMGIC and LPP genes in parosteal lipoma. *Cancer Genet Cytogenet.* 1998;106:18–23.

209. Bui-Mansfield LT, Myers CP, Chew FS. Parosteal lipoma of the fibula. *AJR Am J Roentgenol.* 2000;174:1698.

210. Rodriguez-Peralto JL, Lopez-Barea F, Gonzalez-Lopez J, et al. Case report 821. Parosteal ossifying lipoma of femur. *Skeletal Radiol.* 1994;23:67–69.

211. Kindblom LG, Angervall L, Svendsen P. Liposarcoma: a clinicopathologic, radiographic, and prognostic study. *Acta Pathol Microbiol Scand Suppl.* 1975;253:1–71.

212. Weiss SW, Goldblum JR. Liposarcoma. In: *Enzinger and Weiss's Soft Tissue Tumors.* 4th ed. St. Louis: Mosby; 2001:641–693.

213. Enzinger FM, Winslow DL. Liposarcoma: a study of 103 cases. *Virchows Arch Pathol Anat Physiol.* 1962;335:367–388.

214. Dei Tos AP. Liposarcoma: new entities and evolving concepts. *Ann Diagn Pathol.* 2000;4:252–266.

215. Evans HL. Liposarcomas and atypical lipomatous tumors: a study of 66 cases followed for a minimum of 10 years. *Surg Pathol.* 1988;1:41–54.

216. Meis JM. "Dedifferentiation" in bone and soft-tissue tumors: a histologic indicator of tumor progression. In: Rosen PP, Feckner RE, eds. *Pathology Annual.* Norwalk, Conn: Appleton & Lange; 1991:37–62.

217. Weiss SW, Rao VK. Well-differentiated liposarcoma (atypical lipoma) of the deep soft tissues of the extremities, retroperitoneum and miscellaneous sites: a follow-up study of 92 cases with analysis of "dedifferentiation." *Am J Surg Pathol.* 1992;16:1051–1058.

218. Ippolito V, Brien EW, Menendez LR, et al. Case report 797. "Dedifferentiated" lipoma-like liposarcoma of soft tissue with focal transformation to high-grade "sclerosing" osteosarcoma. *Skeletal Radiol.* 1993;22:604–608.

219. Lucas DR, Nascimento AG, Sabjay KKS, et al. Well-differentiated liposarcoma: the Mayo clinic experience with 58 cases. *Am J Clin Pathol.* 1994;102:677–683.

220. LaQuaglia MP, Spiro SA, Ghavimi F, et al. Liposarcoma in patients younger than or equal to 22 years of age. *Cancer.* 1993;72:3114–3119.

221. Castleberry RP, Kelly DR, Wilson ER, et al. Childhood liposarcoma. Report of a case and review of the literature. *Cancer.* 1984;54:579–584.

222. Reszel PA, Soule EH, Coventry MB. Liposarcoma of the extremities and limb girdles. A study of two hundred twenty-two cases. *J Bone Joint Surg Am.* 1966;48A:229–244.

223. Vezeridis MP, Moore R, Karakousis CP. Metastatic patterns in soft-tissue sarcomas. *Arch Surg.* 1983;118:915–918.

224. Sim FH, Pritchard DJ, Reiman HM, et al. Soft-tissue sarcoma: Mayo clinic experience. *Semin Surg Oncol.* 1988;4:38–44.

225. Pearlstone DB, Pisters PWT, Bold RJ, et al. Patterns of recurrence in extremity liposarcoma. Implications for staging and follow-up. *Cancer.* 1999;85:85–92.

226. Oliveira AM, Nascimento AG. Pleomorphic liposarcoma. *Semin Diagn Pathol.* 2001;18:274–285.

227. Tateishi I, Hasegawa T, Beppu Y, et al. Prognostic significance of MRI findings in patients with myxoid-round cell liposarcoma. *AJR Am J Roentgenol.* 2004;182:725–731.

228. Kransdorf MJ, Meis JM, Jelinek JS. Dedifferentiated liposarcoma of the extremities: imaging findings in four patients. *AJR Am J Roentgenol.* 1993;161:127–130.

229. Brooks JJ, Connor AM. Atypical lipoma of the extremities and peripheral soft tissues with dedifferentiation: implications for management. *Surg Pathol.* 1990;3:169–178.

230. Matsumoto K, Hukuda S, Ishizawa M, et al. Liposarcoma associated with multiple intramuscular lipomas. A case report. *Clin Orthop.* 2000;373:202–207.

231. Yang YJ, Damron TA, Cohen H, et al. Distinction of well-differentiated liposarcoma from lipoma in two patients with multiple well-differentiated fatty masses. *Skeletal Radiol.* 2001;30:584–589.

232. Barkhof F, Melkert P, Meyer S, et al. Derangement of adipose tissue: a case report of multicentric retroperitoneal liposarcomas, retroperitoneal lipomatosis and multiple subcutaneous lipomas. *Eur J Surg Oncol.* 1991;17:547–550.

233. Schiller H. Lipomata in sarcomatous transformation. *Surg Gynecol Obstet.* 1918;27:218–219.

234. Wright CJE. Liposarcoma arising in a simple lipoma. *J Pathol Bacteriol.* 1948;60:483–487.

235. Sampson CC, Saunders EH, Green WE. Liposarcoma developing in a lipoma. *Arch Pathol.* 1960;69:506–510.

236. Sternberg SS. Liposarcoma arising within a subcutaneous lipoma. *Cancer.* 1952;5:975–978.

237. Chew FS, Hudson TM. Radionuclide imaging of lipoma and liposarcoma. *Radiology.* 1980;136:741–745.

238. Munk PL, Lee MJ, Janzen DL, et al. Lipoma and liposarcoma: evaluation using CT and MR imaging. *AJR Am J Roentgenol.* 1997;169:589–594.

239. Bush CH, Spanier SS, Gillespy T. Imaging of atypical lipomas of the extremities: report of three cases. *Skeletal Radiol.* 1988;17:472–475.

240. Jelinek JS, Kransdorf MJ, Shmookler BM, et al. Liposarcoma of the extremities: MR and CT findings of the histologic subtypes. *Radiology.* 1993;186:455–459.

241. Lindahl S, Markhede G, Berlin Ö. Computed tomography of lipomatous and myxoid tumors. *Acta Radiol Diagn.* 1985;26:709–713.

242. Hosono M, Kobayashi H, Fujimoto R, et al. Septum-like structure in lipoma and liposarcoma: MR imaging and pathologic correlation. *Skeletal Radiol.* 1997;26:150–154.

243. Arkun R, Memis A, Akalin T, et al. Liposarcoma of soft tissue: MRI findings with pathologic correlation. *Skeletal Radiol.* 1997;26:167–172.

244. Sung MS, Kang HS, Suh JS, et al. Myxoid liposarcoma: appearance at MR imaging with histologic correlation. *Radiographics.* 2000;20:1007–1019.

245. Bancroft LW, Kransdorf MJ, Menke DM, et al. Intramuscular myxoma: characteristic MR imaging features. *AJR Am J Roentgenol.* 2002;178:1255–1259.

246. O'Connor MI. Surgical management of malignant soft-tissue tumors. In: Simon MA, Springfield DS, eds. *Surgery for Bone and Soft-Tissue Tumors,* ed. Philadelphia: Lippincott-Raven; 1998:555–565.

247. O'Connor MI. Multimodality management of malignant soft-tissue tumors. In: Simon MA, Springfield DS, eds. *Surgery for Bone and Soft-Tissue Tumors,* ed. Philadelphia: Lippincott-Raven; 1998:567–575.

248. Redmonson JH, Peterson IA, Shives TC, et al. Chemotherapy, irradiation, and surgery for function-preserving therapy of primary extremity soft tissue sarcomas. *Cancer.* 2002;94:786–792.

249. Sundaram M, McGuire MH, Herbold DR, et al. High signal intensity soft tissue masses on T1 weighted pulsing sequences. *Skeletal Radiol.* 1987;16:30–36.

250. Greene KM, Brantly PN, Thompson WR. Adenocarcinoma metastatic to the adrenal gland simulating myelolipoma: CT evaluation. *J Comput Assist Tomogr.* 1985;9:820–821.

251. Kumar AJ, Francis FP, Martinez CR, et al. Computed tomography of extracranial nerve sheath tumors with pathologic correlation. *J Comput Assist Tomogr.* 1983;7:857–865.

252. Cohen LM, Schwartz AM, Rockoff SD. Benign schwannomas: pathologic basis for CT inhomogeneities. *AJR Am J Roentgenol.* 1986;147:141–143.

Vascular and Lymphatic Tumors

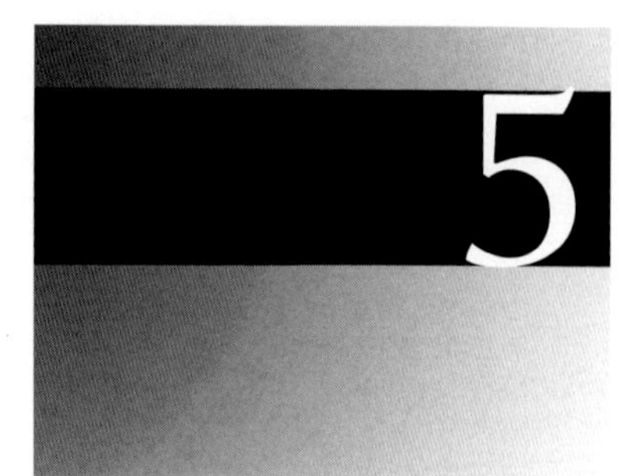

Angiomatous lesions of the musculoskeletal system are common causes of soft tissue masses, particularly in young patients (1,2). These lesions, unfortunately, are frequently confused with other neoplastic masses both clinically and radiologically. However, CT and MR imaging often demonstrate characteristic features that allow radiologic diagnosis. This chapter reviews the spectrum of angiomatous lesions of the musculoskeletal system, including hemangioma, pleomorphic hyalinizing angiectatic tumor of soft parts, reactive vascular lesions, lymphangioma, angiomatosis, angiomatous syndromes and associations, glomus tumor, hemangioendothelioma, hemangiopericytoma, Kaposi sarcoma, and angiosarcoma. This organization is largely based on the categorization by the WHO Committee for the Classification of Soft Tissue Tumors (3).

KEY CONCEPTS
Angiomatous lesions can be divided into the following categories:
- Hemangioma
- Other benign and reactive vascular lesions
- Lymphangioma
- Glomus tumor
- Aggressive and malignant vascular tumor: hemangioendothelioma; hemangiopericytoma/solitary fibrous tumor; Kaposi sarcoma; and angiosarcoma

---

HEMANGIOMA

Hemangiomas are among the most frequent tumors to involve the soft tissue. These vascular lesions comprise 7% of all benign tumors, and hemangioma is the most common tumor of infancy and childhood (1–5). An estimated 1% to 2% of the general population is affected and up to 10% of Caucasians (6). Clinical evaluation often reveals a painful lesion that intermittently changes in size, and superficial lesions may have characteristic overlying bluish skin discoloration (7). The pain associated with intramuscular hemangiomas may be vague and only present after exercise. This is presumably caused by relative hypoxia of surrounding muscle as opposed to increased blood flow to the hemangioma. Soft tissue hemangiomas are usually discovered in the first three decades of life, with 30% discovered at birth (2–6). These lesions are more common in women with an approximate 3:1 ratio (2). Lesions may increase dramatically in size during pregnancy because of both increased blood volume and engorgement, as well as endocrine-related stimulation of growth. Soft tissue hemangiomas may be superficial or deep, with the latter lesions most frequently intramuscular.

We use the term *hemangioma* in its broadest sense, agreeing with Weiss and Goldblum that these lesions represent a benign nonreactive lesion with an increase in the number of normal- or abnormal-appearing vessels (2). We acknowledge that other classifications distinguish vascular malformations (blood or lymphatic vessels with normal endothelial cell mitotic activity) and hemangioma (bloods vessels with endothelial hyperplasia). Pathologically, hemangiomas can be subclassified by the predominant type of vascular channel (capillary, cavernous, arteriovenous, or venous) identified within the lesion (2). There is frequently an admixture of histologic components within hemangiomas, and in some lesions subclassification is not possible. Nonvascular elements are also commonly present in hemangiomas, including fat, smooth muscle, fibrous tissue, bone, hemosiderin, and thrombus. Identification of fat is particularly common in hemangiomas (cavernous lesions most frequently) and deserves specific comment. In almost all cases, overgrowth of adipose tissue should be considered a reactive phenomenon rather than a true neoplastic component (see discussion of angiolipoma) (8–12).

Capillary Hemangioma

Capillary hemangiomas are composed of small vessels lined by a flattened endothelium. They are divided into juvenile, tufted, verrucous, and senile subtypes. *Pyogenic granuloma* is also a type of capillary hemangioma. These hemangiomas, which typically involve the skin and subcutaneous tissue, are discovered in the first years of life. The juvenile variety is particularly common, occurring in 1 to 2 of every 100 to 200 births, and is multiple in 20% of cases (2,6,13). Juvenile capillary hemangiomas are also referred to as *strawberry nevus, infantile hemangioendothelioma,* and *cellular hemangioma of infancy* (14). Clinically juvenile hemangiomas usually present several weeks after birth and enlarge, at times rapidly, for the ensuing several months, reaching their maximal size by 6 to 12 months of age (14). Lesions initially appear as a flat reddish macule that is similar to a birthmark but intensifies its color with crying or straining. The vast majority of juvenile hemangiomas (75% to 90%) involute spontaneously by 7 years of age (15). Additional subtypes of capillary hemangiomas include: acquired tufted angioma (older patients; acquired erythematous macules involving the upper extremity dermis with slow growth); hobnail hemangioma (young adults; extremities revealing a pigmented or exophytic mass); verrucous hemangioma (overlying reactive hyperkeratosis seen in childhood; recur locally and develop satellite lesions if not fully resected); and cherry angioma (also referred to as senile angioma; affects almost all adults eventually with red papules on thumb or upper limb girdle; increases in number with age). Although capillary hemangiomas are overall the most common type of angiomatous lesion, radiologic evaluation is infrequent because of the superficial location, diagnostic appearance clinically and nonsurgical treatment with spontaneous resolution. Capillary hemangiomas involving the deep soft tissues have a predilection to affect the head and neck region (particularly the midcheek, upper lip, and upper eyelid) (Fig. 5.1).

Cavernous Hemangioma

Cavernous hemangiomas are composed pathologically of dilated spaces filled with blood and lined by flattened endothelium. These lesions most frequently affect young children or adults and present clinically as a nonspecific deep intramuscular mass. Overlying skin discoloration is not apparent in deeply seated lesions. In unusual cases located superficially, lesions may reveal bluish skin discoloration. Sinusoidal hemangioma is a distinct variety of a cavernous lesion in which the large vascular spaces ramify extensively with one another. These lesions often present as a solitary purplish well-defined nodule on the trunk (or breast) and are more common in women. Unlike capillary hemangiomas, cavernous lesions do not involute, are often less well circumscribed, and frequently require surgical

resection (16). For these reasons, although cavernous hemangiomas are less common than the capillary variety, they are more frequently imaged by radiologists (Figs. 5.2–5.8). Cavernous hemangiomas commonly calcify, typically containing dystrophic mineralization in organizing thrombus (phlebolith).

Arteriovenous Hemangioma

Arteriovenous hemangiomas are composed of an abnormal communication of arteries and veins, and pathologically they are considered to represent a persistence of the fetal capillary bed (1,2,17). Arteriovenous hemangiomas occur in the soft tissues of young patients in two forms: superficial lesions (cirsoid aneurysm or acral arteriovenous tumor) without arteriovenous shunting (clinically insignificant) and deep lesions with arteriovenous shunting (clinically symptomatic). Superficial arteriovenous hemangiomas commonly affect the head and neck (particularly the oral and lip region) and present as a painful red-blue papule. Deep-seated lesions typically occur in the extremities, head, and neck of children to young adults. High blood flow is characteristic of these lesions, although occasionally stenosis and thrombosis can cause reduced flow (Figs. 5.9 and 5.10). Clinical abnormalities associated with high-flow lesions are a result of the vascular shunt and include enlarged extremity, venous distention, bruit, increased overlying skin temperature, and reflex bradycardia after compression (Branham sign) (2). As previously discussed, some investigators describe these lesions as arteriovenous malformations (AVMs); we prefer the more general term *arteriovenous hemangioma,* implying a benign nonreactive process with increased number of large blood vessels (normal or abnormal) (2,18). In addition, these lesions are not histologically distinct and are frequently associated with other areas composed of capillary and/or cavernous hemangioma.

Venous Hemangioma

Venous hemangiomas are composed of vessels with thick muscular walls and are rare in the musculoskeletal system. They usually occur in adults involving the deep soft tissues, including the retroperitoneum, mesentery, and extremity musculature (Figs. 5.11 and 5.12). Slow blood flow typifies these lesions and phleboliths may also be present. Dystrophic calcification may also occur in these lesions.

Spindle Cell Hemangioma

Weiss and Enzinger first described the spindle cell hemangioma in 1986 as *spindle cell hemangioendothelioma* that typically affects the subcutaneous tissues of the distal extremities (particularly the hand) in young adults (19). Histologically, this benign tumor is composed of cavernous

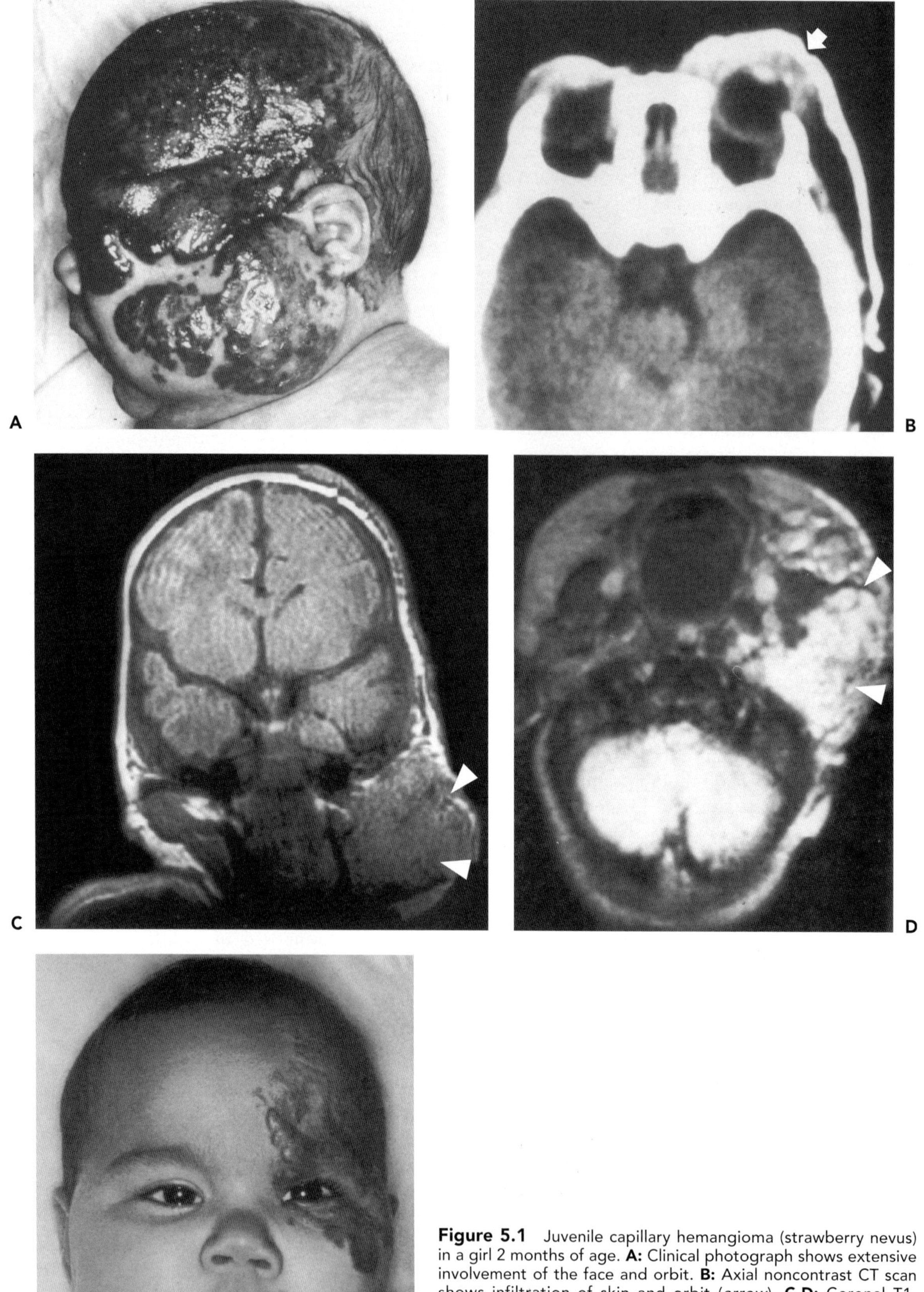

Figure 5.1 Juvenile capillary hemangioma (strawberry nevus) in a girl 2 months of age. **A:** Clinical photograph shows extensive involvement of the face and orbit. **B:** Axial noncontrast CT scan shows infiltration of skin and orbit (*arrow*). **C,D:** Coronal T1-weighted (TR/TE; 500/20) **(C)** and axial T2-weighted (TR/TE; 2000/80) **(D)** spin-echo MR images reveal similar findings, with a mass infiltrating the subcutaneous and deeper soft tissues. The mass (*arrowheads*) shows a nonspecific intermediated signal intensity with T1-weighting and high signal intensity with T2-weighting. **E:** Involution of the hemangioma is depicted by the clinical photograph at 22 months of age with the eye now open and functioning.

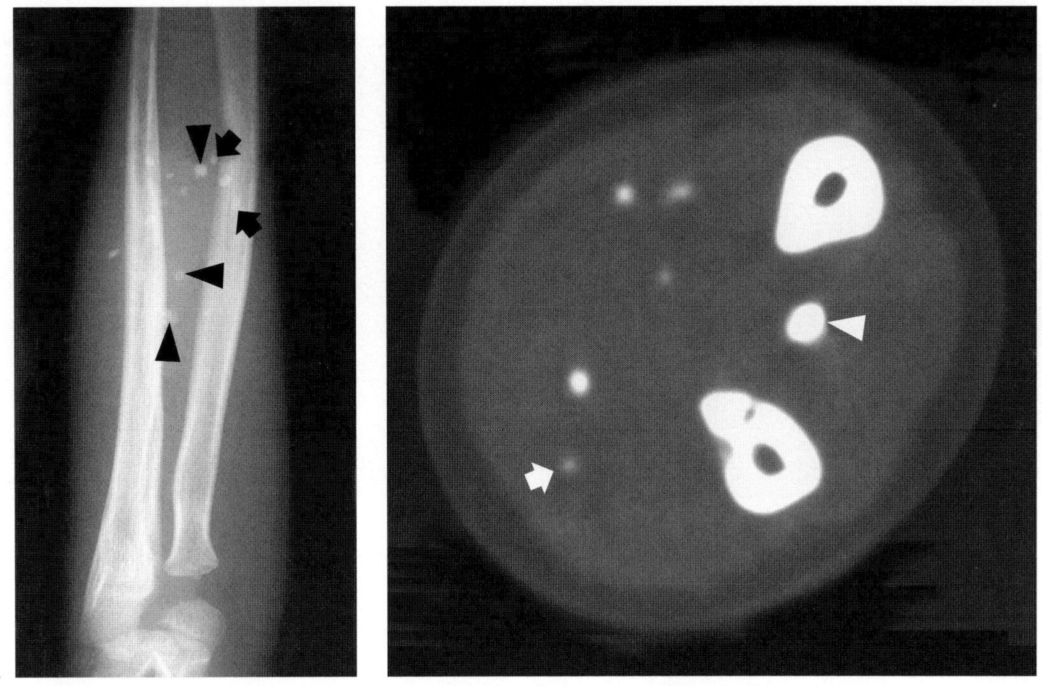

Figure 5.2   Cavernous hemangioma of the forearm in a boy 8 years of age. **A:** Radiograph shows multiple calcifications. Several calcifications have the classic appearance of phleboliths (*arrowheads*); others are more nonspecific (*arrows*). **B:** Axial noncontrast CT displayed at bone windows also shows the calcifications (*arrow* and *arrowhead*).

spaces and spindle cell areas (similar to those seen in Kaposi sarcoma). Treatment is often delayed for a long period of time because of limited initial symptoms. Although most spindle cell hemangiomas begin as a solitary nodule, multiple satellite lesions are frequent. Intravascular growth is seen in approximately 50% of cases and may be responsible for the multifocal lesions and local recurrence in an estimated 60% of cases (20). These lesions may also be associated with Maffucci syndrome and Klippel-Trenaunay-Weber syndrome.

Imaging of Soft Tissue Hemangioma

The vast majority of soft tissue hemangiomas evaluated radiologically are intramuscular lesions. Radiographs are

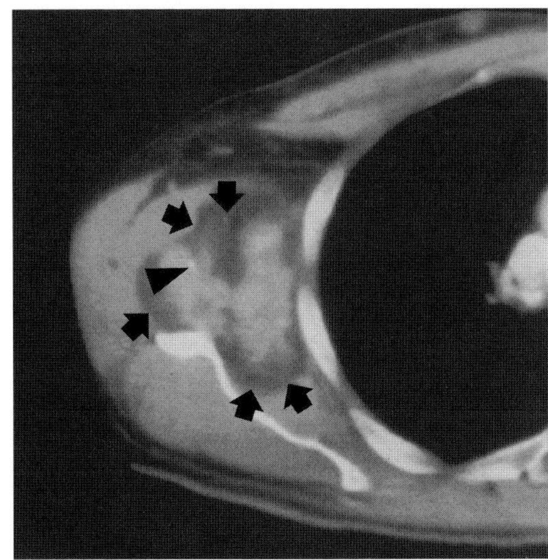
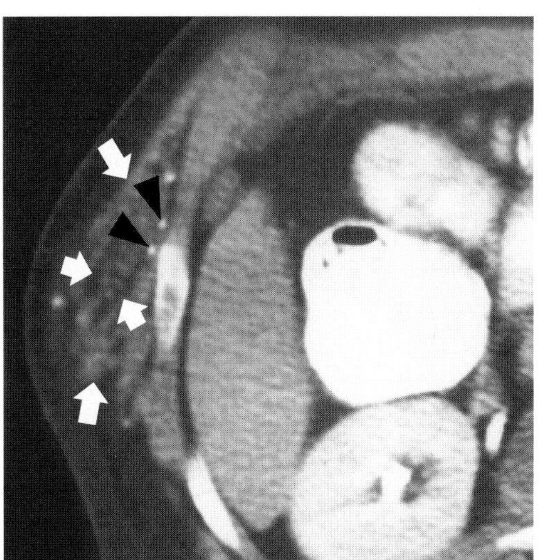

Figure 5.3   Cavernous hemangiomas of the chest wall in two middle-aged patients. **A,B:** Axial CT scans of the chest **(A)** and abdominal wall **(B)** reveal masses (*large arrows,* not seen on radiographs, not shown), and fat overgrowth (*small arrows*). Phleboliths are also seen (*arrowheads*).

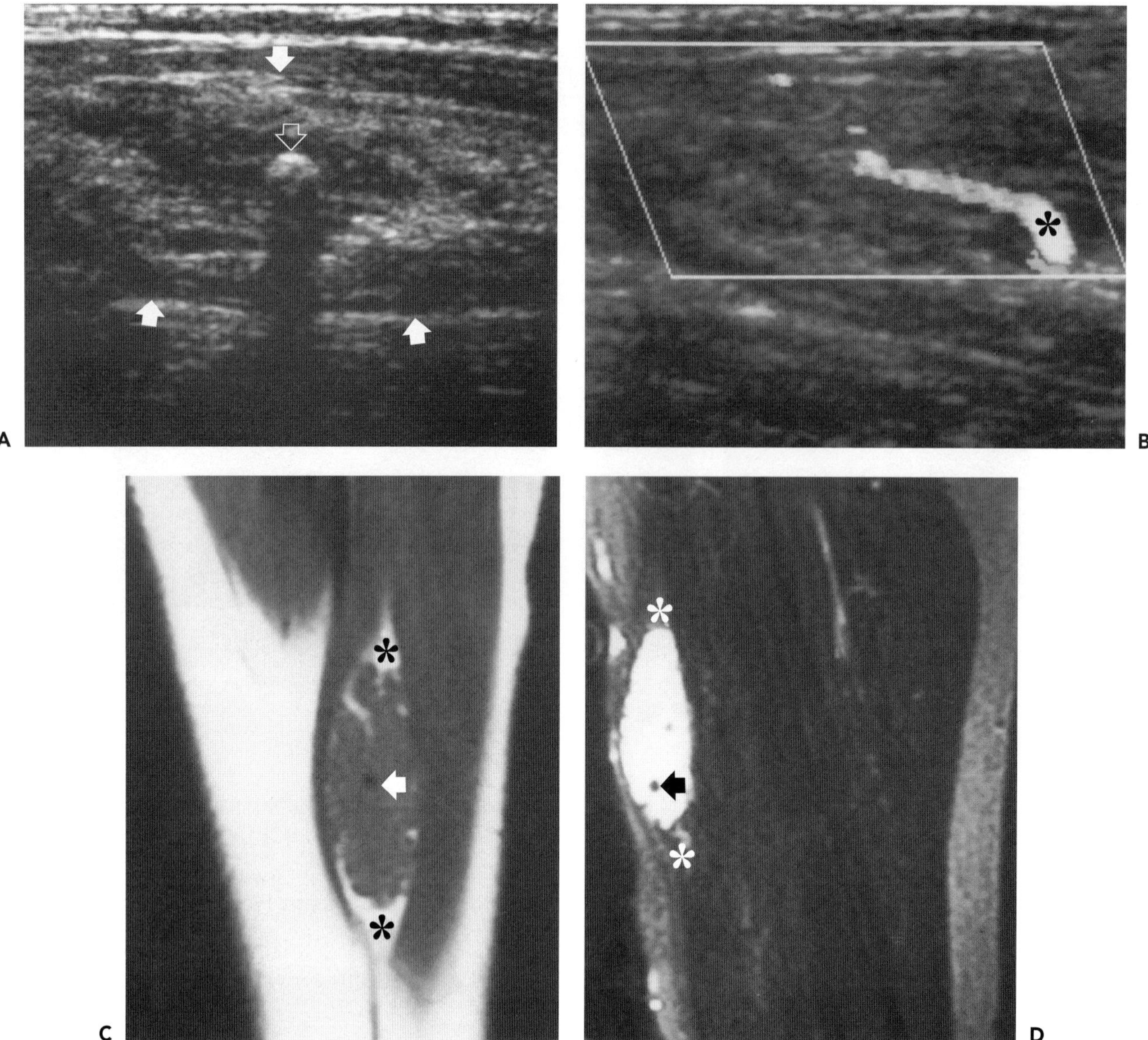

Figure 5.4   Intramuscular cavernous hemangioma in a woman 43 years of age. **A:** Longitudinal image from sonogram reveals a complex mass (*arrows*). Echogenic focus with posterior acoustic shadowing (*open arrow*) represents a phlebolith. **B:** Doppler study demonstrates prominent vascular elements (*asterisk*). **C,D:** Coronal T1-weighted (TR/TE; 500/20) **(C)** and turbo T2-weighted (TR/TE; 3600/102) **(D)** spin-echo MR images reveal a heterogeneous mass that shows areas of high intensity on the long TR image. Phleboliths (*arrow*, low signal intensity all pulse sequences) and peripheral fat overgrowth (*asterisks*) are also present.

often normal or reveal only a nonspecific soft tissue mass. Identification of characteristic calcification in the form of phleboliths is most frequent in cavernous hemangiomas, seen in 20% to 67% of cases (Fig. 5.2), but they are also seen in other angiomatous lesions (1,18,21,22). Nonspecific calcification may also occur in hemangiomas, appearing curvilinear or amorphous (Fig. 5.2). Associated osseous abnormalities are described in 37% of soft tissue hemangiomas on radiographs (22). These bone manifestations include periosteal reaction (23%), cortical abnormality (31%), and medullary abnormality (29%) (22) (Figs. 5.9

and 5.12). These osseous manifestations are best evaluated on radiographs and correspond to a closer proximity of the lesion to bone. Periosteal reaction is typically nonaggressive but rarely spiculated (22). Cortical changes include thickening, erosion, channel-like lucencies (tunneling), and osteopenia (22). Medullary abnormalities include osteopenia, sclerosis, marrow replacement on MR, and rarely serpentine channel-like radiolucencies (22). In addition, chronic hyperemia, resulting from vascular lesions, can lead to bone overgrowth similar to that seen in juvenile chronic arthritis.

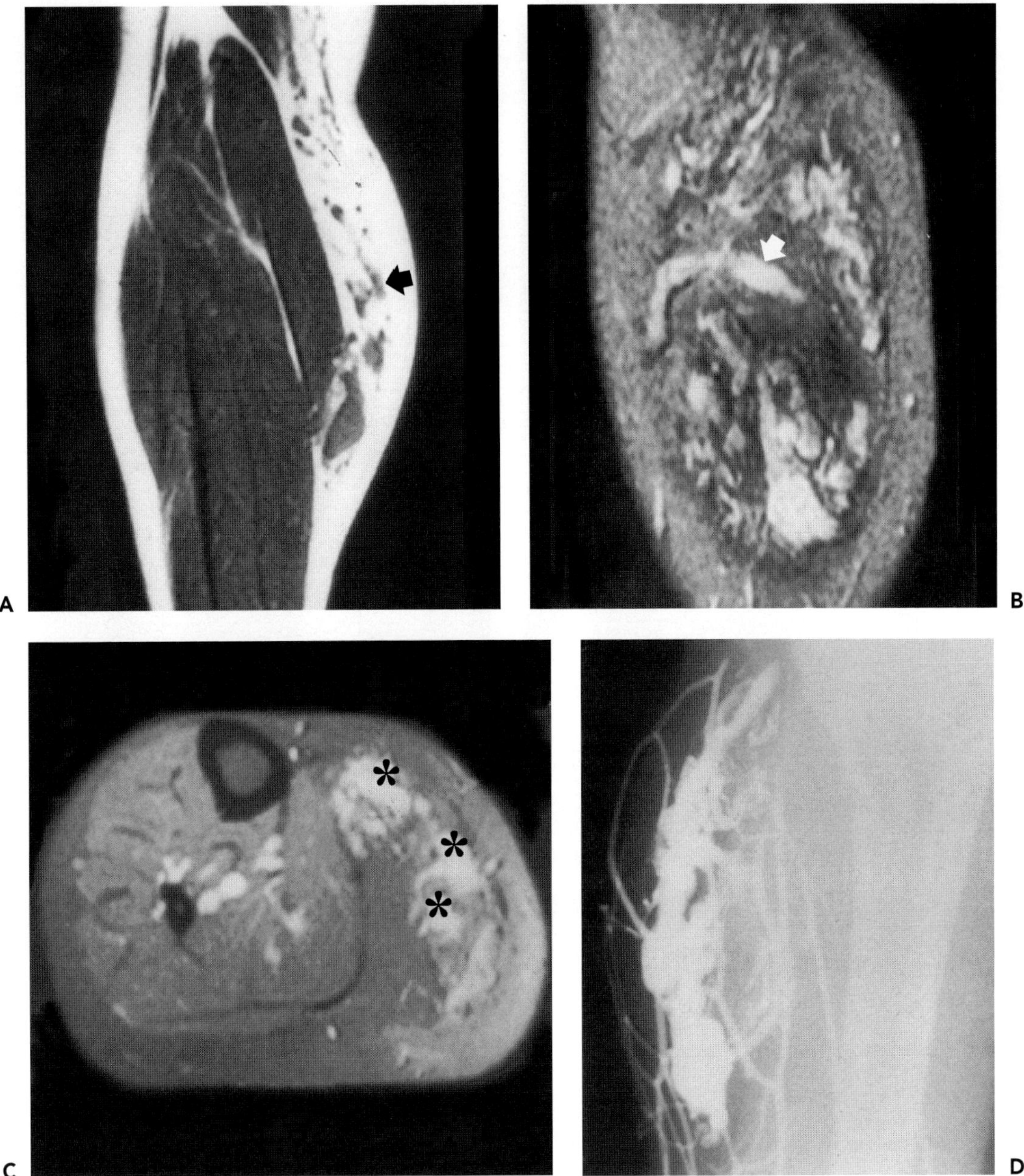

Figure 5.5   Cavernous hemangioma of the calf in a woman 22 years of age with a 10-year history of a slowly enlarging mass. **A,B:** Coronal T1-weighted (TR/TE; 700/20) **(A)** and sagittal T2-weighted (TR/TE; 2250/80) **(B)** spin-echo MR images show a large heterogeneous mass with serpentine vascular channels/spaces (*arrow*) and fat overgrowth. Vascular spaces become markedly high signal on the long TR image **B. C:** Axial T1-weighted (TR/TE; 300/12) MR image with fat suppression following intravenous gadolinium also shows prominent enhancing vascular spaces (*asterisks*). **D:** Large cavernous vascular spaces are also well shown on the angiogram.

Noncontrast CT generally shows a poorly defined lesion of similar attenuation to that of skeletal muscle. Marked enhancement of the serpentine vascular components may be seen after intravenous contrast administration (23,24) (Figs. 5.7 and 5.9). Areas of associated fat overgrowth may be recognized, although in our experience, MR imaging is superior to CT in detecting both the serpentine vessels and adipose tissue (25,26). Phleboliths

are easily detected on CT, even when they are small or obscured by overlying osseous structures or radiographs CT is the most sensitive modality to identify these calcifications (Figs. 5.2 and 5.3).

Ultrasound examination of intramuscular hemangioma typically reveals a complex mass, and acoustic shadowing may be caused by phleboliths, if they are large enough (27–31) (Fig. 5.4). More recently findings on Doppler

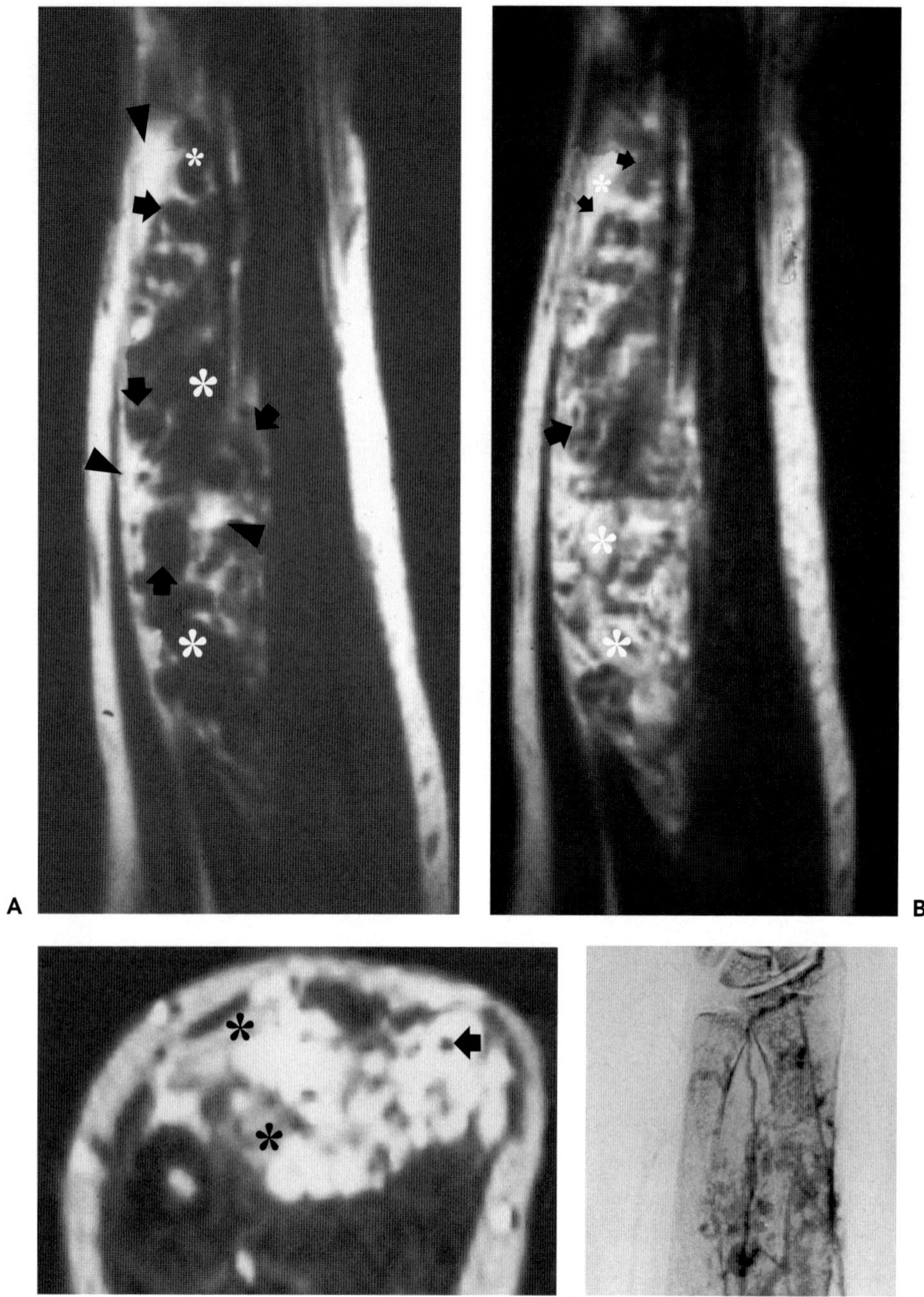

Figure 5.6 Intramuscular cavernous hemangioma of forearm in girl 15 years of age with soft tissue mass. **A,B:** Sagittal T1-weighted (TR/TE; 500/15) MR images before **(A)** and after **(B)** gadolinium administration show fat overgrowth most prominent peripherally and vascular channels/spaces (*white asterisks* in **A**) that enhance with contrast. **C:** Axial T2-weighted (TR/TE; 2442/90) MR image reveals heterogenous signal with very high signal intensity circular foci representing slow-flowing vascular spaces, intermediate-intensity fat overgrowth (*black asterisks*), and low-intensity phlebolith (*arrow*). **D:** Subtraction image from arteriogram shows filling of cavernous spaces.

studies have been reported (30,31). In some cases, no abnormality is present; however, low-resistance Doppler arterial signal with forward flow during both systole and diastole, indicative of abnormal low vascular resistance, may be seen (30,31) (Fig. 5.7). Dubois et al. emphasized the identification of high vessel density (five Doppler signals per square cm) and Doppler shift of greater than 2 kHz, as signs allowing reliable diagnosis of hemangioma (30,31). In our experience, strict application of this rule is not reliable for diagnosis and can also be seen in hemangiopericytoma, hemangioendothelioma, paraganglioma, angiosarcoma, and alveolar soft part sarcoma. In a hemangioma, the entire lesion should be composed of vascular structures, without the other solid nonvascular

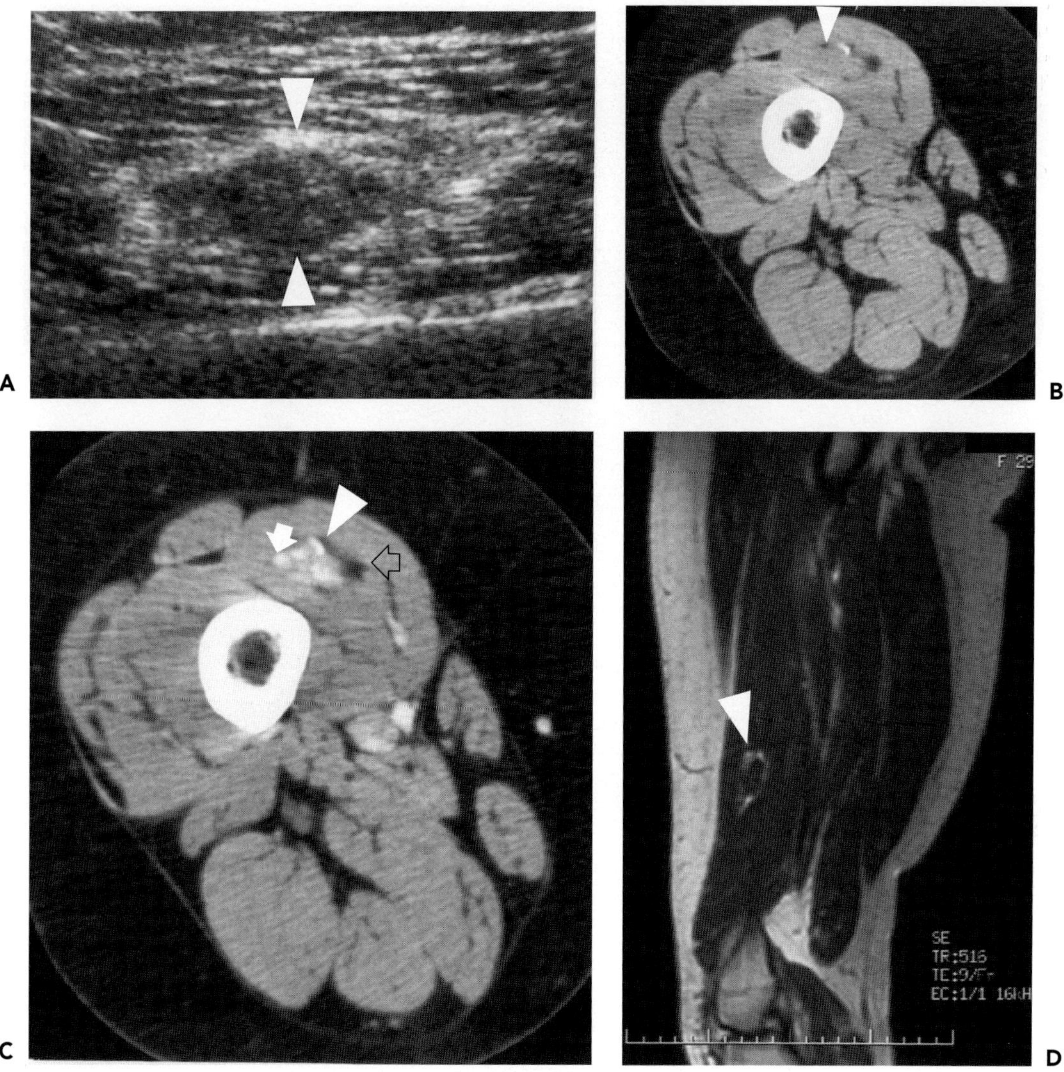

Figure 5.7 Intramuscular cavernous hemangioma of the thigh in a woman 29 years of age with chronic thigh pain exacerbated during exercise. **A:** Ultrasound shows a nonspecific intramuscular soft tissue mass (*large arrowheads*). **B,C:** CT images before **(B)** and following **(C)** intravenous contrast reveal a small focus of calcification (*arrowheads*) and multiple circular areas of enhancement (*arrow* in **C**) in the intramuscular mass. **D:** Sagittal T1-weighted (TR/TE; 516/19) spin-echo MR image shows peripheral fatty overgrowth (*arrow*) to better advantage. (*continued*)

channels or spaces that can be identified in these other lesions.

MR imaging, in our experience, is the best modality to evaluate soft tissue hemangiomas, which often show a characteristic imaging appearance (22,25,26,32–43). On T1-weighted images, the intramuscular hemangioma shows a poorly marginated mass of low-to-intermediate signal intensity (Figs. 5.4–5.12). Areas of high signal intensity are also often present on short TR/TE images. Previous reports suggested this appearance could be related to fat or slow-flowing blood (28,33,34,36,40–42). These high signal intensity regions vary in appearance from fine, delicate, or lacelike strands to thick coarse bands that predominate peripherally, as well as extending into septations (39). In our experience, these areas are almost always caused by

reactive fat overgrowth (Figs. 5.4–5.8). In some cases (particularly cavernous hemangioma), the adipose tissue can be so extensive as to be indistinguishable from lipoma (Fig. 5.8). On T2-weighted MR images, soft tissue hemangiomas reveal either a well-marginated or an infiltrative mass with very high signal intensity in areas of vascular components, whereas regions of adipose tissue are intermediate signal intensity and isointense to subcutaneous fat (Figs. 5.4–5.8). Thus, these lesions are often heterogeneous on all MR pulse sequences, although hemangiomas smaller than 2 cm are reported to be more homogeneous (21). In a study by Levine et al. (21), the ratio of MR signal intensity measurements of hemangioma to skeletal muscle on T2-weighted images (TR = 2000 msec; TR = 90 msec) at 1.0 Tesla was greater than 7. This ratio was higher than

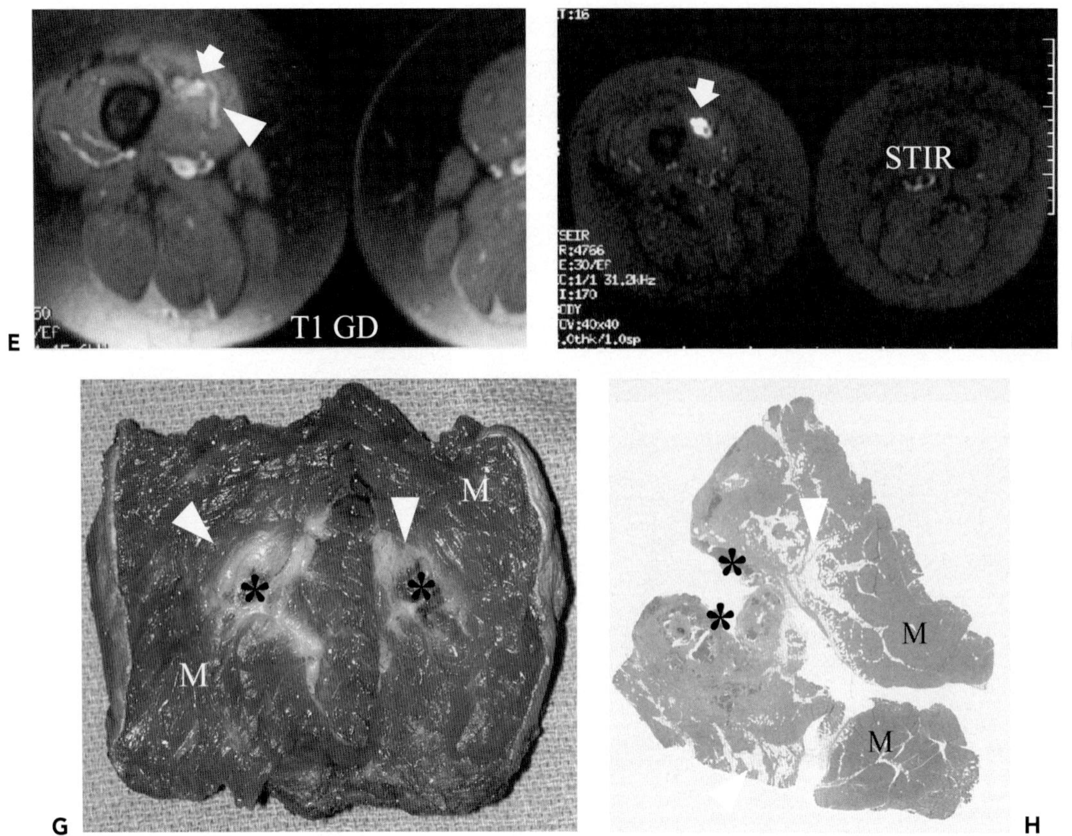

Figure 5.7 *(continued)* **E,F:** Axial enhanced fat-suppressed T1-weighted (TR/TE; 516/9) **(E)** and short-tau inversion recovery (STIR) (TR/TE/TI; 4766/30/170) **(F)** MR images show circular vascular channels and spaces (*arrow*) with serpentine feeding vessels (*arrowhead* in **E**). **G,H:** Corresponding sectioned gross specimen photograph **(G)** and photomicrograph **(H)**, revealing large vascular spaces (*asterisk*) and surrounding muscle atrophy with increased fat (*arrowheads*) compared to normal muscle (*M*).

that seen for other soft tissue masses. In addition to a relatively characteristic signal intensity, hemangiomas show a typical pattern of growth. Rather than displacing or destroying adjacent structures, they frequently tend to infiltrate adjacent tissue.

The areas of high signal intensity on T2-weighted MR images within hemangiomas often have a characteristic appearance when examined more critically and reflect the underlying morphology. Typically, circular (vessels seen en face or cavernous spaces) and/or linear/serpentine (vessels

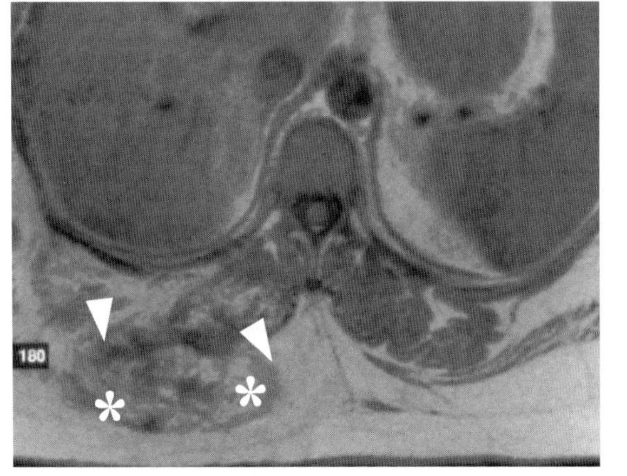
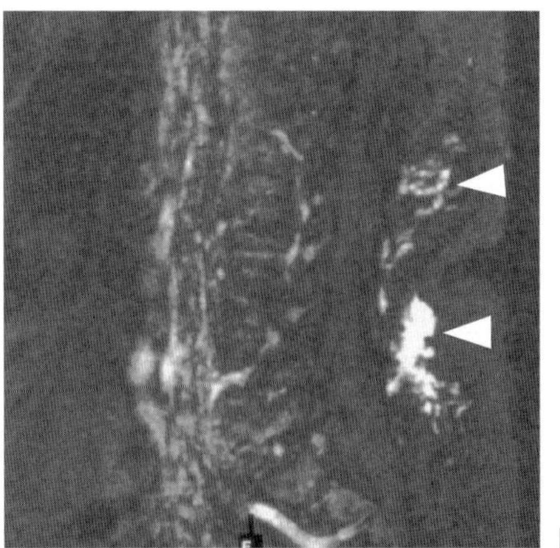

Figure 5.8 Infiltrating cavernous hemangioma of the paraspinal muscles with prominent fat overgrowth in a woman 39 years of age. **A,B:** Axial T1-weighted (TR/TE; 473/17) **(A)** and sagittal STIR (TR/TE/TI; 4000/50/180) **(B)** MR images show a paraspinal mass with predominant adipose signal intensity (*asterisk*) and smaller vascular channels and spaces (*arrowheads*) that reveal marked high signal intensity on the long TR image **B**.

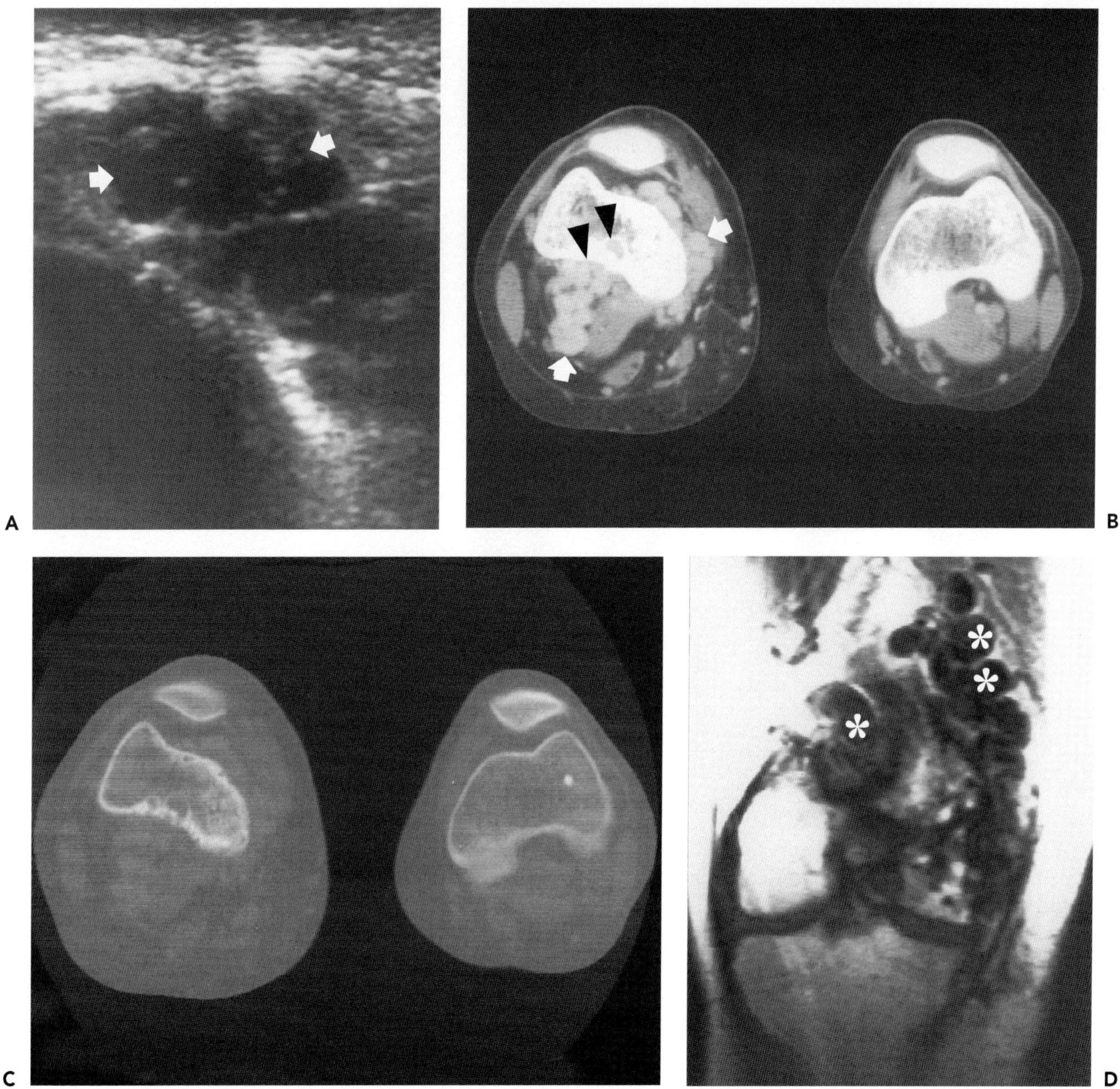

Figure 5.9 Arteriovenous hemangioma with high flow about knee in woman 31 years of age. **A:** sonogram reveals tubular hypoechoic vascular channels (*arrows*). **B:** CT images after intravenous contrast shows intensely enhancing vascular structures (*arrows*) and with secondary osseous involvement (*arrowheads*). **C:** CT displayed at bone windows shows osseous involvement to better advantage. **D:** Coronal T2-weighted (TR/TE; 2000/80) spin-echo MR images show large serpentine arteriovenous channels with low intensity (*asterisks*) from high flow. *(continued)*

seen longitudinally) high signal intensity can be recognized and are caused by slow flow in the vascular channels and spaces (39) (Figs. 5.4–5.12). In our experience, these serpentine vascular channels/spaces and/or fat overgrowth can be recognized in 90% to 95% of hemangiomas at MR imaging and are pathognomonic. Pathologic subtypes of angiomatous lesions can occasionally be recognized by MR imaging. A mass composed primarily of large vascular spaces suggests a cavernous hemangioma (Figs. 5.4–5.8); an arteriovenous or venous hemangioma (Figs. 5.9–5.12) shows pre-

dominantly serpentine vascular channels. Arteriovenous hemangiomas may also demonstrate low-intensity serpentine vascular channels on all MR pulse sequences in lesions with rapid flow (Figs. 5.9 and 5.10). It is important to detect high-flow components in any hemangioma because of the clinical and treatment implications. Hemangiomas typically show prominent enhancement after intravenous gadolinium injection (Figs. 5.5–5.7). Hemorrhage also occurs in hemangiomas, often showing high signal intensity on all pulse sequences, as well as fluid levels (44). Phleboliths are

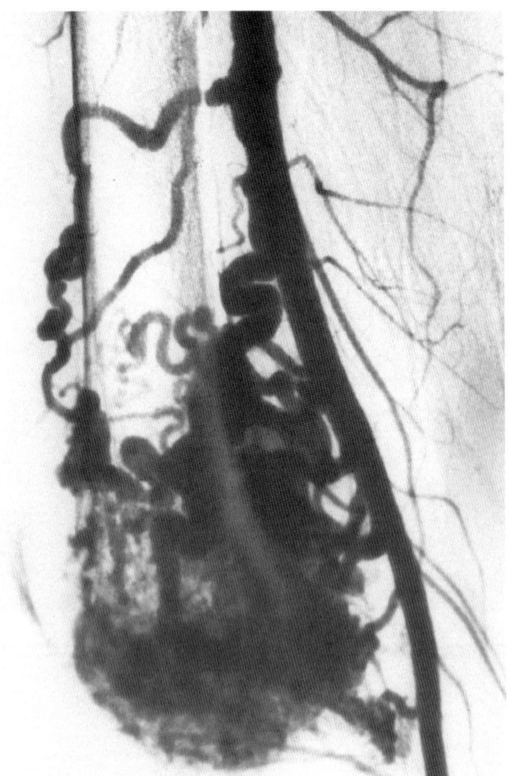

E

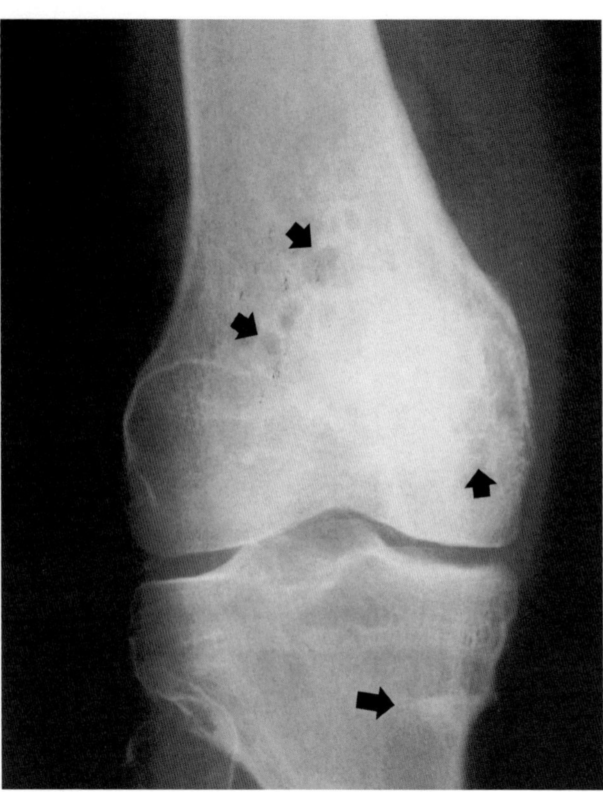

F

Figure 5.9 *(continued)* **E:** Arteriogram reveals marked vascularity with enlarged feeding arteries, staining, and early venous filling. **F:** Radiograph shows multiple osseous erosions (*arrows*). Osteotomy (*long arrow*) was done approximately 15 years earlier when patient was evaluated for a leg length inequality.

more easily detected by radiographs or CT than on MR images; however, on MR they appear as low-intensity circular foci on all pulse sequences (Fig. 5.6).

Interestingly, capillary hemangiomas, unlike cavernous lesions, frequently demonstrate a nonspecific appearance on MR imaging. Capillary hemangiomas show intermediate signal intensity on T1 weighting and intermediate-to-high signal intensity on T2 weighting, without the characteristic presence of serpentine vascular channels and spaces seen with cavernous lesions (Fig. 5.2). Fat overgrowth is also not typically seen because these lesions usually arise in the subcutaneous tissue. This nonspecific imaging appearance is likely directly related to the underlying pathology of these cellular lesions, composed of vascular channels that are too small to detect radiologically. Thus, in contradistinction to cavernous hemangiomas, capillary lesions can be identified on MR imaging, but not specifically diagnosed by intrinsic characteristics. However, these superficial lesions (strawberry nevi) are typically easily diagnosed clinically with confidence, and if imaged, only staging with extent is required for appropriate patient management. This is in distinct contrast to cavernous lesions that are clinically nonspecific but usually reveal a pathognomonic MR imaging appearance.

Angiographic studies show variable findings in evaluation of hemangiomas depending on the histologic subtype (45). Capillary and cavernous hemangiomas demonstrate enlarged feeding vessels with arteriovenous shunting and contrast puddling (Figs. 5.5 and 5.6). Arteriovenous lesions, however, reveal markedly torturous feeding vessels with early draining veins and intense tumor staining (Figs. 5.9 and 5.10). Venous hemangiomas often demonstrate no abnormality in the arterial phase of an angiogram and may only be detected on delayed imaging of the venous phase, after injection of contrast during venography, or following direct puncture of the lesion (46) (Fig. 5.12). Large, slow-flowing vessels are seen in venous hemangiomas after opacification with contrast. These angiographic features of soft tissue hemangiomas are also reflected in nuclear medicine studies. Technetium-99m DTPA or red blood cell studies often show uptake of radionuclide (47–49). Mild increased activity may also be seen on bone scintigraphy, particularly during the dynamic and blood pool stages with less uptake on the static images (47) (Fig. 5.12). These findings on bone scintigraphy are caused by increased blood flow, alterations of capillary permeability, and calcification.

OTHER BENIGN VASCULAR LESIONS

Although hemangioma is the most commonly encountered vascular soft tissue mass, a number of uncommonly encountered variants deserve separate classification.

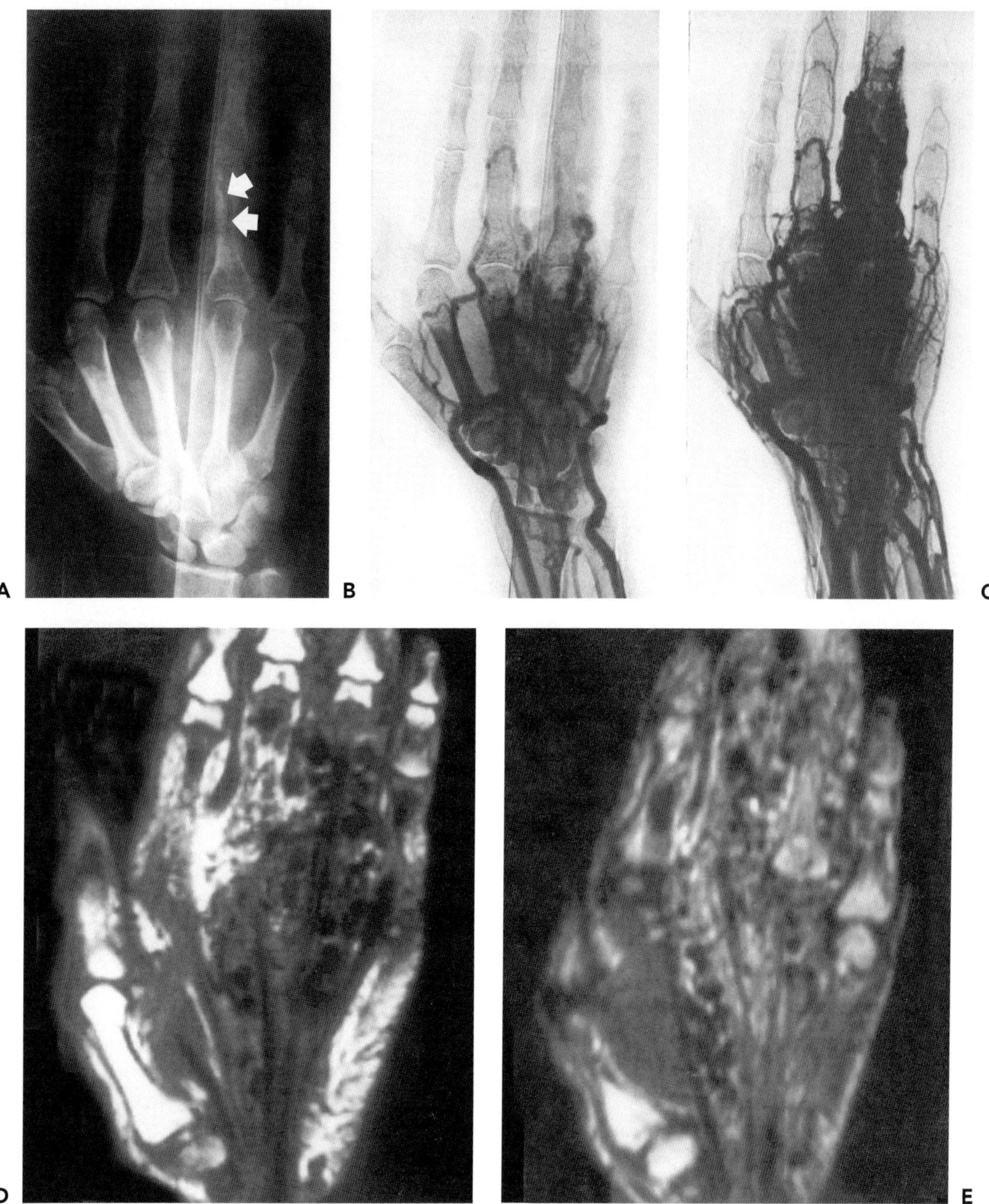

Figure 5.10 Arteriovenous hemangioma in the hand of woman 28 years of age. **A:** Radiograph of the hand shows a soft tissue mass with a serpentine channel-like radiolucency (*arrows*) in the proximal phalanx of the ring finger. **B,C:** Early **(B)** and late arterial **(C)** films show marked vascularity of the lesion, with prominent draining veins. **D,E:** Coronal T1-weighted (TR/TE; 500/20) **(D)** and T2-weighted (TR/TE; 1800/80) **(E)** spin-echo MR images of the hand show multiple serpentine flow voids, representing rapidly flowing blood within large caliber vessels of the lesion.

Synovial Hemangioma

Soft tissue hemangioma arising in the synovium is rare, accounting for less than 1% of all hemangiomas (50). Young adults and adolescents are usually affected, and there is often a long history of joint symptoms. Patients are symptomatic by 16 years of age in approximately 75% of cases. In contradistinction to intramuscular heman-

giomas, almost all patients are symptomatic, presenting with pain, swelling, and decreased range of motion (51). Histologically, 50% of these lesions are cavernous, 25% capillary, 20% arteriovenous, and 5% venous (50–52). The knee is the most commonly affected joint, accounting for approximately 60% of cases, followed by the elbow, involved in 30% of cases (50–52). The majority of lesions

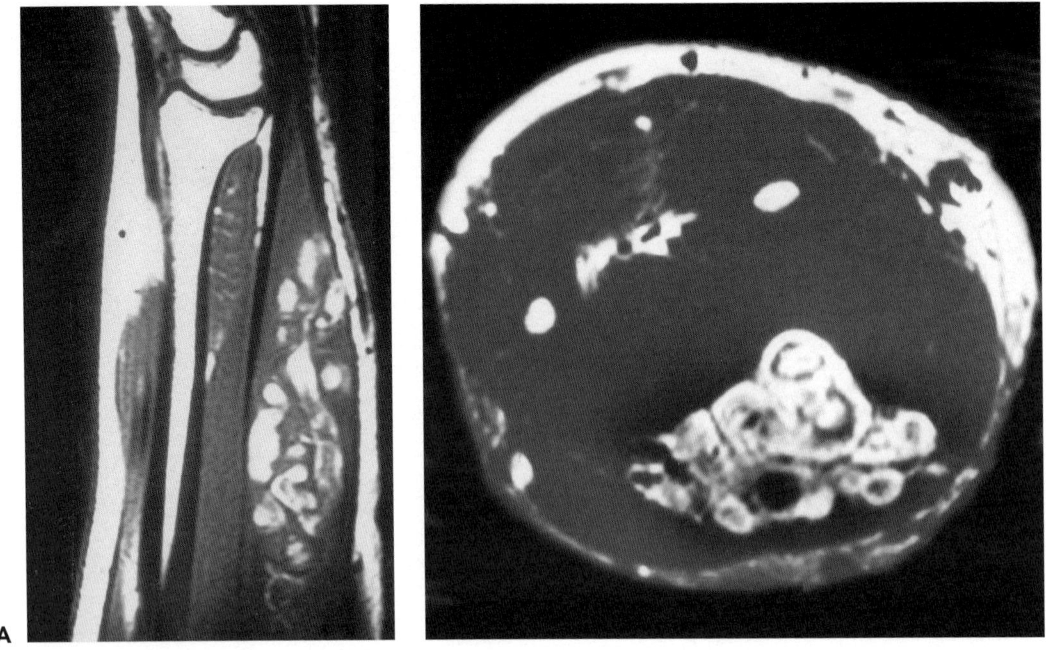

Figure 5.11   Venous hemangioma of the forearm in a man 46 years of age. **A:** Sagittal T1-weighted (TR/TE; 517/20) MR image shows high signal intensity in serpentine vascular channels representing slow flow. **B:** Axial T2-weighted (TR/TE; 1700/90) MR image reveals intermediate intensity in areas of slow flow/thrombus and higher intensity peripherally.

(67%) are intra-articular, with the remainder occurring in a bursa adjacent to a joint (50–52). These lesions have a similar appearance on radiologic studies as that previously described for other soft tissue hemangiomas (51,53) (Figs. 5.13 and 5.14). Chronic hyperemia can also result in focal limb enlargement. However, in addition, synovial hemangioma may cause repetitive episodes of intraarticular bleeding (Fig. 5.14). This may result in a radiologic appearance that can be confused with pigmented villonodular synovitis or the arthropathy associated with hemophilia. In distinction from hemophiliac arthropathy, synovial hemangioma is almost exclusively a monoarticular process.

Epithelioid Hemangioma

Epithelioid hemangioma is a benign vascular tumor, also called *angiolymphoid hyperplasia with eosinophilia, pseudo* or *atypical pyogenic granuloma, inflammatory angiomatous nodule, histiocytoid hemangioma, angioblastic hyperplasia,* or *Kimura disease.* The etiology of these lesions, either reactive or neoplastic, is uncertain and controversial. Features favoring a reactive process include a predilection for the superficial soft tissues and history of trauma in up to 10% of cases (2,3). Epithelioid hemangioma is a lesion of adults, with most patients between 20 and 50 years of age, and there is a female predilection (2,3). It is usually located superficially in the dermis or subcutis of the head (often in the superficial temporal artery distribution) and

neck, with a predilection for the auricular region and the distal extremities (digits). Multiple lesions develop in approximately 50% of patients, often closely associated with one another (2). Peripheral blood eosinophilia and lymphadenopathy are also seen in approximately 20% of patients. Pathologic features of these lesions include prominent proliferation of small-sized (capillary) vessels lined by epithelioid endothelial cells. Clinically, dermal lesions present as dull red, pruritic plaques, which may ulcerate. Subcutaneous lesions are typically asymptomatic. Local recurrence is reported in approximately 30% of lesions.

Angiolymphoid hyperplasia (Kimura disease) is now considered to be a different entity than epithelioid hemangioma, with only superficial pathologic similarities. This entity represents a chronic inflammatory disease that is endemic in the Asian population and infrequent elsewhere. Lymphadenopathy with or without a soft tissue mass is the hallmark of Kimura disease, and there is a marked male predilection (>80%) (54). The subcutaneous tissues of the head and neck are most commonly affected, although the groin, extremities, and chest wall may also be involved. Peripheral eosinophilia almost invariably accompanies this disease. Pathologically, there are dense lymphoid aggregates with prominent surrounding eosinophilic infiltrates. In the later stages of this disease, hyaline fibrosis occurs creating infiltration of surrounding structures, simulating a more aggressive malignant process.

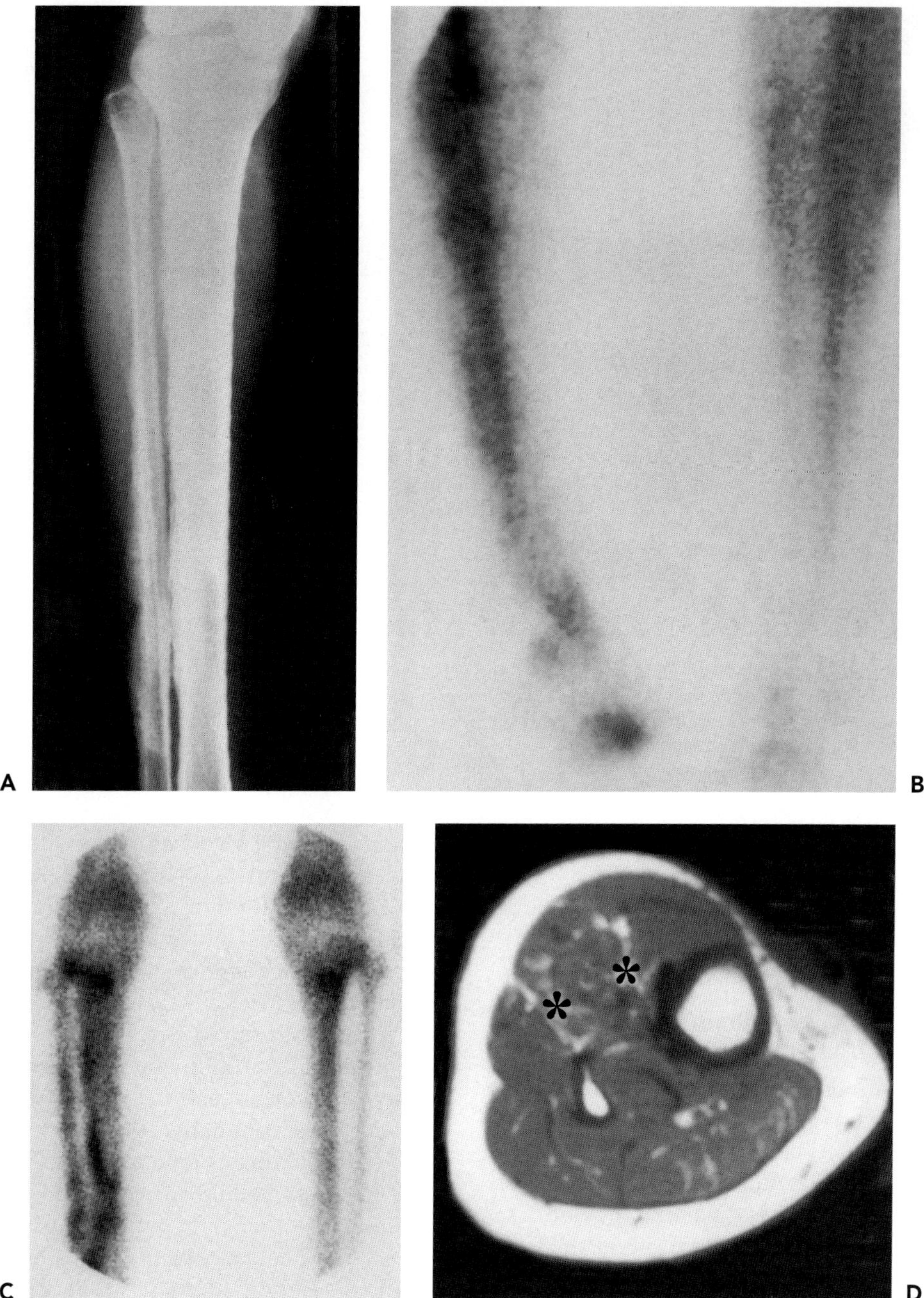

Figure 5.12   Venous hemangioma of the calf in a woman 22 years of age with long-standing lower leg swelling. **A:** Radiograph shows thick periosteal reaction, perhaps related to chronic vascular stasis. **B,C:** Blood-pool **(B)** and static delayed **(C)** images from technetium-99m bone scan reveal increased activity. **D:** Axial T1-weighted (TR/TE; 800/17) spin-echo MR image shows fat overgrowth (*asterisks*) associated with the lesion. *(continued)*

Imaging of epithelioid hemangioma or angiolymphoid hyperplasia is only rarely reported (55). In our experience, these lesions reveal a nonspecific heterogeneous appearance on CT and MR imaging and enhance following contrast administration. Prominent high signal intensity on T2-weighted MR images and irregular infiltrative lesion margins (including the parotid gland in head/neck lesions), with surrounding edema, reflect the pathologic appearance (55,56). Lesions are often along a lymph node distribution.

Sonography reveals round hypoechoic masses with normal hilar lymph node architecture and homogeneous internal echoes. Power Doppler studies reveal prominent intranodal vessels with a hilar pattern and low intranodal resistance (57). The cause of Kimura disease is unknown, although the laboratory abnormalities suggest an immunologic reaction. These benign lesions may recur locally following surgical excision, but have no malignant potential. Other treatment options include steroids and radiation therapy.

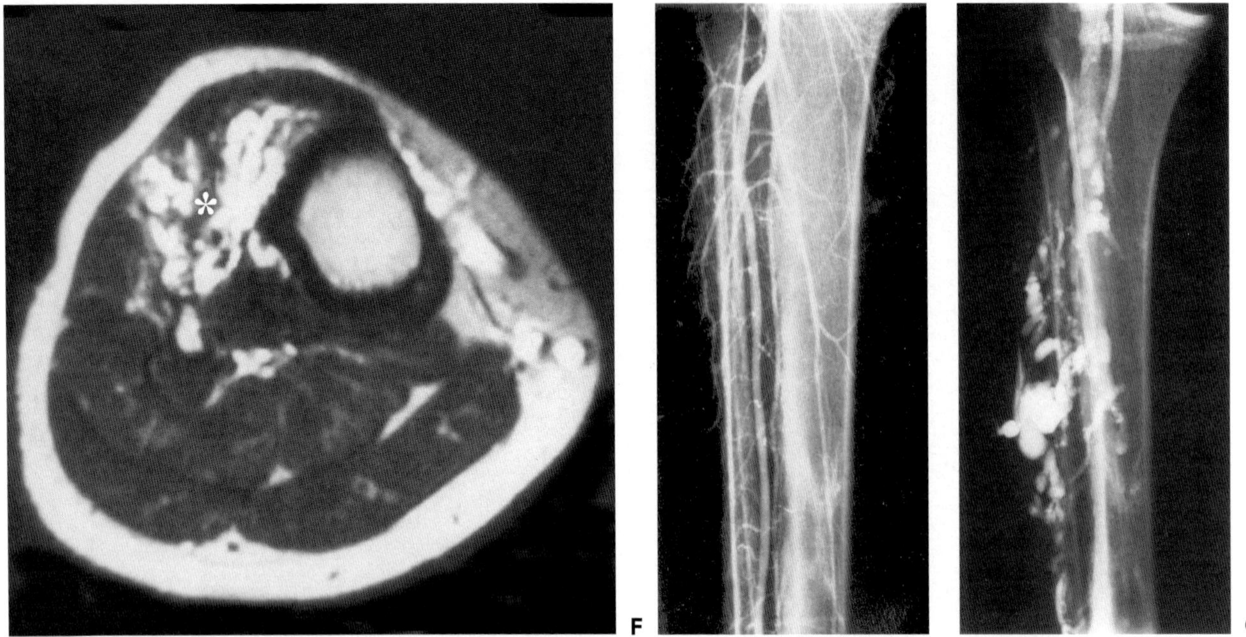

Figure 5.12 *(continued)*   **E:** Axial T2-weighted (TR/TE; 2400/90) spin-echo MR image shows the serpentine high intensity, slow flow vascular component, with fat overgrowth (*asterisk*). Note infiltrative pattern of growth. **F:** Arteriogram of the lower leg is normal. **G:** Direct puncture venogram reveals extensive hemangioma.

Pleomorphic Hyalinizing Angiectatic Tumor of Soft Parts

Smith and colleagues described pleomorphic hyalinizing angiectatic tumor (PHAT) of soft parts in 1997 (58). It represents a nonmetastasizing tumor of uncertain lineage, characterized by clusters of ectatic, fibrin-lined, thin-walled blood vessels surrounded, by a pleomorphic neoplastic stroma. These lesions affect adults with no sex predilection. Clinically, PHAT presents as a slowly enlarging mass of several years' duration (58,59). The most common location of these lesions is the subcutaneous tissue (79%) of the lower extremity (57%), with other sites including the buttock, chest wall, and upper extremity (58,59). Lesions may be more deep-seated as well (21% in skeletal muscle) (58,59). Radiologic features are only rarely reported and typically nonspecific, revealing an irregular enhancing subcutaneous mass on CT or MR imaging. Surgical wide-local excision is the treatment of choice, although local recurrence is reported in approximately 50% of cases, including one case ultimately requiring amputation (58–60). However, no metastases have been described with these lesions.

Reactive Vascular Lesions

A number of additional benign vascular lesions that pathologists encounter are not usually evaluated radiologically, and they are likely reactive in origin. These include pyogenic granuloma, papillary endothelial hyperplasia, vascular transformation of lymph nodes, glomeruloid hemangioma, and bacillary angiomatosis (61). Pyogenic granuloma (granulation tissue–type hemangioma) represents a polypoid form of capillary hemangioma occurring in the skin and mucous membrane (60% of cases), that can be multiple and grow rapidly (2). These lesions are associated with trauma in 30% of cases (2,3). Specific sites of involvement of pyogenic granulomas are the gingiva, finger, lips, face, and tongue, in order of decreasing frequency. Pyogenic granuloma may also occur related to a vein wall, most commonly in the neck and upper extremity. Local recurrence is reported in up to 16% of cases as either a solitary nodule or multiple satellite lesions (2,3). Papillary endothelial hyperplasia likely represents an unusual type of organizing thrombus, and most frequently is seen superficially in the head, neck, trunk, and fingers (2,3,62). These lesions may be confused with angiosarcoma pathologically, and simple excision is usually curative. Vascular lymph node transformation occurs as a result of a variety of conditions, including chronic venous/lymphatic obstruction (nodal angiomatosis) or radiation. This is most frequent in the axillary nodes following treatment related to breast carcinoma. Glomeruloid hemangioma is a reactive vascular proliferation associated with the POEMS (polyneuropathy, organomegaly, endocrinopathy, M protein, and skin lesions) syndrome, involving the dermis. Imaging of these lesions is only rarely reported, typically with nonspecific intrinsic characteristics on MR. High signal intensity on T2-weighting, surrounding edema, and identification of serpentine tubular structures (suggesting a vascular lesion) are described.

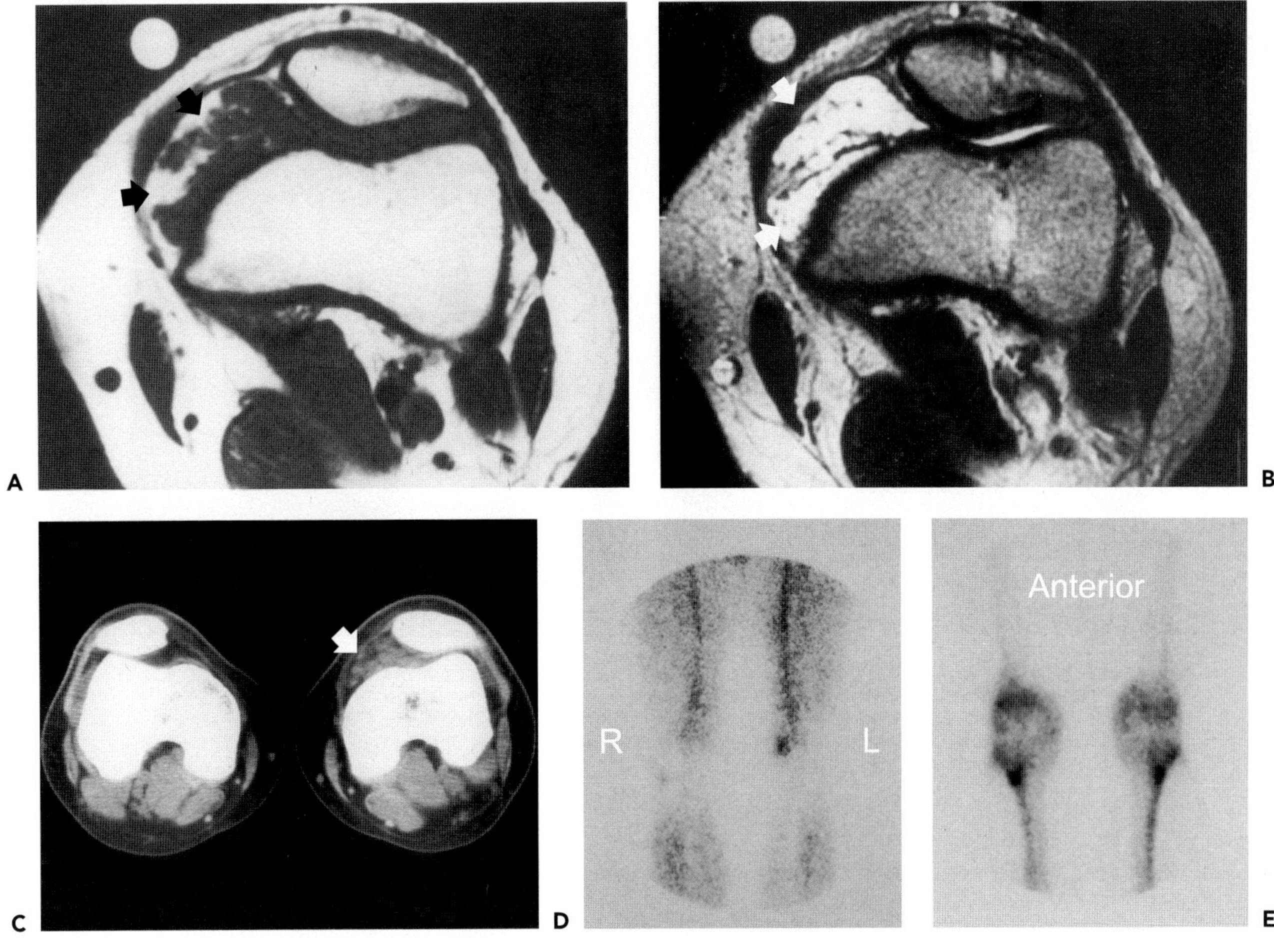

Figure 5.13   Synovial hemangioma of the knee in a man 21 years of age. **A,B:** Axial T1-weighted (TR/TE; 600/20) **(A)** and T2-weighted (TR/TE; 1800/80) **(B)** spin-echo MR images show a soft tissue mass arising from the medial aspect of the knee joint. The associated fat overgrowth (*arrows* in **A**), infiltrative pattern of growth, and serpentine vascular spaces/channels (*arrows* in **B**) with high signal intensity are typical of a hemangioma. **C:** Corresponding axial noncontrast CT shows the multiple, circular, vascular structures (*arrow*) of the lesion, as well as associated adipose tissue. **D:** Blood-pool image from technetium-99m bone scan reveals increased tracer accumulation in the medial aspect of the left knee. **E:** Delayed static image shows minimal increased tracer accumulation on the left.

Bacillary angiomatosis represents an infectious pseudo-neoplastic vascular proliferation caused by the *Bartonella* family of gram-negative bacilli (usually *Bartonella henselae* or *Bartonella quintana*). This disease is seen almost exclusively in immunocompromised patients and specifically associated with AIDS (63–65). Clinically, the lesions may simulate Kaposi sarcoma, with multiple pink elevated skin lesions, although visceral involvement may occur. Pathologically, bacillary angiomatosis consists of capillary-sized vessels. Imaging may reveal multiple nodular regions of skin thickening. Underlying osseous involvement (very unusual in Kaposi sarcoma) is reported with a propensity for cortical lysis (66). Isolated osseous involvement with periosteal reaction most commonly affects the tibia, fibula, femur, humerus, and radius (medullary and/or cortical bone). Antibiotic treatment with either doxycycline or erythromycin is highly effective.

LYMPHANGIOMA

> ### KEY CONCEPTS
>
> - Lymphangiomas are most frequent in the neck (75%) and axilla (20%).
> - Lesions are usually present at birth (50% to 65%) or by 2 years of age (90%).
> - Lymphangiomas are usually cavernous/cystic pathologically.
> - Imaging reflects the pathologic appearance with large, cystic spaces on sonography, CT, and MR.
> - Lymphangiomas with secondary dissection along the chest wall or mediastinum (3% to 10% of cases) may reveal a more complex imaging appearance.

Lymphangioma of the musculoskeletal system, almost exclusively a soft tissue lesion, is composed of sequestered

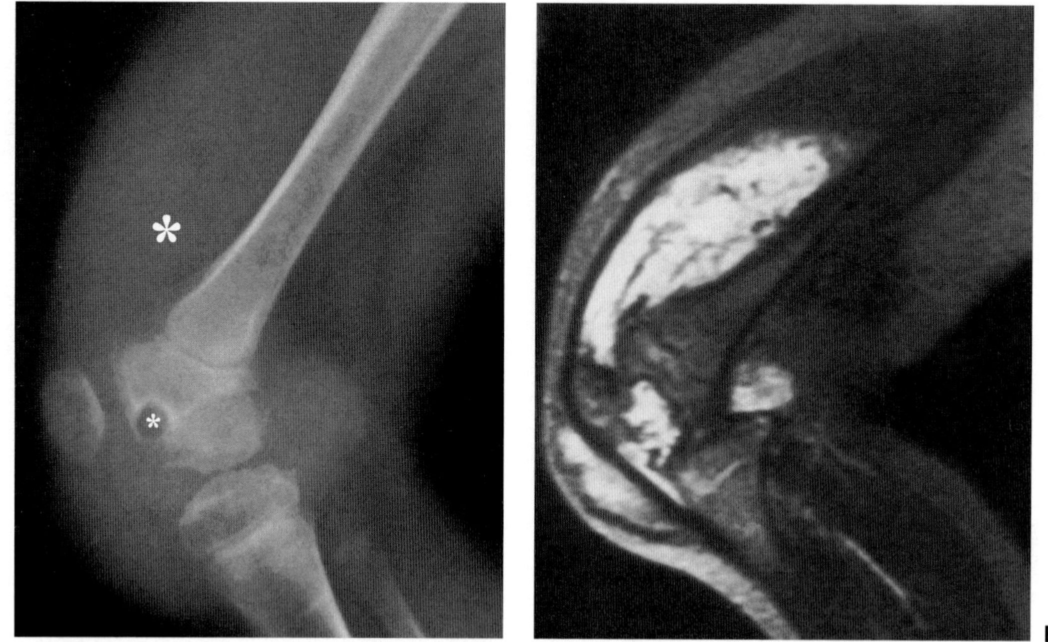

Figure 5.14 Synovial hemangioma of the knee in a girl 3 years of age with joint pain, swelling, and recurrent hemarthrosis. **A:** Lateral radiograph shows soft tissue swelling, joint effusion (*asterisk*), as well as joint narrowing and erosion (*small asterisk*). **B:** Sagittal T2-weighted (TR/TE; 1500/60) MR image reveals heterogeneous serpentine and circular areas of high signal intensity representing a cavernous hemangioma infiltrating the joint.

noncommunicating lymphoid tissue, lined by lymphatic endothelium (67). The underlying cause is believed to be congenital obstruction of lymphatic drainage (68). Pathologically, these lesions are similar to hemangiomas and classified by vessel size, although there is often an admixture of histologic subtypes, and they should be considered a histologic spectrum (68,69).

Capillary lymphangiomas are rare lesions composed of small capillary-sized vessels. They are small, well circumscribed, and located in the subcutaneous tissue (dermis and epidermis), which limits extensive growth (69,70). Because of its superficial location and small size, capillary lymphangioma is rarely imaged. Cavernous lymphangiomas are usually subcutaneous lesions located about the mouth, tongue, salivary glands, and intramuscular septa. The lymphatic spaces are intermediate in size between capillary and cystic lymphangiomas. Cystic lymphangiomas (cystic hygroma) are the most common type and usually located in the neck (75%) or axilla (20%) (71–78). Cystic and cavernous lymphangiomas are composed of unilocular or multilocular spaces (larger in cystic lesions) containing serous or chylous, proteinaceous material (Figs. 5.15 and 5.16). Distinction from cavernous hemangioma may be difficult histologically.

Lymphangiomas are present at birth in 50% to 65% of cases, and 90% are detected in the first 2 years of life (67). The clinical presentation is that of a palpable, soft, fluctuant mass involving the head, neck, or axilla (Figs. 5.15 and 5.16). Other unusual locations for lymphangioma include

mediastinum, retroperitoneum, bone, omentum, and mesentery (79). The retroperitoneal lesions often present in older children and adults (71–75). Cervical cystic hygromas extend into the mediastinum in 3% to 10% of cases and may cause tracheal compression and clinical symptoms of respiratory distress (77) (Fig. 5.16). Acute symptoms may also result from superimposed infection, rupture, hemorrhage, or pressure on adjacent structures. Hydrops fetalis, Turner syndrome, Noonan syndrome, familial pterygium colli, fetal alcohol syndrome, and chromosomal aneuploidies may be associated with cystic lymphangiomas (67,69). These cases may be detected in utero by ultrasonography and are associated with a high mortality rate. Capillary lymphangiomas may be seen in patients of any age, and approximately 25% are found in patients older than 45 years (67,69).

Surgery remains the treatment of choice, although recurrence is as high as 15% (68,69,79,80). Complete excision frequently is not possible because of infiltration of adjacent essential structures (68). The most common postoperative complication is edema and may be seen in up to 50% of cases (68). Seroma and infection occur in 5% to 10% of cases (80).

Radiographs of lymphangioma are nonspecific, typically revealing only a soft tissue mass with rare calcification (70,79,81). Osseous overgrowth in association with isolated lesions is rare but reported in the clavicle (82). Sonography of cystic lymphangiomas reveals a multiloculated cystic mass with septa of variable thickness that

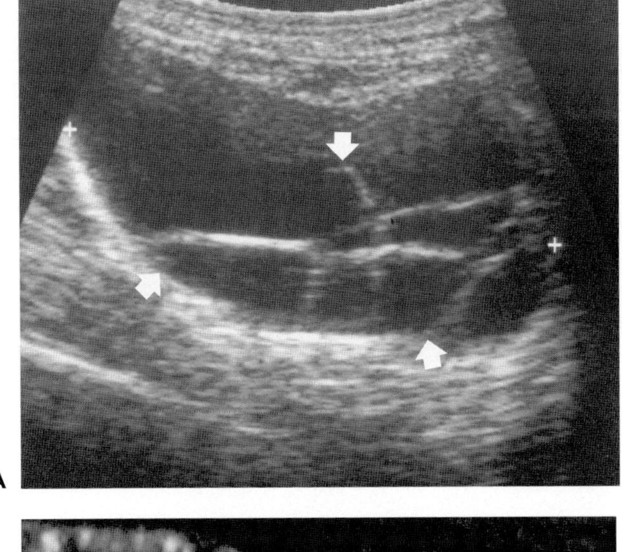

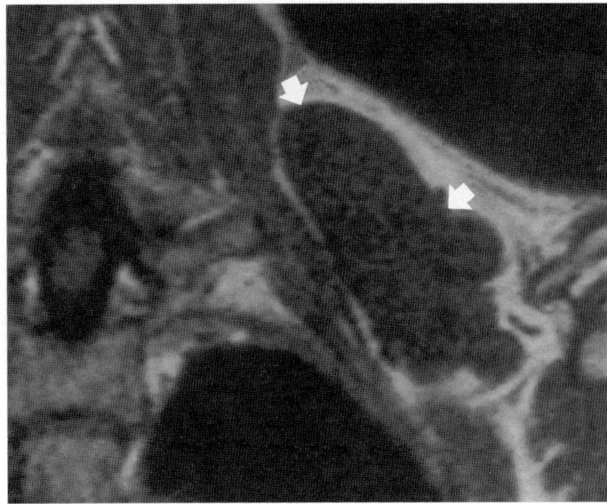

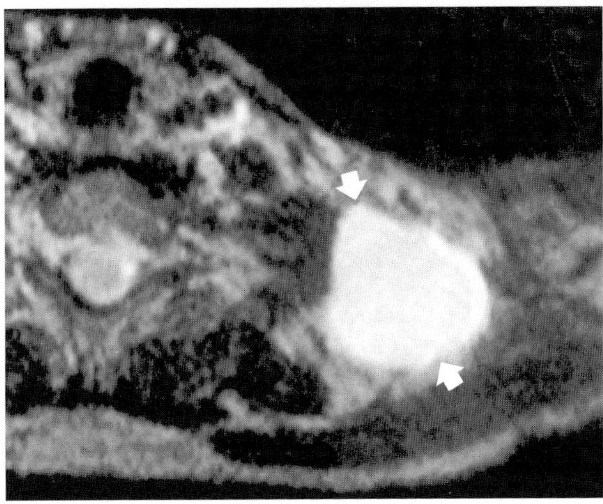

Figure 5.15 Cystic hygroma of the neck in a woman 41 years of age. **A:** Sonogram shows a multiloculated cystic mass with thin septa (*arrows*) in the neck. **B:** Coronal T1-weighted (TR/TE; 500/16) and **(C)** axial T2-weighted (TR/TE; 2000/80) MR images also reveal a homogeneous multilocated cystic mass (*arrows*). The septations seen on ultrasound are not appreciated on MR imaging.

contain solid components arising from the cyst wall or the septa (76) (Fig. 5.15). These echogenic components correspond to clusters of abnormal lymphatic channels, too small to be resolved by ultrasound. Large lesions dissect between normal tissue planes, creating ill-defined margins. The echogenicity of cystic lymphangiomas depends on the nature of the fluid. Typically anechoic or hypoechoic, the fluid may contain low-level echoes (debris) if it is bloody, chylous, or infected. Cystic lesions complicated by hemorrhage or infection may appear as solid lesions (Fig. 5.17).

CT shows a cystic lymphangioma as a unilocular or multilocular mass (Fig. 5.16) of water attenuation (73,74,77,83). Lesion walls and septa are typically of uniform thickness, and enhancement after intravenous contrast may be seen (83). Thin internal septations are better delineated by sonography than by CT. Thicker septations are well delineated on CT. Calcification is rarely seen. Similar to sonography, complicated lymphangiomas may show more prominent solid components (Fig. 5.17).

Siegel et al. reported the MR appearance of 17 lymphangiomas in 15 patients, describing a typical appearance: heterogeneous with a low signal intensity, similar to or

slightly less that of muscle, on T1-weighted images, and high signal intensity, greater than that of fat on T2-weighted images, reflecting the preponderance of fluid-filled cystic spaces (78) (Fig. 5.15). Focal heterogeneity in the lesions is present in nearly all cases and appears as low-intensity linear structures of variable thickness representing fibrous septa. Four of these lymphangiomas demonstrated a signal intensity similar to that of fat on T1-weighted MR images (78) (Fig. 5.18). In two of these cases, the lesions were composed of small lymphatic vessels, separated by thick fibrous, fatty septa (78). One lesion was composed of both small and large cysts filled with fat, and the other was filled with clotted blood and necrotic debris.

These lesions may be associated with secondary bone changes, and consequently, they may cause increased tracer accumulation on bone scintigraphy (74). Lymphangiography can demonstrate a communication between retroperitoneal cystic lymphangiomas and normal lymphatic channels, and lymphangiomas may be opacified during lymphangiography (71). Angiography reveals a space-occupying lesion, displacing normal vessels, but without neovascularity.

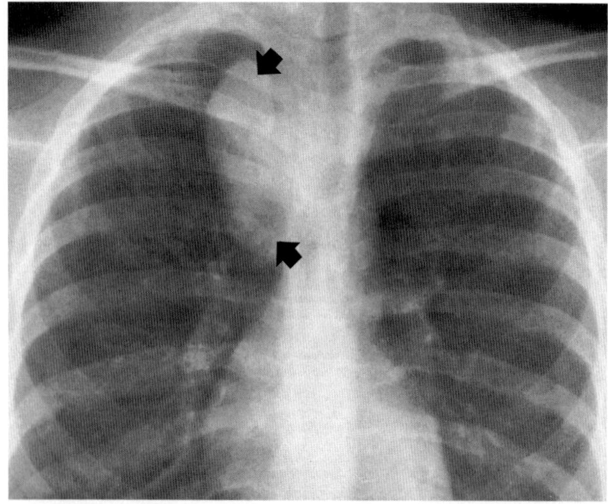

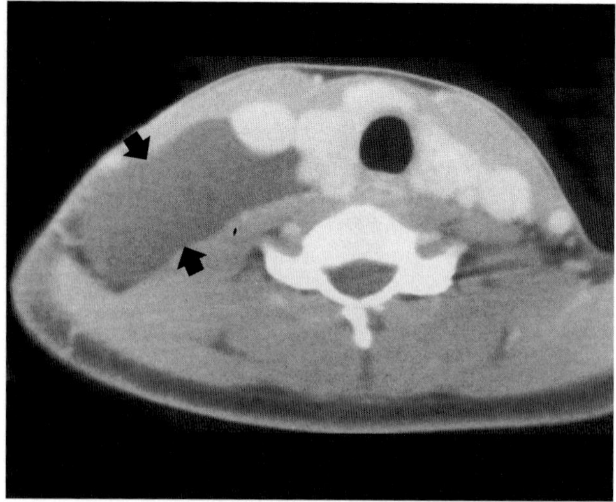

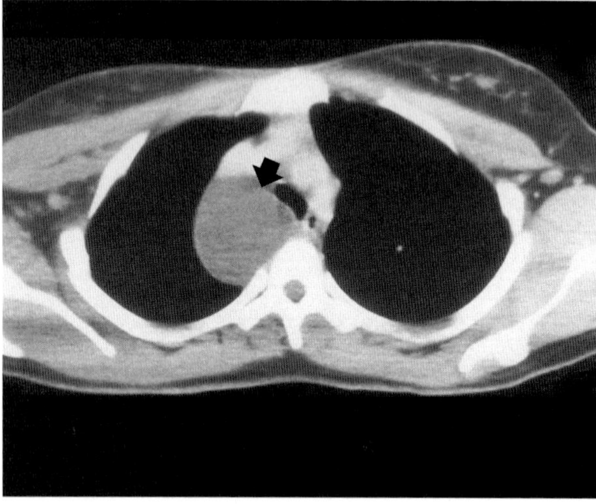

Figure 5.16. Cystic hygroma of the neck in a woman 25 years of age presenting as a mediastinal mass. **A:** Chest radiograph shows a mediastinal mass (*arrows*). **B,C:** Axial contrast-enhanced CT images of the neck **(B)** and upper chest **(C)** show the cystic mass (*arrows*) extending from the neck into the mediastinum.

The differential diagnosis of cystic masses of the retroperitoneum includes cystic pancreatic tumor, pseudocyst, hematoma, abscess, and cystic degeneration of other tumors. Mesenteric cysts and omental cysts are cystic lymphangiomas of the mesentery and omentum, respectively. In the mediastinum, bronchogenic and pericardial cysts may image identically to cystic lymphangiomas.

ANGIOMATOSIS

> ### KEY CONCEPTS
> - Angiomatosis represents diffuse infiltration of hemangiomatous and/or lymphangiomatous tissue.
> - The more extensive the soft tissue involvement, particularly visceral, the poorer the prognosis.
> - Imaging of these lesions is identical to that of solitary hemangioma but much more extensive.
> - Multiple angiomatous syndromes and associations are described, most without malignant potential, with the exception of Maffucci syndrome.

Angiomatosis represents a diffuse infiltration (soft tissue and/or bone) of tissue by hemangiomatous and/or lymphangiomatous lesions (Figs. 5.18–5.21). The disease is recognized in patients in the first three decades of life with more than 50% diagnosed before 20 years of age (84). Clinical symptoms include pain and swelling; skin discoloration may also be present. Gigantism, hypertrophy, and clinical findings of arteriovenous shunting are only rarely apparent. The vascular lesions are benign, without malignant potential, with the exception of Maffucci syndrome (see later discussion).

Pathologically, the hemangiomatous component of the lesion is usually a mixture of arteriovenous, capillary, and cavernous vascular tissue, although occasionally capillary regions predominate. Fat overgrowth frequently accompanies these infiltrative angiomatous lesions, similar to that in focal hemangiomas (Fig. 5.18). There may be a mixture of hemangiomatous and lymphangiomatous tissue that is difficult to distinguish histologically, and thus we prefer the term *angiomatosis* (Fig. 5.19).

Angiomatosis that only involves osseous structures (30% to 40% of cases) usually has a relatively indolent clinical course (85,86). Unfortunately, the majority of

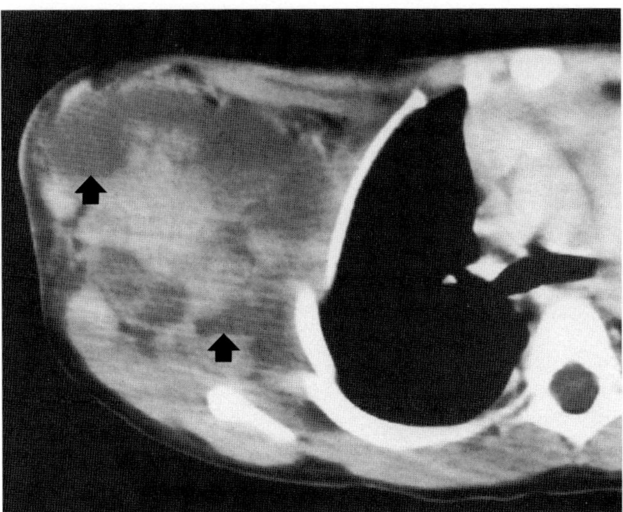

Figure 5.17 Lymphangioma in the axilla in a girl 3 months of age with a mass. CT shows multiloculated complex, partially cystic axillary lesion, with fluid levels (*arrows*). Histology (not shown) was largely that of a lymphangioma. However, there was also an hemangiomatous component that caused the bleeding and resultant fluid levels.

cases of angiomatosis (60% to 70%) have more extensive soft tissue involvement. The identification of visceral involvement is particularly associated with a poorer prognosis (2,84,86). In cases in which lymphangiomatous elements predominate, chylothorax, chyloperitoneum, lymphedema, hepatosplenomegaly, and cystic hygroma may occur. In addition, osseous lesions are seen in the majority of patients (>75%) with lymphangiomatosis (2,7,84) (Fig. 5.20). Congenital lymphangiómatosis, also called

congenital elephantiasis (Nonne-Milroy-Meige syndrome), is caused by severe hypoplasia or absence of lymphatic channels (69,87) (Fig. 5.21). It is an autosomal dominant condition usually associated with a markedly enlarged lower extremity. Bone involvement is common, as opposed to abdominal or retroperitoneal extension, which is rare. Imaging appearance with angiomatosis is similar to that already described for solitary hemangioma. However, these lesions are infiltrative, involving either multiple tissue planes including subcutaneous muscle and bone or extensive vertical involvement of a single tissue plane. Fat overgrowth may also be seen on imaging. Osseous lesions are usually lytic and multifocal, although sclerosis is sometimes described. Lymphangiomatous components may show uptake of contrast after lymphangiography.

ANGIOMATOUS SYNDROMES AND ASSOCIATIONS

Maffucci Syndrome

Maffucci syndrome consists of multiple enchondromas and soft tissue cavernous hemangiomas. Lymphangiomas are also described in association with this syndrome (88) (Figs. 5.22 and 5.23). It was described in 1881, interestingly, 8 years prior to the description of Ollier disease (multiple enchondromatosis) (89). Maffucci syndrome is nonhereditary, has a mild male predilection, and represents a mesodermal dysplasia. Clinical symptoms are present at birth to the first year of life in 25% of patients, before 6 years of age in 45% of patients, and prior to puberty in 75% of patients (90). Enchondromas often are most prominent

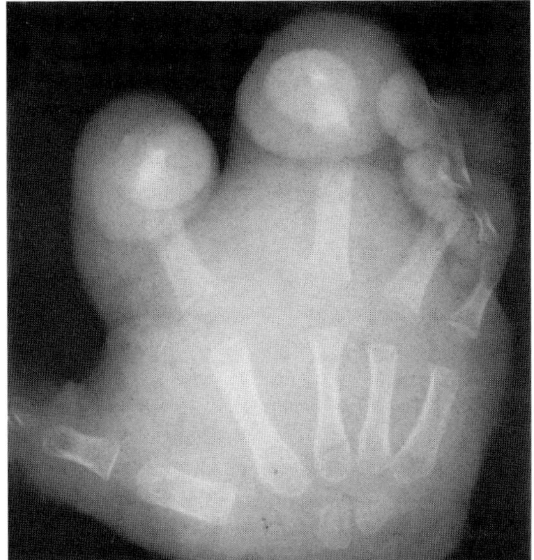
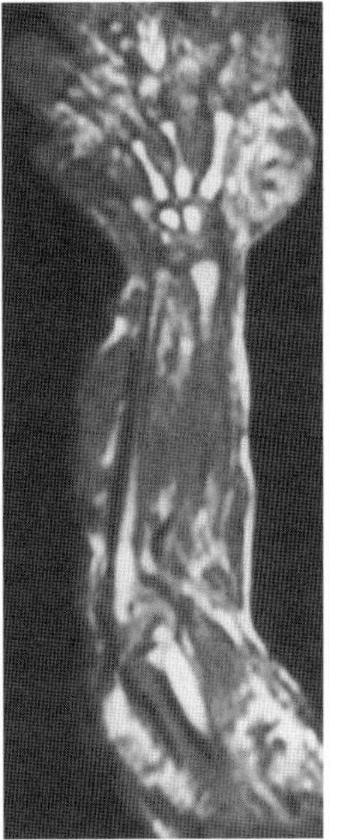
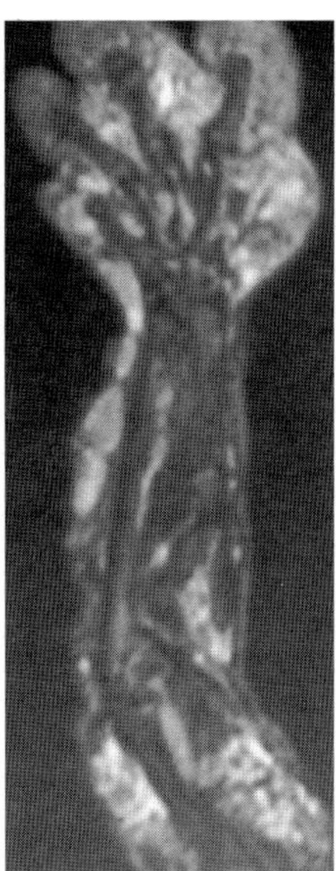

Figure 5.18 Angiomatosis (hemangiomatosis) of the upper extremity in a 3-year-old boy. **A:** Radiograph of the hand and wrist shows extensive soft tissue involvement. **B,C:** Coronal T1-weighted (TR/TE; 600/20) **(B)** and T2-weighted (TR/TE; 2000/80). **(C)** spin-echo MR images show extensive involvement of the upper extremity, with prominent fatty overgrowth.

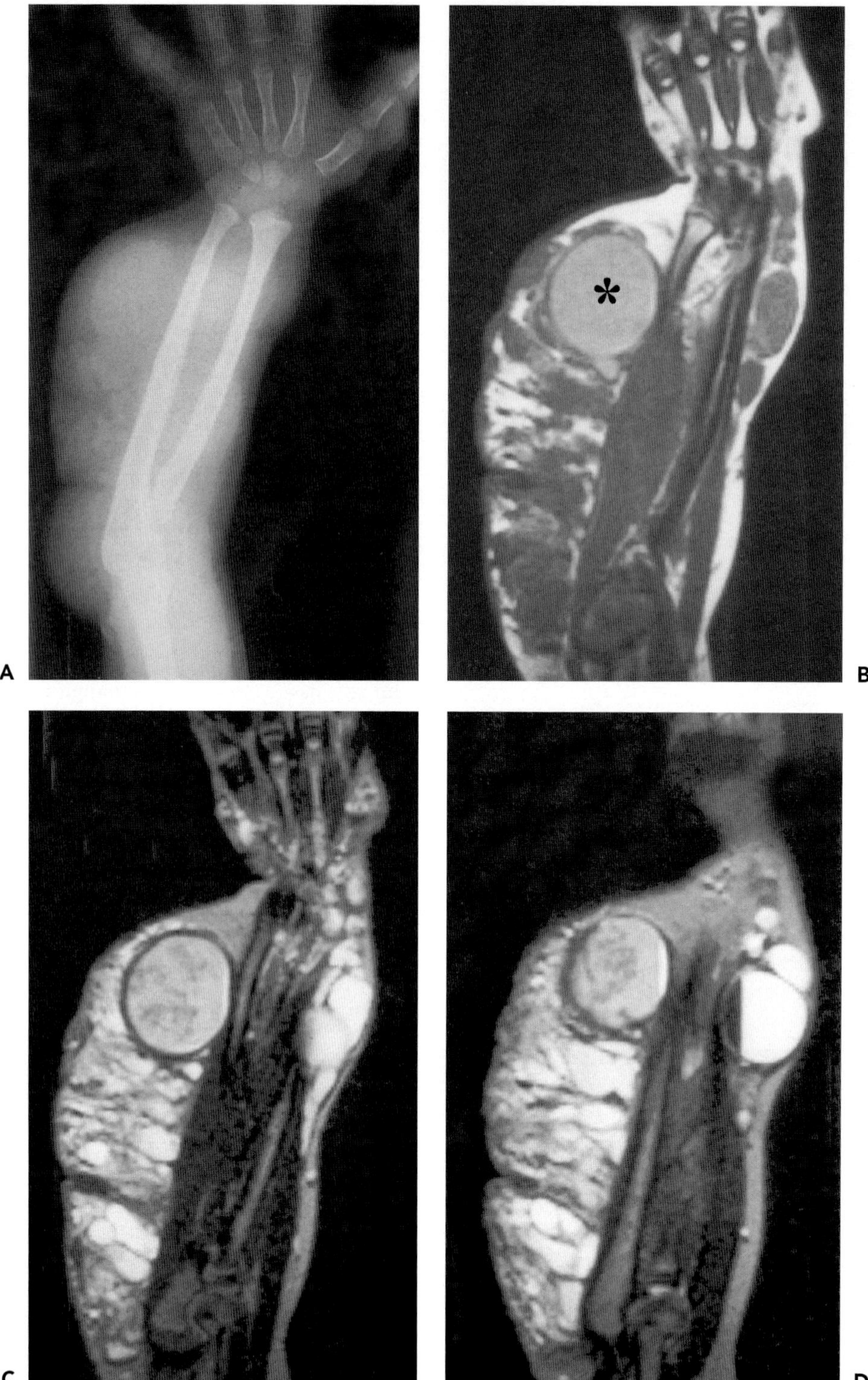

Figure 5.19 Angiomatosis (lymphangiomatosis) of the upper extremity in a girl 3 years of age. **A:** Radiograph of the upper extremity shows extensive soft tissue involvement. **B,C:** Coronal T1-weighted (TR/TE; 450/15) **(B)** and T2-weighted (TR/TE; 2000/80) **(C)** spin-echo MR images show extensive involvement of the upper extremity, predominantly confined to the subcutaneous tissue. The large rounded area (*asterisk* in **B**) contains subacute blood and clot causing the high signal intensity **D:** T2-weighted Image adjacent to **(C)** shows multiple fluid levels from previous hemorrhage. (*continued*)

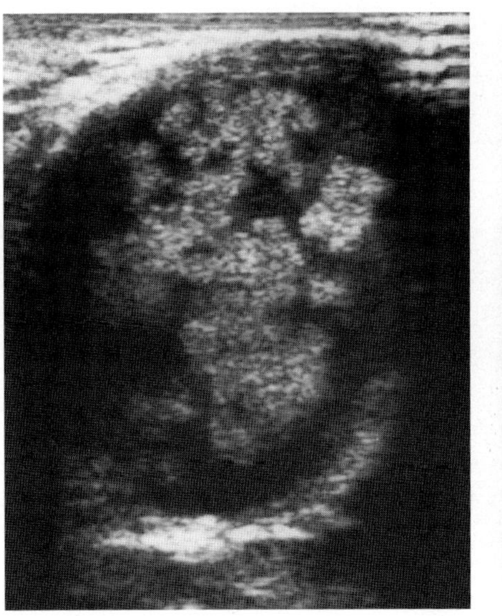
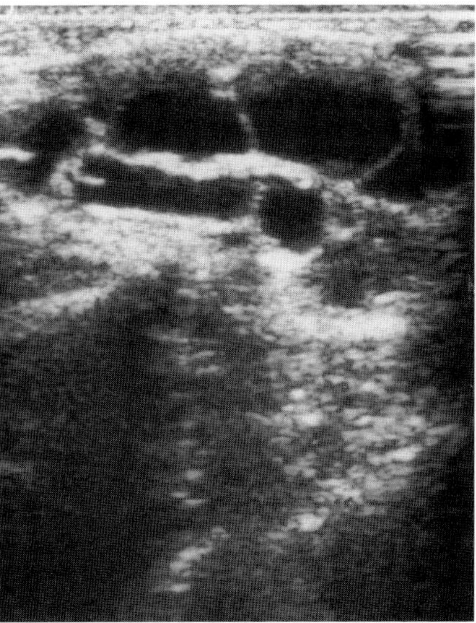

Figure 5.19 *(continued)*   **E:** Ultrasonography of blood-filled area in **B** shows central clot with surrounding fluid. **F:** Ultrasonography of the remainder of the lesion revealed primarily a multiloculated appearance, typical of lymphangioma. At surgery, the lesion was predominantly lymphangioma with a small hemangiomatous component.

in the hands and feet, demonstrating typical ringlike chondroid matrix calcification (7) (Fig. 5.22). Soft tissue cavernous hemangiomas (or spindle cell hemangiomas) have an imaging appearance as previously described, with phleboliths commonly present (91) (Fig. 5.23). Unfortunately, malignant transformation occurs in both lesions. Enchondromas undergo malignant transformation to chondrosarcoma in 15% to 56% of patients, and the hemangioma similarly transforms to vascular sarcoma in 3% to 5% of cases (90,92). In addition, there is a higher incidence of ovarian carcinoma, gastrointestinal adeno-

carcinoma, pancreatic carcinoma, and central nervous system glioma in these patients (92).

Osler-Weber-Rendu Syndrome

The Osler-Weber-Rendu syndrome is also referred to as *hereditary hemorrhagic telangiectasia* (93–95). It is inherited in an autosomal dominant pattern (95). The underlying cause is a systemic fibrovascular dysplasia of all vessels, resulting in aneurysms, telangiectasias, and high-flow arteriovenous hemangiomas (malformations). Lesions

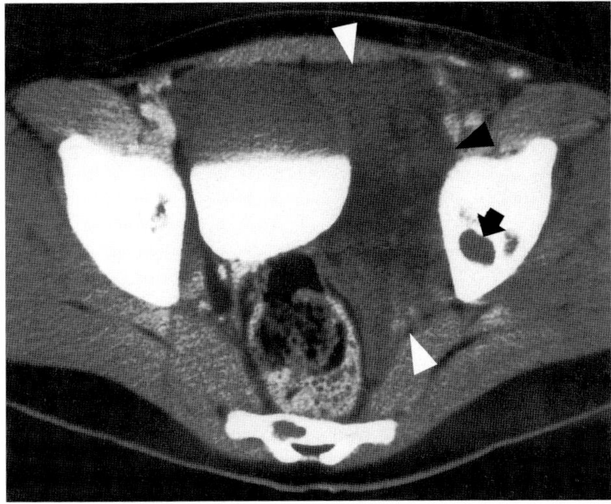
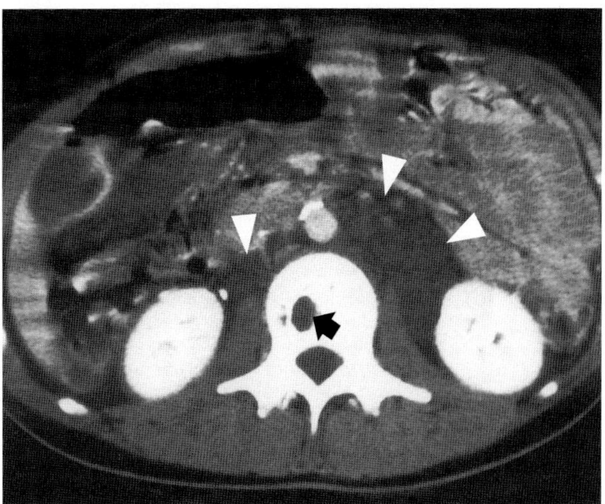

Figure 5.20   Angiomatosis in a boy 16 years of age with groin swelling. **A:** Axial contrast-enhanced CT image of the pelvis and **(B)** lumbar spine show cystic paravertebral and left pelvic masses *(arrowheads)* and areas of bone involvement *(arrow)*. These fluid collections extended superiorly (not shown) to the entrance of the lymphatic channels into the left subclavian vein, and pathologically, this process represented predominantly lymphangiomatosis.

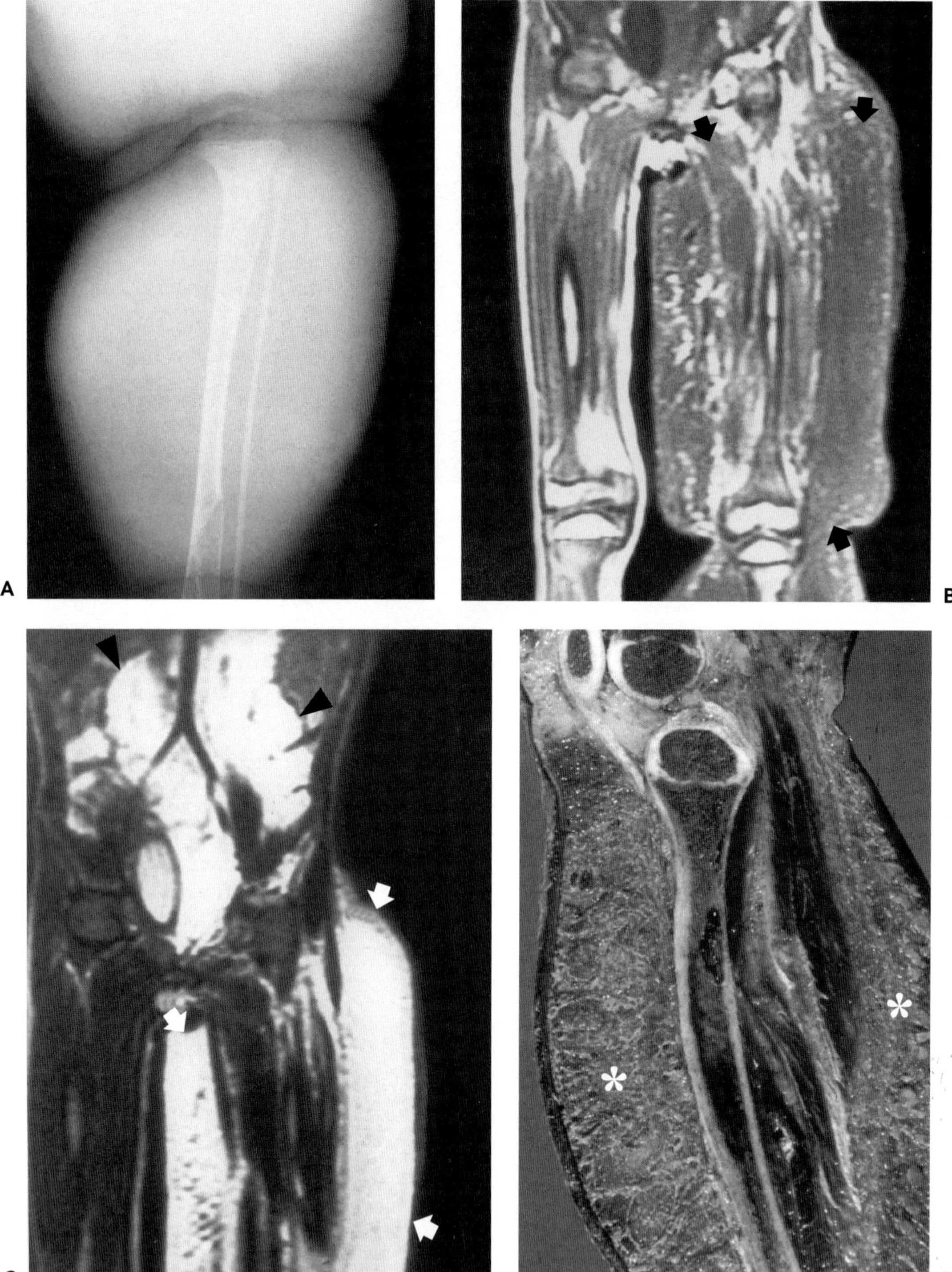

Figure 5.21 Congenital lymphangiomatosis of the lower extremity in a boy 6 years of age. **A:** Anteroposterior radiograph shows elephantiasis with osseous involvement. **B,C:** Coronal T1-weighted (TR/TE; 500/20) **(B)** and T2-weighted (TR/TE; 2500/100) **(C)** MR images reveal replacement of subcutaneous tissue (*arrows*) and extension into the pelvis and abdomen (*arrowheads* in **C**). Note marked enlargement of the left lower extremity. **D:** Sagittal section of gross specimen also shows the extensive lymphangiomatous infiltration (*asterisks*).

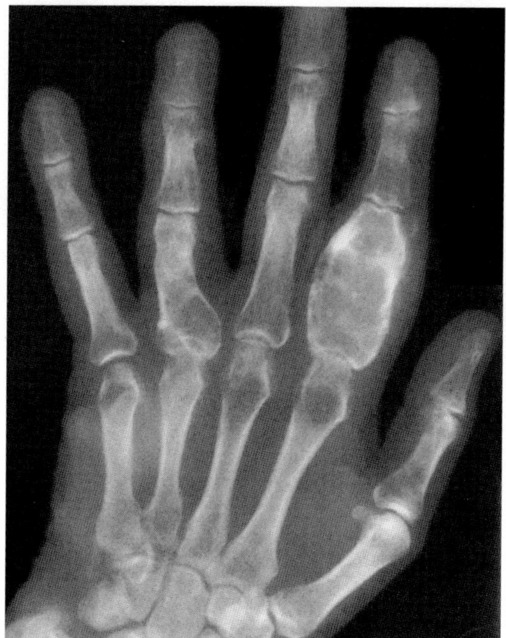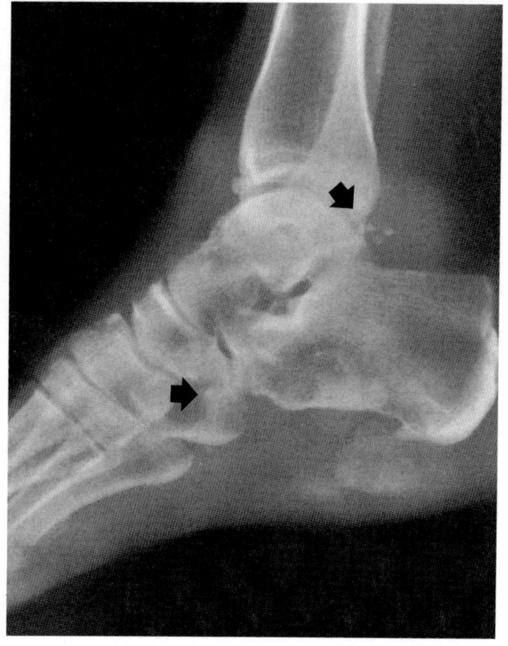

Figure 5.22　Maffucci syndrome in a woman 50 years of age. **A:** Radiograph of the hand shows multiple enchondromas. **B:** Radiograph of foot reveals multiple hemangiomas with phleboliths (*arrows*).

commonly involve the mucous membranes and the skin, lung, genitourinary, and gastrointestinal systems, and they are associated with bleeding from vascular weakness (94).

Klippel-Trenaunay-Weber Syndrome

Klippel-Trenaunay-Weber syndrome, originally described by Klippel and Trenaunay in 1900, consists of a classic triad of bone and soft tissue hypertrophy, varicose veins, and cutaneous hemangioma (96–98) (Figs. 5.24 and 5.25). Additional features are the absence of clinically significant arteriovenous shunting and anomalies of the deep venous system, including atresia, agenesis, hypoplasia, aneurysmal dilation, external compression from fibrous bands, and valvular incompetence (96). A characteristic incompetent lateral vein beginning at the ankle and extending to the infrainguinal or pelvic region is present in approximately 70% of patients (99). This syndrome usually affects the lower extremity unilaterally; there is no sex predilection and it is nonhereditary.

The cutaneous hemangioma, frequently a capillary-type lesion, is usually extensive and infiltrating. Venous varicosities are caused by the deep venous system abnormalities. The hypertrophy involves both bone elongation and circumferential soft tissue enlargement, develops in early childhood or at birth, and can affect the entire extremity or only the distal digits (100). Venography typically reveals extensive enlargement of superficial veins and dilated perforating veins that communicate with the deep veinous systems. Arteriovenous fistula may be associated with this syndrome, and this combination is often termed *Parke-Weber syndrome*. Imaging studies demonstrate the diffuse angiomatous infiltration with similar intrinsic characteristics as previously discussed for solitary hemangiomas (Fig. 5.24). These lesions may show evidence of both rapid and slow blood flow. Phleboliths in varicose veins and thickening of the subcutaneous fat may also be recognized. MR imaging is an ideal way to evaluate patients' bone and/or soft tissue hypertrophy, and it is an effective noninvasive modality to image the deep venous system (Fig. 5.25).

Patients present with a wide spectrum of complications, including cosmetic deformity from limb hypertrophy, bleeding from the diffuse vascular lesions, symptoms from chronic venous insufficiency, thrombophlebitis (and potential for pulmonary embolism), and pain (96).

Most patients do well without any treatment, except for elastic support or pneumatic compression devices, for symptoms of chronic venous insufficiency. It is also useful for treatment to decrease swelling caused by lymphatic stasis (96). Surgery is reserved for cases with significant cosmetic deformity, varicose veins, bleeding, or infection (96). Vein stripping or ligation may worsen symptoms with anomalies of the deep venous system (101).

Kasabach-Merritt Syndrome

Kasabach-Merritt syndrome represents an association of vascular lesions (hemangioma, angiomatosis, hemangioendothelioma, or rarely angiosarcoma) with thrombocytopenia and purpura (102–105). A bleeding diathesis results from intravascular coagulation and platelet sequestration within the angiomatous lesion (osseous or soft tissue) (104). Repetitive intraarticular hemarthrosis has also been reported in association with Kasabach-Merritt

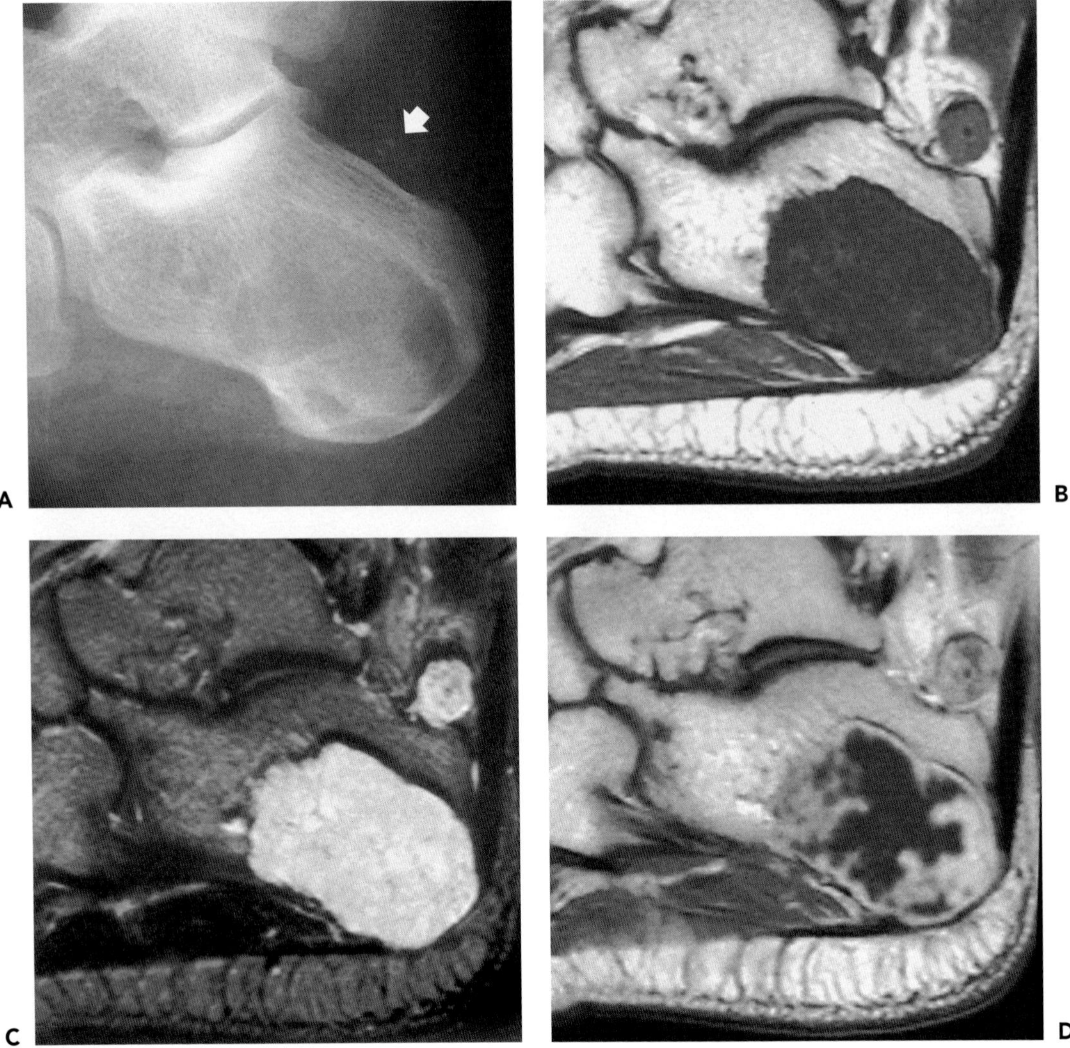

Figure 5.23 Maffucci syndrome in a man 39 years of age presenting with heel pain. **A:** Radiograph of the foot shows large lytic lesion in the posterior calcaneus. Subtle phleboliths are seen just above the calcaneus (*arrow*). **B,C:** Sagittal T1-weighted (TR/TE; 700/16) **(B)** and T2-weighted (TR/TE; 2000/80) **(C)** spin-echo MR images of the soft tissue lesion show typical imaging characteristics of the hemangioma. Note central signal voids from phleboliths. The large calcaneal lesion shows prolonged T1 and T2 relaxation times, typical of hyaline cartilage. **D:** Sagittal T1-weighted (TR/TE; 517/16) spin-echo MR image immediately following gadolinium administration shows marked enhancement of the hemangioma. The calcaneal lesion was a typical enchondroma at surgery.

syndrome and can result in an appearance similar to that of hemophilic arthropathy. Symptoms typically occur in infancy and are associated with rapid enlargement of the vascular lesion. Imaging of the offending vascular lesion is as previously described for solitary hemangioma. Aggressive therapy is usually required because the mortality rate from bleeding and infection is nearly 30% (2). Treatment is usually medical, with steroids and radiation, as well as newer use of recombinant interferon alfa-2a and pentoxifylline, as opposed to surgical intervention (2).

Tumor-Induced Osteomalacia

Numerous neoplasms, both soft tissue and osseous, can cause tumor-induced (oncogenic) osteomalacia. Angio-

matous lesions of the musculoskeletal system, particularly hemangiopericytomas, are most frequently associated with this phenomenon (86,106) (Fig. 5.26). These neoplasms causing oncogenic osteomalacia are frequently referred to as *phosphaturic mesenchymal tumors* (107,108). The neoplasm appears to produce a humoral factor that reduces renal tubular resorption of phosphate, resulting in osteomalacia. This circulation factor has been identified and named phosphatonin (109). Whole-body MR imaging with STIR sequences are used to identify these lesions, when they are otherwise occult, as focal high signal intensity masses that may demonstrate serpentine vascular structures (110). The resulting osteomalacia is often debilitating with multiple insufficiency fractures, and removal of the offending neoplasm is curative (111).

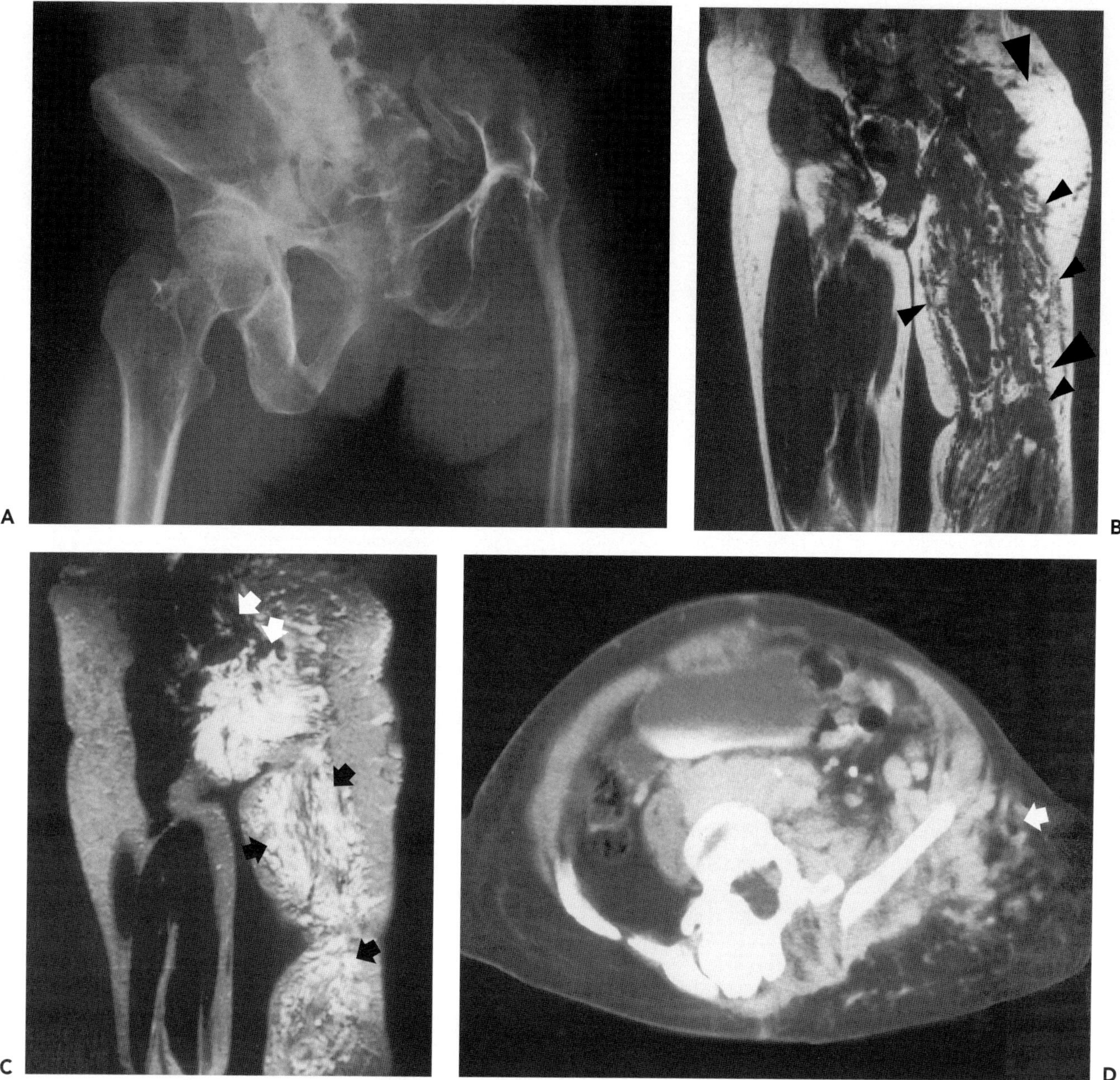

Figure 5.24 Klippel-Trenaunay-Weber syndrome in a woman 37 years of age with extensive cutaneous capillary hemangioma and varicose veins. **A:** Pelvic radiograph shows atrophy of bone on the left with chronic hip dislocation and soft tissue hypertrophy. Atrophy of bone in this unusual case was caused by below-knee amputation required at birth to reduce vascular effects of lower extremity lesion. **B,C:** Coronal T1-weighted (TR/TE; 500/25) **(B)** and T2-weighted (TR/TE; 2000/90) **(C)** spin-echo MR images reveal extensive angiomatous lesions (*small arrowhead* in **B**) of both deep and superficial tissues, and fat overgrowth (*large arrowheads* in **B**). Areas of both slow (high signal intensity: *black arrows* in **C**) and rapid (low signal intensity: *white arrows* in **C**) blood flow are seen on T2-weighted MR image. Soft tissue hypertrophy is caused by infiltration of tissues by angiomatous lesion. **D:** Axial contrast-enhanced CT scan shows extension into the right pelvis and gluteal region (*arrow*).

GLOMUS TUMOR

The glomus tumor is a benign neoplasm (with the rare exception of glomangiosarcoma) derived from the neuromyoarterial plexus. Pathologic variants include glomangioma (20% of cases and lesions with large cavernous spaces); glomangiomyoma (contains a smooth muscle component, less than 10% of cases); and the very rare glomangiosarcoma or malignant glomus tumor (<1% of glomus tumors) (112–116). Glomangiomatosis represents a diffusely infiltrative lesion and is the glomoid counterpart to angiomatosis (113,115). Glomus tumors are usually located about the terminal phalanx of the hand, although other common sites include the wrist, forearm, and foot.

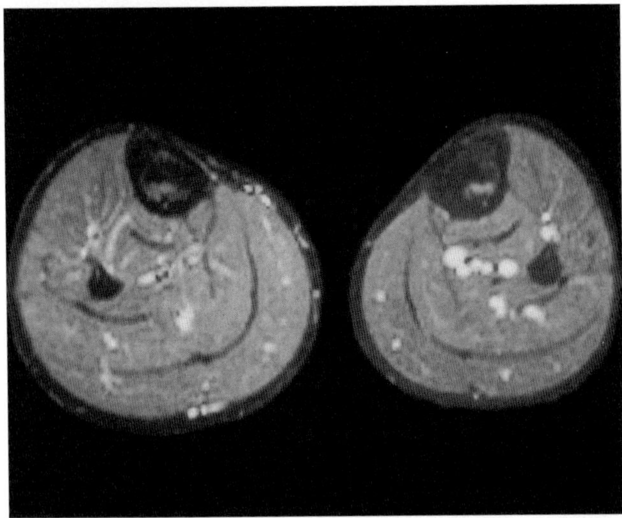

Figure 5.25 Klippel-Trenaunay-Weber syndrome in a boy 15 years of age, presenting with gigantism of the lower extremity. Axial inversion recovery (TR/TE/TI; 2000/30/130) MR image of the lower extremities shows overgrowth of the right lower extremity with hypoplasia of the deep venous system compared to the contralateral side.

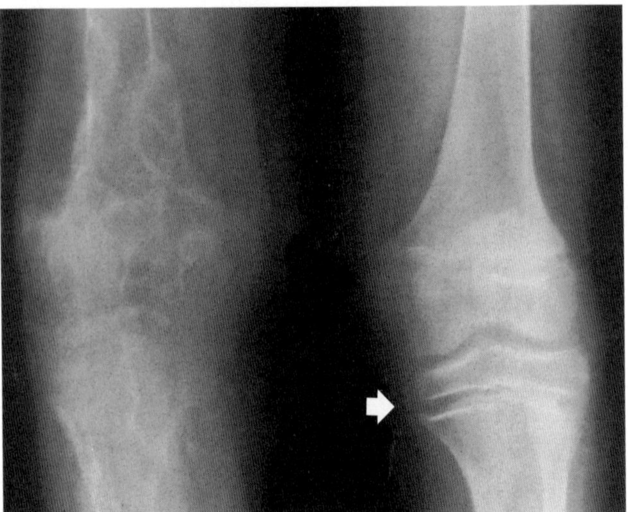

Figure 5.26 Angiomatosis in a boy 15 years of age with tumor-induced osteomalacia. Knee radiographs reveal multifocal osseous and soft tissue hemangiomas around the right knee with changes of osteomalacia (rickets), best seen involving the left knee (*arrow*).

KEY CONCEPTS

- Glomus tumor represents a benign tumor of the neuromyoarterial plexus.
- Most commonly it affects the nail bed of a finger in an adult woman (20 to 40 years of age).
- Clinical symptoms of a small red-blue nodule with paroxysms of pain, caused by temperature change or pressure, is characteristic.
- Imaging reveals a small focal mass related to the nail bed, with erosion of bone in 22% to 82% of cases.

Unusual sites affected include the thigh, bone (patella), stomach, colon, nerve, face, trachea, and mediastinum (117). A striking female predilection (3:1) is observed in subungual lesions, although overall there is no sex predilection. Adults between 20 and 40 years of age are usually affected. Multiple lesions are present in nearly 10% of patients (112). Clinically, the glomus tumor is seen as a small, red-blue, superficial nodule with symptoms of paroxysms of radiating pain, caused by temperature change or pressure. The classic clinical triad of pain, point tenderness, and cold sensitivity is present in approximately 30% of patients (118).

A soft tissue mass is seen on radiographs, located along the dorsal surface of the finger, either laterally or medially, related to the nail bed. In addition, extrinsic erosion of bone, often with a sclerotic margin, can be seen in 22% to 60% of cases (119) (Fig. 5.27).

Advanced imaging appearances of glomus tumor have more recently been described. On sonography, a hypoechoic mass is seen (120). Small subungual masses may go undetected on ultrasound examination. CT scanning

reveals a nonspecific subungual soft tissue mass. MR imaging shows these lesions as small masses with very high signal intensity and homogeneity on T2-weighted images (121,122) (Figs. 5.28 and 5.29). However, Drape et al. demonstrated more variable appearance on long TR images and degree of enhancement after intravenous contrast. Lesions were typically homogeneously hyperintense and enhanced prominently and diffusely (118). Using a high-resolution surface coil for skin imaging, these investigators were able to demonstrate cortical bone erosion on MR imaging in 23 (82%) of 28 cases, whereas radiographs were positive in only 7 (25%) cases. Glomangiomatosis

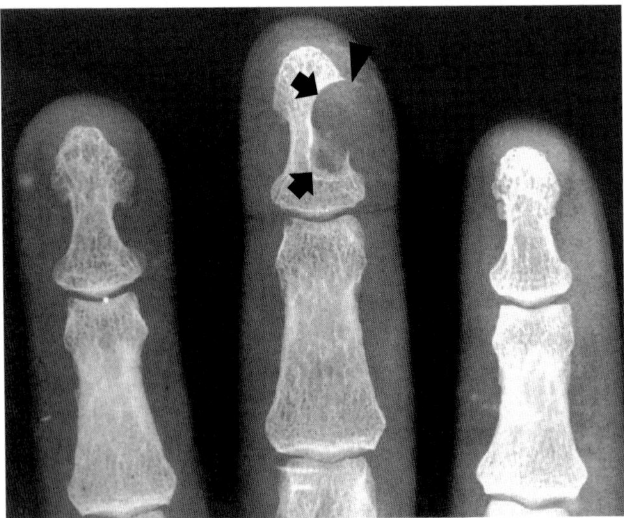

Figure 5.27 Glomus tumor in a man 46 years of age with painful lump on long finger. Radiograph shows extrinsic erosion (*arrows*) of terminal tuft with sclerotic margins and associated soft tissue component (*arrowhead*).

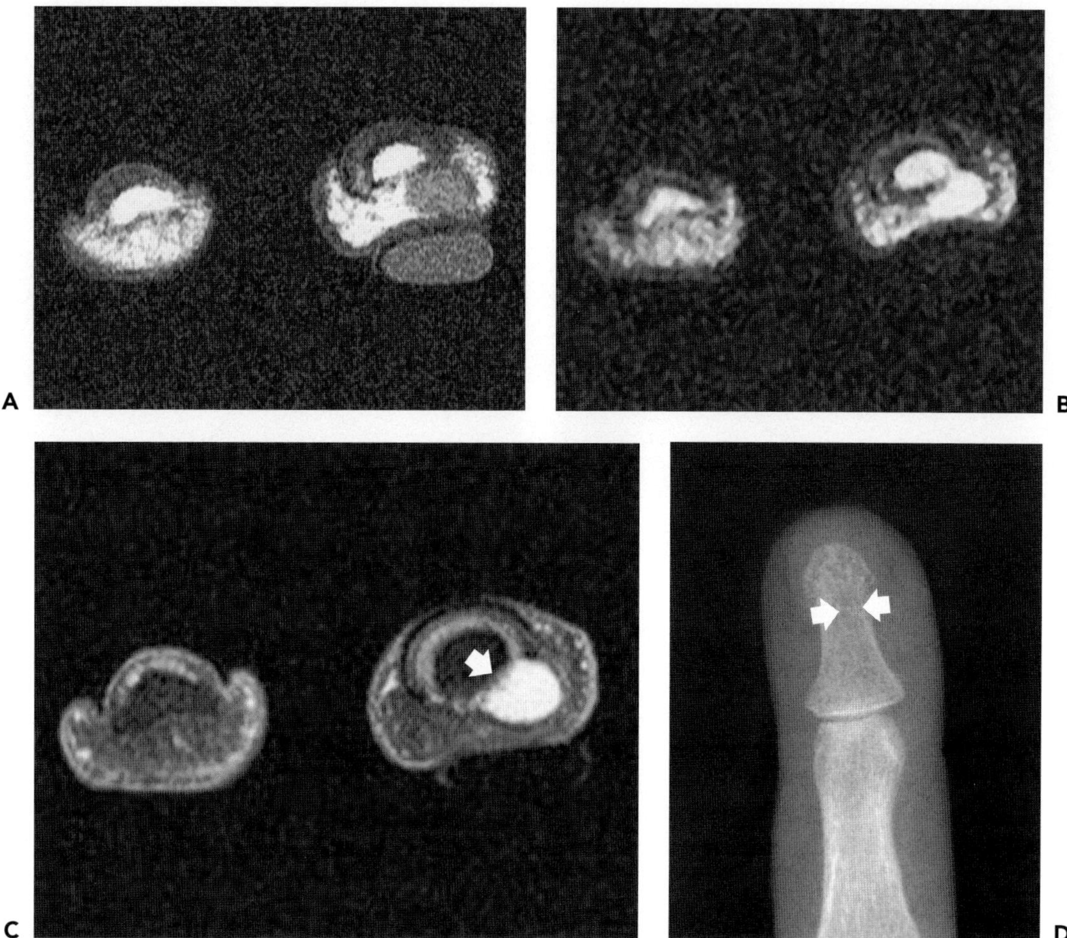

Figure 5.28   Glomus tumor of the middle finger in a woman 69 years of age. **A,B:** Axial T1-weighted (TR/TE; 706/20) **(A)** and T2-weighted (TR,TE; 1800/80) **(B)** spin-echo MR images of the fingertips shows a 4-mm mass along the radial margin of the nail fold. The lesion is markedly hyperintense on T2-weighted image **B. C:** Axial fat-suppressed T1-weighted (TR/TE; 500/20) spin-echo MR image shows the lesion to enhance markedly following contrast administration. Note subtle osseous erosion (*arrow*). **D:** Radiograph shows very subtle bone erosion (*arrows*).

shows multifocal lesions with similar intrinsic characteristics as compared to solitary lesions (113,115). Recurrent glomus tumors can also be detected on MR imaging as focal masses, although signal characteristics are not as uniformly high intensity or enhancing as are lesions preoperatively (116). MR angiography may be useful to differentiate recurrence glomus tumor (strong arterial phase enhancement) versus scar (no enhancement) (116).

AGGRESSIVE AND MALIGNANT VASCULAR TUMORS

Hemangioendothelioma, Hemangiopericytoma, Kaposi Sarcoma, and Angiosarcoma

Hemangioendothelioma is a vascular neoplasm of intermediate aggressiveness, between that of hemangioma and

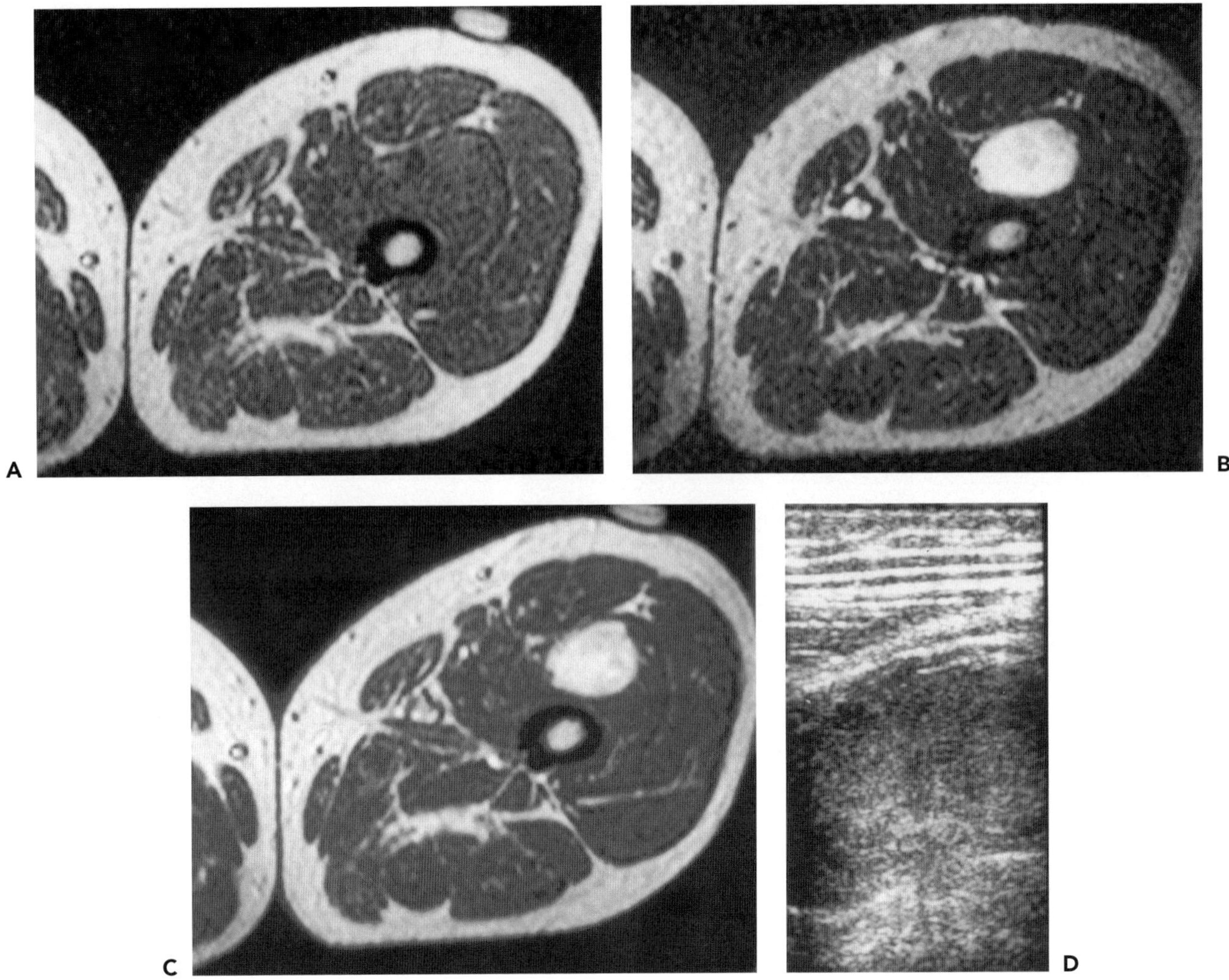

Figure 5.29 Glomus tumor in a man 42 years of age. **A,B:** Axial T1-weighted (TR/TE; 550/20) **(A)** and T2-weighted (TR/TE; 2000/80) **(B)** spin-echo MR images show a well-defined, relatively heterogeneous, nonspecific mass in the anterior aspect of the left thigh. **C:** Axial T1-weighted (TR/TE; 550/20) spin-echo MR image following contrast administration shows marked homogeneous enhancement. **D:** Longitudinal ultrasonography shows as a well-defined nonspecific mass.

angiosarcoma. This neoplasm arises from the vascular endothelial cells, and the WHO subtypes of hemangioendothelioma include epithelioid, kaposiform, retiform, composite, and papillary intralymphatic angioendothelioma (Dabska tumor) (19,20,123–125).

Epithelioid hemangioendothelioma is a rare vascular neoplasm (endothelial cells have an epithelial appearance) usually occurring in the second to ninth decade, and there is no sex predilection. These neoplasms are most frequent in the deep soft tissues of the extremities, and approximately 50% to 70% arise near a vessel, often a vein (123,124). The adjacent vascular structures may be occluded, leading to symptoms of thrombophlebitis. These tumors may also involve bone and viscera (lung and liver). The local recurrence rate is 10% to 15%, the metastatic rate is 20% to 30%, and the mortality rate is 10% to 20% (123,124).

Kaposiform hemangioendothelioma is rare, may involve the superficial or deep soft tissues, and usually affects children and adolescents. This lesion may be associated with Kasabach-Merritt syndrome, particularly when retroperitoneal in location. Lesions involving the deep soft tissues are usually invasive and unresectable, and, although nonmetastasizing, they often lead to patient demise. In contradistinction, lesions in the somatic soft tissues are usually cured by complete resection with only rare recurrences.

Retiform and papillary intralymphatic angioendothelioma (Dabska tumor) appear to be closely related and represent locally aggressive, nonmetastasizing, vascular lesions. These lesions involve the subcutaneous tissues of the lower extremity most frequently, with no sex predilection. Retiform (also known as hobnail) hemangioendothelioma usually affects young adults, whereas Dabska tumor has a predilection for infants and children (25% in adults) (3). Retiform lesions are more likely to recur locally (up to 60% of cases), and wide-local excision is suggested for both lesions (3).

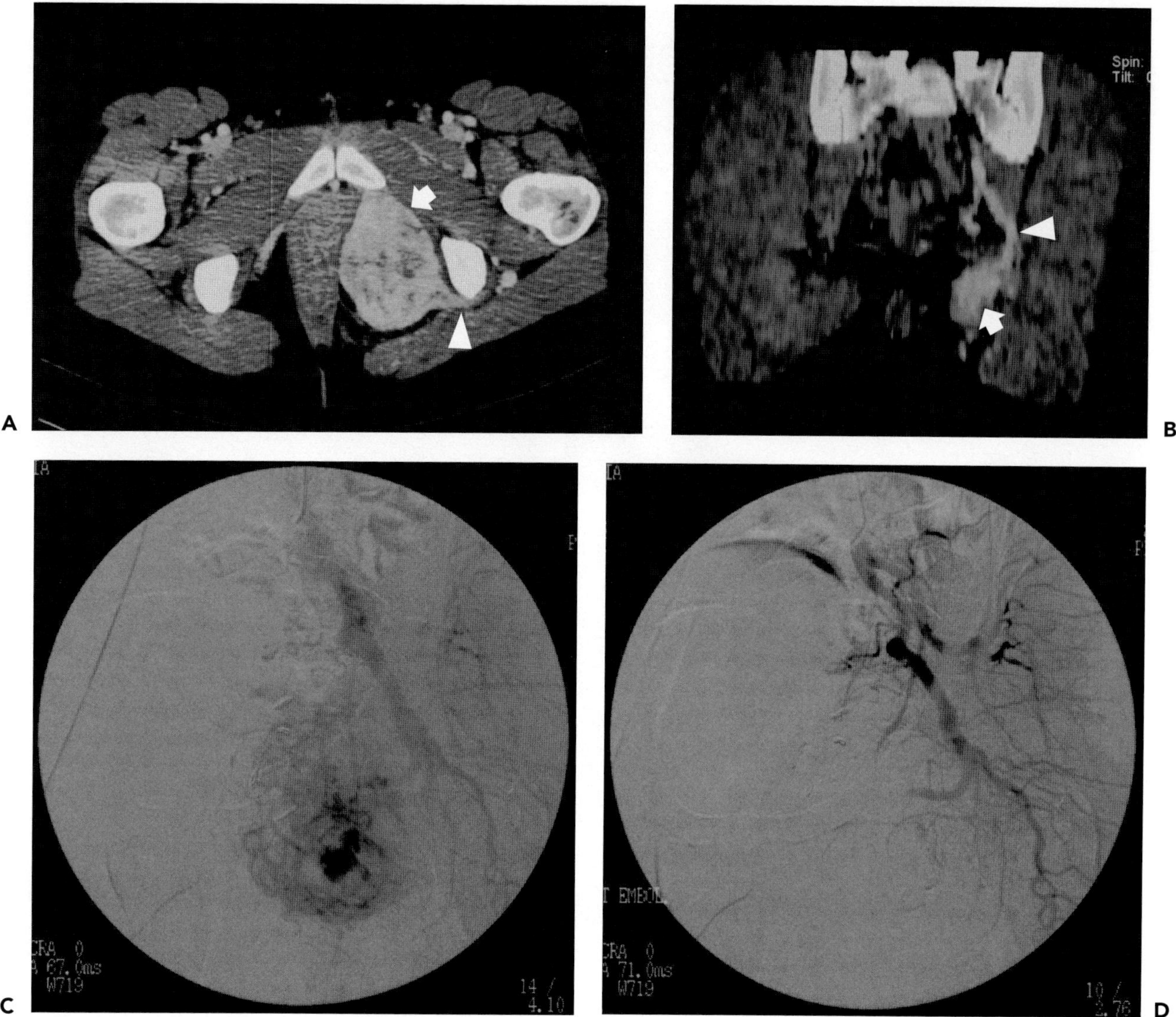

Figure 5.30 Hemangiopericytoma/extrapleural solitary fibrous tumor in a woman 32 years of age with left hip pain. **A,B:** Axial CT **(A)** and coronal CT reconstruction **(B)** show intensively enhancing mass in the ischiorectal region (*arrow*) with feeding gluteal vessels (*arrowhead*). **C,D:** Angiogram prior to **(C)** and following embolization **(D)** reveal marked hypervascular lesion before therapy.

Composite hemangioendothelioma is an extremely aggressive, nonmetastasizing vascular lesion. Adults are most commonly affected, with a particular predilection for the hands and feet. Wide-local excision is the treatment of choice, with an approximately 50% recurrence rate.

Hemangiopericytoma is also a vascular neoplasm of intermediate aggressiveness with both benign and malignant forms (112) (Figs. 5.30, 5.31, and 5.32). These lesions are closely related to and likely synonymous with *solitary fibrous tumor* (extrapleural) according to the WHO. The WHO also designates another lesion as the lipomatous hemangiopericytoma, although we believe these lesions have simply engulfed normal adipose tissue and are not truly distinct neoplasms. During a 10-year period (1980 to 1990), 525 cases of hemangiopericytoma were

seen in consultation by the Department of Soft Tissue Pathology at the AFIP, of which 141 (27%) were malignant (126). This neoplasm arises from pericytes (cells of Zimmerman), contractile spindle cells, surrounding capillaries, and postcapillary venules. Hemangiopericytoma most frequently affects adults in the fifth decade, with 80% of patients between 25 and 65 years of age, except the rare infantile type (first year of life) (112,127). Males and females are equally affected. The most frequent location is the lower extremity (35%), followed by the retroperitoneum (25%), head/neck (16%), trunk (14%), and upper extremity (10%) (112). The typical clinical history is that of a slowly enlarging painless mass, and hypoglycemia may be associated with these tumors (19,20,96, 123–131).

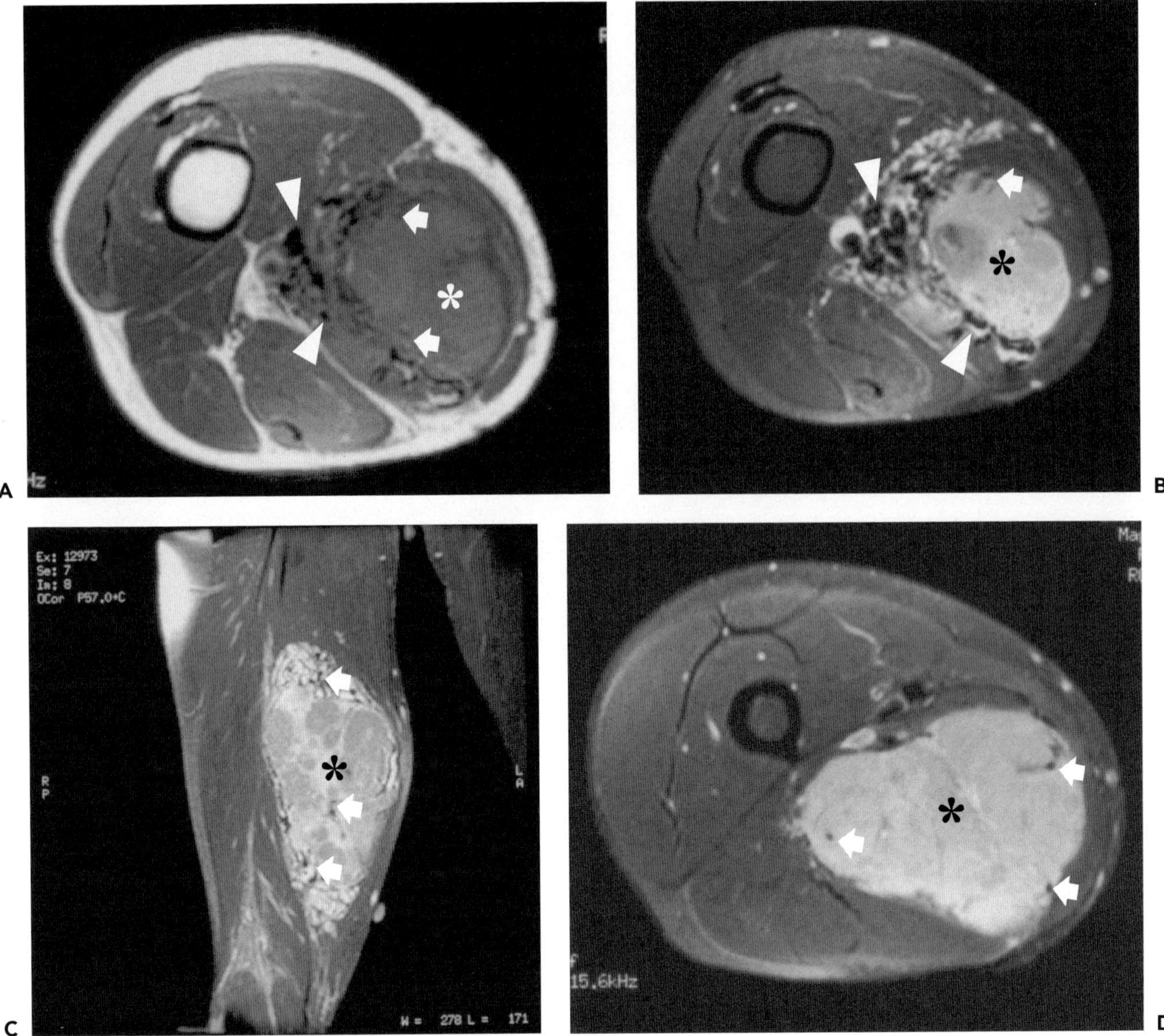

Figure 5.31 Malignant soft tissue hemangiopericytoma in man 35 years of age with enlarging thigh mass. **A,B:** Axial T1-weighted (TR/TE; 500/10) **(A)** and axial enhanced fat-suppressed T1-weighted (TR/TE; 500/8) **(B)** MR images show a large mass (*asterisk*) with prominent serpentine vascular channels. Feeding vessels with rapid blood-flow show signal voids (*arrowheads*), while smaller, less prominent flow voids are also seen within the neoplasm (*arrows*). **C,D:** Sagittal enhanced fat-suppressed T1-weighted (TR/TE; 500/8) **(C)** and axial fat-suppressed T2-weighted (TR/TE; 4000/60) **(D)** show the mass (*asterisk*). Note prominent vascularity (*arrows*). The mass has an intermediate signal intensity on both T1- and T2-weighted MR images.

Kaposi sarcoma is a malignant skin lesion showing prominent vascular proliferation that is viral related (Figs. 5.33 and 5.34). The disease is the result of an inter-relationship of the Kaposi sarcoma–associated herpesvirus and immunologic, genetic, and environmental factors. This disease occurs in four clinical and epidemiologic patterns, including the classic or chronic form, endemic African, iatrogenic, and AIDS-related types (Figs. 5.33 and 5.34). The classic form of Kaposi sarcoma is rare in the United States (predominating in men of Mediterranean or eastern European descent); is associated with lymphoreticular neoplasms (myeloma, lymphoma, leukemia); and occurs in elderly patients. In addition, unlike AIDS-related Kaposi sarcoma, which has a high mortality rate, only 10% to 20% of patients with the classic form die of their disease (132). The iatrogenic form is relatively frequent and associated with solid organ transplantation or immunosuppressive therapy for other conditions. The endemic form is not associated with HIV infection and affects middle-aged adults and children in equatorial Africa, often with a protracted course. AIDS-related Kaposi sarcoma is the most aggressive form and frequently affects the face, genitals, lower extremities, oral mucosa, and lymph nodes.

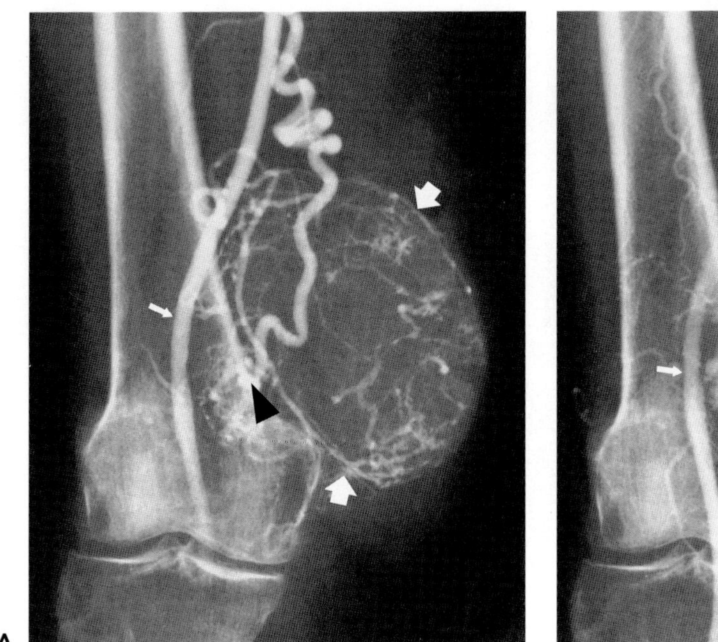

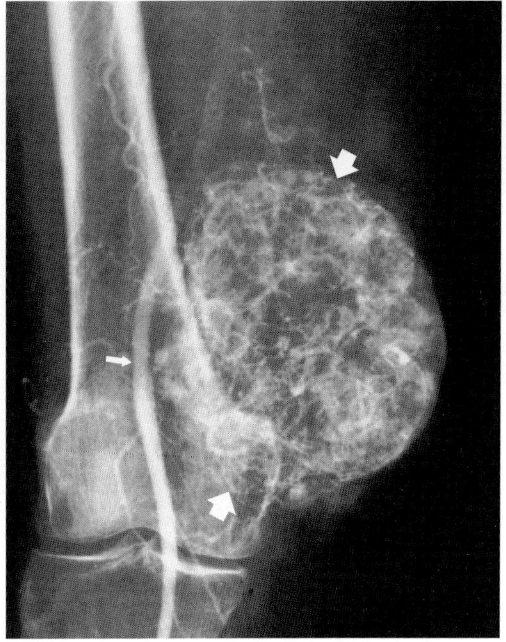

Figure 5.32 Malignant soft tissue hemangiopericytoma of the distal thigh in a woman 73 years of age. **A,B:** Early **(A)** and midphase **(B)** films from arteriogram show neovascularity entering the mass as a pedicle (*arrowhead* in **A**) and then arborizing to supply the tumor with staining (*arrows*). Femoral artery is displaced by the mass (*thin arrow*).

Angiosarcomas are malignant vascular neoplasms (Fig. 5.35). Pathologically, cellular elements may be either hemangiosarcoma and/or lymphangiosarcoma, and distinction is often difficult or impossible, particu-

larly when higher degrees of anaplasia are present. The term *angiosarcoma* is preferable. Angiosarcoma involves the skin (with or without lymphedema, 33% of cases) and deep soft tissues (24%) most frequently, with other sites (breast, liver, bone, spleen, heart, head, and neck) accounting for the remainder of cases (132,133). Older patients are generally affected, and excluding those tumors associated with lymphedema, men are affected twice as commonly as women. Chronic lymphedema is a

Figure 5.33 Kaposi sarcoma of the fingertip in a man 77 years of age. Digital subtraction arteriogram shows marked vascularity of the lesion.

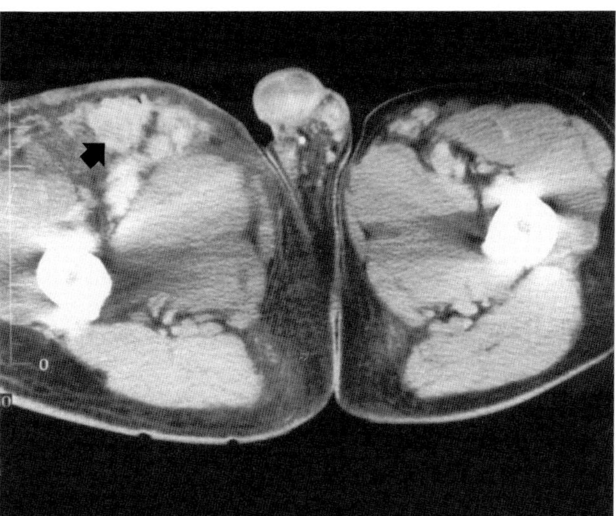

Figure 5.34 Kaposi sarcoma in a man 45 years of age with AIDS. Axial contrast-enhanced CT of the groin shows an enhancing nodular mass (*arrow*) in the right inguinal region. Skin thickening and subcutaneous edema are present.

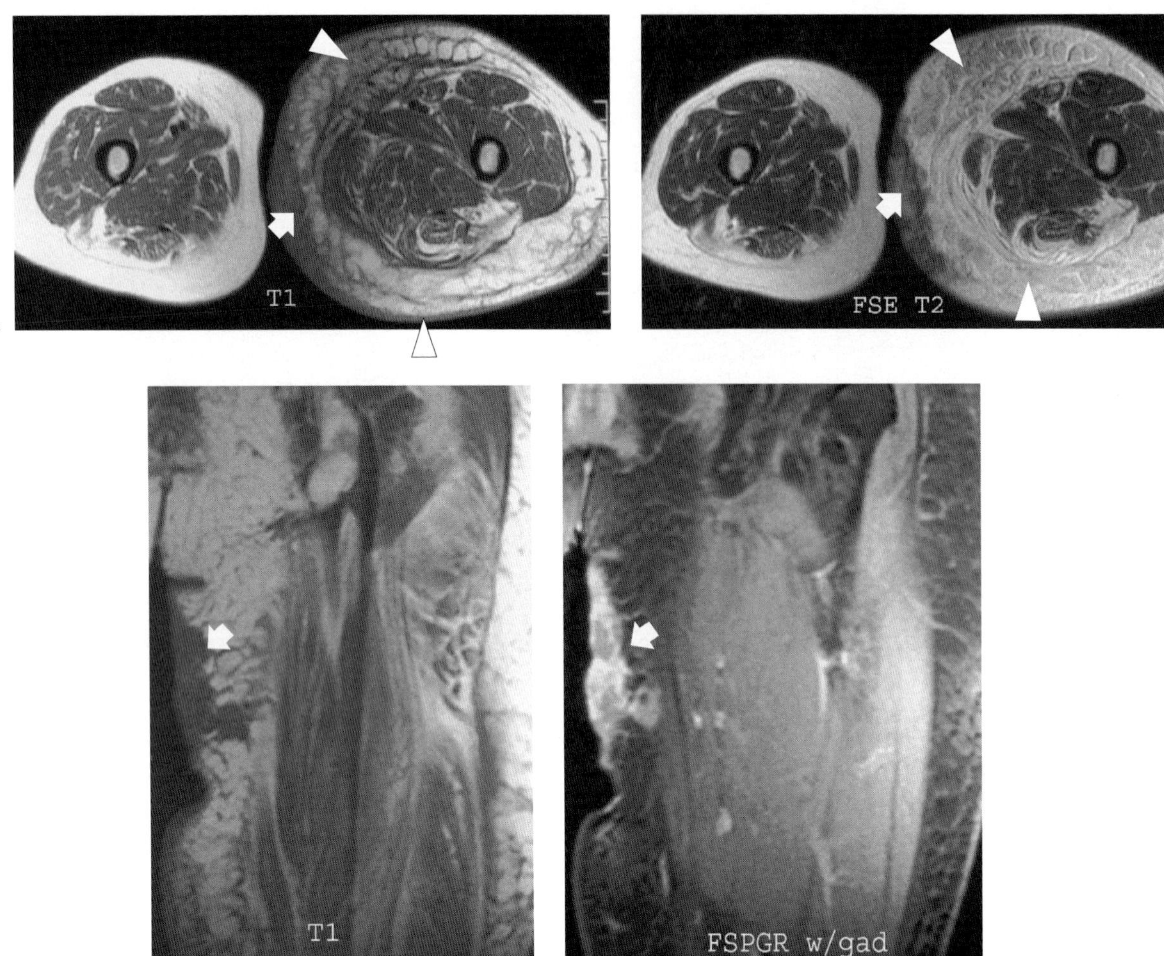

Figure 5.35 Angiosarcoma in a woman 74 years of age with chronic lymphedema of the leg. **A-D:** Axial T1-weighted (TR/TE; 500/15) **(A)**, axial T2-weighted (TR/TE; 4000/60) **(B)**, coronal T1-weighted (TR/TE; 500/20) **(C)**, and coronal enhanced fat-suppressed T1-weighted (TR/TE; 500/20) **(D)** MR images show an enlarged left extremity (*arrowhead*) with subcutaneous edema caused by congenital lymphatic hypoplasia. Lobular enhancing superficial skin mass (*arrow*) represents the development of angiosarcoma.

well-recognized predisposition to angiosarcoma; however, only approximately 10% of cases demonstrate this association (132). The vast majority of these angiosarcomas (90%) are found in postmastectomy patients (Stewart-Treves syndrome), but any cause of chronic lymphedema (congenital, idiopathic, traumatic, or infectious) is also a predisposition (133,134) (Fig. 5.35). A small minority (0.07% to 0.45% of women surviving 5 years) of postmastectomy patients are affected with a latency period of 4 to 27 years (average: 10 years) (132). Angiosarcoma may also be radiation-induced.

The imaging appearance of these more aggressive vascular lesions, including hemangioendothelioma, hemangiopericytoma, Kaposi sarcoma, and angiosarcoma, is particularly dependant on lesion location, either superficial or deep. Kaposi sarcoma and angiosarcoma involving the skin and subcutaneous tissues typically reveal areas of skin thickening with nodularity and focal soft tissue mass on sonography, CT, or MR imaging (134) (Figs. 5.34 and

5.35). The intrinsic characteristics are usually nonspecific, with intermediate echogenicity, soft tissue attenuation, and intermediate intensity on T1-weighting and intermediate-to-high intensity on T2-weighting. In our experience, vascular channels and spaces are not typically apparent by imaging in these superficial lesions. Underlying manifestations of chronic lymphedema are frequently associated with angiosarcoma, including extremity enlargement, diffuse skin thickening, as well as thickening and edema of the subcutaneous connective tissue septae on CT and MR imaging.

Hemangioendothelioma, hemangiopericytoma, and angiosarcoma involving the deep soft tissues have a different imaging appearance compared to their superficial counterparts. Calcification and erosion of adjacent bone have been described on radiographs. These lesions may reveal a nonspecific appearance of a solid soft tissue mass on ultrasound, CT, or MR imaging. However, detection of a prominent serpentine vascular component with other nonspecific solid regions on advanced imaging studies should suggest one of these diagnoses (Figs. 5.30 and 5.31). These lesions typically cannot be distinguished from one other by imaging and are most frequently intermuscular masses, often related to a major neurovascular bundle. Specific description of these lesions on ultrasound, CT, or MR is limited (20,39,128,130). These lesions may be hypo- or hyperechoic at sonography, and cystic areas can be prominent, resulting from hemorrhage. Arteriovenous shunting may be apparent on Doppler studies. CT reveals a soft tissue mass of similar attenuation to that of muscle which enhances, often markedly, after intravenous contrast (Fig. 5.30). MR imaging is best to identify characteristic vascular channels, and these areas are often in the periphery of the mass. This pattern is particularly prominent in hemangiopericytomas, reflecting their vascular supply (39). The serpentine vascular structures show prominent areas of low signal intensity on all MR pulse sequences from rapid blood flow, although other channels become high signal on long TR images, reflecting slow blood flow (Fig. 5.31). A feeding, high-flow, vascular pedicle may also be apparent on MR imaging. Other soft tissue sarcomas, even if hypervascular, do not typically demonstrate definable prominent vessels on MR imaging, with the exception of alveolar soft part sarcoma, rhabdomyosarcoma, and extraskeletal Ewing sarcoma/peripheral neuroectodermal tumor (PNET). The remainder of the mass shows nonspecific MR imaging appearance with intermediate intensity on T1-weighting and high signal on T2-weighting. In contradistinction to hemangioma, these more aggressive vascular neoplasms lack fat overgrowth and are not solely composed of vascular channels and spaces. Fluid levels may be seen as a result of hemorrhage. Angiography of these deep vascular neoplasms show dense areas of well-circumscribed staining, early draining veins, and shunting. Hemangiopericytoma often has a characteristic angiographic appearance, with vessels supplying the tumor forming a pedicle entering the mass (131) (Fig. 5.32). Vessels branch from this vascular pedicle to encircle the tumor, and the mass displaces major vessels.

BIOPSY, TREATMENT AND PROGNOSIS

We believe the identification of serpentine vascular channels or spaces comprising the entire lesion and/or fat overgrowth is pathognomonic in 90% to 95% of intramuscular hemangiomas (39). In lesions in which these features are confidently identified radiologically (optimally by MR imaging), we do not advocate biopsy or treatment, if symptoms are limited and not clinically warranted. In cases with a nonpathognomonic imaging appearance or those requiring treatment based on clinical symptoms, biopsy prior to resection may be performed. However, percutaneous small-needle biopsy of soft tissue angiomatous lesions may not yield diagnosis, particularly in benign cavernous

hemangiomas (39). This is probably related to obtaining predominantly hemorrhage as opposed to solid tissue for histologic analysis. Noncavernous hemangiomas and more aggressive vascular tumors are usually more readily diagnosed via fine-needle aspiration biopsy. Bleeding after biopsy of the vast majority of soft tissue angiomatous lesions has been usually limited and controlled with direct pressure. However, extensive bleeding with death by exsanguination has been rarely reported as a result of biopsy, particularly of deeply seated musculoskeletal angiomatous lesions (i.e., retroperitoneal) and/or those with high/rapid flow components, where control of hemorrhage is more difficult and bleeding may not be clinically obvious (86).

Treatment of hemangioma or lymphangioma is often surgical resection and/or laser photocoagulation. In addition, embolotherapy or sclerotherapy may also be used in the treatment of angiomatous (hemangioma or lymphangioma) lesions (135–138) (Figs. 5.36 and 5.37). This form of therapy may be performed as an adjunct, prior to surgery to lessen blood loss, or may be the sole treatment in unresectable lesions where amputation would be the only other alternative. Various embolic agents may be used, including blood products, Gelfoam, collagen, ethanol, alcohol, coils, and balloons. Embolization is frequently performed with a mixture of polyvinyl alcohol particles, ranging in diameter from 200 to 300 or 300 to 500 μm, and the sclerosing agents (135–138). MR imaging has been used to guide and follow response during and subsequent to hemangioma percutaneous sclerotherapy treatment (139). MR imaging can identify the sclerosant distribution and scar formation following treatment (139). Molitch et al. reported successful palliative treatment by percutaneous sclerotherapy in five patients with unresectable lymphangioma using doxycycline (137). In the series by Gomes, symptomatic control was achieved in 77% of patients with better results in low flow-lesions (136). Other researchers reported some symptomatic relief in 74% to 91% of vascular lesions treated by percutaneous sclerotherapy (140,141). Goyal et al. identified a relationship between lesion size and margin, with response to percutaneous sclerotherapy (140). In their

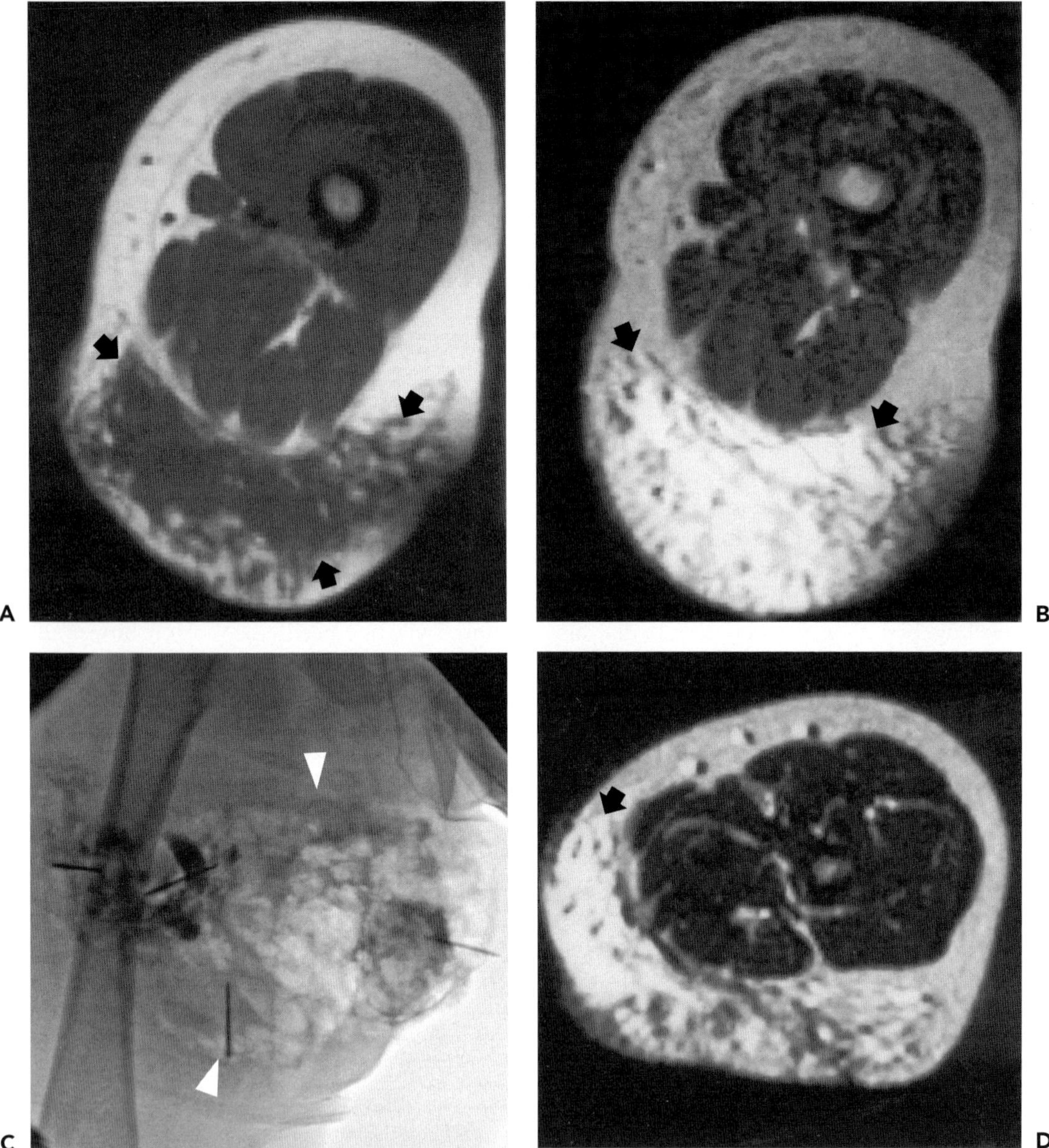

Figure 5.36   Soft tissue lymphangioma of buttock (discovered at birth) in boy 3 years of age. **A,B:** Axial T1-weighted (TR/TE; 500/20) **(A)** and T2-weighted (TR/TE; 2000/90) **(B)** spin-echo MR images show a subcutaneous lesion composed of cavernous spaces (*arrows*), with low-signal intensity on T1-weighted image **A,** and high-signal in T2-weighted image **B.** Hemangioma was suspected; however, arteriogram (not shown) was normal. **C:** Needle puncture aspirated clear milky fluid, and cavernous lymphangioma was distended with air and contrast (*arrowheads*). Subsequent sclerotherapy with alcohol was performed with shrinkage of lesion. **D:** Axial T2-weighted (TR/TE; 2100/100) MR image 6-months following sclerotherapy shows significant reduction in tumor size.

series of venous lesions, size larger than 5 cm and infiltrative margins were associated with a poorer response to percutaneous sclerotherapy, often necessitating multiple episodes of treatment. Complications of embolic agents include ischemia and resulting pain, inflammation, skin sloughing, and recanalization of vessels. In addition, Mason et al. reported dose-related coagulation abnormalities associated with use of dehydrated alcohol or sodium tetradecyl sulfate (141). In cases not amenable to surgery, radiation therapy is also a treatment option (142,143).

Recurrence of angiomatous lesions varies with the specific lesion. Soft tissue hemangiomas recur in approximately 28% of cases (28). Diffuse involvement with angiomatosis, in contrast, is accompanied by a high rate of recurrence (90%) after surgery as reported by Rao and Weiss (144). Vascular neoplasms of intermediate aggressiveness hemangioendothelioma and hemangiopericytoma, have a generally favorable prognosis following wide surgical resection. However, recurrence is relatively frequent, and metastases occur in 10% to 25% of cases, to the lungs, bone, and

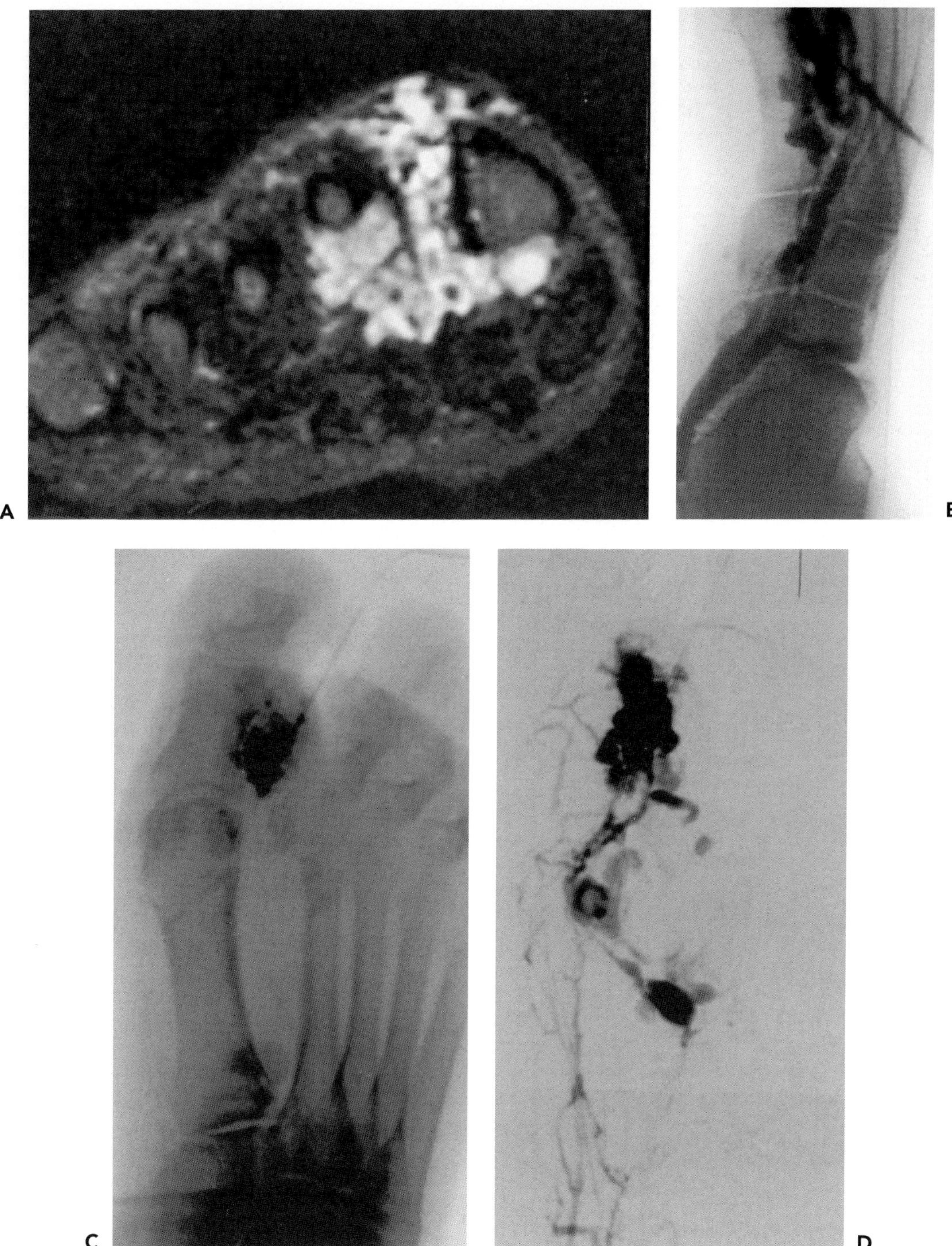

Figure 5.37 Intramuscular hemangioma in the foot of a woman 40 years of age. **A:** Coronal T2-weighted (TR/TE; 1800/80) spin-echo MR image shows the lesion to have a lobular configuration with areas markedly hyperintense to subcutaneous fat. Septations within the lesion are isointense to either fat and/or muscle. Note infiltrative growth pattern, extending between the metatarsals, to the dorsum of the foot. **B:** Direct puncture venogram shows the large cavernous spaces of the lesion with prominent draining veins. **C,D:** Early **(C)** and delayed **(D)** images from venogram done 4 weeks after Sotradecol sclerotherapy shows marked radiographic improvement, with resolution of patient's symptoms.

liver (112,125). The prognosis for Kaposi sarcoma depends on the type of lesion, as previously discussed, and disease extent at diagnosis. Angiosarcoma, however, has a dismal prognosis, despite aggressive wide surgical resection, adjuvant radiation therapy, and chemotherapy. Local recurrence of angiosarcoma is common, with early metastases to lung, bone, and lymph nodes. Angiosarcoma associated with lymphedema showed only a 15% 5-year survival in one study, and deep-seated lesions revealed a 53% mortality within 1 year in another series (3,132).

REFERENCES

1. Allen PW, Enzinger FM. Hemangioma of skeletal muscle. An analysis of 89 cases. *Cancer.* 1972;29:8–22.
2. Weiss S, Goldblum J. Benign tumors and tumor-like lesions of blood vessels. In: *Enzinger and Weiss's Soft Tissue Tumors.* 4th ed. St. Louis: CV Mosby; 2001:837–890.
3. Fletcher C, Unni K, Mertens F. *World Health Organization Classification of Tumors. Pathology and Genetics of Tumors of Soft Tissue and Bone.* Lyon, France: IARC Press; 2002.
4. Kempson R, Fletcher C, Evans H, et al. *Tumors of the Soft Tissues.* Bethesda, MD: Armed Forces Institute of Pathology; 2001.
5. Miettinen M. *Diagnostic Soft Tissue Pathology.* New York: Churchill Livingstone; 2003.
6. Moron FE, Morriss MC, Jones JJ, et al. Lumps and bumps on the head in children: use of CT and MR imaging in solving the clinical diagnostic dilemma. *Radiographics.* 2004;24:1655–1674.
7. Resnick D. Tumors and tumor-like lesions of bone: imaging and pathology of specific lesions. In: *Diagnosis of Bone and Joint Disorders.* 4th ed. Philadelphia: WB Saunders; 2002;4129–4273.
8. Chew FS, Hudson TM, Hawkins IF Jr. Radiology of infiltrating angiolipoma. *AJR Am J Roentgenol.* 1980;135:781–787.
9. De Orchis D, Ozonoff MB. Infiltrating angiolipoma with phlebolith formation. *Skeletal Radiol.* 1986;15:464–467.
10. Gonzalez-Crussi F, Enneking WF, Arean VM. Infiltrating angiolipoma. *J Bone Joint Surg Am.* 1966;48:1111–1124.
11. Lin JJ, Lin F. Two entities in angiolipoma. A study of 459 cases of lipoma with review of literature on infiltrating angiolipoma. *Cancer.* 1974;34:720–727.
12. Pribyl C, Burke SW, Roberts JM, et al. Infiltrating angiolipoma or intramuscular hemangioma? A report of five cases. *J Pediatr Orthop.* 1986;6:172–176.
13. Metry DW, Hebert AA. Benign cutaneous vascular tumors of infancy: when to worry, what to do. *Arch Dermatol.* 2000;136:905–914.
14. Tompkins VN, Walsh TS Jr. Some observations on the strawberry nevus of infancy. *Cancer.* 1956;9:869–904.
15. Walsh TS Jr, Tompkins VN. Some observations on the strawberry nevus of infancy. *Cancer.* 1959;9:869–904.
16. Shallow T, Eger S, Wagner F. Primary hemangiomatous tumours of skeletal muscle. *Ann Surg.* 1944;119:700–704.
17. Cohen JM, Weinreb JC, Redman HC. Arteriovenous malformations of the extremities: MR imaging. *Radiology.* 1986;158:475–479.
18. Mulliken JB, Glowacki J. Hemangiomas and vascular malformations in infants and children: a classification based on endothelial characteristics. *Plast Reconstr Surg.* 1982;69:412–422.
19. Weiss SW, Enzinger FM. Spindle cell hemangioendothelioma. A low-grade angiosarcoma resembling a cavernous hemangioma and Kaposi's sarcoma. *Am J Surg Pathol.* 1986;10:521–530.
20. Steinbach LS, Ominsky SH, Shpall S, et al. MR imaging of spindle cell hemangioendothelioma. *J Comput Assist Tomogr.* 1991;15:155–157.
21. Levine E, Wetzel LH, Neff JR. MR imaging and CT of extrahepatic cavernous hemangiomas. *AJR Am J Roentgenol.* 1986;147:1299–1304.
22. Ly JQ, Sanders TG, Mulloy JP, et al. Osseous change adjacent to soft-tissue hemangiomas of the extremities: correlation with lesion size and proximity to bone. *AJR Am J Roentgenol.* 2003;180:1695–1700.
23. Hill JH, Mafee MF, Chow JM, et al. Dynamic computerized tomography in the assessment of hemangioma. *Am J Otolaryngol.* 1985;6:23–28.
24. Rauch RF, Silverman PM, Korobkin M, et al. Computed tomography of benign angiomatous lesions of the extremities. *J Comput Assist Tomogr.* 1984;8:1143–1146.
25. Ly JQ, Sanders TG. Case 65: hemangioma of the chest wall. *Radiology.* 2003;229:726–729.
26. Olsen KI, Stacy GS, Montag A. Soft-tissue cavernous hemangioma. *Radiographics.* 2004;24:849–854.
27. Derchi LE, Balconi G, De Flaviis L, et al. Sonographic appearances of hemangiomas of skeletal muscle. *J Ultrasound Med.* 1989;8:263–267.
28. Greenspan A, McGahan JP, Vogelsang P, et al. Imaging strategies in the evaluation of soft-tissue hemangiomas of the extremities: correlation of the findings of plain radiography, angiography, CT, MRI, and ultrasonography in 12 histologically proven cases. *Skeletal Radiol.* 1992;21:11–18.
29. Hawnaur JM, Whitehouse RW, Jenkins JP, et al. Musculoskeletal haemangiomas: comparison of MRI with CT. *Skeletal Radiol.* 1990;19:251–258.
30. Dubois J, Garel L, David M, et al. Vascular soft-tissue tumors in infancy: distinguishing features on Doppler sonography. *AJR Am J Roentgenol.* 2002;178:1541–1545.
31. Dubois J, Soulez G, Oliva VL, et al. Soft-tissue venous malformations in adult patients: imaging and therapeutic issues. *Radiographics.* 2001;21:1519–1531.
32. Berquist TH, Ehman RL, King BF, et al. Value of MR imaging in differentiating benign from malignant soft-tissue masses: study of 95 lesions. *AJR Am J Roentgenol.* 1990;155:1251–1255.
33. Buetow PC, Kransdorf MJ, Moser RP Jr, et al. Radiologic appearance of intramuscular hemangioma with emphasis on MR imaging. *AJR Am J Roentgenol.* 1990;154:563–567.
34. Cohen EK, Kressel HY, Perosio T, et al. MR imaging of soft-tissue hemangiomas: correlation with pathologic findings. *AJR Am J Roentgenol.* 1988;150:1079–1081.
35. Crim JR, Seeger LL, Yao L, et al. Diagnosis of soft-tissue masses with MR imaging: can benign masses be differentiated from malignant ones? *Radiology.* 1992;185:581–586.
36. Kaplan PA, Williams SM. Mucocutaneous and peripheral soft-tissue hemangiomas: MR imaging. *Radiology.* 1987;163:163–166.
37. Kransdorf MJ, Jelinek JS, Moser RP Jr, et al. Soft-tissue masses: diagnosis using MR imaging. *AJR Am J Roentgenol.* 1989;153:541–547.
38. Teo ELHT, Strause PJ, Hernandez RJ. MR imaging differentiation of soft-tissue hemangiomas from malignant soft-tissue masses. *AJR.* 2000;174:1623–1628.
39. Murphey MD, Fairbairn KJ, Parman LM, et al. From the archives of the AFIP. Musculoskeletal angiomatous lesions: radiologic-pathologic correlation. *Radiographics.* 1995;15:893–917.
40. Nelson MC, Stull MA, Teitelbaum GP, et al. Magnetic resonance imaging of peripheral soft tissue hemangiomas. *Skeletal Radiol.* 1990;19:477–482.
41. Rak KM, Yakes WF, Ray RL, et al. MR imaging of symptomatic peripheral vascular malformations. *AJR Am J Roentgenol.* 1992;159:107–112.
42. Yuh WT, Kathol MH, Sein MA, et al. Hemangiomas of skeletal muscle: MR findings in five patients. *AJR Am J Roentgenol.* 1987;149:765–768.
43. Bui-Mansfield LT, Myers CP, Fellows D, et al. Bilateral temporal fossa hemangiomas. *AJR Am J Roentgenol.* 2002;179:790.
44. Tsai JC, Dalinka MK, Fallon MD, et al. Fluid-fluid level: a nonspecific finding in tumors of bone and soft tissue. *Radiology.* 1990;175:779–782.
45. Levin DC, Gordon DH, McSweeney J. Arteriography of peripheral hemangiomas. *Radiology.* 1976;121:625–630.
46. Troughton AH, Paxton RM. Direct puncture venography in subcutaneous cavernous hemangiomas. *Clin Radiol.* 1992;45:250–253.
47. Makhija M, Bofill ER. Hemangioma, a rare cause of photopenic lesion on skeletal imaging. *Clin Nucl Med.* 1988;13:661–662.
48. Oshima M, Muramoto H, Sakuma S. Detection of soft tissue hemangioma of the leg by Tc-99m DTPA-HSA blood pool imaging. *Clin Nucl Med.* 1993;18:454.
49. Tupler RH, Turbiner EH. Tc-99m labeled RBC scan in Maffucci's syndrome. *Clin Nucl Med.* 1991;16:872–873.
50. Resnick D, Oliphant M. Hemophilia-like arthropathy of the knee associated with cutaneous and synovial hemangiomas. Report of 3 cases and review of the literature. *Radiology.* 1975;114:323–326.
51. Greenspan A, Azouz EM, Matthews J II, et al. Synovial hemangioma: imaging features in eight histologically proven cases, review of the literature, and differential diagnosis. *Skeletal Radiol.* 1995;24:583–590.
52. Devaney K, Vinh TN, Sweet DE. Synovial hemangioma: a report of 20 cases with differential diagnostic considerations. *Hum Pathol.* 1993;24:737–745.

53. Llauger J, Monill JM, Palmer J, et al. Synovial hemangioma of the knee: MRI findings in two cases. *Skeletal Radiol.* 1995;24: 579–581.

54. Chen H, Thompson LD, Aguilera NS, et al. Kimura disease: a clinicopathologic study of 21 cases. *Am J Surg Pathol.* 2004;28: 505–513.

55. Persaud R, Upile T, Tudge S, et al. Radiology quiz case 2: Kimura disease. *Arch Otolaryngol Head Neck Surg.* 2004;130:1237–1238.

56. Som PM, Biller HF. Kimura disease involving parotid gland and cervical nodes: CT and MR findings. *J Comput Assist Tomogr.* 1992;16:320–322.

57. Ahuja A, Ying M, Mok JS, et al. Gray scale and power Doppler sonography in cases of Kimura disease. *AJNR Am J Neuroradiol.* 2001;22:513–517.

58. Smith ME, Fisher C, Weiss SW. Pleomorphic hyalinizing angiectatic tumor of soft parts. A low-grade neoplasm resembling neurilemoma. *Am J Surg Pathol.* 1996;20:21–29.

59. Temple HT, Fanburg-Smith J, et al. Unusual soft tissue mass in a 43-year-old man. *Clin Orthop Relat Res.* 1998;249–252;255–246.

60. Folpe AL, Weiss SW. Pleomorphic hyalinizing angiectatic tumor: analysis of 41 cases supporting evolution from a distinctive precursor lesion. *Am J Surg Pathol.* 2004;28:1417–1425.

61. Choi YW, Chang MS, Lee JS, et al. Intravascular papillary endothelial hyperplasia of the chest wall. *AJR Am J Roentgenol.* 1994;163:475–476.

62. Clifford PD, Temple HT, Jorda M, et al. Intravascular papillary endothelial hyperplasia (Masson's tumor) presenting as a triceps mass. *Skeletal Radiol.* 2004;33:421–425.

63. Conrad SE, Jacobs D, Gee J, et al. Pseudoneoplastic infection of bone in acquired immunodeficiency syndrome. A case report involving the cat-scratch disease bacillus. *J Bone Joint Surg Am.* 1991;73:774–777.

64. Herts BR, Rafii M, Spiegel G. Soft-tissue and osseous lesions caused by bacillary angiomatosis: unusual manifestations of cat-scratch fever in patients with AIDS. *AJR Am J Roentgenol.* 1991;157:1249–1251.

65. Koehler JE, Quinn FD, Berger TG, et al. Isolation of *Rochalimaea* species from cutaneous and osseous lesions of bacillary angiomatosis. *N Engl J Med.* 1992;327:1625–1631.

66. Baron AL, Steinbach LS, LeBoit PE, et al. Osteolytic lesions and bacillary angiomatosis in HIV infection: radiologic differentiation from AIDS-related Kaposi sarcoma. *Radiology.* 1990; 177:77–81.

67. Weiss S, Goldblum J. Tumors of lymph vessels. In: *Enzinger and Weiss's Soft Tissue Tumors.* 4th ed. St. Louis: Mosby; 2001:955–983.

68. Bill AH Jr, Sumner DS. A unified concept of lymphangioma and cystic hygroma. *Surg Gynecol Obstet.* 1965;120:79–86.

69. Zadvinskis DP, Benson MT, Kerr HH, et al. Congenital malformations of the cervicothoracic lymphatic system: embryology and pathogenesis. *Radiographics.* 1992;12:1175–1189.

70. Kittredge RD, Finby N. The many facets of lymphangioma. *Am J Roentgenol Radium Ther Nucl Med.* 1965;95:56–66.

71. Castellino RA, Finkelstein S. Lymphographic demonstration of a retroperitoneal lymphangioma. *Radiology.* 1975;115:355–356.

72. Leonidas JC, Brill PW, Bhan I, et al. Cystic retroperitoneal lymphangioma in infants and children. *Radiology.* 1978;127:203–208.

73. Munechika H, Honda M, Kushihashi T, et al. Computed tomography of retroperitoneal cystic lymphangiomas. *J Comput Assist Tomogr.* 1987;11:116–119.

74. Pilla TJ, Wolverson MK, Sundaram M, et al. CT evaluation of cystic lymphangiomas of the mediastinum. *Radiology.* 1982;144:841–842.

75. Radin R, Weiner S, Koenigsberg M, et al. Retroperitoneal cystic lymphangioma. *AJR Am J Roentgenol.* 1983;140:733–734.

76. Sheth S, Nussbaum AR, Hutchins GM, et al. Cystic hygromas in children: sonographic-pathologic correlation. *Radiology.* 1987; 162:821–824.

77. Shin MS, Berland LL, Ho KJ. Mediastinal cystic hygromas: CT characteristics and pathogenetic consideration. *J Comput Assist Tomogr.* 1985;9:297–301.

78. Siegel MJ, Glazer HS, St. Amour TE, et al. Lymphangiomas in children: MR imaging. *Radiology.* 1989;170:467–470.

79. Singh S, Baboo ML, Pathak IC. Cystic lymphangioma in children: report of 32 cases including lesions at rare sites. *Surgery.* 1971;69:947–951.

80. Hancock BJ, St-Vil D, Luks FI, et al. Complications of lymphangiomas in children. *J Pediatr Surg.* 1992;27:220–224; discussion 224–226.

81. Buonomo C, Griscom NT. Pediatric case of the day. Cystic lymphangioma (omental cyst). *Radiographics.* 1991;11:1146–1148.

82. Law PJ, Hall CM. Clavicular overgrowth in association with cystic hygroma. *Skeletal Radiol.* 1991;20:597–599.

83. Caro PA, Mahboubi S, Faerber EN. Computed tomography in the diagnosis of lymphangiomas in infants and children. *Clin Imaging.* 1991;15:41–46.

84. Paley D, Evans DC. Angiomatous involvement of an extremity. A spectrum of syndromes. *Clin Orthop.* 1986:215–218.

85. Cutillo DP, Swayne LC, Cucco J, et al. CT and MR imaging in cystic abdominal lymphangiomatosis. *J Comput Assist Tomogr.* 1989;13:534–536.

86. Resnick D, Kyriakos M, Greenway GD. Tumors and tumor-like lesions of bone: imaging and pathology of specific lesions. In: *Diagnosis of Bone and Joint Disorders.* 4th ed. Philadelphia: WB Saunders; 2002:3979–4010.

87. Castillo M, Dominguez R. Congenital lymphangiectatic elephantiasis. *Magn Reson Imaging.* 1992;10:321–324.

88. Zwenneke Flach H, Ginai AZ, Wolter Oosterhuis J. Best cases from the AFIP. Maffucci syndrome: radiologic and pathologic findings. Armed Forces Institutes of Pathology. *Radiographics.* 2001;21:1311–1316.

89. Maffucci A. Di un caso di enchondroma ed angioma multiplo: contribuzione ell eenesi embrionale de: tumor. *Monimento Medico-Chirurgico.* 1881;3:399–412.

90. Schwartz HS, Zimmerman NB, Simon MA, et al. The malignant potential of enchondromatosis. *J Bone Joint Surg Am.* 1987;69: 269–274.

91. Unger EC, Kessler HB, Kowalyshyn MJ, et al. MR imaging of Maffucci syndrome. *AJR Am J Roentgenol.* 1988;150:351–353.

92. Banna M, Parwani GS. Multiple sarcomas in Maffucci's syndrome. *Br J Radiol.* 1969;42:304–307.

93. Abdullah DC, Hallisey MJ, Muraki AS, et al. Diffuse calvarial hemangiomatosis associated with hereditary hemorrhagic telangiectasia. *AJNR Am J Neuroradiol.* 1989;10:S59.

94. Calvo-Alen J, Loza E, Alonso JL, et al. Pseudohaemarthrosis: a new manifestation of Osler-Rendu-Weber disease. *Ann Rheum Dis.* 1992;51:1021.

95. Czerniak P, Schorr S. Hereditary hemorrhagic telangiectasis with involvement of bone. *Am J Roentgenol Radium Ther Nucl Med.* 1955;74:299–303.

96. Gloviczki P, Stanson AW, Stickler GB, et al. Klippel-Trenaunay syndrome: the risks and benefits of vascular interventions. *Surgery.* 1991;110:469–479.

97. Klippel M, Trenaunay P. Du naevus variquex osteohypertrophique. *Arch Gen Med (Paris).* 1900;3:641–672.

98. Phillips GN, Gordon DH, Martin EC, et al. The Klippel-Trenaunay syndrome: clinical and radiological aspects. *Radiology.* 1978;128:429–434.

99. James CA, Allison JW, Waner M. Pediatric case of the day. Klippel-Trenaunay syndrome. *Radiographics.* 1999;19:1093–1096.

100. McGrory BJ, Amadio PC, Dobyns JH, et al. Anomalies of the fingers and toes associated with Klippel-Trenaunay syndrome. *J Bone Joint Surg Am.* 1991;73:1537–1546.

101. Lindenauer SM. The Klippel-Trenaunay syndrome: varicosity, hypertrophy and hemangioma with no arteriovenous fistula. *Ann Surg.* 1965;162:303–314.

102. Kasaback H, Merritt K. Capillary hemangioma with extensive purpura. Report of a case. *Am J Dis Child.* 1940;59:1063–1070.

103. Lee JH Jr, Kirk RF. Pregnancy associated with giant hemangiomata, thrombocytopenia, and fibrinogenopenia (Kasabach-Merritt syndrome). Report of a case. *Obstet Gynecol.* 1967;29:24–29.

104. Milikow E, Asch T. Hemangiomatosis, localized growth disturbance, and intravascular coagulation disorder presenting with an unusual arthritis resembling hemophilia. *Radiology.* 1970;97:387–388.

105. Rodriguez-Erdmann F, Button L, Murray JE, et al. Kasabach-Merritt syndrome: coagulo-analytical observations. *Am J Med Sci.* 1971;261:9–15.

106. Renton P, Shaw D. Hypophosphatemic-osteomalacia secondary to vascular tumors of bone and soft tissue. *Skeletal Radiol.* 1976;1:21–24.

107. Ogose A, Hotta T, Emura I, et al. Recurrent malignant variant of phosphaturic mesenchymal tumor with oncogenic osteomalacia. *Skeletal Radiol.* 2001;30:99–103.

108. Sundaram M, McCarthy EF. Oncogenic osteomalacia. *Skeletal Radiol.* 2000;29:117–124.

109. Weidner N. Review and update: oncogenic osteomalacia-rickets. *Ultrastruct Pathol.* 1991;15:317–333.

110. Avila NA, Skarulis M, Rubino DM, et al. Oncogenic osteomalacia: lesion detection by MR skeletal survey. *AJR Am J Roentgenol.* 1996;167:343–345.

111. Ohashi K, Ohnishi T, Ishikawa T, et al. Oncogenic osteomalacia presenting as bilateral stress fractures of the tibia. *Skeletal Radiol.* 1999;28:46–48.

112. Weiss S, Goldblum J. Perivascular tumors. In: *Enzinger and Weiss's Soft Tissue Tumors.* 4th ed. St. Louis: Mosby; 2001:985–1035.

113. Dalrymple NC, Hayes J, Bessinger VJ, et al. MRI of multiple glomus tumors of the finger. *Skeletal Radiol.* 1997;26:664–666.

114. Hermann G, Klein MJ, Springfield D, et al. Glomus tumor of the thigh: confluent with the periosteum of the femur. *Skeletal Radiol.* 2005;34:116–120.

115. Park EA, Hong SH, Choi JY, et al. Glomangiomatosis: magnetic resonance imaging findings in three cases. *Skeletal Radiol.* 2005;34:108–111.

116. Theumann NH, Goettmann S, Le Viet D, et al. Recurrent glomus tumors of fingertips: MR imaging evaluation. *Radiology.* 2002;223:143–151.

117. Axmann C, Feiden W, Moeller V, et al. Paravertebral glomus tumors. *Skeletal Radiol.* 2005;34:112–115.

118. Drape JL, Idy-Peretti I, Goettmann S, et al. Subungual glomus tumors: evaluation with MR imaging. *Radiology.* 1995;195:507–515.

119. Mathis W, Schulz M. Roentgen diagnosis of glomus tumors. *Radiology.* 1948;51:71–76.

120. Fornage BD. Glomus tumors in the fingers: diagnosis with US. *Radiology.* 1988;167:183–185.

121. Kneeland JB, Middleton WD, Matloub HS, et al. High resolution MR imaging of glomus tumor. *J Comput Assist Tomogr.* 1987;11:351–352.

122. Matloub HS, Muoneke VN, et al. Glomus tumor imaging: use of MRI for localization of occult lesions. *J Hand Surg [Am].* 1992;17:472–475.

123. Weiss SW, Enzinger FM. Epithelioid hemangioendothelioma: a vascular tumor often mistaken for a carcinoma. *Cancer.* 1982;50:970–981.

124. Weiss SW, Ishak KG, Dail DH, et al. Epithelioid hemangioendothelioma and related lesions. *Semin Diagn Pathol.* 1986;3:259–287.

125. Weiss S, Goldblum J. Hemangioendothelioma: vascular tumors of intermediate malignancy. In: *Enzinger and Weiss's Soft Tissue Tumors.* 4th ed. St. Louis: Mosby; 2001:891–915.

126. Kransdorf MJ. Malignant soft-tissue tumors in a large referral population: distribution of diagnoses by age, sex, and location. *AJR Am J Roentgenol.* 1995;164:129–134.

127. Enzinger FM, Smith BH. Hemangiopericytoma. An analysis of 106 cases. *Hum Pathol.* 1976;7:61–82.

128. Alpern MB, Thorsen MK, Kellman GM, et al. CT appearance of hemangiopericytoma. *J Comput Assist Tomogr.* 1986;10:264–267.

129. Goldman SM, Davidson AJ, Neal J. Retroperitoneal and pelvic hemangiopericytomas: clinical, radiologic, and pathologic correlation. *Radiology.* 1988;168:13–17.

130. Lorigan JG, David CL, Evans HL, et al. The clinical and radiologic manifestations of hemangiopericytoma. *AJR Am J Roentgenol.* 1989;153:345–349.

131. Yaghmai I. Angiographic manifestations of soft-tissue and osseous hemangiopericytomas. *Radiology.* 1978;126:653–659.

132. Weiss S, Goldblum J. Malignant vascular tumors. In: *Enzinger and Weiss's Soft Tissue Tumors.* 4th ed. St. Louis: Mosby; 2001:917–954.

133. Coldwell DM, Baron RL, Charnsangavej C. Angiosarcoma. Diagnosis and clinical course. *Acta Radiol.* 1989;30:627–631.

134. Nakazono T, Kudo S, Matsuo Y, et al. Angiosarcoma associated with chronic lymphedema (Stewart-Treves syndrome) of the leg: MR imaging. *Skeletal Radiol.* 2000;29:413–416.

135. Doppman JL, Pevsner P. Embolization of arteriovenous malformations by direct percutaneous puncture. *AJR Am J Roentgenol.* 1983;140:773–778.

136. Gomes AS. Embolization therapy of congenital arteriovenous malformations: use of alternate approaches. *Radiology.* 1994;190:191–198.

137. Molitch HI, Unger EC, Witte CL, et al. Percutaneous sclerotherapy of lymphangiomas. *Radiology.* 1995;194:343–347.

138. Yakes WF, Haas DK, Parker SH, et al. Symptomatic vascular malformations: ethanol embolotherapy. *Radiology.* 1989;170:1059–1066.

139. Hayashi N, Masumoto T, Okubo T, et al. Hemangiomas in the face and extremities: MR-guided sclerotherapy—optimization with monitoring of signal intensity changes in vivo. *Radiology.* 2003;226:567–572.

140. Goyal M, Causer PA, Armstrong D. Venous vascular malformations in pediatric patients: comparison of results of alcohol sclerotherapy with proposed MR imaging classification. *Radiology.* 2002;223:639–644.

141. Mason KP, Neufeld EJ, Karian VE, et al. Coagulation abnormalities in pediatric and adult patients after sclerotherapy or embolization of vascular anomalies. *AJR Am J Roentgenol.* 2001;177:1359–1363.

142. Dutton SC, Plowman PN. Paediatric haemangiomas: the role of radiotherapy. *Br J Radiol.* 1991;64:261–269.

143. Schild SE, Buskirk SJ, Frick LM, et al. Radiotherapy for large symptomatic hemangiomas. *Int J Radiat Oncol Biol Phys.* 1991;21:729–735.

144. Rao VK, Weiss SW. Angiomatosis of soft tissue. An analysis of the histologic features and clinical outcome in 51 cases. *Am J Surg Pathol.* 1992;16:764–771.

Benign Fibrous and Fibrohistiocytic Tumors

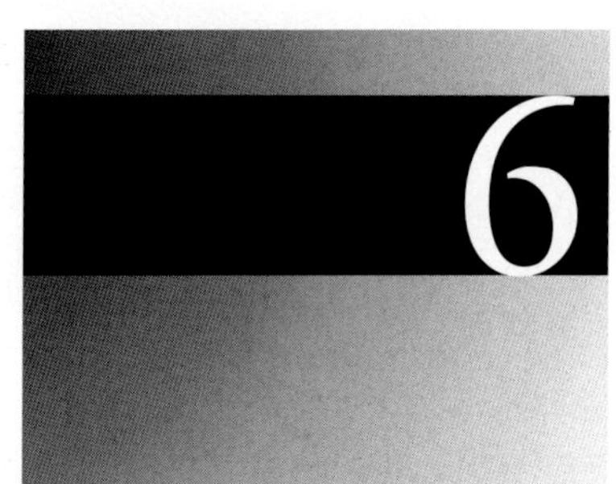

Since the previous edition of this book, there has been significant reorganization of the nomenclature of the fibrous and fibrohistiocytic tumors by the World Health Organization (WHO) Classification of Soft Tissue Tumors, obscuring the histologic lineage of these lesions. We have therefore chosen to divide these lesions into benign and malignant, with chapters reviewing each of these groups. Benign fibrous and fibrohistiocytic tumors of soft tissue are among the most commonly encountered in clinical practice and are seen in all age groups. On the basis of clinical presentation, natural history, and patient age at presentation, fibrous tumors are usually subdivided into several distinct groups: (1) benign fibroblastic proliferations (nodular fasciitis, other types of fasciitis, fibroma of tendon sheath, other types of superficial fibromas, elastofibroma, keloid, desmoplastic fibroblastoma, and mammary-type fibroblastoma); (2) fibroblastic proliferations of infancy and childhood (myofibroma/myofibromatosis, juvenile hyaline fibromatosis, fibromatosis colli, infantile fibromatosis, lipofibromatosis, calcifying aponeurotica fibroma, inclusion body fibromatosis, and fibrous hamartoma of infancy); (3) the fibromatoses (palmar, plantar, and deep); (4) and rare fibroblastic tumors (calcifying fibrous tumor and exuberant cervical fibrosclerosis). Benign fibrohistiocytic lesions include benign fibrous histiocytoma, xanthoma, xanthogranuloma, extranodal Rosai-Dorfman disease, and foreign body reaction.

BENIGN FIBROBLASTIC PROLIFERATIONS

The benign fibroblastic proliferations are a heterogeneous group of lesions that are primarily reactive rather than neoplastic (1). Enzinger et al. (1) note that many of these lesions grow rapidly and may be mistaken clinically and microscopically for a sarcoma, whereas others grow slowly and insidiously. Interestingly, despite these lesions' aggres-

sive clinical and histologic features, local recurrence is rare even after incomplete resection. Lesions discussed in this section include nodular fasciitis and other types of fasciitis (intravascular, ossifying, cranial, and ischemic) and proliferative myositis.

Nodular Fasciitis

KEY CONCEPTS
- Nodular fasciitis is the most benign common tumor or tumor-like lesion of fibrous tissue.
- It affects young adults (20 to 40 years of age).
- The upper extremity is involved in 46% of cases, particularly the volar aspect of the forearm.
- Lesions may grow rapidly, initially suggesting an aggressive tumor, as may the histology of this reactive lesion.
- Complete excision usually curative.
- Lesions are typically subcutaneous, attached to superficial fascia, although deeper locations may be affected.
- MR imaging shows nonspecific low-to-intermediate signal intensity on T1-weighting and intermediate-to-high signal on T2-weighting, with enhancement following intravenous contrast.
- Linear extension along the fascia (fascial tail sign) helps suggest the diagnosis; mild surrounding edema may be seen on MR imaging.

Nodular fasciitis is a benign soft tissue lesion, of unknown cause, composed of proliferating fibroblasts. The lesion, first described in 1955 by Konwaler et al. (2) as *subcutaneous pseudosarcomatous fibromatosis (fasciitis)*, represents a common pseudosarcomatous fibroblastic proliferation that is presumably reactive in nature. Nodular fasciitis is the most frequent tumor or tumorlike lesion of fibrous tissue (3–6). It is also likely the most common reactive lesion misdiagnosed as a sarcoma, reflecting the rapid growth and mitotic activity of this tumor (3–6).

Nodular fasciitis occurs primarily in young adults (20–40 years of age) without a sex predilection (3–6). The upper extremities (46% of cases, particularly the volar aspect of the forearm) are affected most frequently, followed by the lower extremities (16%), head/neck (20% and the most frequent site in children), and trunk (18%) (7,8). However, no age or location is exempt from this lesion, with approximately 14% of cases occurring in patients younger than 10 years of age or older than 60 years of age (2,9–11). This lesion is characterized clinically by a rapid growth phase (first 1–2 weeks) that may arouse suspicion of a sarcoma (12,13). Although not typically associated with a documented traumatic event, nodular fasciitis is believed by many to be initiated by a local injury or reaction to a localized inflammation process. Mild pain or tenderness may be present in approximately 50% of cases (3). Nodular fasciitis occurs in three forms: subcutaneous, fascial and intramuscular (14). The subcutaneous form is most common, followed by the fascial form, with the intramuscular form least common. The subcutaneous form occurs three to ten times more commonly than the other subtypes and typically presents as a subcutaneous nodule (14). The intramuscular form is typically larger in size and therefore, as a result of its size and deep location, is clinically more likely to suggest a soft tissue malignancy. The fascial form is less well-circumscribed, similar to the intramuscular form, and may have a stellate appearance as a result of its growth pattern (1).

At gross pathologic examination nodular fasciitis may be fibrous, myxoid, and even cystic, depending on the predominant component of the extracellular matrix. Although most lesions are 3 to 4 cm in diameter, occasionally they may obtain a much greater size. Grossly, nodular fasciitis cannot be distinguished from a sarcoma. Microscopically, it consists of a cellular fibroblastic and myofibroblastic proliferation in which the cells are uniform and cytologically bland, while displaying a brisk mitotic rate (2,9,10,15). Typically the cells are slender and delicate, mimicking the appearance of fibroblasts in tissue culture and are arranged in whorls, short fascicles, or haphazardly. The amount and type of extracellular matrix associated with the lesion is variable and may reflect the age of the lesion (16). Early lesions may consist of solid proliferations of fibroblasts or be associated with a myxoid matrix rich in acid mucopolysaccharide. The latter may be sufficiently abundant to the extent that microcysts develop and eventually coalesce to form macrocysts. Although microscopic hemorrhage may be present, hemosiderin deposition is virtually never seen. There is a variable amount of collagen deposition, which ranges from delicate fibrils to coarse keloidlike strands of collagen. Occasionally there is heterotopic bone formation and calcification, and metaplastic ossification is also identified histologically. These lesions are often referred to as *ossifying fasciitis* or *fasciitis ossificans* (17). Electron microscopic as well as immunohistochemical studies confirm that this is a fibroblastic and myofibro-

blastic proliferation, similar to that found in granulation tissue (9–11,14,18).

Complete, local excision is usually curative; local recurrences are rare and treated by simple reexcision. Local recurrence rates vary from 0% to 13% with a 1% rate in the largest series of 895 patients by Allen (16). In fact, local recurrence is so rare that it should prompt reevaluation to confirm the diagnosis. Spontaneous regression is reported, and resection of incompletely excised lesions is probably unwarranted (19). We would suggest that biopsy confirmation of this diagnosis may allow observation, without need for resection, in some cases. Metastases do not occur. Response to intralesional steroid injection is also reported (20).

The radiologic description of nodular fasciitis is limited in the literature, with the largest report of 10 cases by Wang et al. (21–23). Radiographs are typically normal or demonstrate a nonspecific soft tissue mass. Calcification or ossification may rarely be seen (particularly in ossifying fasciitis).

On three-phase bone scan, there is no evidence of increased tracer accumulation in the lesion (except in ossifying fasciitis). Arteriography shows the lesion to be markedly hypovascular (17,24). Sonography reveals a nonspecific hypoechoic mass (25) (Figs. 6.1, 6.2, and 6.3).

On CT, lesions may be ill-defined or well-defined, with tissue attenuation similar to or mildly less than that of skeletal muscle (24) (Fig. 6.3). Intramuscular lesions are more often less well-defined as opposed to subcutaneous tumors that are more frequently well-defined, delineated by the surrounding fat (24,26). The relatively decreased CT tissue attenuation coefficients found in the intramuscular cases likely reflect the myxoid character of the lesions imaged. Soft tissue calcification and ossification are rarely observed (17).

On T1-weighted MR images, nodular fasciitis has a signal intensity similar to or slightly higher than that of skeletal muscle (22) (Figs. 6.1–6.4). On T2-weighted MR images, the lesions are frequently high signal intensity, greater than that of subcutaneous fat, although intermediate signal intensity may also be seen (23) (Figs. 6.1–6.4). Lesions are usually more homogeneous on short TR images and heterogeneous on T2-weighted sequences (24,27). Wang et al. reported enhancement following intravenous contrast in all eight patients, most commonly diffuse (63%) or peripheral (25%) (23). This prominent variation in signal intensity on MR imaging is likely related to the distribution and degree of myxoid and fibrous (collagen) components in the lesion and to the cellularity seen pathologically (28) (Figs. 6.2 and 6.4). Subcutaneous and myxoid lesions are usually more homogenous and higher signal intensity on long TR images, whereas deeper cellular and fibrotic lesions are more heterogeneous and intermediate signal on T2-weighting. We believe important findings on MR imaging suggesting this diagnosis are linear extensions either along the superficial fascia (fascial tail sign) in subcutaneous lesions or about the mass in more deeply

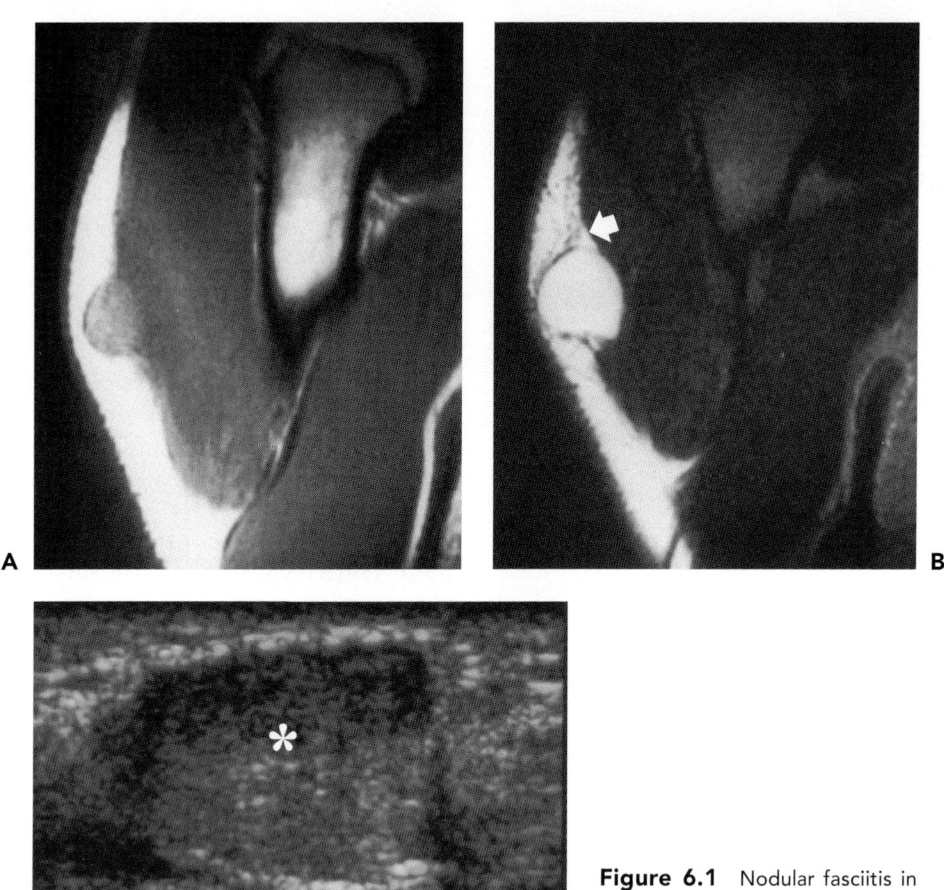

Figure 6.1 Nodular fasciitis in the upper arm of a man 16 years of age. **A,B:** Coronal T1-weighted (TR/TE; 600/20) **(A)** and T2-weighted (TR/TE; 2000/80) **(B)** spin-echo MR images of the shoulder show a well-defined mass superficial to the deltoid muscle with small linear fascial extension proximally (*arrow*). **C:** Ultrasound shows a well-defined hypoechoic mass (*white asterisk*).

located tumors (Figs. 6.1, 6.2, and 6.4). Mild surrounding edema may be seen about these lesions.

Other Types of Fasciitis

Intravascular Fasciitis

Intravascular fasciitis is a relatively rare variant of nodular fasciitis that involves arteries and veins of small-to-medium caliber (29). It primarily affects children and adolescents. The typical presentation is that of a slowly growing subcutaneous mass. The upper extremity is most frequently affected, followed by the trunk and lower extremity (3–6). There is no sex predilection (3–6). Similar to nodular fasciitis, intravascular fasciitis may be confused with a sarcoma because of its marked cellularity, decreased myxoid matrix, intravascular growth, and presence of multinucleated giant cells. The imaging characteristics of intravascular fasciitis have not been described, to the best of our knowledge (Fig. 6.5).

Ossifying Fasciitis

Ossifying fasciitis is a term applied to those cases of nodular fasciitis that contain metaplastic bone and involve the fascia or periosteum (periosteal fasciitis), the imaging of which was discussed earlier (see nodular fasciitis section).

Cranial Fasciitis

Cranial fasciitis is a unique clinicopathologic entity that occurs between birth and the first year of life (5,30,31). It typically is a rapidly enlarging, circumscribed mass that involves the soft tissues of the scalp (32–35). Cranial fasciitis may erode and penetrate the outer and inner tables of the skull, simulating an aggressive sarcomatous lesion (36). It is composed of fibroblasts and myofibroblasts in a myxoid matrix and bears a close pathologic similarity to nodular fasciitis (37). Frequently it is associated with birth trauma and it is believed to arise from the galea aponeurotica (38). Imaging of cranial fasciitis may reveal lytic

---

KEY CONCEPTS

- Other types of fasciitis include intravascular, ossifying, cranial, ischemic, and proliferative (also proliferative myositis).
- Intravascular fasciitis is a rare form of nodular fasciitis occurring in a small-to-medium-sized artery or vein.
- Ossifying fasciitis refers to nodular fasciitis that contains metaplastic bone.
- Cranial fasciitis occurs from birth to the first year of life and involves the scalp soft tissues, although it may penetrate to involve bone and the dura.
- Ischemia fasciitis represents a pseudosarcomatous fibroblastic proliferation over osseous protuberances, most commonly the greater trochanter.
- Proliferative fasciitis and myositis are pseudosarcomatous fibroblastic proliferations that involve either the subcutaneous septae and/or fascia overlying muscle. These masses are often ill-defined on CT or MR imaging, suggesting an inflammatory process.

---

destruction of the calvarium (39,40). CT and MR imaging may show a heterogeneous mass with subgaleal and bone involvement (41,42). There are nonspecific intrinsic features, with attenuation similar to that of muscle on CT scanning, and intermediate signal intensity on T1-weighted and intermediate-to-high signal intensity on T2-weighted MR images (Fig. 6.6). Invasion through the inner table of the calvarium may also be apparent. Similar to nodular fasciitis, treatment is surgical resection, and recurrence is unusual, even if incompletely excised initially.

Ischemic Fasciitis

Ischemic fasciitis is a pseudosarcomatous fibroblastic proliferation that usually occurs over osseous prominences subjected to intermittent pressure (3–6). *Atypical decubital fibroplasia* is a synonymous term for this process. This lesion typically affects elderly (eighth and ninth decades of life), debilitated or immobilized patients and reveals a female predilection (3–6). The most commonly affected sites are the shoulder and hip (over the greater tuberosities and trochanters), as well as the chest wall (3–6). Clinically, patients present with a painless mass of relatively short duration (less than 6 months).

At gross pathologic evaluation, ischemic fasciitis is an ill-defined multinodular mass, involving the subcutaneous tissue. Dermal involvement and ulceration may also be present. Histologically, there is a central zone of liquefaction and/or necrosis surrounded by a peripheral rim of vascular proliferation and fibroblasts. The process is likely related to intermittent ischemia with subsequent repair and tissue regeneration that may simulate a sarcomatous lesion pathologically.

Excision of ischemic fasciitis is usually curative. Local recurrence is rare. There is no malignant potential for this lesion.

The MR imaging of ischemic fasciitis was described by Ilaslan et al. (personal communication, article under review) (Fig. 6.7). There is poorly circumscribed replacement of the subcutaneous fat with intermediate signal intensity on T1-weighted images. On T2-weighted images, high signal intensity is seen, with peripheral edema suggesting an inflammatory process. Images after intravenous contrast frequently reveal a peripheral rind of enhancement. The nonenhancing central region represents the necrosis seen pathologically.

Proliferative Fasciitis and Proliferative Myositis

Proliferative fasciitis and proliferative myositis are pseudosarcomatous fibroblastic proliferations, that occur in the fibrous septa of the subcutaneous adipose tissue (43) and skeletal muscle fascia (44,45), respectively (46). Proliferative fasciitis was described by Chung and Enzinger in 1975 (43). Proliferative myositis was originally described by Kern in 1960 (45). Both lesions occur much less frequently than nodular fasciitis (3–6).

These lesions typically occur in adults, usually in the fifth to seventh decades of life, although rare cases in children are reported (47–50). Patients tend to be older than those affected by nodular fasciitis (3–6). There is no sex predilection. Similar to nodular fasciitis, these lesions are rapidly growing and may be slightly tender masses. A history of trauma may be elicited in approximately 30% of cases of proliferative fasciitis. Proliferative fasciitis occurs frequently in the upper extremity (particularly the forearm), followed by the lower extremity. The trunk and, rarely, the head and neck may also be affected. Proliferative myositis usually affects the muscles of the trunk and shoulder (particularly the pectoral, latissimus, and serratus anterior) and less commonly, the thigh and chest wall.

At gross pathologic examination, these are gray-white, firm, fibrous lesions with ill-defined margins that are attributable to growth along fascial planes. These lesions are usually less than 4 to 5 cm in size (3,5,6). The histologic hallmark of both proliferative fasciitis and myositis is the presence of large, plump, polygonal fibroblasts with abundant eosinophilic to basophilic cytoplasm and large nuclei with inclusionlike nucleoli. Their similarity to ganglion cells and rhabdomyoblasts may cause problems in diagnosis. The ganglionlike fibroblasts are interspersed in a fibromyxoid matrix, and they proliferate along the fascia. In skeletal muscle, these cells are distributed along the epimysium, perimysium, and endomysium and may cause atrophy of the adjacent musculature. Small areas of metaplastic bone or cartilage may be seen in up to 10% of cases of proliferative myositis (31,44,51). Again, both immunohistochemical and ultrastructural studies have confirmed that these are fibroblastic and myofibroblastic proliferations that also share some features of histiocytes (49,52,53).

Proliferative fasciitis and proliferative myositis are self-limited lesions with only rare recurrence following surgical excision. Similar to nodular fasciitis, local recurrence

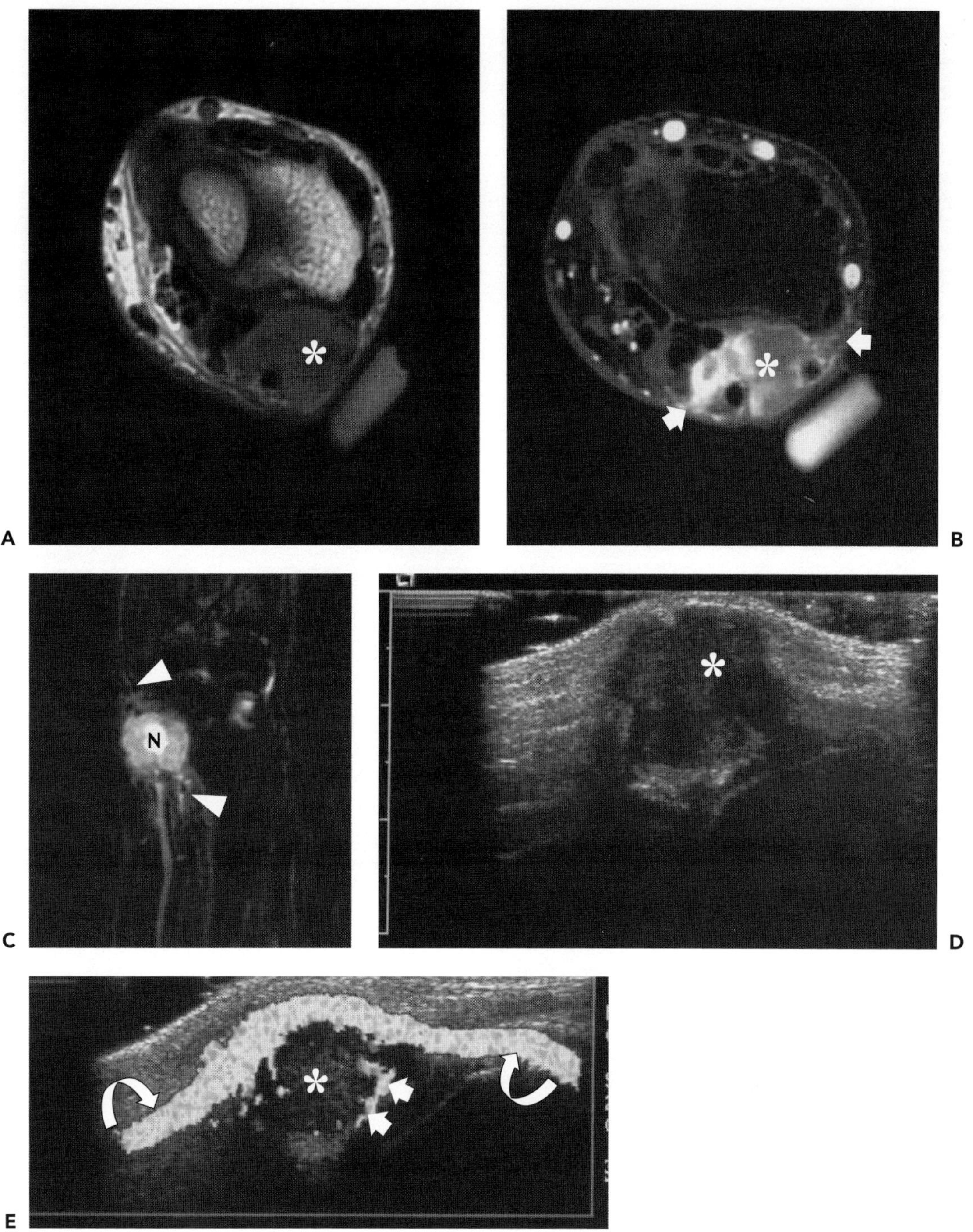

Figure 6.2 Nodular fasciitis involving the wrist of a woman 30 years of age. **A–C:** Axial T1-weighted before (TR/TE; 517/12) **(A)** and after (TR/TE; 600/12) **(B)** intravenous contrast and sagittal T2-weighted (TR/TE; 4000/103) **(C)** MR images of the wrist show a subcutaneous mass, with prolonged T1 and T2 relaxation times (*asterisk*). There is mild surrounding edema (*arrows*) and fascial extension (*arrowheads*). The postcontrast image **B** demonstrates enhancement which is more prominent peripherally, and there is high signal intensity necrosis (*N*) centrally on the T2-weighted image **C.** **D,E:** Sonogram shows the hypoechoic well-defined mass (*asterisk*) and Doppler study **(E)** reveals the radial artery draped over the mass (*curved arrows*) and several intrinsic vessels.

should raise the suspicion of a different diagnosis. These lesions do not metastasize.

There is scant literature characterizing the radiologic appearance of these unusual lesions, and great caution must be exercised not to overemphasize the findings from these individual case reports (54). Increased tracer accumulation on dynamic flow and blood-pool images of a three-phase bone scan was reported in one case, as was a vascular blush suggesting a capillary telangiectasia (48). Sonography shows a heterogeneous mass. Areas of posterior acoustic shadowing

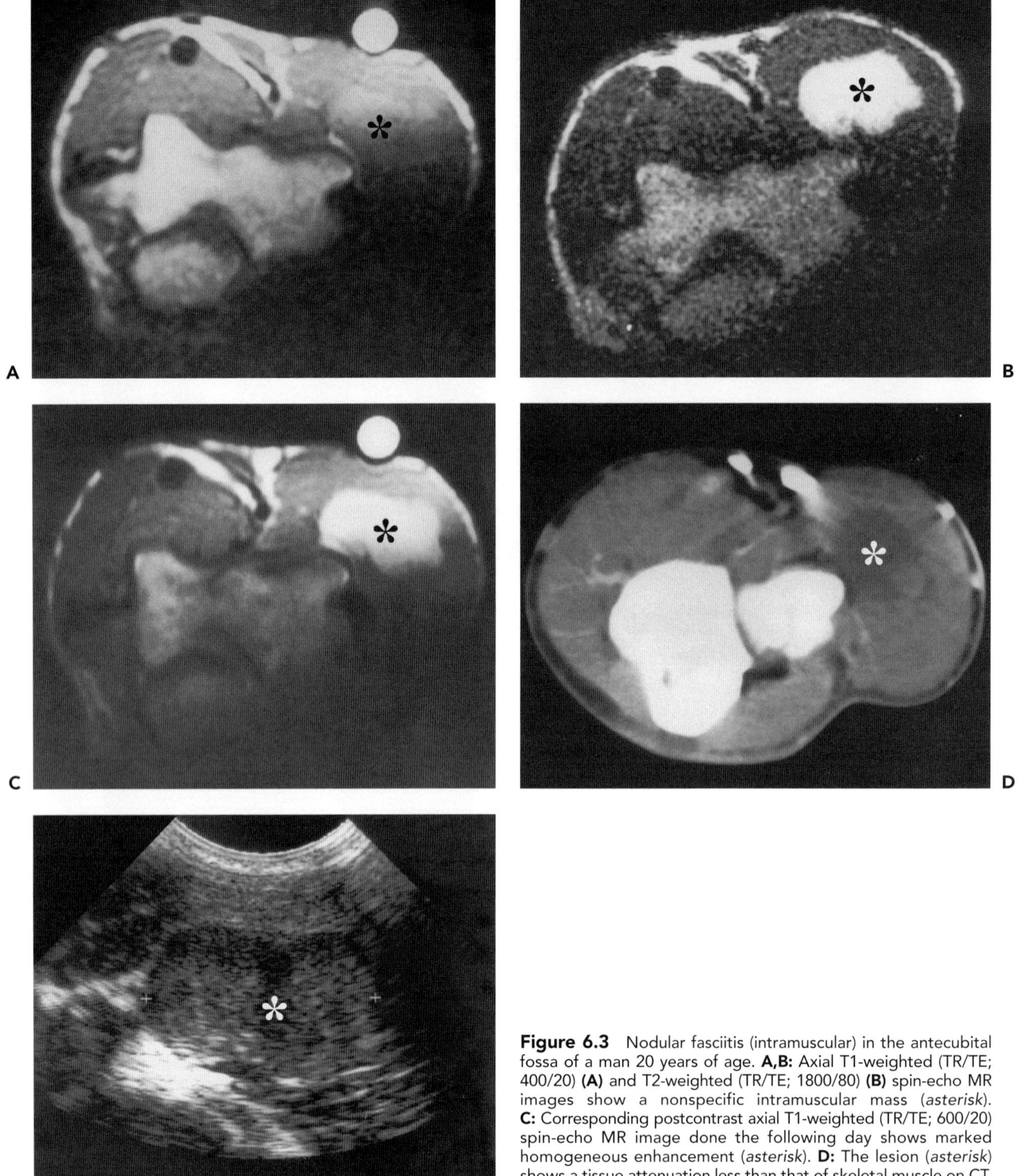

Figure 6.3 Nodular fasciitis (intramuscular) in the antecubital fossa of a man 20 years of age. **A,B:** Axial T1-weighted (TR/TE; 400/20) **(A)** and T2-weighted (TR/TE; 1800/80) **(B)** spin-echo MR images show a nonspecific intramuscular mass (*asterisk*). **C:** Corresponding postcontrast axial T1-weighted (TR/TE; 600/20) spin-echo MR image done the following day shows marked homogeneous enhancement (*asterisk*). **D:** The lesion (*asterisk*) shows a tissue attenuation less than that of skeletal muscle on CT. **E:** Ultrasound shows a well-defined hypoechoic mass (*asterisk*).

may be seen resulting from calcification. CT scanning results have been reported in less than 10 cases and usually reveals a poorly defined mass with attenuation similar to or less than that of muscle (54–56). CT contrast enhancement is variable (homogeneous, heterogeneous, or absent). The MR imaging appearance is typically low signal intensity on T1-weighting and high signal intensity on T2-weighting, with ill-defined margins, suggesting an inflammatory process (56). Enhancement is usually seen following intravenous contrast administration on MR imaging (56).

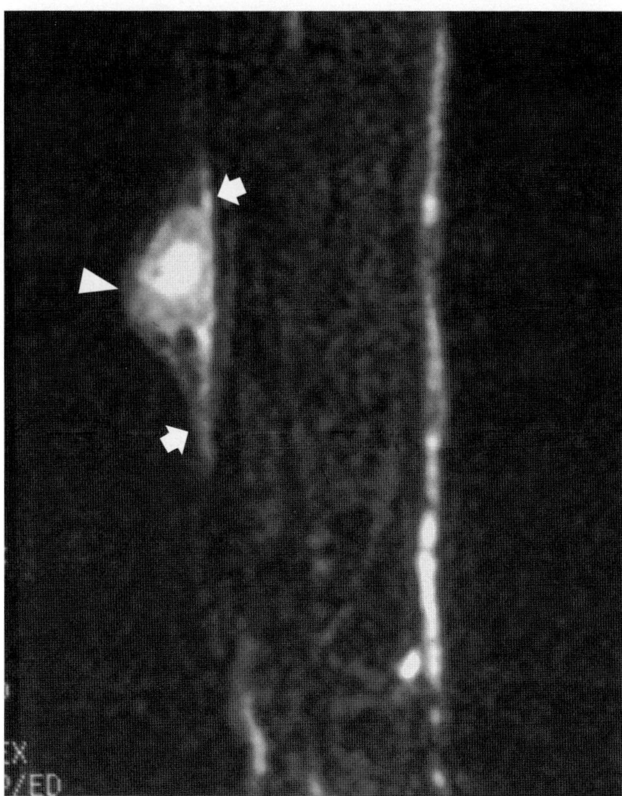

Figure 6.4 Nodular fasciitis of the forearm in a woman 35 years of age. Coronal short-tau inversion recovery (STIR) MR image shows a high signal intensity subcutaneous soft tissue mass (*arrowhead*) with linear extension along the superficial fascia (*arrows*) (fascial tail sign). Central high signal intensity represents necrosis.

Fibroma of Tendon Sheath

KEY CONCEPTS

- Fibroma of tendon sheath represents a benign fibroblastic proliferation that occurs in the distal extremities.
- Patients are most commonly affected in the third to fifth decade, with a male predominance.
- The hand/wrist accounts for 80% of cases.
- Surgical resection is the treatment of choice.
- On MR imaging, these lesions are low-to-intermediate signal intensity on T1-weighting and T2-weighting, intimately related to the tendon sheath, with variable enhancement following intravenous contrast.

Fibroma of tendon sheath is a benign fibroblastic proliferation that occurs in the distal extremities and may represent either a reactive or neoplastic process (57). The lesion was initially described by Geschickter and Copland (58); however, the first detailed description of the lesion was presented by Chung and Enzinger in 1979 (57,58).

Fibroma of tendon sheath affects adults in the third to fifth decades of life, although there is a wide age spectrum and it may occur in infants and the elderly (3–6). There is

a male predominance that ranges from 1.5:1 to 3:1 (57,59,60). The overwhelming majority of cases occur in the hand (particularly the thumb, index, and middle digits) and wrist (80% of cases) (57,59–61). The lesions may consequently simulate a giant cell tumor of tendon sheath clinically. The lower extremity (foot and ankle) is less commonly involved (3–6). The right side is affected more frequently than the left, adding credence to the theory that this lesion is a reactive process (3–6). Fibroma of tendon sheath grows slowly and patients typically present with a painless mass that is present for months to years. Rarely, lesions cause a mechanical block to tendon motion and mild pain is seen in less than 30% of patients (57,59,62). An association with trauma is seen in up to 10% of cases (3–6).

At gross pathologic evaluation, fibroma of tendon sheath is a very firm, whitish-gray nodular mass, that is intimately associated with and attached to the tendon sheath and averages 2 cm in size, but may be as large as 5 cm (57,59,60). Microscopically, it is composed of paucicellular, dense fibrous connective tissue with a lobular configuration. Occasionally, the periphery of the lesion has cellular areas resembling those of nodular fasciitis or fibrous histiocytoma and rarely, chondro-osseous metaplasia is observed. Ultrastructurally, this lesion is also shown to be composed of fibroblasts and myofibroblasts.

Some investigators have suggested that fibroma of tendon sheath and giant cell tumor of tendon sheath comprise a spectrum of histiocytic-fibroblastic-myofibroblastic lesions (63,64). Maluf et al. (63) noted that the lesions have an overlapping clinical presentation with similar patient age, gender, and lesion location. In addition, these lesions share similar growth patterns, showing a lobulated architecture. Although the microscopic appearance varies, both lesions contain spindle cells and multinucleated giant cells and share similar immunohistochemical attributes. Hence, the fibroma and giant cell tumor of tendon sheath may represent end points of a spectrum of cellular proliferation (63).

Initial and recurrent lesions are treated adequately by surgical excision (57,60). Local recurrence is seen in approximately 25% of cases, usually between 1 to 4 months following surgery (61). These lesions do not metastasize.

The superficial location of these lesions allows clinical assessment; therefore, extensive radiologic evaluation is rarely obtained. Radiographs are usually unremarkable or may demonstrate a nonspecific soft tissue mass (65). Bone involvement secondary to remodeling or extrinsic erosion is reported in the phalanges but is very uncommon and occurs in less than 2% of cases (57,66,67).

Fox et al. reported the MR imaging appearance in six cases of fibroma of tendon sheath (Fig. 6.8) (68). Lesions were similar (83%) or slightly greater (7%) in signal intensity compared to that of muscle on T1-weighting. On T2-weighting, lesions were low (50%) or intermediate (50%) in signal

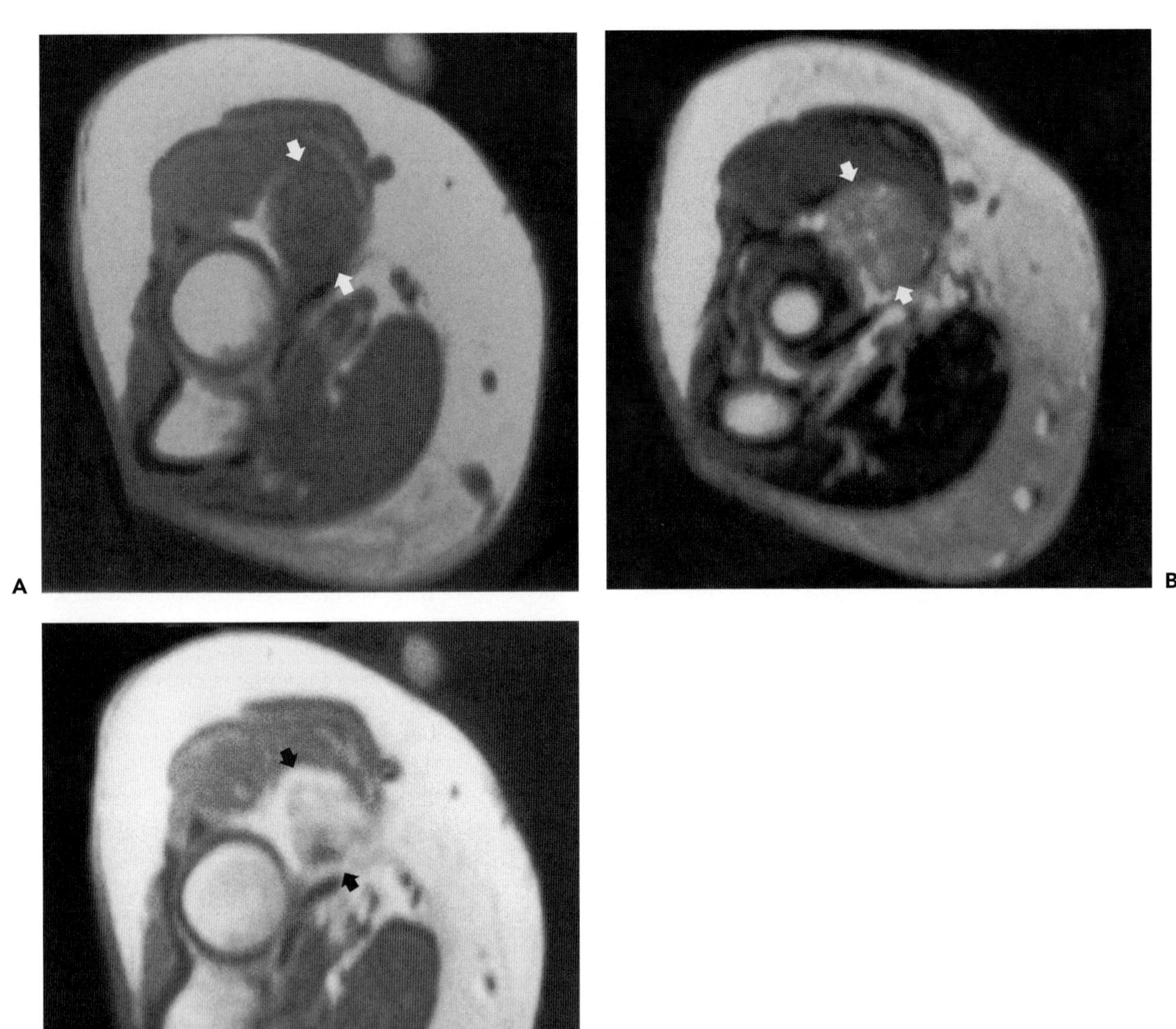

Figure 6.5 Intravascular fasciitis in the forearm of a woman 41 years of age. **A,B:** Axial T1-weighted (TR/TE; 450/15) **(A)** and fast spin-echo T2-weighted (TR/TE; 3000/95) **(B)** MR images show a nonspecific mass in the region of the antecubital fossa (*arrows*). **C:** Axial T1-weighted (TR/TE; 450/15) spin-echo MR image at the level of **A** following intravenous contrast administration reveals marked heterogeneous enhancement (*arrows*).

intensity. Most lesions (83%) were heterogeneous, which was more prominent on long TR images. Enhancement was seen in four of six cases after intravenous contrast.

Other Types of Superficial Fibromas

Multiple other types of superficial fibromas are described, including *pleomorphic fibroma of skin, sclerotic fibroma of skin, nuchal-type fibroma, cellular angiofibroma, giant cell angiofibroma,* and *Gardner fibroma* (Fig. 6.9) (3–6). These lesions are differentiated by their location, mild variations in histology, and associated condition (Table 6.1). The treatment of these benign

lesions is surgical resection with the majority having a low rate of recurrence.

Elastofibroma

Elastofibroma or *elastofibroma dorsi* is a slowly growing, fibroblastic pseudotumor that was originally described at the Twelfth Congress of Scandinavian Pathologists by Järvi and Saxén in 1959 and subsequently reported in 1961 (3–6,69,70). Elastofibroma has received relatively little attention in the radiologic literature and is considered to be a rare lesion. However, it is not uncommon and was found in 24% of women and 11% of men in one autopsy series of patients

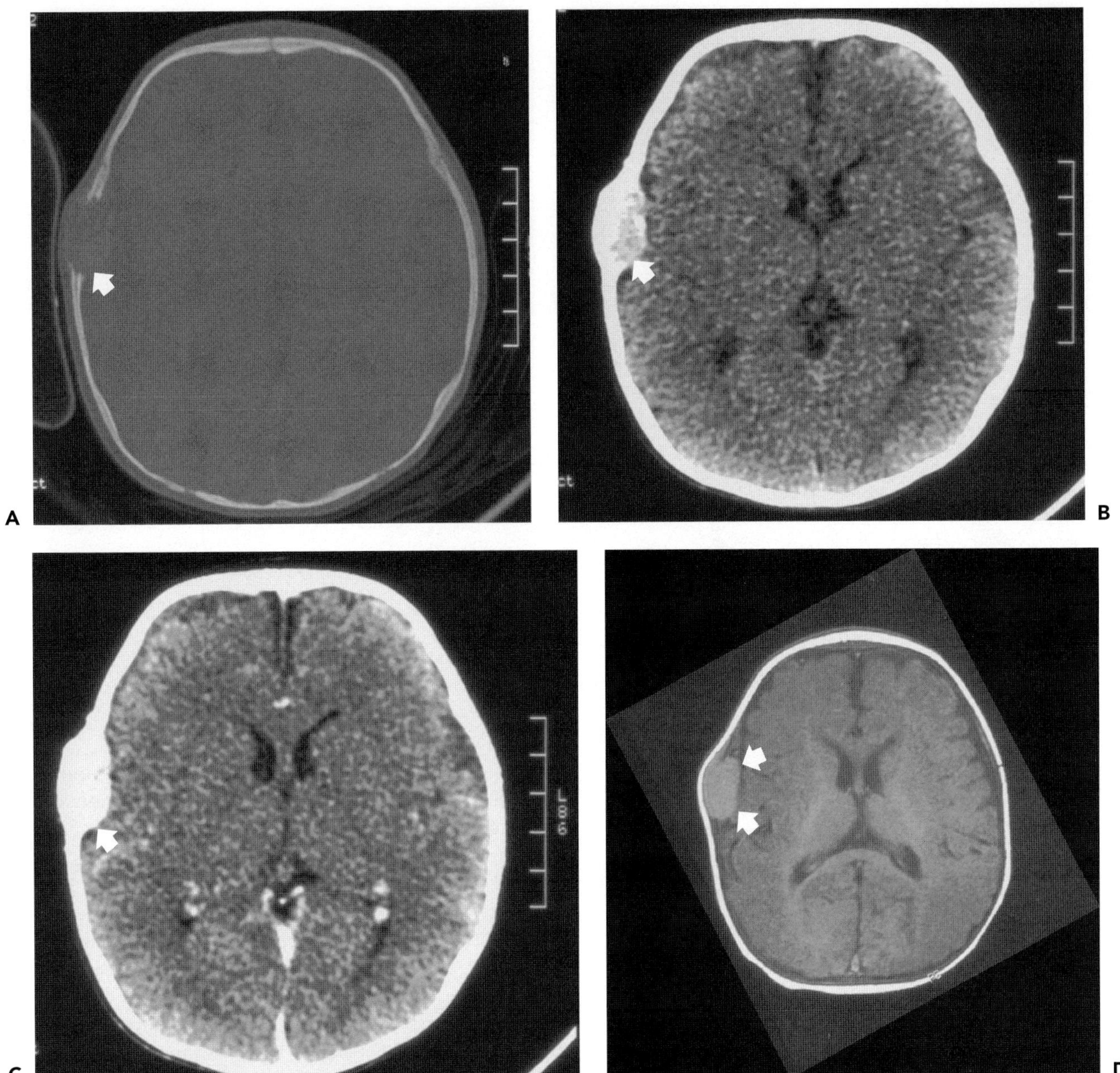

Figure 6.6 Cranial fasciitis in a boy 7 months of age with a rapidly enlarging painless scalp soft tissue mass. **A:** Axial CT scan viewed on bone window shows a large lytic skull lesion (*arrow*). **B,C:** Axial CT scans viewed on soft tissue windows preceding **(B)** and following **(C)** intravenous contrast show that the lesion involves both bone and the subgaleal soft tissue (*arrow*). **D:** Axial enhanced T1-weighted (TR/TE; 530/12) spin-echo MR image shows the intraosseous component (*arrows*), and correlated well with the CT images. (*continued*)

older than 55 years of age (71). In this autopsy study, lesions were 3 cm or smaller, suggesting that most elastofibromas are clinically occult, accounting for the perception that they are rare. Elastofibroma is not a true neoplasm and is generally considered to be a fibroblastic pseudotumor, probably arising from periosteal fibroblasts with deranged elastic fibrillogenesis (3–6,72). Lesions typically occur in a periscapular location, deep to the rhomboid major and latissimus dorsa muscles, at the level of the sixth to eighth ribs (3–6). The etiology is thought to be repeated mechanical friction between the chest wall and the tip of the scapula; hence the elastofibroma is considered reactive, not neoplastic. Patients often have an occupational history of manual labor, such as farming. However, this may be a coincidence (69,70,73,74) in view of the prevalence of elastofibroma at autopsy and its presumed occult clinical

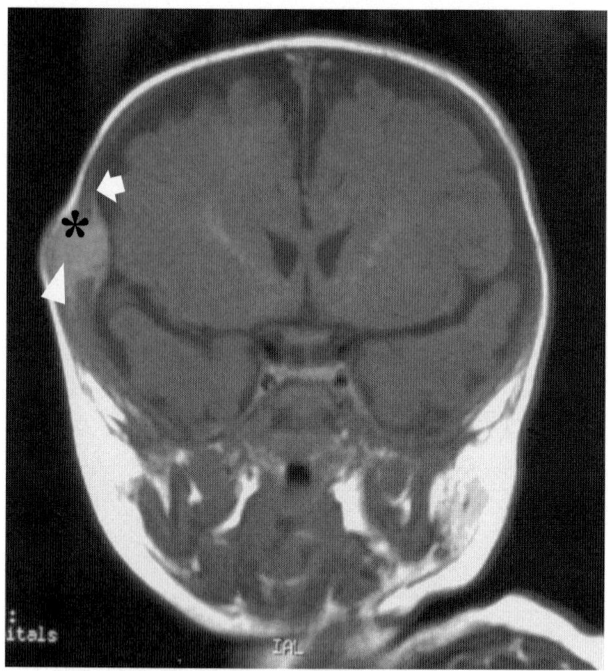
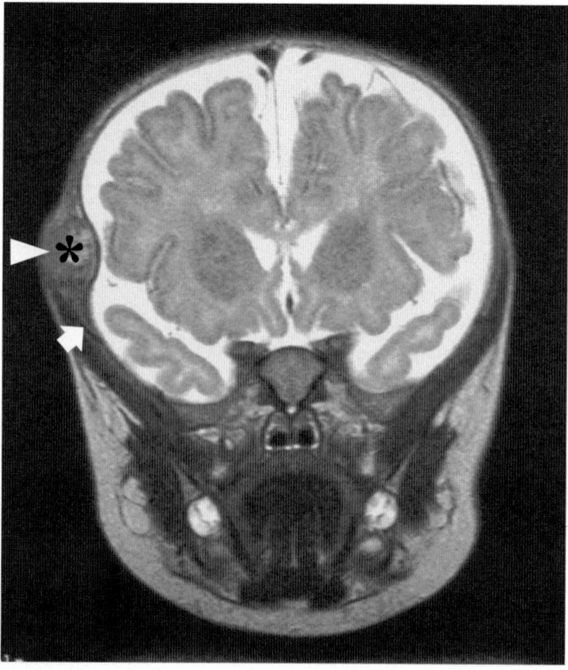

Figure 6.6 *(continued)* **E,F:** Coronal enhanced T1-weighted (TR/TE; 530/12) **(E)** and T2-weighted (TR/TE; 4784/99) **(F)** MR images show the subgaleal (*arrowhead*) and intraosseous (*asterisk*) components, as well as linear dural extension (*arrows*). The lesion shows mild diffuse enhancement and is intermediate in signal intensity on all pulse sequences.

KEY CONCEPTS

- Elastofibroma is a common, reactive fibroblastic pseudo-tumor, seen in 11% of men and 24% of women at autopsy series.
- Elastofibroma occurs in a periscapular location in 95% to 99% of lesions, related to the scapular tip, and may be bilateral in 10% to 66% of cases.
- Patients are older (sixth to seventh decade of life) and lesions are often asymptomatic (>50% of cases).
- CT chest examinations reveal elastofibromas in 2% of cases.
- On CT and MR imaging, the periscapular masses often contain small amounts of entrapped fat with otherwise nonspecific features.
- MR imaging frequently reveals intermediate signal intensity on T1- and T2-weighting.
- The location and imaging appearance with entrapped fat is pathognomonic of elastofibroma.

---

nature (71). Other types of trauma, mechanical stress, chronic irritation, and nutritional derangement are also suggested as etiologic factors (71,75), although these alone may not explain the development of elastofibroma. Some patients may also have a genetic predisposition as suggested in a study by Nagamine et al. (74) of 170 cases of the lesion in Okinawa, in which approximately 33% of patients had a family history of elastofibroma. Barr (76) postulated that "the lesion results from elastic degenera-

tion of collagen following trauma and friction in individuals who possibly have some inherited enzymatic defect related to connective tissue metabolism."

The location between the chest wall and inferior scapular tip is most characteristic of elastofibroma; it is the site of the lesion in 95% to 99% of reported cases (74). Bilateral lesions are common and seen in 10% to 66% of patients (69,70,73,74,76). Synchronous infraolecranon lesions are also common, and the elbow is the second most frequently reported site of involvement (77). Nagamine et al. (74) found the elbow involved in approximately 16% of patients. They also noted isolated synchronous lesions in the thoracic wall and in the area of the ischial tuberosity. One patient in their study had lesions in seven different anatomic locations. Isolated lesions are rarely reported in other locations such as the hand (78), foot (79,80), small bowel, colon, tracheobronchial tree, omentum, stomach, rectum, regions overlying the greater trochanter and ischial tuberosity (76,80,81), deltoid area (75), thigh (80), temporal bulbar conjunctiva (82), and cervical epidural space (83).

Most patients are older adults with a peak incidence in the sixth and seventh decades. The mean age of patients is approximately 70 years (74), although elastofibroma is reported in children as young as 6 years of age (73). Patients are asymptomatic in greater than 50% of cases (73,74). The most common symptom is stiffness, which is seen in approximately 25% of patients (74). Pain is relatively uncommon and the presenting symptom in another

TABLE 6.1
SUPERFICIAL FIBROMAS

Lesion	Age	Location	Size	Associations/Recurrence
Pleomorphic fibroma	Fifth decade Females > males	Skin, extremity, trunk, head/neck	0.5–2 cm	Recurrence rare
Sclerotic fibroma	Adults	No predilection	<1 cm	Cowden disease Rare recurrence
Nuchal fibroma	Third–fifth decades	Dermis/subcutis, upper back	2.5–8 cm	? Gardner syndrome May recur
Cellular angiofibroma	Fifth–seventh decades	Vulva, scrotal	Females: <3 cm; Males: 2.5–14 cm	Hernia/hydrocele Rare recurrence
Giant cell angiofibroma	Middle-aged adults	Orbital, eyelid	Median: 3 cm	Rare recurrence
Gardner fibroma	Infants, children, and adolescents	Superficial and deep paraspinal	1–10 cm	90% develop Gardner syndrome 45% develop desmoids

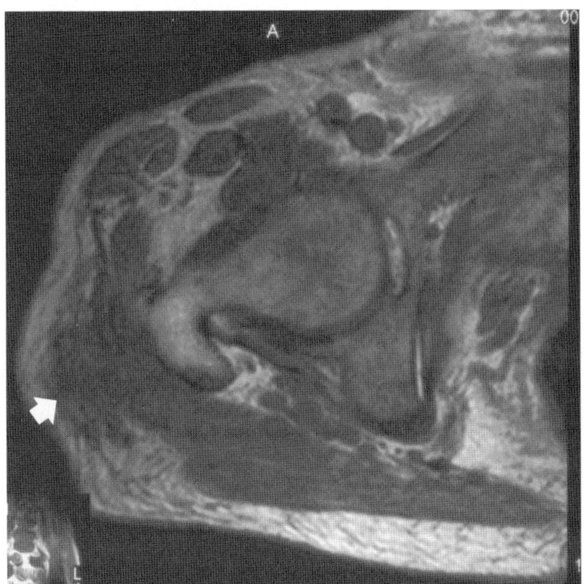

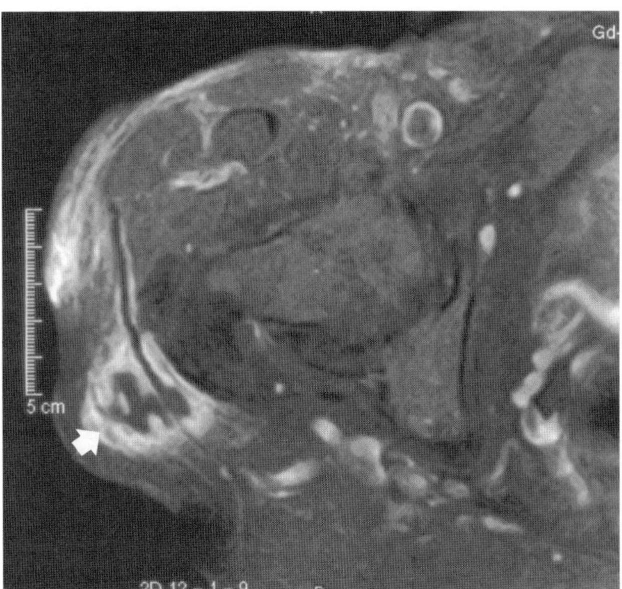

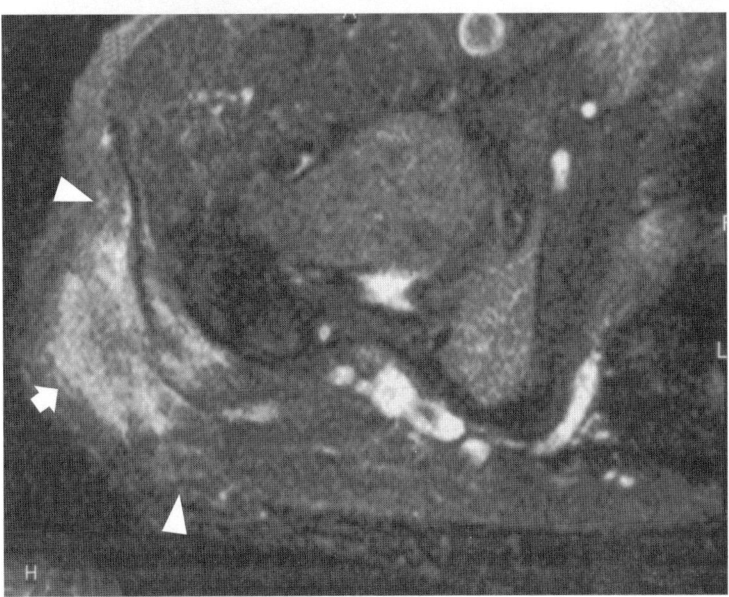

Figure 6.7 Ischemic fasciitis adjacent to the greater trochanter in a woman 70 years of age. **A–C:** Axial T1-weighted (TR/TE; 600/20) **(A)**, enhanced fat-suppressed T1-weighted (TR/TE; 606/18) **(B)** and T2-weighted (TR/TE; 4000/60) **(C)** MR images show a heterogeneous mass in the subcutaneous tissue (*arrow*) extending to the greater trochanter. The mass is intermediate signal intensity on T1-weighting and high signal intensity on T2-weighting with thick peripheral enhancement following contrast. There is also surrounding inflammation (*arrowheads* in **C**). (Case courtesy of Dr. Hakan Ilaslan.)

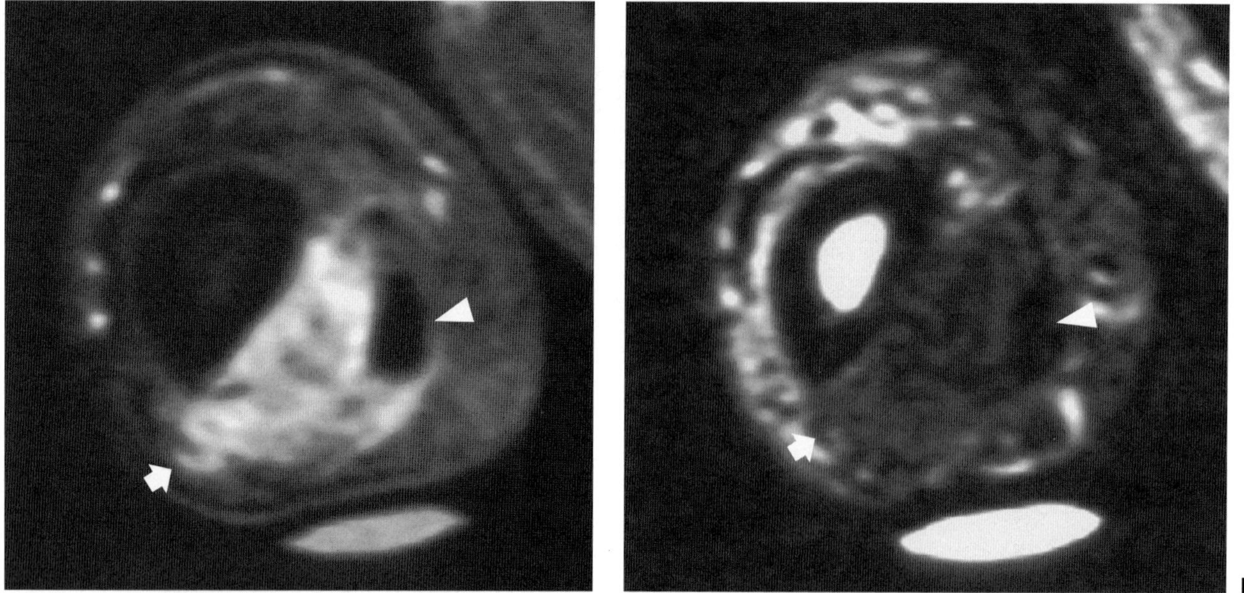

Figure 6.8 Fibroma of the flexor tendon sheath of the thumb in a woman 22 years of age. **A,B:** Axial postcontrast (TR/TE; 750/12) **(A)** and T2-weighted (TR/TE; 4500/103) **(B)** MR images of the hand show a well-defined soft tissue mass (*arrow*) surrounding the flexor tendon of the thumb (*arrowhead*). The mass shows diffuse heterogeneous enhancement and is low signal intensity on the long TR image.

10% of patients (74,84). Large lesions may ulcerate (85). The disorder has a female predominance, usually estimated to be 2:1 (71,75); however, ranges from 1:1 to 13:1 are reported (74,80).

At gross pathologic examination, elastofibroma is a gray-white, poorly defined mass containing entrapped adipose tissue and usually ranging from 5 to 10 cm in dimension, although sizes larger than 20 cm have been reported

(3–6). The great discrepancy between the prevalence of elastofibroma in autopsy series as opposed to clinically apparent lesions is likely related to the great variability in size, with clinically occult lesions only producing a thickened and indurated area of the thoracic fascia or a "streak in the fascia" detected or histologic examination (71,86). Microscopically, it is composed of fibroblasts, mature adipose tissue, abundant collagen, and elastic

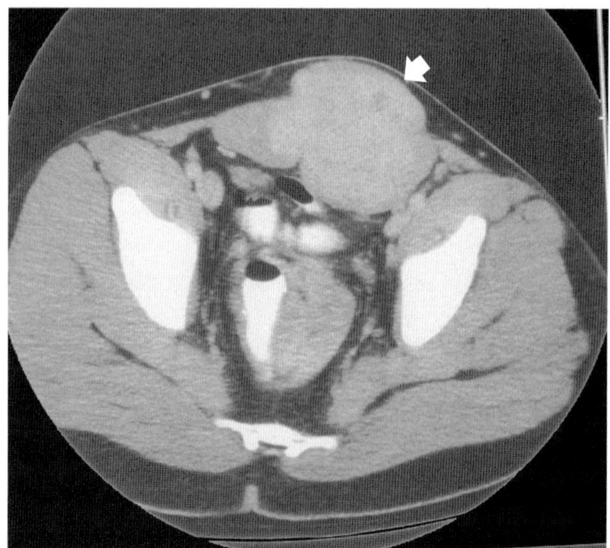

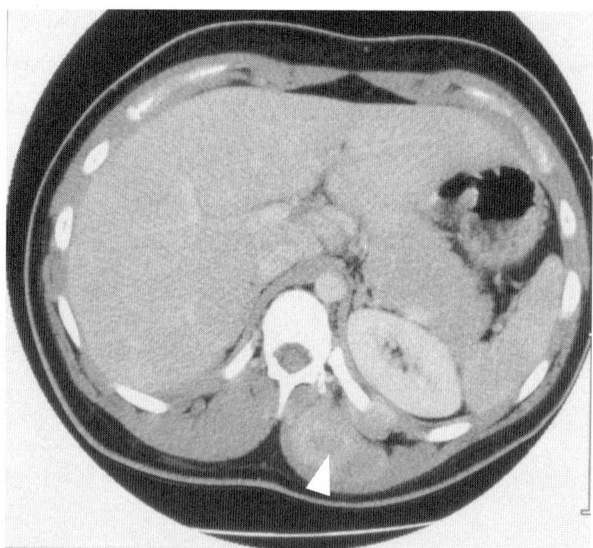

Figure 6.9 Gardner fibroma in a man 22 years of age with multiple soft tissue masses and osteomas at clinical presentation. **A,B:** Axial enhanced CT images of the pelvis **(A)** and upper abdomen **(B)** show masses in the rectus abdominus (*arrow* in **A**) and paraspinal region (*arrowhead* in **B**).

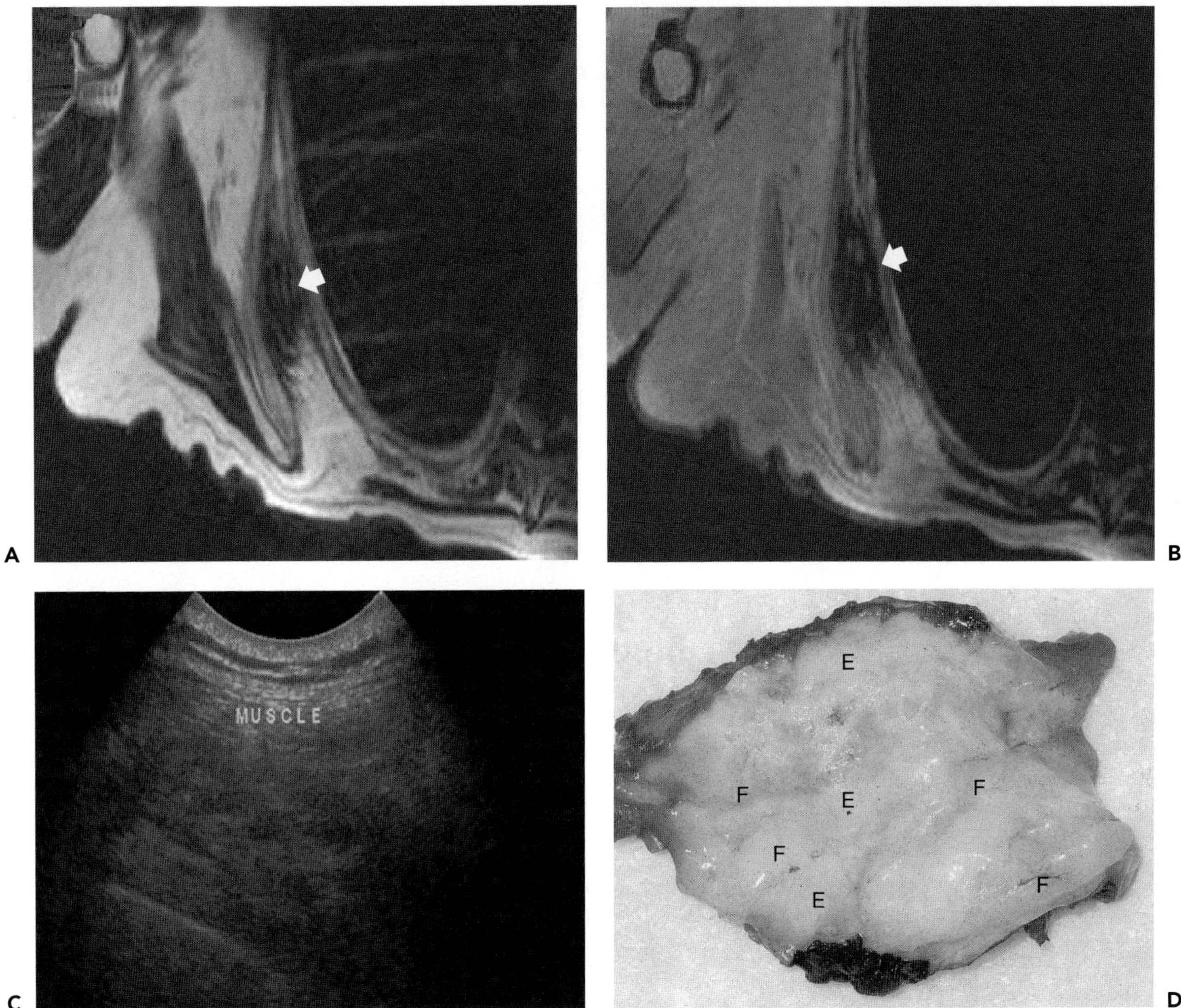

Figure 6.10 Elastofibroma deep to the scapular tip in a woman 81 years of age with breast cancer and a palpable chest wall mass clinically concerning for metastatic disease. **A,B:** Axial T1-weighted (TR/TE; 300/12) **(A)** and T2-weighted (TR/TE; 4500/99) **(B)** MR images show a low signal intensity soft tissue mass with interspersed fat (*arrow*). **C:** Ultrasound reveals a poorly circumscribed, heterogeneous, hypoechoic, nonspecific soft tissue mass (*between* +) that is difficult to identify. **D:** Photograph of the sectioned gross specimen shows the fibrous tissue **(E)** of the elastofibroma with interspersed fat **(F)**.

fibrils (Fig. 6.10). The latter are distinguished by their markedly enlarged diameter, hypereosinophilia, and asterisklike configuration on cross section. Ultrastructural examination discloses the presence of fibroblasts and myofibroblasts containing intracytoplasmic precursors of the elastic material, as well as extracellular, amorphous, fibrillary material corresponding to the thickened elastic fibrils (70,87). Microscopically, lesions are composed primarily of hyalinized collagen, with scattered fibroblasts and entrapped islands of mature adipose tissue. Cystic change within the lesion may be seen (70,74), as may bursalike areas (71,78).

Lesions may be stable or may grow slowly over many years (73,74). Surgery is considered to be curative. Local recurrences (7%) are unusual and probably a result of incomplete excision. One elastofibroma was reported to regress spontaneously. There is no metastatic potential and no reports of malignant transformation.

Radiographs of elastofibroma are usually normal, although rarely bone erosion is reported. The sonographic appearance was described in three patients by Bianchi et al. (88). Elastofibroma reveals interspersed curvilinear hypoechoic strands and an echogenic background corresponding to fibroblastic strands and intervening fat (Fig. 6.10). Color Doppler evaluation does not show significant flow and margins can be defined or ill-defined (88).

A review of CT chest examination revealed a 2% incidence of elastofibromas (89). On CT, elastofibroma is usually a poorly defined, crescent-shaped, heterogeneous soft tissue mass with attenuation approximately the same as that of skeletal muscle and containing linear low attenuation streaks representing entrapped adipose tissue (73,86,90) (Fig. 6.11). Uncommonly, lesions may be relatively homogeneous with an attenuation less than that of muscle (73,80).

On MR imaging, the typical subscapular elastofibroma is a lenticular, well-defined, soft tissue mass with an intermediate signal intensity approximately equal to that of skeletal muscle, interlaced with areas of signal intensity similar to that of fat (usually at the periphery) on both T1- and T2-weighted images (80,91–96) (Figs. 6.10 and 6.11). Gadolinium-enhanced MR images show areas with and without contrast enhancement (80,92,97,98) (Fig. 6.11). The MR imaging features of elastofibroma are different from those of most other

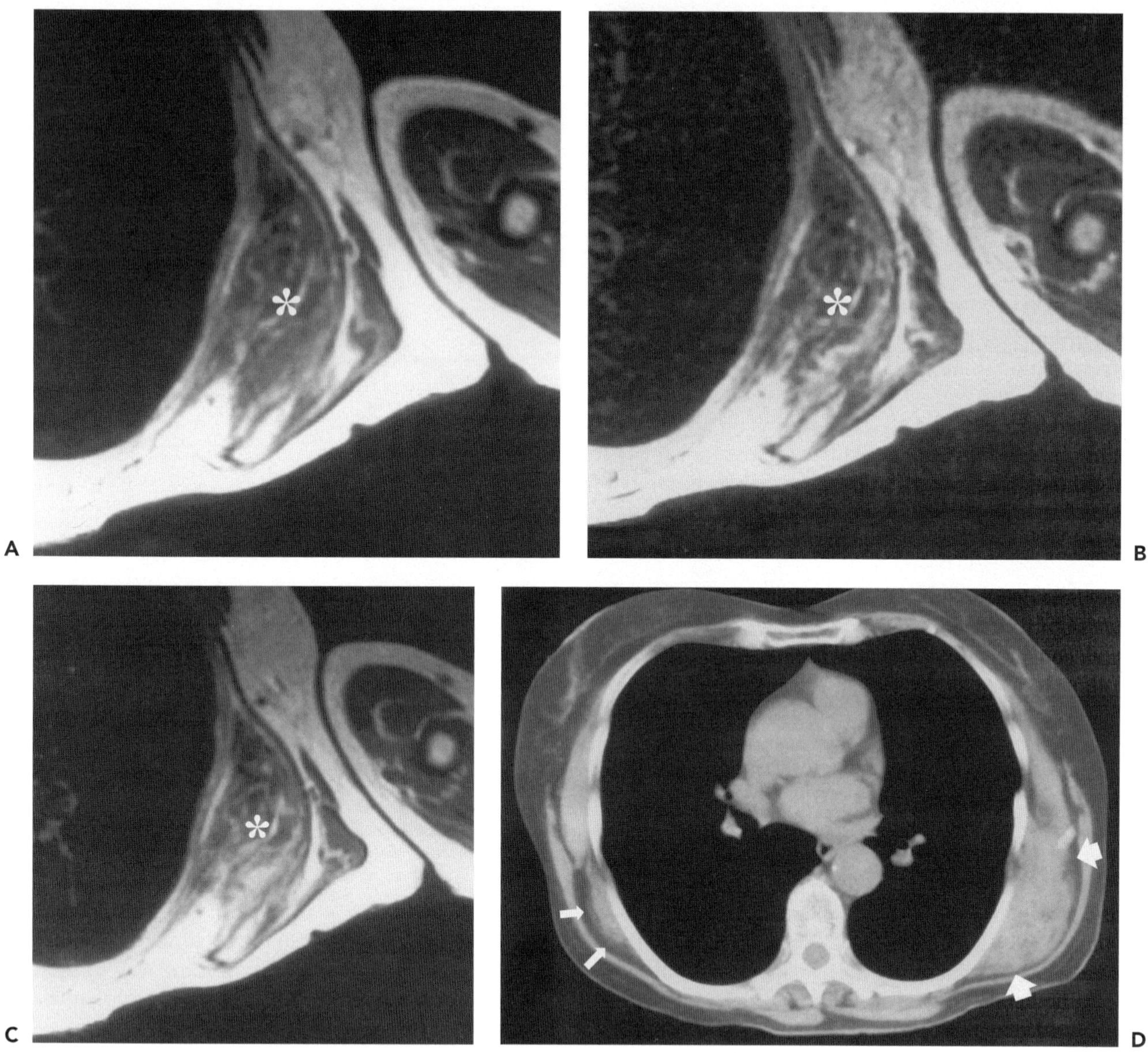

Figure 6.11   Subscapular elastofibroma in a man 72 years of age. **A,B:** Corresponding axial T1-weighted (TR/TE; 767/20) **(A)** and T2-weighted (TR/TE; 2000/90) **(B)** spin-echo MR images show a relatively well-defined, heterogeneous mass (*asterisk*) between the chest wall and the scapular tip. Most of the mass has a signal intensity approximately equal to that of the surrounding skeletal muscle. Interspersed within mass are linear and curvilinear areas of increased signal intensity approximately the same as the intensity of the subcutaneous fat on both T1- and T2-weighted images. **C:** Postcontrast axial T1-weighted (TR/TE; 767/20) spin-echo MR image at the level of **A** shows areas of enhancement (*asterisk*) and other nonenhancing areas. **D:** Corresponding axial noncontrast CT scan shows a larger left subscapular mass (*arrows*). Note subtle areas of decreased attenuation within mass representing adipose tissue. Although well-outlined by fat laterally, lesion cannot be separated from intercostal muscles. Small contralateral elastofibroma (*long arrows*) is also apparent. (*continued*)

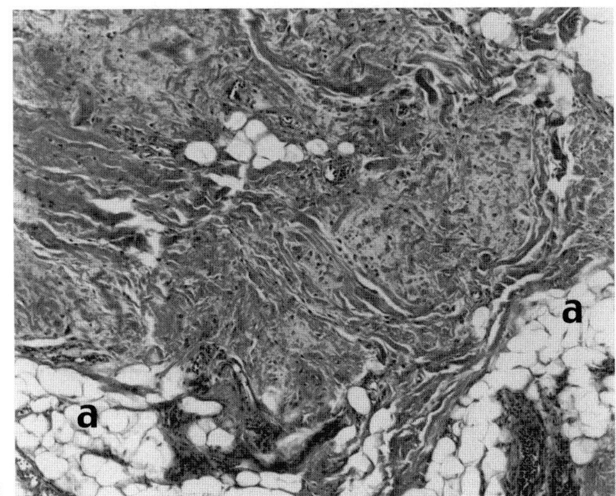
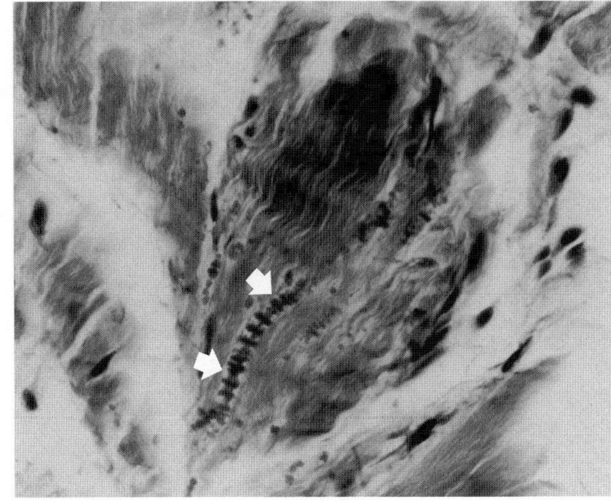

Figure 6.11 *(continued)* **E:** Low-power photomicrograph shows lesion, composed primarily of hyalinized collagen with scattered fibroblasts and entrapped islands of mature adipose tissue, infiltrating adjacent adipose tissue (a). **F:** High-power photomicrograph shows characteristic serrated fibrils *(arrows)*, which resemble a pipe cleaner in longitudinal section and an asterisk or flower in cross-section.

soft tissue tumors, reflecting entrapped fat within a predominantly fibrous mass (99,100).

We believe recognition of these characteristic CT or MR imaging features in a lesion located deep to the scapular tip in an older patient is pathognomonic of elastofibroma. Other soft tissue masses do not generally occur in this specific location. However, these masses are often small and may not be perceived as abnormal, as shown by Naylor et al., where 19% of 21 lesions were not detected at initial radiologic evaluation (101). Biopsy may not be required in asymptomatic lesions or those with limited symptoms. A diligent search for a contralateral lesion may also aid in diagnosis.

Keloid

KEY CONCEPTS

- Keloid represents exuberant dermal scar tissue.
- Keloid usually affects young people aged 15 to 45 years and has a predilection for blacks and those of Chinese descent.
- Common sites of involvement include the face, shoulder, forearms, and hands.
- Local recurrence is common (45% to 100%) following attempts at surgical excision.
- In our experience, MR imaging reveals low signal intensity on all pulse sequences, reflecting the high collagen content of these lesions.

Keloid represents formation of exuberant scar tissue usually centered in the dermis. It is a reactive benign non-neoplastic overgrowth. Keloid generally affects people 15 to 45 years

of age and may be solitary or multiple. Keloid more commonly affects blacks and dark-skinned individuals, as well as those of Chinese descent (3). Clinically, keloid is a well-circumscribed area of scar causing elevation of the skin with frequent linear extensions. Lesions are often painful or tender, and there is no sex predilection. Frequent sites of involvement are the face, shoulders, forearms, and hands. Lesions are likely induced by minor infections or surgical procedures (including tattoos and body piercings). Excess fibrosis-promoting cytokines, such as transforming growth factor-β (TGF-β), also play an important role in keloid development (3). Keloid formation is associated with numerous other conditions, including acne, Ehlers-Danlos syndrome, scleroderma, the superficial fibromatoses, and Rubinstein-Taybi syndrome (3).

Pathologically, keloid represents fibrocollagenous proliferation with abundant collagen fibers. Vascularity may be present initially, but chronic lesions are hypocellular with prominent hyalinization and decreased blood supply. Areas of calcification or osseous metaplasia may be seen.

The rate of local recurrence following surgical excision of keloid formation is high (45% to 100%) (102). Steroid injection typically combined with surgery reduces local recurrence to less than 50% (103). Radiation therapy also lowers local recurrence dramatically, to less than 10% (104,105). Multiple additional methods of treatment, including laser therapy, cryosurgery, pressure pads, and silicone gel, have been attempted (106–109). Cosmetic surgery should be avoided by patients who have a previous history of keloid formation.

Imaging of keloid, similar to many other cutaneous lesions, is not commonly performed. In our limited experiences, MR imaging demonstrates markedly low signal intensity on all pulse sequences. This corresponds to the high collagen content of these lesions.

Desmoplastic Fibroblastoma

Desmoplastic fibroblastoma is a rare, benign, fibrous soft tissue tumor that is also referred to as *collagenous fibroma* (3–6). The lesion usually affects patients in the fifth to seventh decades of life (70% of cases) and is more frequent in men (3–4:1 ratio) (110–112). Lesions are most common in the subcutaneous tissue of the upper extremity (shoulder 19%, upper arm 24%, forearm, and hand), followed by the lower extremity (particularly the lateral thigh), head/neck region, back, and feet (3–6).

At gross pathologic examination, more than 50% of lesions are larger than 5 cm, although neoplasms ranging from 1 to 20 cm are described (3–6). Desmoplastic fibro-

blastoma is a well-circumscribed, white to gray, subcutaneous mass, although infiltration of the surrounding fat (70%), superficial fascia and muscle (25%), and occasional deep-seated lesions are reported (3–6). Microscopically, lesions are hypocellular, with bland stellate spindle cells, in a dense collagenous stroma. Hemorrhage, necrosis, mitoses, and prominent vascularity are absent. Small calcifications are described as a characteristic feature. Cytogenetic studies in a few patients have shown abnormalities at 11q12 and a 2:11 translocation, identical to that seen in fibroma of tendon sheath (4).

Treatment of desmoplastic fibroma is simple excision. Neither local recurrence nor metastases are reported.

Imaging of desmoplastic fibroma is described in only a limited number of case reports (110–112) (Fig. 6.12). As would be expected for lesions composed of primarily hypocellular collagen, MR imaging reveals prominent

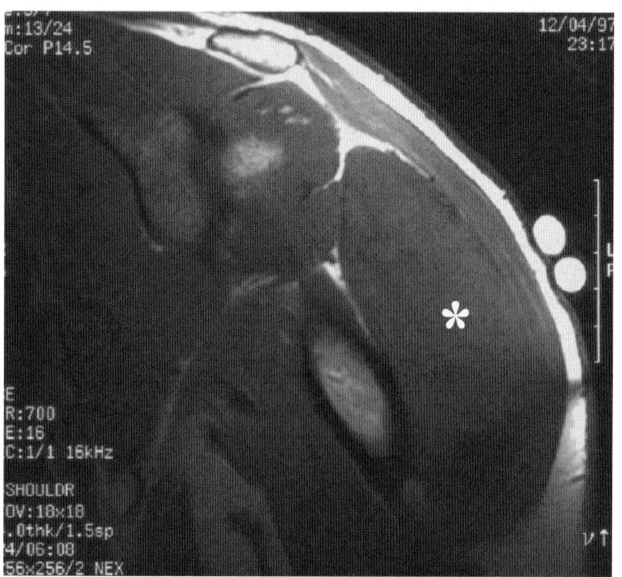

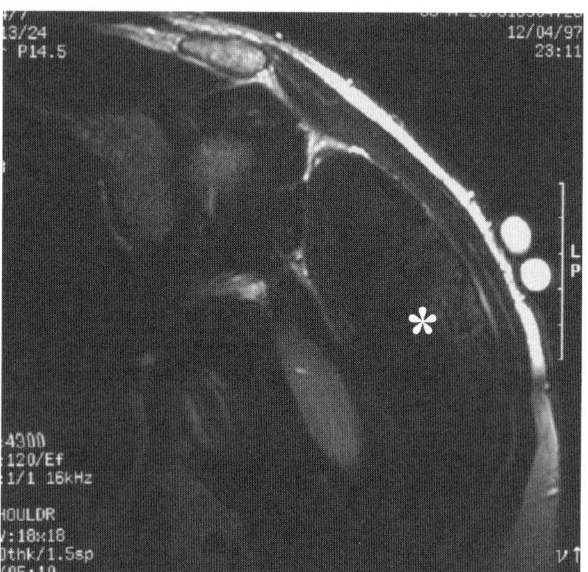

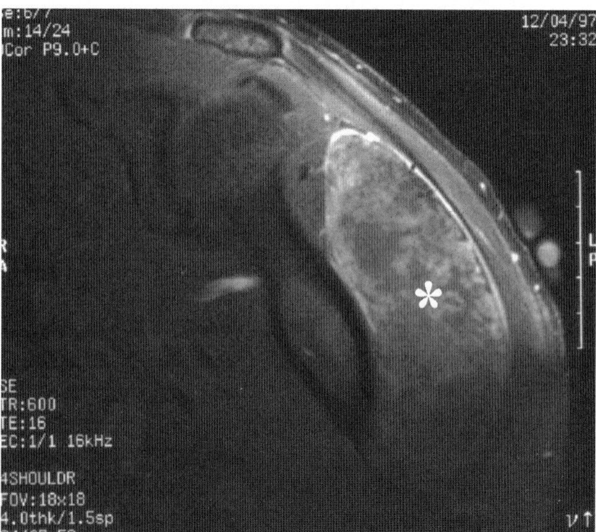

Figure 6.12 Desmoplastic fibroblastoma of the shoulder in a man 25 years of age. **A,B:** Coronal T1-weighted (TR/TE; 700/16) **(A)** and T2-weighted (TR/TE; 4300/120) **(B)** MR images show a large soft tissue mass (*asterisk*) lateral to the humerus. The mass is heterogeneous with intermediate signal intensity on T1-weighting and low signal intensity on T2-weighting. **C:** Enhanced fat-suppressed T1-weighted (TR/TE; 600/16) MR image shows only mild enhancement.

low signal intensity on all pulse sequences. Only mild contrast enhancement is seen, paralleling the limited vascularity, which is in marked distinction from the majority of fibromatoses.

Mammary-Type Myofibroblastoma

Mammary-type myofibroblastoma represents a benign mesenchymal neoplasm that occurs in the inguinal and groin area and is identical histologically to its counterpart in the breast (4,113,114). Other reported locations include the abdominal wall, buttock, paraspinal area, and vaginal wall (113,114). These extramammary sites are very rare, and the fact that they commonly affect older men (35 to 67 years of age; mean 56 years, with a 4:1 ratio) with gynecomastia or on antiandrogen treatment, and occur along the milk line (extending from the axilla to the groin), suggests a hormonal stimulation etiology (4,115).

Lesions range in size from 2 to 13 cm (median: 6 cm) on gross pathologic examination (4). Mammary-type myofibroblastoma of the soft tissue is a well-circumscribed but nonencapsulated lesion composed of spindle cells resembling myofibroblasts. There are prominent broad bands of collagen with variable intermixed fat. Marginal resection is curative.

We are unaware of any reports of the imaging appearance of mammary-type myofibroblastoma but would expect nonspecific characteristics with intermediate-to-high signal intensity on T2-weighted MR images. We would postulate that the interspersed fat may be apparent on MR imaging as areas isointense to fat on all pulse sequences.

FIBROBLASTIC PROLIFERATIONS OF INFANCY AND CHILDHOOD

There is a group of fibrous proliferative processes that are relatively specific to infancy and childhood. Generally, these have no clinical or morphologic adult counterpart (1). Of these, myofibroma/myofibromatosis is the most frequent, although it is still quite uncommon in comparison to fibrous lesions in adults. Other rare lesions, such as fibrous hamartoma of infancy and infantile digital fibromatosis, are typically superficial, and similar to other subcutaneous lesions, they are only rarely subject to radiologic imaging.

Myofibroma/Myofibromatosis

Myofibromatosis is a term used to describe a distinct, benign, fibrous proliferation characteristically seen in infants and children (4,5,31,116,117). Infantile myofibromatosis is the most common fibrous tumor of infancy (118). This lesion was originally described by Williams and Schrum in 1951 (119). Initially termed *congenital generalized fibromatosis* by

Stout in 1954 (120), this disease process is characterized by numerous nodular lesions that affect multiple organ systems including skin, bone, skeletal muscle, and visceral organs (121). The deep soft tissues and viscera are involved in 15% to 20% of cases of myofibromatosis (122). Subsequent reports documented that both solitary (myofibroma) and multicentric forms (myofibromatosis) exist (123). The designation *generalized hamartomatosis* was proposed by Morettin et al. (124); the name *infantile myofibromatosis* was coined by Chung and Enzinger in a report of 61 cases in 1981 (121). The WHO designated these lesions as *myofibroma* (solitary form) and *myofibromatosis* (multicentric form) because these terms emphasize the dual histologic features of this entity, which is characterized by spindle cells having features of both smooth muscle and fibroblasts (4,121).

The solitary myofibroma occurs as a small (less than 2 cm) subcutaneous mass most commonly affecting the head and neck (50% of lesions frequently located in the scalp, forehead, orbit, oral cavity, and parotid area) followed by the thumb, and lower and upper extremities (125). The prevalence of solitary versus multiple lesions varies from 4:1 to 1:2 (126). Although these lesions typically affect infants and children, myofibromas have also been reported in adults (127). Fletcher et al. suggested that myofibroma and infantile hemangiopericytoma may be the same or closely related lesions (128).

Both autosomal recessive and autosomal dominant patterns of inheritance are suggested for infantile myofibromatosis (129–131). An autosomal-dominant inheritance pattern would require reduced penetrance, with many gene carriers being nonpenetrant or else overlooked through regression of solitary small nodules at birth (132). The relationship to estrogen is unclear. Myofibromatosislike lesions were produced in the uterus and abdominal and thoracic cavities of guinea pigs treated with estrogen (130).

The vast majority of cases of myofibromatosis occur in infants and children, with 90% of cases presenting before 2 years of age (120). Lesions are present at birth in 70% of cases (4,5,31,117). Uncommonly, older children and, rarely, adults may be affected, either primarily or with recurrence (132,133). Myofibromatosis is the most common fibroblastic-myofibroblastic soft tissue tumor of childhood and adolescents (newborn to 20 years of age), accounting for 24 (22%) of 108 tumors reported by Coffin and Dehner, on reviewing the files of the University of Minnesota Hospital and Clinics, between 1960 and 1984 (4,5,31,117,134). The mean age of diagnosis was 5 months, with 90% of patients diagnosed within the first year of life (4,5,31,117). In the Armed Forces Institute of Pathology (AFIP) experience, 114 (64%) of 178 patients were 10 years or younger (4,5,31,117). Interestingly, 25 (14%) patients were 40 years or older. In a review of 170 cases by Wiswell et al., there was a male predominance in both forms (1.7:1) (118,121,135). There is a similar male predominance in the AFIP cases, with a ratio of 1.6:1 (121,135). Earlier reports suggested that the solitary form is more common in males; in contradistinction, the multicentric form more typically affected females, involving the soft tissue, bones, and viscera (121). The number of nodules present is variable with myofibromatosis and may number from only a few to more than 100 (4,5,31,117). Lesions are typically not painful and may have an appearance of a purple macule, suggesting a vascular lesion.

At gross pathologic examination, subcutaneous lesions are well-marginated and may measure several centimeters in diameter; deeper intramuscular nodules may be more poorly defined (121). On microscopic examination, the nodules tend to be well-circumscribed, although infiltration of the adjacent tissue may also be seen (132). Lesions are biphasic, with one component composed of short bundles of plump spindle-shaped cells displaying characteristics intermediate between those of fibroblasts and those of smooth muscle cells (121,132), and the other element composed of less differentiated small round cells, demonstrating a hemangiopericytoma pattern. Necrosis may be seen (121). Skin lesions may resemble hemangiomas because of the prominent vascularity (118). Mitoses are usually rare but in some cases are more numerous (8–10 per high power field [HPF]) (4,5,31,117).

In patients with multicentric disease, spontaneous regression may be seen in approximately 33% of cases (118,123). Visceral involvement, seen in approximately 40% of cases, is invariably present at birth (118,123). In these patients there is a 75% mortality rate with respiratory distress and diarrhea (123), usually caused by extensive involvement of visceral organs, particularly the cardiopulmonary or gastrointestinal systems (118,121,123,136). These patients may be treated aggressively, including the

use of chemotherapy. Visceral involvement may not portend the grave prognosis once thought, and outcome may be more a function of the extent and specific location of lesions within the affected viscera (137). The exception to this may be pulmonary involvement, which is still associated with a poor outcome (137). Rarely, multifocal cases with visceral involvement spontaneously regress. Rare involvement of the central nervous system was also reported in a handful of cases (137,138). The overall mortality rate, however, is less than 15% to 20% (118). Without visceral involvement the disease is benign, the prognosis is uniformly good (118,123), and the typical course for these lesions is spontaneous regression (61%), although the number and size of lesions may increase prior to regression (118,139). When solitary lesions are excised, local recurrence is seen in approximately 9% to 11% of cases (118,121). No features are known to predict local recurrence. Solitary lesions may be adequately treated by biopsy only, to document diagnosis, without the need of resection. A single case with associated major malformations, including esophageal atresia, annular pancreas, vertebral anomalies, and hypoplastic kidney, has been reported (140).

On radiographs, extraskeletal lesions may present as nonspecific soft tissue masses, often with small foci of calcification (121,139,141) (Figs. 6.13 and 6.14). When bone is involved, lesions are lytic with lobulated, geographic (well-defined) margins, often with sclerosis at the time of radiographic evaluation (121,124) (Figs. 6.13 and 6.14). Initially, there may be no sclerosis in the margin, as sclerosis is considered to indicate healing (137). Lesions are typically eccentrically located in the metaphyseal regions of long bones, and involvement may be symmetric (124). The femur, tibia, rib, spine, and pelvis are frequently involved. Calvarial lesions are reported as common in some studies (121), but distinctly unusual in others (124). Early lesions demonstrate cortical erosion, suggesting that these lesions may arise from the periosteum (124). Periosteal reaction is unusual and rarely may be extensive (124,137). Pathologic fracture has been reported as well (124). Calcifications may be seen within lesions and are described as having multiple foci, a peripheral rim, multiple nodules, or "cornflake" appearance (142) (Fig. 6.13). Bone destruction may not develop for days or weeks after birth, and these lesions heal without sequela during regression (124,139,143). Scintigraphy may be normal or may show increased tracer accumulation (137,139). Sonography is nonspecific, typically revealing a well-defined, hypoechoic-to-isoechoic soft tissue mass (Fig. 6.13). Calcific foci show high echogenicity and posterior acoustic shadowing (Fig. 6.13).

CT scanning demonstrates the soft tissue, bone, and visceral lesions (Fig. 6.14). Lesions may demonstrate increased attenuation compared to that of skeletal muscle both before and after intravenous contrast administration (144). MR imaging may provide an ideal means of detecting and

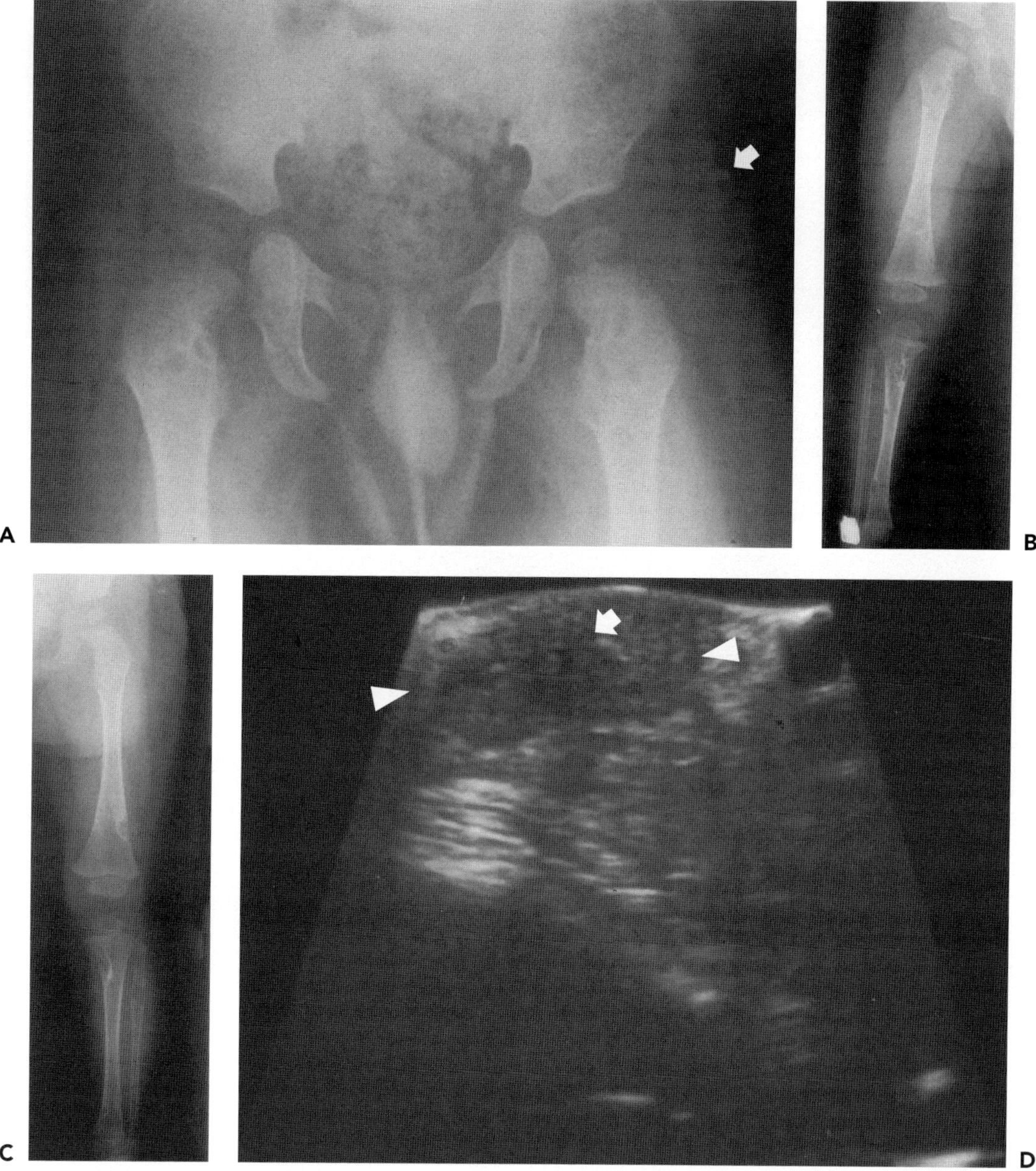

Figure 6.13 Multifocal myofibromatosis in a boy 3 months of age. **A:** Anteroposterior radiograph of the pelvis shows symmetric, well-defined, geographic lytic lesions with sclerotic margins in the metaphyseal regions of proximal femurs. There is a soft tissue mass in the left buttocks with subtle calcification (*arrow*). **B,C:** Anteroposterior radiographs of the lower extremities also shows multiple relatively symmetric, excentric, metaphyseal lesions. **D:** Ultrasound also reveals the mass (*arrowheads*) with small focus of increased echogenicity and posterior acoustic shadowing resulting from calcification (*arrow*).

following individual lesions (123), and it may be the best radiologic method of accurately accessing the location and extent of visceral lesions (137) (Fig. 6.15).

Pulmonary involvement may appear radiologically as interstitial fibrosis, a reticulonodular infiltrate, or generalized bronchopneumonia (124,144). Barium studies of the gastrointestinal tract may demonstrate diffuse narrowing with numerous small filling defects (136). The radiographic differential diagnosis of cases with multiple skeletal lesions includes Langerhans cell histiocytosis, angiomatosis, lymphangiomatosis, hematogenous osteomyelitis, enchondromatosis, lipomatosis, and metastatic neuroblastoma (139, 145).

Juvenile Hyaline Fibromatosis

Juvenile hyaline fibromatosis is an extremely rare, nonneoplastic, hereditary (autosomal recessive) disorder that

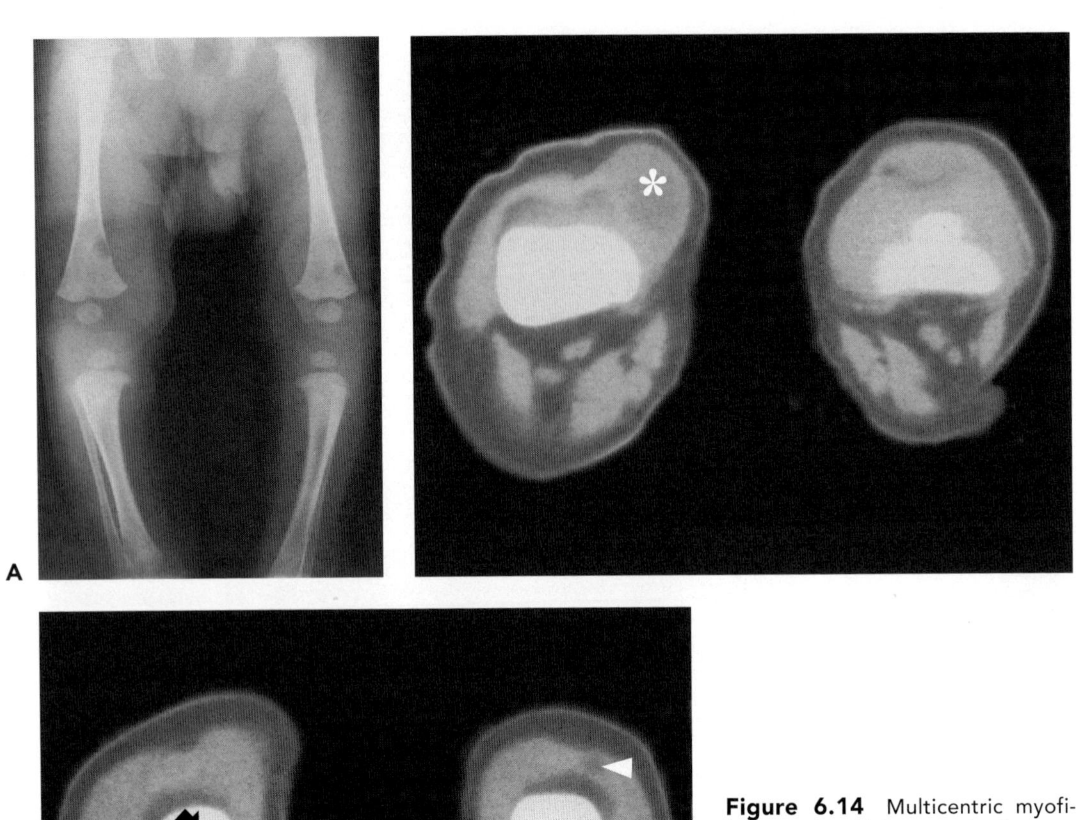

Figure 6.14 Multicentric myofibromatosis with bone and soft tissue involvement in a boy 1 month of age. **A:** Anteroposterior radiograph of the lower extremities shows lytic lesions in the distal metaphysis of both femura. **B:** Noncontrast axial CT scan of the distal thighs shows a soft tissue mass in the anteromedial aspect of the right thigh (*asterisk*). **C:** Noncontrast axial CT scan of the distal thighs, just proximal to **B,** shows a lytic lesion in the distal right femur (*arrow*) as well as an additional soft tissue lesion anteriorly on the left (*arrowhead*).

resembles myofibromatosis, with fewer than 50 reported cases (4,5,31,117). Murray first described this correlation in 1873 as *molluscum fibrosum* in children (146). Synonymous terms for this entity also include *mesenchymal dysplasia, fibromatosis hyaline multiplex, systemic hyalinosis,* and *disseminated painful fibromatosis* (4,5,31,117). The term *juvenile hyaline fibromatosis* was described by Kitano et al. in 1972 (147). This entity may be related to Winchester syndrome.

Patients are affected from birth to 5 years of age, and there is a mild male predilection (4,5,31,117). Clinical presentation is of skin papules on the face, neck, and around the ears and perianal region. Periarticular deposits may cause joint contractures. Larger subcutaneous lesions also develop in the scalp, trunk, and limbs. Additional features include gingival hypertrophy, muscle weakness, and poorly developed muscle. The number of cutaneous lesions is variable but may be greater than 100, and they can continue to develop into adulthood (4,5,31,117).

At gross pathologic examination, the nodules are poorly circumscribed with a solid white, waxy appearance, and range from several millimeters to 5 cm in size (1). Histologically, the nodules are composed of a mixture of fibroblastic cells with extracellular hyaline material. Biochemical evaluation suggests increased chondroitin sulfate and types 1 and 6 collagen (4).

The treatment of the multiple lesions is surgical resection, depending on their location. Unfortunately, local recurrence is frequent (4,5,31,117). Lesions are not radiosensitive. Physical therapy and steroids may improve contractures that are often severely disabling.

Radiographs reveal multifocal lytic bone lesions in more than 60% of cases (117). These frequently affect the distal phalanges of the toes and fingers and may progress to extensive destruction. Flexion contractures may also be apparent on radiographs. The cross-sectional imaging appearance of the subcutaneous lesion has not been

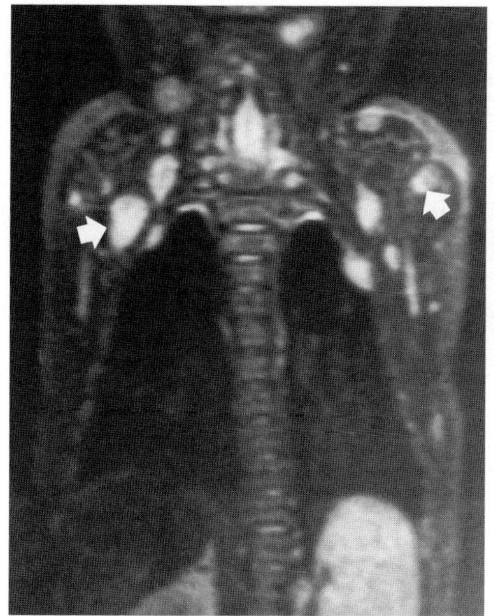
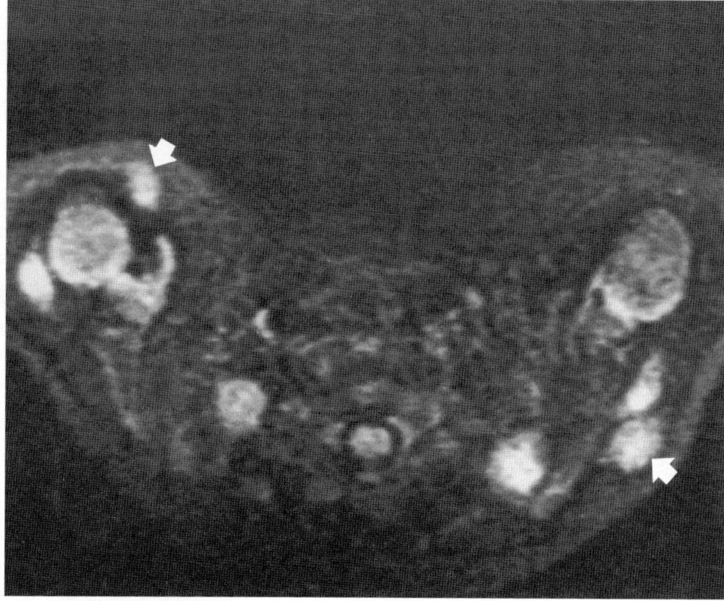
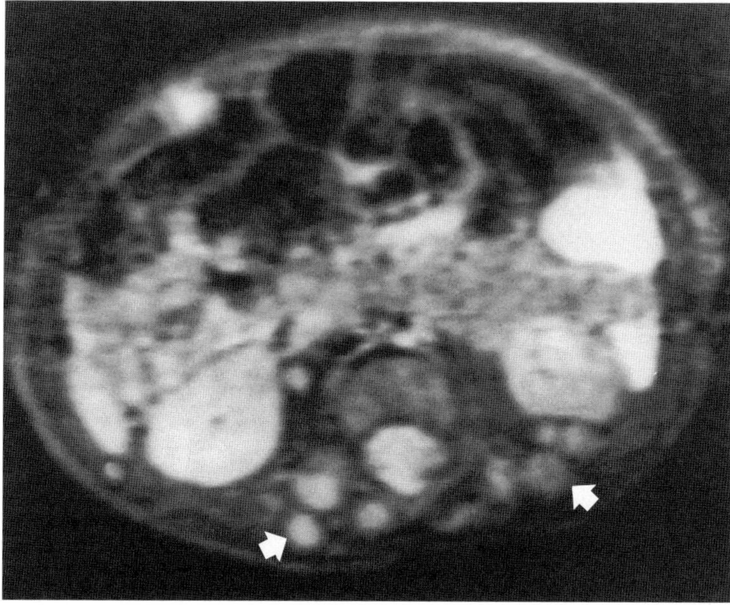

Figure 6.15 Multifocal myofibromatosis in a boy 2 months of age. **A–C:** T2-weighted (TR/TE; 2000/80) spin-echo MR images of the chest **(A)** shoulders **(B)** and abdomen **(C)** show multiple high signal intensity nodules in the soft tissue of the neck, axilla, and back (*arrows*).

described, to the best of our knowledge. We would expect the high water content of the hyaline material to be reflected as low attenuation on CT scanning, hypoechogenic on sonography, low signal on T1-weighted, and very high signal intensity on T2-weighted MR images.

Fibromatosis Colli

Fibromatosis colli is a relatively rare, distinct form of infantile fibromatosis, characterized by fibrous proliferation in the sternocleidomastoid muscle, usually presenting within the first few weeks of life (1). Additional terms for this lesion include *congenital muscle torticollis, sternocleidomastoid tumor of infancy,* and *pseudotumor of infancy* (4,5,31,117). The

KEY CONCEPTS

- Fibromatosis colli represents a distinct form of infantile fibromatosis involving the sternocleidomastoid muscle.
- The lesion is usually associated with difficult birth and presents at 2 to 4 weeks of age with a firm mass in the lower neck.
- Regression occurs spontaneously in 70% of cases after 1 to 2 years.
- Ultrasonography and MR imaging reveal an enlarged sternocleidomastoid muscle with mildly abnormal intrinsic appearance; hypoechoic on sonography and increased signal intensity on long TR MR images.

most widely quoted prevalence is from a study of infants born at the Mayo Clinic between January 1, 1944, and December 31, 1954, in which the lesion was identified in 35 (0.4%) of 7,835 resident-born infants (148). Although the cause is unclear, it is thought to be related to birth trauma with subsequent pressure necrosis and secondary fibrosis in the sternocleidomastoid muscle (149). Cases are associated with a difficult delivery, often requiring forceps in more than 90% of cases, or abnormal intrauterine positioning (149,150). Armstrong et al. (151), in reviewing 92 cases collected at Duke University over 20 years, noted breech delivery in approximately 51% of cases in which the delivery method was known. Davids et al. (150) suggested the changes are caused by selective injury of the sternocleidomastoid muscle in utero because of the position of the fetal head, with a secondary compartment syndrome within the muscle. Familial cases are rarely reported (151); however, Isigkeit et al. reported an 11% familial history (152).

Patients are typically normal at birth, but present between 2 and 4 weeks of age with a firm mass in the lower neck (1,148–151). The lesion is typically in the lower third of the sternocleidomastoid muscle (less than 5 cm in length), affecting both the sternal and clavicular heads, but either may be spared as well (153). It is rarely bilateral, shows a mild predilection for the right side, and initially the lesion grows rapidly (151). There is a reduced growth rate over time, and eventually the mass remains static in size. Fibromatosis colli regresses in approximately 70% of cases, usually after 1 to 2 years (1,148), but this phenomenon may occur as early as 5 to 8 months (151). There is a mild male predilection (1,148). Associated torticollis, caused by contracture of the sternocleidomastoid muscle, is seen in 14% to 30% of cases and may be transient (154). Patients presenting with congenital muscular torticollis, but with no history of a focal mass, probably represent cases of unrecognized fibromatosis colli (155). Infants who typically sleep in a prone position are most comfortable with the affected side down. This results in pressure on the growing cranium, resulting in progressive deformity of the skull and facial asymmetry referred to as *plagiocephaly* (150). Patients may also develop a compensatory thoracic scoliosis. Associated abnormalities were seen in 13 (14%) of 92 patients reported by Armstrong et al. (151), with the most common being mental retardation (4 cases) and seizure disorder (2 cases). There is also an increased incidence of metatarsus adductus, rib anomalies, developmental dysplasia of the hip, and talipes equinovarus (150).

At gross pathologic evaluation, most lesions are small, measuring 2 to 3 cm in diameter, and show a glistening gray-white appearance (1). The mass blends imperceptibly and infiltrates the surrounding skeletal muscle (1). Microscopy reveals replacement of muscle by a fibroblastic process of varying cellularity, although often limited (1). This lesional tissue is intermixed with skeletal muscle that has undergone atrophy or degeneration.

Treatment is often conservative in patients younger than 1 year, using exercise, because of the high incidence of spontaneous (70%) regression (148,156,157). Fibromatosis colli does not recur. Clinical features associated with poor outcome include marked facial asymmetry and significant neck rotation limitation (148,156,157). Treatment delay also adversely effects outcome. Surgery is reserved for those lesions that fail conservative therapy, typically after 1 year of age and may include resection or muscle release (149).

Radiographs are typically normal, although lytic lesions in the clavicle at the insertion of the clavicular head of the sternocleidomastoid muscle may occasionally be seen (153). Sartoris et al. (153) suggest that the associated bone lesion is more frequent than appreciated, since radiographs are often not obtained. Other skeletal abnormalities reported with fibromatosis colli include ipsilateral lateral mandibular asymmetry, ipsilateral mastoid process hypertrophy, scoliosis capitis, facial deformities, elevation of the ipsilateral clavicle and shoulder, and postural cervicothoracic scoliosis (153).

Ultrasonography remains the modality of choice for the evaluation of fibromatosis colli because it is inexpensive and uses no ionizing radiation in these infants (Fig. 6.16). Fibromatosis colli demonstrates varying findings from a homogeneously enlarged sternocleidomastoid muscle to a hypoechoic mass, with ill-defined to well-defined margins within the substance of the sternocleidomastoid muscle (149,158,159) (Fig. 6.16). The echogenicity of the mass varies with the age of the lesion (149). Typically, the lesion affects the lower two-thirds of the muscle. If the mass extends beyond the boundaries of the muscle or there is significant lymphadenopathy, other diagnoses should be considered (149,158).

On unenhanced CT scan, fibromatosis colli appears as a homogeneously enlarged sternocleidomastoid muscle without a focal mass (158). Davids et al. (150) reported the MR imaging appearance in ten cases, noting that in no case was a discrete mass seen in the sternocleidomastoid muscle. The muscle was enlarged (two to four times normal size) and showed diffuse, abnormal signal intensity that was greater than that of fat on T2-weighted MR images (Figs. 6.16 and 6.17). Whyte et al. (155) reported a case in which T1-weighted MR images showed an enlarged, abnormally shaped sternocleidomastoid muscle, with poorly defined, decreased signal intensity. In a single patient with a chronic lesion, the MR imaging was compatible with atrophy and fibrosis, without inflammation or edema.

Infantile Fibromatosis

Infantile fibromatosis is the childhood equivalent of the adult desmoid tumor and was first described by Stout in 1954 (120). This lesion is also referred to as *aggressive infantile fibromatosis*. The WHO includes this lesion in the group of desmoid-type fibromatoses (4). The majority of cases present as a firm, solitary, nodular mass, usually in

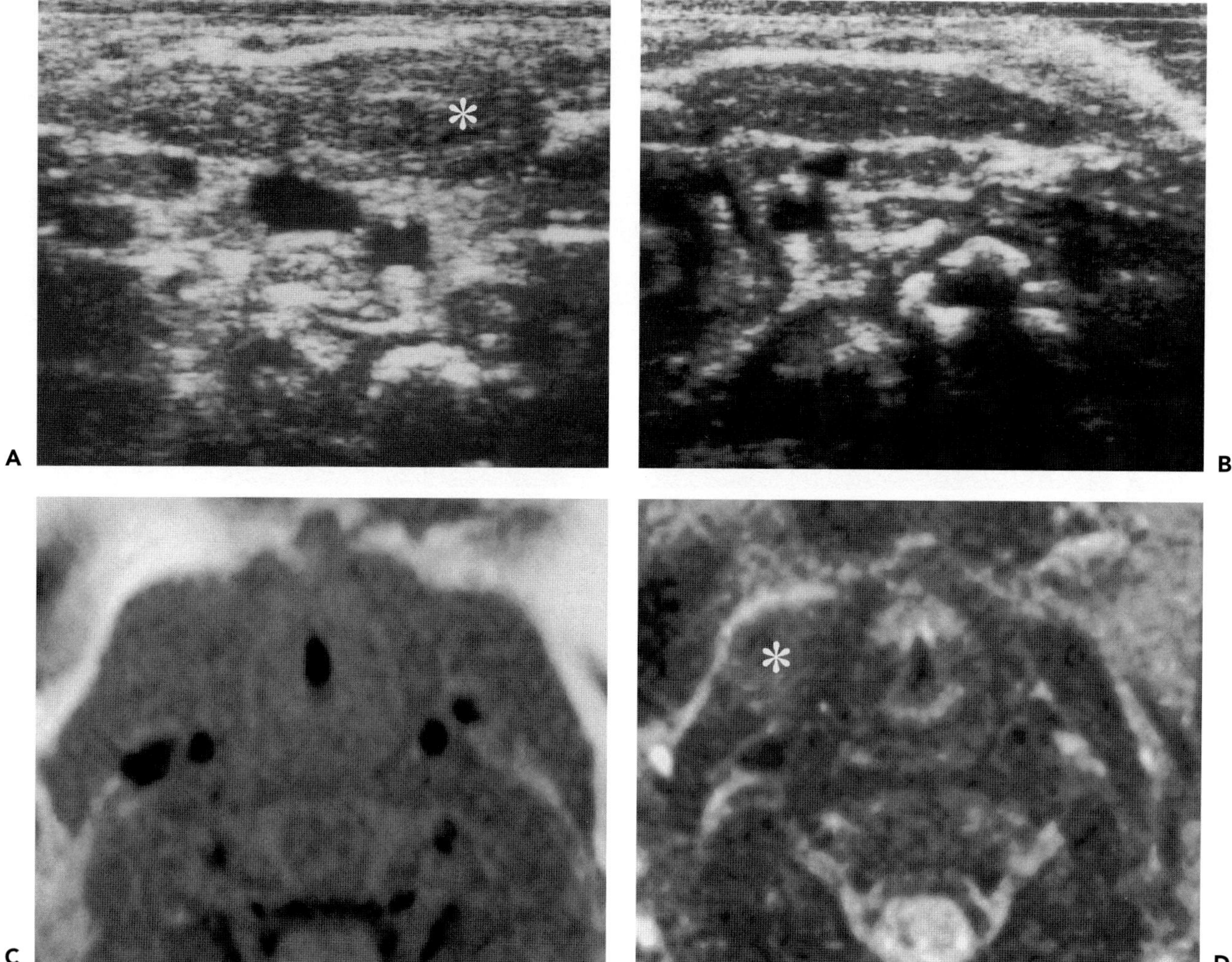

Figure 6.16   Fibromatosis colli in a girl 6 weeks of age. **A,B:** Axial ultrasound of the affected right **(A)** and normal left **(B)** sternocleudomastoid muscle show a diffusely enlarged right sternocleido-mastoid muscle (*asterisk* in **A**) without a focal mass. **C,D:** Axial T1-weighted (TR/TE; 800/15) **(C)** and T2-weighted (TR/TE; 2000/90) **(D)** spin-echo MR images of the neck show a poorly defined mass (*asterisk* in **D**) in the anterior aspect of the sternocleidomastoid muscle. Note some increased signal intensity at the periphery of the muscle. The lesion is not defined on T1-weighted images and shows a signal intensity similar to that of skeletal muscle.

> ## KEY CONCEPTS
> - Infantile fibromatosis is the child equivalent to adult desmoid tumor.
> - It most commonly affects the head/neck, shoulder, and thigh in the first 2 years of life.
> - Lesions are benign with no metastatic potential, but high local recurrence rate (up to 65% in one study).
> - Treatment is surgical resection.
> - Cross-sectional imaging appearance is similar to desmoid tumor.

skeletal muscle or adjacent fascia, aponeurosis, or periosteum (160). The lesion is most common in the head and neck (particularly the tongue, mandible region, maxilla, and mastoid process), shoulder, and thigh (1). Infantile fibro-matosis typically presents in the first 2 years of life and rarely after 8 years of age (1,160). The lesion is slightly more common in boys (1). Clinically, the typical presentation is that of a solitary ill-defined mass that initially rapidly enlarges, often without pain. No familial pattern is described. Antecedent trauma is reported in up to 17% of patients (161).

At gross pathologic evaluation, the lesion appears as a gray-white nodular mass. Infantile fibromatosis is not encapsulated and infiltrates the surrounding muscle and fat, often measuring 1 to 10 cm (160). Microscopy reveals several histologic patterns that reflect the differentiation of fibroblasts from a primitive mesenchymal form to a lesion that closely resembles the adult desmoid tumor (1,160). The immature form, sometimes referred to as the *diffuse (mesenchymal) type of infantile fibromatosis,* is most frequent and characterized by small, haphazardly arranged

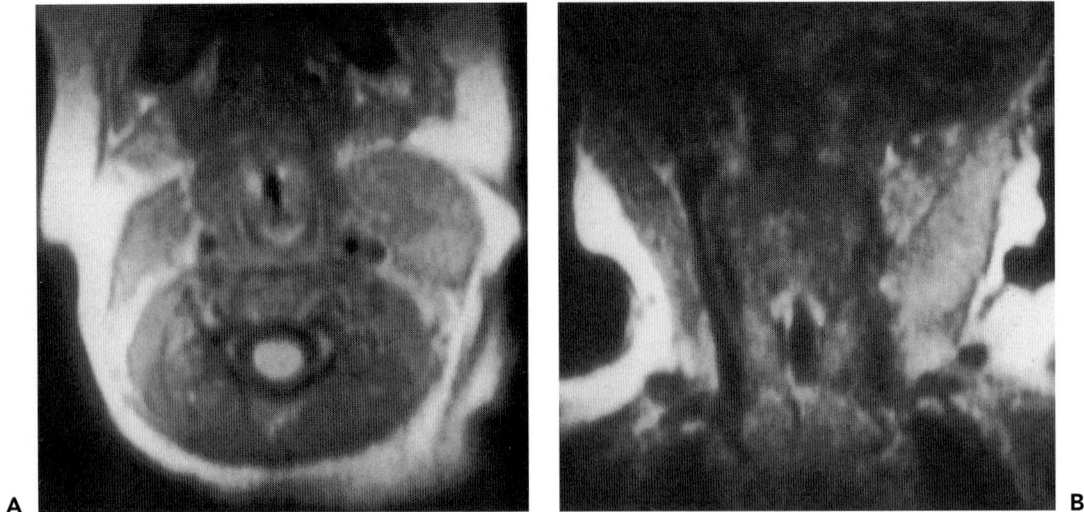

Figure 6.17 Fibromatosis colli. Axial **(A)** and coronal **(B)** T1-weighted spin-echo MR images show diffuse enlargement of the left sternocleidomastoid muscle, without discrete mass. (Courtesy of Wendy R. K. Smoker, MD.)

cells associated with reticulin fibers and mucoid material (1). This type of infantile fibromatosis may also be quite cellular, with mitoses and may mimic infantile fibrosarcoma. It is also referred to as *cellular fibromatosis, fibrosarcomalike fibromatosis,* and *aggressive infantile fibromatosis* (1). The less common form of infantile fibromatosis demonstrates more mature-appearing spindle-shaped fibroblasts that are arranged in a fascicular pattern, identical to that of desmoid-type fibromatosis (1). These histologic forms may coexist in a single lesion (1).

Infantile fibromatosis has no metastatic potential but has a high rate of local recurrence (65% in one study), particularly if not adequately resected (134,162,163). Most local recurrences are seen in the first year (51%) following resection, with 90% in the first 3 postoperative years (163). Complete resection with wide margins is the treatment of choice for infantile fibromatosis. Chemotherapy or radiation therapy are of uncertain benefit in unresectable or recurrent cases (164,165).

Radiographs reveal a soft tissue mass that may be associated with osseous bowing and deformity (166) (Fig. 6.18). Facial lesions frequently involve bone, and the origin is difficult to identify, as is exclusion of desmoplastic fibroma (167). Cintora et al. (160) reported ultrasonography in a single case. This lesion was homogeneous and hypoechoic to adjacent skeletal muscle (167). CT of the lesion demonstrated an ill-defined, homogeneous tumor with attenuation similar to or slightly greater than that of skeletal muscle (Fig. 6.18). Extensive ossification has been reported but is likely rare (168). In our experience, cross-sectional imaging of infantile fibromatosis is similar to that of desmoid tumors (see subsequent discussion) (Figs. 6.18 and 6.19).

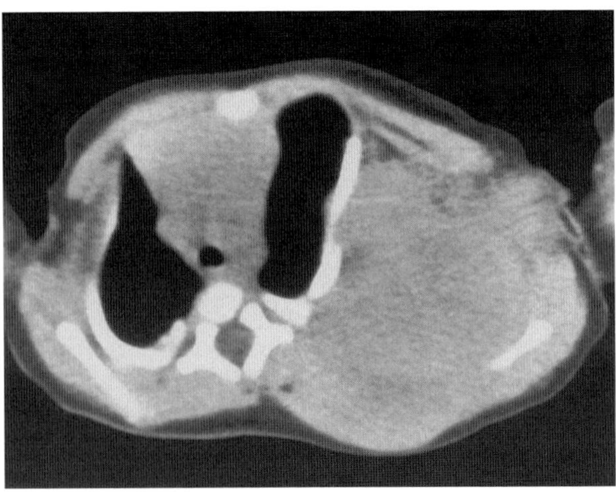
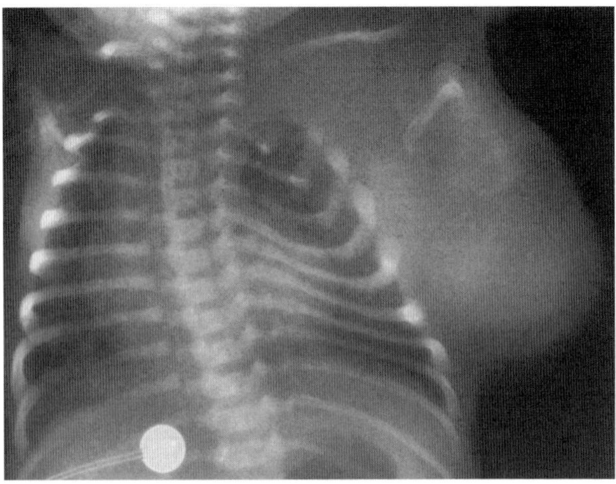

Figure 6.18 Infantile fibromatosis of the chest wall in a newborn infant. **A:** Axial CT of the chest shows a large mass without calcification. **B:** Anteroposterior radiograph of the chest shows a large mass with associated deformity of the chest wall and displacement of the scapula.

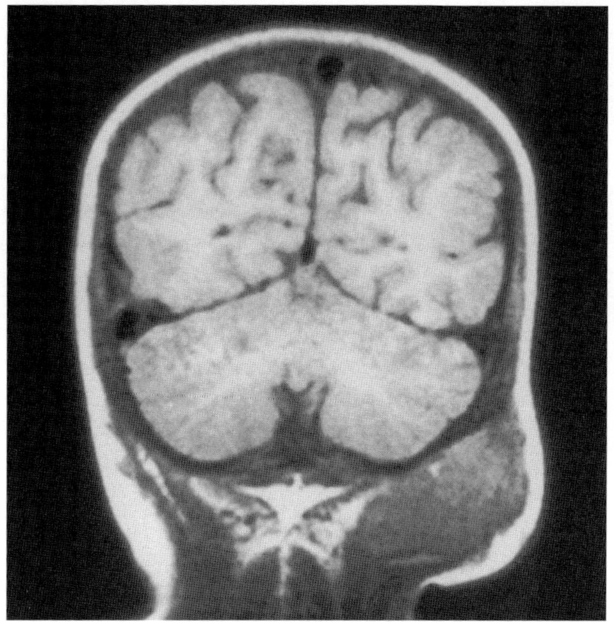
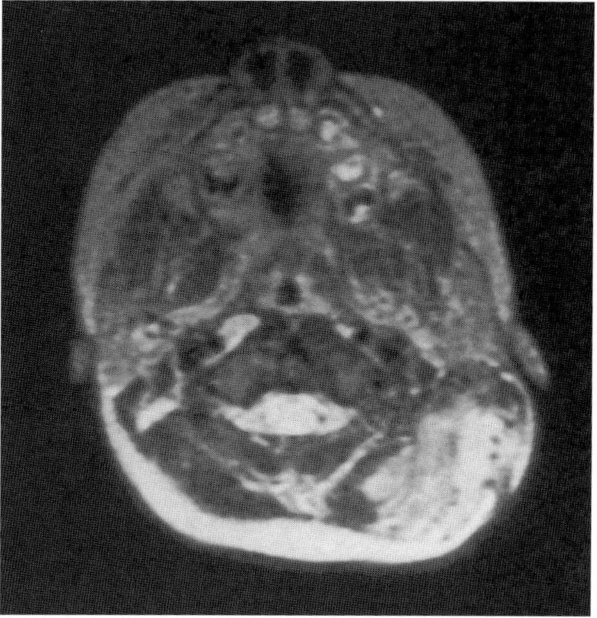

Figure 6.19 Infantile fibromatosis in a girl 3 years of age. **A,B:** Coronal T1-weighted (TR/TE; 800/20) **(A)** and T2-weighted (TR/TE; 3000/18) **(B)** MR images of the neck show a relatively well-defined superficial mass.

Lipofibromatosis

Lipofibromatosis, a rare fibrofatty tumor of childhood, was described by Fetsch et al. and is also known as *infantile fibromatosis, nondesmoid type* (169). Lipofibromatosis most commonly affects the hands and feet in infants (including newborns) and children, with a male predilection (2:1 ratio) (4,169). Other reported sites of involvement include the thigh, trunk, and head (4,169).

At gross pathologic examination, these lesions usually measure 1 to 3 cm (median: 2 cm) with a yellowish fatty component and whitish fibrous streaks (4). Histologically, the fat is mature adipose tissue with the cellular fibrous tissue along septae. These lesions were likely previously diagnosed as infantile fibromatosis or fibrous hamartoma of infancy.

This lesion has a high rate of local recurrence following attempts at surgical excision. There is no metastatic potential.

Imaging of lipofibromatosis has not been reported, to the best of our knowledge. We would expect MR imaging to identify an infiltrative, intermixed lesion of fat and non-specific soft tissue intensity, affecting the hands and feet.

Calcifying Aponeurotic Fibroma

Calcifying aponeurotic fibroma was initially described by Keasbey in 1953 as a very rare, distinctive, locally aggressive but self-limiting fibroblastic lesion in the palms and soles of small children (170). Because of the age group affected, this lesion is also referred to as *juvenile aponeurotic fibroma* (4,5,31,117). Patients typically are young, and the majority present in the first two decades of life (peak incidence: 8 to 14 years of age) (4,5,31,117). However,

> ### KEY CONCEPTS
> - Calcifying aponeurotic fibroma is a locally aggressive but self-limiting benign fibroblastic lesion.
> - It most frequently affects the palms of the hand (67% to 75%) and soles of the feet in the first two decades of life.
> - Males are more commonly affected than females (2:1 ratio).
> - Treatment includes conservative surgical resection but local recurrence is seen in up to 52% of cases.
> - Imaging shows a mass with frequent fine-stippled calcification and additional features similar to other fibromatoses.

patients in their fifth and sixth decades have been reported with this lesion (4,5,31,117,171). Males are affected twice as often as females (171,172). The lesion is relatively rare and represented only 0.4% of all benign soft tissue tumors seen by the Department of Soft Tissue Pathology at the AFIP during the 10-year period starting January 1, 1980 (135). The lesion has a predilection for the deep volar fascia, tendons, and aponeuroses, particularly those involving the hand, with 67% to 75% of lesions occurring in this location (170–174). The foot is the second most commonly involved site with other locations (neck, forearm, thigh, popliteal fossa, and lumbosacral region) only rarely affected (4,5,31,117). Clinical presentation is usually that of an asymptomatic, poorly circumscribed, firm mass, which develops slowly over a period of months to years. The lesion is typically painless and does not limit range of motion. The growth rate is variable and seems to be less in older patients (171,175). There is no reported familial incidence.

At gross pathologic examination, calcifying aponeurotic fibroma is usually a poorly defined, gray to white subcutaneous nodule that is less than 3-cm in size (4,5,31,117). Microscopically, the lesion is characterized by a diffuse proliferation of mesenchymal fibroblastlike elements with blunt nuclei and abundant ill-defined cytoplasm (171,173). Cells show a parallel orientation, in sharp contrast to the "herringbone" pattern seen in many fibroblastic lesions, with rare mitoses (170). Calcification is usually more centrally located and appears to be more common in cases affecting older patients.

Conservative initial resection is the treatment of choice, despite the high local recurrence rate of 52% (175). Local recurrence is usually seen within 3 years and more likely in younger patients (175). Reexcision of local recurrence, rather than more aggressive resection, is preferred to maintain function. Rare malignant transformation with metastases has been reported.

Radiographs may reveal a nonspecific soft tissue mass that shows fine stippled calcification (170,171,173,176) (Figs. 6.20 and 6.21). The mass rarely causes extrinsic erosion of the adjacent bone (173). The appearance of the lesion is not characteristic, although our limited MR imaging experience reveal features similar to those of the other fibromatoses (Figs. 6.20 and 6.21).

Inclusion Body Fibromatosis

KEY CONCEPTS

- Inclusion body fibromatosis is a unique lesion distinguished from other types of fibromatosis by the age group affected and peculiar intracytoplasmic perinuclear inclusion bodies.
- It is congenital in up to 33% of cases, with more than 80% of patients diagnosed before the age of 1 year.
- The fingers (particularly the third through fifth rays) account for 60% of cases, with 40% involving the toes.
- Local excision is the treatment of choice, with a 60% local recurrence rate. Spontaneous regression may occur.
- Imaging appearance is similar to that of other forms of fibromatosis.

Inclusion body fibromatosis is a unique tumor that occurs almost exclusively in the fingers and toes of infants. The lesion was likely first described by Jensen et al. in 1957 but referred to as *digital neurofibrosarcomas* (177). Subsequently, Reye and Enzinger, both in 1965, reported nine and seven lesions, respectively (178). The lesion is separated from other infantile fibromatoses by its characteristic location and age group, as well as a peculiar intracytoplasmic perinuclear inclusion body from which its name is derived (179). Former synonymous terms for this entity include *infantile digital fibromatosis, Reye tumor, digital fibrous tumor of infancy and childhood, infantile digital fibroma,* and *infantile digital myofibroblastoma* (4,5,31,117, 179,180). The

lesion is congenital in up to 33% of cases and more than 80% of cases are diagnosed within the first year of life (178,180,181). Involvement in older patients is rare. Girls appear to be affected slightly more than boys, unlike other fibromatoses (178,180–182). There is no familial tendency.

Patients usually present with an asymptomatic, smooth, dome-shaped nodular nontender mass involving the extensor surface of the digits, usually the dorsal or lateral aspect at the level of the distal or middle phalangeal joint of the digit (179). The fingers are affected in approximately 60% of cases (particularly the third, fourth, and fifth rays); 40% involve the toes (4,5,31,117). Involvement of the thumb is rare, and no cases of a great toe location have been reported, to the best of our knowledge. Simultaneous involvement of both fingers and toes has also been reported (181). Nodules may be single or multifocal and multiple digits may be involved (183,184). An equal number of patients have single or multiple lesions (182). Superficial ulceration may rarely occur, as may digit deformities.

At gross pathologic examination, lesions are almost invariably smaller than 2 cm, nodular, poorly circumscribed, and involve the subcutaneous tissue (4,5,31,117). Microscopically, the lesion is similar to other fibromatoses, with interdigitating fascicles of uniform spindle cells. It is composed of proliferating spindle-shaped cells, with ultrastructural features of myofibroblasts (185). The characteristic eosinophilic intracytoplasmic inclusion bodies are related to contractile proteins, likely composed of actin filaments, and derived from degradation products of actomyosin (179,180,183). The cytoplasmic inclusions appear to be specific and are not found in the other childhood fibromatoses.

Local excision is the treatment of choice. The prognosis is excellent, despite a 60% local recurrence rate (180,181). In a review of the literature by Beckett and Jacobs in 1977 (181), spontaneous regression was noted in 5 (8%) of 60 cases. The natural course of untreated lesions is unclear; however, the documented lack of metastatic potential and the possibility of spontaneous regression suggest conservative initial management as the optimal course. If surgery is required, the lesion must be removed totally because of the substantial risk of local recurrence (181). Angular deformities or contractures may persist following operative removal and require surgical correction. These lesions have no malignant potential (179,181).

Radiographs may be normal or show a soft tissue mass. The underlying bone is typically normal, although cases of osseous erosion and invasion are reported. We would expect cross-sectional imaging to reveal features similar to those of other superficial fibromatoses (Fig. 6.22).

Fibrous Hamartoma of Infancy

The fibrous hamartoma of infancy is a rare, benign lesion first described in 1956 by Reye (186) in a report of six

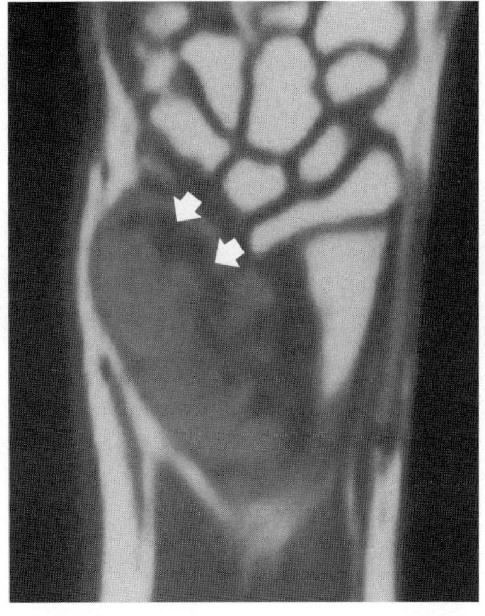

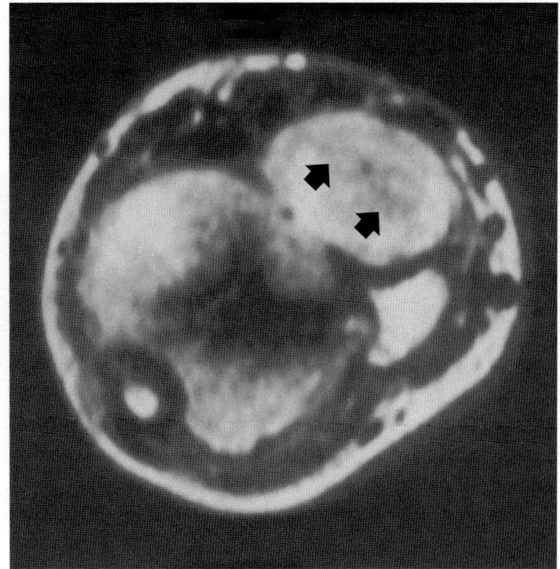

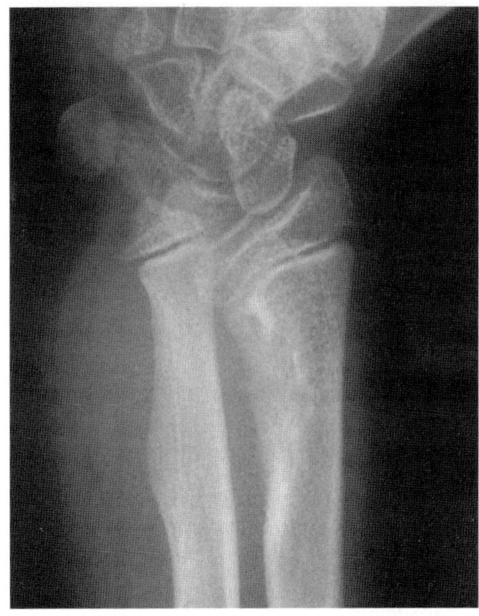

Figure 6.20 Calcifying aponeurotic fibroma of the forearm in a girl 11 years of age. **A,B:** Coronal T1-weighted (TR/TE; 800/20) **(A)** and axial T2-weighted (TR/TE; 2000/70) **(B)** spin-echo of the forearm show a lobulated, heterogeneous, soft tissue mass. The signal intensity of the lesion is greater than that of skeletal muscle on T1-weighted image and similar to that of fat on corresponding T2-weighted image. Within the mass are areas of decreased signal intensity on both pulse sequences, several of which have a band-like appearance (*arrows*). Although not pathognomonic, this MR appearance suggests a fibrous lesion, specifically a fibromatosis. **C:** Radiograph, corresponding to **A,** shows well-defined osseous remodeling and extrinsic erosion of bone.

KEY CONCEPTS

- Fibrous hamartoma of infancy represents a rare benign tumor recapitulating embryonic stages of connective tissue development.
- Lesions are congenital in 17% to 33% of cases and are seen before the age of 2 years.
- Boys are more frequently affected (3:1 ratio).
- The most common location is the subcutaneous fat of the axilla and upper extremity, accounting for 50% to 67% of cases.
- Surgical resection is the treatment of choice, with local recurrence reported in 10% to 16% of cases.
- MR imaging shows a nonspecific mass with low-to-intermediate signal intensity on all pulse sequences and interspersed adipose tissue.

infants with subcutaneous tumors. He termed these lesions *subdermal fibromatous tumors of infancy,* noting they were probably a reparative process rather than a true neoplasm (186). The term *fibrous hamartoma of infancy* was coined by Enzinger in 1965, in a report of 30 cases from the AFIP, to emphasize that the tumor is best categorized among the dysontogenic lesions and as a hamartoma (187). The concept that the lesion is a hamartoma was confirmed by ultrastructural studies, with the components of the tumor recapitulating embryonic stages of connective tissue development (188). Overall, this lesion is rare and accounts for only 0.02% of all benign soft tissue tumors, but is relatively more frequent in early childhood (4,5,31,117).

Fibrous hamartoma of infancy usually affects patients younger than 2 years (median: 10 months) (4,5,31,117).

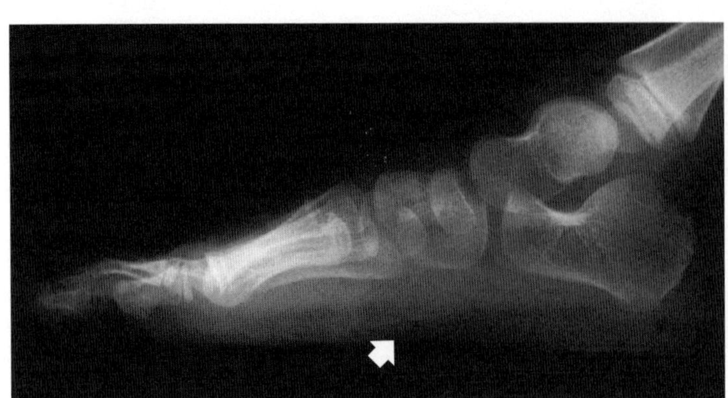

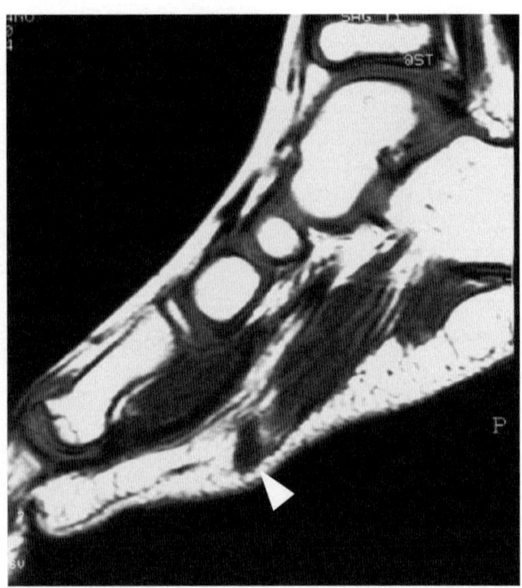

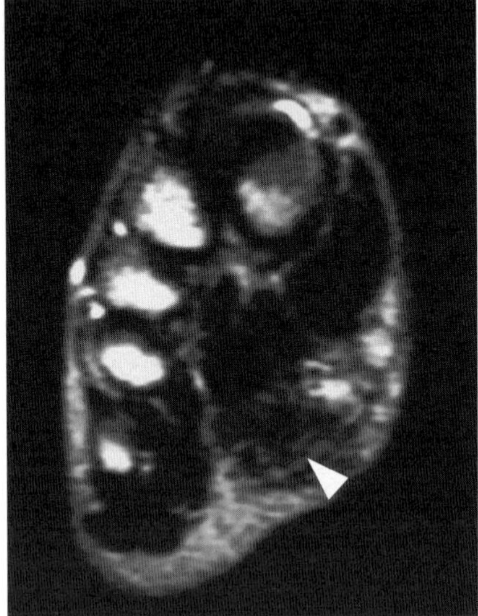

Figure 6.21   Calcifying aponeurotic fibroma in the foot of a boy 5 years of age. **A:** Lateral foot radiograph shows a vague plantar soft tissue mass (*arrow*) with faint calcification. **B,C:** Sagittal T1-weighted (TR/TE; 600/34) **(B)** and coronal T2-weighted (TR/TE; 2000/100) spin-echo MR images reveal the soft tissue mass (*arrowheads*) related to the plantar aponeurosis with intermediate signal intensity on T1-weighting and predominantly low signal intensity on T2-weighting.

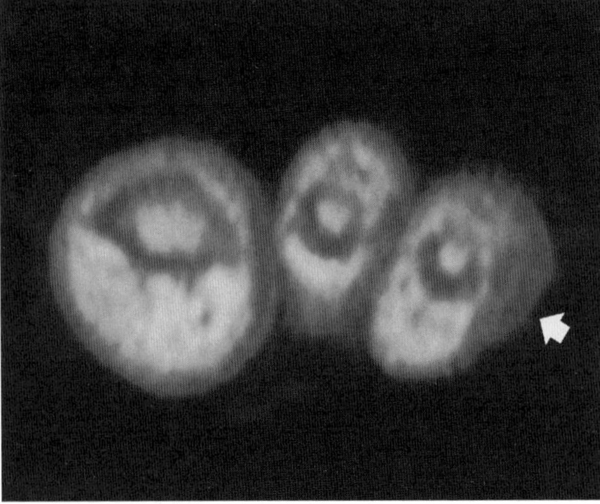

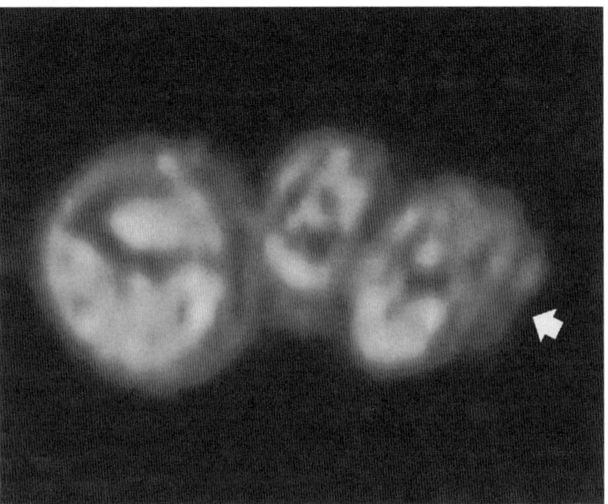

Figure 6.22   Inclusion body fibromatosis in the third toe of a girl 10 months of age with previous amputations of the fourth and fifth toes. **A,B:** Coronal T1-weighted (TR/TE; 600/15) **(A)** and T2-weighted (TR/TE; 2300/90) **(B)** MR images of the foot show a small superficial nodule in the lateral dorsal aspect of the third toe (*arrow*).

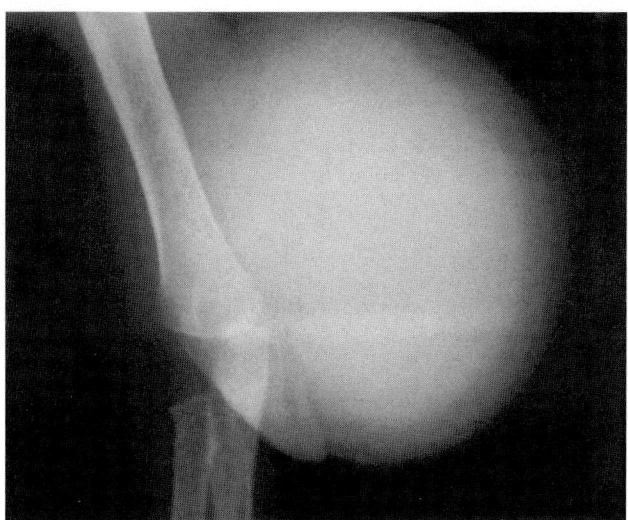

Figure 6.23   Fibrous hamartoma of infancy in the soft tissues of the elbow of a boy 12 months of age. The mass had grown rapidly over the preceding 6 months.

Lesions are congenital in 17% to 33% of cases and not reported to occur after puberty (186,187). As in the other fibrous proliferations of infancy, boys are much more commonly affected, by as much as a 3:1 ratio (189). Clinical presentation is that of a solitary soft tissue mass that is usually freely movable. These lesions initially may grow rapidly, with subsequent reduction in growth rate (187). The most common locations are the axilla and the upper extremity, with 50% to 67% of lesions occurring in these locations (187). Other reported sites include the thigh, inguinal area, pubic region, and back. No familial tendency is reported.

Fibrous hamartoma of infancy is located in the dermis or subcutaneous fat (187). At gross pathologic examination, these lesions are firm, rounded nodules (usually 3 to 5 cm in size, although larger lesions have been reported), with grayish-white tissue intermixed with small islands of adipose tissue (187). These lesions are typically not well-circumscribed. Macroscopic cysts were seen in 3 (10%) of 30 patients reported by Enzinger (187). Microscopically, the lesion consists of dense fibrocollagenous tissue, resembling fetal tendon, immature-appearing, loose textured cellular areas, and mature fat interposed between the two areas (187,190). The amount of fat may vary from scant to the majority of the lesion, suggesting a lipoma (187).

Local excision is the treatment of choice, with local recurrence seen in approximately 10% to 16% of cases (187). This local recurrence rate is much lower than that seen in many other types of fibromatoses. Local recurrence is usually early, within a few months of initial surgery, and cured by reexcision (187). Lesions do not regress spontaneously or metastasize.

As one would suspect, there is a paucity of literature depicting the imaging appearance of fibrous hamartoma of infancy, because this lesion is rare, small, and subcutaneous. Radiographs may show a soft tissue mass or appear normal (Fig. 6.23). The cross sectional imaging appearance reflects the histologic composition of the lesion. Lesions involve the subcutaneous tissue, showing nonspecific low-to-intermediate signal intensity on T1- and T2-weighted MR images, with interspersed tissue imaging similar to that of fat (191,192) (Fig. 6.24).

THE FIBROMATOSES

Fibromatosis refers to a family of soft tissue lesions characterized by a proliferation of benign fibrous tissue, composed of uniform, elongated, fusiform, or spindle-shaped cells surrounded and separated by variable degrees of collagen (1). Their biologic behavior is intermediate between that of benign fibrous lesions (such as fibroma or fasciitis) and that of fibrosarcoma, although they never metastasize (1,189,193). Synonymous terms include *nonmetastasizing fibrosarcoma* or *aggressive fibromatosis,* but these may be misleading because the clinical course of any individual tumor is unpredictable (1).

The fibromatoses are classified on the basis of their anatomic location as either superficial or deep by the WHO (4). The superficial group includes *palmar fibromatosis (Dupuytren contracture), plantar fibromatosis (Ledderhose disease), penile fibromatosis (Peyronie disease)* and *knuckle pads.* The deep, or musculoaponeurotic, fibromatoses include *extra-abdominal fibromatosis (aggressive fibromatosis), abdominal fibromatosis,* and *intra-abdominal fibromatosis.* In the study by Reitamo et al., abdominal wall lesions represented 49% of deep fibromatosis, while extra-abdominal and intra-abdominal lesions were 43% and 8%, respectively (194). The descriptive term *desmoid tumor* was coined in 1838 to emphasize the "bandlike or tendonlike" character of the lesions (from the Greek *desmos* meaning "band" or "tendon") (1,195–198). This chapter extensively discusses extra-abdominal fibromatoses with more limited evaluation of abdominal wall and intra-abdominal lesions.

Superficial Fibromatosis

The superficial fibromatoses are, in general, small lesions that usually arise from fascia or aponeuroses. These lesions are typically slowly growing, in sharp contrast to the deep fibromatoses that usually grow rapidly and are larger and more aggressive in their biologic behavior.

Palmar Fibromatosis

Fibromatosis arising from the palmar aponeurosis and its extensors is referred to as *Dupuytren contracture* or *Dupuytren disease,* named for the French physician who described it in 1831 (199,200). Dupuytren contracture is the most common type of fibromatosis, with an incidence ranging between 1% and 2% of the general population (4–6,201).

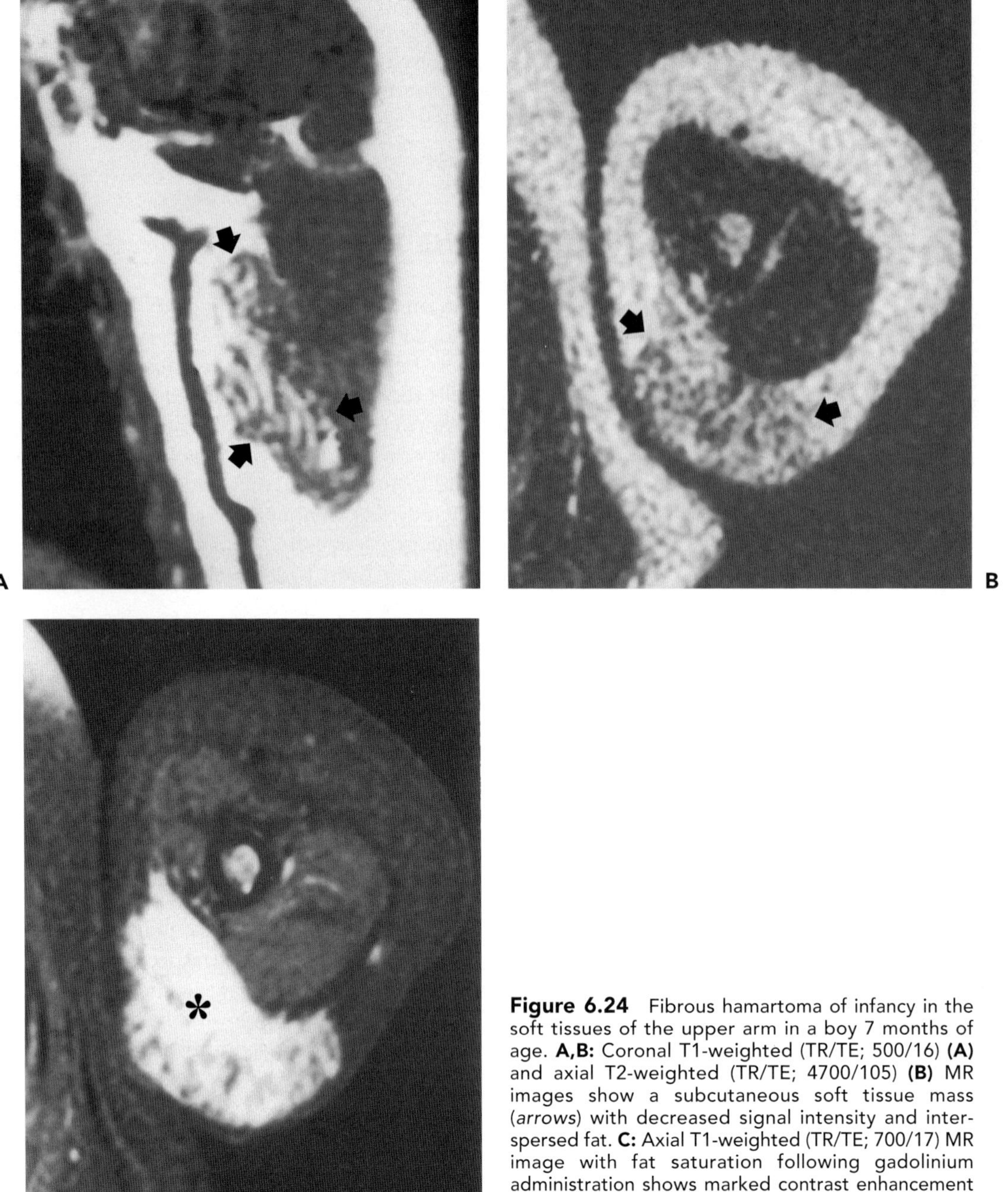

Figure 6.24 Fibrous hamartoma of infancy in the soft tissues of the upper arm in a boy 7 months of age. **A,B:** Coronal T1-weighted (TR/TE; 500/16) **(A)** and axial T2-weighted (TR/TE; 4700/105) **(B)** MR images show a subcutaneous soft tissue mass (*arrows*) with decreased signal intensity and interspersed fat. **C:** Axial T1-weighted (TR/TE; 700/17) MR image with fat saturation following gadolinium administration shows marked contrast enhancement (*asterisk*).

The incidence increases significantly with age and is reported as high as in 20% of those 65 years and older (4–6,201). Men are three to four times more commonly affected than women (199,202,203). The disease is particularly frequent in northern Europe and those lands settled by this population (4–6,201,204). Palmar fibromatosis is rare in the black population (4–6,201,205,206). There is a mild predilection to right-sided involvement, although bilateral involvement is seen in 40% to 60% of patients (4–6,201). The cause of palmar fibromatosis is not known, but theories of associations include genetic, trauma, microvascular injury, and an immunologic process (4–6,201).

Patients typically present with a slowly progressive, subcutaneous nodule in the palm of the hand, at the level of the distal palmar crease (Fig. 6.25). The fourth digit is the most commonly affected, followed by the fifth, third, and second rays (200). The nodules are frequently relatively asymptomatic. Intervening cords may develop between the nodules over the ensuing months or years, with associated contractures and puckering of the overlying skin. Progressive deformity results in significant functional impairment. Patients with palmar fibromatosis have additional areas of plantar fibromatosis in 5% to 20% of cases and penile fibromatosis in 2% to 4% of cases (207–209).

KEY CONCEPTS

- Palmar fibromatosis is the cause of Dupuytren contracture and affects 1% to 2% of the general population.
- The incidence of palmar fibromatosis significantly increases with age (reported as high as 20% in those older than 65 years).
- Men are affected more commonly (3–4:1 ratio).
- Bilateral involvement is seen in 40% to 60% of cases.
- Clinically there is a slowly progressive nodule- to cord-like mass causing contracture, most frequently affecting the ulnar digits.
- Surgical release/resection is the treatment of choice, although surgery in early lesions is to be avoided as local recurrence (up to 30% to 40% of patients) is increased.
- Ultrasonography and MR imaging reveal palmar masses adjacent to and causing contraction of the flexion tendons.
- Lesions are hypoechoic on sonography and low-to-intermediate signal intensity on all MR imaging pulse sequences. Intermediate signal intensity on long TR MR images is associated with more cellular lesions and a higher local recurrence rate following surgical resection.

Additional associations include diabetes mellitus (type 1 or 2), epilepsy, alcoholism (particularly those with liver disease), smoking, and patients with elevated cholesterol and triglycerides (210–213).

At gross pathologic examination, nodules are usually small, less than 1 cm, and poorly circumscribed, with interconnecting collagenized bands. The microscopic appearance depends on the lesion stage, with the earliest lesions being proliferative with whorls of fibroblasts, myofibroblasts, and fibrocytes. Mitoses may be prominent with a lesser extent of collagen. Chronic lesions contain much more collagen and lesser degrees of cellularity. Cytogenetic aberrations are described, particularly gains at chromosomes 7 and 8 (4).

Surgery remains the primary mode of therapy, with release of the flexion contracture. Early resection is generally avoided because of an increased tendency for lesions in the early proliferative stage to recur locally (200). Local recurrence is common, affecting 30% to 40% of patients (203). Fasciectomy may improve symptoms in patients not amenable to surgical resection. The lowest rate of local recurrence (<10%) is associated with dermato-fasciectomy with skin grafting, although this represents extensive surgical intervention (214,215). Radiation therapy was also used successfully in advanced disease by Keilholz et al. (216). These lesions have no metastatic potential.

Radiographs of palmar fibromatosis are usually normal other than visible flexion contractures. Ultrasonography reveals a hypoechoic mass in the palmar subcutaneous tissue, directly superficial to the flexor tendons, with skin retraction (217,218). Color Doppler imaging may show prominent vascularity (219). Flexion tendon function can be evaluated on real-time examination with the tendons smoothly sliding in their sheaths initially (25).

Yacoe et al. (200) reported the MR findings in 22 lesions of Dupuytren contracture in ten patients. They noted the lesions (cords) arise from the proximal palmar aponeurosis and extend distally and superficially, parallel to the flexor tendons (Fig. 6.25). The lesions varied in length from 10 to 55 mm and most often terminated in fine strands extending into the subcutaneous tissue at the level of the distal metacarpals. Less commonly, the lesion terminated as a nodule or other branching configuration. Associated subcutaneous nodules were seen in approximately 64% of cases (200). Yacoe et al. correlated the cellularity of lesions with their MR appearance. They noted all lesions had low signal intensity on T2-weighted MR images: 18 (82%) of 22 cords had uniform decreased signal intensity, and 4 (18%) had a low-to-intermediate signal on T1-weighted images. These lesions were hypocellular and mostly dense collagen. Eleven nodules that demonstrated intermediate signal intensity on both T1- and T2-weighted MR images were all either cellular or demonstrated a mixed histologic picture, with hypocellular and cellular regions. Interestingly, active cellular lesions have a higher local recurrence rate following surgical resection than do hypocellular lesions. This information is important for our clinical colleagues in planning surgery, to ensure optimal results. We strongly believe imaging of these patients should be performed more frequently, particularly with improved surface coil technology and resulting better resolution, to direct which lesions are optimal for surgical removal and to lessen the likelihood of local recurrence. Lesions with intermediate signal intensity on T1-weighted and T2-weighted MR images may well be more appropriately managed by delaying surgical resection, allowing maturation prior to excision (220). Follow-up MR imaging may be useful to identify maturation with increasing collagenization as evidenced by progressive decreased signal intensity, particularly on long TR images.

Plantar Fibromatosis

Plantar fibromatosis was first established as a distinct clinical entity by Ledderhose in 1897 (221), although it was reported by Dupuytren in 1832, who observed both palmar and plantar lesions in laborers (222,223). This disease is at times referred to as *Ledderhose disease*. It is characterized by a proliferation of fibrous tissue within the plantar aponeurosis, which eventually may extend into the skin or adjacent deep structures (222). Anatomically, the plantar aponeurosis may be divided into a medial and lateral compartment (222). The lateral portion, the *aponeurosis plantaris fibularis*, is rudimentary and absent in approximately 10% of the population (222). The medial portion, the *aponeurosis plantaris*

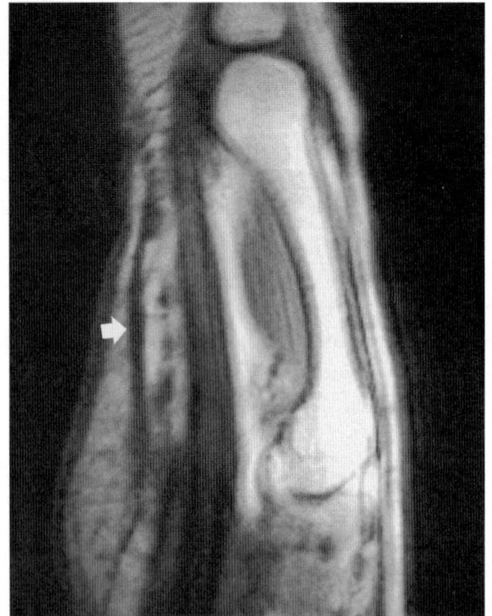
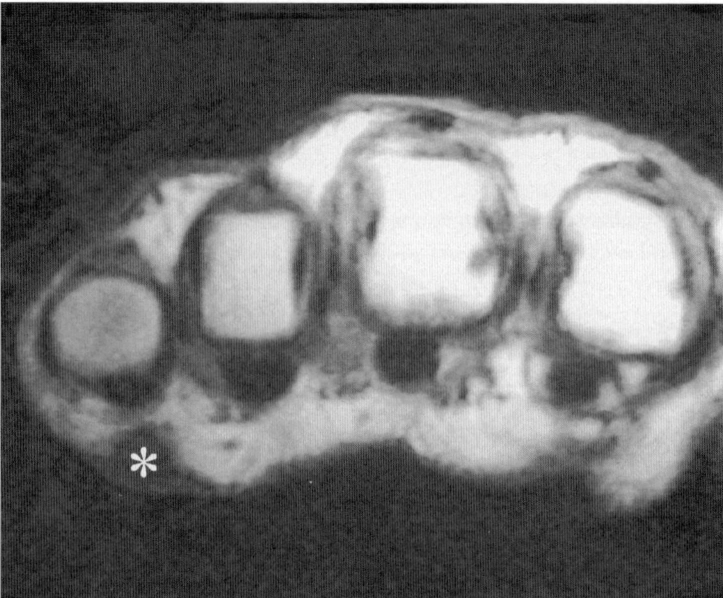

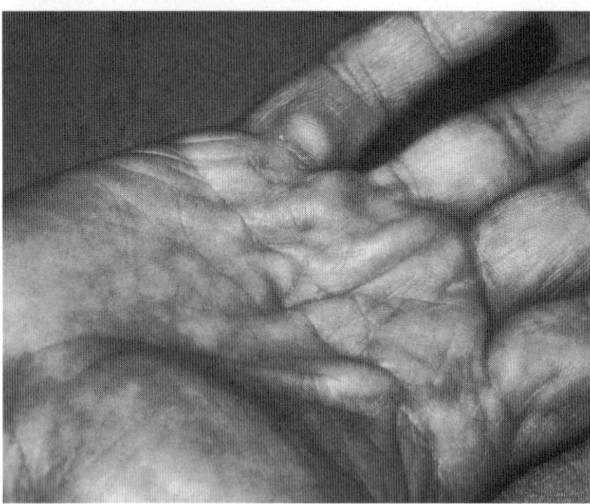

Figure 6.25 Palmar fibromatosis (Dupuytren contracture) in a man 62 years of age. **A:** Sagittal T1-weighted (TR/TE; 633/20) MR image of the fifth metacarpal shows a low-signal intensity cord (*arrow*) in the superficial palmar soft tissues. **B:** Axial Tl-weighted (TR/TE; 633/20) MR image shows a subcutaneous nodule (*asterisk*) which was the termination of the subcutaneous cord. **C:** Clinical photograph shows subcutaneous nodule at the base of the middle and little fingers as well as prominent subcutaneous cords.

KEY CONCEPTS

- Plantar fibromatosis (Ledderhose disease) represents a benign proliferation of fibrous tissue about the plantar aponeurosis (more common medially).
- The incidence increases with patient age and is reported to affect 0.23% of patients.
- There is a male predilection and involvement is bilateral in 20% to 50% in patients.
- Concomitant palmar involvement is seen in approximately 50% of patients.
- Clinically, patients reveal firm subcutaneous nodules on the soles of the feet that are multiple in 33% of cases.
- Surgical treatment is not usually required; modified footwear is the typical therapy.
- Sonography reveals hypoechoic to mixed echogenic elongated mass.
- MR imaging typically reveals intermediate signal intensity mass with linear tails of extension along the plantar aponeurosis. Contrast enhancement is common.

tibialis, is the primary constituent of the plantar aponeurosis (222). Plantar fibromatosis usually involves the non–weight-bearing medial portion of the aponeurosis. Plantar fibromatosis is much less frequent than palmar disease and was reported in 0.23% of patients by Yost et al. (203). The incidence also increases with age, similar to that of palmar disease, although there is a higher incidence in patients younger than 30 years compared to that of Dupuytren contracture (4–6,201). In fact, in one series, 35% of patients were younger than 30 years (4–6,201). Patients are typically adults or young adults, in the third through fifth decades, although there is a wide age spectrum. There is a male predilection but not as great as that seen with palmar fibromatosis (222). Bilateral involvement is seen in 20% to 50% (usually metachronous with an interval of 2 to 7 years), and concomitant palmar involvement is seen in approximately 50% (range: 9% to 69%) of patients (222,224). The palmar and plantar fibromatoses also usually occur metachronously with an interval of 5 to 40 years

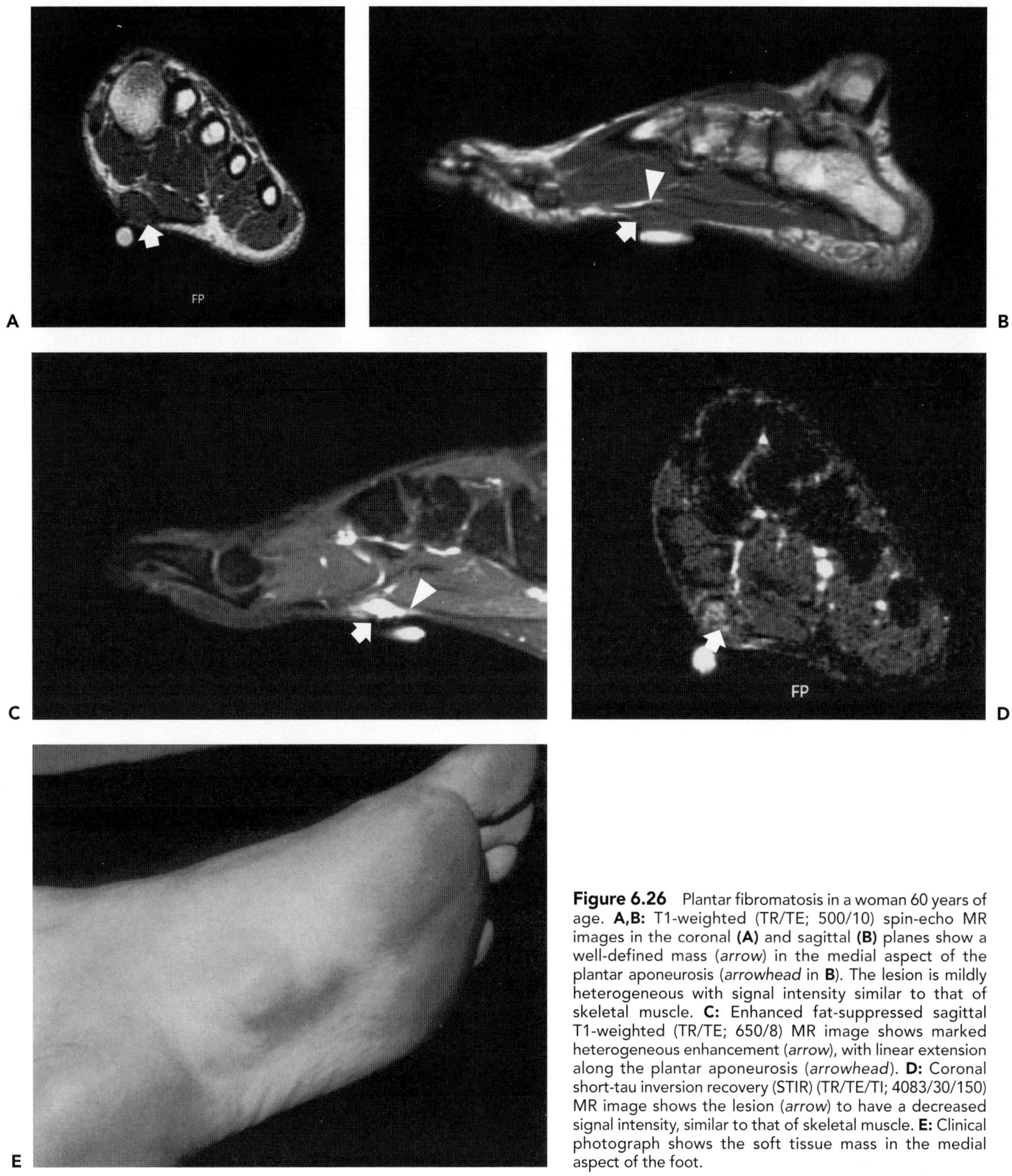

Figure 6.26 Plantar fibromatosis in a woman 60 years of age. **A,B:** T1-weighted (TR/TE; 500/10) spin-echo MR images in the coronal **(A)** and sagittal **(B)** planes show a well-defined mass (*arrow*) in the medial aspect of the plantar aponeurosis (*arrowhead* in **B**). The lesion is mildly heterogeneous with signal intensity similar to that of skeletal muscle. **C:** Enhanced fat-suppressed sagittal T1-weighted (TR/TE; 650/8) MR image shows marked heterogeneous enhancement (*arrow*), with linear extension along the plantar aponeurosis (*arrowhead*). **D:** Coronal short-tau inversion recovery (STIR) (TR/TE/TI; 4083/30/150) MR image shows the lesion (*arrow*) to have a decreased signal intensity, similar to that of skeletal muscle. **E:** Clinical photograph shows the soft tissue mass in the medial aspect of the foot.

(4–6,201). Knuckle pads are seen in 42% of patients (225). Associated Peyronie disease is quite uncommon and seen in no more than 1% to 4% of patients (222). Similar etiologic factors for palmar disease are implicated with plantar fibromatosis, including genetic and traumatic causes. Plantar fibromatosis, similar to palmar disease, is more common in diabetics (type 1 and 2), epileptics, and alcoholics with liver disease (4–6,201).

Patients typically present with one or more firm subcutaneous nodules on the plantar aspect of the foot (222) (Fig. 6.26). Plantar fibromatosis is more common medially. Multiple lesions are seen in approximately

33% of patients (223). Lesions may remain asymptomatic until late in the course of the disease, and symptoms may be secondary to mass effect or local invasion of adjacent muscles or neurovascular structures (222). In contradistinction to palmar disease, contractures are a rare sequela.

Pathologically (both grossly and microscopically), plantar fibromatosis is identical to palmar fibromatosis as previously described. Lesion size is usually 2 to 3 cm (4–6,201). Differences with palmar disease include less frequent multinodularity, lack of intervening fibrous cords, and less mitotic activity. Similar to palmar lesions, the degree of cellularity is variable. Cytogenetic aberrations include trisomies at chromosomes 8 and 14 (4).

Conservative treatment with molded shoes or inserts may be useful in patients with mild symptoms (226).

Unlike the treatment of palmar lesions, surgical resection is not usually required unless the lesions are large, infiltrating, or cause continued pain or disability. Intralesional steroid injection has been successful in the treatment of some cases (227). Simple surgical excision is associated with a high rate of local recurrence, most within 1 year following resection (228). More extensive resection with fasciectomy lowers the local recurrence rate. A higher local recurrence rate is associated with multiple nodules, bilateral lesions, family history, and those that develop a postoperative neuroma (4–6,201). Wide resection is augmented by radiation in cases with local recurrence (216). These lesions have no metastatic potential (222).

Radiographs are invariably normal in patients with plantar fibromatosis. Ultrasonography is reported to demonstrate a well-defined (64%) or ill-defined (36%),

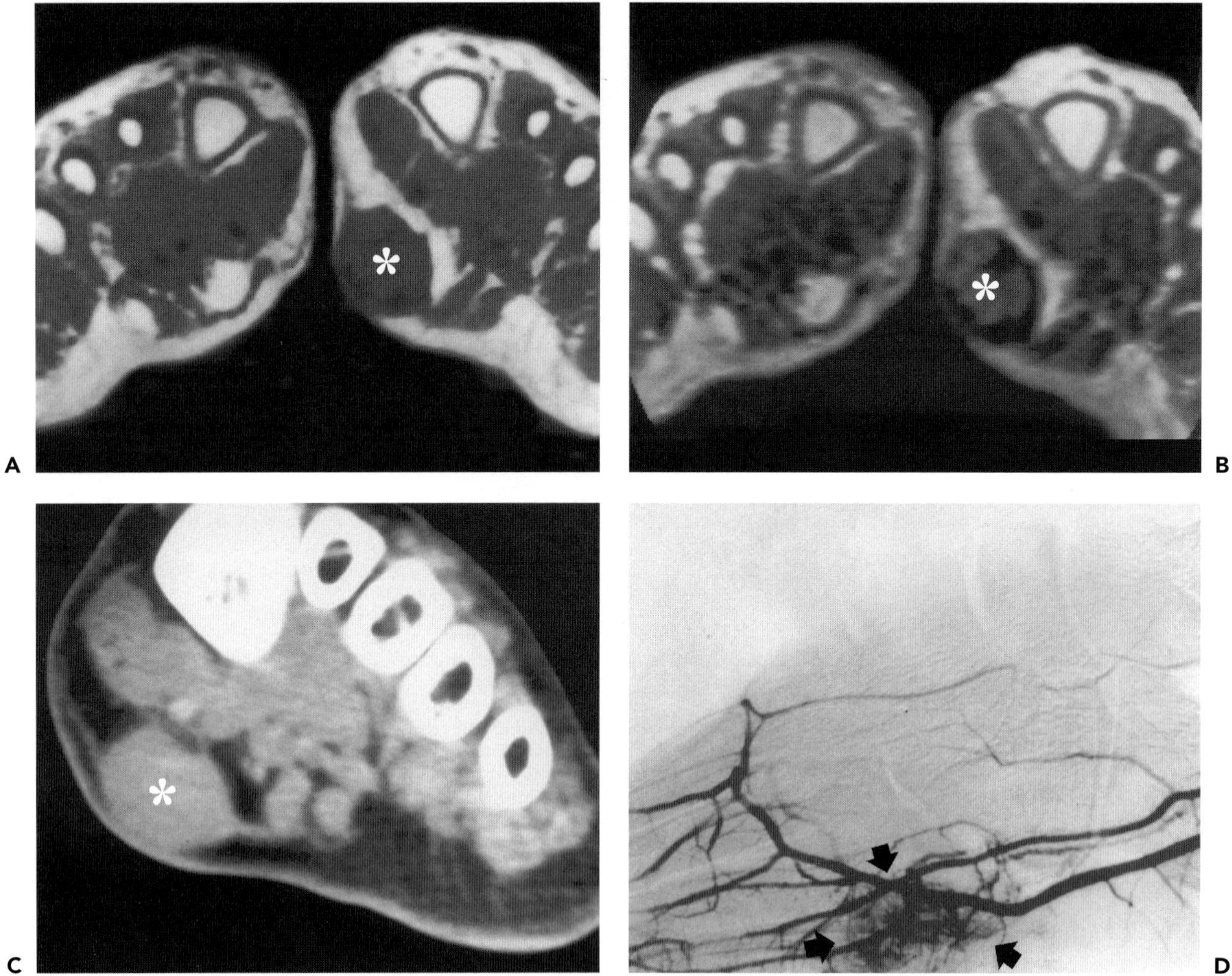

Figure 6.27   Plantar fibromatosis in a woman 27 years of age. **A,B:** Coronal T1-weighted (TR/TE; 550/26) **(A)** and T2-weighted (TR/TE; 1800/80) **(B)** spin-echo MR images show a well-defined heterogeneous soft tissue mass (*asterisk*) in the medial aspect of the plantar aponeurosis, with signal intensity similar to that of skeletal muscle on all pulse sequences. **C:** Corresponding short axis CT shows a nonspecific soft tissue mass (*asterisk*) in the medial aspect of the plantar aponeurosis. **D:** The lesion is hypervascular on arteriography (*arrows*).

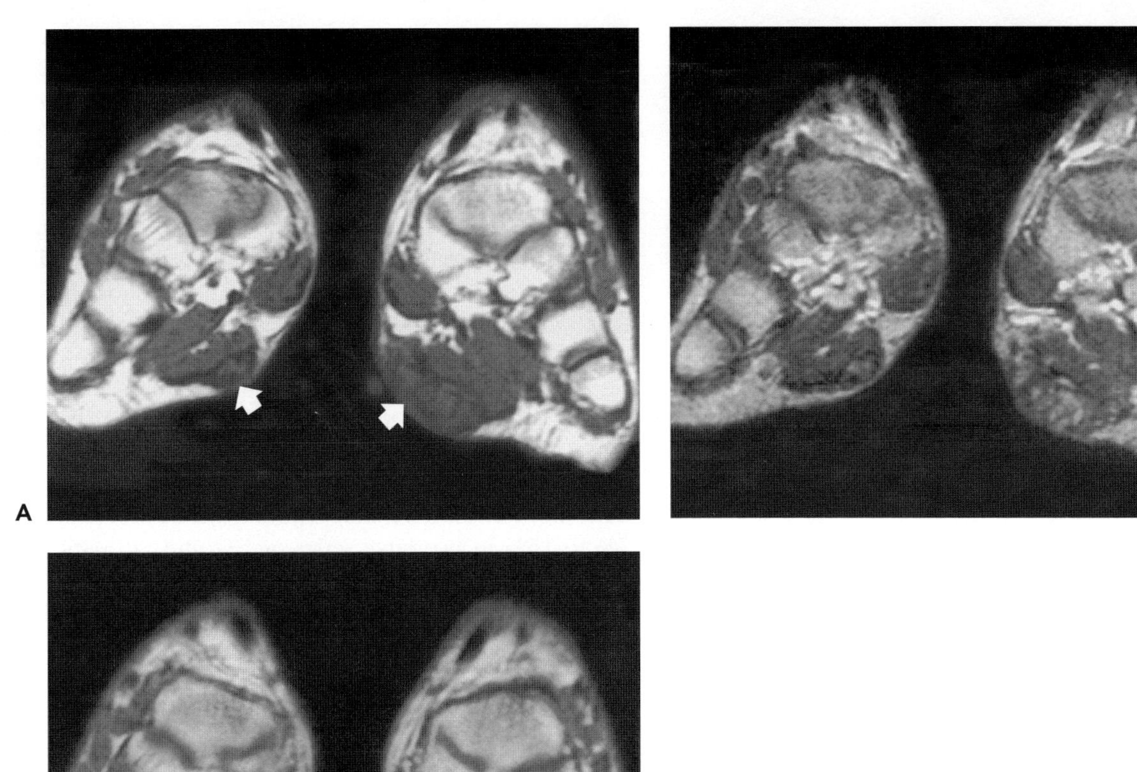

Figure 6.28 Bilateral plantar fibromatosis in a man 39 years of age. **A,B:** Coronal T1-weighted (TR/TE; 700/15) **(A)** and T2-weighted (TR/TE; 2500/80) **(B)** spin-echo MR images show heterogeneous masses in the medial aspect of the plantar aponeuroses (*arrows*). The lesions are well-defined by the adjacent subcutaneous fat but not well-delineated from the adjacent muscle. **C:** Coronal T1-weighted (TR/TE; 700/15) MR image following contrast administration shows moderate enhancement.

elongated, hypoechoic or mixed echoic, fusiform (76%) mass in the subcutaneous tissues superficial to the echogenic plantar fascia, either medially (60%) or centrally (40%) (219,229–231). Similar to palmar lesions, color Doppler sonography may reveal marked vascularity (92%) (218,219,232). Coexistent thickening of the plantar fascia at the calcaneal insertion was reported by Griffith et al. (232). CT shows a soft tissue mass with attenuation similar to or slightly higher that of muscle (Fig. 6.27).

On MR imaging, plantar fibromatosis demonstrates a relatively characteristic appearance (Figs. 6.26–6.28). Morrison et al. (223) described the MR findings in 27 lesions (in 16 patients). They noted lesions were typically located in the medial aspect of the plantar aponeurosis, with the lateral aspect affected in only 6 (22%) of 27 patients (223). Lesions were well-defined superficially against the subcutaneous fat, but they were inseparable from the muscle underlying the deep aponeurosis. The deep tissues were invaded in four (15%) patients (223).

On T1- and T2-weighted images, lesions were typically heterogeneous, with an overall signal intensity equal to or less than that of skeletal muscle (223). Five of six lesions evaluated with short-tau inversion recovery (STIR) images demonstrated a signal intensity hyperintense to that of muscle but less than that of fat, with the remaining lesion showing a signal intensity similar to that of muscle (223). Contrast enhancement was seen in 15 lesions, was heterogeneous, and varied from marked in nine (60%), mild in five (33%), to none in one (7%) (223) (Figs. 6.26 and 6.28). This appearance is similar to that noted by Wetzel and Levine (233) in reviewing the MR imaging of the foot, in which they reported one case of plantar fibromatosis that appeared as a nodular thickening of plantar aponeurosis and demonstrated decreased signal intensity on all pulse sequences. We have noted linear tails of extension (fascial tail sign) along the plantar aponeurosis are best seen after intravenous contrast administration, creating a fusiform shape (Fig. 6.26).

Deep Fibromatosis

KEY CONCEPTS

- The deep fibromatoses are benign fibrous lesions divided into extra-abdominal, abdominal wall, and intra-abdominal.
- These lesions are relatively common (2 to 4 per million people).
- Young adults (30 to 40 years) are most frequently affected, with a female predilection.
- Common locations include shoulder/upper arm (28%), chest wall/paraspinal (17%), and head/neck (10% to 23%).
- Deep fibromatosis is multicentric in 5% to 15% of cases and clinically presents as a slowly growing soft tissue mass. Lesions may invade neurovascular structures.
- Surgical resection is the usual treatment but local recurrence is common (19% to 77%). Radiation therapy may also be employed in treatment.
- CT shows a nonspecific soft tissue mass that may have ill-defined margins with enhancement.
- MR imaging appearance is variable with low-to-high signal intensity on T2-weighting, corresponding to the degree of collagenization in the lesion. Low signal intensity bands, extension along the superficial fascia (fascial tail sign), and enhancement are common.
- Signal intensity on long TR MR images may have an implication on tumor recurrence, with greater recurrence rate in lesions with high signal intensity.

The deep fibromatoses typically affect the fascia, septae, and aponeuroses between muscles. Historically, these lesions were divided into extra-abdominal, abdominal wall, and intra-abdominal. The WHO now refers to all of these lesions as the *desmoid-type fibromatoses* (4). We limit our discussion in this section to extra-abdominal lesions. Synonymous terms for these lesions include *musculoaponeurotic fibromatosis, extra-abdominal desmoid, desmoid tumor,* and *aggressive fibromatosis*. These lesions are relatively common, with an estimated incidence of 2 to 4 per million in the United States (700 to 900 new cases annually) (194,234). The deep fibromatoses are less common than their superficial counterparts. The deep musculoaponeurotic fibromatoses typically present in young adults between puberty and 40 years of age, with a peak incidence between 25 and 35 years of age (4,6,8,201). Cases are reported in infants and children, although this age group is less frequently affected (197,235). These lesions are more common in women (1,195). The deep fibromatoses may occur anywhere, with approximately 70% of cases involving the extremities (4,6,8,201). Specific locations for these lesions include the shoulder and upper arm (28%), chest wall/paraspinal (17%), thigh (12%), head/neck (10% to 23%), knee (7%), buttock/hip (6%), lower leg (5%), and forearm (4%) (4,6,8,201). Lesions in the head and neck often behave more aggres-

sively. These deep fibromatoses, particularly those in the axilla, often surround vital neurovascular structures, such as the brachial plexus, and are not amenable to complete resection. Lesion distribution is also affected by age. Juvenile lesions occur more frequently in girls and are typically in an extra-abdominal location. Young adults show a marked female predilection and affect the abdominal wall. In middle-aged adults, lesions show an equal sex distribution and are most common in an intra-abdominal location, while in older adults, lesions are seen in intra- and extra-abdominal sites, also with an equal sex distribution (194). The cause of these lesions is multifactorial, but likely involve genetic, endocrine and traumatic factors (4,6,8,201).

These tumors are usually solitary. However, synchronous multicentric lesions are reported, with a prevalence of 5% to 15% in two large series of 192 and 110 patients, respectively (195,236). Synchronous lesions are confined to the same extremity in 75% to 100% of cases (195,236); therefore, a second soft tissue mass in the extremity of a patient with a previously confirmed desmoid tumor should be regarded as a second desmoid tumor until proven otherwise (237).

Very rarely the lesion may be juxtacortical or periosteal. Dong et al. (238) reported a juxtacortical lesion in the forearm of a boy 14 years of age, noting it was impossible to determine if the tumor arose from the region of the interosseous membrane or within the periosteum of the adjacent bone.

Disler et al. (195) reported a skeletal dysplasia in 3 (18.8%) of 16 patients with multicentric fibromatosis. In two of these cases, the dysplastic changes were seen in all long bones and consisted predominantly of undertubulation similar to that seen in Pyle disease or the Erlenmeyer flask deformity of Gaucher disease. In the remaining case, these changes were seen only in the involved limb. Unlike Pyle disease, the skull was normal in all of these three patients, and in none of the cases was a marrow abnormality detected. Hayry et al. found an even higher incidence (80%) of associated osseous abnormalities, including cortical thickening, focal lucencies, bone islands, and osseous excrescences (239). Familial cases of fibromatosis have also been reported (1,237).

The clinical presentation of the deep fibromatoses is typically a poorly defined, firm, painless, slowly growing soft tissue mass. Limitation of range of motion, neurologic symptoms, and pain are unusual but are reported.

At gross pathologic examination, most tumors are between 5 and 10 cm in size and are firm, with a gritty consistency similar to that of scar tissue. Lesions are usually deep to the fascia or aponeurosis and growth may extend along these areas with poorly circumscribed margins. All fibromatoses show infiltrative growth and are indistinguishable on both gross and microscopic inspection (1) (Fig. 6.29). The growth pattern consists of relatively uniform fibroblasts with bland nuclei proliferating in parallel

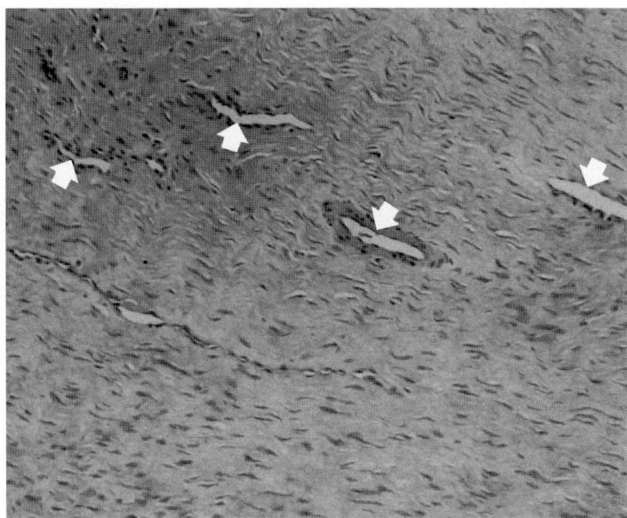

Figure 6.29 Histologic appearance of deep-type fibromatosis (extra-abdominal desmoid). Medium-power photomicrograph shows relatively uniform fibroblasts with bland nuclei proliferating in parallel arrays with a variable amount of intermingled collagen (original magnification 200×, hematoxylin and eosin). Vascular channels are also prominent (*arrows*).

arrays. There is a variable amount of intermingled collagen, in some cases relatively scant, in others more abundant (Fig. 6.29). In addition, other changes may be seen, including myxoid change, focal hemorrhage, vascularity (Fig. 6.29), and focal inflammation, perhaps induced by chronic trauma or injury (240). The relationship to surrounding tissue (subcutaneous fat and skeletal muscle) is marked by interdigitating, infiltrative growth. This last mentioned feature and extension along fascial planes likely accounts for the difficulty in establishing adequate margins of resection, thereby creating a predisposition for local recurrence due to incomplete excision. Cytogenetic aberrations, particularly trisomies at chromosomes 8 and 20, are identified in up to 30% of cases of deep fibromatosis (239,241,242).

The deep fibromatoses have no potential to metastasize but frequently recur locally (243,244). The local recurrence rate varies from 19% to 77% (average: approximately 40%), usually within the first 2 postoperative years (4,6,8,201,245). Features increasing the likelihood of local recurrence include large initial tumor size, patient age older than 30 years, female gender, and marginal/intralesional resection (4,6,8,201). Recurrence with wide-local excision is approximated at 20% to 50% compared to 90% with incomplete resection (236,245,246). Spontaneous regression is rarely reported. Although the treatment of choice for the deep fibromatoses is wide surgical excision, radiation therapy is also performed both as an adjunct and as the sole therapy in patients or lesions not amenable to resection. Local control is reported with adjunct radiation therapy in patients with positive surgical margins in 79% to 90% of cases (247). Radiation therapy alone is successful in treatment of deep fibromatoses

in several series with outcomes similar to those reported after surgery (248–250). Long-term risk of radiation-induced sarcomas is not reliably assessed in this group of patients. Chemotherapy is also proven effective in some aggressive cases. Other modes of therapy, including anti-inflammatory (prostaglandin-inhibiting) and anti-estrogen medications, are also used successfully in treatment of nonresponsive lesions (251–259). The overall 5-year survival is greater than 90% (236,260,261). However, despite this lesion's nonmalignant potential, local recurrence and involvement of vital local structures can lead to patient demise (particularly with neck and chest wall lesions). In extremity lesions, amputation may ultimately be required for local control.

Radiographs are usually normal, but may reveal a nonspecific soft tissue mass. Bone involvement is seen in approximately 6% to 37% of patients (116,166,262). Osseous involvement usually reveals pressure erosion or scalloping, without invasion or destruction, or stimulation of the bone surface producing a "frondlike" periosteal reaction (236,262–266) (Fig. 6.30). Bone involvement is more common in patients with multiple recurrences (236) (Fig. 6.30). Juxtacortical or periosteal lesions may cause lysis and saucerize or extrinsically erode the adjacent bone (238). Rare cases with calcification or ossification may be seen.

The sonographic appearance of extra-abdominal desmoids is not extensively described (267). These lesions typically demonstrate an ill-defined hypoechoic mass. Large desmoid tumors are described as being associated with prominent posterior acoustic shadowing. Color Doppler evaluation reflects the hypervascularity of the majority of these lesions.

Scintigraphy shows focal tracer accumulation on blood pool and delayed static images and may be useful in detecting lesions (262) (Fig. 6.31). Scintigraphy may also identify loss of the tissue plane between the tumor and bone (268). However, this information is more readily obtained from other modalities (266). On arteriography, extra-abdominal desmoid tumors are often hypervascular, with either a capillary blush or venous hypervascularity, although these features may be absent and arteriography may be normal (193,269) (Figs. 6.31 and 6.32).

On CT, the deep fibromatoses frequently appear as nonspecific soft tissue masses (Figs. 6.31–6.35). Unless outlined by fat, the margins of the masses are often poorly defined (193), and the attenuation relative to skeletal muscle is variable, reported as lower, similar, or higher (140,189,193). Lesions enhance following intravenous contrast (140,189, 193,270) (Fig. 6.33). Hudson et al. (193) noted a case in which a low attenuation lesion became similar to muscle attenuation following contrast administration. Such cases underscore the need to obtain a few CT images prior to contrast administration. Subtle bone involvement may be better evaluated on radiographs because of beam-hardening artifact

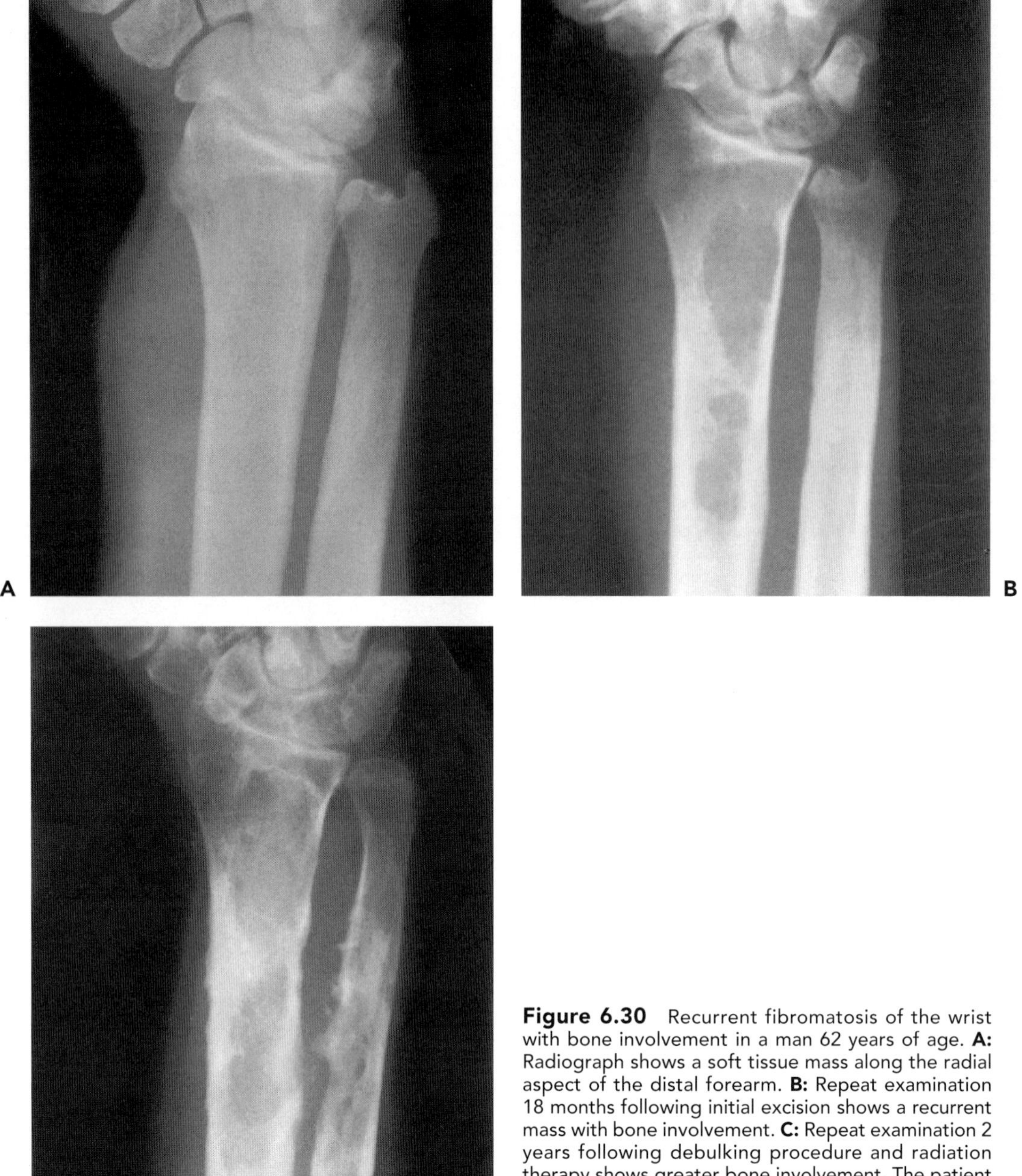

Figure 6.30 Recurrent fibromatosis of the wrist with bone involvement in a man 62 years of age. **A:** Radiograph shows a soft tissue mass along the radial aspect of the distal forearm. **B:** Repeat examination 18 months following initial excision shows a recurrent mass with bone involvement. **C:** Repeat examination 2 years following debulking procedure and radiation therapy shows greater bone involvement. The patient underwent subsequent amputation for intractable pain.

(193). Investigators attempts to correlate the CT appearance of the tumors with the underlying histology and collagen content (189), and to correspond contrast enhancement with microscopic or angiographic vascularity, have been unsuccessful (193). The abundant capillary network of these fibrous tumors is suggested as an explanation of the increased attenuation following contrast administration (140).

The best radiologic modality to evaluate and stage the deep fibromatoses is MR imaging (Figs. 6.31–6.37). These lesions are usually centered in the intermuscular region, although invasion of muscle is frequent. On MR imaging,

the deep musculoaponeurotic fibromatoses were initially described as demonstrating decreased signal intensity on all pulse sequences, reflecting the fibrous nature of the tumor (193,271,272). Sundaram et al. described three cases of "aggressive fibromatosis," two demonstrating a decreased signal on T2-weighted pulse sequences and one showing a paradoxical increased signal (273). Two of these three tumors were hypocellular and had abundant collagen. The lesion that showed high signal on T2-weighted MR images had marked cellularity as well as abundant collagen. Sundaram et al. concluded that the combination of

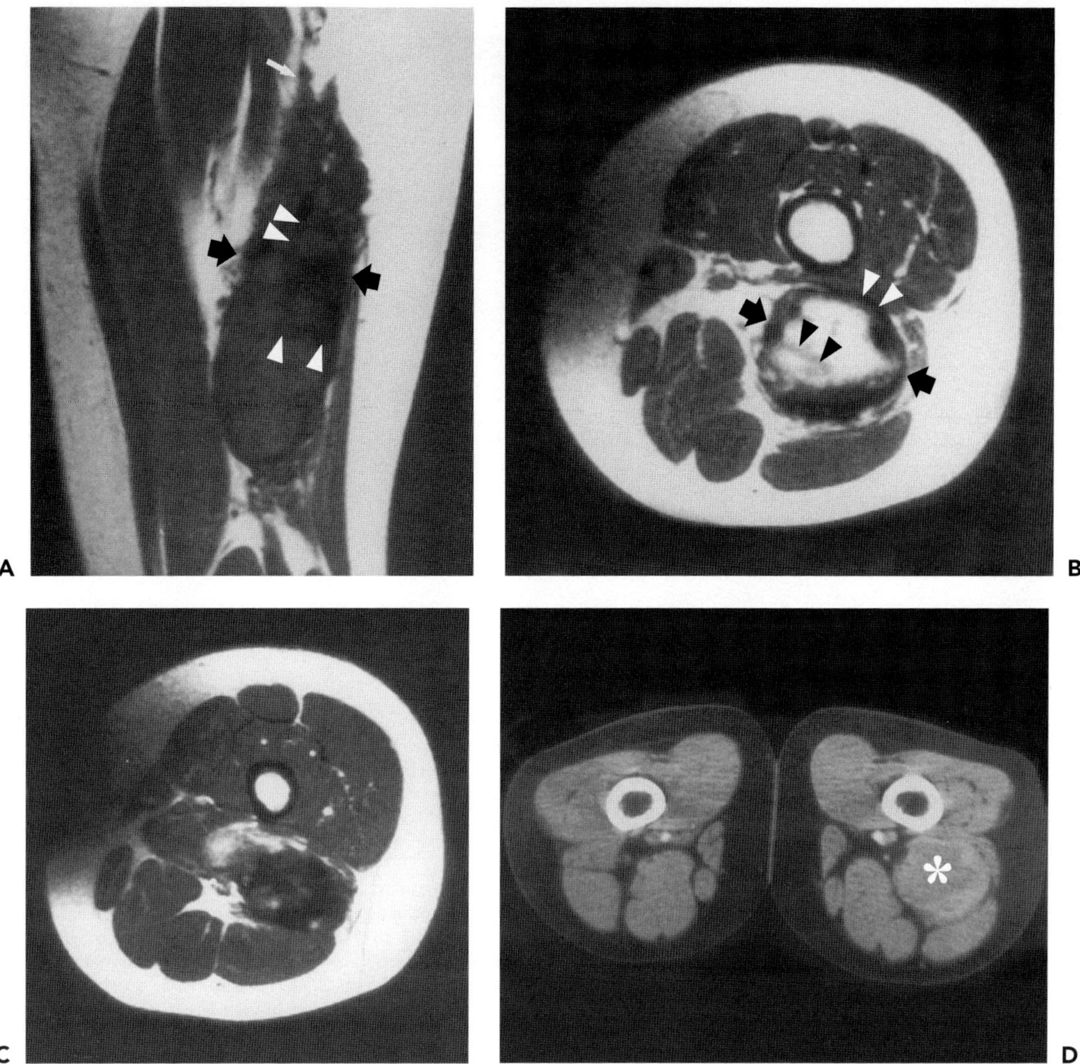

Figure 6.31 Extra-abdominal desmoid of the lower thigh in a woman 19 years of age with a history of a mass progressively enlarging over 2 years. **A,B:** Coronal T1-weighted (TR/TE; 800/20) **(A)** and axial T2-weighted (TR/TE; 2000/60) **(B)** spin-echo MR image show a well-defined intermuscular soft tissue mass (*arrows*) in the thigh, with signal intensity similar to that of skeletal muscle on T1-weighted images and fat on T2-weighted images. Note areas of bandlike, low signal intensity (*arrowheads*) on both pulse sequences that are predominantly peripheral and the linear extension (*long arrow* **A**) along the superficial fascia (fascial tail sign). **C:** Axial T2-weighted (TR/TE; 2000/60) MR image superior to **B** shows similar findings, with predominantly decreased signal intensity. **D:** Contrast-enhanced axial CT scan shows a heterogeneous soft tissue mass (*asterisk*). (*continued*)

marked hypocellularity and abundant collagen produces decreased signal on T2-weighted pulse sequences and that the decreased cellularity is of prime importance (273) (Figs. 6.31–6.37).

Subsequent reports showed great variability in the MR imaging characteristics of these deep fibromatoses (193,270,274–277) (Figs. 6.31–6.36). More typically, the lesion has a heterogeneous signal intensity approximating that of fat on T2-weighted and that of skeletal muscle on T1-weighted spin-echo images. The heterogeneous signal likely reflects varying proportions and distribution of collagen, spindle cells, and mucopolysaccharide within the tumor.

Corresponding areas of decreased signal intensity are noted on all pulse sequences, likely reflecting areas of dense collagen within the lesions. Extra-abdominal desmoids typically demonstrate moderate to marked enhancement following the administration of intravenous contrast on MR imaging, with enhancement corresponding to the cellular portions of the lesion (270) (Figs. 6.34 and 6.36). No significant enhancement is seen in approximately 10% of lesions (278). Tumor margins vary greatly, although they are usually well-defined at initial presentation (275,277). Infiltrative margins are reported to be more common in young patients (278) (Fig. 6.36). Extension of the tumor

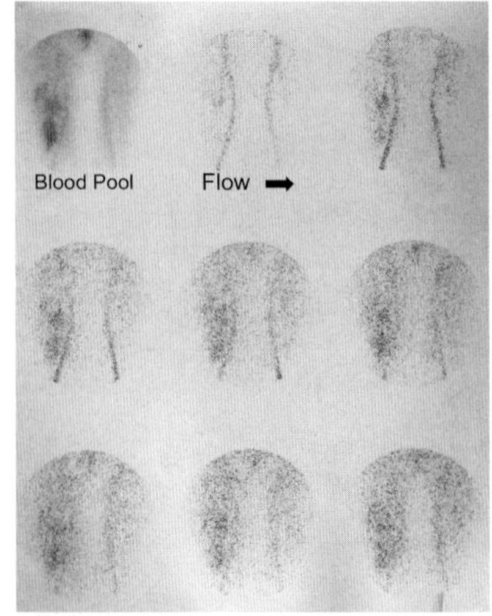

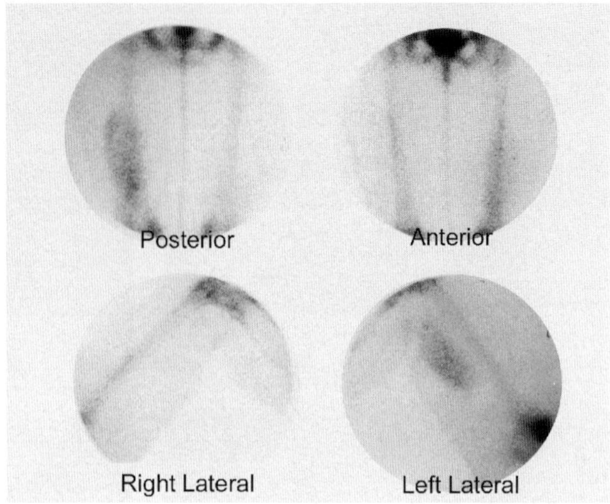

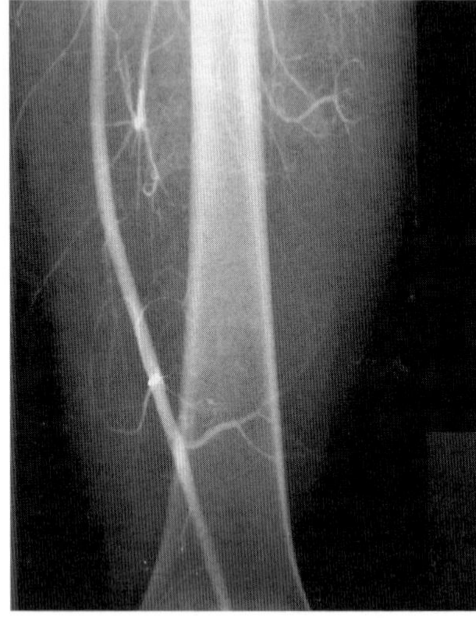

Figure 6.31 *(continued)* **E,F:** Flow and blood pool **(E)** and delayed static **(F)** images from technetium-99m methylene diphosphonate (MDP) bone scan show increased tracer on all phases. **G:** Anteroposterior film from conventional arteriogram shows mild displacement of the superficial femoral artery as well as a minimal tumor blush, predominantly from the profunda femoris.

along the fascia (particularly the superficial fascia) as a linear band is very suggestive of extra-abdominal desmoid (Figs. 6.33 and 6.37). This is described as the *fascial tail sign* and is very unusual with other masses, except nodular fasciitis. However, nodular fasciitis is usually a subcutaneous lesion. To ensure adequate resection, these extensions are vital to detect because they may protrude significantly beyond the other portions of the lesions (Fig. 6.37). It must be emphasized that decreased signal intensity on all pulse sequences only reflects the gross morphology of a lesion and is not specific for the fibromatoses. There are multiple other causes of decreased signal intensity on long TR images that include dense mineralization, air, foreign bodies, rapidly flowing blood, hemosiderin-laden tissue (such as pigmented villonodular synovitis [PVNS]), and other fibrous lesions with a high collagen content (273,279) (including malignant fibrous histiocytoma as well as other malignancies) (279). The morphology of these low signal intensity regions in fibromatosis as promi-

nent bandlike areas may be more important to suggest diagnosis than the intrinsic signal intensity (Figs. 6.31, 6.34, and 6.36). These collagenized bands do not enhance significantly following intravenous contrast (Figs. 6.34 and 6.36).

We believe MR imaging features of a heterogeneous intramuscular mass (well-defined or ill-defined), with nonenhancing bands of low signal on all pulse sequences, and linear fascial extensions, are nearly pathognomic of extra-abdominal desmoid. Two other MR imaging features deserve mention. First, we believe the signal intensity on long TR images has a significant implication on the likelihood of local recurrence. High signal intensity on these images (and these enhance more dramatically as well) corresponds to relatively more cellular and less collagenized lesions (280). In our experience, extra-abdominal desmoids with this appearance are far more likely to recur locally, and we suggest more extensive surgical margins at initial resection to lessen this possibility. Second, patients

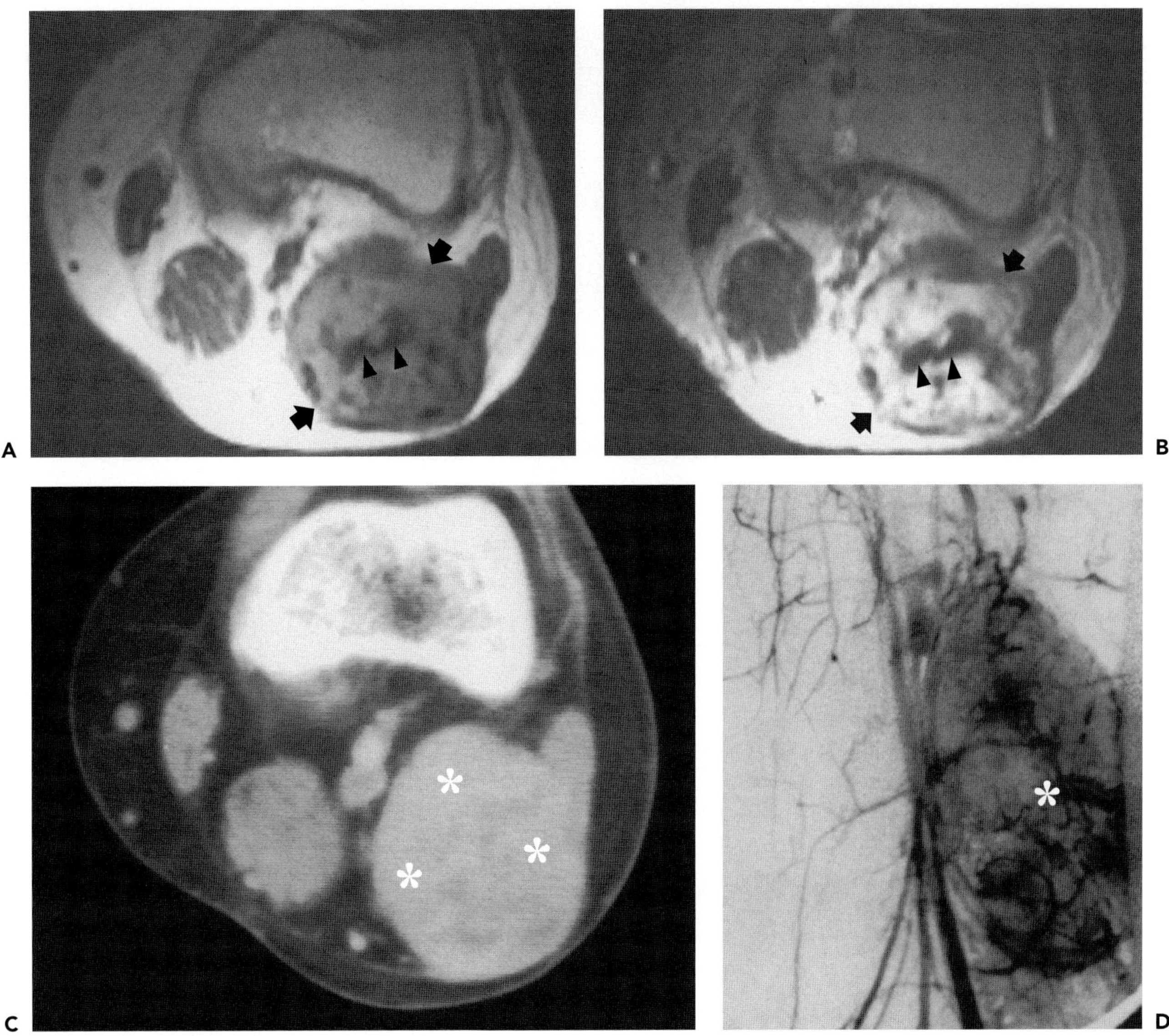

Figure 6.32   Deep-type fibromatosis in the popliteal fossa in a man 22 years of age. **A,B:** Axial T1-weighted (TR/TE; 700/34) **(A)** and T2-weighted (TR/TE; 2000/80) **(B)** spin-echo MR image show a well-defined intermuscular soft tissue mass (*arrows*) in the popliteal fossa with signal intensity similar to that of skeletal muscle on T1-weighted images and fat on T2-weighted images. Within the mass are bandlike areas of low signal intensity on both pulse sequences (*arrowheads*). **C:** Corresponding contrast-enhanced axial CT scan shows a heterogeneous intermuscular soft tissue mass with mildly higher attenuation compared to that of muscle (*asterisks*). **D:** Collimated lateral projection from digital subtraction arteriogram shows marked tumor blush (*asterisk*).

treated with radiation may be followed with MR imaging to detect response to therapy. Lesions that positively respond to radiation therapy demonstrate progressive collagenization and show dramatic low signal intensity on long TR images, as well as decreased size (Fig. 6.38). In our opinion and experience, extra-abdominal desmoids that are markedly low signal on all pulse sequences following this therapy probably do not require surgical resection (Fig. 6.38). In contradistinction, lesions that remain high signal intensity or reveal increased size following radiation therapy have not responded; therefore, they require surgical resection.

Fibromatosis of the Abdominal Wall

Fibromatosis of the abdominal wall (abdominal desmoid) is distinguished from the other deep musculoaponeurotic fibromatoses because of its distinct predilection to develop in women of child-bearing age (usually 20 to 30 years) (281–284). These lesions were initially described in 1832 (4,6,8,201). Typically, the

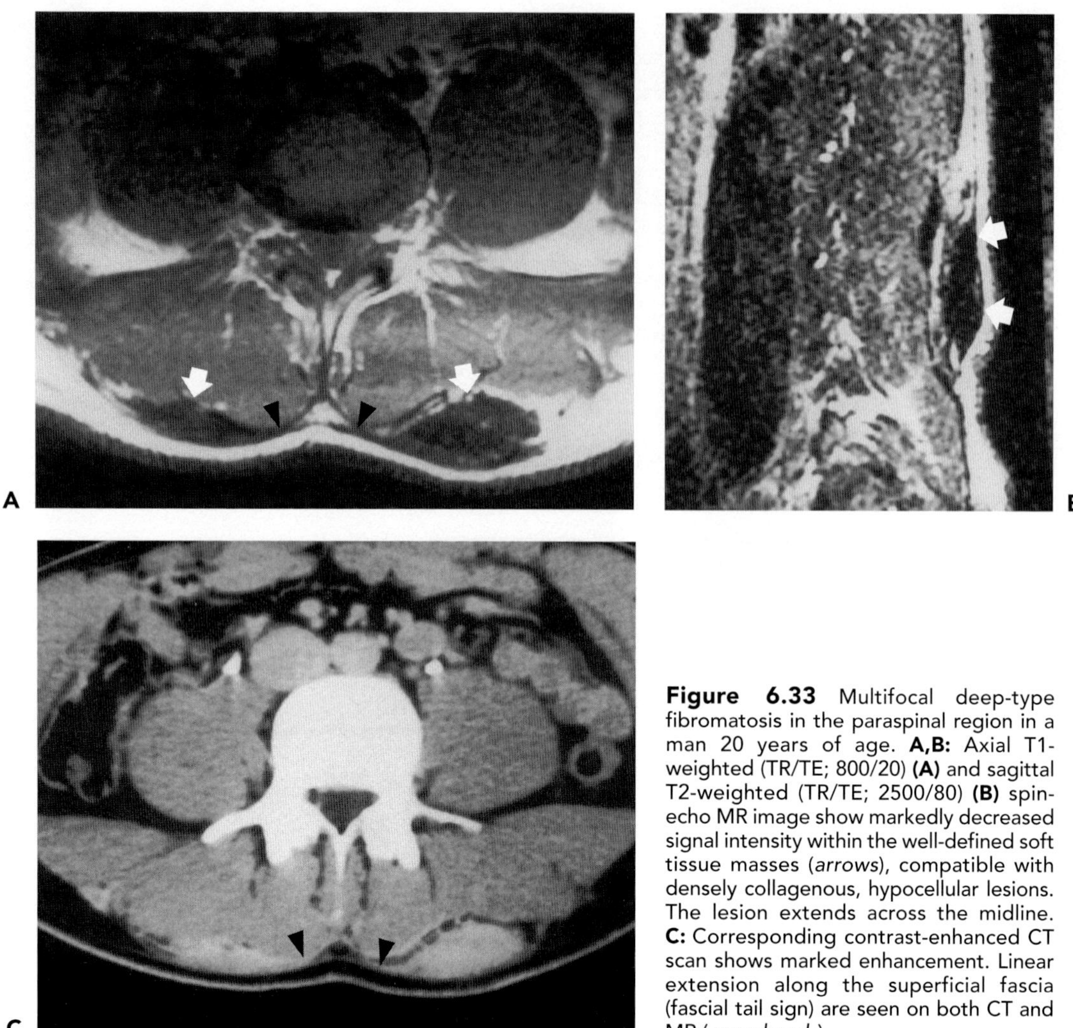

Figure 6.33 Multifocal deep-type fibromatosis in the paraspinal region in a man 20 years of age. **A,B:** Axial T1-weighted (TR/TE; 800/20) **(A)** and sagittal T2-weighted (TR/TE; 2500/80) **(B)** spin-echo MR image show markedly decreased signal intensity within the well-defined soft tissue masses (*arrows*), compatible with densely collagenous, hypocellular lesions. The lesion extends across the midline. **C:** Corresponding contrast-enhanced CT scan shows marked enhancement. Linear extension along the superficial fascia (fascial tail sign) are seen on both CT and MR (*arrowheads*).

lesion develops following, or less often during, pregnancy. Desmoids of the abdominal wall affect women in approximately 87% of cases, and 95% of those patients have had at least one child (1,244). The rectus abdominus and internal oblique muscles and overlying fascia are most commonly affected. These lesions are often smaller at detection than other deep fibromatoses (average size: 3 to 7 cm). The local recurrence rate of abdominal wall lesions is 15% to 30% (lower than that of extra-abdominal lesions) (285). Estrogen receptors were found in 79% of these lesions in the study by Lim et al. (258). Antiestrogen or testosterone therapy may be effective in treatment of abdominal wall lesions (251–259). Abdominal wall fibromatosis may also be associated with polyposis syndromes (286–288). These lesions have a similar imaging appearance to that described for other deep-type fibromatoses (Fig. 6.39).

Intra-Abdominal Fibromatosis and Fibromatosis Associated with Gardner Syndrome

Intra-abdominal fibromatosis (intra-abdominal desmoid) refers to those lesions occurring in the pelvis, mesentery, and retroperitoneum. Of these, the latter two are associated with Gardner syndrome in approximately 15% of patients (287,289–291). Pelvic fibromatosis shows a female predilection, whereas mesenteric lesions are more variable. These lesions, as expected because of the location, are often large (>10 cm) at detection (4,6,8,201). Local recurrences are thus common because the initial resection is often incomplete (292). As a group, these lesions are usually not within the realm of the musculoskeletal radiologist and therefore are largely beyond the scope of our discussion. Patients with Gardner syndrome may demonstrate both intra-abdominal fibromatosis as well as coincident deep musculoaponeurotic lesions, and these are estimated

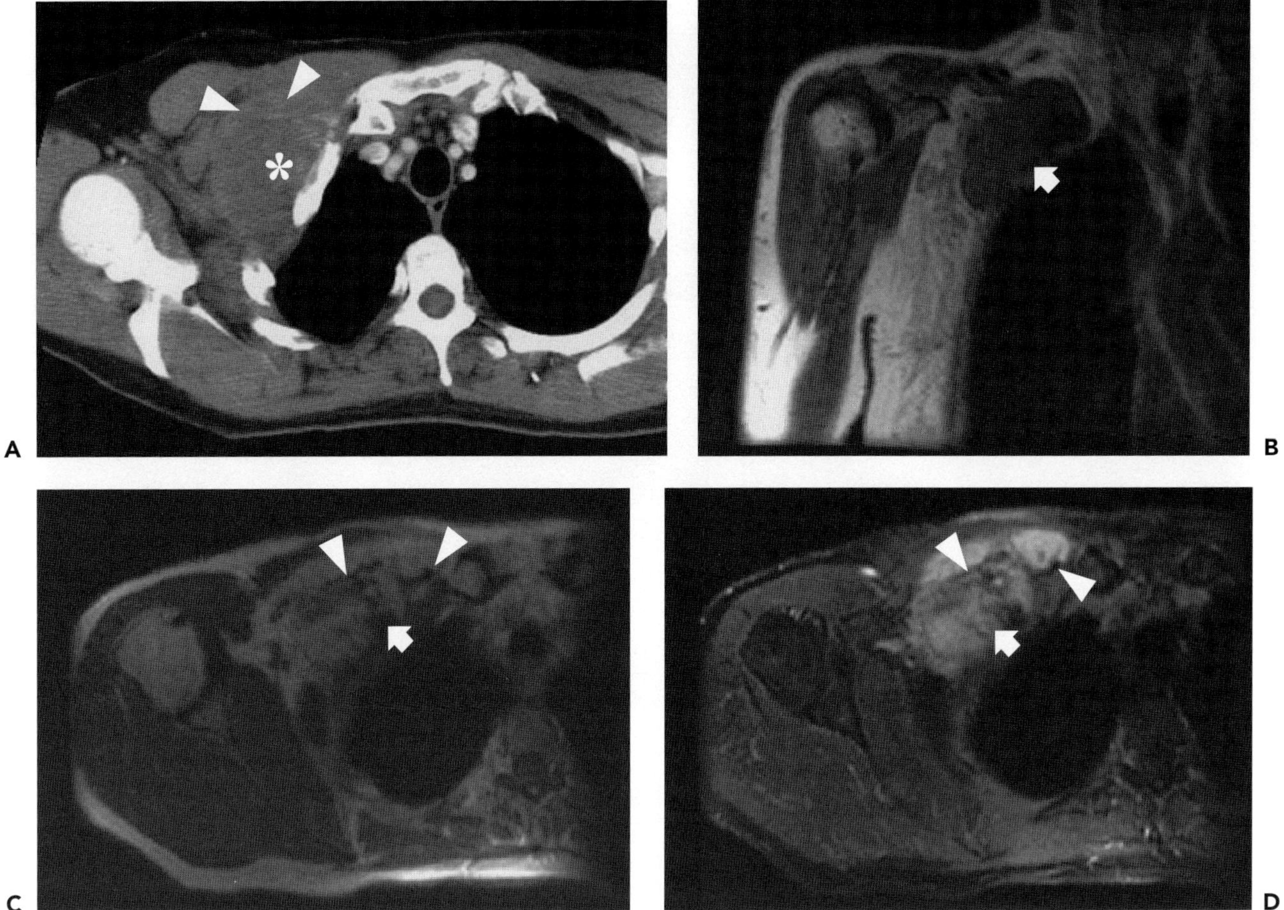

Figure 6.34 Deep-type fibromatosis in the chest wall of a woman 54 years of age. **A:** Axial CT scan shows a large heterogeneous soft tissue mass in the axilla (*asterisk*) with higher attenuation areas representing collagenized bands (*arrowheads*). **B,C:** Coronal T1-weighted (TR/TE; 600/10) **(B)** and axial T2-weighted (TR/TE; 2000/100) **(C)** spin-echo MR images show a well-defined soft tissue mass (*arrow*) in the axilla, with low to intermediate signal intensity. Note low signal intensity collagenized bands in **C** (*arrowheads*). **D:** Axial fat-suppressed enhanced T1-weighted (TR/TE; 500/8) MR image shows prominent enhancement following intravenous contrast (*arrow*). Note nonenhancing collagenized bands (*arrowheads*).

to occur in approximately 10% of patients (293). Intra-abdominal fibromatosis and desmoid tumors associated with Gardner syndrome cannot be differentiated from other lesions of deep fibromatosis on the basis of imaging findings (Figs. 6.40 and 6.41), although the former are smaller, more likely to be multiple and occur in younger patients (294).

RARE FIBROBLASTIC TUMORS

Calcifying Fibrous Tumor

Calcifying fibrous tumor, a distinctive benign fibrous lesion described in 1993 by Fetsch et al. (295), was for-

> **KEY CONCEPTS**
> - Calcifying fibrous tumor is a distinct benign fibrous lesion affecting children and young adults (second to third decades of life).
> - There is a mild female predilection; lesions most frequently involve the extremities.
> - Simple excision is the treatment of choice with only rare local recurrence.
> - Calcification may be seen and MR imaging shows low-to-intermediate signal intensity on all pulse sequences.

merly known as *calcifying fibrous pseudotumor*. This lesion is similar to the childhood fibrous tumor with psammoma bodies reported by Rosenthal and Abdul-Karim

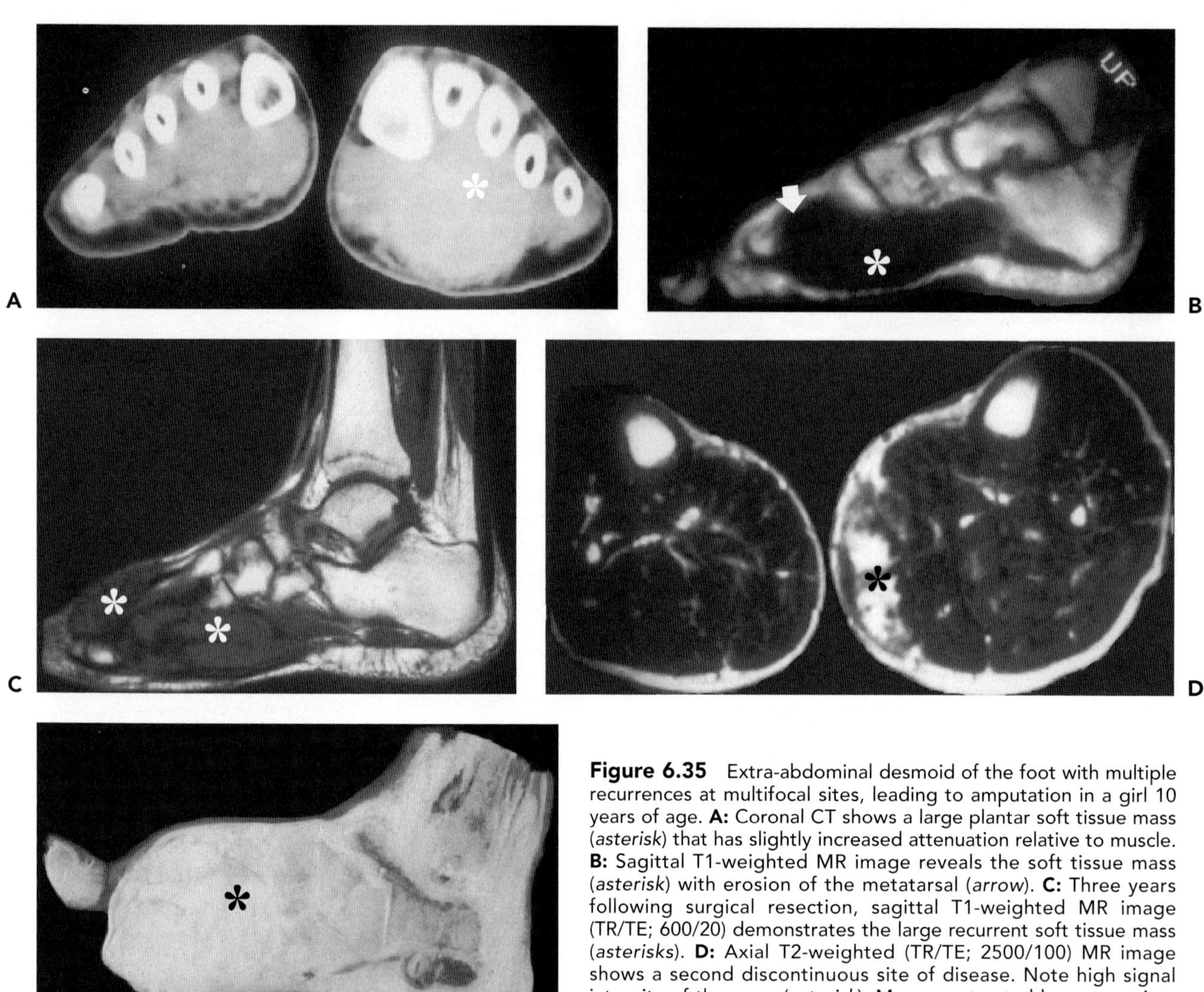

Figure 6.35 Extra-abdominal desmoid of the foot with multiple recurrences at multifocal sites, leading to amputation in a girl 10 years of age. **A:** Coronal CT shows a large plantar soft tissue mass (*asterisk*) that has slightly increased attenuation relative to muscle. **B:** Sagittal T1-weighted MR image reveals the soft tissue mass (*asterisk*) with erosion of the metatarsal (*arrow*). **C:** Three years following surgical resection, sagittal T1-weighted MR image (TR/TE; 600/20) demonstrates the large recurrent soft tissue mass (*asterisks*). **D:** Axial T2-weighted (TR/TE; 2500/100) MR image shows a second discontinuous site of disease. Note high signal intensity of the mass (*asterisk*). Mass was treated by amputation. **E:** Sagittally sectioned gross specimen shows the recurrent aggressive fibromatosis (*asterisk*).

(296), although the former designation is preferred because the lesion is seen in a wide range of ages. The lesion is most commonly seen in young adults in the second or third decade of life (ranging from 1 to 33 years of age), with a mild female predilection (295). Of the 12 reported cases, 5 occurred in the extremities, 2 occurred in the trunk, 2 in the scrotum, and 1 each in the groin, neck, and axilla (295). Rare involvement of the pleura, mediastinum, and visceral peritoneum have also been reported (297–300). Patients present with a subcutaneous or deep-seated soft tissue mass that varies in duration from months to years. These lesions are associated with Castleman disease and inflammatory myofibroblastic tumors (4,5,117).

At gross pathologic examination, lesions range in size from 2 to 15 cm with a 3 to 5 cm average (4,5,117). They are well-circumscribed, gray/white, and often have a gritty consistency because of the calcification. Microscopically, the calcifying fibrous pseudotumor is characterized by abundant hyalinized collagen with psammomatous or dystrophic calcifications and a lymphoplasmacytic infiltrate (295).

Simple excision appears to be adequate management. Of six patients with follow-up, only one had local recurrence that was seen 7.5 years after initial surgery (295). This lesion has no malignant or metastatic potential.

Radiologic characteristics of this rare lesion are quite limited, and one can only speculate to the full spectrum of imaging findings, although an appearance similar to that of the musculoaponeurotic fibromatoses would be expected. The calcification may be seen on radiographs and CT as thick and bandlike or punctate (301). MR imaging reflects the fibrous nature of the lesion with low-to-intermediate signal intensity on all pulse sequences (Fig. 6.42).

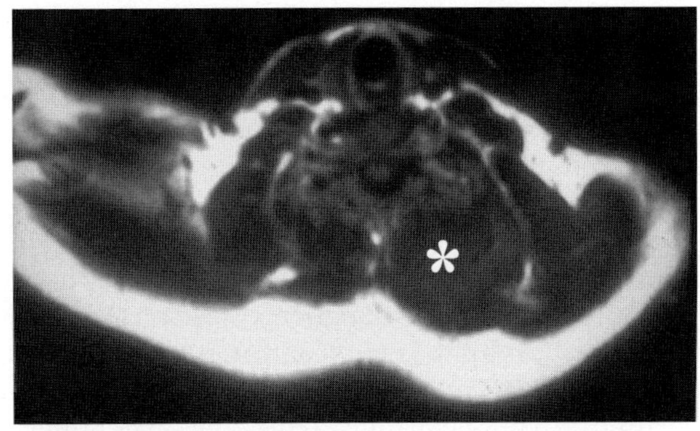

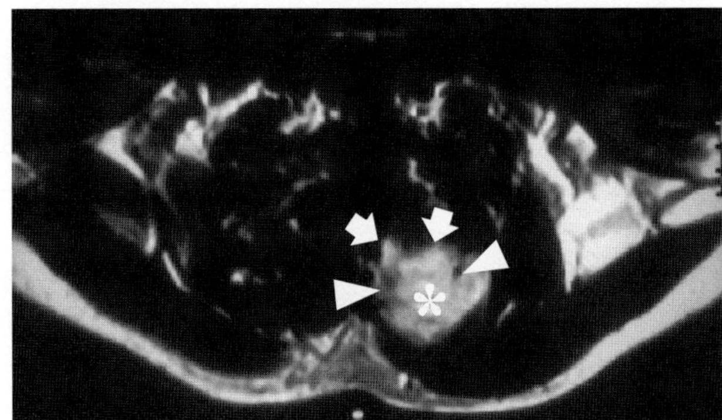

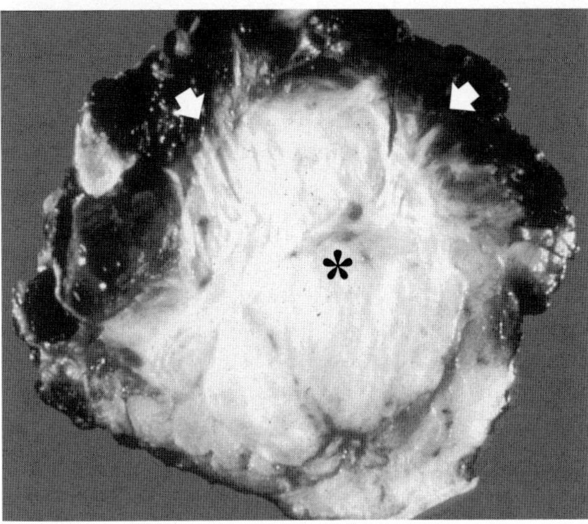

Figure 6.36 Extra-abdominal desmoid of the paraspinal region in a man 30 years of age. **A:** Axial T1-weighted (TR/TE; 500/15) MR image shows a paraspinal mass (*asterisk*) that is isointense to skeletal muscle. **B:** Axial postcontrast T1-weighted (TR/TE; 500/20) MR image shows prominent enhancement (*asterisk*), with two nonenhancing collagenized bands (*arrowheads*). Note spiculated, infiltrating margin (*arrows*). High signal intensity was seen on T2-weighted, not show. **C:** Photograph of the sectioned mass (*asterisk*) shows irregular, spiculated margins (*arrows*).

Exuberant Cervical Fibrosclerosis

Cervical fibrosclerosis is a very rare fibrous lesion (117). Initially called *sclerosing cervicitis*, it is the cervical equivalent of mediastinal and retroperitoneal fibrosis (302,303). Signs and symptoms such as pain, headache, dysphagia, hoarseness, trismus, epistaxis, painless swelling, nasal obstruction, and airway obstruction have been reported (304). The lesion may grow slowly over many years (303).

Microscopically, the lesion is characterized by dense fibrous tissue infiltrated by lymphocytes, plasma cells, macrophages, and scattered eosinophils and neutrophils (303).

CT of a single case in the literature (303) showed a large, enhancing, soft tissue mass infiltrating the deep and superficial soft tissue of the neck. The lesion compressed the hypopharynx and extended from the clavicles to the level

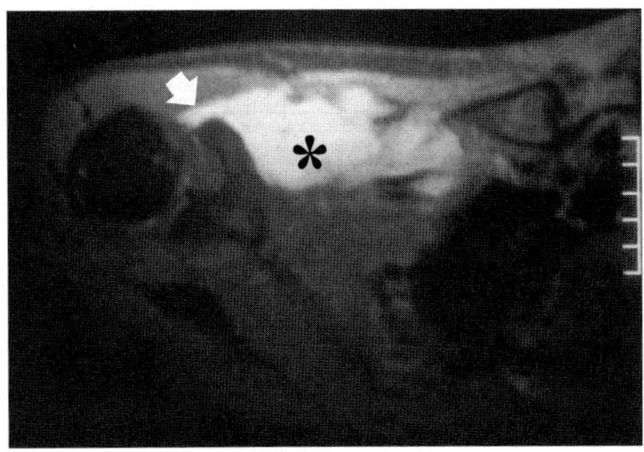

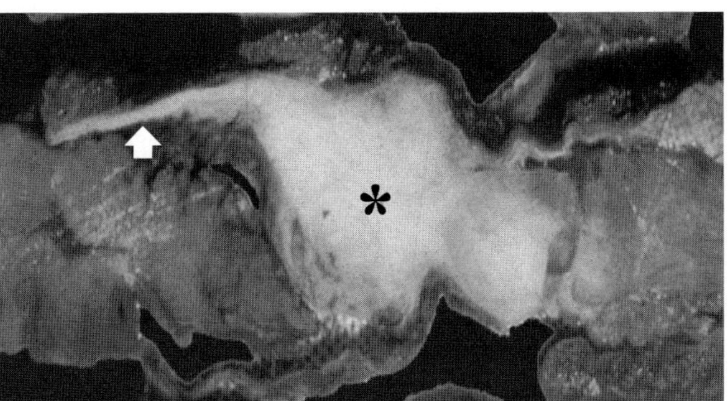

Figure 6.37 Extra-abdominal desmoid about the shoulder in a man 35 years of age. **A:** Axial fat-suppressed T2-weighted (TR/TE; 4000/100) MR image shows a high signal intensity intermuscular soft tissue mass (*asterisk*) with fascial extension (*arrow: fascial tail sign*). **B:** Photograph of sectioned gross specimen shows an extra-abdominal desmoid (*asterisk*) and the prominent fascial extension (*arrow*).

of the zygomas. Involvement was largely symmetric, involving the anterior and lateral neck.

Benign Fibrohistiocytic Lesions

> ### KEY CONCEPTS
> - Benign fibrous histiocytoma is rare and may affect the skin and subcutaneous or deeper soft tissues.
> - It is most frequently seen in the skin and subcutaneous tissue of the lower extremities and head/neck.
> - Deep benign fibrous histiocytoma presents as a painless mass in patients between the ages of 20 and 40 years; lesions are often larger than 5 cm.
> - Treatment is surgical excision with local recurrence in less than 5% of superficial cases and 50% to 60% of deep-seated lesions.
> - Cross-sectional imaging appearance is nonspecific; there are only limited reports.

The benign fibrous histiocytoma is rare, representing less than 1% of all fibrohistiocytic tumors (3,4,6,305). Benign fibrous histiocytoma is also referred to as *sclerosing hemangioma, dermatofibroma, dermal histiocytoma, fibroxanthomas, histiocytoma cutis,* and *nodular subepidermal fibrosis* (3,4,6,305,306). This lesion occurs most frequently in the skin and subcutaneous tissue in the lower limb and head and neck (307). However, they can also involve deeper soft tissues and occasionally the viscera (3,4,308,

309). The lesion is currently referred to by the WHO as *deep benign fibrous histiocytoma* in any location including a subcutaneous site (4). Cutaneous, benign, fibrous histiocytomas affect young to middle-aged adults and are most common in the extremities. These protuberant or pedunculated, red-brown, painless, nodular masses are several millimeters to centimeters in size and are multiple in up to 33% of cases, either metachronously or synchronously (in immunocompromised patients) (310). Deep benign fibrous histiocytoma is rare compared to its cutaneous counterpart (311). Deep benign fibrous histiocytoma is usually intramuscular, involving the extremities or paraspinal regions, although viscera can be involved. The orbit is also not an uncommon site. Clinically, deep benign fibrous histiocytoma usually presents as a painless mass, affecting patients ranging from 20 to 40 years of age (Fig. 6.43) (3,4,6,305). As opposed to its cutaneous counterpart, almost 50% of these lesions are larger than 5 cm in size at diagnosis (3,4,6,305).

At gross pathologic examination, benign fibrous histiocytomas are well-circumscribed, yellow to white masses. Microscopically, these lesions are composed of fibrocytes, fibroblasts, myofibroblasts, and histiocytes, often with a storiform pattern. The histiocytic or xanthomatous elements are variable in their extent, and focal hemorrhage may be seen. The benign features of these neoplasms are usually apparent, allowing distinction from malignant fibrous histiocytomas. Histologic subtypes of benign fibrous histiocytoma include cellular, aneurysmal, epithelioid, myxoid, lipidized, palisaded, and clear cell.

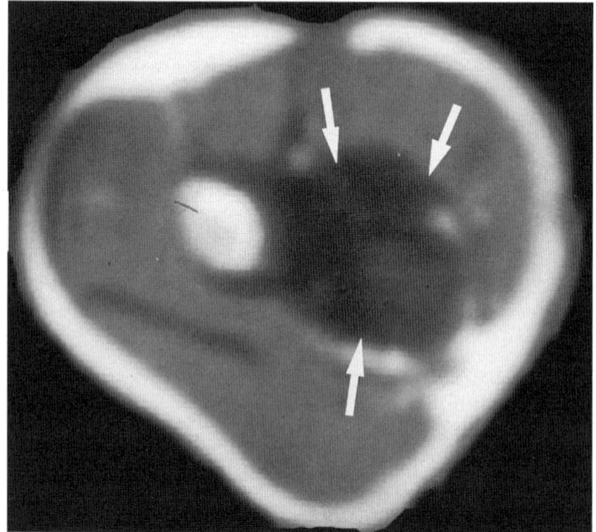
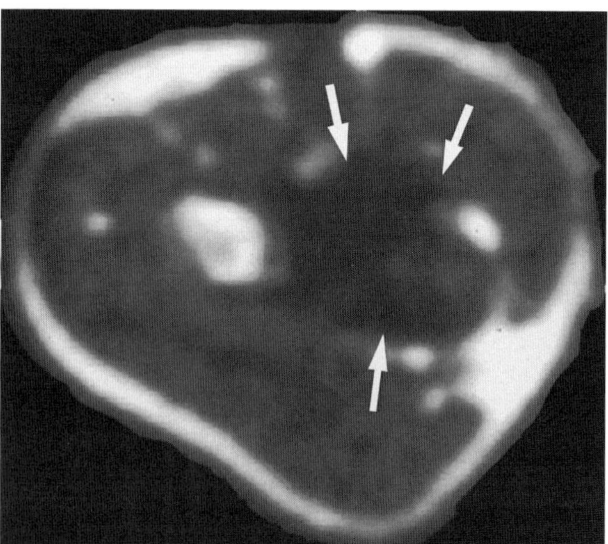

Figure 6.38 Extra-abdominal desmoid recurrence treated with radiation therapy (RT). **A,B:** Axial T1-weighted (TR/TE; 500/20) **(A)** and T2-weighted (TR/TE; 2500/90) **(B)** MR images show marked low signal intensity in the soft tissue mass (*arrows*), resulting from successful treatment and response of the lesion to RT. The mass had mild decrease in size and had significantly lower signal intensity than pre-RT MR images (not shown) and remained stable over multiple years without the need for surgical excision.

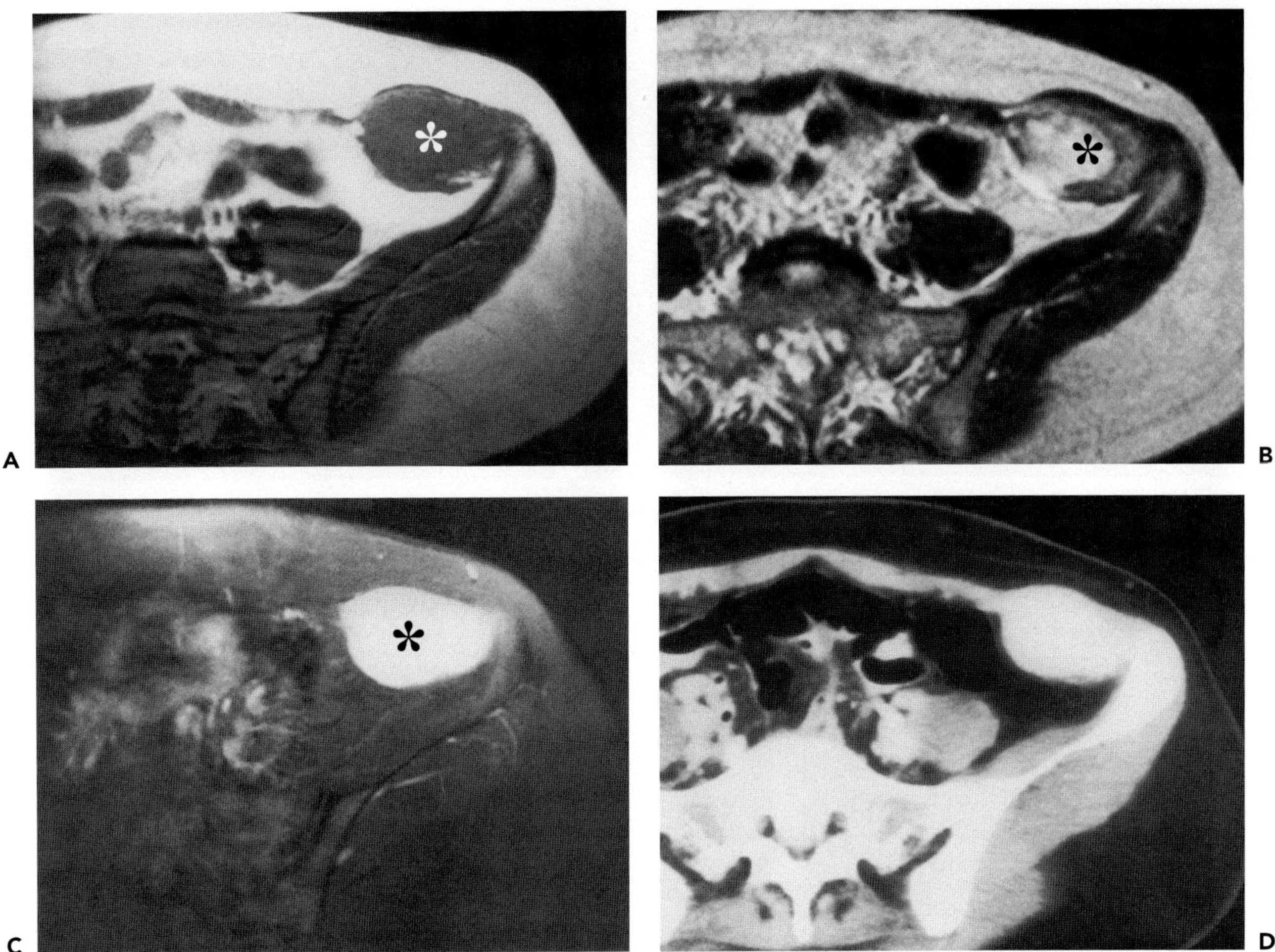

Figure 6.39 Fibromatosis of the abdominal wall in a woman 29 years of age. **A:** Axial T1-weighted (TR/TE; 544/18) **(A)** and T2-weighted (TR/TE; 1800/80) **(B)** MR images show a soft tissue mass (*asterisk*) in the anterior abdominal wall. The mass is homogeneous on the T1-weighted image with signal intensity similar to that of skeletal muscle. The lesion (*asterisk*) is heterogeneous and better defined on T2-weighted image with signal intensity between that of skeletal muscle and fat. **C:** Axial fat-suppressed postcontrast T1-weighted MR image (TR/TE; 600/15) MR image shows the lesion (*asterisk*) to enhance markedly. **D:** Axial contrast-enhanced CT shows the lesion to enhance homogeneously and markedly.

The treatment of benign fibrous histiocytoma is surgical resection. Local recurrence of cutaneous fibrous histiocytoma is uncommon and is seen in less than 5% of cases following surgical resection (306,308,312). Deep lesions, as would be expected, have a higher likelihood of recurrence following attempts at surgical resection, and in some series approach 50% to 60% (308,311). This presumably reflects the larger size of these lesions and the resulting lack of complete surgical excision. Very rare reports of metastases to regional lymph nodes and lung are reported in these lesions (313). The pathologic appearance of these metastatic deposits is similar to the primary focus and has not led to patient demise following resection. These may represent benign metastases, similar to those seen in benign giant cell tumor of bone.

There are only very limited radiologic reports in the literature concerning the appearance of benign fibrous histiocytoma (Figs. 6.43, 6.44, and 6.45). This likely reflects the distribution, with the vast majority of lesions located superficially, not leading to radiologic investigation. In our limited experience, CT and MR imaging features are nonspecific. On CT scanning, lesions show an attenuation similar to that of muscle. Tumors located in the subcutaneous fat are well seen, outlined by fat, in contrast to deep seated lesions. On MR imaging, benign fibrous histiocytoma is low-to-intermediate signal intensity on short TR images (Figs. 6.44 and 6.45). There is a variable appearance on T2-weighted MR images ranging from low-to-high signal intensity, and heterogeneity is also often present (Figs. 6.44 and 6.45). In addition, lesion margins may not be well-defined.

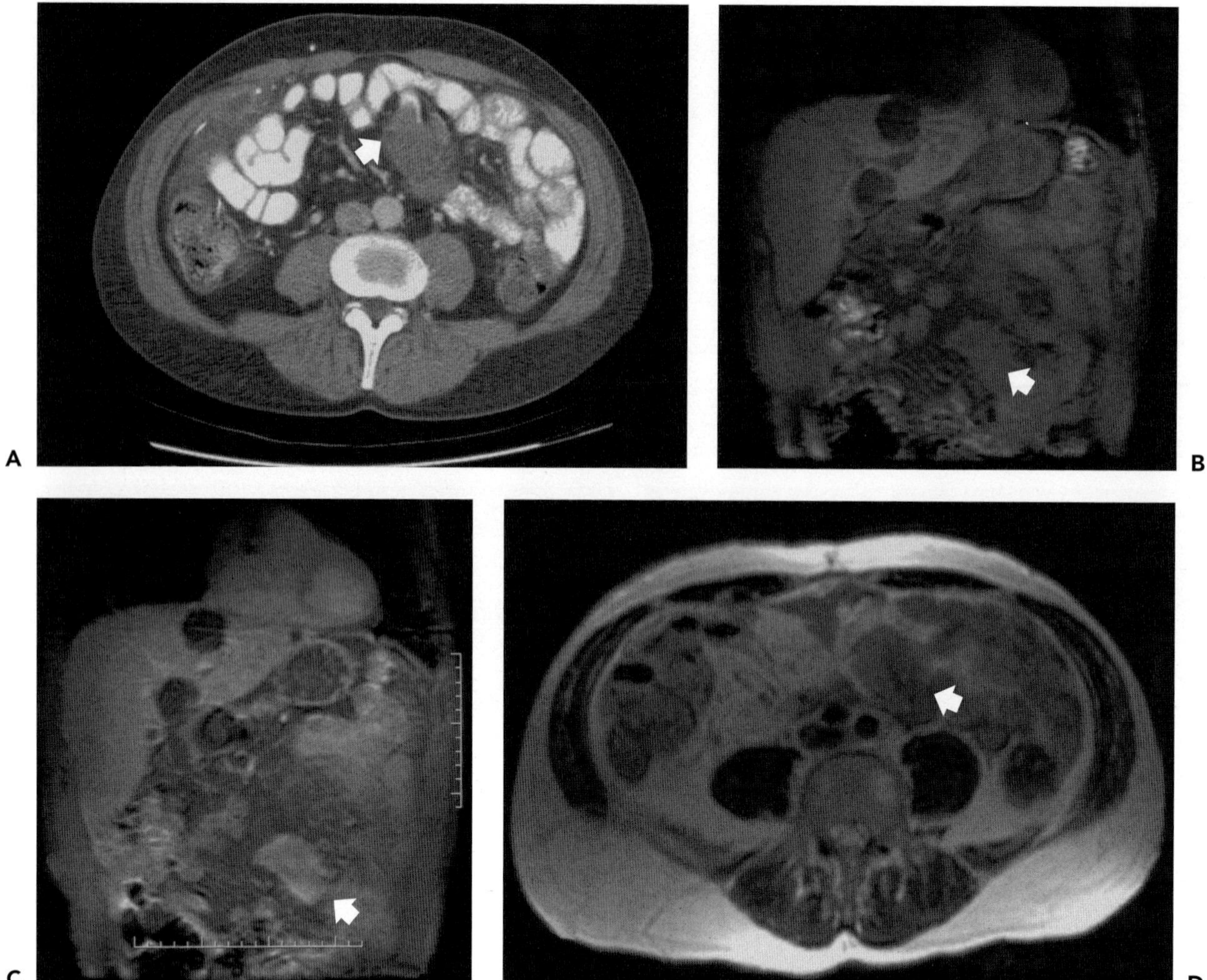

Figure 6.40   Intra-abdominal desmoid in a man 57 years of age. **A:** CT shows a soft tissue attenuation mass in the abdominal cavity (*arrow*). **B,C:** Coronal gradient-echo (TR/TE/Flip; 170/1.4/80) MR images before **(B)** and after **(C)** intravenous contrast reveal the mass (*arrow*) and mild heteregenous enhancement. **D:** Axial T2-weighted (TR/TE; 2500/90) MR image demonstrate low-to-intermediate signal intensity in the mass (*arrow*).

Xanthoma

A xanthoma represents a focal accumulation of histiocytes containing prominent amounts of lipids (3,31,305). These lesions generally occur in association with primary (essential hyperlipidemia) or secondary causes of hyperlipoproteinemia (primary biliary cirrhosis or diabetes mellitus) and only rarely in the normolipemic population (3,31, 305). As such, the xanthomas are reactive, rather than true neoplastic processes.

Xanthomas most frequently involve the skin and subcutaneous tissue; however, tendon, synovium, and, rarely, bone can also be affected. These lesions may be solitary or multiple, are usually painless, and are common about the fingers, wrists, and ankles (3,31,305). The masses may grow slowly, and although they are commonly less than several centimeters in size, diffuse extensive involvement of tendon also occurs. The extent of involvement is usually directly related to the degree and duration of the increased

KEY CONCEPTS

- Xanthoma represents focal accumulation of histiocytes containing prominent lipids, associated with hyperlipoproteinemia.
- It most frequently affects the skin and subcutaneous tissue, but may involve tendons, synovium, and bone.
- Clinically, patients present with a solitary or multiple painless nodules, commonly about the fingers, wrists or ankles.
- Treatment is conservative: often medical to reduce the hyperlipidemia, with surgical resection reserved for larger lesions.
- Sonography of deep lesions reveals single or multiple hypoechoic masses or a diffusely enlarged tendon.
- MR imaging shows a speckled pattern on T1- and T2-weighting with low-to-intermediate signal intensity often diffusely enlarging a tendon (most frequently the Achilles tendon).

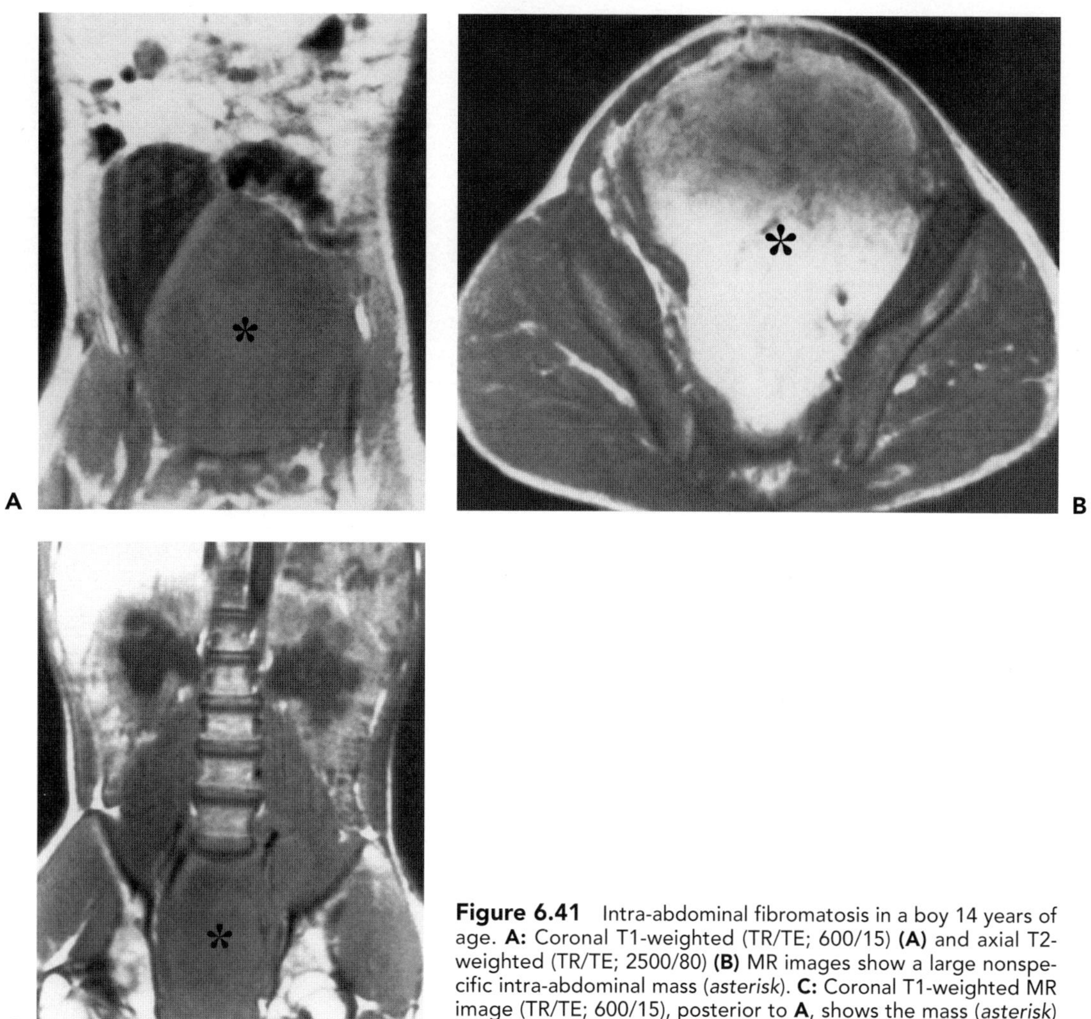

Figure 6.41 Intra-abdominal fibromatosis in a boy 14 years of age. **A:** Coronal T1-weighted (TR/TE; 600/15) **(A)** and axial T2-weighted (TR/TE; 2500/80) **(B)** MR images show a large nonspecific intra-abdominal mass (*asterisk*). **C:** Coronal T1-weighted MR image (TR/TE; 600/15), posterior to **A**, shows the mass (*asterisk*) to be causing bilateral hydronephrosis.

cholesterol levels. Eruptive xanthomas are associated with types 1, 3, and 5 hyperlipidemia and are small, cutaneous lesions most frequently affecting the buttock (3,31,305). Tuberous xanthomas are seen with type 2a and 3 hyperlipidemia, and cause plaquelike lesions of the subcutis, commonly affecting the elbows, buttock, knees, and fingers (3,31,305). Plane xanthomas affect the palmar skin creases. Tendon xanthomas are most frequently associated with type 2a hyperlipidemia (314). In addition, cerebrotendinous xanthomatosis represents a rare inherited (autosomal recessive) defect of bile acid synthesis in which xanthomas commonly occur localized to the Achilles tendon (315,316). Other abnormalities in patients with cerebrotendinous xanthomatosis include dementia, ataxia, and cataracts, and are associated with cholesterol deposition in nerve myelin both centrally, peripherally, and in the spinal cord (3,315).

Pathologically, these lesions are characterized by sheets of foamy histiocytes, and some inflammatory component may be present. Cholesterol collections (clefts) are seen under polarized light as birefringent crystals with surrounding giant cells. There are variable amounts of associated fibrosis. Focal cystic and degenerative change with calcification can also be seen.

Xanthomas are usually treated conservatively and they may regress with medical therapy for the hyperlipidemia (3,31,305). Surgical excision is reserved for large lesions, and tendon reconstruction is usually required for xanthoma involvement (317). Xanthomas may recur slowly, although additional surgical intervention is usually not necessary.

Imaging of superficial lesions is usually not performed. Radiographs may reveal a focal soft tissue mass, and occasionally adjacent extrinsic bone erosion (phalangeal) may be apparent, with lesions involving the finger (318,319). Rarely, calcification can be detected on radiographs (Fig. 6.46). Both sonography and MR imaging are helpful to evaluate tendon xanthomas (320–331) (Figs. 6.46–6.48).

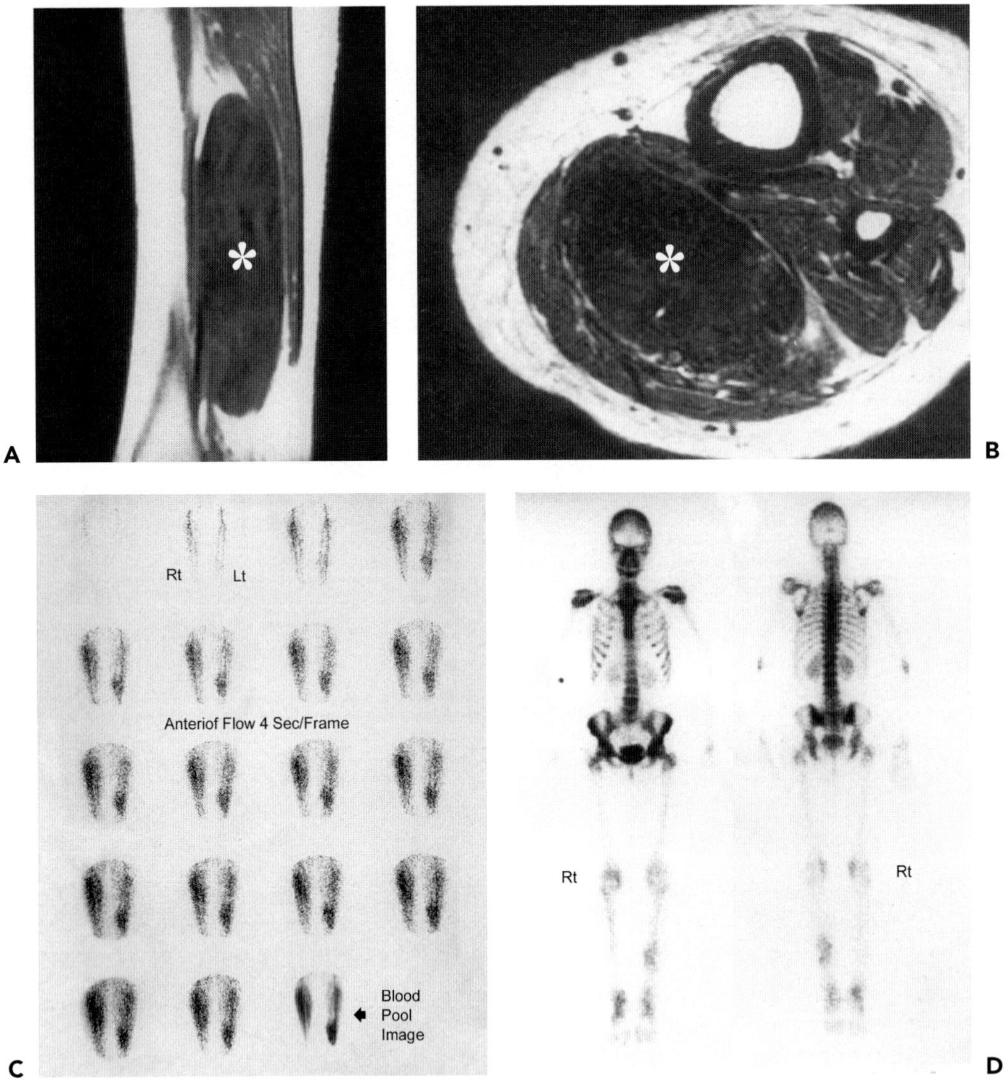

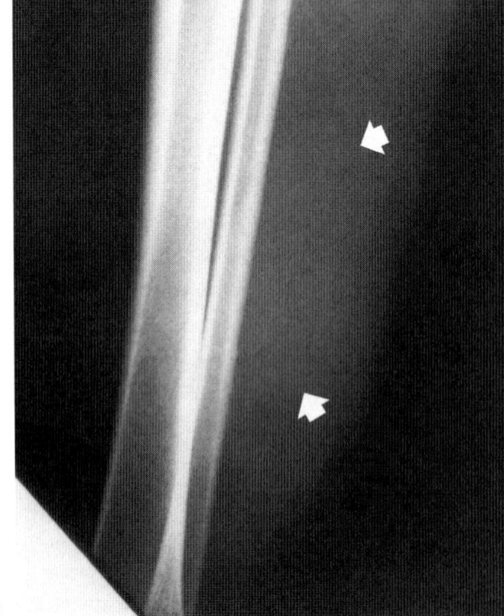

Figure 6.42 Calcifying fibrous pseudotumor in a man 25 years of age presenting with an enlarging painful mass of 4 to 5 years' duration. **A:** Sagittal T1-weighted (TR/TE; 600/12) **(A)** and axial T2-weighted (TR/TE; 2700/80) **(B)** MR images show a well-defined soft tissue mass (*asterisk*), with signal intensity less than that of skeletal muscle on both T1- and T2-weighted images. **C,D:** Anterior flow and blood pool **(C)** and delayed static images **(D)** from bone scan reveal increased tracer accumulation within the mass. **E:** Lateral radiograph shows the mass in the posterior soft tissues (*arrows*) with subtle calcification.

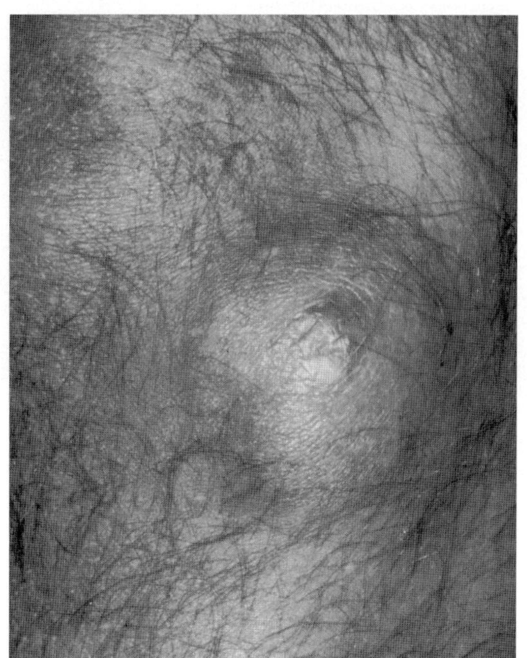
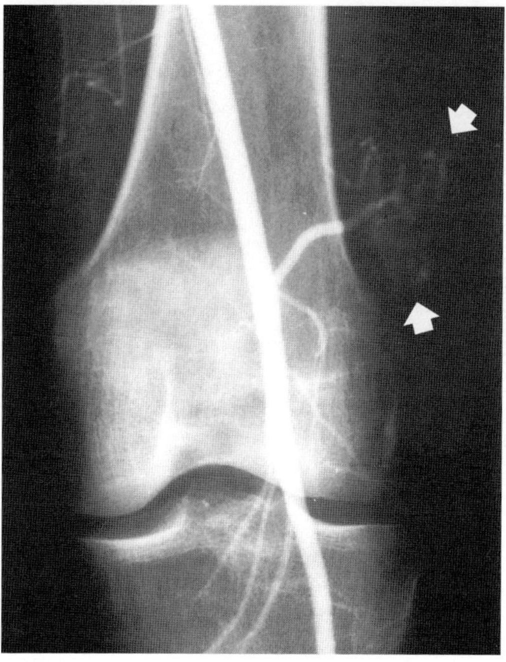

Figure 6.43 Cutaneous benign fibrous histiocytoma in a man 46 years of age with a 10-year history of enlarging protuberant cutaneous nodule. **A:** Clinical photograph of the knee shows a protuberant cutaneous nodule. **B:** Angiogram of the lower extremity shows a hypervascular lesion (*arrows*).

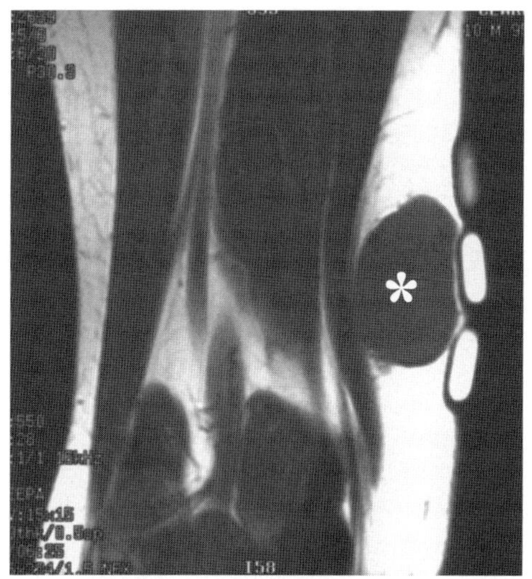
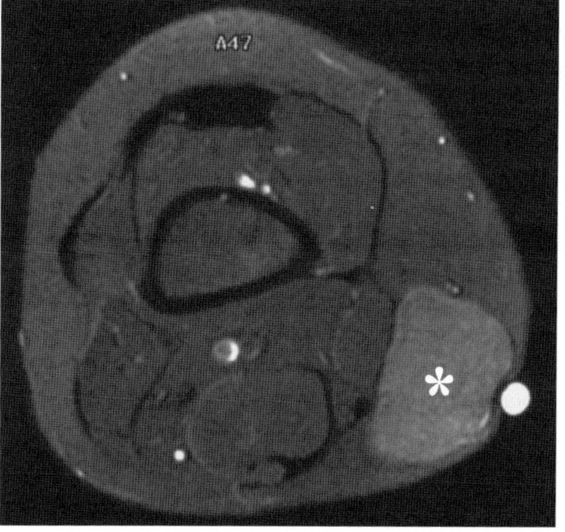
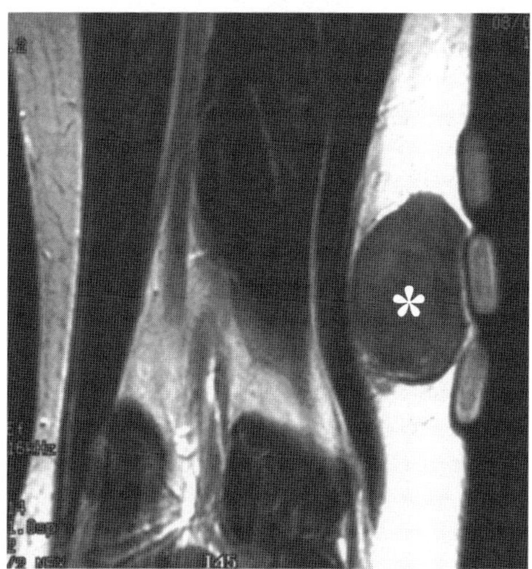

Figure 6.44 Benign fibrous histiocytoma in the subcutaneous tissues about the knee. **A:** Coronal T1-weighted (TR/TE; 550/28) MR image shows a well-defined, intermediate signal intensity, subcutaneous soft tissue mass (*asterisk*). **B:** Axial fat-suppressed T1-weighted (TR/TE; 600/29) MR image following contrast reveals moderate diffuse enhancement (*asterisk*). **C:** Coronal T2-weighted (TR/TE; 4000/120) MR image shows the mass to remain low signal intensity (*asterisk*).

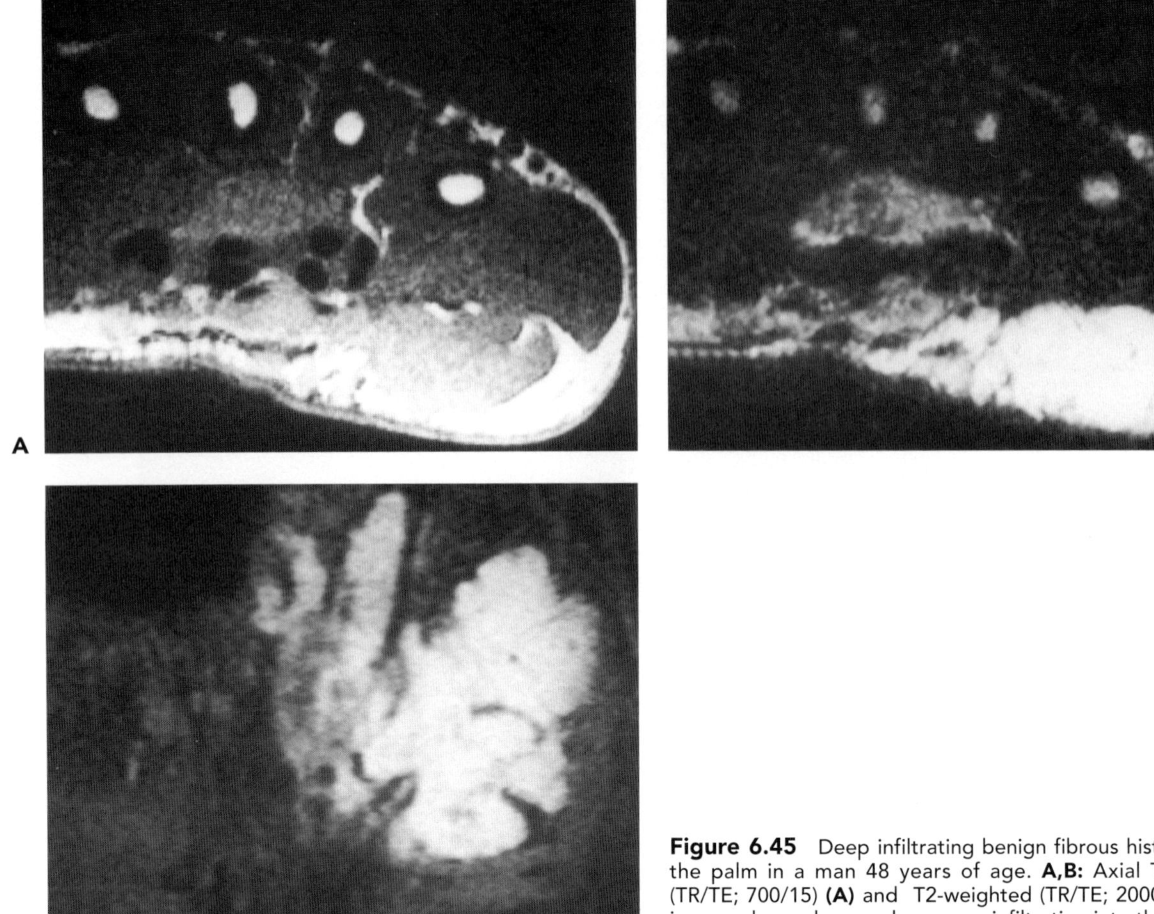

Figure 6.45 Deep infiltrating benign fibrous histiocytoma of the palm in a man 48 years of age. **A,B:** Axial T1-weighted (TR/TE; 700/15) **(A)** and T2-weighted (TR/TE; 2000/90) **(B)** MR images show a large palmar mass infiltrating into the carpal tunnel. **C:** Coronal STIR (TR/TE/TI; 1800/25/160) MR image also shows a high-intensity infiltrating mass.

Sonography was reported by Bude et al. to demonstrate single or multiple, focal, hypoechoic lesions representing tendon xanthomas or a diffusely enlarged heterogeneous tendon (320,321). Similar features were reported by Bureau et al. in a large population of 94 patients, and sonographic detection of xanthomas was more sensitive than physical examination (332). On MR imaging, a speckled or reticulated appearance was described on both T1- and T2-weighted images, diffusely involving the tendon (323,326,327). This is better seen on fat-suppressed T1-weighted or gradient-echo images (323). The overall signal intensity is low-to-intermediate on long TR images (Figs. 6.46, 6.47, and 6.48). Diffuse enlargement of the tendon is often apparent (normal Achilles tendon is less than 7 mm thick in men and 6 mm in women) as is bilateral involvement on both CT and MR images (Figs. 6.47 and 6.48). Most imaging studies are performed on the Achilles tendon because of its size, easy accessibility, and common involvement by xanthomas (Figs. 6.47 and 6.48). These imaging changes can usually be distinguished

from trauma or tendonitis, although as suggested by Dussault et al., a significant overlap in imaging appearance can be observed (323). Patients with cerebrotendinous xanthomatosis often reveal abnormal deposition in the brain and spinal cord on CT and MR imaging (333–336).

Xanthogranuloma

KEY CONCEPTS

- Xanthogranuloma represents a benign histiocytic lesion that usually affects children, but may be seen in adults as well (10% to 40% of cases).
- Common sites are the head/neck (50%), trunk, and extremities; lesions are usually cutaneous.
- Lesions often spontaneously resolve.
- Simple excision is curative.
- Imaging would be expected to reveal similar features to those seen with focal xanthomas.

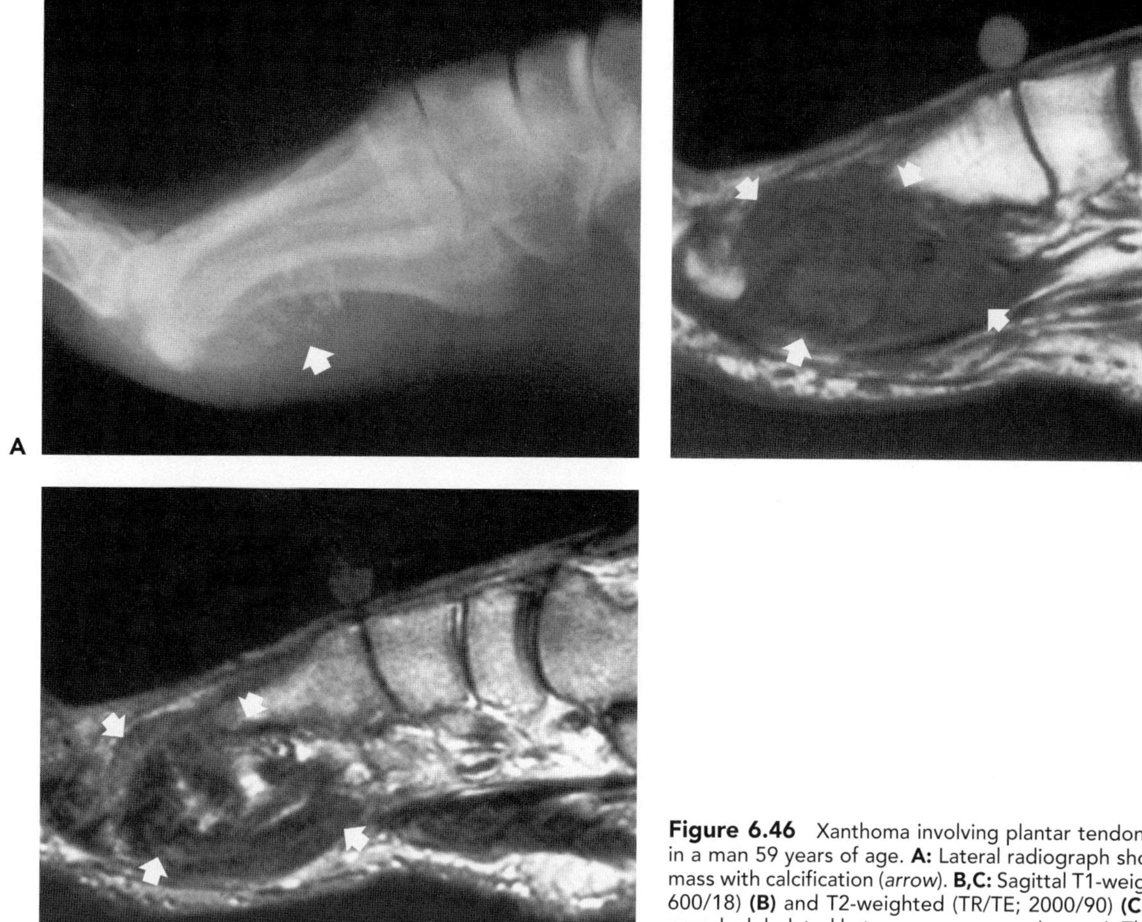

Figure 6.46 Xanthoma involving plantar tendons of the foot in a man 59 years of age. **A:** Lateral radiograph shows a plantar mass with calcification (*arrow*). **B,C:** Sagittal T1-weighted (TR/TE; 600/18) **(B)** and T2-weighted (TR/TE; 2000/90) **(C)** MR images reveal a lobulated heterogeneous mass (*arrows*). The majority of the mass remains low signal intensity, likely reflecting the effects of calcification.

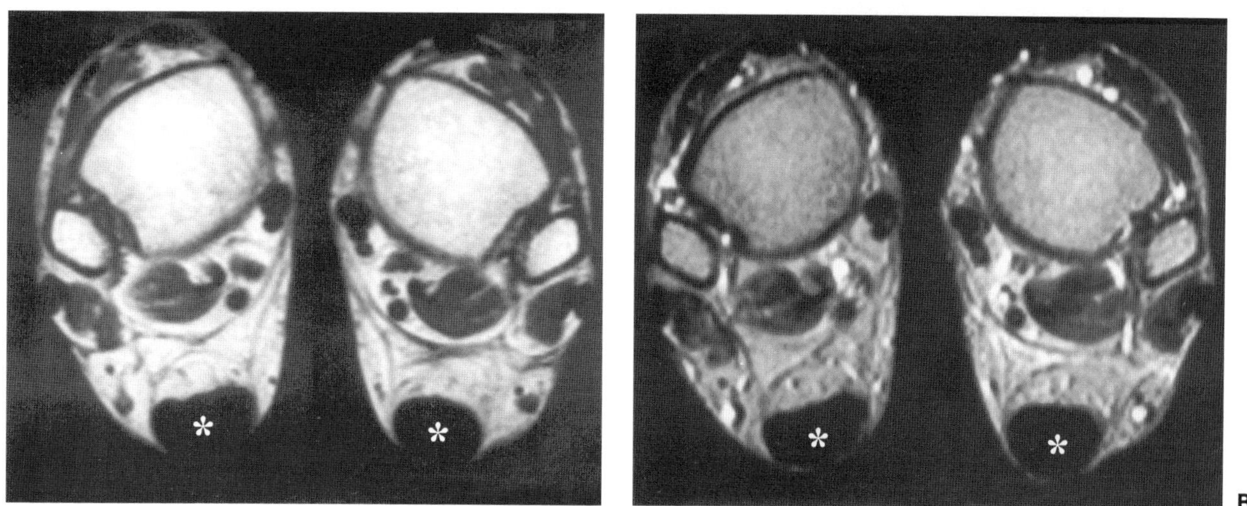

Figure 6.47 Xanthoma of tendon sheaths in a woman 70 years of age with familial hypercholesterolemia. **A,B:** Axial T1-weighted (TR/TE; 712/25) **(A)** and T2-weighted (TR/TE; 1800/90) **(B)** MR images of the ankles show marked enlargement of both Achilles tendons (*asterisks*).

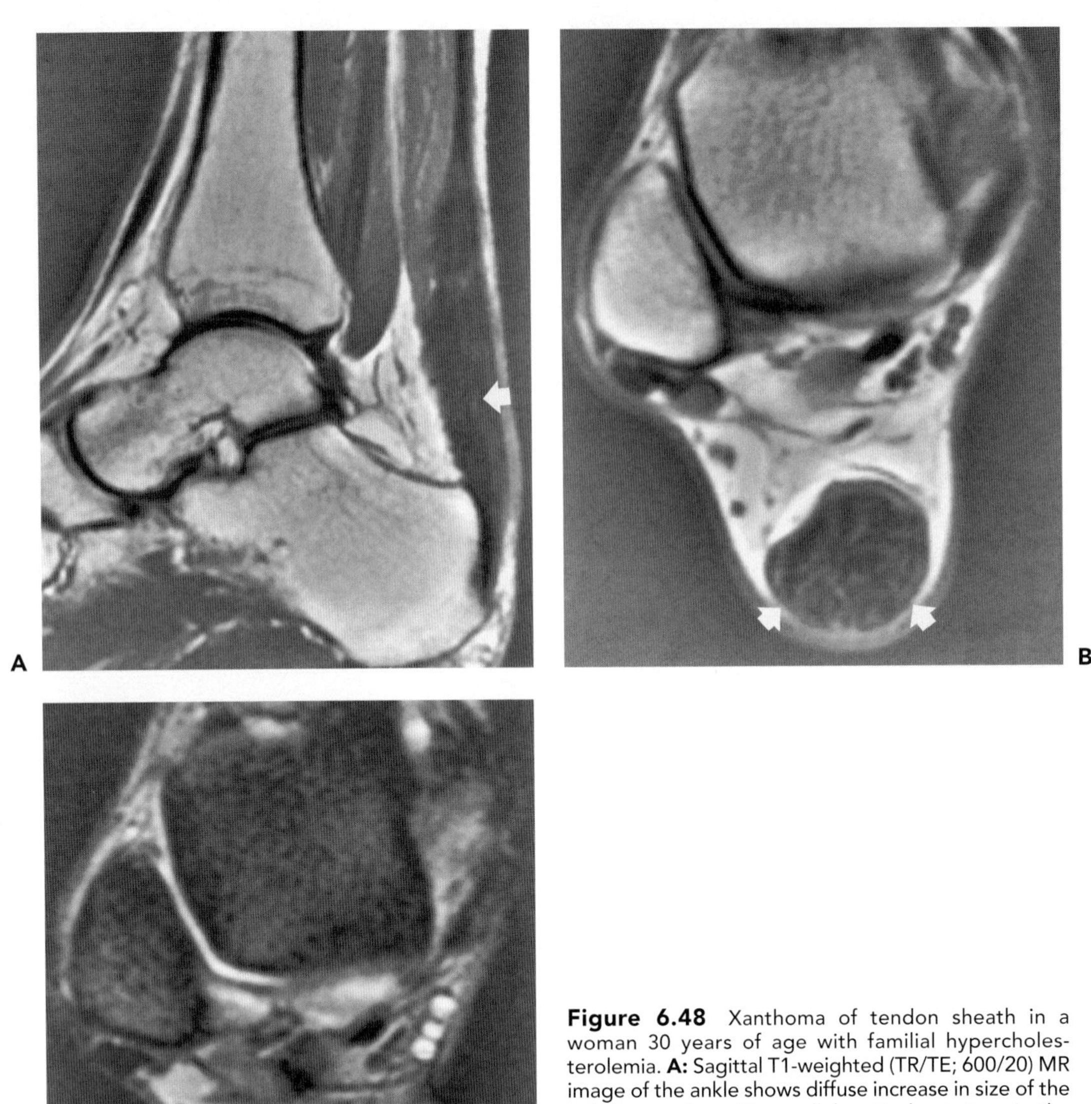

Figure 6.48 Xanthoma of tendon sheath in a woman 30 years of age with familial hypercholesterolemia. **A:** Sagittal T1-weighted (TR/TE; 600/20) MR image of the ankle shows diffuse increase in size of the Achilles tendon with parallel vertical striations in the substance of the tendon (*arrow*). **B:** Axial T1-weighted (TR/TE; 600/20) MR image shows an enlarged tendon with a diffuse stippled pattern, presumably caused by low signal collagen surrounded by higher signal foamy histiocytes and inflammatory reaction (*arrow*). **C:** Axial gradient-echo (TR/TE/Flip; 500/20/20 degrees) MR image shows these findings to better advantage (*arrows*). (Case courtesy of Robert G. Dussault, MD, and Phoebe A. Kaplan, MD.)

Xanthogranuloma is a histiocytic lesion that usually occurs in childhood (juvenile xanthogranuloma), but up to 10% to 40% of cases occur in adults (older than 20 years) (3,31,305,337). These lesions may be present at birth (20% of cases: congenital xanthogranulomas), while juvenile lesions usually present before 2 years of age (3,31,305). Cutaneous lesions are seen as red papules which may be multiple, and may regress spontaneously. Common sites of involvement are the head and neck (approximately 50% of cases), followed by the trunk and extremities. Unlike xanthomas, there is no association with hyperlipidemia; however, there is an association with neurofibromatosis and urticaria pigmentosa (338,339).

Cutaneous lesions are smaller (less than 1 cm) than deep-seated lesions. Sheets of histiocytes are seen microscopically, particularly in early lesions. Chronic lesions contain more extensive xanthomatous areas.

Xanthogranulomas is benign and self-limited. Simple excision is curative. Local recurrence is uncommon, and there is no malignant potential. Imaging of these lesions is not

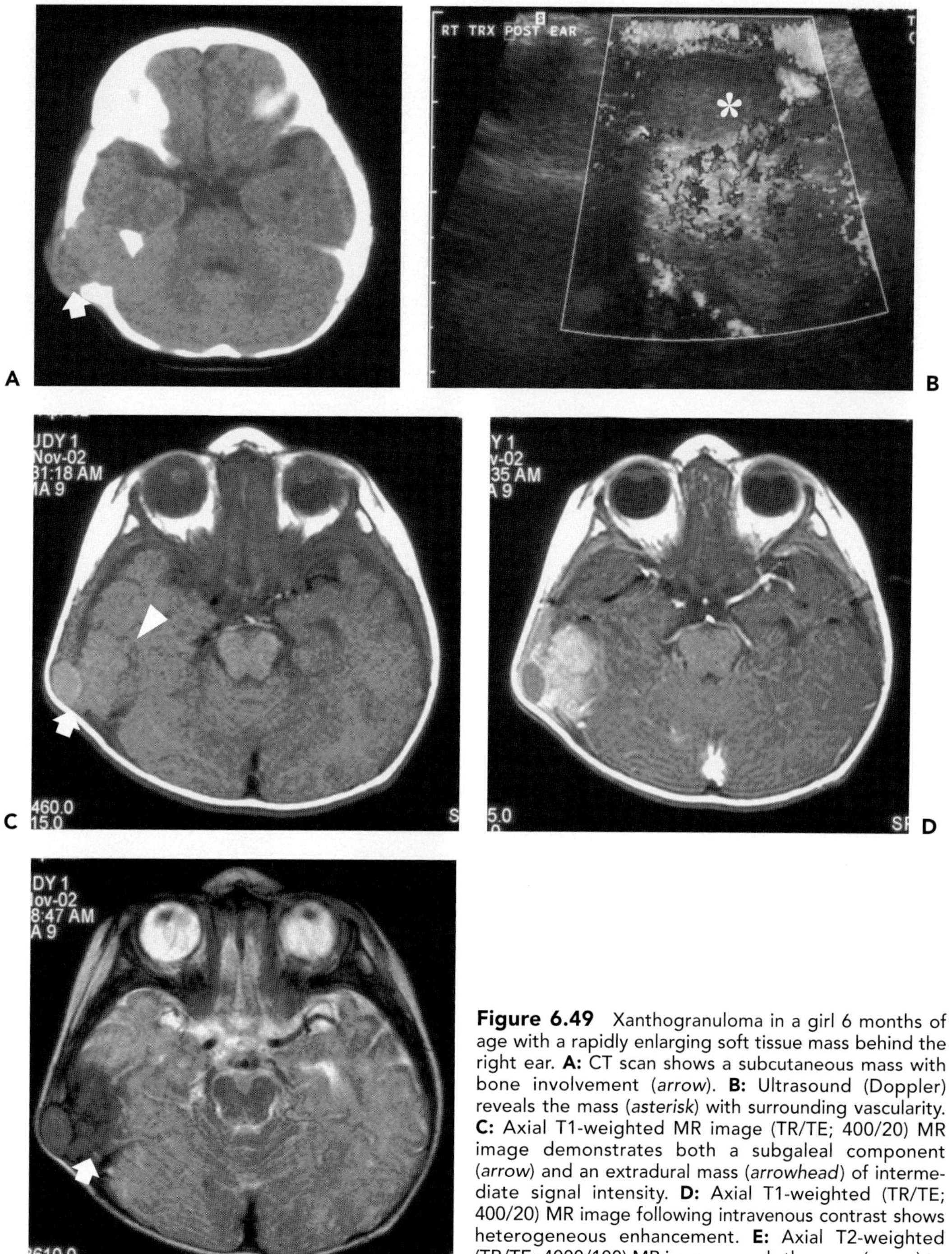

Figure 6.49 Xanthogranuloma in a girl 6 months of age with a rapidly enlarging soft tissue mass behind the right ear. **A:** CT scan shows a subcutaneous mass with bone involvement (*arrow*). **B:** Ultrasound (Doppler) reveals the mass (*asterisk*) with surrounding vascularity. **C:** Axial T1-weighted MR image (TR/TE; 400/20) MR image demonstrates both a subgaleal component (*arrow*) and an extradural mass (*arrowhead*) of intermediate signal intensity. **D:** Axial T1-weighted (TR/TE; 400/20) MR image following intravenous contrast shows heterogeneous enhancement. **E:** Axial T2-weighted (TR/TE; 4000/100) MR image reveals the mass (*arrow*) to show a low-to-intermediate signal intensity.

reported, to the best of our knowledge, but would likely show similar characteristics to those seen in xanthomas (Fig. 6.49).

Extranodal Rosai-Dorfman Disease

Sinus histiocytosis with massive lymphadenopathy (SHML) was described by Rosai and Dorfman in 1969 (340) with a subsequent report in 1972 (341). However,

the disease can occur in extranodal sites (43% of cases), both with or without lymph node involvement (342). Soft tissue involvement is most frequent in the proximal limbs and trunk and occurs in approximately 9% to 10% of cases of Rosai-Dorfman disease (343). It may be the sole manifestation (3% of patients) (1,344–346). Bone involvement may occur. Patients with extranodal disease are generally older than those with SHML (3,31). Skin and

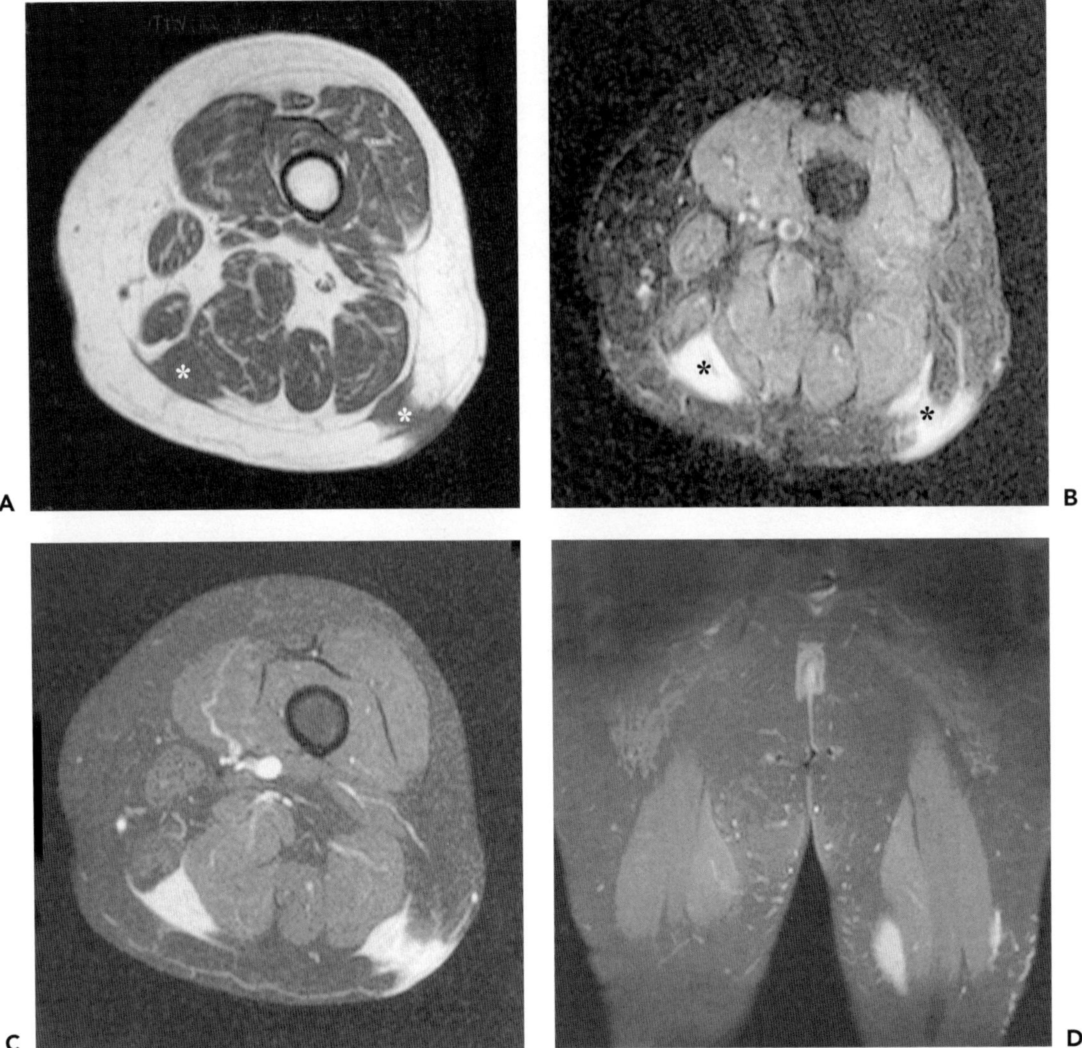

Figure 6.50   Rosai-Dorfman disease: MR imaging in a woman 40 years of age presenting with a soft tissue mass. **A,B:** Axial T1-weighted (TR/TE; 537/12) **(A)** and short-tau inversion recovery (STIR) (TR/TE/TI; 4003/18/120) **(B)** MR images show two nonspecific soft tissue masses in the posterior subcutaneous adipose tissue (*asterisks*). The lateral mass extends to the skin. **C,D:** Fat-suppressed, enhanced, axial **(C)** and coronal **(D)** T1-weighted (TR/TE; 504/12) MR images show intense homogeneous enhancement and surrounding edema.

KEY CONCEPTS

- Extranodal Rosai-Dorfman disease is seen in 43% of cases of sinus histiocytosis with massive lymphadenopathy.
- Soft tissue involvement is most frequent in the proximal limbs and trunk, and occurs in about 10% of patients.
- Surgical resection reveals residual or recurrent disease in approximately 50% of cases.
- Imaging is only rarely reported and shows intermediate signal intensity on T1-weighted images and high signal intensity on T2-weighted images. PET imaging has been reported to reveal the lesion to be hypermetabolic.

subcutaneous involvement are likely underreported. The soft tissue masses range from 0.5 to 10 cm, and histologically the masses contain sheets of histiocytes (3,31). Prognosis in these patients is good following surgical resection, although residual or recurrent disease is reported in approximately 50% of patients (3,31). Steroid therapy, radiation, and chemotherapy are reserved for patients with refractory disease (3,31). Imaging are only rarely reported and demonstrate a nonspecific soft tissue mass with or without associated adenopathy. Radiographs are typically normal. Lymph node involvement is reported to show increased metabolic activity on fluorodeoxyglucose-positron emission tomography (FDG-PET)

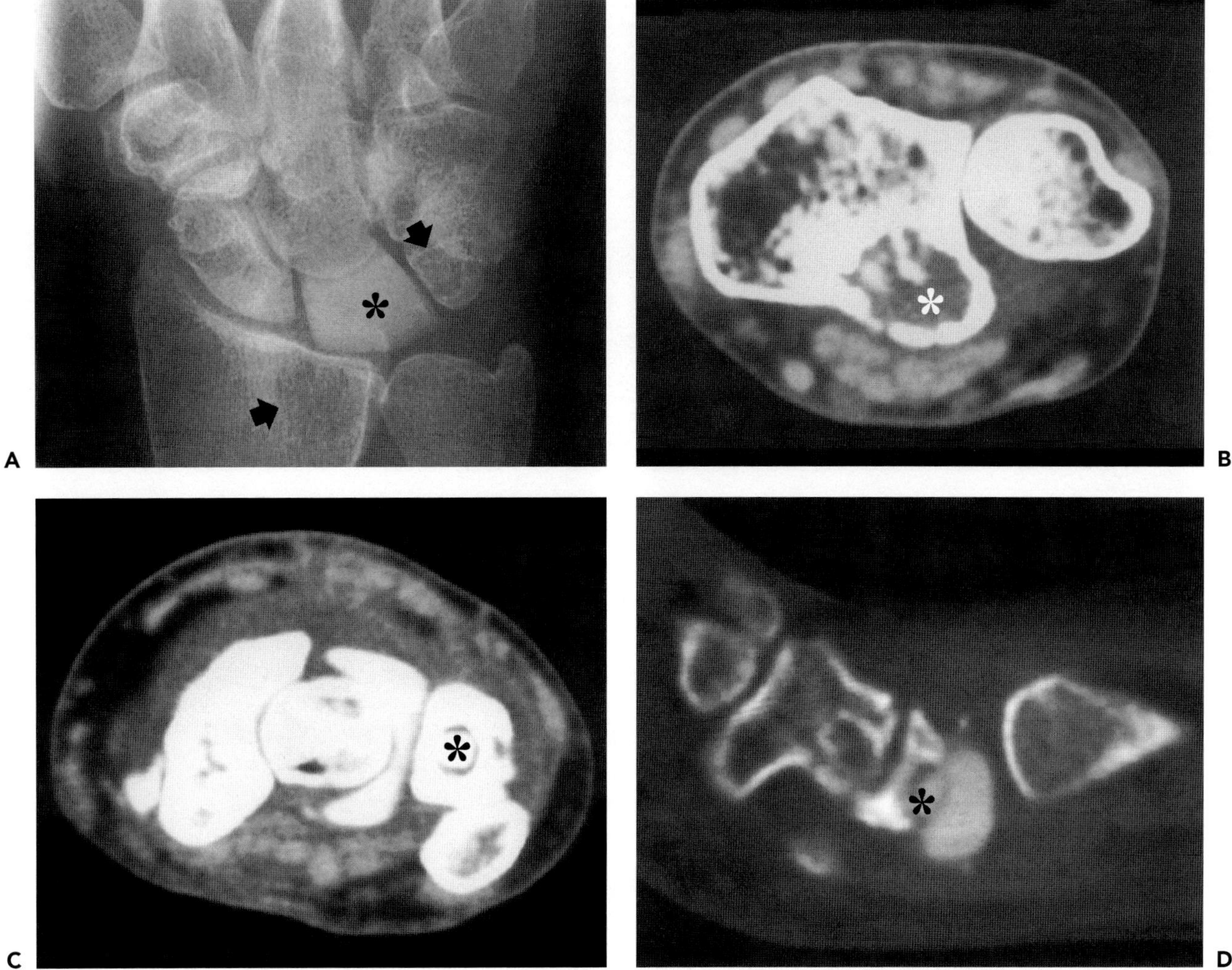

Figure 6.51 Silastic arthropathy 1 year after implant replacing lunate in a woman 34 years of age. **A:** Radiograph shows silastic implant (*asterisk*) and subtle lucencies in surrounding subchondral bone (*arrows*). **B,C:** Axial CT scans at the level of the distal radius **(B)** and lunate **(C)** reveal marked soft tissue thickening from foreign body reaction and distal radial cyst containing silastic fragments (*asterisk*). **D:** Direct sagittal CT image also shows these changes. Silastic lunate (*asterisk*) is well seen.

(343). Young et al. reported a patient with two lesions in the subcutaneous tissue of the thigh (347). MR imaging of this patient's mass revealed homogenous and intermediate signal intensity on T1-weighting, high signal intensity on STIR, and homogeneous intense enhancement following intravenous contrast administration (Fig. 6.50).

Foreign Body Reaction

Fibrohistiocytic and giant cell granulomatous reaction to foreign bodies within the soft tissues can simulate a neoplastic process both radiologically and pathologically (3,348) (Figs. 6.51–6.54). The foreign material can originate from endogenous sources (lipid extruded from cells: lipogranuloma, urate, or cholesterol) or exogenous substances (metal, wood, metallic, joint prostheses, silica, paraffin, implants, plastic, suture material, glass, thorns,

---

KEY CONCEPTS

- Fibrohistiocytic and giant cell granulomatous reaction to foreign bodies may simulate a neoplastic process.
- The foreign material may be from an endogenous or exogenous source.
- Silicone prostheses, because of their inherent weakness, may fragment and lead to an extensive synovitis.
- The hand and foot are the most common locations for foreign bodies and many are readily apparent on radiography.
- Nonopaque foreign bodies (particularly wood and glass) are well-seen on sonography as echogenic foci with posterior acoustic shadowing.
- The surrounding granulomatous reaction may simulate a nonspecific soft tissue mass with intermediate-to-high signal intensity on long TR MR images. The foreign body is usually low signal intensity on all MR pulse sequences, but may be quite subtle.

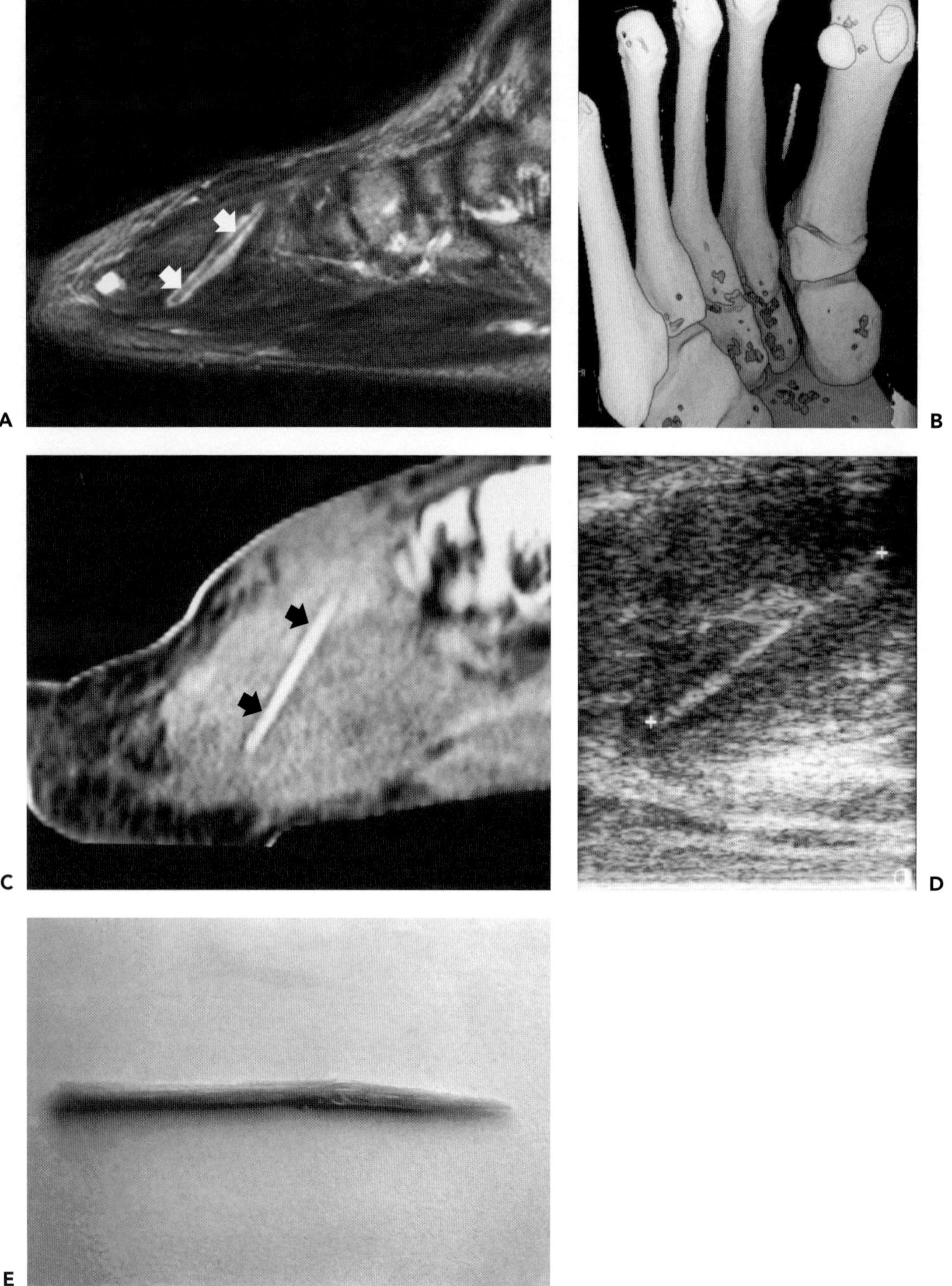

Figure 6.52   Retained wooden foreign body: Imaging in a girl 11 years of age who presented with a 2-year history of intermittently draining sinus on dorsum of foot, at site of previous surgery for a "ganglion cyst." **A:** Sagittal short-tau inversion recovery (STIR) (TR/TE/TI; 4500/96/150) MR image shows hypointense retained wooden foreign body (*arrows*) with surrounding high signal inflammatory response. **B:** Three-dimensional surface-rendered CT scan of foot shows retained wooden foreign body within soft tissue between first and second metatarsals. **C:** Sagittal reformatted CT shows increased attenuation of the foreign body (*arrows*). **D:** Gray-scale sonogram shows hyperechoic retained wooden foreign body with associated acoustic shadowing. Image is positioned to correspond to MR image **A**. **E:** Gross specimen photograph depicts toothpick removed at surgery.

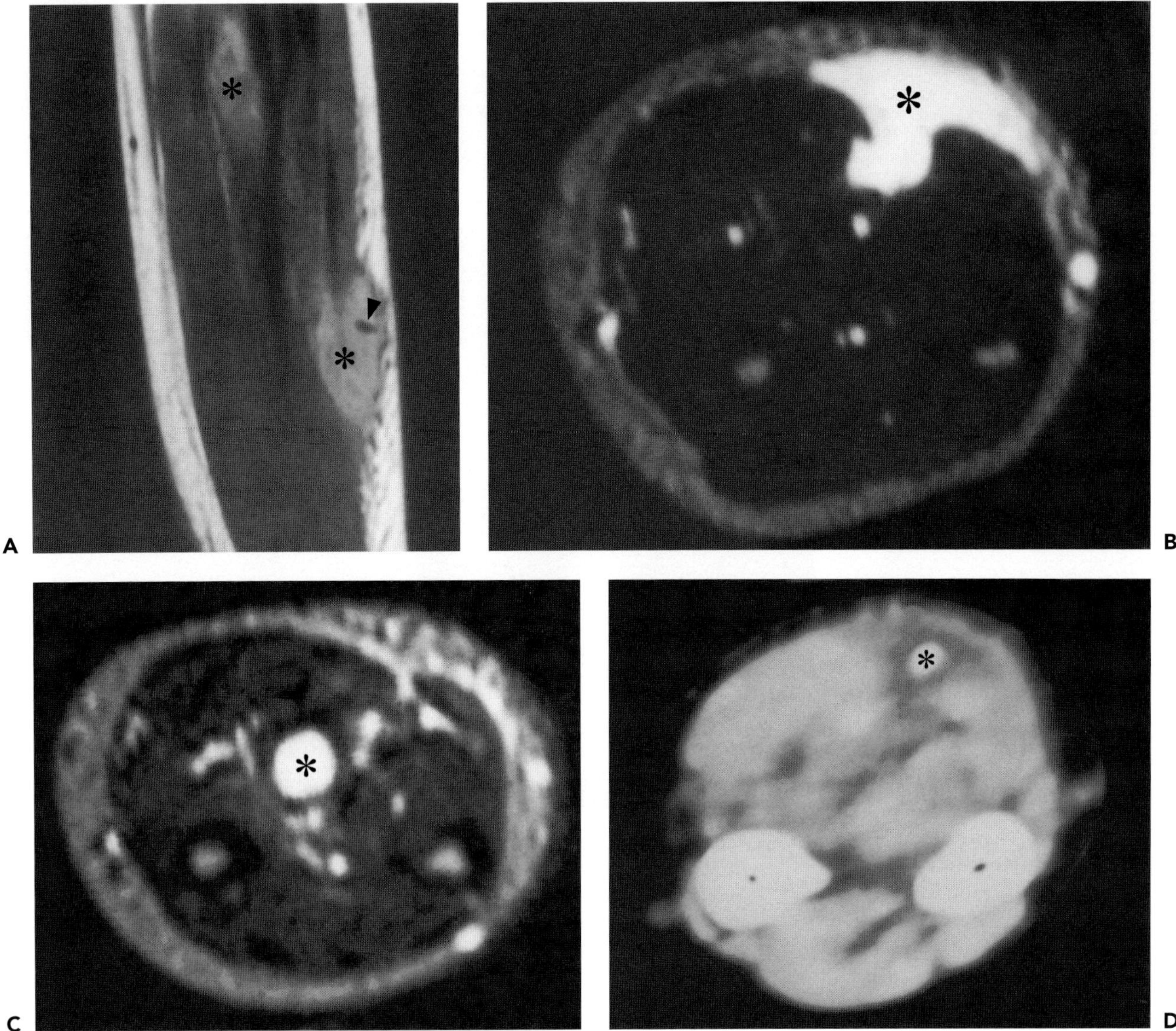

Figure 6.53 Granulomatous foreign body reaction around pencil fragment imbedded in upper arm of a woman 19 years of age who initially did not remember puncture incident. **A-C:** Coronal proton density (TR/TE; 2000/20) **(A)** and axial T2-weighted (TR/TE; 2500/80) MR images in the proximal **(B)** and distal **(C)** forearm show an alongated tubular soft tissue mass (*asterisks*), suggesting a neoplasm beginning superficially and extending into the deep soft tissues. Foreign body is seen as a low intensity tubular structure (*arrowhead* in **A**). **D:** Axial noncontrast CT demonstrates high attenuation foreign body (*asterisk*) and surrounding low attenuation foreign body reaction. (*continued*)

hemostatic agents) (3,31,349,350). Localized masses resulting from fibrohistiocytic reactions are also reported with silica and polyvinylpyrrolidone administered in focal injections (3) or ingestion substances such as clofazimine (351). In addition, silicone prostheses have been used extensively for replacement of small joints (particularly in rheumatoid arthritis patients) of the hands, wrists, feet, and temporomandibular joints (352–355). The inherent weakness of this material allows progressive fragmentation and debris from the shedding of silicone particles. The associated foreign body reaction can result in extensive synovitis, and regional adenopathy has also been reported (355). The incidence of silicone synovitis ranges from very low to 75% of patients and appears to be most frequent in carpal prostheses (356). The synovitis occurs from months to years after surgery, and classic radiographic changes may be present in asymptomatic patients. Radiologic changes of synovitis are apparent, with soft tissue thickening and swelling about the involved joints on CT or MR imaging (Fig. 6.51) (357,358). There may be low signal intensity on both T1- and T2-weighted

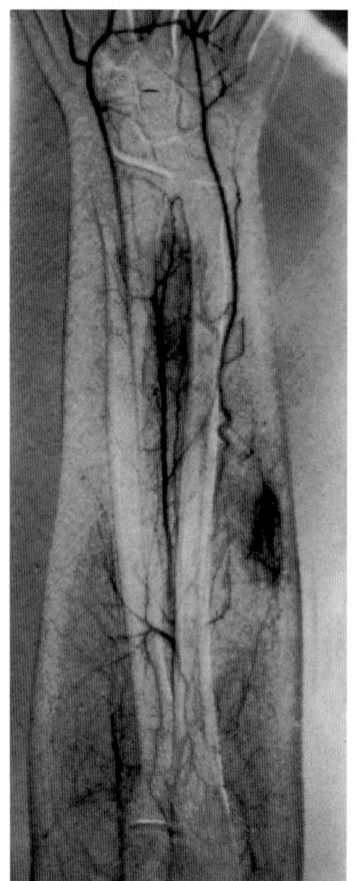

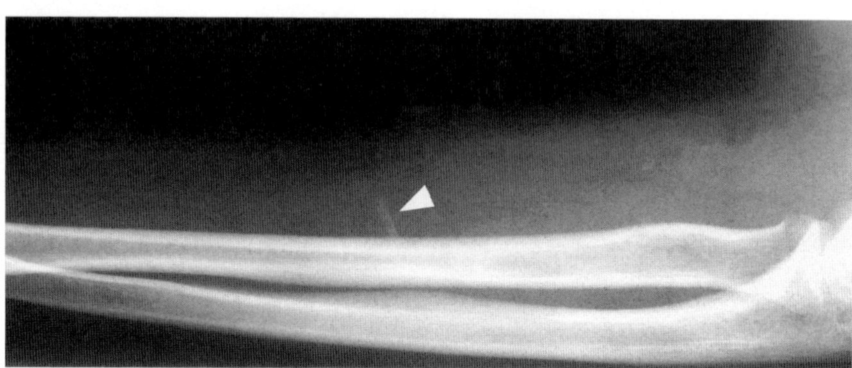

Figure 6.53 *(continued)*   **E:** Angiogram reveals staining and neovascularity along granulomatous foreign body reaction. **F:** Radiograph, subsequently obtained, shows opaque pencil fragment (*arrowhead*) in volar soft tissues.

MR images because of the collagen content of the fibrohistiocytic reaction. Osseous changes are also often present and include subchondral lucencies, erosions, lack of osteopenia, maintained joint spaces, and fractured or subluxed silicone prostheses (Fig. 6.51) (357,358).

Multiple additional foreign bodies in the soft tissue may result in a giant cell granulomatous reaction largely composed of histiocytes and a background of inflammatory cells (Figs. 6.52, 6.53, and 6.54). Although any site can be involved, the hand and foot are most frequent. Many foreign bodies are readily apparent on radiographs, and associated secondary infection of bone may also be recognized (359). However, wood and glass may be very difficult to detect on routine radiography and may be better appreciated with xeroradiography, computed radiography, or CT (Fig. 6.53) (359–361). Other foreign bodies, such as plastic and thorns, typically cannot be seen on radiographs (349). Sonography may be the most sensitive modality to detect these subtle foreign bodies (Figs. 6.52 and 6.54) (362–370). Echogenic foci with shadowing are typically seen on ultrasound exami-

nation (Figs. 6.52 and 6.54). Sonography or CT may also be used in directing removal of the foreign body, obviating the need for surgery (371,372). CT of foreign bodies usually reveals high attenuation areas, although fragments of wood may initially have air attenuation (for approximately 1 week) (361,363,370,371). Prominent focal soft tissue masses may also be detected with imaging and are not infrequently misdiagnosed as neoplasms, if the foreign body is not recognized (348). MR imaging of these masses usually reveals masses of low-to-intermediate intensity with T1-weighting and intermediate-to-high intensity with T2-weighting (Fig. 6.53) (220,362, 364,373,374). Surrounding changes of inflammation may or may not be identified. The foreign body is usually linear and low intensity on all MR pulse sequences (Fig. 6.53) (361,370,375). However, the foreign body is often small and relatively inconspicuous within the soft tissue mass. Angiography in these cases reveals hypervascularity and staining, further simulating a neoplastic process. Clinical correlation and comparison with radiographs is vital to ensure accurate diagnosis of these lesions.

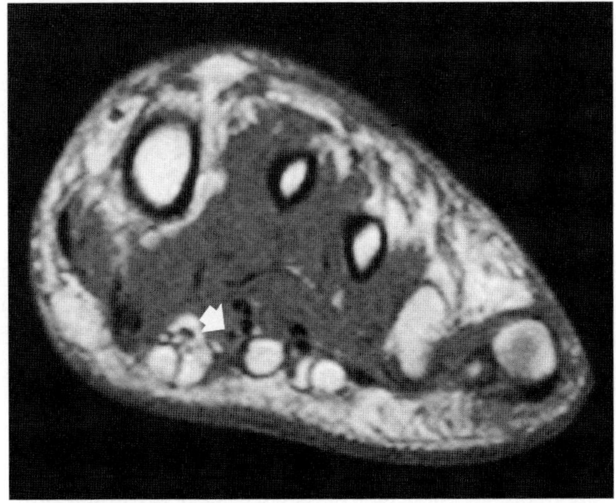

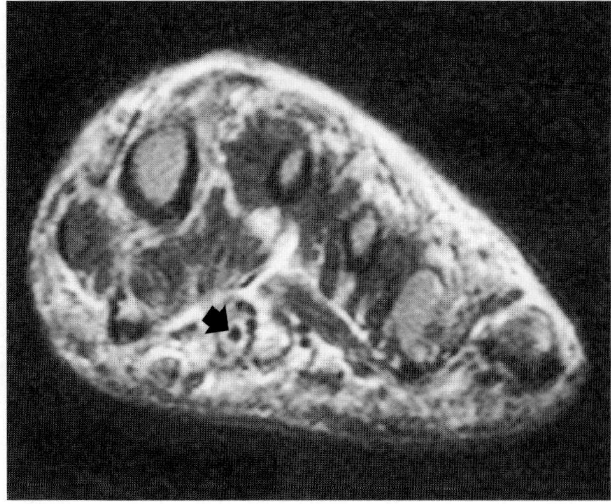

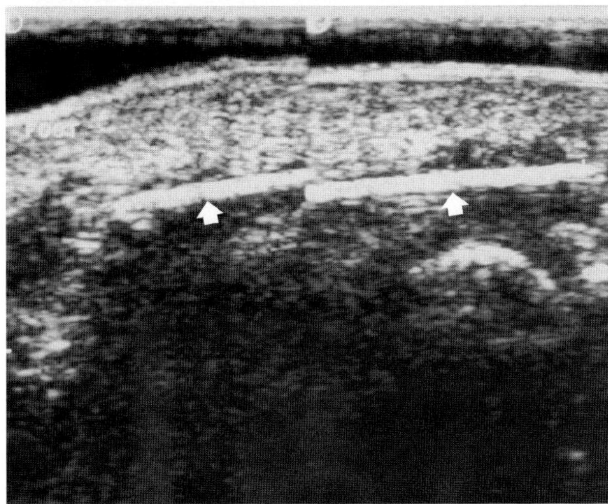

Figure 6.54 Retained wooden foreign body: MR and ultrasound imaging in a woman 49 years of age presenting 1 month following suspected puncture injury. **A,B:** Coronal T1-weighted (TR/TE; 700/20) **(A)** and T2-weighted (TR/TE; 2000/90) **(B)** spin-echo MR images show a toothpick (*arrow*) in the plantar aspect of the foot. The foreign body is difficult to distinguish from adjacent tendons. Note surrounding rind of high signal intensity representing inflammatory response **(B)**. **C:** Sonogram done to confirm MR findings shows hyperechoic retained wooden foreign body (*arrows*).

REFERENCES

1. Enzinger F, Weiss S, Goldblum J. *Enzinger and Weiss's Soft Tissue Tumors*. 4th ed. St. Louis: Mosby; 2001.
2. Konwaler BE, Keasbey L, Kaplan L. Subcutaneous pseudosarcomatous fibromatosis (fasciitis). *Am J Clin Pathol*. 1955;25:241–252.
3. Enzinger F, Weiss SW. Benign fibrohistiocytic tumors. In: Weiss SW and Goldblum JR, eds. *Soft Tissue Tumors*. 4th ed. St. Louis: Mosby; 2001:441–490.
4. Fletcher C, Unni K, Mertens F. *World Health Organization Classification of Tumors. Pathology and Genetics of Tumors of Soft Tissue and Bone*. Lyon, France: IARC Press; 2002.
5. Kempson R, Fletcher C, Evans H, et al. Fibrous and myofibroblastic tumors. In: Rosai J, ed. *Tumors of the Soft Tissues*. 3rd ed. Bethesda, MD: Armed Forces Institute of Pathology; 2001:23–112.
6. Miettinen M. Benign fibroblastic and myofibroblastic proliferations. In: *Diagnostic Soft Tissue Pathology*. New York: Churchill Livingstone; 2003:143–172.
7. Katz MA, Beredjiklian PK, Wirganowicz PZ. Nodular fasciitis of the hand: a case report. *Clin Orthop*. 2001;108–111.
8. Kempson RL, Fletcher CM, Evans HL, et al. *Tumors of the Soft Tissues*. Bethesda, MD: Armed Forces Institute of Pathology; 2001.
9. Montgomery EA, Meis JM. Nodular fasciitis. Its morphologic spectrum and immunohistochemical profile. *Am J Surg Pathol*. 1991;15:942–948.
10. Price EB Jr, Silliphant WM, Shuman R. Nodular fasciitis: a clinicopathologic analysis of 65 cases. *Am J Clin Pathol*. 1961;35:122–136.
11. Batsakis JG, Rice DH, Howard DR. The pathology of head and neck tumors: spindle cell lesions (sarcomatoid carcinomas, nodular fasciitis, and fibrosarcoma) of the aerodigestive tracts, Part 14. *Head Neck Surg*. 1982;4:499–513.
12. Rankin G, Kuschner SH, Gellman H. Nodular fasciitis: a rapidly growing tumor of the hand. *J Hand Surg [Am]*. 1991;16:791–795.
13. Samaratunga H, Searle J, O'Loughlin B. Nodular fasciitis and related pseudosarcomatous lesions of soft tissues. *Aust N Z J Surg*. 1996;66:22–25.
14. Shimizu S, Hashimoto H, Enjoji M. Nodular fasciitis: an analysis of 250 patients. *Pathology*. 1984;16:161–166.
15. Bernstein KE, Lattes R. Nodular (pseudosarcomatous) fasciitis, a nonrecurrent lesion: clinicopathologic study of 134 cases. *Cancer*. 1982;49:1668–1678.
16. Allen PW. Nodular fasciitis. *Pathology*. 1972;4:9–26.
17. Broder MS, Leonidas JC, Mitty HA. Pseudosarcomatous fasciitis: an unusual cause of soft-tissue calcification. *Radiology*. 1973;107:173–174.
18. Wirman JA. Nodular fasciitis, a lesion of myofibroblasts: an ultrastructural study. *Cancer*. 1976;38:2378–2389.
19. Stanley MW, Skoog L, Tani EM, et al. Nodular fasciitis: spontaneous resolution following diagnosis by fine-needle aspiration. *Diagn Cytopathol*. 1993;9:322–324.
20. Graham BS, Barrett TL, Goltz RW. Nodular fasciitis: response to intralesional corticosteroids. *J Am Acad Dermatol*. 1999;40:490–492.
21. Kijima H, Okada K, Ito H, Shimada Y, et al. Nodular fasciitis of the finger. *Skeletal Radiol*. 2005;34:121–123.

22. Leung LY, Shu SJ, Chan AC, et al. Nodular fasciitis: MRI appearance and literature review. *Skeletal Radiol.* 2002;31:9–13.

23. Wang XL, De Schepper AM, Vanhoenacker F, et al. Nodular fasciitis: correlation of MRI findings and histopathology. *Skeletal Radiol.* 2002;31:155–161.

24. Meyer CA, Kransdorf MJ, Jelinek JS, et al. MR and CT appearance of nodular fasciitis. *J Comput Assist Tomogr.* 1991;15:276–279.

25. Wilson DJ. Ultrasonic imaging of soft tissues. *Clin Radiol.* 1989;40:341–342.

26. Toledo AS, Rodriguez J, Cuasay NS, et al. Nodular fasciitis of the facial region: CT characteristics. *J Comput Assist Tomogr.* 1988;12:898–899.

27. Frei S, de Lange EE, Fechner RE. Case report 690. Nodular fasciitis of the elbow. *Skeletal Radiol.* 1991;20:468–471.

28. Meduri S, Zuiani C, Del Frate C, et al. Retroperitoneal nodular fasciitis: magnetic resonance imaging (MRI) and pathological features. *Adv Clin Path.* 1998;2:225–229.

29. Patchefsky AS, Enzinger FM. Intravascular fasciitis: a report of 17 cases. *Am J Surg Pathol.* 1981;5:29–36.

30. Lauer DH, Enzinger FM. Cranial fasciitis of childhood. *Cancer.* 1980;45:401–406.

31. Miettinen M. Lymphoid, myeloid, and histiocytic neoplasms involving soft tissues. In: *Diagnostic Soft Tissue Pathology.* New York: Churchill Livingstone; 2003:505–569.

32. Adler R, Wong CA. Cranial fasciitis simulating histiocytosis. *J Pediatr* 1986;109:85–88.

33. Pagenstecher A, Emmerich B, van Velthoven V, et al. Exclusively intracranial cranial fasciitis in a child. Case report. *J Neurosurg.* 1995;83:744–747.

34. Sajben FP, Eichenfield LF, O'Grady TC, et al. Cranial fasciitis of childhood. *Pediatr Dermatol.* 1999;16:232–234.

35. Sayama T, Morioka T, Baba T, et al. Cranial fasciitis with massive intracranial extension. *Childs Nerv Syst.* 1995;11:242–245.

36. Clapp CG, Dodson EE, Pickett BP, et al. Cranial fasciitis presenting as an external auditory canal mass. *Arch Otolaryngol Head Neck Surg.* 1997;123:223–225.

37. Hoya K, Usui M, Sugiyama Y, et al. Cranial fasciitis. *Childs Nerv Syst.* 1996;12:556–558.

38. Kumon Y, Sakaki S, Sakoh M, et al. Cranial fasciitis of childhood: a case report. *Surg Neurol.* 1992;38:68–72.

39. Boddie DE, Distante S, Blaiklock CT. Cranial fasciitis of childhood: an incidental finding of a lytic skull lesion. *Br J Neurosurg.* 1997;11:445–447.

40. Martinez-Lage JF, Torroba A, Lopez F, et al. Cranial fasciitis of the anterior fontanel. *Childs Nerv Syst.* 1997;13:626–628.

41. Hoeffel JC, Galloy MA, Palau R, et al. Case report: cranial fasciitis in childhood. *Br J Radiol.* 1993;66:1058–1060.

42. Hunter NS, Bulas DI, Chadduck WM, et al. Cranial fasciitis of childhood. *Pediatr Radiol.* 1993;23:398–399.

43. Chung EB, Enzinger FM. Proliferative fasciitis. *Cancer.* 1975;36:1450–1458.

44. Enzinger FM, Dulcey F. Proliferative myositis. Report of thirty-three cases. *Cancer.* 1967;20:2213–2223.

45. Kern WH. Proliferative myositis; a pseudosarcomatous reaction to injury: a report of seven cases. *Arch Pathol.* 1960;69:209–216.

46. Choi SS, Myer CM III. Proliferative myositis of the mylohyoid muscle. *Am J Otolaryngol.* 1990;11:198–202.

47. Kleinman GM, Zelem JD, Sanders FJ. Proliferative myositis in a two-year-old child. *Pediatr Pathol.* 1987;7:71–75.

48. Lorenc ZP, Brourman S, Imbriglia JE. Proliferative fasciitis of the hand in a child. *J Hand Surg [Am].* 1987;12:1066–1070.

49. Meis JM, Enzinger FM. Proliferative fasciitis and myositis of childhood. *Am J Surg Pathol.* 1992;16:364–372.

50. Pasquel P, Salazar M, Marvan E. Proliferative myositis in an infant: report of a case with electron microscopic observations. *Pediatr Pathol.* 1988;8:545–551.

51. Scher N, Dobleman TJ, Poe DS, et al. Proliferative myositis of the masseter muscle. *Laryngoscope.* 1987;97:591–593.

52. Craver JL, McDivitt RW. Proliferative fasciitis: ultrastructural study of two cases. *Arch Pathol Lab Med.* 1981;105:542–545.

53. Rose AG. An electron microscopic study of the giant cells in proliferative myositis. *Cancer.* 1974;33:1543–1547.

54. Mulier S, Stas M, Delabie J, et al. Proliferative myositis in a child. *Skeletal Radiol.* 1999;28:703–709.

55. Pollock L, Fullilove S, Shaw DG, et al. Proliferative myositis in a child. A case report. *J Bone Joint Surg Am.* 1995;77:132–135.

56. Wlachovska B, Abraham B, Deux JF, et al. Proliferative myositis in a patient with AIDS. *Skeletal Radiol.* 2004;33:237–240.

57. Chung EB, Enzinger FM. Fibroma of tendon sheath. *Cancer.* 1979;44:1945–1954.

58. Geschickter CF, Copeland MM. *Tumors of Bone.* Philadelphia: JB Lippincott; 1949.

59. Humphreys S, McKee PH, Fletcher CD. Fibroma of tendon sheath: a clinicopathologic study. *J Cutan Pathol.* 1986;13:331–338.

60. Pulitzer DR, Martin PC, Reed RJ. Fibroma of tendon sheath. A clinicopathologic study of 32 cases. *Am J Surg Pathol.* 1989;13:472–479.

61. Greene TL, Strickland JW. Fibroma of tendon sheath. *J Hand Surg [Am].* 1984;9:758–760.

62. Feinberg MS. Fibroma of a tendon causing limited finger motion: a case report. *J Hand Surg [Am].* 1979;4:386.

63. Maluf HM, DeYoung BR, Swanson PE, et al. Fibroma and giant cell tumor of tendon sheath: a comparative histological and immunohistological study. *Mod Pathol.* 1995;8:155–159.

64. Satti MB. Tendon sheath tumours: a pathological study of the relationship between giant cell tumour and fibroma of tendon sheath. *Histopathology.* 1992;20:213–220.

65. Sarma DP, Townsend GH, Rodriguez FH Jr. Fibroma of tendon sheath. *J Foot Surg.* 1987;26:422–424.

66. Lourie JA, Lwin KY, Woods CG. Case report 734. Fibroma of tendon sheath eroding 3rd metatarsal bone. *Skeletal Radiol.* 1992;21:273–275.

67. Southwick GJ, Karamoskos P. Fibroma of tendon sheath with bone involvement. *J Hand Surg [Br].* 1990;15:373–375.

68. Fox MG, Kransdorf MJ, Bancroft LW, et al. MR imaging of fibroma of the tendon sheath. *AJR Am J Roentgenol.* 2003;180:1449–1453.

69. Järvi O, Saxén E. Elastofibroma dorse. *Acta Pathol Microbiol Scand.* 1961;51(suppl 144):83–84.

70. Järvi OH, Saxén AE, Hopsu-Havu VK, et al. Elastofibroma—a degenerative pseudotumor. *Cancer.* 1969;23:42–63.

71. Järvi OH, Lansimies PH. Subclinical elastofibromas in the scapular region in an autopsy series. *Acta Pathol Microbiol Scand [A].* 1975;83:87–108.

72. Kumaratilake JS, Krishnan R, Lomax-Smith J, et al. Elastofibroma: disturbed elastic fibrillogenesis by periosteal-derived cells? An immunoelectron microscopic and in situ hybridization study. *Hum Pathol.* 1991;22:1017–1029.

73. Marin ML, Perzin KH, Markowitz AM. Elastofibroma dorsi: benign chest wall tumor. *J Thorac Cardiovasc Surg.* 1989;98:234–238.

74. Nagamine N, Nohara Y, Ito E. Elastofibroma in Okinawa. A clinicopathologic study of 170 cases. *Cancer.* 1982;50:1794–1805.

75. Mirra JM, Straub LR, Järvi OH. Elastofibroma of the deltoid. A case report. *Cancer.* 1974;33:234–238.

76. Barr JR. Elastofibroma. *Am J Clin Pathol.* 1966;45:679–683.

77. Nishida A, Uetani M, Okimoto T, et al. Bilateral elastofibroma of the thighs with concomitant subscapular lesions. *Skeletal Radiol.* 2003;32:116–118.

78. Kapff PD, Hocken DB, Simpson RH. Elastofibroma of the hand. *J Bone Joint Surg Br.* 1987;69:468–469.

79. Cross DL, Mills SE, Kulund DN. Elastofibroma arising in the foot. *South Med J.* 1984;77:1194–1196.

80. Kransdorf MJ, Meis JM, Montgomery E. Elastofibroma: MR and CT appearance with radiologic-pathologic correlation. *AJR Am J Roentgenol.* 1992;159:575–579.

81. Waisman J, Smith D. Fine structure of an elastofibroma. *Cancer.* 1968;22:671–677.

82. Austin P, Jakobiec FA, Iwamoto T, et al. Elastofibroma oculi. *Arch Ophthalmol.* 1983;101:1575–1579.

83. Prete PE, Henbest M, Michalski JP, et al. Intraspinal elastofibroma. A case report. *Spine.* 1983;8:800–802.

84. Pechman D, Kenan S, Abdelwahab IF, et al. Case report 839: elastofibroma of the right shoulder causing brachial plexus impingement. *Skeletal Radiol.* 1994;23:459–461.

85. Schwarz T, Oppolzer G, Duschet P, et al. Ulcerating elastofibroma dorsi. *J Am Acad Dermatol.* 1989;21:1142–1144.

86. Ghiatas AA, Armstrong S, Tio FO. Case report 583: elastofibroma dorsi. *Skeletal Radiol.* 1989;18:619–622.

87. Winkelmann RK, Sams WM Jr. Elastofibroma. Report of a case with special histochemical and electron-microscopic studies. *Cancer.* 1969;23:406–415.

88. Bianchi S, Martinoli C, Abdelwahab IF, et al. Elastofibroma dorsi: sonographic findings. *AJR Am J Roentgenol.* 1997;169:1113–1115.

89. Brandser EA, Goree JC, El-Khoury GY. Elastofibroma dorsi: prevalence in an elderly patient population as revealed by CT. *AJR Am J Roentgenol.* 1998;171:977–980.

90. Berthoty DP, Shulman HS, Miller HA. Elastofibroma: chest wall pseudotumor. *Radiology.* 1986;160:341–342.

91. Gould ES, Javors BR, Morrison J, et al. MR appearance of bilateral periscapular elastofibromas. *J Comput Assist Tomogr.* 1989; 13:701–703.

92. Massengill AD, Sundaram M, Kathol MH, et al. Elastofibroma dorsi: a radiological diagnosis. *Skeletal Radiol.* 1993;22:121–123.

93. Bui-Mansfield LT, Chew FS, Stanton CA. Elastofibroma dorsi of the chest wall. *AJR Am J Roentgenol.* 2000;175:244.

94. Devaney D, Livesley P, Shaw D. Elastofibroma dorsi: MRI diagnosis in a young girl. *Pediatr Radiol.* 1995;25:282–283.

95. Nakano T, Tsutsumi Z, Hada T, et al. Radiological manifestation of elastofibroma: a case report and review of the literature. *Br J Radiol.* 1991;64:1069–1072.

96. Yu JS, Weis LD, Vaughan LM, et al. MRI of elastofibroma dorsi. *J Comput Assist Tomogr.* 1995;19:601–603.

97. Schick S, Zembsch A, Gahleitner A, et al. Atypical appearance of elastofibroma dorsi on MRI: case reports and review of the literature. *J Comput Assist Tomogr.* 2000;24:288–292.

98. Soler R, Requejo I, Pombo F, et al. Elastofibroma dorsi: MR and CT findings. *Eur J Radiol.* 1998;27:264–267.

99. Bae SJ, Shin MJ, Kim SM, et al. Intra-articular elastofibroma of the shoulder joint. *Skeletal Radiol.* 2002;31:171–174.

100. Vande Berg B, Malghem J, Leflot JL, et al. Case report: elastofibroma dorsi: a pseudomalignant lesion. *Clin Radiol.* 1996;51: 67–69.

101. Naylor MF, Nascimento AG, Sherrick AD, et al. Elastofibroma dorsi: radiologic findings in 12 patients. *AJR Am J Roentgenol.* 1996;167:683–687.

102. Berman B, Bieley HC. Adjunct therapies to surgical management of keloids. *Dermatol Surg.* 1996;22:126–130.

103. Lawrence WT. In search of the optimal treatment of keloids: report of a series and a review of the literature. *Ann Plast Surg.* 1991;27:164–178.

104. Klumpar DI, Murray JC, Anscher M. Keloids treated with excision followed by radiation therapy. *J Am Acad Dermatol.* 1994;31:225–231.

105. Sallstrom KO, Larson O, Heden P, et al. Treatment of keloids with surgical excision and postoperative X-ray radiation. *Scand J Plast Reconstr Surg Hand Surg.* 1989;23:211–215.

106. Alster TS, Williams CM. Treatment of keloid sternotomy scars with 585 nm flashlamp-pumped pulsed-dye laser. *Lancet.* 1995;345:1198–1200.

107. Katz BE. Silicone gel sheeting in scar therapy. *Cutis.* 1995;56: 65–67.

108. Lawrence WT. Treatment of earlobe keloids with surgery plus adjuvant intralesional verapamil and pressure earrings. *Ann Plast Surg.* 1996;37:167–169.

109. Zouboulis CC, Blume U, Buttner P, et al. Outcomes of cryosurgery in keloids and hypertrophic scars. A prospective consecutive trial of case series. *Arch Dermatol.* 1993;129:1146–1151.

110. Beggs I, Salter DS, Dorfman HD. Synovial desmoplastic fibroblastoma of hip joint with bone erosion. *Skeletal Radiol.* 1999;28:402–406.

111. Shuto R, Kiyosue H, Hori Y, et al. CT and MR imaging of desmoplastic fibroblastoma. *Eur Radiol.* 2002;12:2474–2476.

112. Walker KR, Bui-Mansfield LT, Gering SA, et al. Collagenous fibroma (desmoplastic fibroblastoma) of the shoulder. *AJR Am J Roentgenol.* 2004;183:1766.

113. McMenamin ME, DeSchryver K, Fletcher CD. Fibrous lesions of the breast: a review. *Int J Surg Pathol.* 2000;8:99–108.

114. McMenamin ME, Fletcher CD. Mammary-type myofibroblastoma of soft tissue: a tumor closely related to spindle cell lipoma. *Am J Surg Pathol.* 2001;25:1022–1029.

115. Wargotz ES, Weiss SW, Norris HJ. Myofibroblastoma of the breast. Sixteen cases of a distinctive benign mesenchymal tumor. *Am J Surg Pathol.* 1987;11:493–502.

116. Robbin MR, Murphey MD, Temple HT, et al. Imaging of musculoskeletal fibromatosis. *Radiographics.* 2001;21:585–600.

117. Enzinger F, Weiss SW. Fibrous tumors of infancy and childhood. In: Weiss SW and Goldblum JR, eds. *Soft Tissue Tumors.* 4th ed. St. Louis: Mosby; 2001: 347–408.

118. Wiswell TE, Davis J, Cunningham BE, et al. Infantile myofibromatosis: the most common fibrous tumor of infancy. *J Pediatr Surg.* 1988;23:315–318.

119. Williams JO, Schrum D. Congenital fibrosarcoma; report of a case in a newborn infant. *AMA Arch Pathol.* 1951;51:548–552.

120. Stout A. Juvenile fibromatosis. *Cancer.* 1954;7:953–978.

121. Chung EB, Enzinger FM. Infantile myofibromatosis. *Cancer.* 1981;48:1807–1818.

122. Parker RK, Mallory SB, Baker GF. Infantile myofibromatosis. *Pediatr Dermatol.* 1991;8:129–132.

123. Wiswell TE. Infantile myofibromatosis and the use of magnetic resonance imaging. *Am J Dis Child.* 1988;142:486.

124. Morettin LB, Mueller E, Schreiber M. Generalized hamartomatosis (congenital generalized fibromatosis). *Am J Roentgenol Radium Ther Nucl Med.* 1972;114:722–734.

125. Queralt JA, Poirier VC. Solitary infantile myofibromatosis of the skull. *AJNR Am J Neuroradiol.* 1995;16:476–478.

126. Thunnissen BT, Bax NM, Rovekamp MH, et al. Infantile myofibromatosis: an unusual presentation and a review of the literature. *Eur J Pediatr Surg.* 1993;3:179–181.

127. Stautz CC. CT of infantile myofibromatosis of the orbit with intracranial involvement: a case report. *AJNR Am J Neuroradiol.* 1991;12:184–185.

128. Mentzel T, Calonje E, Nascimento AG, et al. Infantile hemangiopericytoma versus infantile myofibromatosis. Study of a series suggesting a continuous spectrum of infantile myofibroblastic lesions. *Am J Surg Pathol.* 1994;18:922–930.

129. Bartlett RC, Otis RD, Laakso AO. Multiple congenital neoplasms of soft tissues. Report of 4 cases in 1 family. *Cancer.* 1961;14:913–920.

130. Salamah MM, Hammoudi SM, Sadi AR. Infantile myofibromatosis. *J Pediatr Surg.* 1988;23:975–977.

131. Venencie PY, Bigel P, Desgruelles C, et al. Infantile myofibromatosis. Report of two cases in one family. *Br J Dermatol.* 1987;117:255–259.

132. Jennings TA, Duray PH, Collins FS, et al. Infantile myofibromatosis. Evidence for an autosomal-dominant disorder. *Am J Surg Pathol.* 1984;8:529–538.

133. Daimaru Y, Hashimoto H, Enjoji M. Myofibromatosis in adults (adult counterpart of infantile myofibromatosis). *Am J Surg Pathol.* 1989;13:859–865.

134. Coffin CM, Dehner LP. Fibroblastic-myofibroblastic tumors in children and adolescents: a clinicopathologic study of 108 examples in 103 patients. *Pediatr Pathol.* 1991;11:569–588.

135. Kransdorf MJ. Benign soft-tissue tumors in a large referral population: distribution of specific diagnoses by age, sex, and location. *AJR Am J Roentgenol.* 1995;164:395–402.

136. Stenzel P, Fitterer S. Gastrointestinal multicentric infantile myofibromatosis: characteristic histology on rectal biopsy. *Am J Gastroenterol.* 1989;84:1115–1119.

137. Soper JR, De Silva M. Infantile myofibromatosis: a radiological review. *Pediatr Radiol.* 1993;23:189–194.

138. Adickes ED, Goodrich P, AuchMoedy J, et al. Central nervous system involvement in congenital visceral fibromatosis. *Pediatr Pathol.* 1985;3:329–340.

139. Gold RH, Mirra JM. Case report 339: congenital multiple fibromatosis. *Skeletal Radiol.* 1985;14:309–311.

140. Michel M, Ninane J, Claus D, et al. Major malformations in a case of infantile myofibromatosis. *Eur J Pediatr.* 1990;149: 251–252.

141. Davies RS, Carty H, Pierro A. Infantile myofibromatosis—a review. *Br J Radiol.* 1994;67:619–623.

142. Chateil JF, Brun M, Lebail B, et al. Infantile myofibromatosis. *Skeletal Radiol.* 1995;24:629–632.

143. Rubenstein WA, Gray G, Auh YH, et al. CT of fibrous tissues and tumors with sonographic correlation. *AJR Am J Roentgenol.* 1986;147:1067–1074.

144. Baer JW, Radkowski MA. Congenital multiple fibromatosis. A case report with review of the world literature. *Am J Roentgenol Radium Ther Nucl Med.* 1973;118:200–205.

145. Present DA, Abdelwahab IF, Zwass A, et al. Case report 575. Infantile myofibromatosis. *Skeletal Radiol.* 1989;18:557–560.

146. Murray J. On three peculiar cases of molluscum fibrosum in children. *Med Chir Trans.* 1873;38:235.

147. Kitano Y, Horiki M, Aoki T, et al. Two cases of juvenile hyalin fibromatosis. Some histological, electron microscopic, and tissue culture observations. *Arch Dermatol.* 1972;106:877–883.

148. Coventry MB, Harris LE, Bianco AJ Jr et al. Congenital muscular torticollis (wryneck). *Postgrad Med.* 1960;28:383–392.

149. Campbell RE, Barone CA, Makris AN, et al. Image interpretation session: 1993. Fibromatosis colli. *Radiographics.* 1994;14:208–209.

150. Davids JR, Wenger DR, Mubarak SJ. Congenital muscular torticollis: sequela of intrauterine or perinatal compartment syndrome. *J Pediatr Orthop.* 1993;13:141–147.

151. Armstrong D, Pickrell K, Fetter B, et al. Torticollis: an analysis of 271 cases. *Plast Reconstr Surg.* 1965;35:14–25.

152. Isigkeit E. Untersuchungen uber die Hereditat orthopadischer leiden. *Arch Orthop Unfallchir.* 1931;30:459.

153. Sartoris DJ, Mochizuki RM, Parker BR. Lytic clavicular lesions in fibromatosis colli. *Skeletal Radiol.* 1983;10:34–36.

154. Gruhn J, Hurwitt ES. Fibrous sternomastoid tumor of infancy. *Pediatrics.* 1951;8:522–526.

155. Whyte AM, Lufkin RB, Bredenkamp J, et al. Sternocleidomastoid fibrosis in congenital muscular torticollis: MR appearance. *J Comput Assist Tomogr.* 1989;13:163–164.

156. Binder H, Eng GD, Gaiser JF, et al. Congenital muscular torticollis: results of conservative management with long-term follow-up in 85 cases. *Arch Phys Med Rehabil.* 1987;68:222–225.

157. Hulbert K. Congenital torticollis. *J Bone Joint Surg Br.* 1950;32:50.

158. Crawford SC, Harnsberger HR, Johnson L, et al. Fibromatosis colli of infancy: CT and sonographic findings. *AJR Am J Roentgenol.* 1988;151:1183–1184.

159. Kraus R, Han BK, Babcock DS, et al. Sonography of neck masses in children. *AJR Am J Roentgenol.* 1986;146:609–613.

160. Cintora E, del Cura JL, Ruiz JC, et al. Case report 807: infantile desmoid-type fibromatosis. *Skeletal Radiol.* 1993;22:533–535.

161. Fisher C. Fibromatosis and fibrosarcoma in infancy and childhood. *Eur J Cancer.* 1996;32A:2094–2100.

162. Connolly NK. Juvenile fibromatosis. A case report showing invasion of the bone. *Arch Dis Child.* 1961;36:171–175.

163. Faulkner LB, Hajdu SI, Kher U, et al. Pediatric desmoid tumor: retrospective analysis of 63 cases. *J Clin Oncol.* 1995;13:2813–2818.

164. Goepfert H, Cangir A, Ayala AG, et al. Chemotherapy of locally aggressive head and neck tumors in the pediatric age group. Desmoid fibromatosis and nasopharyngeal angiofibroma. *Am J Surg.* 1982;144:437–444.

165. Raney B, Evans A, Granowetter L, et al. Nonsurgical management of children with recurrent or unresectable fibromatosis. *Pediatrics.* 1987;79:394–398.

166. Griffiths HJ, Robinson K, Bonfiglio TA. Aggressive fibromatosis. *Skeletal Radiol.* 1983;9:179–184.

167. Dentino CM, Frush DP, Bisset GS III. Pediatric radiology case of the day. Multifocal infantile fibromatosis. *AJR Am J Roentgenol.* 1995;165:209–210.

168. Fromowitz FB, Hurst LC, Nathan J, et al. Infantile (desmoid type) fibromatosis with extensive ossification. *Am J Surg Pathol.* 1987;11:66–75.

169. Fetsch JF, Miettinen M, Laskin WB, et al. A clinicopathologic study of 45 pediatric soft tissue tumors with an admixture of adipose tissue and fibroblastic elements, and a proposal for classification as lipofibromatosis. *Am J Surg Pathol.* 2000;24:1491–1500.

170. Keasbey LE. Juvenile aponeurotic fibroma (calcifying fibroma); a distinctive tumor arising in the palms and soles of young children. *Cancer.* 1953;6:338–346.

171. Goldman RL. The cartilage analogue of fibromatosis (aponeurotic fibroma). Further observations based on 7 new cases. *Cancer.* 1970;26:1325–1331.

172. Specht EE, Konkin LA. Juvenile aponeurotic fibroma. The cartilage analogue of fibromatosis. *JAMA.* 1975;234:626–628.

173. Karasick D, O'Hara AE. Juvenile aponeurotic fibroma. A review and report of a case with osseous involvement. *Radiology.* 1977;123:725–726.

174. Rosenberg HS, Stenback WA, Spjut HJ. The fibromatoses of infancy and childhood. *Perspect Pediatr Pathol.* 1978;4:269–348.

175. Carroll RE. Juvenile aponeurotic fibroma. *Hand Clin.* 1987;3:219–224.

176. Pringle J, Stoker D. Juvenile aponeurotic fibroma. *Skeletal Radiol.* 1980;5:53–55.

177. Jensen AR, Martin LW, Longino LA. Digital neurofibrosarcoma in infancy. *J Pediatr.* 1957;51:566–570.

178. Reye RD. Recurring digital fibrous tumors of childhood. *Arch Pathol.* 1965;80:228–231.

179. Fringes B, Thais H, Bohm N, et al. Identification of actin microfilaments in the intracytoplasmic inclusions present in recurring infantile digital fibromatosis (Reye tumor). *Pediatr Pathol.* 1986;6:311–324.

180. Bhawan J, Bacchetta C, Joris I, et al. A myofibroblastic tumor. Infantile digital fibroma (recurrent digital fibrous tumor of childhood). *Am J Pathol.* 1979;94:19–36.

181. Beckett JH, Jacobs AH. Recurring digital fibrous tumors of childhood: a review. *Pediatrics.* 1977;59:401–406.

182. McKenzie AW, Innes FL, Rack JM, et al. Digital fibrous swellings in children. *Br J Dermatol.* 1970;83:446–458.

183. Iwasaki H, Kikuchi M, Mori R, et al. Infantile digital fibromatosis. Ultrastructural, histochemical, and tissue culture observations. *Cancer.* 1980;46:2238–2247.

184. Battifora H, Hines JR. Recurrent digital fibromas of childhood. An electron microscope study. *Cancer.* 1971;27:1530–1536.

185. Viale G, Doglioni C, Iuzzolino P, et al. Infantile digital fibromatosis-like tumour (inclusion body fibromatosis) of adulthood: report of two cases with ultrastructural and immunocytochemical findings. *Histopathology.* 1988;12:415–424.

186. Reye RD. A consideration of certain subdermal fibromatous tumours of infancy. *J Pathol Bacteriol.* 1956;72:149–154.

187. Enzinger FM. Fibrous hamartoma of infancy. *Cancer.* 1965;18:241–248.

188. Greco MA, Schinella RA, Vuletin JC. Fibrous hamartoma of infancy: an ultrastructural study. *Hum Pathol.* 1984;15:717–723.

189. Francis IR, Dorovini-Zis K, Glazer GM, et al. The fibromatoses: CT-pathologic correlation. *AJR Am J Roentgenol.* 1986;147:1063–1066.

190. Mitchell ML, di Sant'Agnese PA, Gerber JE. Fibrous hamartoma of infancy. *Hum Pathol.* 1982;13:586–588.

191. Loyer EM, Shabb NS, Mahon TG, et al. Fibrous hamartoma of infancy: MR-pathologic correlation. *J Comput Assist Tomogr.* 1992;16:311–313.

192. Patrick LE, O'Shea P, Simoneaux SF, et al. Fibromatoses of childhood: the spectrum of radiographic findings. *AJR Am J Roentgenol.* 1996;166:163–169.

193. Hudson TM, Vandergriend RA, Springfield DS, et al. Aggressive fibromatosis: evaluation by computed tomography and angiography. *Radiology.* 1984;150:495–501.

194. Reitamo JJ, Hayry P, Nykyri E, et al. The desmoid tumor. I. Incidence, sex-, age- and anatomical distribution in the Finnish population. *Am J Clin Pathol.* 1982;77:665–673.

195. Disler DG, Alexander AA, Mankin HJ, et al. Multicentric fibromatosis with metaphyseal dysplasia. *Radiology.* 1993;187:489–492.

196. Mueller J. Uber den feineren Bau der Krankhaften Geschwukste. *Breicht.* 1836;107–113.

197. Taylor LJ. Musculoaponeurotic fibromatosis. A report of 28 cases and review of the literature. *Clin Orthop.* 1987:294–302.

198. Macfarlane J. Clinical reports of the surgical practice of the Glasgow Royal Infirmary. In: Glasgow, Scotland: Robertson; 1832:63–66.

199. Laskin W, Weiss SW. Benign fibrous lesions. In: Bogumill G, Fleegler E, eds. *Tumors of the Hand and Upper Limb.* Edinburgh: Churchill Livingstone; 1993:224–243.

200. Yacoe ME, Bergman AG, Ladd AL, et al. Dupuytren's contracture: MR imaging findings and correlation between MR signal intensity and cellularity of lesions. *AJR Am J Roentgenol.* 1993;160: 813–817.

201. Weiss SW, Goldblum JR. Fibromatoses. In: Weiss SW and Goldblum JR, eds. *Soft Tissue Tumors,* 4th ed. St. Louis, Mosby; 2001;309–346.

202. Mikkelsen OA. Dupuytren's disease—initial symptoms, age of onset and spontaneous course. *Hand.* 1977;9:11–15.

203. Yost J, Winters T, Fett HC Sr. Dupuytren's contracture; a statistical study. *Am J Surg.* 1955;90:568–571.

204. Hill NA. Dupuytren's contracture. *J Bone Joint Surg Am.* 1985;67:1439–1443.

205. Mitra A, Goldstein RY. Dupuytren's contracture in the black population: a review. *Ann Plast Surg.* 1994;32:619–622.

206. Sladicka MS, Benfanti P, Raab M, et al. Dupuytren's contracture in the black population: a case report and review of the literature. *J Hand Surg [Am].* 1996;21:898–899.

207. Billig R, Baker R, Immergut M, et al. Peyronie's disease. *Urology.* 1975;6:409–418.

208. Gossrau G, Selle W. On the coincidence of induration penis plastica, Dupuytren's contracture and knuckle pads [in German]. *Dermatol Wochenschr.* 1965;151:1039–1043.

209. Williams JL, Thomas GG. The natural history of Peyronie's disease. *J Urol.* 1970;103:75–76.

210. Attali P, Ink O, Pelletier G, et al. Dupuytren's contracture, alcohol consumption, and chronic liver disease. *Arch Intern Med.* 1987;147:1065–1067.

211. Burge P, Hoy G, Regan P, et al. Smoking, alcohol and the risk of Dupuytren's contracture. *J Bone Joint Surg Br.* 1997;79:206–210.

212. Lund M. Dupuytren's contracture and epilepsy: clinical connection between Dupuytren's contracture, fibroma plantae, periarthrosis humeri, halodermia, induratio penis plastica and epilepsy with attempt at pathogenetic evaluation. *Acta Psychiatr Neurol.* 1941;16:465.

213. Noble J, Arafa M, Royle SG, et al. The association between alcohol, hepatic pathology and Dupuytren's disease. *J Hand Surg [Br].* 1992;17:71–74.

214. Brotherston TM, Balakrishnan C, Milner RH, et al. Long term follow-up of dermofasciectomy for Dupuytren's contracture. *Br J Plast Surg.* 1994;47:440–443.

215. Hall PN, Fitzgerald A, Sterne GD, et al. Skin replacement in Dupuytren's disease. *J Hand Surg [Br].* 1997;22:193–197.

216. Keilholz L, Seegenschmiedt MH, Sauer R. Radiotherapy for prevention of disease progression in early-stage Dupuytren's contracture: initial and long-term results. *Int J Radiat Oncol Biol Phys.* 1996;36:891–897.

217. Moschilla G, Breidahl W. Sonography of the finger. *AJR Am J Roentgenol.* 2002;178:1451–1457.

218. Pham H, Fessell DP, Femino JE, et al. Sonography and MR imaging of selected benign masses in the ankle and foot. *AJR Am J Roentgenol.* 2003;180:99–107.

219. Sintzoff SA Jr, Gillard I, Van Gansbeke D, et al. Ultrasound evaluation of soft tissue tumors. *J Belge Radiol.* 1992;75:276–280.

220. Jabra AA, Taylor GA. MRI evaluation of superficial soft tissue lesions in children. *Pediatr Radiol.* 1993;23:425–428.

221. Ledderhose G. Zur pathoogie der aponeurose des fusses und der hand. *Arch Klin Chir.* 1897;55:694–712.

222. Lee TH, Wapner KL, Hecht PJ. Plantar fibromatosis. *J Bone Joint Surg Am.* 1993;75:1080–1084.

223. Morrison WB, Schweitzer ME, Wapner KL, et al. Plantar fibromatosis: a benign aggressive neoplasm with a characteristic appearance on MR images. *Radiology.* 1994;193:841–845.

224. Aviles E, Arlen M, Miller T. Plantar fibromatosis. *Surgery.* 1971;69:117–120.

225. Snyder M. Dupuytren's contracture and plantar fibromatosis: is there more than a causal relationship? *J Am Podiatry Assoc.* 1980;70:410–415.

226. Durr HR, Krodel A, Trouillier H, et al. Fibromatosis of the plantar fascia: diagnosis and indications for surgical treatment. *Foot Ankle Int.* 1999;20:13–17.

227. Pentland AP, Anderson TF. Plantar fibromatosis responds to intralesional steroids. *J Am Acad Dermatol.* 1985;12:212–214.

228. Allen RA, Woolner LB, Ghormley RK. Soft-tissue tumors of the sole; with special reference to plantar fibromatosis. *J Bone Joint Surg Am.* 1955;37-A:14–26.

229. Gibbon WW, Long G. Ultrasound of the plantar aponeurosis (fascia). *Skeletal Radiol.* 1999;28:21–26.

230. Reed M, Gooding GA, Kerley SM, et al. Sonography of plantar fibromatosis. *J Clin Ultrasound.* 1991;19:578–582.

231. Solivetti FM, Luzi F, Bucher S, et al. Plantar fibromatosis: ultrasonography results [in Italian]. *Radiol Med (Torino).* 1999;97:341–343.

232. Griffith JF, Wong TY, Wong SM, et al. Sonography of plantar fibromatosis. *AJR Am J Roentgenol.* 2002;179:1167–1172.

233. Wetzel LH, Levine E. Soft-tissue tumors of the foot: value of MR imaging for specific diagnosis. *AJR Am J Roentgenol.* 1990;155:1025–1030.

234. Dahn I, Jonsson N, Lundh G. Desmoid tumours. A series of 33 cases. *Acta Chir Scand.* 1963;126:305–314.

235. Brockman D. Congenital desmoid of the abdominal wall. *J Pediatr.* 1947;31:217.

236. Rock MG, Pritchard DJ, Reiman HM, et al. Extra-abdominal desmoid tumors. *J Bone Joint Surg Am.* 1984;66:1369–1374.

237. Sundaram M, Duffrin H, McGuire MH, et al. Synchronous multicentric desmoid tumors (aggressive fibromatosis) of the extremities. *Skeletal Radiol.* 1988;17:16–19.

238. Dong PR, Seeger LL, Eckardt JJ, et al. Case report 847. Juxtacortical aggressive fibromatosis (desmoplastic fibroma) of the forearm. *Skeletal Radiol.* 1994;23:560–563.

239. Hayry P, Reitamo JJ, Totterman S, et al. The desmoid tumor. II. Analysis of factors possibly contributing to the etiology and growth behavior. *Am J Clin Pathol.* 1982;77:674–680.

240. Lee YS, Sen BK. Dystrophic and psammomatous calcifications in a desmoid tumor. A light microscopic and ultrastructural study. *Cancer.* 1985;55:84–90.

241. Bridge JA, Sreekantaiah C, Mouron B, et al. Clonal chromosomal abnormalities in desmoid tumors. Implications for histopathogenesis. *Cancer.* 1992;69:430–436.

242. Hayry P, Reitamo JJ, Vihko R, et al. The desmoid tumor. III. A biochemical and genetic analysis. *Am J Clin Pathol.* 1982;77:681–685.

243. Musgrove J, McDonald J. Extra-abdominal desmoid tumors. Their differential diagnosis and treatment. *Arch Pathol.* 1948;45:513–540.

244. Pfeiffer C. Desmoide der Bauchdecken und igre prognose. *Beitr Klin Chir.* 1904;44:334.

245. Enzinger FM, Shiraki M. Musculo-aponeurotic fibromatosis of the shoulder girdle (extra-abdominal desmoid). Analysis of thirty cases followed up for ten or more years. *Cancer.* 1967;20:1131–1140.

246. Pritchard DJ, Nascimento AG, Petersen IA. Local control of extra-abdominal desmoid tumors. *J Bone Joint Surg Am.* 1996;78:848–854.

247. Karakousis CP, Mayordomo J, Zografos GC, et al. Desmoid tumors of the trunk and extremity. *Cancer.* 1993;72:1637–1641.

248. Kamath SS, Parsons JT, Marcus RB, et al. Radiotherapy for local control of aggressive fibromatosis. *Int J Radiat Oncol Biol Phys.* 1996;36:325–328.

249. Kiel KD, Suit HD. Radiation therapy in the treatment of aggressive fibromatoses (desmoid tumors). *Cancer.* 1984;54:2051–2055.

250. McCollough WM, Parsons JT, van der Griend R, et al. Radiation therapy for aggressive fibromatosis. The Experience at the University of Florida. *J Bone Joint Surg Am.* 1991;73:717–725.

251. Jadrijevic D, Mardones E, Lipschutz A. Antifibromatogenic activity of 19-nor-alpha-ethinyltestosterone in the guinea pig. *Proc Soc Exp Biol Med.* 1956;91:38–39.

252. Kinzbrunner B, Ritter S, Domingo J, et al. Remission of rapidly growing desmoid tumors after tamoxifen therapy. *Cancer.* 1983;52:2201–2204.

253. Lipschutz A, Grismali J. On the antifibromatogen activity of synthetic progesterone in experiments with the 17-caprylic and dipropionic esters of estradiol. *Cancer.* 1944;4:186.

254. Patel SR, Evans HL, Benjamin RS. Combination chemotherapy in adult desmoid tumors. *Cancer.* 1993;72:3244–3247.

255. Seiter K, Kemeny N. Successful treatment of a desmoid tumor with doxorubicin. *Cancer.* 1993;71:2242–2244.

256. Tsukada K, Church JM, Jagelman DG, et al. Noncytotoxic drug therapy for intra-abdominal desmoid tumor in patients with familial adenomatous polyposis. *Dis Colon Rectum.* 1992;35:29–33.

257. Wilcken N, Tattersall MH. Endocrine therapy for desmoid tumors. *Cancer.* 1991;68:1384–1388.

258. Lim CL, Walker MJ, Mehta RR, et al. Estrogen and antiestrogen binding sites in desmoid tumors. *Eur J Cancer Clin Oncol.* 1986;22:583–587.

259. Waddell WR, Kirsch WM. Testolactone, sulindac, warfarin, and vitamin K1 for unresectable desmoid tumors. *Am J Surg.* 1991;161:416–421.

260. Brodsky JT, Gordon MS, Hajdu SI, et al. Desmoid tumors of the chest wall. A locally recurrent problem. *J Thorac Cardiovasc Surg.* 1992;104:900–903.

261. Posner MC, Shiu MH, Newsome JL, et al. The desmoid tumor. Not a benign disease. *Arch Surg.* 1989;124:191–196.

262. Terui S, Terauchi T, Abe H, et al. Role of technetium-99m pertechnetate scintigraphy in the management of extra-abdominal fibromatosis. *Skeletal Radiol.* 1995;24:331–336.

263. Abramowitz D, Zornoza J, Ayala AG, et al. Soft-tissue desmoid tumors: radiographic bone changes. *Radiology.* 1983;146:11–13.

264. Capusten BM, Azouz EM, Rosman MA. Fibromatosis of bone in children. *Radiology.* 1984;152:693–694.

265. Hartman TE, Berquist TH, Fetsch JF. MR imaging of extraabdominal desmoids: differentiation from other neoplasms. *AJR Am J Roentgenol.* 1992;158:581–585.

266. Hudson TM, Bertoni F, Enneking WF. Scintigraphy of aggressive fibromatosis. *Skeletal Radiol.* 1985;13:26–32.

267. Kingston CA, Owens CM, Jeanes A, et al. Imaging of desmoid fibromatosis in pediatric patients. *AJR Am J Roentgenol.* 2002; 178:191–199.

268. Enneking WF, Chew FS, Springfield DS, et al. The role of radionuclide bone-scanning in determining the resectability of soft-tissue sarcomas. *J Bone Joint Surg Am.* 1981;63:249–257.

269. Totterman S, Reitamo JJ. Desmoid tumour: an angiographic study of five cases. *Br J Radiol.* 1979;52:936–941.

270. Hawnaur JM, Jenkins JP, Isherwood I. Magnetic resonance imaging of musculoaponeurotic fibromatosis. *Skeletal Radiol.* 1990; 19:509–514.

271. Aisen AM, Martel W, Braunstein EM, et al. MRI and CT evaluation of primary bone and soft-tissue tumors. *AJR Am J Roentgenol.* 1986;146:749–756.

272. Wetzel LH, Levine E, Murphey MD. A comparison of MR imaging and CT in the evaluation of musculoskeletal masses. *Radiographics.* 1987;7:851–874.

273. Sundaram M, McGuire MH, Schajowicz F. Soft-tissue masses: histologic basis for decreased signal (short T2) on T2-weighted MR images. *AJR Am J Roentgenol.* 1987;148:1247–1250.

274. Feld R, Burk DL Jr, McCue P, et al. MRI of aggressive fibromatosis: frequent appearance of high signal intensity on T2-weighted images. *Magn Reson Imaging.* 1990;8:583–588.

275. Kransdorf MJ, Jelinek JS, Moser RP Jr, et al. Magnetic resonance appearance of fibromatosis. A report of 14 cases and review of the literature. *Skeletal Radiol.* 1990;19:495–499.

276. Petasnick JP, Turner DA, Charters JR, et al. Soft-tissue masses of the locomotor system: comparison of MR imaging with CT. *Radiology.* 1986;160:125–133.

277. Quinn SF, Erickson SJ, Dee PM, et al. MR imaging in fibromatosis: results in 26 patients with pathologic correlation. *AJR Am J Roentgenol.* 1991;156:539–542.

278. Romero JA, Kim EE, Kim CG, et al. Different biologic features of desmoid tumors in adult and juvenile patients: MR demonstration. *J Comput Assist Tomogr.* 1995;19:782–787.

279. Sundaram M, McLeod RA. MR imaging of tumor and tumorlike lesions of bone and soft tissue. *AJR Am J Roentgenol.* 1990;155: 817–824.

280. Vandevenne JE, De Schepper AM, De Beuckeleer L, et al. New concepts in understanding evolution of desmoid tumors: MR imaging of 30 lesions. *Eur Radiol.* 1997;7:1013–1019.

281. Shiu MH, Flancbaum L, Hajdu SI, et al. Malignant soft-tissue tumors of the anterior abdominal wall. *Arch Surg.* 1980;115: 152–155.

282. Caldwell EH. Desmoid tumor: musculoaponeurotic fibrosis of the abdominal wall. *Surgery.* 1976;79:104–106.

283. Pack G. Neoplasms of the anterior abdominal wall with special consideration of desmoid tumors: experience with 391 cases and collective review of the literature. *Surgery.* 1959;45:77.

284. Salmon M, Payan H, Lavaurs G, et al. Desmoid tumor (invasive fibroma of Lecene and Delamare) of the abdominal wall in a young boy [in French]. *Ann Chir Infant.* 1964;108:107–117.

285. Bach C, Esteve P, Sarrut S, Cloup M. Desmoid tumors of the abdominal wall (or invasive fibromas of Lecene and Delamare) in children. Apropos of a case. *Ann Pediatr (Paris).* 1964;11: 239–246.

286. Gurbuz AK, Giardiello FM, Petersen GM, et al. Desmoid tumours in familial adenomatous polyposis. *Gut.* 1994;35:377–381.

287. Heiskanen I, Jarvinen HJ. Occurrence of desmoid tumours in familial adenomatous polyposis and results of treatment. *Int J Colorectal Dis.* 1996;11:157–162.

288. Rodriguez-Bigas MA, Mahoney MC, Karakousis CP, et al. Desmoid tumors in patients with familial adenomatous polyposis. *Cancer.* 1994;74:1270–1274.

289. Burke AP, Sobin LH, Shekitka KM. Mesenteric fibromatosis. A follow-up study. *Arch Pathol Lab Med.* 1990;114:832–835.

290. McAdam WA, Goligher JC. The occurrence of desmoids in patients with familial polyposis coli. *Br J Surg.* 1970;57: 618–631.

291. Nichols R. Desmoid tumors: a report of 31 cases. *Arch Surg.* 1923;7:227–236.

292. Bauernhofer T, Stoger H, Schmid M, et al. Sequential treatment of recurrent mesenteric desmoid tumor. *Cancer.* 1996;77:1061–1065.

293. Bessler W, Egloff B, Sulser H. Case report 253. Gardner syndrome with aggressive fibromatosis. *Skeletal Radiol.* 1984;11:56–59.

294. Kawashima A, Goldman SM, Fishman EK, et al. CT of intraabdominal desmoid tumors: is the tumor different in patients with Gardner's disease? *AJR Am J Roentgenol.* 1994;162:339–342.

295. Fetsch JF, Montgomery EA, Meis JM. Calcifying fibrous pseudotumor. *Am J Surg Pathol.* 1993;17:502–508.

296. Rosenthal NS, Abdul-Karim FW. Childhood fibrous tumor with psammoma bodies. Clinicopathologic features in two cases. *Arch Pathol Lab Med.* 1988;112:798–800.

297. Dumont P, de Muret A, Skrobala D, et al. Calcifying fibrous pseudotumor of the mediastinum. *Ann Thorac Surg.* 1997;63: 543–544.

298. Hainaut P, Lesage V, Weynand B, et al. Calcifying fibrous pseudotumor (CFPT): a patient presenting with multiple pleural lesions. *Acta Clin Belg.* 1999;54:162–164.

299. Pinkard NB, Wilson RW, Lawless N, et al. Calcifying fibrous pseudotumor of pleura. A report of three cases of a newly described entity involving the pleura. *Am J Clin Pathol.* 1996;105: 189–194.

300. Weynand B, Draguet AP, Bernard P, et al. Calcifying fibrous pseudotumour: first case report in the peritoneum with immunostaining for CD34. *Histopathology.* 1999;34:86–87.

301. Erasmus JJ, McAdams HP, Patz EF Jr, et al. Calcifying fibrous pseudotumor of pleura: radiologic features in three cases. *J Comput Assist Tomogr.* 1996;20:763–765.

302. Rice DH, Batsakis JG, Coulthard SW. Sclerosing cervicitis: homologue of sclerosing retroperitonitis and mediastinitis. *Arch Surg.* 1975;110:120–122.

303. Smith M, Castillo M, Weissler M. CT findings in a case of exuberant cervical fibrosclerosis. *AJR Am J Roentgenol.* 1992;159: 1263–1264.

304. Wold LE, Weiland LH. Tumefactive fibro-inflammatory lesions of the head and neck. *Am J Surg Pathol.* 1983;7:477–482.

305. Kempson R, Fletcher C, Evans H, et al. Fibrous histiocytomas. In: Rosai J, ed. *Tumors of the Soft Tissues.* 3rd ed. Bethesda, MD: Armed Forces Institute of Pathology; 2001:113–186.

306. Niemi KM. The benign fibrohistiocytic tumours of the skin. *Acta Derm Venereol Suppl (Stockh).* 1970;50:(Suppl 63):1–66.

307. Font RL, Hidayat AA. Fibrous histiocytoma of the orbit. A clinicopathologic study of 150 cases. *Hum Pathol.* 1982;13:199–209.

308. Franquemont DW, Cooper PH, Shmookler BM, et al. Benign fibrous histiocytoma of the skin with potential for local recurrence: a tumor to be distinguished from dermatofibroma. *Mod Pathol.* 1990;3:158–163.

309. Meister P, Konrad E, Krauss F. Fibrous histiocytoma: a histological and statistical analysis of 155 cases. *Pathol Res Pract.* 1978; 162:361–379.

310. Newman DM, Walter JB. Multiple dermatofibromas in patients with systemic lupus erythematosus on immunosuppressive therapy. *N Engl J Med.* 1973;289:842–843.

311. Smith NM, Davies JB, Shrimankar JS, et al. Deep fibrous histiocytoma with giant cells and bone metaplasia. *Histopathology.* 1990;17:365–367.

312. Calonje E, Fletcher CD. Cutaneous fibrohistiocytic tumors: an update. *Adv Anat Pathol.* 1994;1:2.

313. Colome-Grimmer MI, Evans HL. Metastasizing cellular dermatofibroma. A report of two cases. *Am J Surg Pathol.* 1996;20:1361–1367.

314. Marcoval J, Moreno A, Bordas X, et al. Diffuse plane xanthoma: clinicopathologic study of 8 cases. *J Am Acad Dermatol.* 1998;39:439–442.

315. Burnstein M, Buckwalter KA, Martel W, et al. Case report 427: Cerebrotendinous xanthomatosis. *Skeletal Radiol.* 1987;16:346–349.

316. Cruysberg JR, Wevers RA, van Engelen BG, et al. Ocular and systemic manifestations of cerebrotendinous xanthomatosis. *Am J Ophthalmol.* 1995;120:597–604.

317. Fahey JJ, Stark HH, Donovan WF, et al. Xanthoma of the Achilles tendon. Seven cases with familial hyperbetalipoproteinemia. *J Bone Joint Surg Am.* 1973;55:1197–1211.

318. Blankenhorn DH, Meyers HI. Radiographic determination of Achilles tendon xanthoma size. *Metabolism.* 1969;18:882–886.

319. Gattereau A, Davignon J, Langelier M, et al. An improved radiological method for the evaluation of Achilles tendon xanthomatosis. *Can Med Assoc J.* 1973;108:39–42.

320. Bude RO, Adler RS, Bassett DR. Diagnosis of Achilles tendon xanthoma in patients with heterozygous familial hypercholesterolemia: MR vs sonography. *AJR Am J Roentgenol.* 1994;162:913–917.

321. Bude RO, Adler RS, Bassett DR, et al. Heterozygous familial hypercholesterolemia: detection of xanthomas in the Achilles tendon with US. *Radiology.* 1993;188:567–571.

322. Durrington PN, Adams JE, Beastall MD. The assessment of Achilles tendon size in primary hypercholesterolaemia by computed tomography. *Atherosclerosis.* 1982;45:345–358.

323. Dussault RG, Kaplan PA, Roederer G. MR imaging of Achilles tendon in patients with familial hyperlipidemia: comparison with plain films, physical examination, and patients with traumatic tendon lesions. *AJR Am J Roentgenol.* 1995;164:403–407.

324. Ebeling T, Farin P, Pyorala K. Ultrasonography in the detection of Achilles tendon xanthomata in heterozygous familial hypercholesterolemia. *Atherosclerosis.* 1992;97:217–228.

325. Koblik PD, Freeman DM. Short echo time magnetic resonance imaging of tendon. *Invest Radiol.* 1993;28:1095–1100.

326. Liem MS, Leuven JA, Bloem JL, et al. Magnetic resonance imaging of Achilles tendon xanthomas in familial hypercholesterolemia. *Skeletal Radiol.* 1992;21:453–457.

327. Quinn SF, Murray WT, Clark RA, et al. Achilles tendon: MR imaging at 1.5 T. *Radiology.* 1987;164:767–770.

328. Steinmetz A, Schmitt W, Schuler P, et al. Ultrasonography of Achilles tendons in primary hypercholesterolemia. Comparison with computed tomography. *Atherosclerosis.* 1988;74:231–239.

329. Yuzawa K, Yamakawa K, Tohno E, et al. An ultrasonographic method for detection of Achilles tendon xanthomas in familial hypercholesterolemia. *Atherosclerosis.* 1989;75:211–218.

330. Koivunen-Niemela T, Viikari J, Niinikoski H, et al. Sonography in the detection of Achilles tendon xanthomata in children with familial hypercholesterolaemia. *Acta Paediatr.* 1994;83:1178–1181.

331. Kelman CG, Disler DG, Kremer JM, et al. Xanthomatous infiltration of ankle tendons. *Skeletal Radiol.* 1997;26:256–259.

332. Bureau NJ, Roederer G. Sonography of Achilles tendon xanthomas in patients with heterozygous familial hypercholesterolemia. *AJR Am J Roentgenol.* 1998;171:745–749.

333. Barkhof F, Verrips A, Wesseling P, et al. Cerebrotendinous xanthomatosis: the spectrum of imaging findings and the correlation with neuropathologic findings. *Radiology.* 2000;217:869–876.

334. Berginer VM, Berginer J, Korczyn AD, et al. Magnetic resonance imaging in cerebrotendinous xanthomatosis: a prospective clinical and neuroradiological study. *J Neurol Sci.* 1994;122:102–108.

335. Dotti MT, Federico A, Signorini E, et al. Cerebrotendinous xanthomatosis (van Bogaert-Scherer-Epstein disease): CT and MR findings. *AJNR Am J Neuroradiol.* 1994;15:1721–1726.

336. Verrips A, Nijeholt GJ, Barkhof F, et al. Spinal xanthomatosis: a variant of cerebrotendinous xanthomatosis. *Brain.* 1999;122 (Pt 8):1589–1595.

337. Tahan SR, Pastel-Levy C, Bhan AK, et al. Juvenile xanthogranuloma. Clinical and pathologic characterization. *Arch Pathol Lab Med.* 1989;113:1057–1061.

338. De Villez RL, Limmer BL. Juvenile xanthogranuloma and urticaria pigmentosa. *Arch Dermatol.* 1975;111:365–366.

339. Jensen NE, Sabharwal S, Walker AE. Naevoxanthoendothelioma and neurofibromatosis. *Br J Dermatol.* 1971;85:326–330.

340. Rosai J, Dorfman RF. Sinus histiocytosis with massive lymphadenopathy. A newly recognized benign clinicopathological entity. *Arch Pathol.* 1969;87:63–70.

341. Rosai J, Dorfman RF. Sinus histiocytosis with massive lymphadenopathy: a pseudolymphomatous benign disorder. Analysis of 34 cases. *Cancer.* 1972;30:1174–1188.

342. Carbone A, Passannante A, Gloghini A, et al. Review of sinus histiocytosis with massive lymphadenopathy (Rosai-Dorfman disease) of head and neck. *Ann Otol Rhinol Laryngol.* 1999;108:1095–1104.

343. Lim R, Wittram C, Ferry JA, Shepard JA. FDG PET of Rosai-Dorfman disease of the thymus. *AJR Am J Roentgenol.* 2004;182:514.

344. Foucar E, Rosai J, Dorfman R. Sinus histiocytosis with massive lymphadenopathy (Rosai-Dorfman disease): review of the entity. *Semin Diagn Pathol.* 1990;7:19–73.

345. Montgomery EA, Meis JM, Frizzera G. Rosai-Dorfman disease of soft tissue. *Am J Surg Pathol.* 1992;16:122–129.

346. Wenig BM, Abbondanzo SL, Childers EL, et al. Extranodal sinus histiocytosis with massive lymphadenopathy (Rosai-Dorfman disease) of the head and neck. *Hum Pathol.* 1993;24:483–492.

347. Young PM, Kransdorf MJ, Temple HT, et al. Rosai-Dorfman disease presenting as multiple soft tissue masses. *Skeletal Radiol.* 2005;34:665–669.

348. Jelinek J, Kransdorf MJ. MR imaging of soft-tissue masses. Mass-like lesions that simulate neoplasms. *Magn Reson Imaging Clin North Am.* 1995;3:727–741.

349. Borup LH, Meehan JJ, Severson JM, et al. Terminal spine of agave plant extracted from patient's spinal cord. *AJR Am J Roentgenol.* 2003;181:1155–1156.

350. Zaloudek C, Treseler PA, Powell CB. Postarthroplasty histiocytic lymphadenopathy in gynecologic oncology patients. A benign reactive process that clinically may be mistaken for cancer. *Cancer.* 1996;78:834–844.

351. Sukpanichnant S, Hargrove NS, Kachintorn U, et al. Clofazimine-induced crystal-storing histiocytosis producing chronic abdominal pain in a leprosy patient. *Am J Surg Pathol.* 2000;24:129–135.

352. Comstock CP, Louis DS, Eckenrode JF. Silicone wrist implant: long-term follow-up study. *J Hand Surg [Am].* 1988;13:201–205.

353. Fatti JF, Palmer AK, Greenky S, et al. Long-term results of Swanson interpositional wrist arthroplasty: Part II. *J Hand Surg [Am].* 1991;16:432–437.

354. Jolly SL, Ferlic DC, Clayton ML, et al. Swanson silicone arthroplasty of the wrist in rheumatoid arthritis: a long-term follow-up. *J Hand Surg [Am].* 1992;17:142–149.

355. Sammarco GJ, Tabatowski K. Silicone lymphadenopathy associated with failed prosthesis of the hallux: a case report and literature review. *Foot Ankle.* 1992;13:273–276.

356. Carter PR, Benton LJ, Dysert PA. Silicone rubber carpal implants: a study of the incidence of late osseous complications. *J Hand Surg [Am].* 1986;11:639–644.

357. Bansal M, Goldman AB, Bullough PG, et al. Case report 706: silicone-induced reactive synovitis. *Skeletal Radiol.* 1992;21:49–51.

358. Rosenthal DI, Rosenberg AE, Schiller AL, et al. Destructive arthritis due to silicone: a foreign-body reaction. *Radiology.* 1983;149:69–72.

359. Laor T, Barnewolt CE. Nonradiopaque penetrating foreign body: "a sticky situation." *Pediatr Radiol.* 1999;29:702–704.

360. Murphey MD, Quale JL, Martin NL, et al. Computed radiography in musculoskeletal imaging: state of the art. *AJR Am J Roentgenol.* 1992;158:19–27.

361. McGuckin JF Jr, Akhtar N, Ho VT, et al. CT and MR evaluation of a wooden foreign body in an in vitro model of the orbit. *AJNR Am J Neuroradiol.* 1996;17:129–133.

362. Bodne D, Quinn SF, Cochran CF. Imaging foreign glass and wooden bodies of the extremities with CT and MR. *J Comput Assist Tomogr.* 1988;12:608–611.

363. Firooznia H, Bjorkengren A, Hofstetter SR, et al. Computed tomography in localization of foreign bodies lodged in the extremities. *Comput Radiol.* 1984;8:237–239.

364. Oikarinen KS, Nieminen TM, Makarainen H, et al. Visibility of foreign bodies in soft tissue in plain radiographs, computed tomography, magnetic resonance imaging, and ultrasound. An in vitro study. *Int J Oral Maxillofac Surg.* 1993;22:119–124.

365. Russell RC, Williamson DA, Sullivan JW, et al. Detection of foreign bodies in the hand. *J Hand Surg [Am].* 1991; 16:2–11.

366. Fornage B. Soft-tissue masses: the case for increased utilization of sonography. *Appl Radiol.* 2000;29:8–22.

367. Fornage BD, Schernberg FL. Sonographic diagnosis of foreign bodies of the distal extremities. *AJR Am J Roentgenol.* 1986;147: 567–569.

368. Horton LK, Jacobson JA, Powell A, et al. Sonography and radiography of soft-tissue foreign bodies. *AJR Am J Roentgenol.* 2001;176:1155–1159.

369. Jacobson JA, Powell A, Craig JG, et al. Wooden foreign bodies in soft tissue: detection at US. *Radiology.* 1998;206:45–48.

370. Mizel MS, Steinmetz ND, Trepman E. Detection of wooden foreign bodies in muscle tissue: experimental comparison of computed tomography, magnetic resonance imaging, and ultrasonography. *Foot Ankle Int.* 1994;15:437–443.

371. Peterson JJ, Bancroft LW, Kransdorf MJ. Wooden foreign bodies: imaging appearance. *AJR Am J Roentgenol.* 2002;178: 557–562.

372. Shiels WE II, Babcock DS, Wilson JL, et al. Localization and guided removal of soft-tissue foreign bodies with sonography. *AJR Am J Roentgenol.* 1990;155:1277–1281.

373. LoBue TD, Deutsch TA, Lobick J, et al. Detection and localization of nonmetallic intraocular foreign bodies by magnetic resonance imaging. *Arch Ophthalmol.* 1988;106:260–261.

374. Varma DG, Ro JY, Guo SQ, et al. Magnetic resonance imaging appearance of foreign body granulomas of the upper arms. *Clin Imaging.* 1994;18:39–42.

375. Monu JU, McManus CM, Ward WG, et al. Soft-tissue masses caused by long-standing foreign bodies in the extremities: MR imaging findings. *AJR Am J Roentgenol.* 1995;165:395–397.

Malignant Fibrous and Fibrohistiocytic Tumors

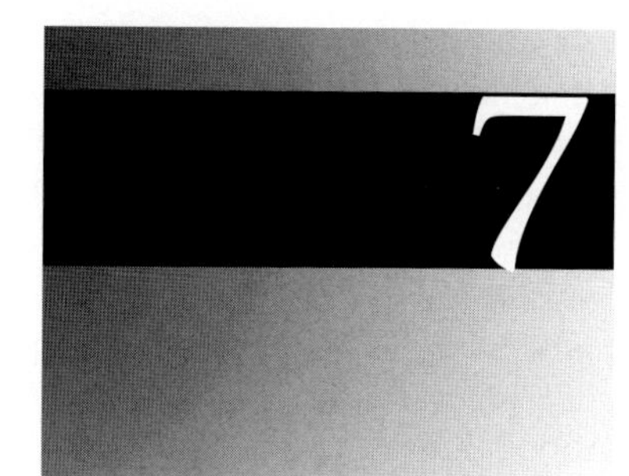

As it did with their benign counterparts, the World Health Organization (WHO) Classification of Soft Tissue Tumors has significantly reorganized the nomenclature of the malignant fibrous and fibrohistiocytic tumors since the previous edition of this book, obscuring the histologic lineage of these lesions. Entities discussed in this chapter are either malignant or potentially malignant and include dermatofibrosarcoma protuberans, giant cell fibroblastoma, atypical fibroxanthoma, myxoinflammatory fibroblastic sarcoma, plexiform histiocytic tumor, angiomatoid fibrous histiocytoma, infantile fibrosarcoma, adult fibrosarcoma, low-grade fibromyxoid sarcoma, sclerosing epithelioid fibrosarcoma, and malignant fibrous histiocytoma (MFH). The malignant fibrous and fibrohistiocytic neoplasms are particularly common; therefore, it is important to understand the spectrum of imaging appearances of this diverse group of lesions.

DERMATOFIBROSARCOMA PROTUBERANS

KEY CONCEPTS

- Dermatofibrosarcoma protuberans constitutes 6% of all soft tissue sarcomas.
- Men are affected more frequently than women, and the lesion occurs most commonly in the third to fifth decade of life.
- This subcutaneous mass affects the trunk (50%) and proximal upper and lower extremities (35% to 40%).
- Imaging shows a subcutaneous protuberant mass with skin involvement: satellite nodules less common.
  - Nonspecific intrinsic characteristic ultrasonography, CT, MRI
  - Extension along skin surface is seen on long TR images
- Local recurrence is common (20% to 55%); metastatic rate is low (3% to 6%).

Dermatofibrosarcoma protuberans (DFSP) accounts for approximately 6% of all soft tissue sarcomas (1). Darier and Ferrand originally described DFSP as a distinct clinicopathologic entity in 1924 (2). The term *dermatofibrosarcoma protuberans* was coined for this entity in 1925 by Hoffman (3).

DFSP usually occurs in the third to fifth decade of life, although there are increasing reports of pediatric involvement (4–6). These lesions may begin in childhood, but because of the indolent growth, they only become clinically apparent in early adulthood. The clinical presentation is a slowly growing, redish-brown to bluish, firm, superficial nodule fixed to the skin. Prior trauma, including a scar or burn, is reported in 10% to 20% of cases, although this may be coincidental (7). Lesions may be multiple, and small nodules may coalesce to form a plaque. Growth rate is variable and periods of accelerated growth may also occur. Large lesions may invade underlying structures, ulcerate, bleed, or become painful. Men are affected more commonly than women. Lesions most frequently involve the trunk, with up to 50% occurring in this location (8). The upper and lower extremities (usually proximally) are affected in 35% to 40% of cases, followed by the head and neck (14%) (8–12). The central body cavity and retroperitoneum are rarely involved (8,13).

At gross pathologic examination, this lesion is most commonly seen as a protuberant mass involving the subcutaneous tissue and skin with an average size of 5 cm (8). This solid solitary mass represents a coalescence of the initial plaquelike foci. Multiple nodules may also be apparent initially, although coalescence of these nodules into a single mass is more frequent. Local recurrence with multiple nodules may also occur. Invasion of underlying muscle is uncommon. In rare cases the skin is unaffected (14). The lesion is generally composed of a uniform population of fibroblasts, arranged in a distinct storiform pattern (5,15,16). Lesions may contain myxoid or densely collagenous regions. Areas of hemorrhage or necrosis are unusual, in contrast to MFH. Areas of higher grade sarcoma (most commonly fibrosarcoma) may arise within a conventional DFSP, and these areas may be focally necrotic (17–19). Cytogenetic aberrations include the presence of supernumerary ring chromosomes 11 and 15 with amplification sequences from chromosomes 17 and 22, as well as t12:22 translocation (9,11).

Areas of fibrosarcomatous transformation (and rarely MFH) are found in 17% to 27% of DFSP (17–19). Although not firmly established, the criteria for fibrosarcomatous transformation in DFSP include that at least 5% to 10% of the lesion is composed of this higher grade tissue with increased mitotic activity (8). In one study, patients with associated fibrosarcoma were approximately a decade older than patients with conventional DFSP (20,21). Fibrosarcomatous transformation may occur at initial presentation or with recurrence. The significance of fibrosarcoma in local recurrences and distant metastases is unclear and controversial. In some series, such lesions reportedly had a more aggressive clinical course with increased local recurrence (42% to 58%) and metastases (14% to 33%) (20,21). However, other investigations, including a study by Connelly and Evans, suggested the only factor strongly related to local recurrence is the adequacy of surgical margins (17). It is likely that differences among various scientific studies may reflect this lack of control of the adequacy of initial surgical resection.

In 1957, Bednar described a tumor now considered a variant of DFSP that has melanin within the dendritic cells of the tumor (22). This pigmented form of DFSP (Bednar tumor) accounts for 5% to 10% of these lesions (8,22). The clinical manifestations and anatomic locations of the lesion are similar to conventional DFSP, although it is less likely to recur locally.

Local recurrence is seen in 20% to 55% of cases of DFSP (8). This high local recurrence rate is likely a result of infiltration of the lesion which was not detected at initial surgical resection. The relationship of recurrence to lack of prompt aggressive resection is supported by the significant reduction in local recurrence with aggressive local treatment to an average of 18% (23). An excision margin of greater than 3 cm is associated with a 20% local recurrence rate as compared to a 2 cm or less margin with resultant increase of local recurrence to 41% (24). Lesions in the head and neck have a higher recurrence rate, ranging from 50% to 75% (25–27). Most recurrences are seen within 3 years of primary excision. The rate of distant metastases is low (3% to 6%) despite the local aggressiveness of DFSP (7,28). Radiation therapy is advocated for large lesions not amenable to surgical resection or in patients with positive margins following initial resection. Metastases most often affect the lungs (75% of metastases), with less common reported sites including the brain, bones, and heart (8). Regional lymph node involvement occurs in approximately 25% of patients with metastases (29). Metastases are not described at patient presentation but may be seen following biopsy or local recurrence (29). The treatment of choice is wide-local excision with a margin of at least 3 cm and en bloc removal of the underlying subcutaneous tissue and fascia (30). Similar to melanoma, Mohs micrographic surgical resection technique is gaining popularity in treatment of DFSP with a resultant decreased local recurrence rate of 6% to 7% (23).

The radiologic appearance of DFSP is typically that of an unmineralized, nodular soft tissue mass involving the skin and subcutaneous adipose tissue (31–33) (Fig. 7.1).

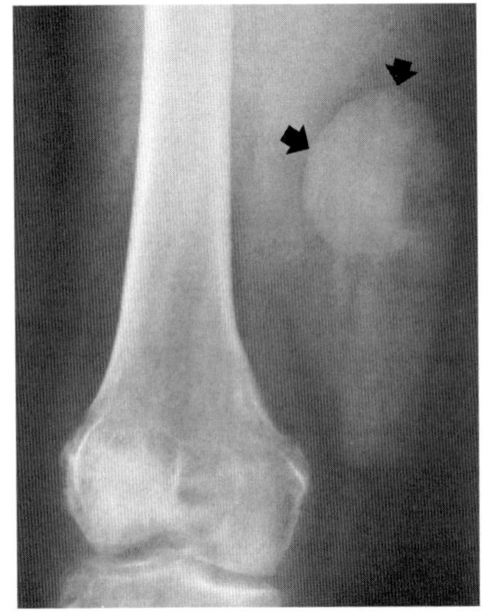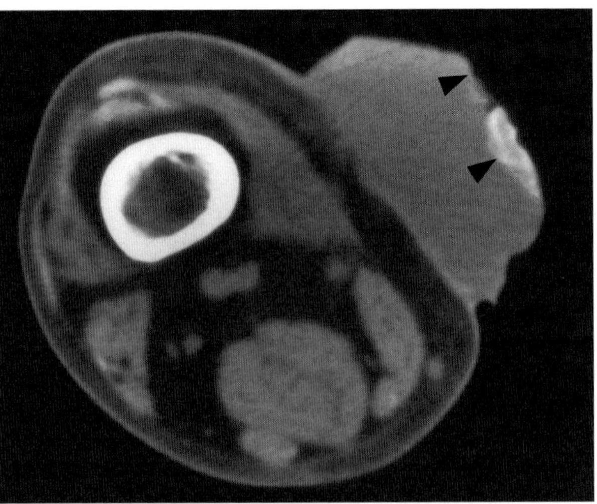

Figure 7.1   Large exophytic dermatofibrosarcoma protuberans arising from the skin of the distal thigh in a man 45 years of age. **A:** Radiograph reveals large medial mass (*arrows*). **B:** Axial noncontrast CT shows the large mass with ulceration at the surface (*arrowheads*).

The lesion also causes focal protuberance of the skin. CT or MR images are well suited to demonstrate this location and the distinct lobular or nodular architecture (Figs. 7.1–7.6). Perhaps more importantly, the relationship of the lesion to the underlying structures is well delineated. The intrinsic signal intensity of the lesion on MR imaging is nonspecific (signal intensity similar to that of skeletal muscle on T1-weighted images and similar to or greater than that of fat on T2-weighted images) as is the tissue attenuation on CT (similar to that of muscle) (31,34) (Figs. 7.2–7.6). Fat-suppressed T2-weighted or short-tau inversion recovery (STIR) sequences typically reveal high

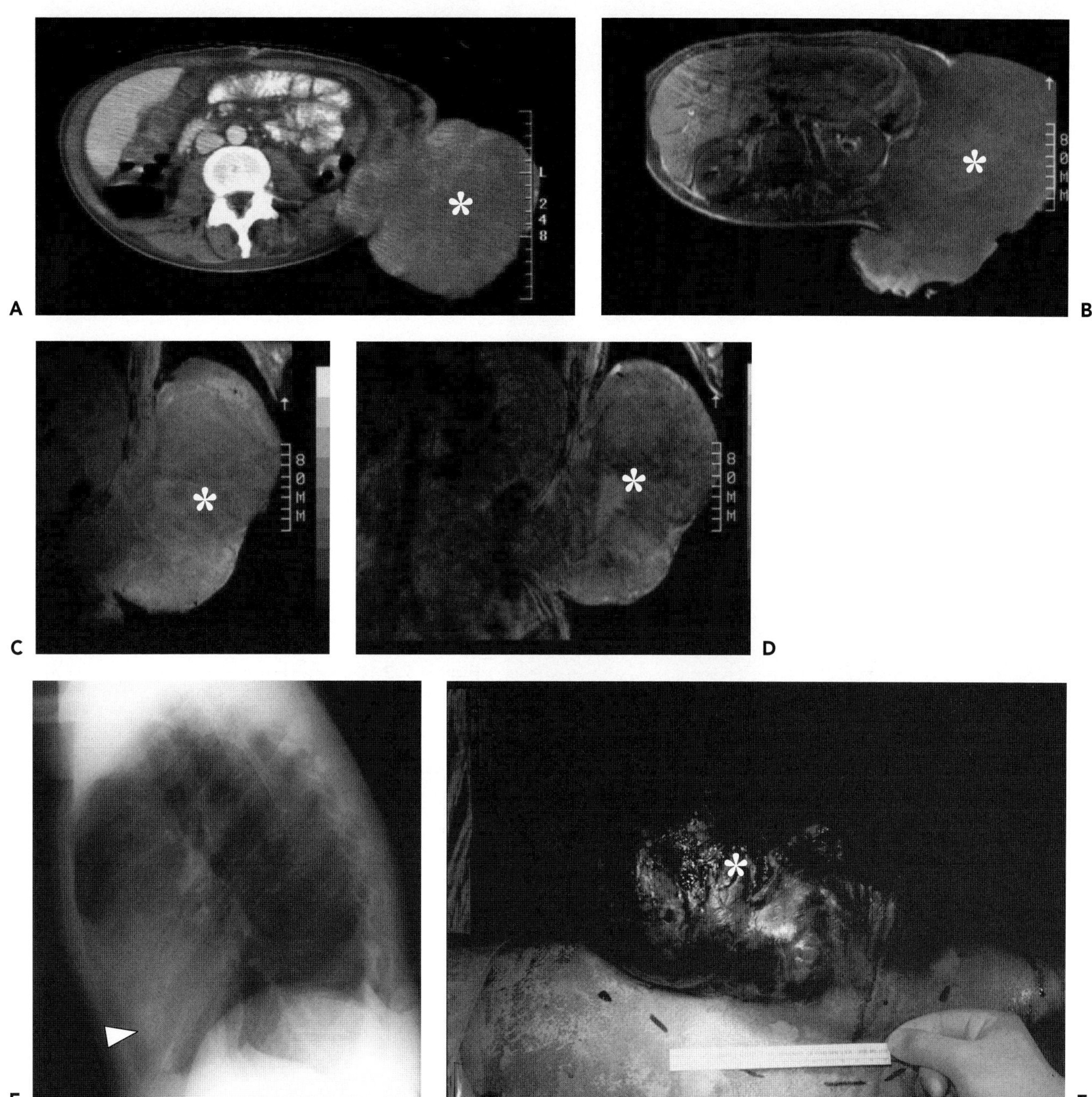

Figure 7.2 Dermatofibrosarcoma protuberans of the abdominal wall with fibrosarcomatous transformation in a man 28 years of age. **A–D:** CT **(A)** and multiple MR images, including axial T1-weighted (TR/TE; 400/10) **(B)**, coronal STIR (TR/TE/TI; 3100/13/150) **(C)**, and coronal fast T2-weighted (TR/TE; 3200/120) **(D)**, show a large fungating, protuberant, and ulcerating abdominal wall mass (*asterisk*) with predominantly low to intermediate signal intensity on the long TR images. **E:** Lateral chest radiograph reveals pulmonary metastasis (*arrowhead*). **F:** Clinical photograph also demonstrates the large fungating mass (*asterisk*).

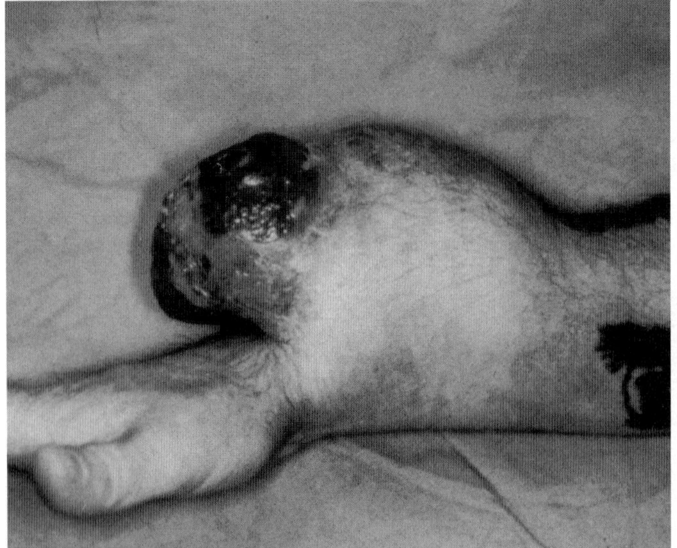

A

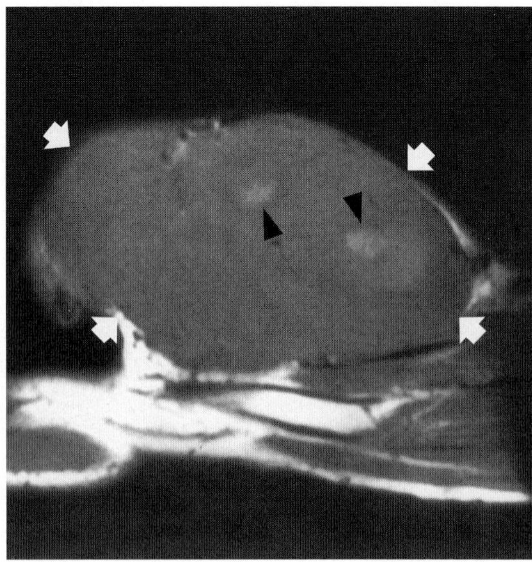

B

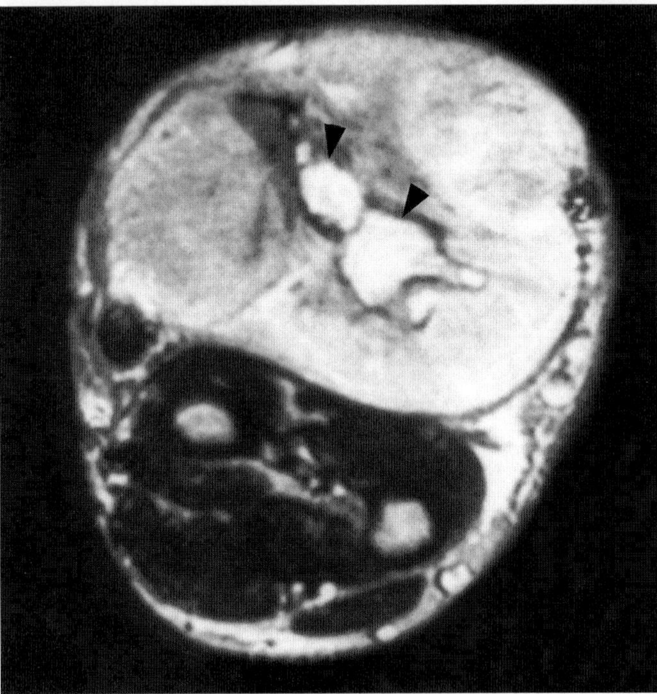

C

Figure 7.3 Dermatofibrosarcoma protuberans of the distal forearm in a man 36 years of age with a 23-year history of an expanding mass. **A:** Clinical photograph shows a large fungating mass. **B,C:** Sagittal T1-weighted (TR/TE; 600/19) **(B)** and axial T2-weighted (TR/TE; 2400/80) **(C)** MR images show a large protuberant mass (*arrows* in **B**) involving the skin and subcutaneous tissue. Central high signal intensity represents focal necrosis and hemorrhage (*arrowheads*).

signal intensity (Figs. 7.2–7.4). Imaging may show heterogeneity compatible with hemorrhage and/or necrosis as seen pathologically within the lesion (Fig. 7.3). Satellite nodules in the adjacent subcutaneous tissues may be seen on CT or MR imaging (Fig. 7.6). In our experience, linear extensions along the skin surface can also be detected (Fig. 7.4). These focal areas of extension must be identified to direct complete surgical resection without residual tumor. Mild-to-moderate hypervascularity is reported at arteriography (31). This hypervascularity is likely responsible for the moderate enhancement seen on CT scan or MR images obtained after injection of intravenous contrast material and the increased radiopharmaceutical accumulation on bone scan (35). Lesions are rarely more deeply seated.

GIANT CELL FIBROBLASTOMA

KEY CONCEPTS

- Giant cell fibroblastoma is the juvenile form of dermatofibrosarcoma protuberans with the identical cytogenetic aberration.
- Ninety percent of cases occur before 4 years of age; boys are affected more than girls (3:1).
- It is characterized by a subcutaneous mass with skin involvement.
- Imaging is likely similar to DFSP.
- Local recurrence is noted up to 50%; metastases are not reported.

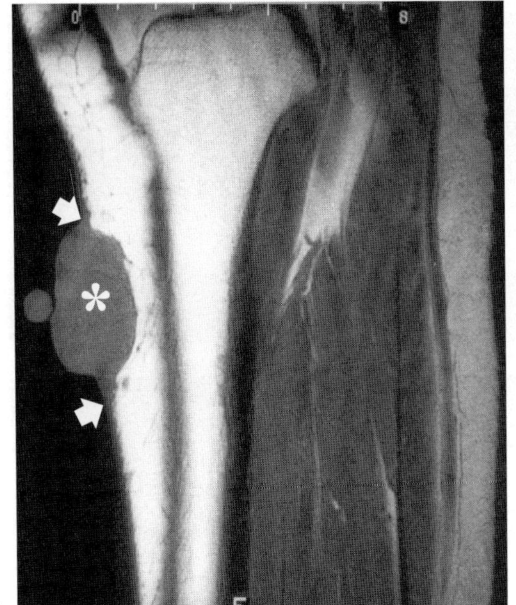

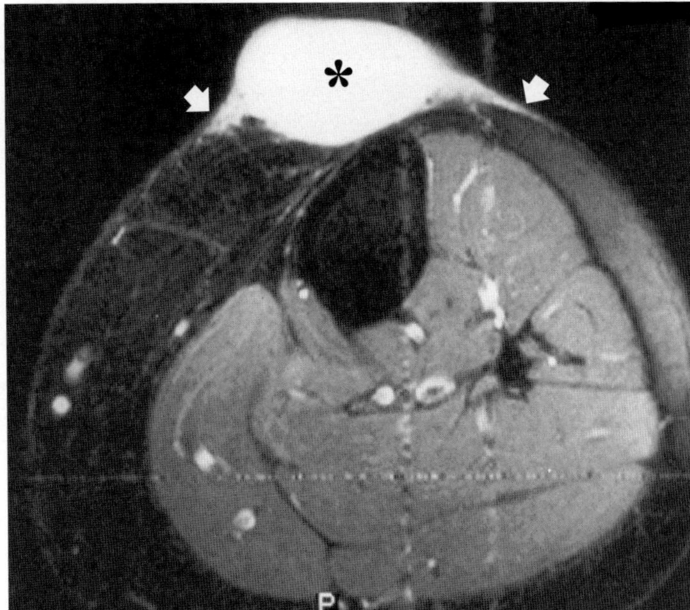

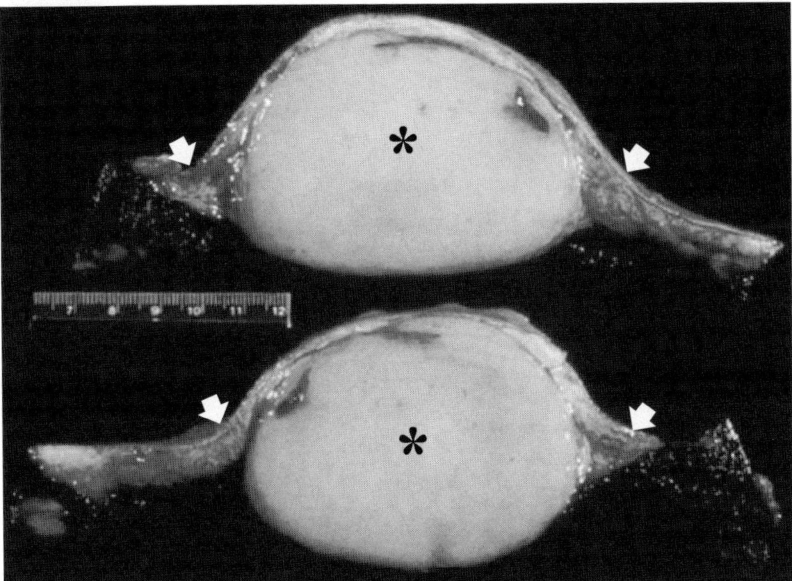

Figure 7.4 Dermatofibrosarcoma protuberans involving the lower leg in a man 45 years of age. **A,B:** Sagittal T1-weighted (TR/TE; 500/20) **(A)** and axial STIR (TR/TE/TI; 4000/20/150) **(B)** MR images show a protuberant mass involving the skin and subcutaneous fat (*asterisk*). There is linear skin extension (*arrows*) isointense with the remainder of the lesion. **C:** Photograph of the sectioned gross specimen reveals the mass (*asterisk*) and skin extension (*arrows*) identical to the imaging appearance.

Giant cell fibroblastoma is a distinctive lesion first described by Shmookler and Enzinger in 1982 (36). These authors suggested this lesion represents a juvenile form of DFSP as a mildly different expression of the same neoplasm (37). Further studies of the cytogenetic abnormalities in giant cell fibroblastoma confirm this similarity with supernumerary ring chromosomes 17 and 22 (38). This lesion typically occurs in young children as a slowly growing, painless, subcutaneous or intracutaneous solitary nodule, and 31 cases were reported through 1986 (39).

Giant cell fibroblastoma most commonly involves the chest wall, inguinal region, and back of the thigh areas (39), although it may be seen on the trunk and extremities. The vast majority of patients are infants and children, with lesions usually discovered before 4 years of age (range: 0.3 to 55 years of age) (8). In fact, 90% of lesions are diagnosed before 10 years of age, with less than 20% of cases occurring in adults (39). Boys are affected more frequently (3:1 ratio) (40). Lesions recur locally in approximately 50% of cases, however, metastases have not been reported (39), to the best of our knowledge.

The histologic features of giant cell fibroblastoma are quite similar to DFSP, although the cellularity is usually lower, collagen content is higher, and mitoses are scant. The imaging characteristics of giant cell fibroblastoma have also not been reported (to the best of our knowledge), although we suspect its appearance would be similar to that of DFSP (see preceding discussion) (Fig. 7.7).

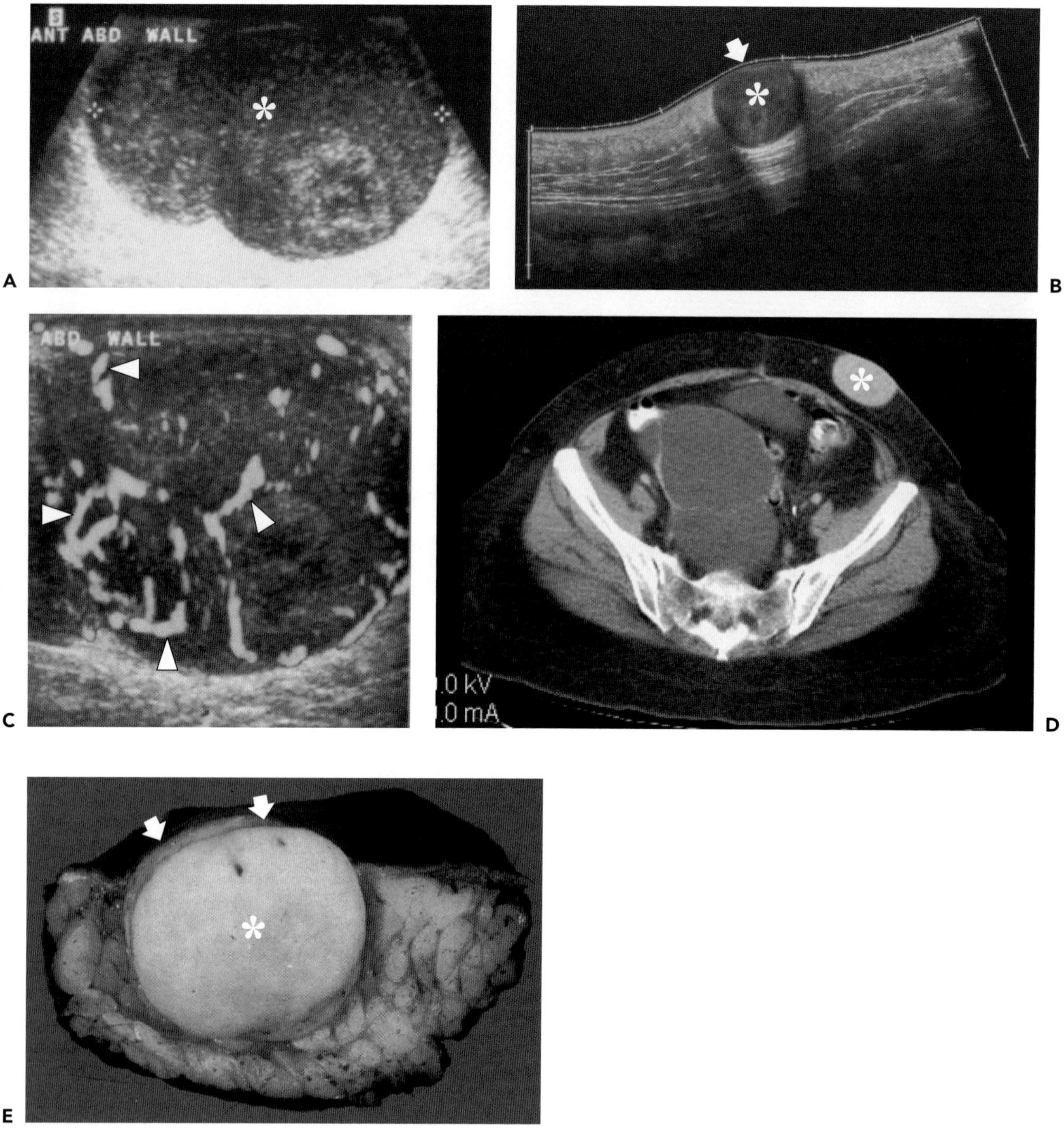

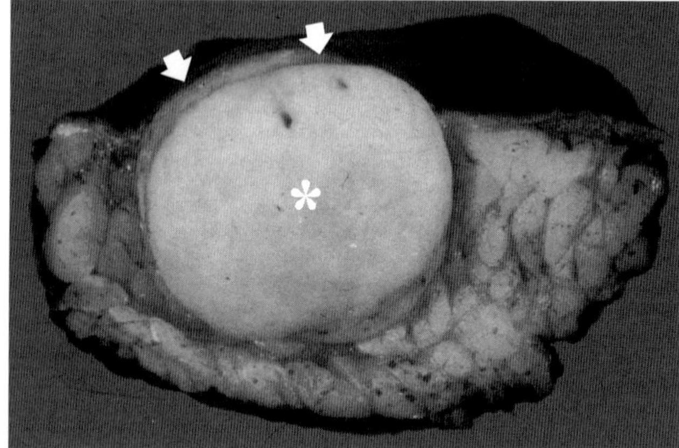

Figure 7.5 Dermatofibrosarcoma protuberans of the abdominal wall in a woman 54 years of age. **A–C:** Multiple ultrasound images including short axis **(A)**, extended view long axis **(B)**, and Doppler examination **(C)** reveal the echogenic subcutaneous mass (*asterisk*). Skin involvement and mild protuberance are well depicted on the long axis image (*arrow* in **B**) and vascular structures on the Doppler study (*arrowheads* in **C**). **D:** Axial CT reveals the diffusely enhancing DFSP. **E:** Photograph of the sectioned gross specimen demonstrates the DFSP (*asterisk*) with mild protuberance and skin involvement (*arrows*) correlating to imaging appearance.

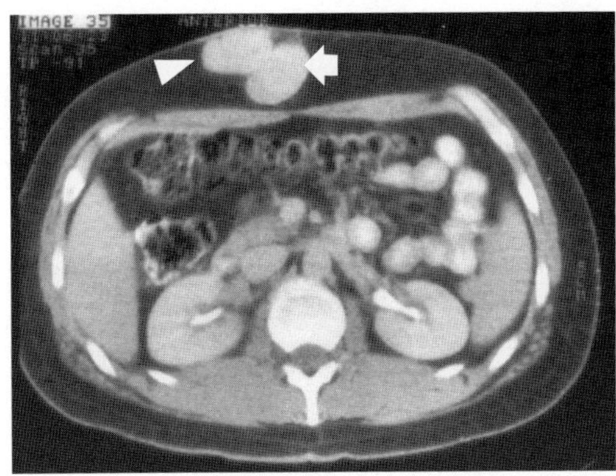
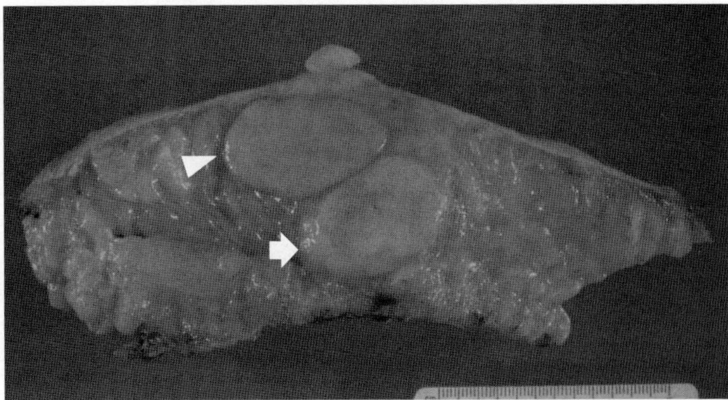

Figure 7.6. Dermatofibrosarcoma protuberans of the anterior abdominal wall in a man 33 years of age with satellite nodules. **A:** CT shows a subcutaneous nodule with skin involvement (*arrowhead*) and adjacent satellite nodule in the deep subcutaneous tissue (*arrow*). **B:** Photograph of gross specimen reveals both nodules identical to the appearance on the CT scan (*arrowhead* and *arrow*).

ATYPICAL FIBROXANTHOMA

> ### KEY CONCEPTS
> - Atypical fibroxanthoma is a subcutaneous mass in the elderly related to actinically damaged areas (head and neck: 75%) or previous radiation.
> - It is identical histologically to MFH.
> - Typically it is confined to subcutaneous tissue; if there is any deep invasion, it should be called MFH.
> - Imaging is not described but should show a nonspecific subcutaneous mass arising from the skin.
> - Local recurrence is 7%; lymph node spread/metastases are very rare.

Atypical fibroxanthoma, a pleomorphic superficial neoplasm, is histologically indistinguishable from MFH (see later discussion) and consequently is sometimes referred to as *superficial MFH*. Clinically, however, its behavior is usually nonaggressive, justifying distinction from MFH. This lesion was also referred to previously as *pseudosarcoma of the skin, pseudosarcoma dermatofibroma, paradoxical fibrosarcoma*, or *pseudosarcoma reticulohistiocytoma*. These solitary skin nodules or ulcerations are most frequently seen in elderly patients in actinically damaged areas (75% of cases), such as exposed regions of the head and neck (41–45). In 25% of cases, young adults are affected, with the most common locations being the limbs or trunk (42). Previous radiation may also play a role in development of these lesions, with the incidence varying from 5% to 50% (43,46). There is a long latent period (at least 10 years) between radiation exposure and atypical fibroxanthoma formation (43,46). Atypical fibroxanthoma is confined to the subcutaneous tissues without invasion of deeper structures. In contradistinction, a subcutaneous lesion with this histology that violates the fascia, invades muscle, or demonstrates vascular invasion

should be designated MFH (47). Local recurrence after surgical resection is unusual (7% of cases). Although rare, regional lymph node spread and metastases have been reported (42,48).

We are unaware of any description of the radiologic appearance of atypical fibroxanthoma. Our limited experience shows imaging to depict a small, well-defined mass with nonspecific intrinsic features similar to those of subcutaneous MFH (Fig. 7.8).

MYXOINFLAMMATORY FIBROBLASTIC SARCOMA

> ### KEY CONCEPTS
> - Myxoinflammatory fibroblastic sarcoma affects adults in the fourth to sixth decade of life.
> - Clinically, it is an ill-defined subcutaneous mass in the distal extremities (upper 56%; lower 30%).
> - Pathologically, it simulates the inflammatory/infectious process.
> - Imaging reveals a subcutaneous mass with nonspecific intrinsic characteristics (CT/MRI) but with surrounding edema in an acral location.
> - Local recurrence is 22% to 67%, with rare metastases.

Myxoinflammatory fibroblastic sarcoma was originally described in 1997 and 1998 by Montgomery et al. (49–51) as a distinct low-grade sarcoma, and these authors designated the term *inflammatory myxohyaline tumor* of the distal extremity with virocyte or Reed-Sternberg–like cells (49,50). Meis-Kindblom and Kindblom subsequently reported a series of patients and used the term *acral myxoinflammatory fibroblastic sarcoma* (51). An additional synonym for this lesion used in the literature is *inflammatory myxoid tumor* of the soft parts with bizarre giant cells.

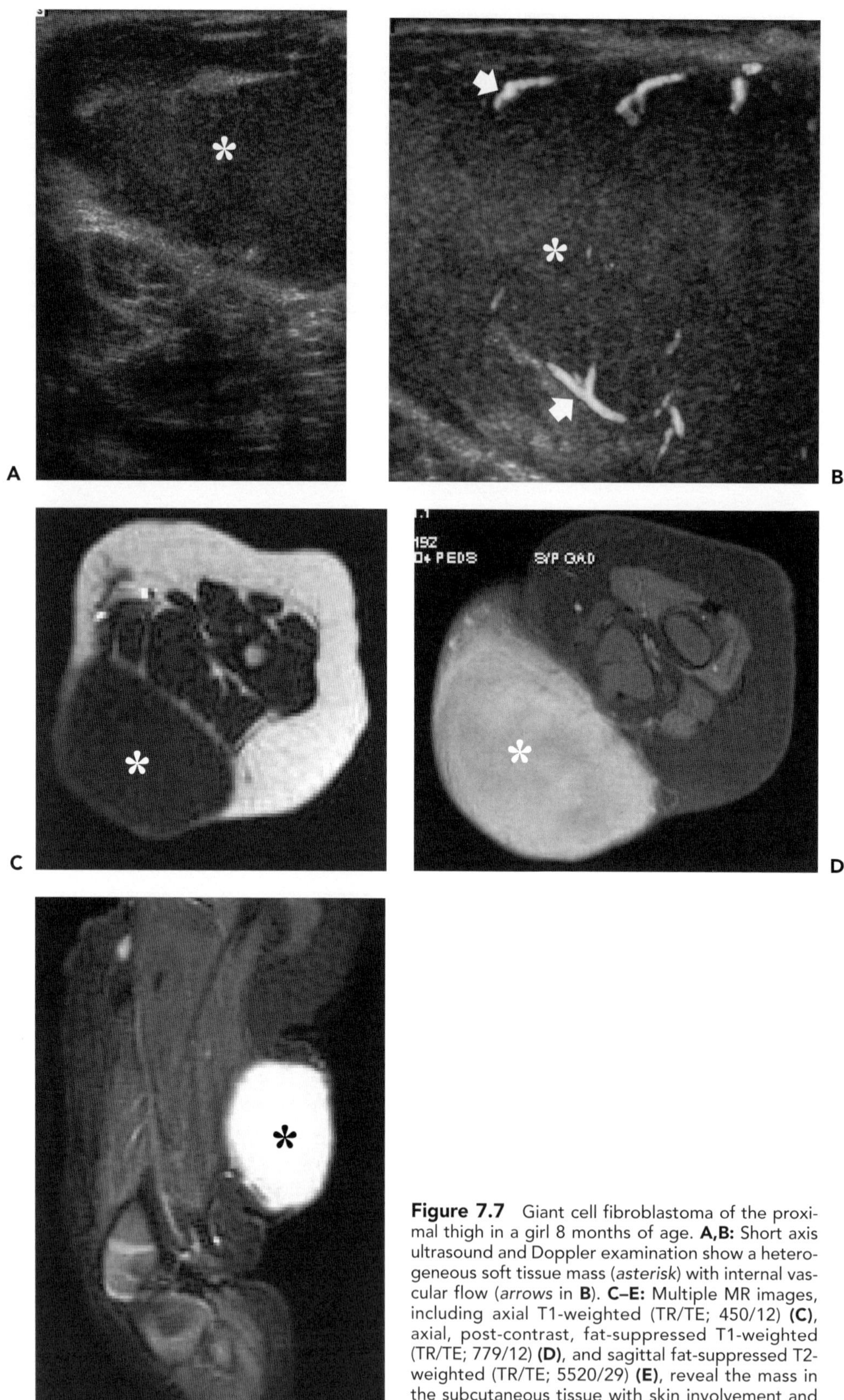

Figure 7.7 Giant cell fibroblastoma of the proximal thigh in a girl 8 months of age. **A,B:** Short axis ultrasound and Doppler examination show a heterogeneous soft tissue mass (*asterisk*) with internal vascular flow (*arrows* in **B**). **C–E:** Multiple MR images, including axial T1-weighted (TR/TE; 450/12) **(C)**, axial, post-contrast, fat-suppressed T1-weighted (TR/TE; 779/12) **(D)**, and sagittal fat-suppressed T2-weighted (TR/TE; 5520/29) **(E)**, reveal the mass in the subcutaneous tissue with skin involvement and protuberance (*asterisk*). There is high signal intensity on the long TR image and diffuse enhancement.

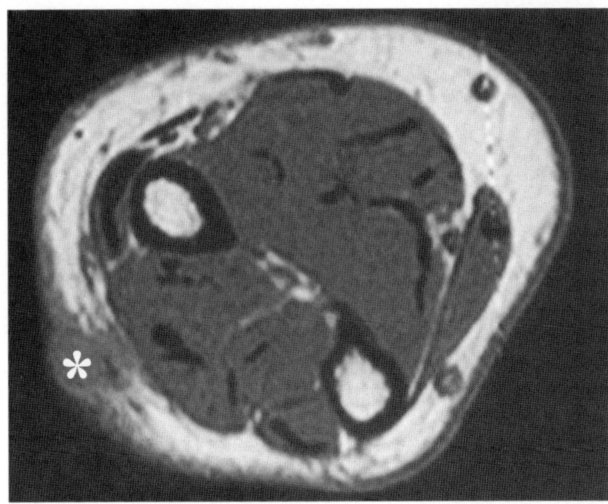
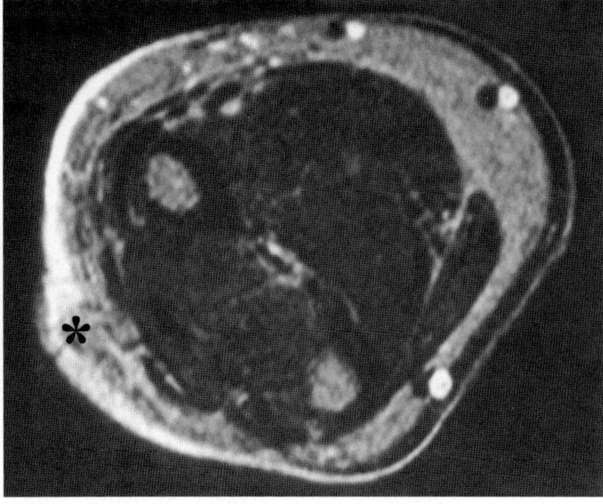

Figure 7.8   Recurrent atypical fibroxanthoma in the forearm of a woman 81 years of age with multiple previous resections. **A,B:** Axial T1-weighted (TR/TE; 850/20) **(A)** and T2-weighted (TR/TE; 2017/90) **(B)** spin-echo MR images show a mass (*asterisk*) in the dorsal subcutaneous tissue. The lesion is well seen on the T1-weighted image, but it is not well delineated from the adjacent fat and operative changes on the T2-weighted image.

Myxoinflammatory fibroblastic sarcoma most commonly affects adults in the fourth to sixth decades of life with an equal sex distribution. Clinically, patients present with a slow-growing, painless subcutaneous mass with ill-defined margins. The distal extremities are most frequently affected with the upper extremity (70% of cases; hands and fingers: 56%, followed by the lower arm and wrist: 11%) mildly more common than the lower extremity (30% of cases; toes and feet: 17%; ankles and lower legs: 14%) (52–56). The clinical presentation suggests an inflammatory process, such as tenosynovitis, as opposed to neoplasm.

At gross examination these lesions are usually multinodular, nonencapsulated, and poorly circumscribed, ranging in size from 1 to 8 cm (average 3 to 4 cm) (57). There is frequent involvement of the surrounding tendon sheaths, adjacent joint synovium, or deep invasion of muscle. Histologically, these lesions consist of a myxoid to hyaline stroma with prominent acute and chronic inflammatory infiltrate and virocytelike cells (58). These features often cause pathologic misdiagnosis of an inflammatory or infectious process.

The current treatment advocated for myxoinflammatory fibroblastic sarcoma is wide-local excision without adjuvant therapy. Local recurrence rates vary from 22% to 67%, with at least 31% demonstrating persistent disease (49–51). The difference in these studies is likely based on referral bias in retrospective studies, in which many of these lesions were misdiagnosed as non-neoplastic, with less aggressive resection. The lower figure of 22% local recurrence rate is likely more accurate because it was based on a prospective study (49,50). Multiple local recurrences are common (30%) (51). Two patients of the nearly 100 in the two largest series developed metastases: one in the inguinal lymph nodes and the other involving the lung (51).

MR imaging findings of these rare lesions was reported by Tateishi et al. (59). In a report of four patients they noted the lesions to show nonspecific low-to-intermediate signal intensity on T1-weighted, and intermediate-to-high signal intensity on T2-weighted MR images, with moderate homogeneous enhancement after intravenous contrast administration (Fig. 7.9). Lesions margins were ill-defined with frequent infiltration of surrounding structures, particularly tendon sheaths, reflecting the inflammatory components seen pathologically. In our experience, the inflammatory appearance and acral location are the only imaging features suggestive of this diagnosis (Fig. 7.9).

ANGIOMATOID FIBROUS HISTIOCYTOMA

> **KEY CONCEPTS**
> - Angiomatoid fibrous histiocytoma was formerly referred to as *angiomatoid malignant fibrous histiocytoma*.
> - Children and young adults are affected; 90% of patients are younger than 30 years.
> - The lesion presents as a slowly growing, cutaneous mass, with 65% to 85% of cases appearing in the extremities.
> - Pathologically hemorrhagic spaces show histiocytic cells and surrounding chronic inflammation.
> - Imaging shows a subcutaneous mass with fluid levels, mild surrounding edema, and a thick peripheral rim of enhancement.
> - Local recurrence rate is 20%, with only one reported case of metastases.

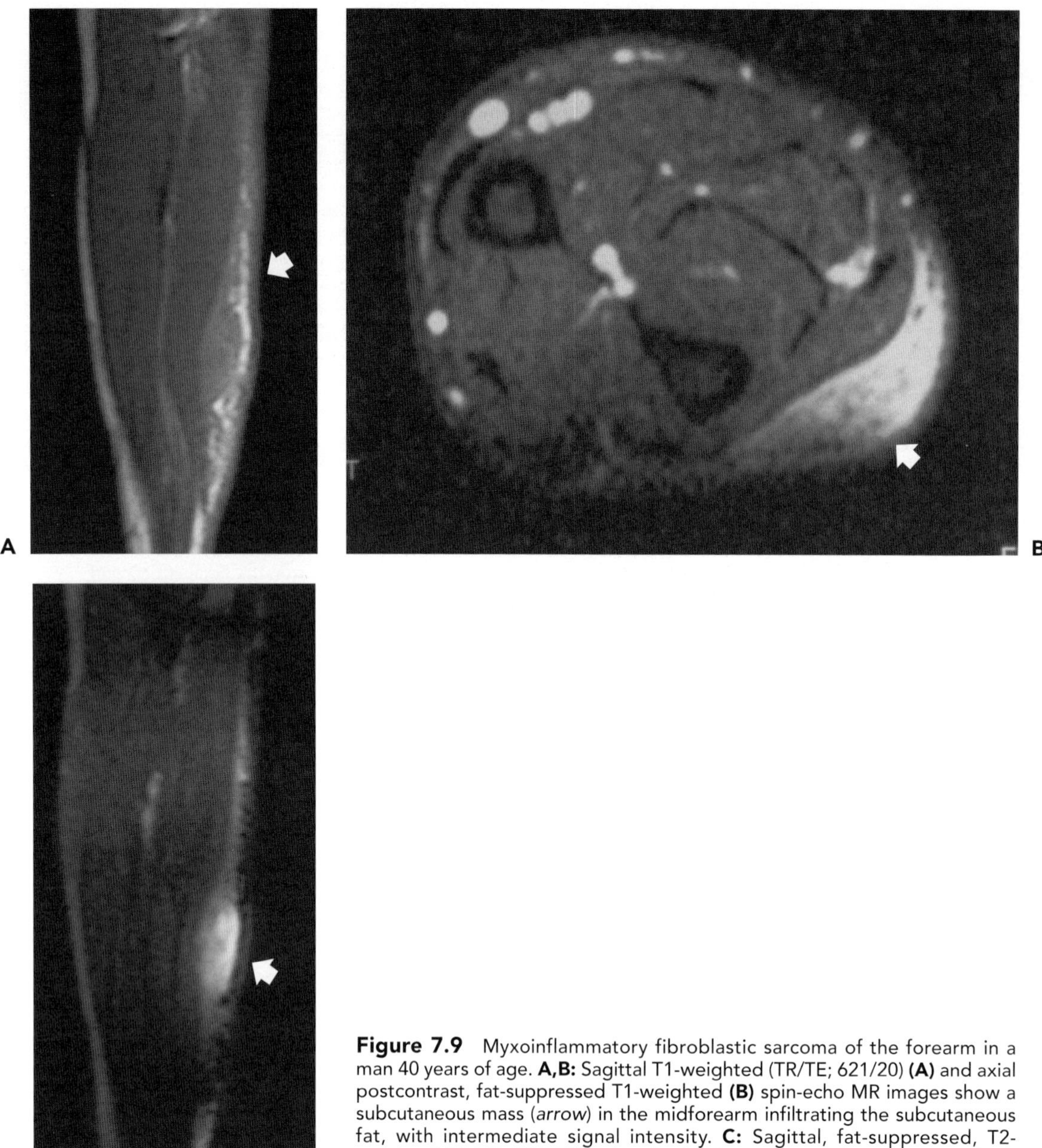

Figure 7.9 Myxoinflammatory fibroblastic sarcoma of the forearm in a man 40 years of age. **A,B:** Sagittal T1-weighted (TR/TE; 621/20) **(A)** and axial postcontrast, fat-suppressed T1-weighted **(B)** spin-echo MR images show a subcutaneous mass (*arrow*) in the midforearm infiltrating the subcutaneous fat, with intermediate signal intensity. **C:** Sagittal, fat-suppressed, T2-weighted (TR/TE; 2125/60) spin-echo MR image reveals heterogeneous high signal intensity in the mass (*arrow*).

Angiomatoid fibrous histiocytoma was formerly referred to as *angiomatoid malignant fibrous histiocytoma* but renamed by the WHO Classification of Soft Tissue Tumors (9,42,60,61). This change of nomenclature better reflects the low metastatic potential of angiomatoid fibrous histiocytoma. Children and young adults are generally affected, with nearly 90% of cases discovered before 30 years of age (8–12,62,63). Angiomatoid fibrous histiocytoma presents as a slowly growing subcutaneous mass most frequently in the extremities (65% to 85% of cases) (8–12,62–64). Systemic symptoms of fever, anemia, and weight loss are occasionally apparent, suggesting production of cytokines by the lesion.

As suggested by the name, angiomatoid fibrous histiocytoma is often composed of irregular blood-filled cystic spaces at gross inspection (Fig. 7.10). This feature may be so prominent as to suggest hematoma. Solid areas showing histiocytic-like cells and surrounding chronic inflammation are also apparent. The histiocytic cells are usually interspersed in the hemorrhagic area; the peripheral inflammatory component blends with the surrounding pseudocapsule.

The treatment for angiomatoid fibrous histiocytoma is complete surgical excision without the need for adjunct therapy. Although originally believed to be a more aggressive neoplasm, experience with larger numbers of lesions supports a favorable prognosis in the vast majority of

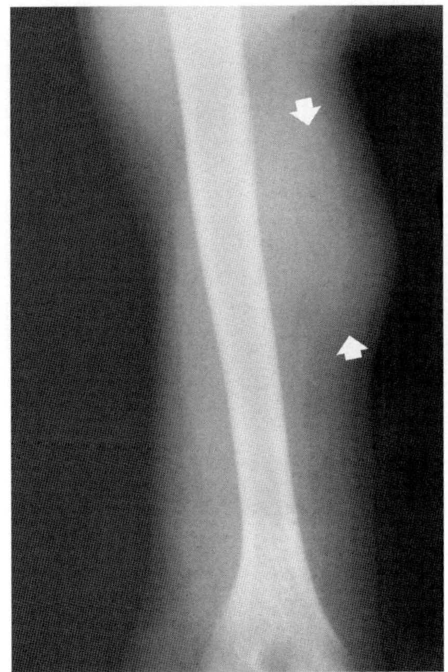
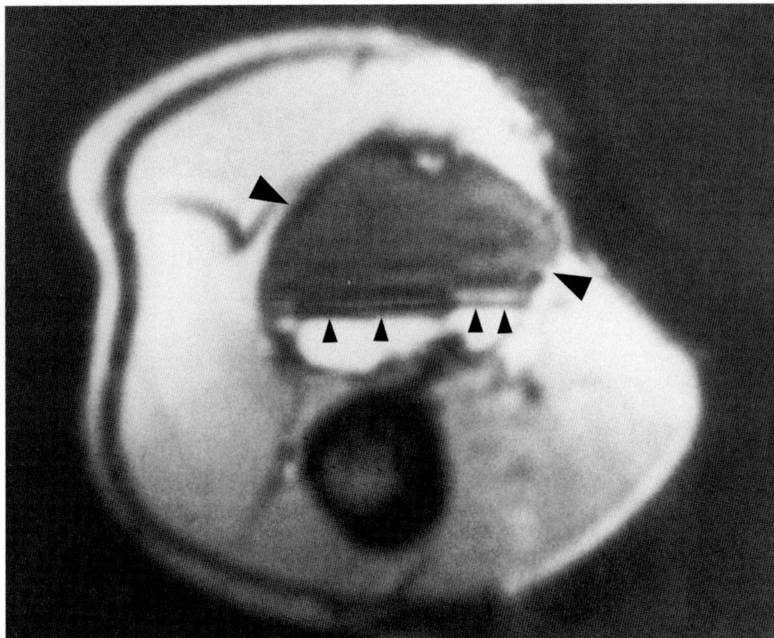
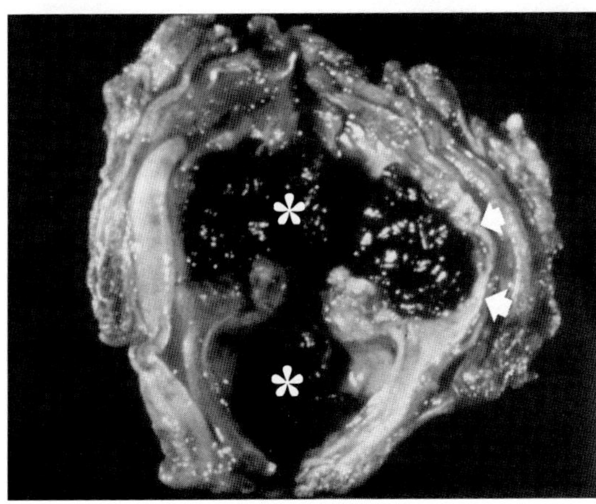

Figure 7.10 Angiomatoid fibrous histiocytoma of the upper arm in a boy 10 years of age. **A:** Radiograph of the humerus shows a medial soft tissue mass (*arrows*). **B:** Axial T1-weighted MR image reveals an intermuscular mass (*large arrowheads*) between the triceps and biceps muscles, with multiple fluid levels (*small arrowheads*) indicating hemorrhage. **C:** Photograph of the gross specimen shows a multiloculated cystic mass with thickened walls (*arrows*) and central blood clot (*asterisks*).

patients. Local recurrence is seen in 20% of patients with only one reported case of distant metastases (65).

Radiographs of patients with angiomatoid fibrous histiocytoma are normal or reveal a nonspecific soft tissue mass (Fig. 7.10). In our experience, MR imaging shows low-to-intermediate signal intensity on T1-weighting with high signal intensity on T2-weighting (Figs. 7.10 and 7.11). Fluid levels are commonly identified, reflecting the hemorrhagic spaces seen pathologically (Figs. 7.10 and 7.11). A thick, peripheral enhancing rim is seen following intravenous contrast administration on MR imaging. Mild surrounding edema, reflecting the histologic inflammatory component, may also be apparent on long TR images.

PLEXIFORM HISTIOCYTIC TUMOR

Plexiform histiocytic tumor was originally described by Enzinger and Zhang in an analysis of 65 cases in 1988 (66).

> **KEY CONCEPTS**
> - Plexiform histiocytic tumor occurs almost exclusively in children and young adults; 70% are younger than 20 years.
> - It is a subcutaneous, slowly growing mass; upper (63% to 65%) or lower (14% to 27%) extremity are the most commonly affected.
> - Hands/wrists represent 45% of cases.
> - Local recurrence occurs in 12% to 38% of cases; metastases occur in 5% to 15%.
> - Imaging is not described but likely would show nonspecific intrinsic features.

This lesion occurs almost exclusively in children and young adults, with 30% younger than 10 years, 70% younger than 20 years, and a mean of 14.5 years of age (66). Clinically, plexiform histiocytic tumor presents as a slowly growing (months to years) subcutaneous mass most commonly

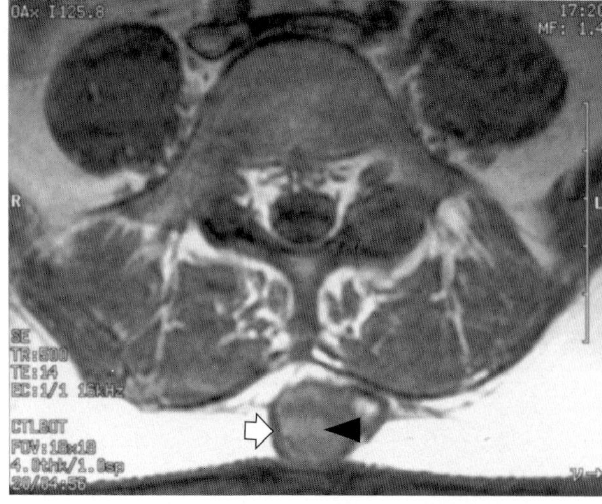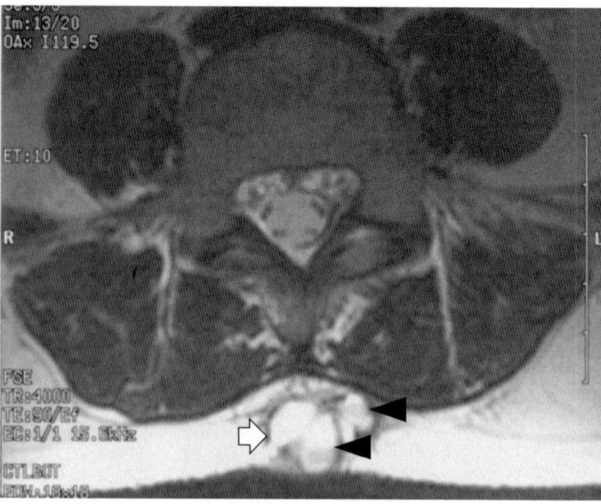

Figure 7.11 Subcutaneous angiomatoid fibrous histiocytoma in a boy 11 years of age with a palpable mass. **A,B:** Axial T1-weighted (TR/TE; 520/14) **(A)** and T2-weighted (TR/TE; 4000/90) **(B)** MR images show a subcutaneous mass (*arrow*) with multiple fluid levels (*arrowheads*) resulting from prominent hemorrhage.

affecting the upper (63% to 65% of cases) or lower (14% to 27% of cases) extremities (8,62,67). The hands and wrists account for 45% of cases (8,62,67). Less commonly affected sites include the trunk, head, and neck. Females are involved more often than males (2–5:1 ratio) (68).

At gross pathologic examination, plexiform histiocytic tumor is usually small, ranging from 1 to 3 cm in size (9–12). The lesion is multinodular and interconnected in a plexiform pattern. The lesion may extend in a radiating fashion into the surrounding subcutaneous fat. The three distinct cellular components in variable amounts include mononuclear histiocytes, spindle cell fibroblastlike cells, and multinucleated giant cells. Mitoses are infrequent and necrosis is absent, although vascular invasion is seen in 10% to 20% of cases (9–12).

Plexiform histiocytic tumor is a low-grade neoplasm. However, the metastatic rate is an estimated 5% to 15% (69–71). Lymph node metastases have been reported in two patients (69–71). Pulmonary metastases have been described in three patients (one leading to patient demise) and may be seen at the time of diagnosis (69–71). Local recurrence is seen in 12% to 38% of cases, typically within 1 to 2 years of initial presentation (69–71). The treatment of these lesions is wide surgical excision without adjuvant therapy because the risk of local or distant disease is low. No clinicopathologic features are described to allow distinction from more aggressive lesions.

Imaging of plexiform histiocytic tumor is not described, to the best of our knowledge. We would expect a nonspecific solid, subcutaneous mass on ultrasound, CT, or MR imaging with intermediate to high signal intensity on long TR images. The plexiform extensions into subcutaneous fat seen pathologically may cause irregular margins on cross-sectional imaging.

INFANTILE FIBROSARCOMA

> ### KEY CONCEPTS
> - Infantile fibrosarcoma almost always occurs in the first two years of life; up to 80% of cases are congenital.
> - This neoplasm accounts for 12% of soft tissue malignancies in infants.
> - Extremities represent nearly 50% of cases; the head and neck account for 16% and the trunk 19% of cases.
> - Treatment is complete resection but may require amputation.
> - Overall prognosis, unlike adult fibrosarcoma, is favorable.
> - Masses may infiltrate multiple tissue planes extensively and are often very large.
> - Cross-sectional imaging demonstrates this extensive multiplane tissue infiltration with nonspecific intrinsic features, although hemorrhage, necrosis, and high-flow vessels are common.

Fibrosarcoma occurring during the first years of life is considered a distinct entity and designated infantile fibrosarcoma by the WHO (9). The terms *congenital fibrosarcoma* and *juvenile fibrosarcoma* are used synonymously with *infantile desmoplastic fibrosarcoma* (67,72,73). Infantile fibrosarcoma was initially described by Stout in 1962, although the largest series were not reported until the 1970s (74). Infantile fibrosarcoma accounts for 12% of soft tissue malignancies in infants (75,76), and is congenital in approximately 36% to 80% of cases, with a biologic behavior and natural history quite different from that of fibrosarcoma occurring in adolescents and adults (77,78).

Infantile fibrosarcoma usually presents during the first 2 years of life (77). In various series, 36% to 100% of lesions are seen in patients younger than 1 year (77,79). The lesion has a predilection for the distal aspect of the extremities and usually presents as a painless mass (77,80,81). There is a slight predilection for boys (3:2 ratio) (77,82). In the series at the Armed Forces Institute of Pathology (AFIP), approximately 48% of the cases occurred in the distal extremities, with 31 (33%) of 94 lesions in the lower extremity (foot, ankle, lower leg) and 14 (15%) in the upper extremity (hand, wrist, and forearm) (77). The head and neck account for 16% of cases and the trunk 19% (77). Clinically, patients present with a nontender soft tissue mass or swelling at birth or developing soon thereafter (83). Lesions may grow rapidly and reach a large grotesque size (1 to 20 cm) (67,72,73). Superficial lesions may cause a purplish discoloration of the skin, suggesting a vascular lesion.

Infantile fibrosarcoma tends to be poorly circumscribed, infiltrating multiple tissue planes, including the subcutaneous fat, muscle, and fascia (76). The lesion is typically firm and rubbery, although occasionally areas of hemorrhage and necrosis are seen (75). Microscopically, the tumor is composed of immature-appearing spindle-shaped cells, with high cellularity and prominent mitotic activity arranged in intertwining fascicles, sometimes exhibiting the characteristic herringbone pattern (77) (Fig. 7.12). The lesion is more cellular and exhibits more prominent cellular activity than infantile fibromatosis, but it may be difficult to separate from the cellular form of fibromatosis (82). Cytogenetic analysis of tumor cells in patients with infantile fibrosarcoma shows trisomies of chromosomes 11, 20, 17, and 8 (in order of decreasing

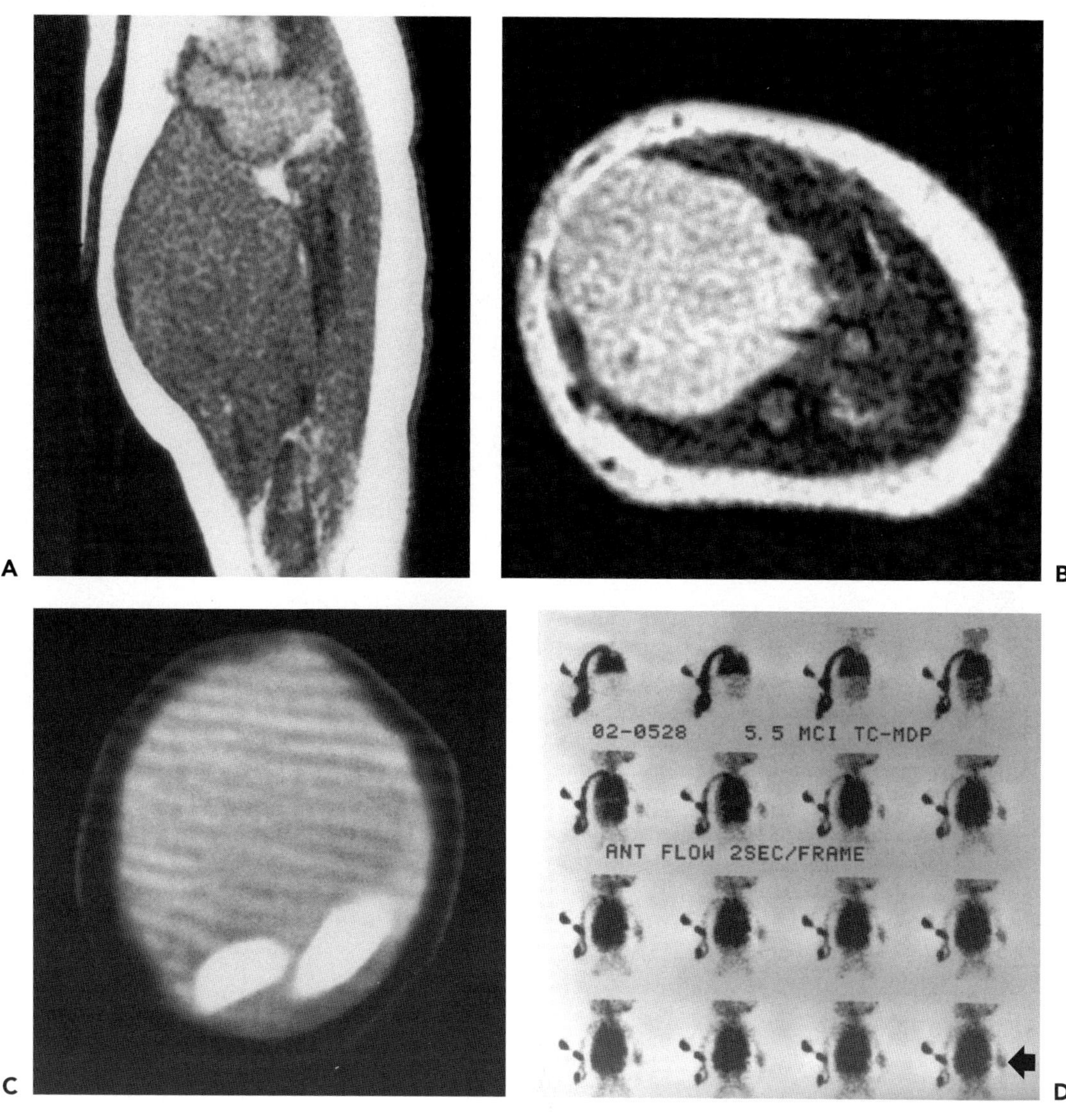

Figure 7.12 Infantile fibrosarcoma in the forearm of a girl 3.5 months of age. **A,B:** Coronal T1-weighted (TR/TE; 400/17) **(A)** and axial T2-weighted (TR/TE; 2000/80) **(B)** spin-echo MR images show a well-defined mass, with signal intensity similar to that of fat on T2-weighted images and similar to that of skeletal muscle on T1-weighted images. **C:** Axial noncontrast CT shows a large mass in the forearm without mineralization. **D:** Flow images from three-phase bone scan show increased tracer accumulation in the left forearm (*arrow*). (*continued*)

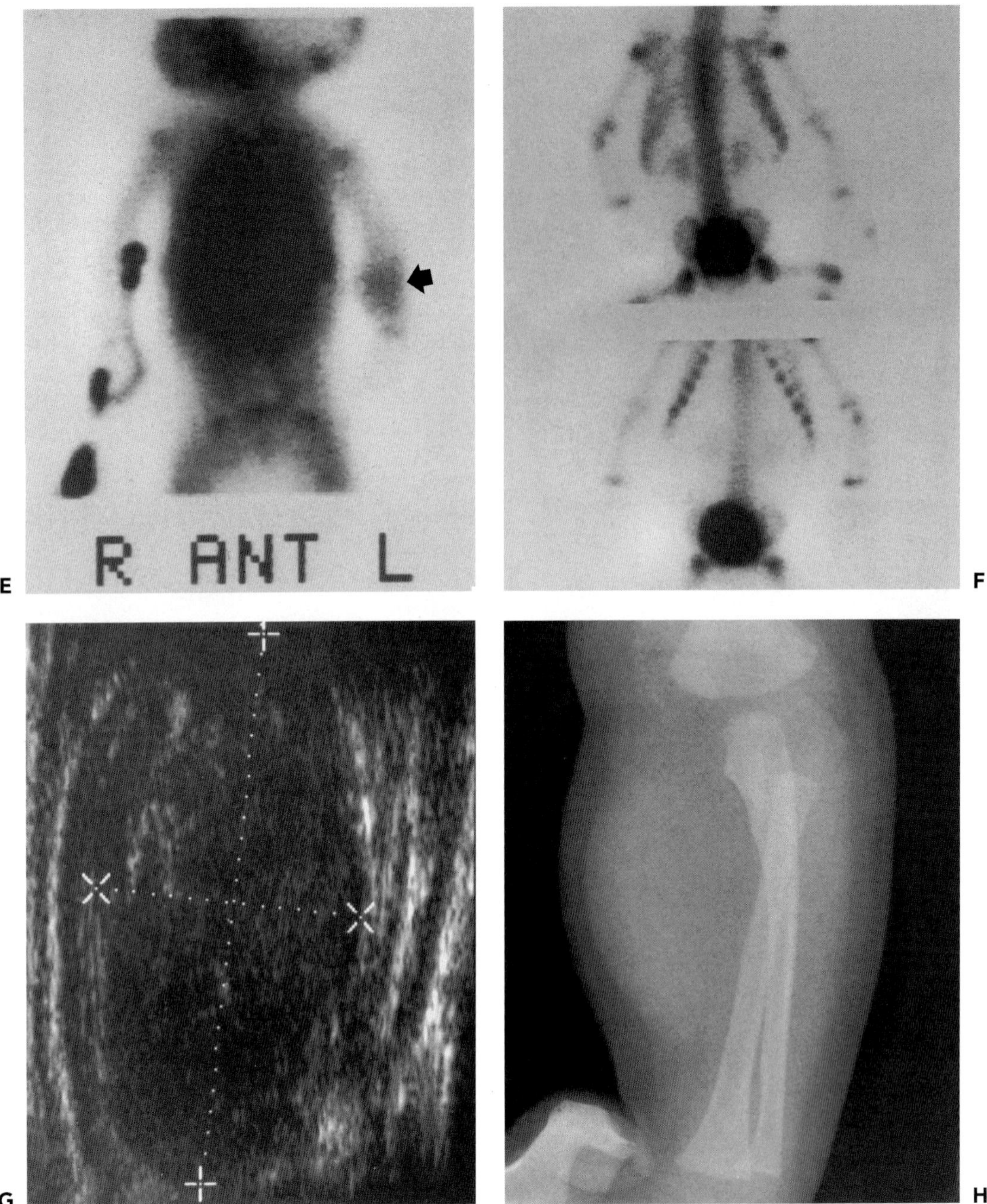

Figure 7.12 *(continued)*   **E,F:** Blood-pool **(E)** and delayed static **(F)** images from a three-phase bone scan show increased tracer accumulation on the blood-pool phase (*arrow* in **E**), but only minimal increased uptake on delayed images. **G:** Ultrasound shows a nonspecific hypoechoic mass. **H:** Corresponding radiograph shows a nonspecific mass. *(continued)*

frequency) in various combinations, as well as DNA content suggesting specific aneusomies (78,84,85). In addition, chromosomal translocation—t(12;15) (p13;q26)—was described in infantile fibrosarcoma identical to that seen in mesoblastic nephroma (86,87). These cytogenetic aberrations are not found in fibrosarcomas in older children and adults (78). Gene mutations at p53 are rare in infantile fibrosarcoma compared to adult fibrosarcoma (12).

The treatment of choice for infantile fibrosarcoma is complete surgical resection (88). Some lesions may not progress or recur, even if only partially resected. Unfortunately, no known morphologic features predict the clinical behavior of infantile fibrosarcoma (to determine which lesions are more aggressive) and help direct the appropriate method of treatment. However, local recurrence following surgery is common, seen in 5% to 50% of cases (76,79,81,82); multiple recurrences are not

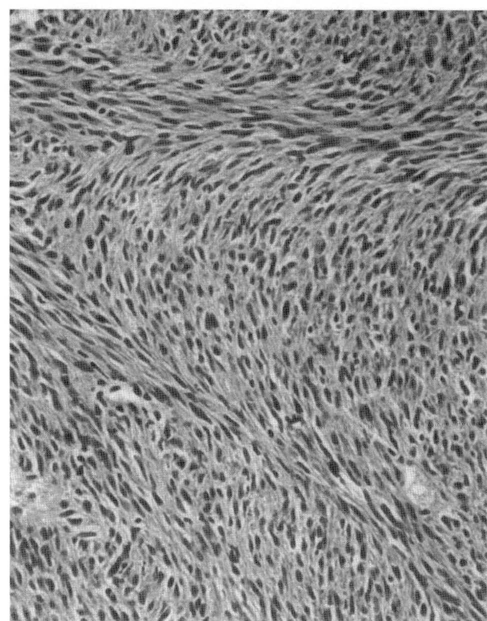

Figure 7.12 *(continued)*   **I:** The tumor is highly cellular, composed of immature-appearing spindle-shaped cells with intertwining fascicles, exhibiting a characteristic herringbone pattern.

infrequent. Amputation may be required for local control, either initially or following recurrence (80). Local recurrence is usually at the site of prior surgery but may be at some distance from the original lesion (80). Chemotherapy before or after surgery or as the sole treatment in unresectable lesions may also be employed. The overall prognosis is favorable, in contradistinction to adult fibrosarcoma. Metastases are uncommon, particularly in young patients (<8% of patients <5 years of age) (76,81). Patients with the primary tumor in the trunk, head, or neck have a slightly worse prognosis than patients with lesions located in the distal extremity (82). The overall 5-year survival was 84% in one series (77). The mortality varies from 4% to 25% (77,79), which may relate to hemorrhage and involvement of vital structures. The survival of older children is similar to that for adults.

Radiographs typically reveal a nonspecific soft tissue mass (83) (Figs. 7.12–7.14). There may be evidence of bone deformity or erosion secondary to the soft tissue mass (83). Discrete bone destruction is reported as rare, occurring in less than 5% of cases, although it is more common in our experience (77). CT and MR imaging are useful in demonstrating the amount of bone and soft tissue involvement by tumor (83) (Figs. 7.12–7.14). The intrinsic appearance on ultrasound, CT or MR imaging is nonspecific. Heterogeneity is common, likely reflecting hemorrhage and necrosis (Figs. 7.12–7.14). High-flow, serpentine vascular structures can be identified on MR and Doppler evaluation, in our experience (Fig. 7.14). Overall, the diagnosis of infantile fibrosarcoma should be suggested in an infant with a large distal extremity soft tissue

mass showing foci of hypervascularity. Lesions may also be markedly vascular on angiography, suggesting an angiomatous lesion.

FIBROSARCOMA AND MALIGNANT FIBROUS HISTIOCYTOMA

The nomenclature of the malignant fibrous and fibrohistiocytic lesions has changed significantly since the previous edition of this book. We follow the current (2002) WHO classification of these lesions in describing the clinical presentation, pathology, treatment and prognosis of each lesion (a). The only exception will be the use of the more common terminology of *malignant fibrous histiocytoma* (MFH) instead of *undifferentiated pleomorphic* sarcoma. These lesions include adult fibrosarcoma, low-grade fibromyxoid sarcoma, sclerosing epithelioid fibrosarcoma, and MFH. Although these lesions are pathologically distinct, the imaging of these neoplasms largely overlaps without features to allow distinction among fibrosarcoma and MFH and their variants. Therefore the radiologic features of these lesions are discussed together.

Adult Fibrosarcoma

> **KEY CONCEPTS**
> - The incidence of adult fibrosarcoma is decreasing (approximately 5% currently) with improved immunohistochemistry and more specific classification of soft tissue tumors.
> - Adults are affected, with 60% of patients between 40 and 70 years of age.
> - This lesion most commonly involves deep soft tissues of the extremities or trunk.
> - Treatment is wide excision; chemotherapy is used for higher grade lesions.
> - Overall, the 5-year survival rates are 39% to 54% but is improved with lower grade tumors.

Fibrosarcoma is a malignant tumor of fibroblasts, composed of a relatively uniform population of spindle cells. It demonstrates variable anaplasia and lacks further differentiating features (89–91). Fibrosarcoma has become a diagnosis of exclusion and must be differentiated from other spindle cell tumors to include monophasic synovial sarcoma, malignant peripheral nerve sheath tumor, leiomyosarcoma, and malignant fibrous histiocytoma. The recognition of these latter spindle cell lesions as distinct entities has significantly decreased the incidence of fibrosarcoma as a diagnosis. This phenomenon is well illustrated by the Mayo Clinic experience, with the incidence of fibrosarcoma (as a percentage of soft tissue sarcomas) decreasing from 65% in 1936 to 12% in 1974

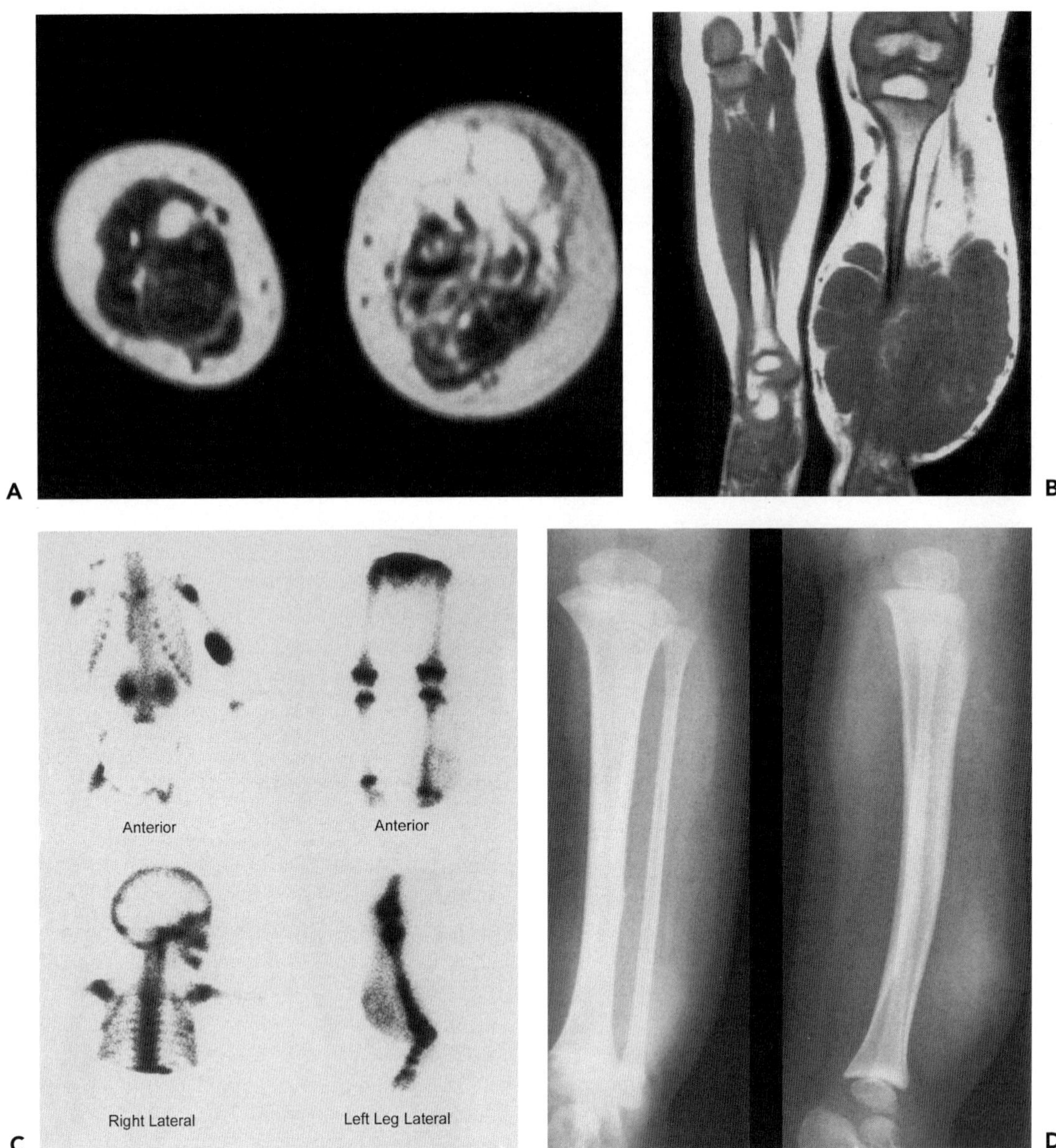

Figure 7.13 Infantile fibrosarcoma in the leg of a girl 2 years of age. **A:** Axial T2-weighted (TR/TE; 3000/90) MR image shows a well-defined lobulated mass in the distal aspect of the left lower leg with high signal intensity. **B:** Coronal T1-weighted (TR/TE; 600/15) MR image approximately 7 weeks later, shows significant increase in size of the mass. **C:** Delayed images from bone scan show increased tracer accumulation in the anterior soft tissue of the lower leg. **D:** Corresponding radiographs show poorly defined mass in the anterior soft tissues. The adjacent bone is normal.

and even further reduction in the review by Scott et al. in 1989 (89,92,93). Whereas fibrosarcoma was previously considered the most commonly occurring soft tissue malignancy, it is now considered uncommon, comprising approximately 5% of soft tissue sarcomas (9–12,40, 73,94). However, we believe the overall trend may well be reversed in the future, with the identification and acceptance of multiple fibrosarcoma variants (Figs. 7.15 and 7.16).

Fibrosarcoma occurs primarily in adults, with approximately 60% of patients between 40 and 70 years of age (81,93). The lesion typically involves the deep soft tissues

of the extremities and trunk (76,81,93). As with most soft tissue sarcomas, the clinical symptoms are nonspecific. Patients often present with a slowly enlarging painless mass over several months' duration. A dull aching pain or tenderness is reported in approximately 30% of patients (81). There is a mild male predilection (61% of cases) (89). Systemic symptoms are unusual, although hypoglycemia, likely related to a humoral insulinlike substance, is rarely reported. Fibrosarcoma typically arises de novo, although development in burn scars, related to foreign bodies, and following radiation (with a typical long latent period) is also reported (9–12,40,73,94).

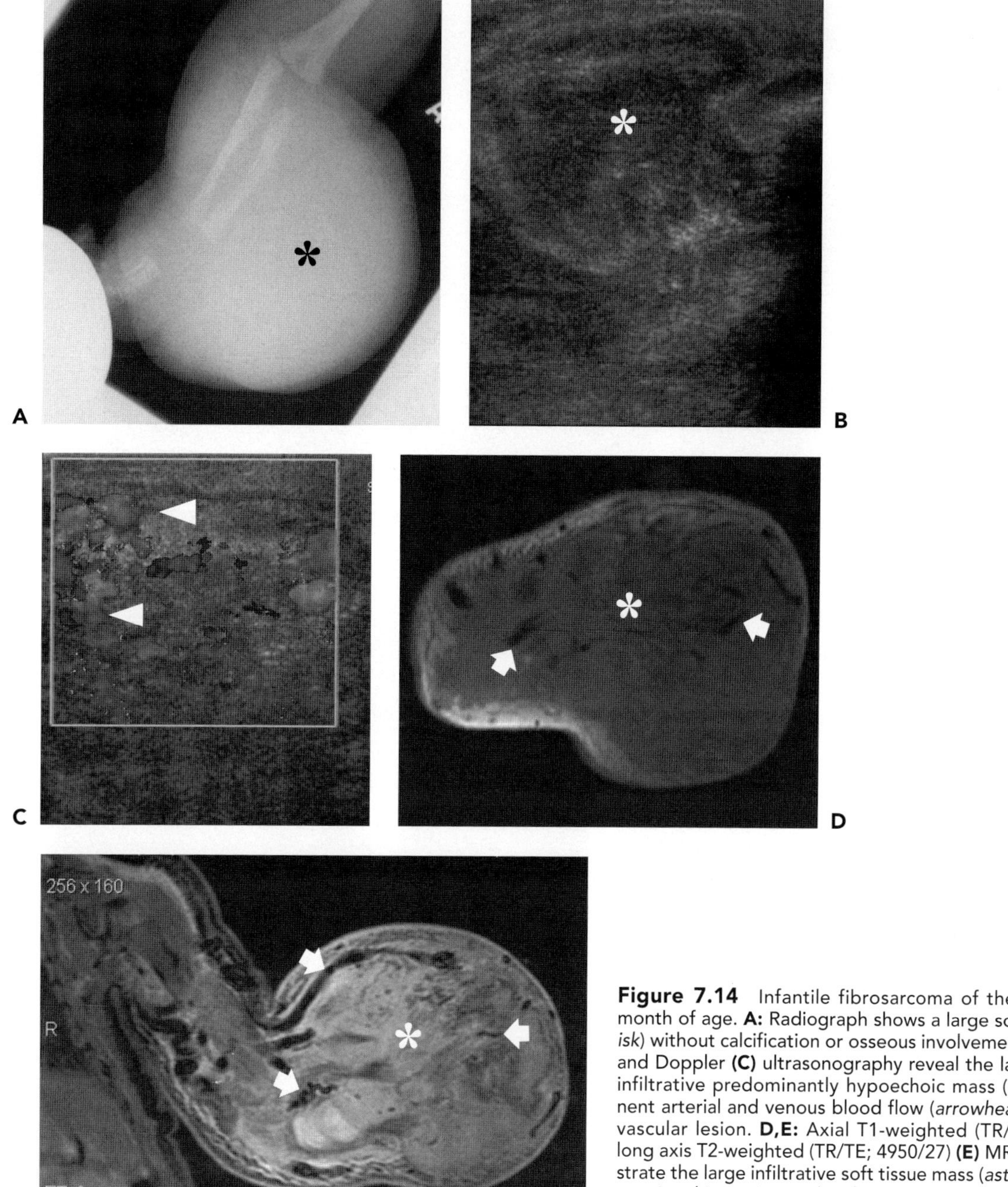

Figure 7.14 Infantile fibrosarcoma of the forearm in a girl 1 month of age. **A:** Radiograph shows a large soft tissue mass (*asterisk*) without calcification or osseous involvement. **B,C:** Short axis (**B**) and Doppler (**C**) ultrasonography reveal the large, heterogeneous, infiltrative predominantly hypoechoic mass (*asterisk*) with prominent arterial and venous blood flow (*arrowheads* in **C**) simulating a vascular lesion. **D,E:** Axial T1-weighted (TR/TE; 750/10) (**D**) and long axis T2-weighted (TR/TE; 4950/27) (**E**) MR images also demonstrate the large infiltrative soft tissue mass (*asterisk*) with intermediate signal intensity on the short TR image and high signal intensity on the long TR image. Multiple serpentine high-flow vascular structures are also seen (*arrows*).

The tumor is usually a solitary gray, lobulated, firm, fleshy mass (3 to 8 cm) with a surrounding pseudocapsule (81). Microscopically, the tumor is composed of anaplastic spindle cells with varying degrees of differentiation. At microscopy, a fascicular or so-called herringbone pattern is frequently identified, as well as a minor myxoid component (89). Fibrosarcoma is differentiated from fibromatosis (desmoid tumor) by the increased collagen and absence of atypia in the latter (89). Myofibroblastic components may also be apparent, and these lesions are often referred to as low-grade myofibroblastic sarcomas (21,95,96). Lesions are generally considered low-to-intermediate-grade tumors with higher grade lesions often diagnosed as MFH.

Fibrosarcoma is best treated by wide-marginal resection and limb salvage. In cases in which complete resection is not possible because of lesion size, location, or involvement of neurovascular structures, adjuvant radiation therapy is used. Chemotherapy is typically reserved for higher grade lesions. The long-term prognosis of

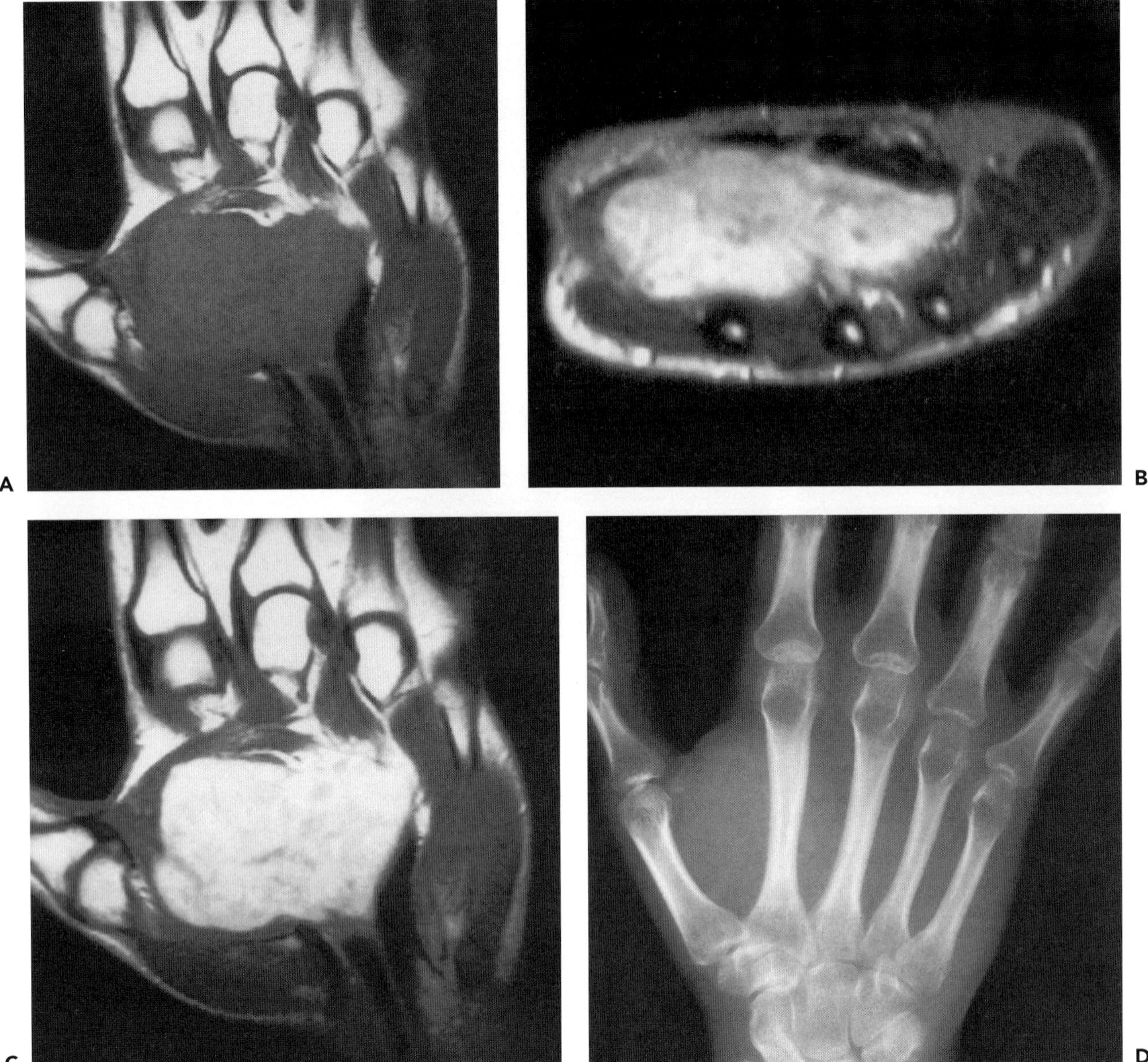

Figure 7.15 Fibrosarcoma in the thenar eminence of the left hand in a woman 22 years of age. **A,B:** Coronal T1-weighted (TR/TE; 480/15) **(A)** and axial T2-weighted (TR/TE; 1800/90) **(B)** MR images show a well-defined intramuscular mass in the thenar eminence of the hand. **C:** Postcontrast T1-weighted (TR/TE; 480/15) MR image reveals marked homogeneous contrast enhancement. **D:** Corresponding radiograph shows a nonspecific nonmineralized soft tissue mass.

fibrosarcoma is difficult to determine accurately because of the changes in nomenclature and advances in immuno-histo-chemical stains. Comparison of studies is even more problematic, reflected by the wide variation of local recurrence and metastatic rates. Despite these limitations, several general statements can be made concerning the prognosis of adult fibrosarcoma. First, higher grade lesions are associated with a poorer prognosis. Second, the adequacy of the initial surgical treatment in obtaining tumor-free margins with aggressive resection is important to improve patient outcome. This is reflected in the study by Scott et al.

that showed a 79% recurrence with inadequate surgical margins versus 18% with wide-margin resection (89). Overall, the local recurrence rate varies between 12% and 79%, likely averaging in the 40% to 50% range (89,97). Metastatic rates in the study by Scott et al. were 63% at 5 years but varied from 43% with low-grade tumors (grade 1 or 2) to 82% with high-grade lesions (grade 4) (89). Metastases are most common to the lung and bone and usually occur in the first 2 years following initial treatment (97). However, delayed metastases more than a decade after the initial treatment have been described (97).

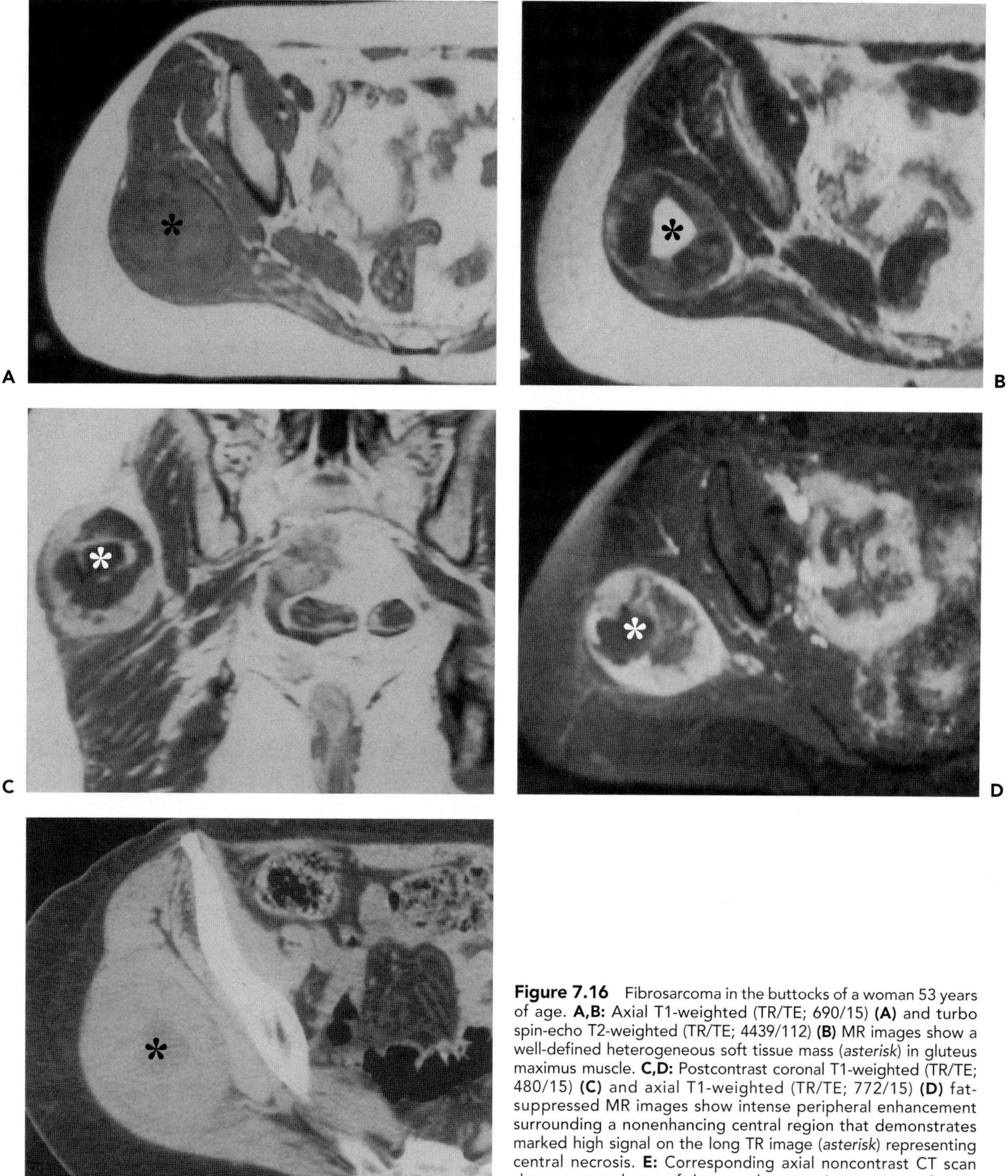

Figure 7.16   Fibrosarcoma in the buttocks of a woman 53 years of age. **A,B:** Axial T1-weighted (TR/TE; 690/15) **(A)** and turbo spin-echo T2-weighted (TR/TE; 4439/112) **(B)** MR images show a well-defined heterogeneous soft tissue mass (*asterisk*) in gluteus maximus muscle. **C,D:** Postcontrast coronal T1-weighted (TR/TE; 480/15) **(C)** and axial T1-weighted (TR/TE; 772/15) **(D)** fat-suppressed MR images show intense peripheral enhancement surrounding a nonenhancing central region that demonstrates marked high signal on the long TR image (*asterisk*) representing central necrosis. **E:** Corresponding axial noncontrast CT scan shows a central area of decreased attenuation corresponding to the area of central necrosis (*asterisk*).

Lymph node metastases occur in 0.5% to 8% of cases (90,91). Survival rates also vary by tumor grade and initial surgery performed. Overall, 5-year survival rates are 39% to 54% (89,98). Patients with low-grade tumors (grades 1 and 2), have a 5-year survival rate ranging from 55% to 82%, whereas the 5-year survival rate for high-grade tumors (grades 3 and 4) range from 21% to 68% (89,98). The 5-year survival rate for fibrosarcoma treated by local excision was 30% as compared to 78% in lesions treated with radical excision in the study by Bizer et al. (99).

Low-Grade Fibromyxoid Sarcoma

> **KEY CONCEPTS**
> - Low-grade fibromyxoid sarcoma is a rare tumor that affects young to middle-aged adults (median: 34 years of age).
> - Deep soft tissues of the lower extremity, particularly the thigh, are most commonly affected.
> - The lesion is a slow-growing, painless soft tissue mass.
> - Treatment is wide-local excision.
> - Local recurrence is 8%; metastases, 6%; death rate, 2% in recent studies.

The low-grade fibromyxoid sarcoma was first described by Evans et al. in 1987 in a report of two cases (100). Other terms for this lesion include *hyalinizing spindle cell tumor with giant rosettes* and *fibromyxoid-type fibrosarcoma*. This is a rare tumor with fewer than 150 reported cases (9–12,40,73,94); but it is probably more common than the literature suggests because many tumors of this type are unrecognized.

Low-grade fibromyxoid sarcoma affects young to middle-aged adults with a median of 34 years of age. Reports vary as to an equal sex distribution or a mild male predilection (9–12). The most commonly affected site is the deep soft tissue of the lower extremity, particularly the thigh. Additional sites of involvement include the chest wall/axilla, shoulder, inguinal areas, buttock, neck, and retroperitoneum, in order of decreasing frequency (9–12) (Fig. 7.17). Subcutaneous tissues may also be involved as the site of origin. Patients typically present with a very slowly growing, painless soft tissue mass.

At gross pathologic examination, most lesions are intramuscular (less commonly subcutaneous) and relatively large (8 to 10 cm) (9–12). The tumor is well-circumscribed, although microscopically the lesion often infiltrates muscle. Histologically, low-grade fibromyxoid sarcomas reveal an admixture of heavily collagenized areas that are hypocellular (usually the more prominent component) and cellular myxoid regions. Giant rosettes formed by epithelioid fibroblasts may be present as a variant of this lesion. There is a low mitotic rate. This deceptively bland pathologic appearance may initially suggest a benign lesion.

The treatment of low-grade fibromyxoid sarcoma is wide excision. Initial reports of local recurrence (68%), metastatic rate (41%), and death rate (18%) likely overestimate the aggressiveness of this lesion as a result of incomplete excision (treated as a benign lesion) (100–103). Subsequent prospective studies with appropriate initial surgical management show a much less aggressive clinical course (100–103). These studies demonstrate local recurrence of 9%, metastases of 6%, and death rate of 2% (100–103). Metastatic disease affects the lungs and pleura almost exclusively and may occur at the time of presentation or develop after a long delay (45 years in one patient) (100–103).

Sclerosing Epithelioid Sarcoma

> **KEY CONCEPTS**
> - Sclerosing epithelioid sarcoma is a very rare and distinct variant of fibrosarcoma.
> - Adults (average: 40 to 45 years of age) are most frequently affected.
> - Proximal lower extremities are most commonly involved.
> - Wide surgical excision is the treatment of choice.
> - Local recurrence is 53%; metastases, 43%; death rate more than 50%.

Sclerosing epithelioid sarcoma is a very rare, distinct variant of fibrosarcoma. The initial description was by Meis-Kindblom et al. in 1995 in a report of 25 cases (104). These lesions affect a wide age range of patients, with the mean age between 40 and 45 years (104–107). Men are reported to be slightly more commonly affected than women. The most frequent location is the deep soft tissues of the proximal lower extremity, followed by the trunk, upper extremities, head, and neck (104–108).

Sclerosing epithelioid fibrosarcomas are often large at detection with a mean size of 7 to 10 cm (9–12,94). These lesions are lobulated or multinodular and well-circumscribed. They typically arise in muscle and may invade underlying bone. These lesions are composed of epithelioid nests and cords within a collagenous matrix and may simulate lymphoma. Myxoid, cystic, and calcified areas may be seen, although necrosis is uncommon.

Wide surgical excision is the treatment of choice. Local recurrence is common (53%). Metastatic disease is also frequent (43%) (104). Metastases typically affect the lung, pleura, and bone, with a median interval of 8 years (104, 106–108). Patient demise occurs in more than 50% of cases in this highly malignant tumor (104).

Malignant Fibrous Histiocytoma

Malignant fibrous histiocytoma (MFH) is a pleomorphic sarcoma described initially by Ozzello et al. in 1963 and subsequently by O'Brien and Stout in 1964 (109,110). It is composed of histiocytelike and fibroblastlike elements, although with refinement of immunohistochemical studies, MFH now appears more related to the fibroblasts, myofibroblasts, or undifferentiated mesenchymal cells (42,109, 111–127). Complex, nonuniform cytogenetic aberrations are common in these lesions. Pathologically, MFH is a diagnosis of exclusion, similar to fibrosarcoma. Pathologically distinct from fibrosarcoma, MFH is based on a relatively variable histologic appearance and the presence of giant cells. Pathologic subtypes of MFH include storiform/pleomorphic, myxoid, giant cell, and inflammatory (9–12, 40,42,62).

The WHO classification of these historic subtypes of MFH has changed to reflect the lack of histiocytic differen-

> **KEY CONCEPTS**
> - Current WHO Classification:
>   - Storiform/Pleomorphic MFH (50% to 60%): Undifferentiated high-grade pleomorphic sarcoma.
>   - Myxoid MFH (25%): Myxofibrosarcoma.
>   - Giant cell MFH (5% to 10%): Undifferentiated pleomorphic sarcoma with giant cells.
>   - Inflammatory MFH (<5%): Undifferentiated pleomorphic sarcoma with prominent inflammation.
> - Use of the term *MFH* is still maintained by many (most?) pathologists and clinicians.
> - MFH is the most common soft tissue sarcoma of late adult life, accounting for 20% to 30% of all soft tissue sarcomas.
> - Peak incidence is in the fifth decade; men account for 70% of lesions.
> - Most commonly affected sites are lower extremity (50%) upper extremity (25%) and retroperitoneum (15%).
> - These are usually deep intramuscular lesions (70%); 5% to 10% are subcutaneous.

tiation (9). The WHO nomenclature designates storiform/pleomorphic MFH as *undifferentiated high-grade pleomorphic sarcoma*; myxoid MFH as *myxofibrosarcoma*; giant cell MFH as *undifferentiated pleomorphic sarcoma* with giant cells; and inflammatory MFH as *undifferentiated pleomorphic sarcoma with prominent inflammation* (9). We and many of our pathologic colleagues (we suspect the majority, in fact) find this terminology cumbersome and awkward and retain the use of MFH in both our daily workload and for purposes of this text, as synonymous with the current WHO classification (9). Fletcher et al. argue that subtle immunohistochemical differentiation in these lesions justifies their recategorization (118). As an example, should minimal positive muscle markers (desmin positive) in a largely pleomorphic lesion be specific for the diagnosis of leiomyosarcoma? If so, the incidence of leiomyosarcoma increases at the expense of pleomorphic MFH, which accounts for statistical variation on incidence. Importantly, this distinction currently does not alter therapy or prognosis and requires application of relatively costly technology. We believe the term *MFH* still serves a useful purpose in clearly communicating to our clinical colleagues. In addition, the radiologic appearance of MFH and adult fibrosarcoma is identical, regardless of the subtleties of histologic variations.

MFH is the most common soft tissue sarcoma of late adult life, accounting for 20% to 30% of all soft tissue sarcomas (9–12,42). This percentage increases to 40% to 45% if nonspecific spindle cell sarcomas are included in this group (1,9–12). The annual incidence in the Swedish population is 0.42 of 100,000 people (126,128). The peak incidence is in the fifth decade with a range of 10 to 90 years of age (most patients are between 50 and 70 years of age) (9–12). Men account for 70% of lesions (42). Sites of involvement with soft tissue MFH vary widely; however, the

vast majority occur in the extremities (70% to 75%) (129). The lower extremity accounts for 50% of all cases (particularly the thigh), whereas the upper extremity is involved in 25% of cases (130,131). Additional locations include retroperitoneum (15%), head/neck (5%), and other unusual sites (5% to 10%) within the thorax, abdomen, and pelvis (132–140). MFH involves the subcutaneous tissue in 5% to 10% of cases (129). Clinically, patients present with an enlarging, painless, soft tissue mass (average size: 5 to 10 cm). Retroperitoneal lesions are even larger at detection; subcutaneous lesions are usually much smaller. Hypoglycemia related to production by the tumor of an insulinlike substance is rarely reported in association with MFH (42). These lesions are deep intramuscular masses in approximately 70% of cases (129). Soft tissue MFH may also be radiation induced (42). MFH is the most common postradiation sarcoma, representing more than 67% of 52 cases reported by Laskin et al. (45), with extraskeletal osteosarcoma representing 13% and fibrosarcoma 11% (45). The latent period between radiation and tumor development is typically long (10 to 12 years) (45). In addition, MFH may be associated with previous shrapnel injury. It may occur adjacent to metallic fixation devices, including total joint replacements, and in patients exposed to phenoxyl acids (141) (Fig. 7.18). MFH was also induced in laboratory animals in association with the SV40 virus and with exposure to tea extract (42,142–145).

Storiform/Pleomorphic Malignant Fibrous Histiocytoma (Undifferentiated High-Grade Pleomorphic Sarcoma)

The storiform/pleomorphic type of MFH is the most frequent histologic type, accounting for between 50% and 60% of lesions (42). Other former terms for this lesion include *fibroxanthosarcoma* and *malignant fibrous xanthoma*. At gross pathologic examination, lesions are multilobulated and often circumscribed, although microscopically infiltrative. The spindle cells classically are arranged in a cartwheel (storiform) pattern around vessels, although the appearance is highly variable. Large numbers of giant cells, hemorrhage, and necrosis are common. This subtype of MFH is most frequent in the extremities, followed by the retroperitoneum (9–12). It is also the most common subtype associated with prior radiation.

Myxoid Malignant Fibrous Histiocytoma (Myxofibrosarcoma)

The second most common histologic type of MFH, myxoid MFH, is sometimes referred to as *myxofibrosarcoma*. Gross pathologic appearance of these lesions reveals a largely gelatinous, lobulated mass. The nonmyxoid areas are typically indistinguishable from the storiform/pleomorphic type of MFH. Myxoid tissue contains a prominent amount of mucoid material rich in extracellular mucopolysaccharide and hyaluronic acid. Although criteria of the extent of

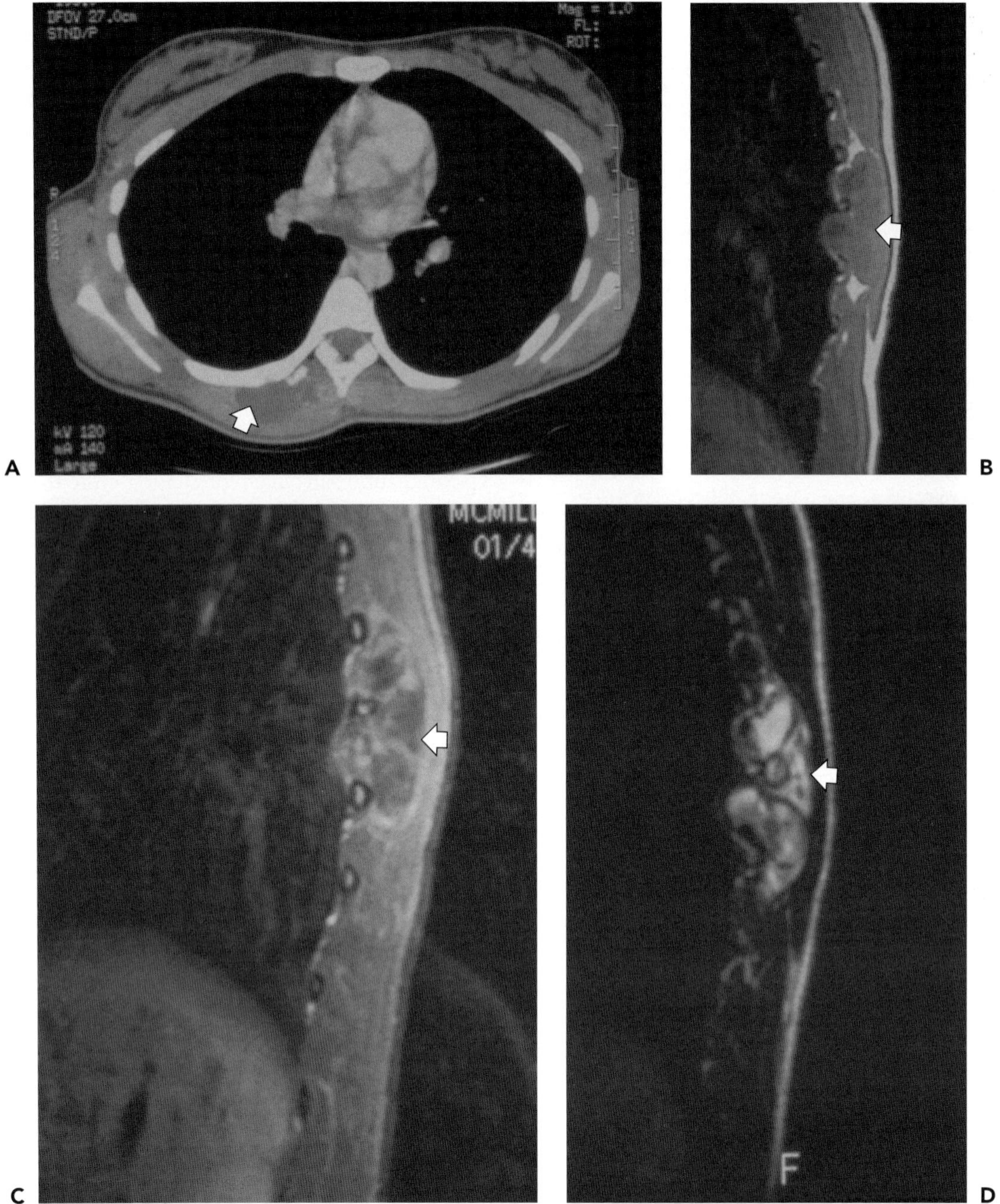

Figure 7.17   Low-grade fibromyxoid sarcoma in the paraspinal region of a girl 17 years of age. **A:** CT shows a low attenuation soft tissue mass in the thoracic paraspinal musculature (*arrow*). **B–D:** Sagittal T1-weighted (TR/TE; 600/11) **(B)** before and (TR/TE; 500/11) **(C)** after intravenous contrast, and T2-weighted (TR/TE; 3000/136) **(D)** MR images reveal the paraspinal mass (*arrow*) with intermediate signal intensity on the short TR image, predominantly peripheral enhancement, and heterogeneous high signal intensity on the long TR image.

myxoid tissue required for the diagnosis varies (10% to 50%), we believe more than 50% of the tumor must have this appearance to be characterized as this type of MFH. Overall, 25% of MFHs are of the myxoid variety (42). Myxoid MFH also involves the extremities, most frequently followed by the retroperitoneum. This subtype of MFH is the most frequent to involve the subcutaneous tissue (in some series approximately 70% of cases).

Giant Cell Malignant Fibrous Histiocytoma (Undifferentiated Pleomorphic Sarcoma with Giant Cells)

The giant cell type of MFH accounts for 5% to 10% of these lesions (9–12). This lesion is also referred to as *malignant giant cell tumor of soft parts, malignant osteoclastoma,* and *giant cell sarcoma* (121,146). The WHO distinguishes giant cell tumor of soft parts and giant cell type of

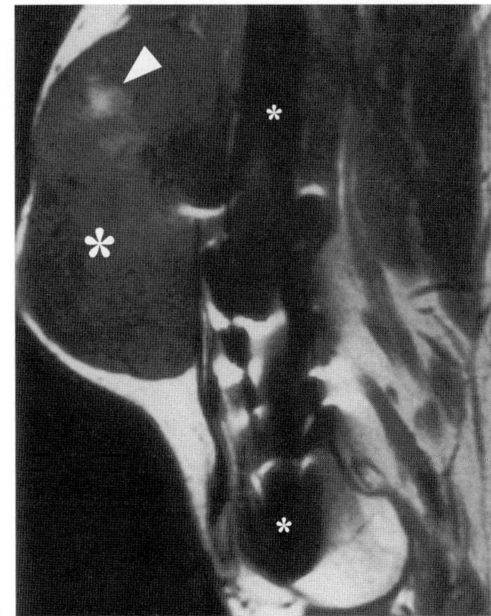
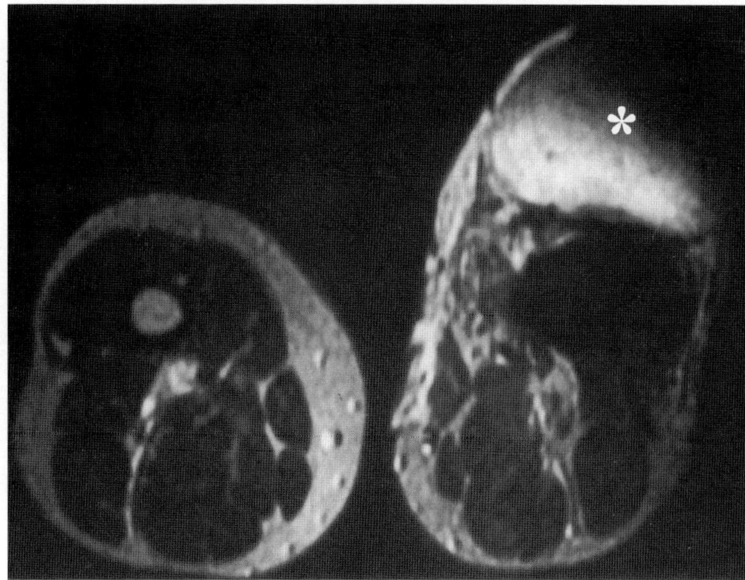

Figure 7.18   Malignant fibrous histiocytoma induced by long-standing metallic fixation device in a man 38 years of age. The fixation plate was placed 15 years previously, and an enlarging soft tissue mass is now present. **A:** Sagittal T1-weighted (TR/TE; 800/20) spin-echo MR image shows a large anterior mass (*large asterisk*) and its intimate relationship to the signal void of the fixation device (*small asterisks*). Focal areas of hemorrhage show high signal intensity (*arrowhead*). **B:** Axial T2-weighted (TR/TE; 2000/80) MR image at the inferior extent of the mass reveals moderate increased signal intensity within the mass (*asterisk*).

MFH (undifferentiated pleomorphic sarcoma with giant cells) as separate neoplasms within a spectrum of giant cell–rich lesions (9). The giant cell tumor of soft parts is a low-grade lesion with limited metastatic potential, whereas giant cell MFH is reserved for high-grade lesions (147,148) (Fig. 7.19). Gross pathologic appearance of giant cell MFH is identical to that of pleomorphic lesions. Histologically, there are prominent osteoclastlike giant cells and frequent areas of necrosis, hemorrhage, and focal osteoid (50% of cases) formation (9–12). These lesions occur in the extremities almost exclusively, and although usually intramuscular, subcutaneous location can also be seen. Giant cell tumor of soft parts is subcutaneous in 60% and may affect the trunk (20%) and head and neck (7% of cases).

Inflammatory Malignant Fibrous Histiocytoma (Undifferentiated Pleomorphic Sarcoma with Prominent Inflammation)

The inflammatory MFH is the rarest type, accounting for less than 5% of these malignancies (9–12,42). Additional terms for this lesion include *xanthosarcoma, malignant xanthogranuloma,* and *retroperitoneal xanthogranuloma.* At gross pathologic evaluation, these large lobulated lesions are often yellow in color because of the xanthomatous elements. Histologically, inflammatory (acute and chronic) and foam (xanthoma) cells are prominent features. Typical storiform/pleomorphic areas are often inconspicuous if present. Areas of necrosis and hemorrhage are unusual. Clinically, this type of MFH may present with fever, leukocytosis, neu-

trophilia, and eosinophilia, simulating infection that may be related to cytokine production by the tumor (9–12). Inflammatory MFH is most common in the retroperitoneum, followed by the extremities (9–12) (Fig. 7.20).

Imaging of Fibrosarcoma and MFH

> ### KEY CONCEPTS
>
> - Cross-sectional imaging features of adult fibrosarcoma, low-grade fibromyxoid sarcoma, sclerosing epithelioid fibrosarcoma, and MFH are indistinguishable.
> - Lesions typically present as a solid, large, intramuscular mass with nonspecific intrinsic characteristics on ultrasound, CT, or MR imaging.
> - MR imaging appearance depends on variable amount of collagen, myxoid tissue, necrosis, and hemorrhage, and may be predominantly high (most common) or low signal intensity on T2-weighted MR images.
> - Margin often is well-defined because of pseudocapsule.
> - One must beware of a history of a spontaneous hematoma and suspect bleeding tumor, and look for nodular, solid or enhancing peripheral areas of tumor.
> - High water content of myxoid lesions (particularly myxoid MFH or low-grade fibromyxoid sarcoma) can often be identified on cross-sectional imaging.
> - At presentation, retroperitoneal tumors are often larger than extremity lesions, whereas subcutaneous tumors are smaller.

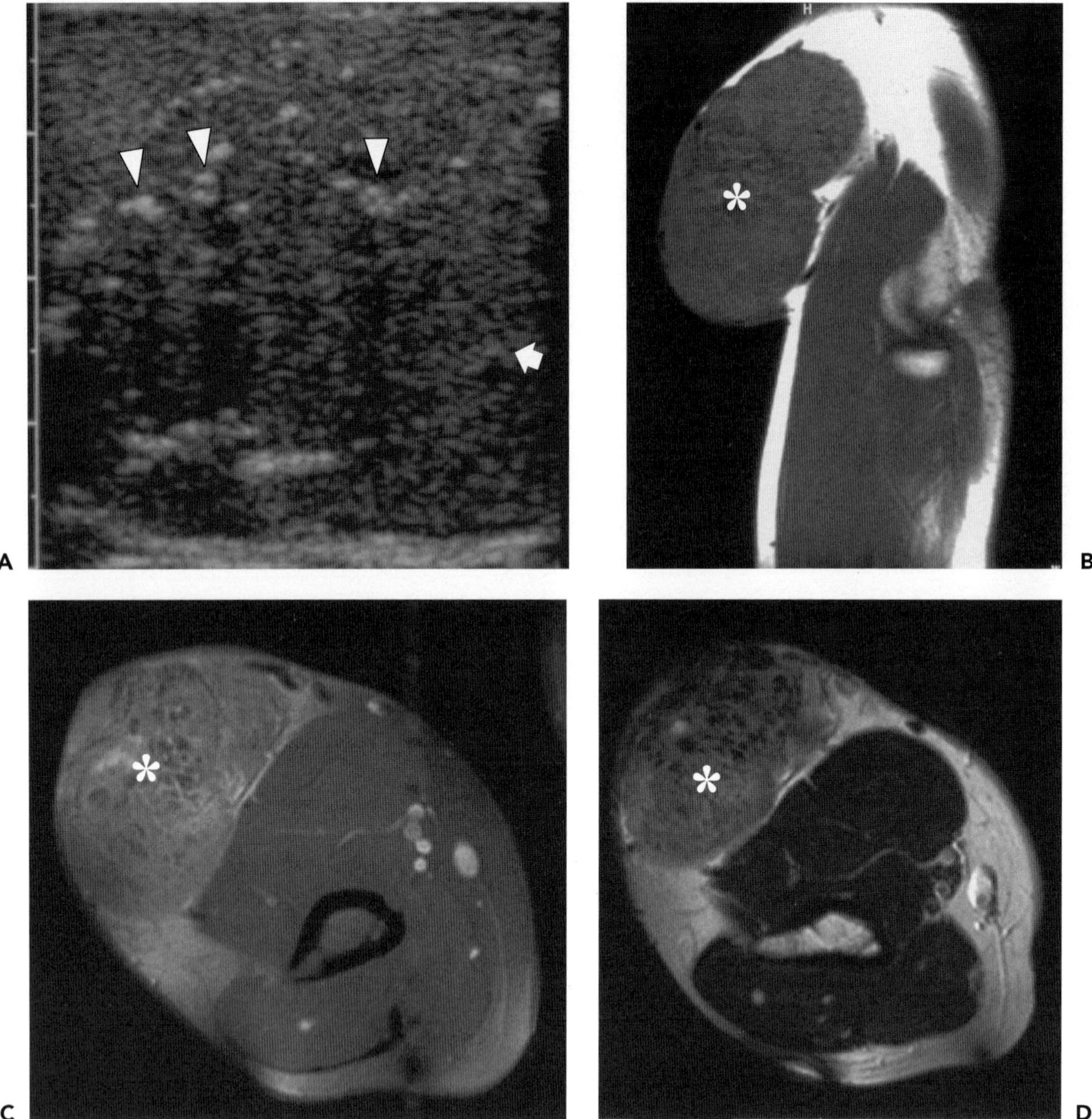

Figure 7.19 Giant cell tumor of soft parts in a man 28 years of age involving the subcutaneous tissues about the elbow. **A:** Short axis sonogram shows a heterogeneous soft tissue mass (*arrow*) with areas of calcification (*arrowheads*; also seen on radiographs; not shown) causing posterior acoustic shadowing (*arrowheads*). **B,C:** Sagittal T1-weighted (TR/TE; 430/16) **(B)** and axial postcontrast T1-weighted (TR/TE; 656/12) **(C)** MR images reveal the subcutaneous, heterogeneous, soft tissue mass (*asterisk*) with intermediate signal intensity and mild enhancement. **D:** Axial T2-weighted MR image demonstrates heterogeneous, but predominantly low signal intensity soft tissue mass (*asterisk*).

As stated previously, imaging characteristics of adult fibrosarcoma (including variations of this lesion, such as low-grade fibromyxoid sarcoma and sclerosing epithelioid sarcoma) and MFH are indistinguishable. We are unaware of any radiologic literature that suggests the ability to distinguish these lesions by imaging characteristics; therefore, we discuss the imaging features together.

Radiographs of soft tissue MFH and adult fibrosarcoma are often nonspecific, only revealing a soft tissue mass (129,149,150). Small lesions and retroperitoneal tumors are typically not identified by radiography. Mineralization (calcification or ossification) can be detected in 5% to 20% of cases of MFH and is frequently seen as punctate or curvilinear, nonspecific densities in the periphery of the mass (151,152) (Fig. 7.21). An appearance similar to that of heterotopic bone formation (myositis ossificans) occasionally can be seen with a zonal pattern of a cortical bone rim and trabecular bone centrally. MFH or fibrosarcoma in the deep intramuscular soft tissue often is adjacent to long bone diaphysis. Extrinsic erosion or actual invasion is not unusual in MFH, and detection of this finding on radiographs is highly suggestive (129) (Fig. 7.22). Other common soft tissue sarcomas, such as liposarcoma, do not demonstrate

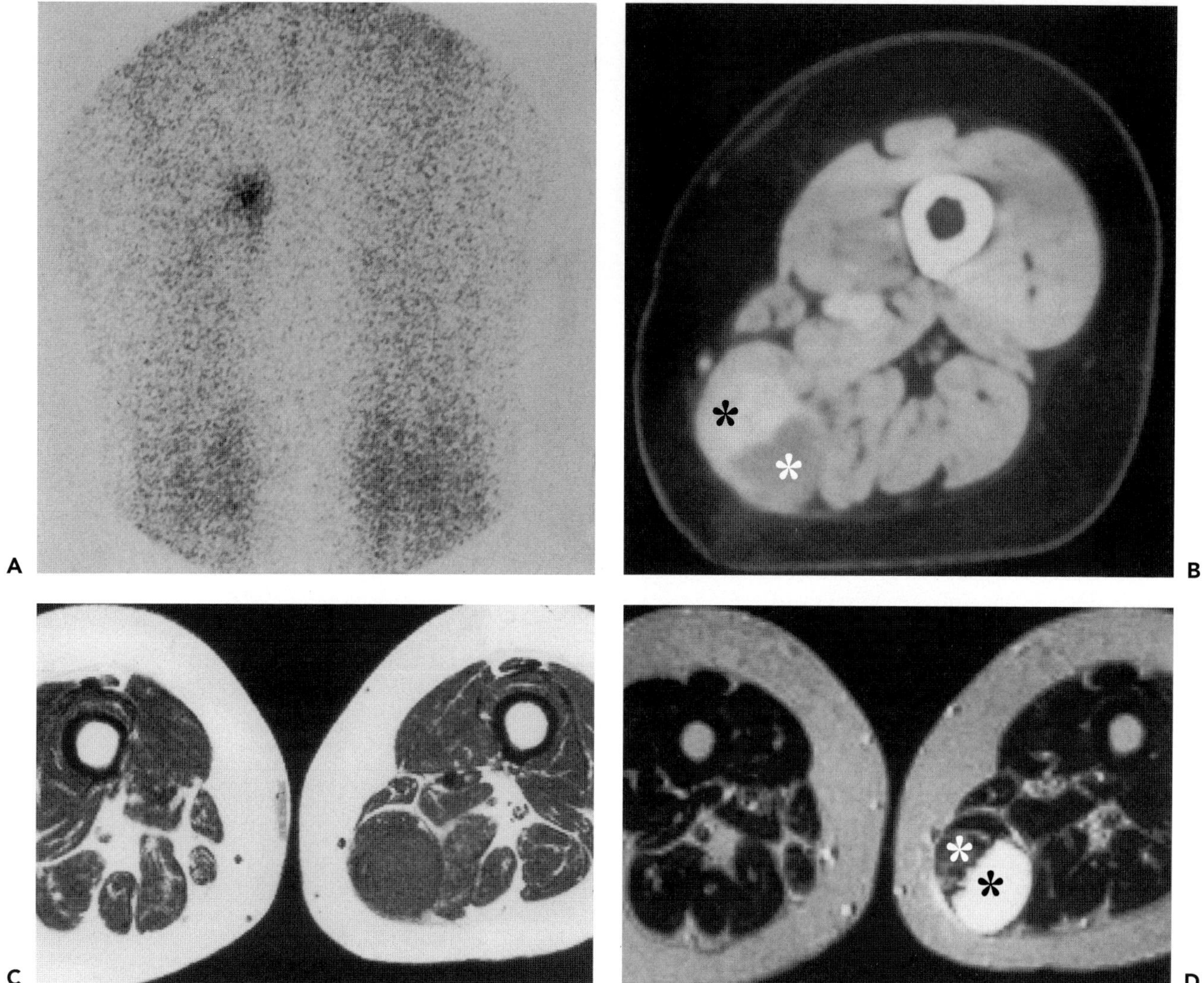

Figure 7.20 Inflammatory malignant fibrous histiocytoma medially in the thigh of a woman 49 years of age. **A:** Gallium scan shows increased uptake of radionuclide in the small mass. **B:** Axial CT following contrast administration reveals both enhancing solid (*black asterisk*) and cystic (*white asterisk*) components. **C,D:** Axial T1-weighted (TR/TE; 500/17) **(C)** and T2-weighted (TR/TE; 2100/90) **(D)** spin-echo MR images also show small mass with solid (*white asterisk*) and cystic (*black asterisk*) components. The solid component has a signal intensity similar to that of muscle on all pulse sequences.

this propensity for cortical involvement. Synovial sarcoma is the other soft tissue sarcoma that has a significant incidence of invading underlying bone, although the involvement of younger patients and location near a joint usually allows distinction from MFH. Cortical involvement also affects surgical management in these patients, often requiring a subperiosteal dissection or more extensive resection of adjacent bone.

Soft tissue MFH and adult fibrosarcoma may be hypovascular or hypervascular at angiography, and findings are nonspecific (153) (Fig. 7.21). Hypervascular lesions show increased radionuclide uptake at bone scintigraphy on both dynamic and blood-pool images. Static images from bone scintigraphy may also reveal mild increased activity caused by calcification, bone invasion, and hypervascularity

(151,152) (Fig. 7.21). Gallium-67 scans may similarly show increased activity, particularly in inflammatory MFH (154) (Fig. 7.20). These high-grade sarcomas are also glucose-avid lesions on positron emission tomography (PET) images (155).

Sonography of MFH or adult fibrosarcoma reveals a large heterogeneous, deep-seated mass of intermediate-to-low echogenicity. Lesion margins are frequently relatively well-defined. Areas of calcification cause posterior shadowing (Fig. 7.19). In our experience, Doppler studies show increased lesion vascularity.

CT scans demonstrate MFH and adult fibrosarcoma as large, lobulated, soft tissue masses of similar attenuation to muscle (129,156) (Figs. 7.20 and 7.21). Areas of decreased attenuation frequently are apparent within the mass more

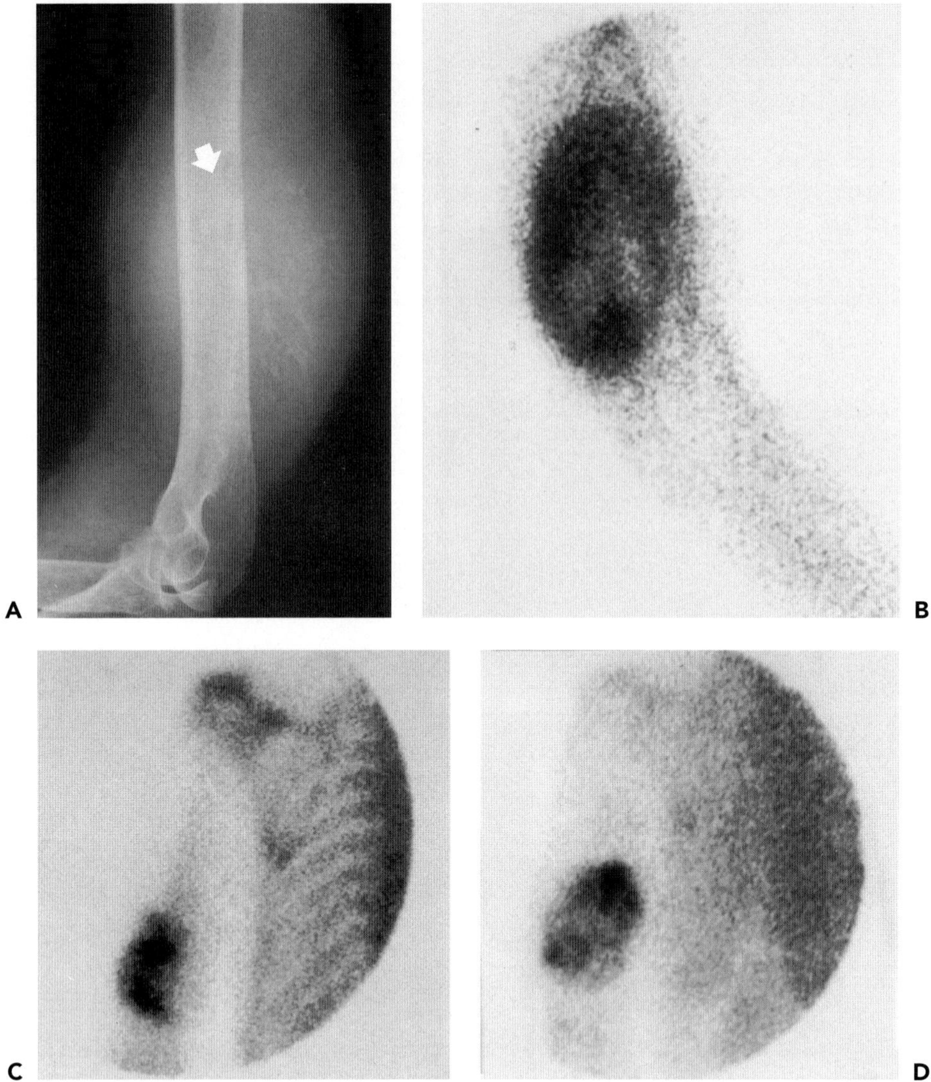

Figure 7.21 Intramuscular malignant fibrous histiocytoma of the upper extremity in a man 84 years of age. **A:** Radiograph shows a calcified mass posteriorly with evidence of osseous involvement (*arrow*). **B,C:** Blood-pool **(B)** and delayed static **(C)** images from technetium-99m bone scan show intense tracer accumulation. **D:** Gallium scan also shows intense uptake of radionuclide. (*continued*)

centrally, corresponding to myxoid regions, hemorrhage, or necrosis. Areas of calcification or cortical erosion are well evaluated by CT. Enhancement of solid portions of MFH is seen on CT following administration of intravenous contrast.

MR imaging of MFH and adult fibrosarcoma typically reveals an intramuscular mass with intermediate intensity on T1-weighting and intermediate-to-high signal intensity (greater than that of fat) on T2 weighting (Figs. 7.15, 7.16, 7.18, 7.20–7.24). MR images often show heterogeneous signal intensity on all pulse sequences, reflecting the variable pattern seen histologically (129,156–159). These variations include regions with prominent fibrous tissue (high collagen content; low signal intensity); calcification (low signal foci); hemorrhage

(high signal on all pulse sequences; fluid levels), necrosis (low signal on T1-weighted and high signal on T2-weighted MR images); and areas of tumor with lower collagen content (intermediate on T1-weighted MR image; high signal on T2-weighted MR image) (Figs. 7.15, 7.16, 7.18, 7.20–7.24). Invasion of the underlying cortical bone and medullary canal may also be detected on MR imaging (Fig. 7.22). The intermixture of these components is particularly reflected in the degree of heterogeneity and variable predominant signal intensity on long TR images, regardless of the specific histologic variation of diagnosis (including adult fibrosarcoma, low-grade fibromyxoid sarcoma, sclerosing epithelioid fibrosarcoma, and MFH). Small areas of calcification are better evaluated by CT or radiographs. Soft tissue MFH

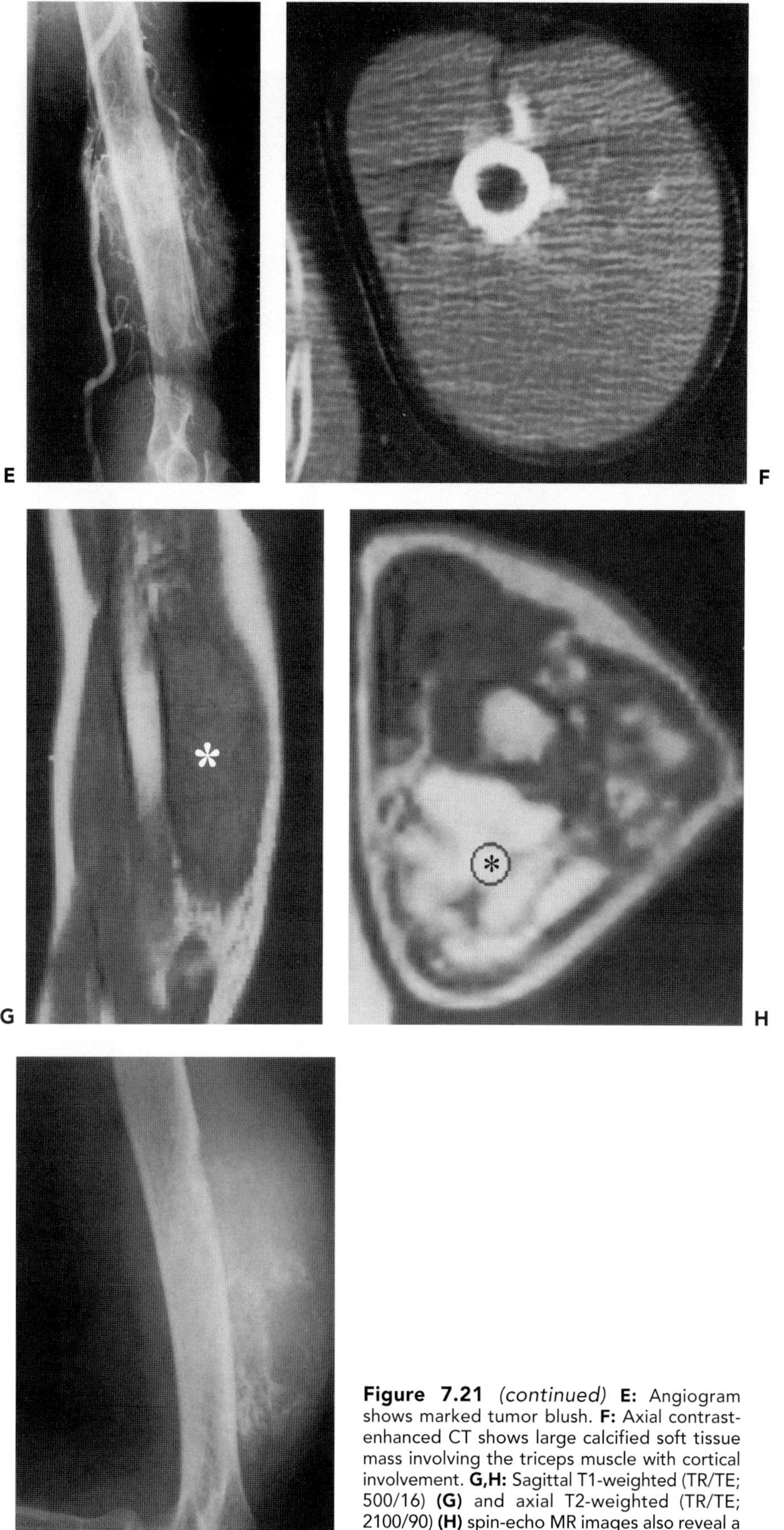

Figure 7.21 *(continued)* **E:** Angiogram shows marked tumor blush. **F:** Axial contrast-enhanced CT shows large calcified soft tissue mass involving the triceps muscle with cortical involvement. **G,H:** Sagittal T1-weighted (TR/TE; 500/16) **(G)** and axial T2-weighted (TR/TE; 2100/90) **(H)** spin-echo MR images also reveal a large mass (*asterisk* in **G**) extensively infiltrating the triceps muscle. **I:** Follow-up radiograph shows progressive mineralization of the mass following chemotherapy and radiation therapy.

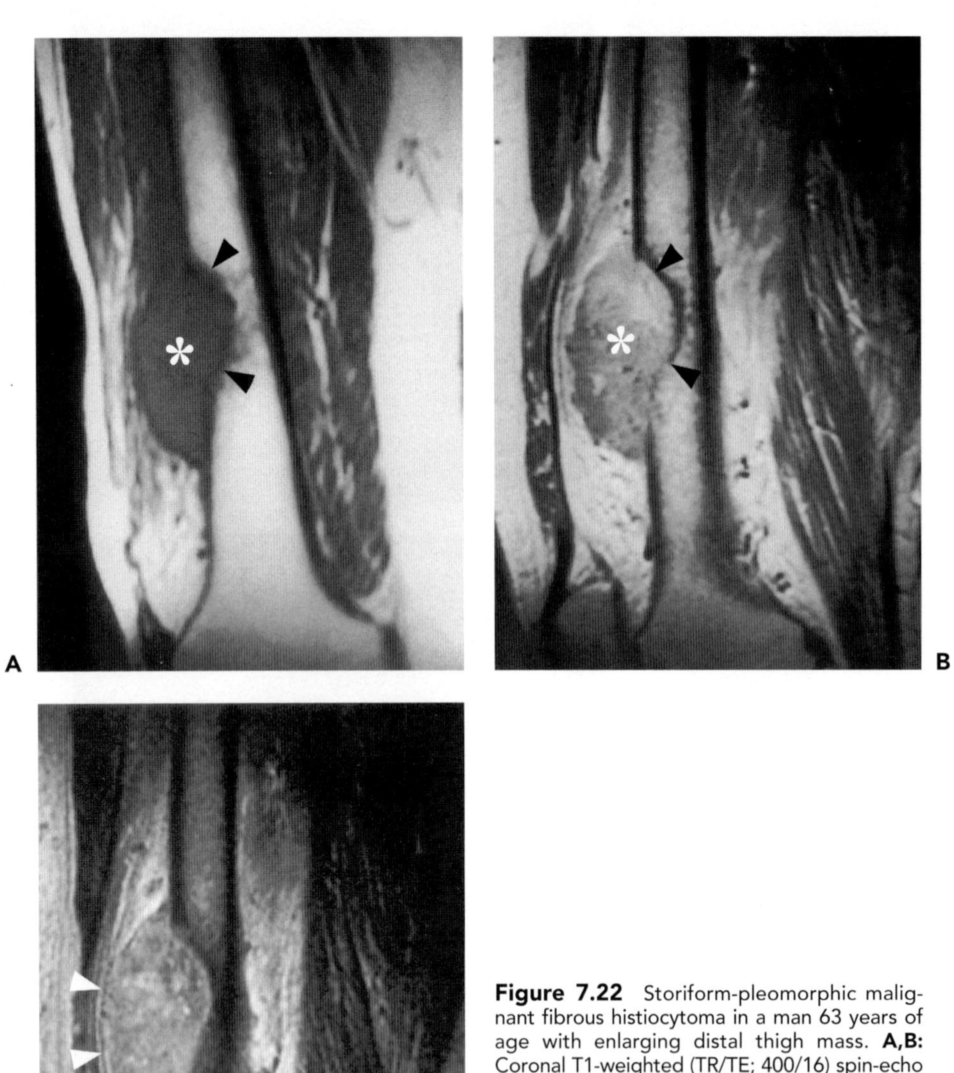

Figure 7.22 Storiform-pleomorphic malignant fibrous histiocytoma in a man 63 years of age with enlarging distal thigh mass. **A,B:** Coronal T1-weighted (TR/TE; 400/16) spin-echo MR image before **(A)** and sagittal image after **(B)** intravenous gadolinium show an intermediate signal intensity, deep, intramuscular thigh mass (*asterisk*) with bone invasion (*arrowheads*). Enhancement is seen on postcontrast images. **C:** Sagittal T2-weighted (TR/TE; 2000/80) spin-echo MR image reveals predominantly low-to-intermediate intensity within the mass, presumably corresponding to high collagen content. Low-intensity periphery (*arrowheads*) represents pseudocapsule.

and adult fibrosarcoma are often large and lobulated, and tumor margins on MR imaging are usually relatively well-defined. A thin low-intensity rim is common, reflecting the pseudocapsule around focal areas of the mass or the majority of the lesion (129) (Figs. 7.22 and 7.23). Occasionally, soft tissue MFH or fibrosarcoma remains relatively low-to-intermediate signal intensity, similar to that of muscle, on T2-weighted MR images (Fig. 7.22). Low signal intensity on T2-weighting was reported in a case of sclerosing epithelioid fibrosarcoma by Christensen et al. (105). This MR appearance is presumably caused by a higher collagen content. MFH and fibrosarcoma (solid components) typically show enhance-ment after the administration of intravenous gadolinium (Figs. 7.22 and 7.23).

The high water content of myxoid MFH and adult fibrosarcoma (with significant myxoid elements or low-grade fibromyxoid sarcoma) are reflected in the imaging appearance (Figs. 7.25–7.27). Sonography, CT, and MR imaging frequently reveal predominantly low echogenicity, low attenuation, or low signal intensity areas on T1-weighted MR, respectively (Figs. 7.25–7.27). Enhancement of the more cellular regions, which are often nodular and peripheral, is frequently apparent after the administration of intravenous contrast material on either CT or MR imaging (129,160) (Fig. 7.25). In our

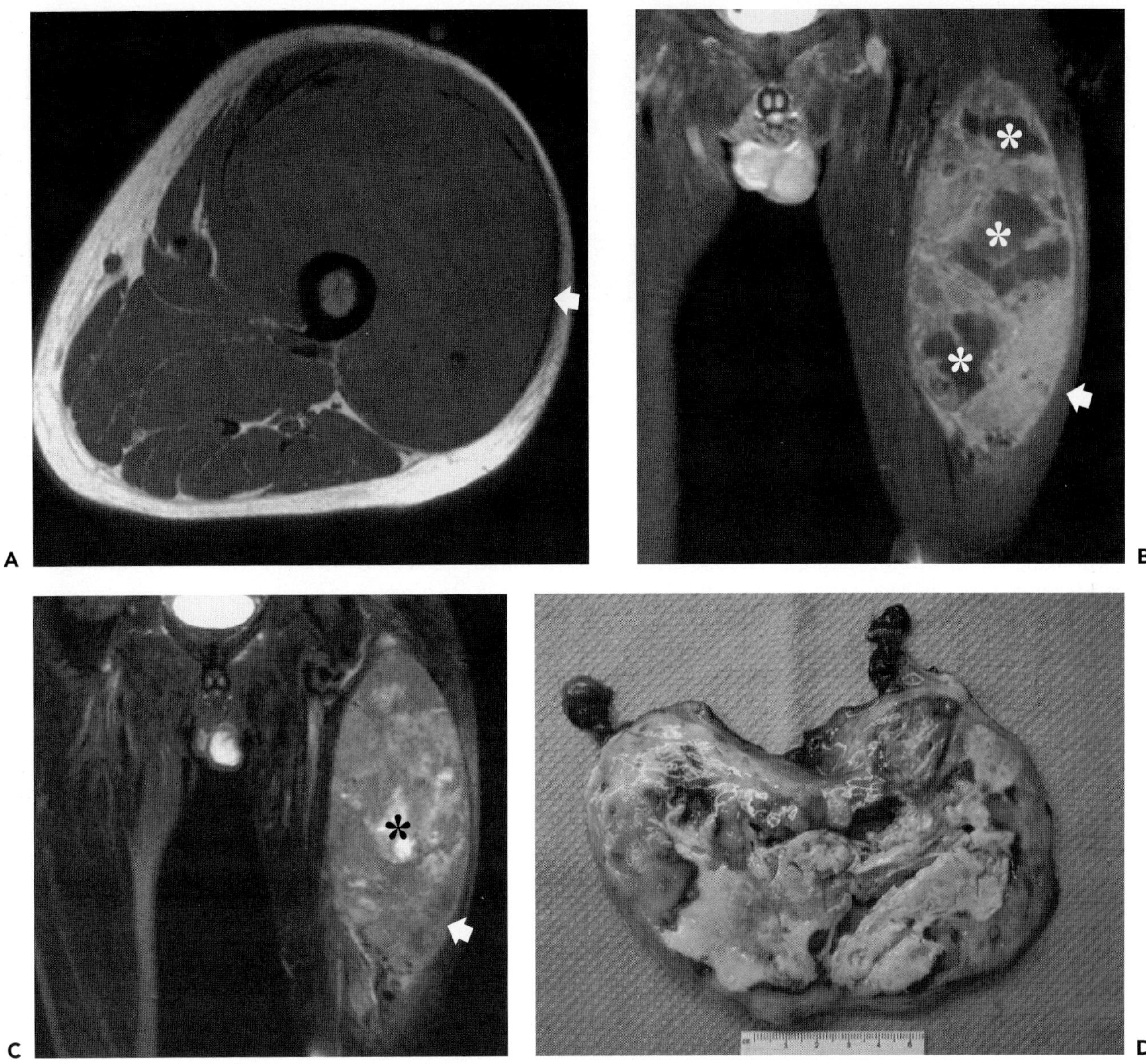

Figure 7.23 Storiform-pleomorphic malignant fibrous histiocytoma in a man 49 years of age with a large thigh mass. **A,B:** Axial T1-weighted (TR/TE; 500/20) **(A)** and coronal T1-weighted (TR/TE; 400/15) **(B)** post-enhanced fat-suppression MR images reveal a large, intramuscular soft tissue mass (*arrow*) that shows intermediate signal intensity and heterogeneous contrast enhancement. Note nonenhancing central areas of necrosis (*asterisks* in **B**). **C:** Coronal fat-suppressed T2-weighted (TR/TE; 4000/50) MR image reveals heterogeneous, predominantly intermediate signal intensity mass (*arrow*) with foci of high signal centrally corresponding to central necrosis (*asterisk*) also seen on the photograph of the sectioned gross specimen **(D)**. Defined margin of the mass is caused by the pseudocapsule.

experience, the rim of solid tissue about the more central high water component is not as thick in myxoid MFH as compared to areas of hemorrhage or necrosis. Long TR MR images show very high signal intensity throughout myxoid MFH, low-grade fibromyxoid sarcomas, or fibrosarcoma with prominent myxoid components (Figs. 7.25 and 7.27). A more nonspecific imaging appearance may also occasionally be seen with myxoid MFH. In these cases the myxoid tissue is more vascular and shows a higher degree of

cellularity (Fig. 7.26). MR imaging or CT in these cases demonstrates a more homogeneous soft tissue mass with diffuse contrast enhancement. Other soft tissue neoplasms with a myxoid appearance include liposarcoma, neurogenic tumor, myxoma, extraskeletal chondrosarcoma, and leiomyosarcoma (necrosis, simulating myxoid tissue) (160). Soft tissue chondrosarcoma and leiomyosarcoma are unusual soft tissue tumors. Myxoid neurogenic tumors usually have a unique morphologic appearance

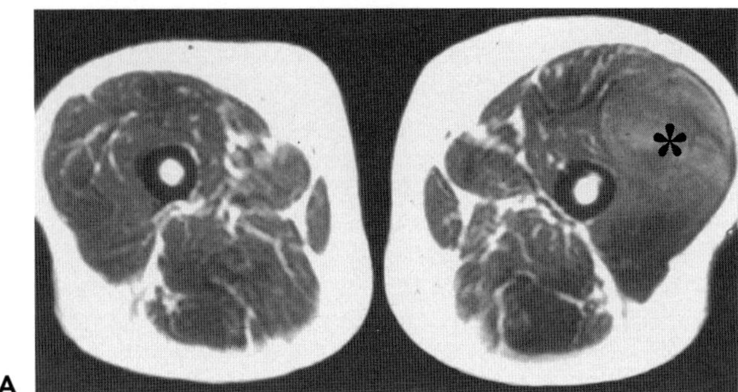 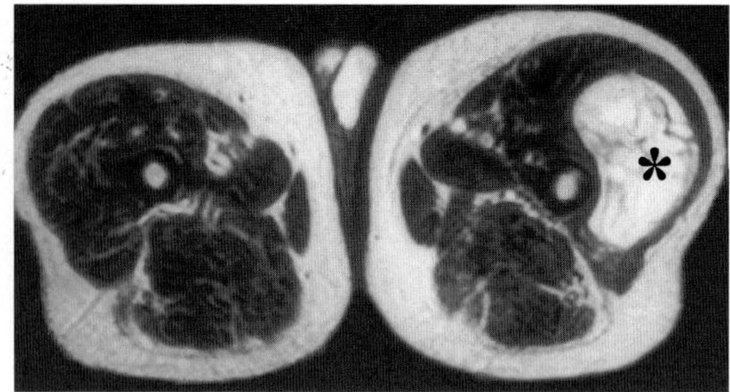

Figure 7.24 Storiform/pleomorphic malignant fibrous histiocytoma of the thigh in a man 65 years of age. **A,B:** Axial T1-weighted (TR/TE; 500/30) **(A)** and T2-weighted (TR/TE; 2000/90) **(B)** MR images show a soft tissue mass (*asterisk*). The mass has nonspecific intermediate signal intensity on T1-weighting and high signal intensity on T2-weighting. It is well-defined and intramuscular, replacing the normal vastus lateralis muscle architecture.

and are located along a neurovascular bundle with a fusiform shape, caused by the entering and exiting involved nerve. Myxoma generally demonstrates only mild rim and septal enhancement after intravenous contrast injection, as opposed to nodular enhancement in myxoid MFH. Myxoid liposarcoma (40% to 50% of all intermediate- and high-grade liposarcomas) is the most difficult lesion to distinguish from myxoid MFH (161). Close attenuation should be directed to the detection of any component of fat within the lesion in these cases. In at least 40% to 50% of cases of myxoid liposarcoma, areas of adipose tissue can be identified, although adipose tissue may represent a small (10% or less) component of the mass (162).

Hemorrhagic components are common in soft tissue MFH (less frequent in adult fibrosarcoma). These are usually recognized on CT as areas of increased attenuation acutely, and decreased attenuation in subacute and chronic hemorrhage. On MR imaging, hemorrhage will also show time dependent changes, however areas of subacute blood demonstrating high signal on both T1- and T2- weighted images are often seen. These hemorrhagic areas can be so extensive as to obscure the underlying neoplasm and simulate a hematoma (Figs. 7.28 and 7.29). This leads to a crucial tenet of imaging soft tissue masses: "Any patient with an apparent spontaneous musculoskeletal hemorrhage should always be suspected of harboring a neoplasm," particularly MFH (129). Contrast-enhanced CT or MR images are often extremely helpful by identifying small tumor nodules as the cause of the hemorrhage (Fig. 7.29). These nodular foci (usually peripheral) reveal significant enhancement and *should not be seen in a hematoma*. These are also foci that harbor diagnostic tissue pathologically; therefore, biopsy should be directed at these regions (Figs. 7.28 and 7.29). Fluid levels may be seen on ultrasonography, CT, or MR imaging after hemorrhage, representing sedimentation of blood products (129,163) (Fig. 7.29). This radiologic finding is certainly nonspecific and can be

seen in many soft tissue neoplasms, benign or malignant, including MFH and fibrosarcoma (163). In addition, edema is often seen surrounding a hematoma from irritation of the tissue. In contradistinction, tumors bleed inside the pseudocapsule, not allowing the blood products to extend into the surrounding tissue; therefore, edema is not a prominent feature of a hemorrhagic neoplasm (Figs. 7.28 and 7.29).

In summary, imaging findings of a large, deep intramuscular mass of the extremities in an older patient (greater than 50 years of age), without other distinguishing features, should suggest the diagnosis of MFH or fibrosarcoma (including low-grade fibromyxoid sarcoma and sclerosing epithelioid fibrosarcoma). A diligent search for evidence of adipose tissue should be made because the second most frequent soft tissue sarcoma in this age group is liposarcoma. The myxoid variety of MFH or fibrosarcoma, and its variants with predominant myxoid components, can often be distinguished because of their diffuse high fluid content and nodular peripheral enhancement pattern after intravenous contrast administration.

In contrast to extremity MFH that is apparent as a palpable mass, retroperitoneal lesions usually present clinically with constitutional symptoms including fever, malaise, and weight loss. Retroperitoneal MFH, are generally larger at the time of identification because of the delay in diagnosis as compared to extremity lesions, with the majority greater than 10 cm in diameter (135,138) (Fig. 7.30). These lesions cause displacement of bowel, kidney, ureter, and bladder on intravenous urogram or barium enema. Sonography reveals a hypoechoic solid mass, although occasionally there is a more heterogenous appearance. Calcification, focal or diffuse, seen in approximately 10% of retroperitoneal MFH, is usually coarse in appearance (135). CT and MR imaging show a heterogeneous mass with areas of hemorrhage and/or necrosis (Fig. 7.30). Angiography may show a hypervascular or

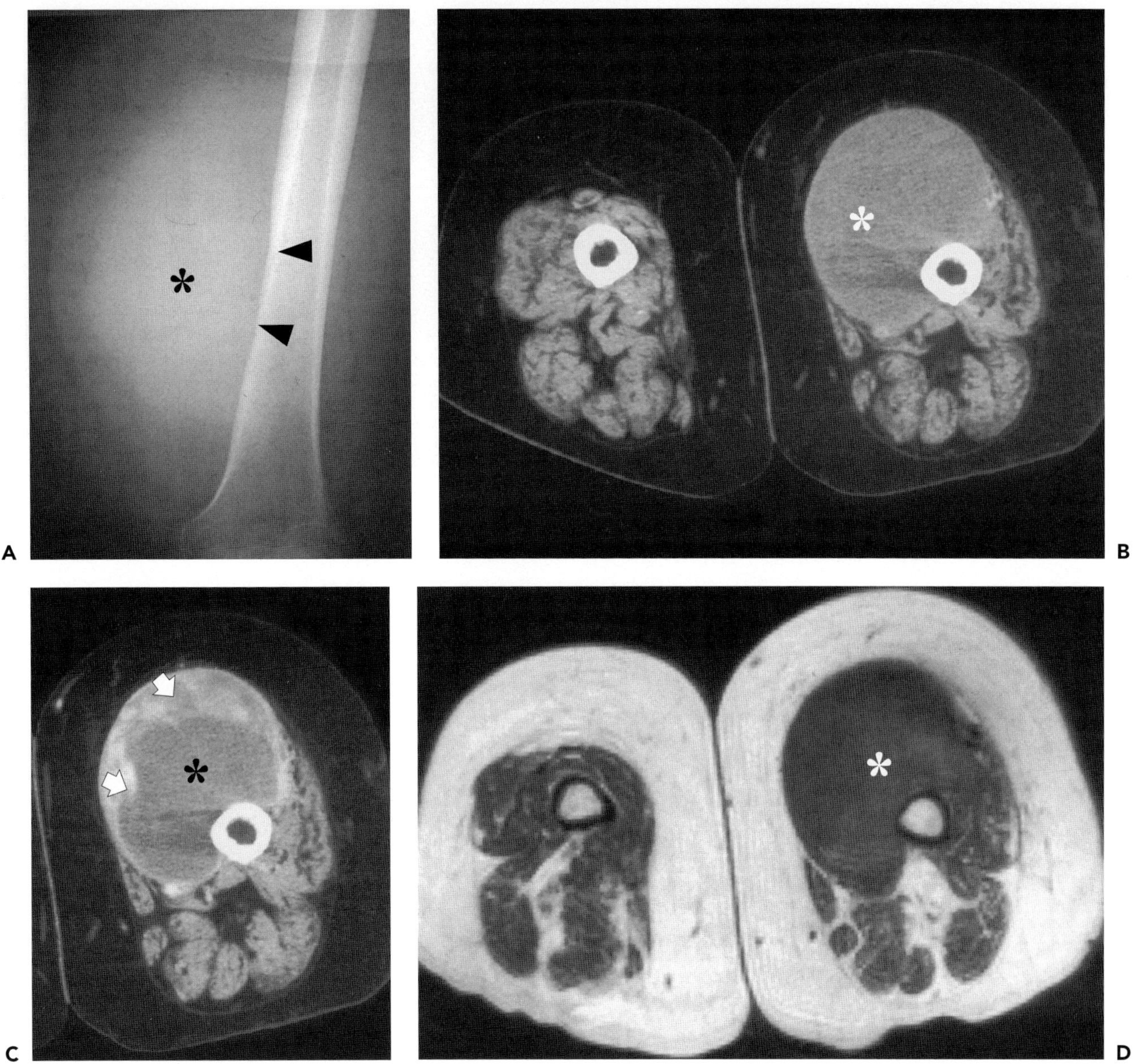

Figure 7.25   Myxoid malignant fibrous histiocytoma in a woman 65 years of age with a 3-month history of an enlarging thigh mass. **A:** Anteroposterior radiograph shows a large soft tissue mass (*asterisk*) and extrinsic erosion of the femur (*arrowheads*). **B,C:** Axial CT scan before **(B)** and after **(C)** intravenous contrast show a largely low-attenuation fluid mass (*asterisk*) with peripheral enhancing nodules representing solid tissue (*arrows*). **D:** Axial T1-weighted (TR/TE; 500/17) spin-echo MR image shows a similar appearance. Note heterogeneous appearance to the mass (*asterisk*) with lower peripheral signal intensity. (*continued*)

hypovascular lesion with vascular supply from lumbar, celiac, iliac, renal, renal capsular, and inferior adrenal arteries. Differential diagnosis primarily includes liposarcoma and leiomyosarcoma.

Subcutaneous MFH (5% to 10% of lesions) or fibrosarcoma reveals an intrinsically nonspecific soft tissue mass replacing the normal subcutaneous fat on sonography, CT, or MR imaging (Figs. 7.19 and 7.31). These patients frequently present earlier than those with deep-seated lesions. Subsequently, the neoplasms are smaller at initial clinical detection and have an overall better prognosis. The small initial lesion size frequently suggests a benign diagnosis to both radiologist and clinician, leading to inappropriate marginal excision and local recurrence. These lesions commonly invade the underlying muscle and may cause overlying skin ulceration.

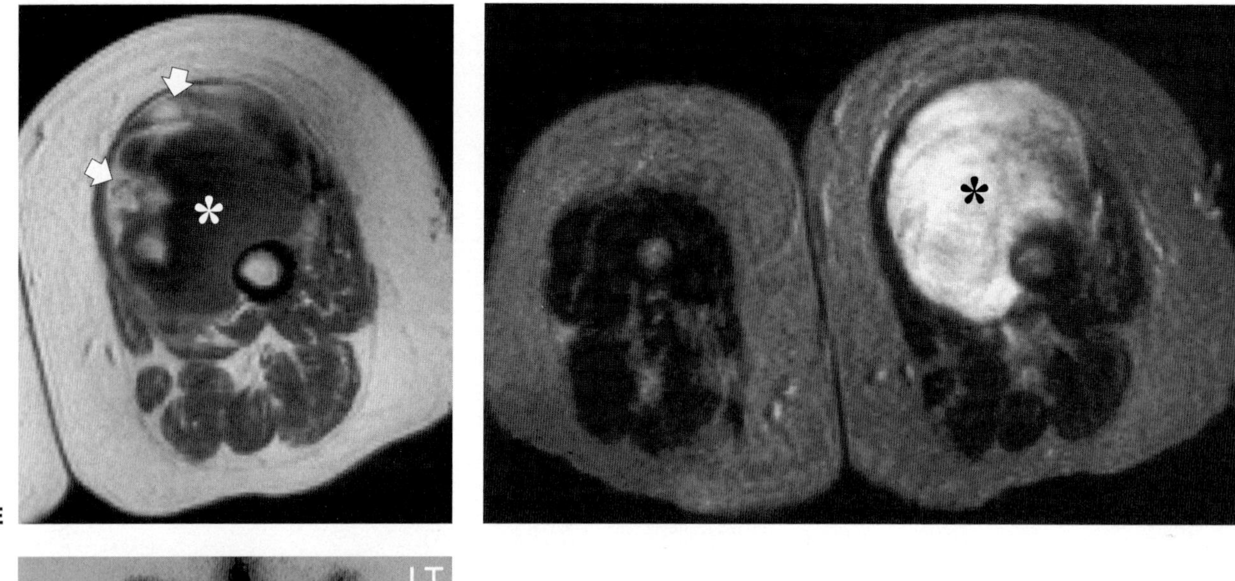

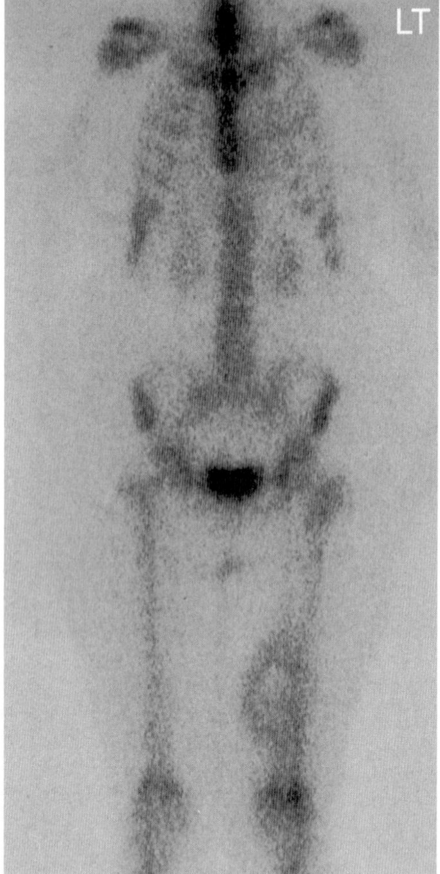

Figure 7.25 *(continued)*   **E:** Corresponding enhanced axial T1-weighted (TR/TE; 500/17) spin-echo MR image shows an appearance similar to **(C)**, with enhancing peripheral nodules *(arrows)* and non-enhancing center *(asterisk)*. **F:** Axial T2-weighted (TR/TE; 2100/90) spin-echo MR image shows the majority of the mass is high intensity because of the high water content. **G:** Delayed image from technetium-99m bone scan reflects vascularity of peripheral portion of the tumor by showing uptake of radionuclide in this region.

Treatment, Follow-up, and Prognosis

Soft tissue MFHs are usually treated with preoperative chemotherapy for 3 to 4 months prior to surgical resection. The mass may remain similar in size, shrink, or enlarge during preoperative treatment (Fig. 7.32). Enlargement of tumor may be caused by true tumor growth; however, this appearance can also result from neoplasm necrosis or hemorrhage, in response to chemotherapy (159) (Fig. 7.32). Areas of mineralization may increase in extent during preoperative therapy (Fig. 7.21). Successful treatment of MFH is reported with selective transcatheter intra-arterial chemotherapy (164,165). This method allows a marked increase in the delivered dose of chemotherapy to the tumor without concomitant systemic effects. Tumor response is seen angiographically as well as with Doppler sonography and contrast-enhanced MR imaging as reduced neovascularity and tumor stain. Loss of early draining veins may also be seen on angiography. Radiation therapy is also frequently used in the treatment of MFH both before and after surgery (166).

The surgical treatment of MFH is usually a wide en bloc resection. Deep intramuscular masses often require a composite reconstruction, including muscle flap and skin graft. In addition, the propensity of MFH to involve adjacent bone requires a more aggressive surgical resection to obtain a margin free of tumor. This frequently leads to a subperiosteal dissection or even more extensive resection of bone, requiring a limb-salvage procedure. Thus, dramatic changes are seen postoperatively, which empha-

sizes the need for a baseline imaging study, preferably MR imaging. This first imaging study after surgery should be obtained within 3 to 6 months, well before local tumor recurrence typically occurs. This study is vital to allow comparison to future images for determination of which changes are postsurgical or related to radiation therapy versus tumor recurrence (167–170) (Fig. 7.33).

The overall prognosis for soft tissue MFH is unfavorable. Important features related to prognosis primarily include tumor depth and size, histologic subtype, grade, and type of initial surgical treatment. Larger and deeper soft tissue MFHs generally have a worse prognosis. MFH involving the subcutaneous tissue alone or with additional fascial extension, metastasize in only 10% and 27% of cases, respectively (115). In contradistinction, deep intramuscular MFHs metastasize in 43% of cases (41,42). Salo et al. correlated the size, depth, and histologic grade of extremity MFH to prognosis, with 5-/10-year survival rates ranging from 100%/100% (low-grade lesions <5 cm), 83%/79% (low-grade lesions >5 cm), 59%/48% (deep high-grade lesions 5–10 cm), and 34%/31% (deep high-grade lesions >10 cm) (127). The prognosis of retroperitoneal MFH is worse than that of peripheral lesions, with a dismal 5-year survival of 15% to 20% (138). The histologic subtype of MFH also has an effect on prognosis, with the local recurrence as follows: storiform/pleomorphic, 50% to 60%; myxoid, 50% to 70%; and both giant cell and inflammatory approximately 50% to 70% (42,125,128,171,172). The 5-year survival of patients with storiform/pleomorphic MFH is 50% to 70%, as compared to myxoid MFH, with a 5-year survival of 60% to 70% (128,171, 172). However, myxoid lesions are typically lower grade and demonstrate a generally wider spectrum in their degree of anaplasia. In the study

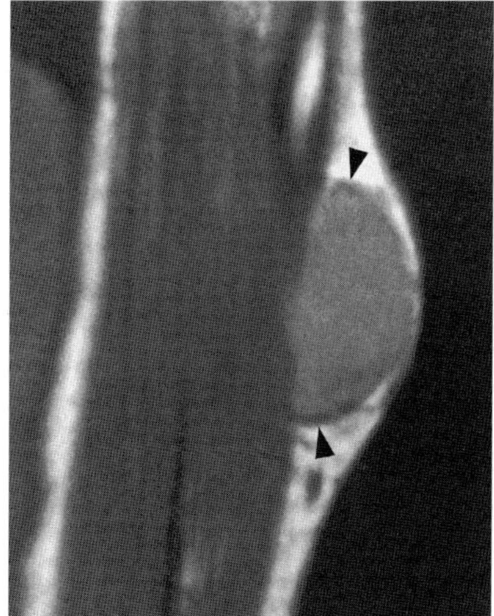
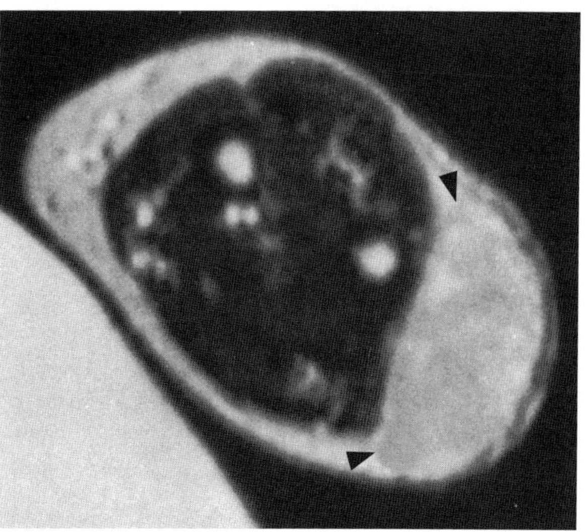

Figure 7.26 Myxoid malignant fibrous histiocytoma of the forearm in a woman 81 years of age with a rapidly enlarging mass. **A,B:** Coronal T1-weighted **(A)** and axial T2-weighted **(B)** spin-echo MR images show a nonspecific soft tissue mass (*arrowheads*) with intermediate signal intensity. This suggests that the myxoid tissue has a higher degree of cellularity than is often present.

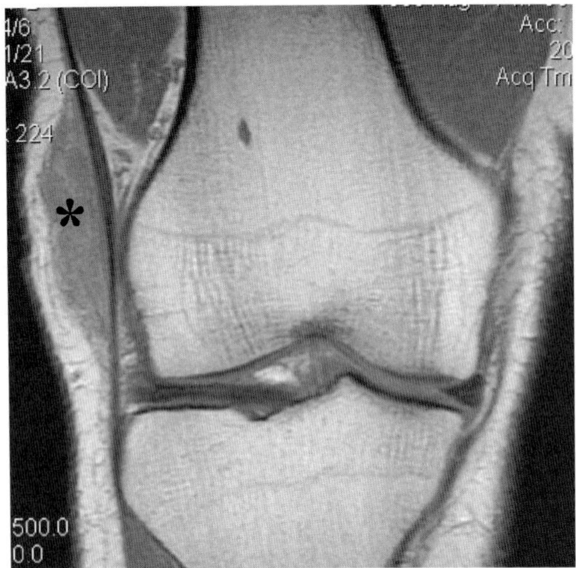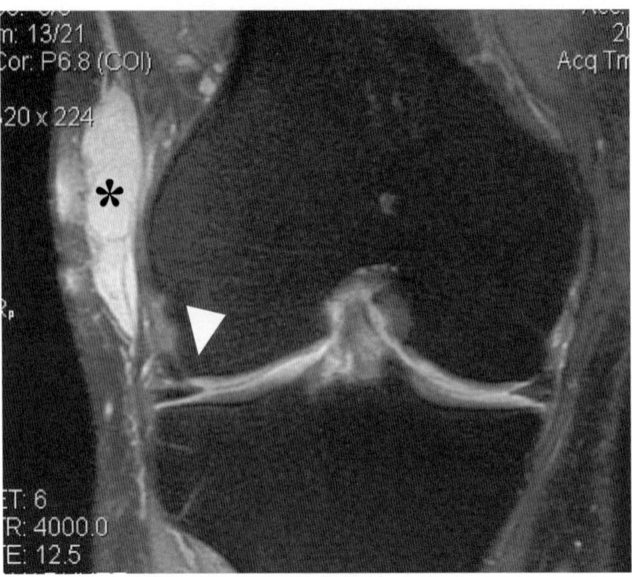

Figure 7.27 Myxoid malignant fibrous histiocytoma of the subcutaneous tissues about the knee, simulating a meniscal cyst because of the high water content. **A,B:** Coronal proton density (TR/TE; 2500/10) **(A)** and fat-suppressed fluid-sensitive proton density (TR/TE; 4000/12) **(B)** MR images reveal a soft tissue mass (*asterisk*) in the subcutaneous tissue about the knee, abutting the iliotibial band, with very high signal intensity on the long TR image. Lateral meniscal tear is also present (*arrowhead*) but does not communicate with the mass.

by Merck et al. of myxoid MFH, no grade I lesions metastasized (173). Giant cell tumor of soft parts, reflecting its lower grade compared to giant cell MFH, also shows a low rate of local recurrence (12%) and only rarely metastasizes. Local recurrence also depends on the type of surgery performed. Local excision invariably (100%) results in recurrence (173), as opposed to wide excision or amputation, which has a 51% local recurrence rate (157). The relatively high local recurrence rate is related to microscopic extension of these tumors beyond the pseudocapsule. Overall 5-year survival for MFH ranges from 36% to 50% (42,125,127, 128,171,172).

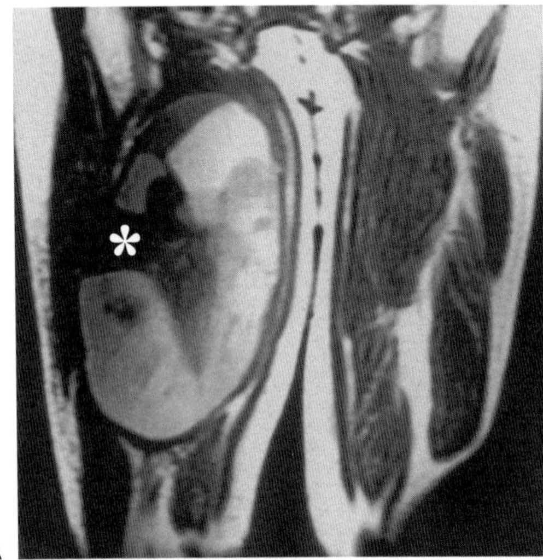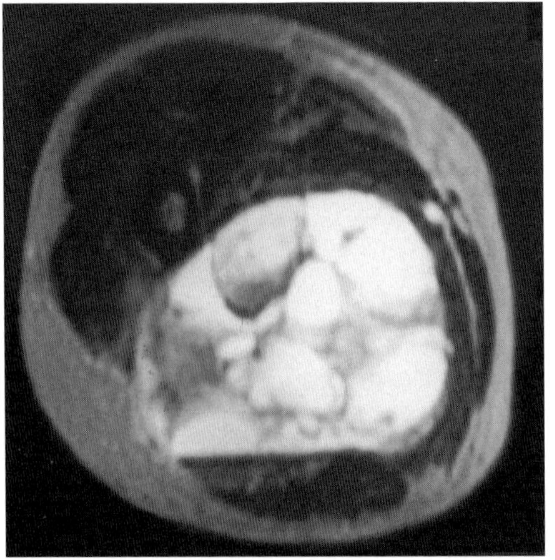

Figure 7.28 Storiform malignant fibrous histiocytoma presenting as a "spontaneous hematoma" of the thigh in a man 45 years of age. **A:** Coronal T1-weighted (TR/TE; 500/16) spin-echo MR image demonstrates a large complex mass with fluid levels and high intensity, representing hemorrhage. Solid portion of the mass is also seen (*asterisk*). **B:** Axial T2-weighted (TR/TE; 2500/80) spin-echo MR image shows the entire mass to have a high signal intensity, and differentiation of hemorrhage from neoplasm is not possible.

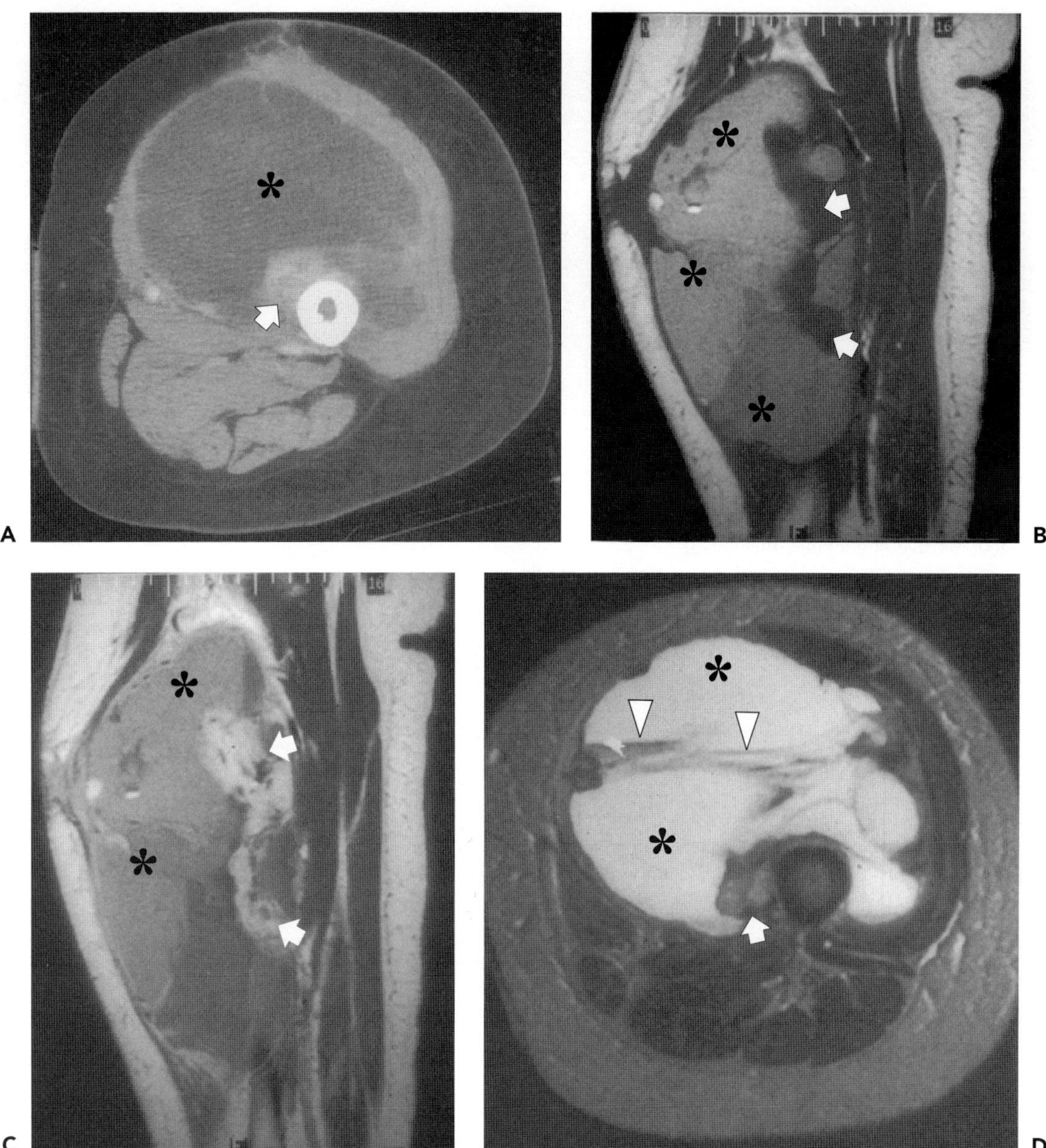

Figure 7.29 Storiform/pleomorphic malignant fibrous histiocytoma presenting as a "spontaneous hematoma" in a man 50 years of age. **A:** Axial postcontrast CT shows a large, well-defined, predominantly low attenuation, intramuscular, soft tissue mass (*asterisk*) with focal nodule of enhancing viable tumor (*arrow*). **B,C:** Sagittal T1-weighted (TR/TE; 500/20) spin-echo MR images before **(B)** and following **(C)** intravenous contrast show areas of subacute hemorrhage (*asterisks*) and enhancing tumor (*arrows*). **D:** Axial T2-weighted (TR/TE; 2500/100) spin-echo MR image reveals the mass to be predominantly composed of hemorrhage (*asterisks*) with multiple fluid levels (*arrowheads*). Solid focus of viable MFH (site that should be biopsied) enhances after contrast and is intermediate in signal intensity on T2-weighting (*arrows*). (*continued*)

The metastatic rate varies with the histologic subtype of MFH, seen in 20% to 65% of storiform/pleomorphic MFH, 23% to 30% of myxoid MFH, approximately 50% of giant cell MFH, and approximately 25% to 30% of inflammatory MFH (with 70% leading to patient demise) (42,127,128,171,172). Regional lymph node metastases occur in between 4% and 17% of cases (42,115,125, 130,131). Distant metastases are most common, involving the lung (90%), bone (8%), and liver (1%) (42,125,127, 128,171,172).

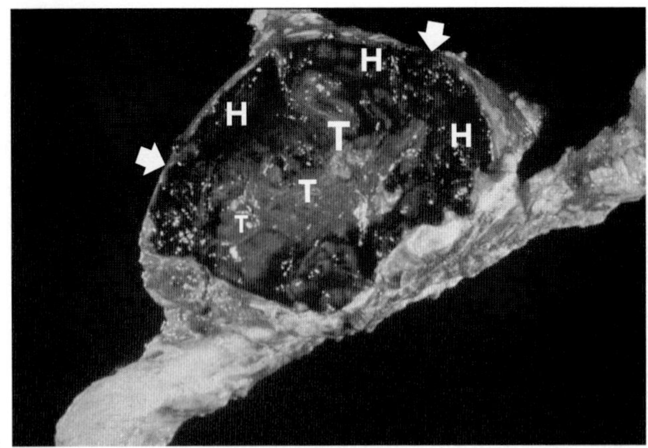

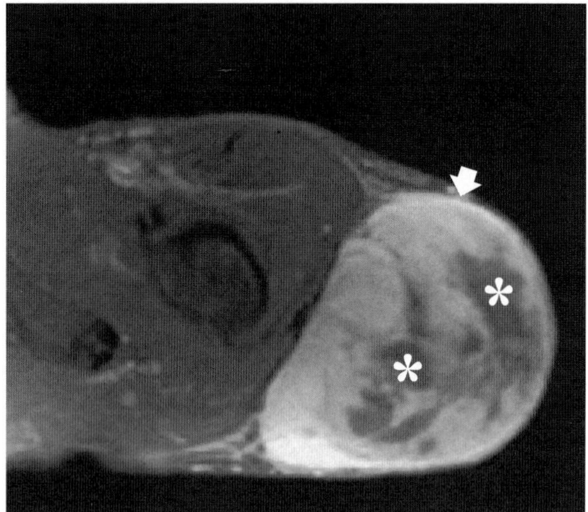

Figure 7.29 *(continued)* **E:** Photograph of sectioned gross specimen also demonstrates the hemorrhagic component (**H**) surrounding the viable portion of the tumor (**T**) and peripheral pseudocapsule (*arrows*) that contained the hemorrhage, causing the well-defined margin and lack of surrounding edema on imaging.

Figure 7.30   Retroperitoneal malignant fibrous histiocytoma in a woman 65 years of age. CT shows the large retroperitoneal mass (*asterisk*) of soft tissue attenuation adjacent to the psoas muscle.

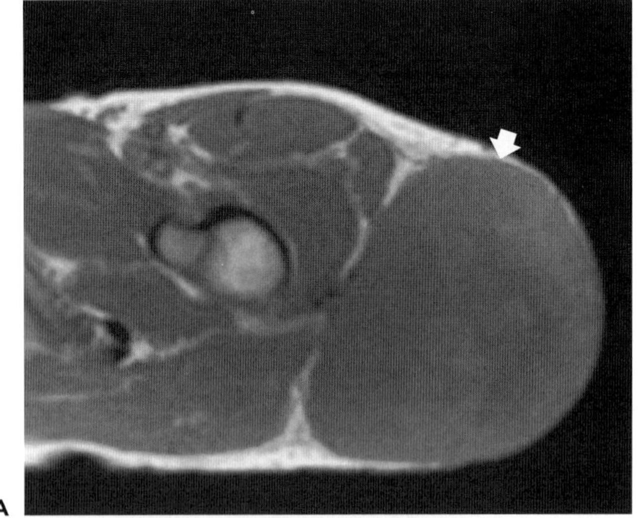

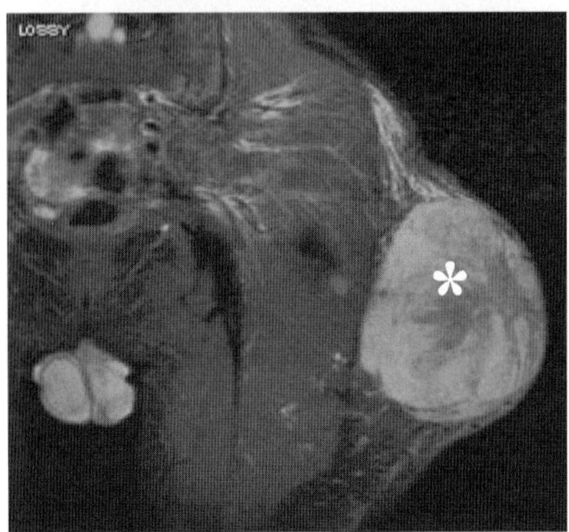

Figure 7.31   Subcutaneous malignant fibrous histiocytoma in the buttock of a man 40 years of age. **A,B:** Axial T1-weighted (TR/TE; 500/20) MR images before **(A)** and after **(B)** intravenous contrast show a large subcutaneous soft tissue mass (*arrow*) with intermediate signal intensity and diffuse enhancement except for central areas of necrosis (*asterisks* in **B**). **C:** Coronal fat-suppressed T2-weighted (TR/TE; 4000/100) MR image reveals heterogeneous intermediate-to-high signal intensity in the MFH (*asterisk*).

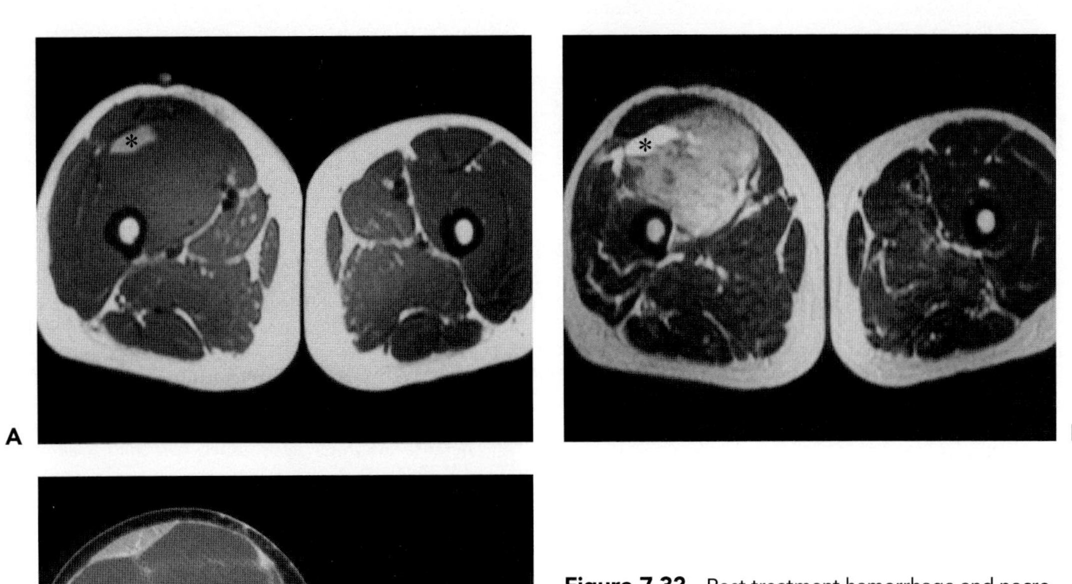

Figure 7.32   Post treatment hemorrhage and necrosis: Imaging feature in man 50 years of age following radiation and chemotherapy for a malignant fibrous histiocytoma. **A,B:** Pre-therapy axial T1-weighted (TR/TE; 600/12) **(A)** and T2-weighted (TR/TE; 2000/80) **(B)** spin-echo MR image shows a heterogeneous anterior compartment mass with focal hemorrhage (*asterisk*). **C:** Axial contrast-enhanced CT after preoperative therapy reveals enlargement of the mass with predominantly low attenuation from necrosis/hemorrhage. However, enhancing portions are also seen, representing viable tumor. At pathologic examination, necrosis was less than 70%.

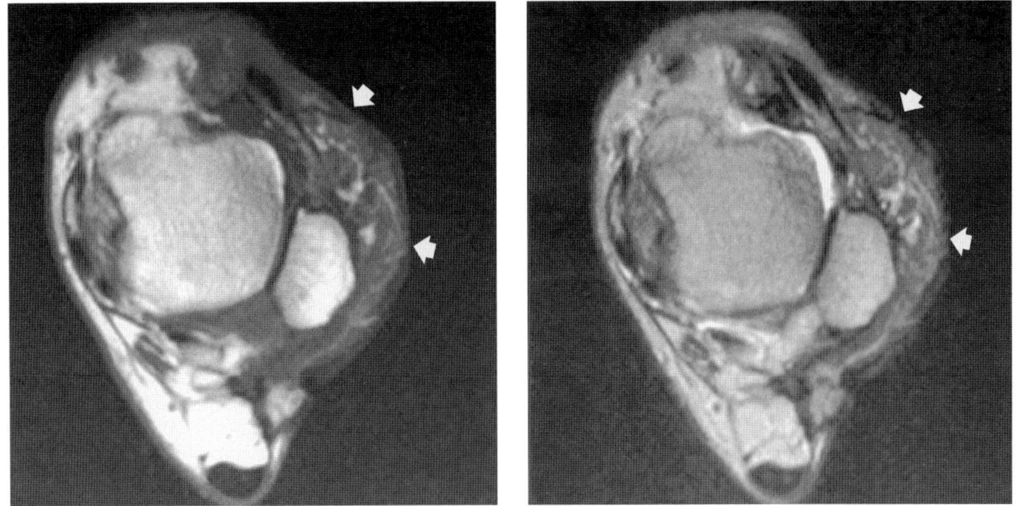

Figure 7.33   Postoperative myocutaneous free flap simulating tumor recurrence: MR imaging in a woman 59 years of age following resection of a high-grade malignant fibrous histiocytoma (undifferentiated pleomorphic sarcoma). **A,B:** Axial T1-weighted (TR/TR; 400/16) **(A)** and fast T2-weighted (TR/TE; 3000/80) **(B)** spin-echo MR images show the lateral free flap (*arrows*). Note the normal so-called marbled muscle texture and absence of focal mass.

REFERENCES

1. Kransdorf MJ. Malignant soft-tissue tumors in a large referral population: distribution of diagnoses by age, sex, and location. *AJR Am J Roentgenol.* 1995;164:129–134.
2. Darier S, Ferrand M. Dermatofibrosarcomes progressifs et recidivantes ou fibrosarcomes de la peau. *Ann Dermatol Venereol.* 1924;5:545–562.
3. Hoffman E. Liber das knollentrichencle fibrokom der hout. *Acta Derm Venereol Suppl (Stockh).* 1925;32.
4. McKee PH, Fletcher CD. Dermatofibrosarcoma protuberans presenting in infancy and childhood. *J Cutan Pathol.* 1991;18:241–246.
5. Taylor HB, Helwig EB. Dermatofibrosarcoma protuberans. A study of 115 cases. *Cancer.* 1962;15:717–725.
6. Thornton SL, Reid J, Papay FA, et al. Childhood dermatofibrosarcoma protuberans: role of preoperative imaging. *J Am Acad Dermatol.* 2005;53:76–83.
7. McPeak CJ, Cruz T, Nicastri AD. Dermatofibrosarcoma protuberans: an analysis of 86 cases—five with metastasis. *Ann Surg.* 1967;166:803–816.
8. Enzinger F, Weiss SW. Fibrohistiocytic tumors of intermediate malignancy. In: Weiss SW and Goldblum JR, eds. *Soft Tissue Tumors.* 4th ed. St. Louis: Mosby; 2001:491–534.
9. Fletcher C, Unni K, Mertens F. *World Health Organization Classification of Tumors. Pathology and Genetics of Tumors of Soft Tissue and Bone.* Lyon, France: IARC Press; 2002.
10. Kempson RL, Fletcher CM, Evans HL, et al. In: Rosai J, ed. *Tumors of the Soft Tissues.* 3rd ed. Bethesda, MD: Armed Forces Institute of Pathology; 2001:23–112.
11. Miettinen M. *Diagnostic Soft Tissue Pathology.* New York: Churchill Livingstone; 2003.
12. Weiss S, Goldblum J. *Enzinger and Weiss's Soft Tissue Tumors.* 4th ed. St. Louis: Mosby; 2001.
13. Simstein NL, Tuthill RJ, Sperber EE, et al. Dermatofibrosarcoma protuberans—case reports and review of literature. *South Med J.* 1977;70:487–489.
14. Diaz-Cascajo C, Weyers W, Rey-Lopez A, et al. Deep dermatofibrosarcoma protuberans: a subcutaneous variant. *Histopathology.* 1998;32:552–555.
15. Burkhardt BR, Soule EH, Winkelmann RK, et al. Dermatofibrosarcoma protuberans. Study of fifty-six cases. *Am J Surg.* 1966;111:638–644.
16. Hashimoto K, Brownstein MH, Jakobiec FA. Dermatofibrosarcoma protuberans. A tumor with perineural and endoneural cell features. *Arch Dermatol.* 1974;110:874–885.
17. Connelly JH, Evans HL. Dermatofibrosarcoma protuberans. A clinicopathologic review with emphasis on fibrosarcomatous areas. *Am J Surg Pathol.* 1992;16:921–925.
18. Ding J, Hashimoto H, Enjoji M. Dermatofibrosarcoma protuberans with fibrosarcomatous areas. A clinicopathologic study of nine cases and a comparison with allied tumors. *Cancer.* 1989;64:721–729.
19. Wrotnowski U, Cooper PH, Shmookler BM. Fibrosarcomatous change in dermatofibrosarcoma protuberans. *Am J Surg Pathol.* 1988;12:287–293.
20. Goldblum JR, Reith JD, Weiss SW. Sarcomas arising in dermatofibrosarcoma protuberans: a reappraisal of biologic behavior in eighteen cases treated by wide local excision with extended clinical follow up. *Am J Surg Pathol.* 2000;24:1125–1130.
21. Mentzel T, Beham A, Katenkamp D, et al. Fibrosarcomatous ("high-grade") dermatofibrosarcoma protuberans: clinicopathologic and immunohistochemical study of a series of 41 cases with emphasis on prognostic significance. *Am J Surg Pathol.* 1998;22:576–587.
22. Bednar B. Storiform neurofibromas of the skin, pigmented and nonpigmented. *Cancer.* 1957;10:368–376.
23. Gloster HM Jr, Harris KR, Roenigk RK. A comparison between Mohs micrographic surgery and wide surgical excision for the treatment of dermatofibrosarcoma protuberans. *J Am Acad Dermatol.* 1996;35:82–87.
24. Roses DF, Valensi Q, LaTrenta G, et al. Surgical treatment of dermatofibrosarcoma protuberans. *Surg Gynecol Obstet.* 1986;162:449–452.
25. Barnes L, Coleman JA Jr, Johnson JT. Dermatofibrosarcoma protuberans of the head and neck. *Arch Otolaryngol.* 1984;110:398–404.
26. Batsakis JG, Manning JT. Soft tissue tumors: unusual forms. *Otolaryngol Clin North Am.* 1986;19:659–683.
27. Rockley PF, Robinson JK, Magid M, et al. Dermatofibrosarcoma protuberans of the scalp: a series of cases. *J Am Acad Dermatol.* 1989;21:278–283.
28. Petoin DS, Verola O, Banzet P, et al. Darier-Ferrand dermatofibrosarcoma. Study of 96 cases over 15 years [in French]. *Chirurgie.* 1985;111:132–138.
29. Brenner W, Schaefler K, Chhabra H, et al. Dermatofibrosarcoma protuberans metastatic to a regional lymph node. Report of a case and review. *Cancer.* 1975;36:1897–1902.
30. Phelan JT, Juardo J. Dermatofibrosarcoma protuberans. *Am J Surg.* 1963;106:943–948.
31. Kransdorf MJ, Meis-Kindblom JM. Dermatofibrosarcoma protuberans: radiologic appearance. *AJR Am J Roentgenol.* 1994;163:391–394.
32. Ehara S, Oda Y. Deep dermatofibrosarcoma protuberans. *AJR Am J Roentgenol.* 2002;179:1643; author reply 1643.
33. Taleb A, Fahoume K, Hommadi A, et al. Contribution of imaging to the diagnosis of Darier-Ferrand's cranio-facial dermatofibrosarcoma. Report of 2 cases. *J Neuroradiol.* 2001;28:272–277.
34. Torreggiani WC, Al-Ismail K, Munk PL, et al. Dermatofibrosarcoma protuberans: MR imaging features. *AJR Am J Roentgenol.* 2002;178:989–993.
35. Daly BD, Currie AR, Choi PC. Case report: computed tomographic and scintigraphic appearances of dermatofibrosarcoma protuberans. *Clin Radiol.* 1993;48:63–65.
36. Shmookler BM, Enzinger FM, Weiss SW. Giant cell fibroblastoma. A juvenile form of dermatofibrosarcoma protuberans. *Cancer.* 1989;64:2154–2161.
37. Enzinger F, Weiss SW. Benign fibrohistiocytic tumors. In: Weiss SW and Goldblum JR, eds. *Soft Tissue Tumors.* 4th ed. St. Louis: Mosby; 2001:441–490.
38. Cin PD, Sciot R, de Wever I, et al. Cytogenetic and immunohistochemical evidence that giant cell fibroblastoma is related to dermatofibrosarcoma protuberans. *Genes Chromosomes Cancer.* 1996;15:73–75.
39. Barr RJ, Young EM Jr, Liao SY. Giant cell fibroblastoma: an immunohistochemical study. *J Cutan Pathol.* 1986;13:301–307.
40. Miettinen M. Malignant and potentially malignant fibroblastic and myofibroblastic tumors. In: *Diagnostic Soft Tissue Pathology.* New York: Churchill Livingstone; 2003:189–206.
41. Alguacil-Garcia A, Unni KK, Goellner JR, et al. Atypical fibroxanthoma of the skin: an ultrastructural study of two cases. *Cancer.* 1977;40:1471–1480.
42. Enzinger F, Weiss SW. Malignant fibrohistiocytic tumors. In: Weiss SW and Goldblum JR, eds. *Soft Tissue Tumors.* 4th ed. St. Louis: Mosby; 2001: 535–570.
43. Fretzin DF, Helwig EB. Atypical fibroxanthoma of the skin. A clinicopathologic study of 140 cases. *Cancer.* 1973;31:1541–1552.
44. Kroe DJ, Pitcock JA. Atypical fibroxanthoma of the skin. Report of ten cases. *Am J Clin Pathol.* 1969;51:487–492.
45. Laskin WB, Silverman TA, Enzinger FM. Postradiation soft tissue sarcomas. An analysis of 53 cases. *Cancer.* 1988;62:2330–2340.
46. Hudson AW, Winkelmann RK. Atypical fibroxanthoma of the skin: a reappraisal of 19 cases in which the original diagnosis was spindle-cell squamous carcinoma. *Cancer.* 1972;29:413–422.
47. Galant J, Marti-Bonmati L, Soler R, et al. Grading of subcutaneous soft tissue tumors by means of their relationship with the superficial fascia on MR imaging. *Skeletal Radiol.* 1998;27:657–663.
48. Helwig EB, May D. Atypical fibroxanthoma of the skin with metastasis. *Cancer.* 1986;57:368–376.
49. Montgomery EA, Devaney KO, Giordano TJ, et al. Inflammatory myxohyaline tumor of distal extremities with virocyte or Reed-Sternberg–like cells: a novel entity with features simulating myxoid malignant fibrous histiocytoma, inflammatory conditions and Hodgkin's disease. *Mod Pathol.* 1997;10:47A.
50. Montgomery EA, Devaney KO, Giordano TJ, et al. Inflammatory myxohyaline tumor of distal extremities with virocyte or Reed-

Sternberg–like cells: a distinctive lesion with features simulating inflammatory conditions, Hodgkin's disease, and various sarcomas. *Mod Pathol.* 1998;11:384–391.

51. Meis-Kindblom JM, Kindblom LG. Acral myxoinflammatory fibroblastic sarcoma: a low-grade tumor of the hands and feet. *Am J Surg Pathol.* 1998;22:911–924.

52. Fetsch JF, Laskin WB, Miettinen M. Superficial acral fibromyxoma: a clinicopathologic and immunohistochemical analysis of 37 cases of a distinctive soft tissue tumor with a predilection for the fingers and toes. *Hum Pathol.* 2001;32:704–714.

53. Lambert I, Debiec-Rychter M, Guelinckx P, et al. Acral myxoinflammatory fibroblastic sarcoma with unique clonal chromosomal changes. *Virchows Arch.* 2001;438:509–512.

54. Michal M. Inflammatory myxoid tumor of the soft parts with bizarre giant cells. *Pathol Res Pract.* 1998;194:529–533.

55. Sakaki M, Hirokawa M, Wakatsuki S, et al. Acral myxoinflammatory fibroblastic sarcoma: a report of five cases and review of the literature. *Virchows Arch.* 2003;442:25–30.

56. Jurcic V, Zidar A, Montiel MD, et al. Myxoinflammatory fibroblastic sarcoma: a tumor not restricted to acral sites. *Ann Diagn Pathol.* 2002;6:272–280.

57. Enzinger F, Weiss SW. Malignant soft tumors of uncertain type. In: Weiss SW and Goldblum JR, eds. *Soft Tissue Tumors.* 4th ed. St. Louis: Mosby; 2001:1483– 1572.

58. Pohar-Marinsek Z, Flezar M, Lamovec J. Acral myxoinflammatory fibroblastic sarcoma in FNAB samples: can we distinguish it from other myxoid lesions? *Cytopathology.* 2003;14:73–78.

59. Tateishi U, Hasegawa T, Onaya H, et al. Myxoinflammatory fibroblastic sarcoma: MR appearance and pathologic correlation. *AJR Am J Roentgenol.* 2005;184:1749–1753.

60. Enzinger FM. Angiomatoid malignant fibrous histiocytoma: a distinct fibrohistiocytic tumor of children and young adults simulating a vascular neoplasm. *Cancer.* 1979;44:2147–2157.

61. Kanter MH, Duane GB. Angiomatoid malignant fibrous histiocytoma. Cytology of fine-needle aspiration and its differential diagnosis. *Arch Pathol Lab Med.* 1985;109:564–566.

62. Kempson R, Fletcher C, Evans H, et al. Fibrous histiocytomas. In: Rosai J, ed. *Tumors of the Soft Tissues.* 3rd ed. Bethesda, MD: Armed Forces Institute of Pathology; 2001:113–186.

63. Miettinen M. Miscellaneous soft tissue tumors of unknown histogenesis. In: *Diagnostic Soft Tissue Pathology.* New York: Churchill Livingstone; 2003:489–503.

64. Daw NC, Billups CA, Pappo AS, et al. Malignant fibrous histiocytoma and other fibrohistiocytic tumors in pediatric patients: the St. Jude Children's Research Hospital experience. *Cancer.* 2003;97:2839–2847.

65. Costa MJ, Weiss SW. Angiomatoid malignant fibrous histiocytoma. A follow-up study of 108 cases with evaluation of possible histologic predictors of outcome. *Am J Surg Pathol.* 1990;14: 1126–1132.

66. Enzinger FM, Zhang RY. Plexiform fibrohistiocytic tumor presenting in children and young adults. An analysis of 65 cases. *Am J Surg Pathol.* 1988;12:818–826.

67. Miettinen M. Fibroblastic proliferation in children. In: *Diagnostic Soft Tissue Pathology.* New York: Churchill Livingstone; 2003:173–188.

68. Salomao DR, Nascimento AG. Plexiform fibrohistiocytic tumor with systemic metastases: a case report. *Am J Surg Pathol.* 1997;21:469–476.

69. Angervall L, Kindblom LG, Lindholm K, et al. Plexiform fibrohistiocytic tumor. Report of a case involving preoperative aspiration cytology and immunohistochemical and ultrastructural analysis of surgical specimens. *Pathol Res Pract.* 1992;188:350–356; discussion 356–359.

70. Giard F, Bonneau R, Raymond GP. Plexiform fibrohistiocytic tumor. *Dermatologica.* 1991;183:290–293.

71. Redlich GC, Montgomery KD, Allgood GA, et al. Plexiform fibrohistiocytic tumor with a clonal cytogenetic anomaly. *Cancer Genet Cytogenet.* 1999;108:141–143.

72. Enzinger F, Weiss SW. Fibrous tumors of infancy and childhood. In: *Soft Tissue Tumors.* 4th ed. St. Louis: Mosby; 2001: 347–408.

73. Kempson R, Fletcher C, Evans H, et al. Fibrous and myofibroblastic tumors. In: Rosai J, ed. *Tumors of the Soft Tissues.* 3rd ed.

Bethesda, MD: Armed Forces Institute of Pathology; 2001: 23–112.

74. Stout AP. Fibrosarcoma in infants and children. *Cancer.* 1962;15:1028–1040.

75. Balsaver AM, Butler JJ, Martin RG. Congenital fibrosarcoma. *Cancer.* 1967;20:1607–1616.

76. Ninane J, Gosseye S, Panteon E, et al. Congenital fibrosarcoma reoperative chemotherapy and conservative surgery. *Cancer.* 1986;58:1400–1406.

77. Chung EB, Enzinger FM. Infantile fibrosarcoma. *Cancer.* 1976; 38:729–739.

78. Schofield DE, Fletcher JA, Grier HE, et al. Fibrosarcoma in infants and children. Application of new techniques. *Am J Surg Pathol.* 1994;18:14–24.

79. Soule EH, Pritchard DJ. Fibrosarcoma in infants and children: a review of 110 cases. *Cancer.* 1977;40:1711–1721.

80. Exelby PR, Knapper WH, Huvos AG, et al. Soft-tissue fibrosarcoma in children. *J Pediatr Surg.* 1973;8:415–420.

81. Pritchard DJ, Sim FH, Ivins JC, et al. Fibrosarcoma of bone and soft tissues of the trunk and extremities. *Orthop Clin North Am.* 1977;8:869–881.

82. Fink AM, Stringer DA, Cairns RA, et al. Pediatric case of the day. Congenital fibrosarcoma (CFS). *Radiographics.* 1995;15:243–246.

83. Vinnicombe SJ, Hall CM. Infantile fibrosarcoma: radiological and clinical features. *Skeletal Radiol.* 1994;23:337–341.

84. Argani P, Fritsch M, Kadkol SS, et al. Detection of the ETV6-NTRK3 chimeric RNA of infantile fibrosarcoma/cellular congenital mesoblastic nephroma in paraffin-embedded tissue: application to challenging pediatric renal stromal tumors. *Mod Pathol.* 2000;13:29–36.

85. Sankary S, Dickman PS, Wiener E, et al. Consistent numerical chromosome aberrations in congenital fibrosarcoma. *Cancer Genet Cytogenet.* 1993;65:152–156.

86. Knezevich SR, Garnett MJ, Pysher TJ, et al. ETV6-NTRK3 gene fusions and trisomy 11 establish a histogenetic link between mesoblastic nephroma and congenital fibrosarcoma. *Cancer Res.* 1998;58:5046–5048.

87. Rubin BP, Chen CJ, Morgan TW, et al. Congenital mesoblastic nephroma t(12;15) is associated with ETV6-NTRK3 gene fusion: cytogenetic and molecular relationship to congenital (infantile) fibrosarcoma. *Am J Pathol.* 1998;153:1451–1458.

88. Cofer BR, Vescio PJ, Wiener ES. Infantile fibrosarcoma: complete excision is the appropriate treatment. *Ann Surg Oncol.* 1996;3: 159–161.

89. Scott SM, Reiman HM, Pritchard DJ, et al. Soft tissue fibrosarcoma. A clinicopathologic study of 132 cases. *Cancer.* 1989;64: 925–931.

90. Stout AP. Fibrosarcoma: the malignant tumor of fibroblasts. *Cancer.* 1948;1:30.

91. Stout AP. The fibromatoses and fibrosarcoma. *Bull Hosp Joint Dis.* 1951;12:126–130.

92. Meyerding H, Broders A, Hargrave R. Clinical aspects of fibrosarcoma of the soft tissues of the extremities. *Surg Gynecol Obstet.* 1936;62:1010.

93. Pritchard DJ, Soule EH, Taylor WF, et al. Fibrosarcoma—a clinicopathologic and statistical study of 199 tumors of the soft tissues of the extremities and trunk. *Cancer.* 1974;33:888–897.

94. Enzinger F, Weiss SW. Fibrosarcoma. In: Weiss SW and Goldblum JR, eds. *Soft Tissue Tumors.* 4th ed. St. Louis: Mosby; 2001:409–440.

95. Montgomery E, Fisher C. Myofibroblastic differentiation in malignant fibrous histiocytoma (pleomorphic myofibrosarcoma): a clinicopathological study. *Histopathology.* 2001;8:499–509.

96. Montgomery E, Goldblum JR, Fisher C. Myofibrosarcoma: a clinicopathologic study. *Am J Surg Pathol.* 2001;25:219–228.

97. Montgomery E, Devaney KO. Low-grade fibroblastic sarcomas and their distinction from deep fibromatoses. *Mod Pathol.* 1996;9:42A.

98. Mackenzie DH. Fibroma: a dangerous diagnosis: a review of 205 cases of fibrosarcoma of soft tissues. *Br J Surg.* 1964;51: 607–612.

99. Bizer LS. Fibrosarcoma. Report of sixty-four cases. *Am J Surg.* 1971;121:586–587.

100. Evans HL. Low-grade fibromyxoid sarcoma. A report of two metastasizing neoplasms having a deceptively benign appearance. *Am J Clin Pathol.* 1987;88:615–619.

101. Evans HL. Low-grade fibromyxoid sarcoma. A report of 12 cases. *Am J Surg Pathol.* 1993;17:595–600.

102. Folpe AL, Lane KL, Paull G, et al. Low-grade fibromyxoid sarcoma and hyalinizing spindle cell tumor with giant rosettes: a clinicopathologic study of 73 cases supporting their identity and assessing the impact of high-grade areas. *Am J Surg Pathol.* 2000;24:1353–1360.

103. Goodlad JR, Mentzel T, Fletcher CD. Low grade fibromyxoid sarcoma: clinicopathological analysis of eleven new cases in support of a distinct entity. *Histopathology.* 1995;26:229–237.

104. Meis-Kindblom JM, Kindblom LG, Enzinger FM. Sclerosing epithelioid fibrosarcoma. A variant of fibrosarcoma simulating carcinoma. *Am J Surg Pathol.* 1995;19:979–993.

105. Christensen DR, Ramsamooj R, Gilbert TJ. Sclerosing epithelioid fibrosarcoma: short T2 on MR imaging. *Skeletal Radiol.* 1997;26:619–621.

106. Eyden BP, Manson C, Banerjee SS, et al. Sclerosing epithelioid fibrosarcoma: a study of five cases emphasizing diagnostic criteria. *Histopathology.* 1998;33:354–360.

107. Reid R, Barrett A, Hamblen DL. Sclerosing epithelioid fibrosarcoma. *Histopathology.* 1996;28:451–455.

108. Antonescu CR, Rosenblum MK, Pereira P, et al. Sclerosing epithelioid fibrosarcoma: a study of 16 cases and confirmation of a clinicopathologically distinct tumor. *Am J Surg Pathol.* 2001;25:699–709.

109. O'Brien JE, Stout AP. Malignant fibrous xanthomas. *Cancer.* 1964;17:1445–1455.

110. Ozzello L, Stout AP, Murray MR. Cultural characteristics of malignant histiocytomas and fibrous xanthomas. *Cancer.* 1963;16:331–344.

111. Dehner LP. Malignant fibrous histiocytoma. Nonspecific morphologic pattern, specific pathologic entity, or both? *Arch Pathol Lab Med.* 1988;112:236–237.

112. Enzinger FM. Malignant fibrous histiocytoma 20 years after Stout. *Am J Surg Pathol.* 1986;10(suppl 1):43–53.

113. Harris M. The ultrastructure of benign and malignant fibrous histiocytomas. *Histopathology.* 1980;4:29–44.

114. Walaas L, Angervall L, Hagmar B, et al. A correlative cytologic and histologic study of malignant fibrous histiocytoma: an analysis of 40 cases examined by fine-needle aspiration cytology. *Diagn Cytopathol.* 1986;2:46–54.

115. Weiss SW, Enzinger FM. Malignant fibrous histiocytoma: an analysis of 200 cases. *Cancer.* 1978;41:2250–2266.

116. Rosenberg AE. Malignant fibrous histiocytoma: past, present, and future. *Skeletal Radiol.* 2003;32:613–618.

117. Fanburg-Smith JC, Miettinen M. Angiomatoid "malignant" fibrous histiocytoma: a clinicopathologic study of 158 cases and further exploration of the myoid phenotype. *Hum Pathol.* 1999;30:1336–1343.

118. Fletcher CD. Pleomorphic malignant fibrous histiocytoma: fact or fiction? A critical reappraisal based on 159 tumors diagnosed as pleomorphic sarcoma. *Am J Surg Pathol.* 1992;16:213–228.

119. Fletcher CD, Gustafson P, Rydholm A, et al. Clinicopathologic re-evaluation of 100 malignant fibrous histiocytomas: prognostic relevance of subclassification. *J Clin Oncol.* 2001;19:3045–3050.

120. Gibbs JF, Huang PP, Lee RJ, et al. Malignant fibrous histiocytoma: an institutional review. *Cancer Invest.* 2001;19:23–27.

121. Guccion JG, Enzinger FM. Malignant giant cell tumor of soft parts. An analysis of 32 cases. *Cancer.* 1972;29:1518–1529.

122. Kyriakos M, Kempson RL. Inflammatory fibrous histiocytoma. An aggressive and lethal lesion. *Cancer.* 1976;37:1584–1606.

123. Mentzel T, Calonje E, Wadden C, et al. Myxofibrosarcoma. Clinicopathologic analysis of 75 cases with emphasis on the low-grade variant. *Am J Surg Pathol.* 1996;20:391–405.

124. Patel SR. Radiation-induced sarcoma. *Curr Treat Options Oncol.* 2000;1:258–261.

125. Pezzi CM, Rawlings MS Jr, Esgro JJ, et al. Prognostic factors in 227 patients with malignant fibrous histiocytoma. *Cancer.* 1992;69:2098–2103.

126. Rooser B, Willen H, Gustafson P, et al. Malignant fibrous histiocytoma of soft tissue. A population-based epidemiologic and prognostic study of 137 patients. *Cancer.* 1991;67:499–505.

127. Salo JC, Lewis JJ, Woodruff JM, et al. Malignant fibrous histiocytoma of the extremity. *Cancer.* 1999;85:1765–1772.

128. Rydholm A, Syk I. Malignant fibrous histiocytoma of soft tissue. Correlation between clinical variables and histologic malignancy grade. *Cancer.* 1986;57:2323–2324.

129. Murphey MD, Gross TM, Rosenthal HG. From the archives of the AFIP. Musculoskeletal malignant fibrous histiocytoma: radiologic-pathologic correlation. *Radiographics.* 1994;14:807–826; quiz 827–828.

130. Bertoni F, Capanna R, Biagini R, et al. Malignant fibrous histiocytoma of soft tissue. An analysis of 78 cases located and deeply seated in the extremities. *Cancer.* 1985;56:356–367.

131. Kearney MM, Soule EH, Ivins JC. Malignant fibrous histiocytoma: a retrospective study of 167 cases. *Cancer.* 1980;45:167–178.

132. Barnes L, Kanbour A. Malignant fibrous histiocytoma of the head and neck. A report of 12 cases. *Arch Otolaryngol Head Neck Surg.* 1988;114:1149–1156.

133. Cole AT, Straus FH, Gill WB. Malignant fibrous histiocytoma: an unusual inguinal tumor. *J Urol.* 1972;107:1005–1007.

134. Faragher IG, Bennett TM, Cass AJ. Primary malignant fibrous histiocytoma of the retroperitoneum. *Aust N Z J Surg.* 1988;58:915–917.

135. Goldman SM, Hartman DS, Weiss SW. The varied radiographic manifestations of retroperitoneal malignant fibrous histiocytoma revealed through 27 cases. *J Urol.* 1986;135:33–38.

136. Joseph TJ, Becker DI, Turton AF. Renal malignant fibrous histiocytoma. *Urology.* 1991;37:483–489.

137. Restrepo JP, Handler SD, Saull SC, et al. Malignant fibrous histiocytoma. *Otolaryngol Head Neck Surg.* 1987;96:362–365.

138. Vera-Donoso CD, Llopis B, Froufe A, et al. Retroperitoneal malignant fibrous histiocytoma. *Eur Urol.* 1988;15:302–305.

139. Yousem SA, Hochholzer L. Malignant fibrous histiocytoma of the lung. *Cancer.* 1987;60:2532–2541.

140. Bruneton JN, Drouillard J, Rogopoulos A, et al. Extra-retroperitoneal abdominal malignant fibrous histiocytoma. *Gastrointest Radiol.* 1988;13:299–305.

141. Cole BJ, Schultz E, Smilari TF, et al. Malignant fibrous histiocytoma at the site of a total hip replacement: review of the literature and case report. *Skeletal Radiol.* 1997;26:559–563.

142. Haag M, Adler CP. Malignant fibrous histiocytoma in association with hip replacement. *J Bone Joint Surg Br.* 1989;71:701.

143. Lindeman G, McKay MJ, Taubman KL, et al. Malignant fibrous histiocytoma developing in bone 44 years after shrapnel trauma. *Cancer.* 1990;66:2229–2232.

144. Nelson JP, Phillips PH. Malignant fibrous histiocytoma associated with total hip replacement. A case report. *Orthop Rev.* 1990;19:1078–1080.

145. Tait NP, Hacking PM, Malcolm AJ. Malignant fibrous histiocytoma occurring at the site of a previous total hip replacement. *Br J Radiol.* 1988;61:73–76.

146. Folpe AL, Morris RJ, Weiss SW. Soft tissue giant cell tumor of low malignant potential: a proposal for the reclassification of malignant giant cell tumor of soft parts. *Mod Pathol.* 1999;12:894–902.

147. O'Connell JX, Wehrli BM, Nielsen GP, et al. Giant cell tumors of soft tissue: a clinicopathologic study of 18 benign and malignant tumors. *Am J Surg Pathol.* 2000;24:386–395.

148. Oliveira AM, Dei Tos AP, Fletcher CD, et al. Primary giant cell tumor of soft tissues: a study of 22 cases. *Am J Surg Pathol.* 2000;24:248–256.

149. Feldman F, Norman D. Intra- and extraosseous malignant histiocytoma (malignant fibrous xanthoma). *Radiology.* 1972;104:497–508.

150. Fischer HJ, Lois JF, Gomes AS, et al. Radiology and pathology of malignant fibrous histiocytomas of the soft tissues: a report of ten cases. *Skeletal Radiol.* 1985;13:202–206.

151. Bhagavan BS, Dorfman HD. The significance of bone and cartilage formation in malignant fibrous histiocytoma of soft tissue. *Cancer.* 1982;49:480–488.

152. Dorfman HD, Bhagavan BS. Malignant fibrous histiocytoma of soft tissue with metaplastic bone and cartilage formation: a new radiologic sign. *Skeletal Radiol.* 1982;8:145–150.

153. Burgener FA, Landman S. Angiographic features of malignant fibrous histiocytomas. *Radiology.* 1976;121:581–583.

154. Harrowe DJ, Kessler S, Jansen AA, et al. Gallium-67 uptake by a malignant fibrous histiocytoma: case report. *J Nucl Med.* 1976;17:630–632.

155. Eary JF, Conrad EU. Positron emission tomography in grading soft tissue sarcomas. *Semin Musculoskelet Radiol.* 1999;3:135–138.

156. Aisen AM, Martel W, Braunstein EM, et al. MRI and CT evaluation of primary bone and soft-tissue tumors. *AJR Am J Roentgenol.* 1986;146:749–756.

157. Mahajan H, Kim EE, Wallace S, et al. Magnetic resonance imaging of malignant fibrous histiocytoma. *Magn Reson Imaging.* 1989;7:283–288.

158. Miller TT, Hermann G, Abdelwahab IF, et al. MRI of malignant fibrous histiocytoma of soft tissue: analysis of 13 cases with pathologic correlation. *Skeletal Radiol.* 1994;23:271–275.

159. Panicek DM, Casper ES, Brennan MF, et al. Hemorrhage simulating tumor growth in malignant fibrous histiocytoma at MR imaging. *Radiology.* 1991;181:398–400.

160. Peterson KK, Renfrew DL, Feddersen RM, et al. Magnetic resonance imaging of myxoid containing tumors. *Skeletal Radiol.* 1991;20:245–250.

161. Jelinek JS, Kransdorf MJ, Shmookler BM, et al. Liposarcoma of the extremities: MR and CT findings in the histologic subtypes. *Radiology.* 1993;186:455–459.

162. Kransdorf MJ, Moser RP Jr, Meis JM, et al. Fat-containing soft-tissue masses of the extremities. *Radiographics.* 1991;11:81–106.

163. Tsai JC, Dalinka MK, Fallon MD, et al. Fluid-fluid level: a nonspecific finding in tumors of bone and soft tissue. *Radiology.* 1990;175:779–782.

164. Sanchez RB, Quinn SF, Walling A, et al. Musculoskeletal neoplasms after intraarterial chemotherapy: correlation of MR images with pathologic specimens. *Radiology.* 1990;174:237–240.

165. Shuman LS, Chuang VP, Wallace S, et al. Intra-arterial chemotherapy of malignant fibrous histiocytoma of the pelvis. *Radiology.* 1982;142:343–346.

166. Fagundes HM, Lai PP, Dehner LP, et al. Postoperative radiotherapy for malignant fibrous histiocytoma. *Int J Radiat Oncol Biol Phys.* 1992;23:615–619.

167. Biondetti PR, Ehman RL. Soft-tissue sarcomas: use of textural patterns in skeletal muscle as a diagnostic feature in postoperative MR imaging. *Radiology.* 1992;183:845–848.

168. Erlemann R, Reiser MF, Peters PE, et al. Musculoskeletal neoplasms: static and dynamic Gd-DTPA–enhanced MR imaging. *Radiology.* 1989;171:767–773.

169. Vanel D, Lacombe MJ, Couanet D, et al. Musculoskeletal tumors: follow-up with MR imaging after treatment with surgery and radiation therapy. *Radiology.* 1987;164:243–245.

170. Vanel D, Shapeero LG, Tardivon A, et al. Dynamic contrast-enhanced MRI with subtraction of aggressive soft tissue tumors after resection. *Skeletal Radiol.* 1998;27:505–510.

171. Le Doussal V, Coindre JM, Leroux A, et al. Prognostic factors for patients with localized primary malignant fibrous histiocytoma: a multicenter study of 216 patients with multivariate analysis. *Cancer.* 1996;77:1823–1830.

172. Zagars GK, Mullen JR, Pollack A. Malignant fibrous histiocytoma: outcome and prognostic factors following conservation surgery and radiotherapy. *Int J Radiat Oncol Biol Phys.* 1996;34:983–994.

173. Merck C, Angervall L, Kindblom LG, et al. Myxofibrosarcoma. A malignant soft tissue tumor of fibroblastic-histiocytic origin. A clinicopathologic and prognostic study of 110 cases using multivariate analysis. *Acta Pathol Microbiol Immunol Scand Suppl.* 1983;282:1–40.

Muscle Tumors

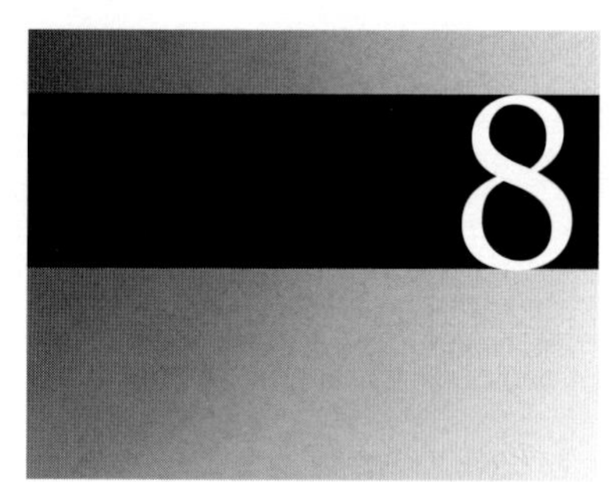

Muscle tumors of the soft tissue are uncommon. It is difficult to establish their prevalence, but it is estimated that benign muscle tumors make up less than 2% of all benign soft tissue tumors (1), and rhabdomyosarcoma and leiomyosarcoma account for approximately 2% to 12% and 8% to 9%, respectively, of all classified soft tissue sarcomas (2,3). This chapter discusses the spectrum of benign and malignant muscle tumors, including leiomyoma, rhabdomyoma, leiomyosarcoma, and rhabdomyosarcoma. Although not considered a musculoskeletal lesion, the gastrointestinal stromal tumor (GIST) is also discussed briefly.

BENIGN MUSCLE TUMORS

Leiomyoma

Leiomyomas are quite unusual outside of the uterus and gastrointestinal tract (4,5). In a study of 7,748 lesions by Farman (6), approximately 95% of leiomyomas occurred in the female genital tract. The remainder were scattered over various anatomic locations, although almost 75% of these occurred in the skin. These results, based on surgical material, likely underestimate the large number of asymptomatic gastrointestinal and genitourinary lesions identified at autopsy (7). When in the soft tissues, leiomyomas are usually small and cutaneous or subcutaneous; consequently, they are not the subject of radiologic imaging. Rarely, leiomyoma may be encountered in the deep soft tissue. These deep lesions are much larger than their superficial counterparts and much more likely to be confused with leiomyosarcoma, which is considerably more common.

It is difficult to estimate the incidence of soft tissue leiomyoma accurately, but in the Armed Forces Institute of Pathology (AFIP) experience, these tumors accounted for approximately 1.7% of 18,667 benign soft tissue tumors (1). Hachisuga et al. reported an incidence of 4.4% in a review of 12,663 benign soft tissue tumors in the pathology registry of Kyushu University (8).

Classification

Soft tissue leiomyomas are usually subdivided into several distinct clinical groups (7). The most common form is the

Leiomyoma for musculoskeletal purposes is classified into three groups, although others are described:
- Leiomyoma cutis (cutaneous leiomyoma): small lesions arising in skin.
- Vascular leiomyoma (angioleiomyoma): small to moderate sized lesions arising in subcutaneous tissue.
- Deep leiomyoma of soft tissue: large lesions in deep soft tissue.

cutaneous leiomyoma (*leiomyoma cutis*). These lesions arise from the arrector pili muscle of the skin and the deep dermis of the scrotum (dartoic muscles), labia majora, and nipple (7). Lesions arising from the deep dermis are collectively termed *genital leiomyomas* (7). The second group of leiomyoma is the angioleiomyoma, also known as *angiomyoma* or *vascular leiomyoma*. This lesion is differentiated from the cutaneous form by its subcutaneous location and histology, which is dominated by a conglomeration of thick-walled vessels associated with smooth muscle tissue (7). The leiomyoma of deep soft tissue is the final group and the one that more typically presents as a musculoskeletal mass. This lesion is much larger than the cutaneous and subcutaneous forms and the most likely to be confused with a leiomyosarcoma (7).

Weiss and Goldblum (7) also note that *leiomyomatosis peritonealis disseminata* and intravenous *leiomyomatosis* are also classified as benign leiomyomas. They note that the former is considered a metaplastic response of the peritoneal surface, characterized by multiple smooth muscle nodules, whereas the latter represents intravenous extension of uterine leiomyoma. These lesions are clearly outside the realm of the musculoskeletal radiologist and are not discussed here.

With the exception of the leiomyoma of the deep soft tissue, these lesions are superficial (dermal or subcutaneous), and they are usually removed without preoperative imaging. The subsequent discussion mentions these superficial lesions only briefly, emphasizing the deep leiomyoma, which is more likely to be confused with a sarcoma.

Superficial Leiomyoma

Superficial (cutaneous) leiomyomas typically arise in association with the smooth muscle of the skin. Those lesions arising from the pilar arrector muscles are termed *piloleiomyoma*. They typically occur as clustered papules or less commonly as single nodules ranging in size from a few millimeters to 2 cm (9). Single lesions tend to be larger (9). Pilar leiomyomas are most common in young adults, on the extensor surfaces of the arms and legs on hair-bearing surfaces (9,10). Lesions are typically painful, eliciting a burning or pinching sensation (7,9,10). Superficial leiomyomas may also arise from the deep dermis of the scrotum, nipple, areola, and vulva, and in these areas they are termed *genital leiomyomas* (7). Superficial leiomyomas are usually considered to be dermatologic lesions and rarely evaluated radiologically (11).

Angioleiomyoma (Angiomyoma, Vascular Leiomyoma)

Angioleiomyoma is a solitary lesion, probably arising from the tunica media of the vein (10,12), composed of a conglomerate of thick-walled vessels associated with smooth muscle (7). Angiomyoma is subcutaneous and represents approximately half of all superficial leiomyomas (7). The term *vascular leiomyoma* was adopted by Stout (13) in 1937 to distinguish these subcutaneous lesions from the cutaneous form, which is characterized histologically by thin-walled, inconspicuous vessels (7).

Angioleiomyoma is most common in adults, with two-thirds occurring in patients in the fourth through sixth decades of life (8). Women are reported to be affected more commonly than men (1.7–2.2:1) (8,12), although there is a male predilection (2.1:1) in the AFIP experience (1). The lesion is typically small (<2 cm) and located in the extremities in 89% to 94% of cases, with the lower extremity most frequently involved (approximately 50% to 75% of extremity cases) (1,8,12,14). Because the foot is a common location, patients may present with complaints related to problems with footwear (15,16). Pain and tenderness are found in more than half of patients and may be initiated with changes in temperature, pressure, pregnancy, or menses (14,17). Symptoms may be initiated by light touching or scratching (14). Lesions are often slowly growing and may be present for 10 to 15 years prior to presentation (15,18).

Leiomyoma of the Deep Soft Tissue

Leiomyoma of the deep soft tissue is quite uncommon in comparison to the superficial forms. The existence of this rare entity is now questioned because long-term follow-up reveals that some lesions demonstrate an aggressive behavior (19). Although evidence supports the existence of this lesion, the diagnosis must be made in accordance with strict histologic criteria (19).

Leiomyoma of the deep soft tissue is a lesion of adults and is typically located in the deep soft tissue of the extremities or retroperitoneum (7,20). Billings et al. (20) reviewed their experience with 36 cases of leiomyoma seen in consultation at Emory University. These investigators confirmed that deep leiomyoma occurs in two distinct locations: the deep somatic soft tissue of the extremities (*n* = 13) and the retroperitoneum (*n* = 23; 3 of which occurred in the abdomen). They also noted that extremity lesions affected both sexes equally, whereas retroperitoneal lesions occurred almost exclusively in women (22 women, 1 man), suggesting two distinct subtypes: the deep leiomyoma of somatic soft tissue and the retroperitoneal-abdominal leiomyoma. This latter form likely arises from hormonally sensitive smooth muscle and is similar to uterine leiomyoma. Deep leiomyomas are usually large at presentation, suggesting that they produce few symptoms (7).

In a review of the literature in 2000, Misumi et al. (21) found 21 previously reported cases. They found a mean patient age of 25 years (range: 3 to 62 years), with men affected twice as often as women. Almost half of the lesions (48%) were located in the extremities, and only a single patient had multiple lesions.

Grossly, leiomyoma of the deep soft tissues is a well-defined, circumscribed, nodular, gray-white mass that may have a gelatinous appearance (22). Microscopy shows a lesion composed of smooth muscle that may demonstrate rich vascularization (22). The lesion is histologically similar to its superficial counterparts, except it is larger and more prone to undergo regressive change, including fibrosis, calcification, and, rarely, ossification (7). It must be emphasized that most deep smooth muscle tumors are leiomyosarcomas, and the diagnosis of leiomyoma requires the absence of microscopic evidence of significant cellular pleomorphism or mitotic activity (7).

Imaging of Leiomyoma

KEY CONCEPTS

- Subcutaneous leiomyoma:
  - MR imaging shows a well-defined mass.
  - T1-weighted images show a signal intensity similar to or slightly hyperintense to that of skeletal muscle.
  - T2-weighted images show heterogeneous high or mixed signal intensity with areas ranging from isointense to hyperintense to that of skeletal muscle.
- Deep soft tissue leiomyoma:
  - Radiographs frequently show calcification. The three distinct patterns are scattered small flecks or sandlike calcification, plaquelike calcification, and large mulberry-like calcification (similar to a fibroid).
  - T1-weighted images show intermediate signal intensity.
  - T2-weighted images show low, intermediate, or high signal intensities.
  - Marked contrast enhancement is observed.
  - Large calcifications within the lesion appear as signal voids within the mass on MR imaging.

Superficial Leiomyoma

As previously noted, superficial leiomyomas, those in the skin and subcutaneous tissue, are only rarely evaluated radiologically. Limited experience with the imaging appearance of angioleiomyoma shows the lesion to be a well-defined, round to oval, subcutaneous or dermal mass with signal intensity similar to or slightly hyperintense to that of skeletal muscle on T1-weighted images. On T2-weighted images, lesions demonstrate a heterogeneous high signal intensity or mixed signal intensity with areas isointense to hyperintense to that of skeletal muscle (14,15,18,23). Both homogeneous and heterogeneous enhancement following contrast administration is reported (14,15,18,23). In 3 of 4 patients reported by Hwang et al. (14), hyperintense areas on T2-weighted images showed intense enhancement following contrast administration (Figs. 8.1 and 8.2). In the remaining patient, multiple vascular tubular and round signal voids were noted (14). Radiographs in patients with angioleiomyoma are typically nonspecific. Calcifications may rarely be seen in a superficial lesion but are more characteristically seen in deep leiomyoma of soft tissue (see next paragraph) (Fig. 8.3).

Deep Leiomyoma of Soft Tissue

There is little radiologic literature on the appearance of deep soft tissue leiomyoma. Scattered calcification, which is likely dystrophic (24,25) and secondary to involutional change, is not uncommon and was observed by Misumi et al. in 7 of 10 cases (21). Three distinct patterns of calcification are noted, although they may coexist within a single lesion (4): scattered small flecks or sandlike calcification, plaquelike calcification, and large mulberry-like calcification (similar to that noted in uterine leiomyoma) (Fig. 8.4). Lubbers et al. (4) suggested this may represent a spectrum of regressive change, with the sandlike calcification representing the earliest change and the mulberry-like calcification representing more advanced degeneration. The mulberry-like calcification is the most common and the most characteristic (21).

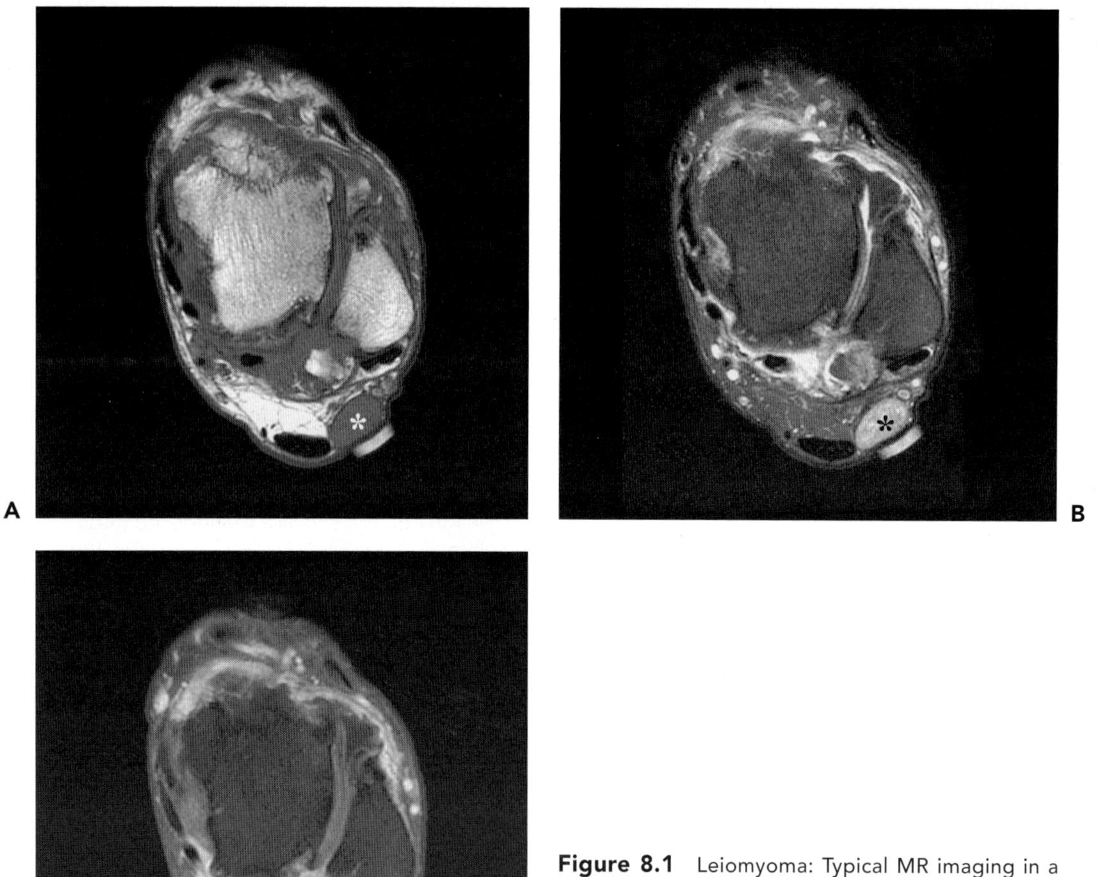

Figure 8.1 Leiomyoma: Typical MR imaging in a man 59 years of age presenting with a superficial ankle mass. **A,B:** Axial T1-weighted **(A)** and fat-suppressed fast T2-weighted **(B)** spin-echo MR images shows a well-defined, rounded soft tissue mass (*asterisk*) arising in association with the skin. **C:** Enhanced axial fat-suppressed spoiled gradient recalled (SPGR) image shows intense homogeneous enhancement of the mass (*asterisk*).

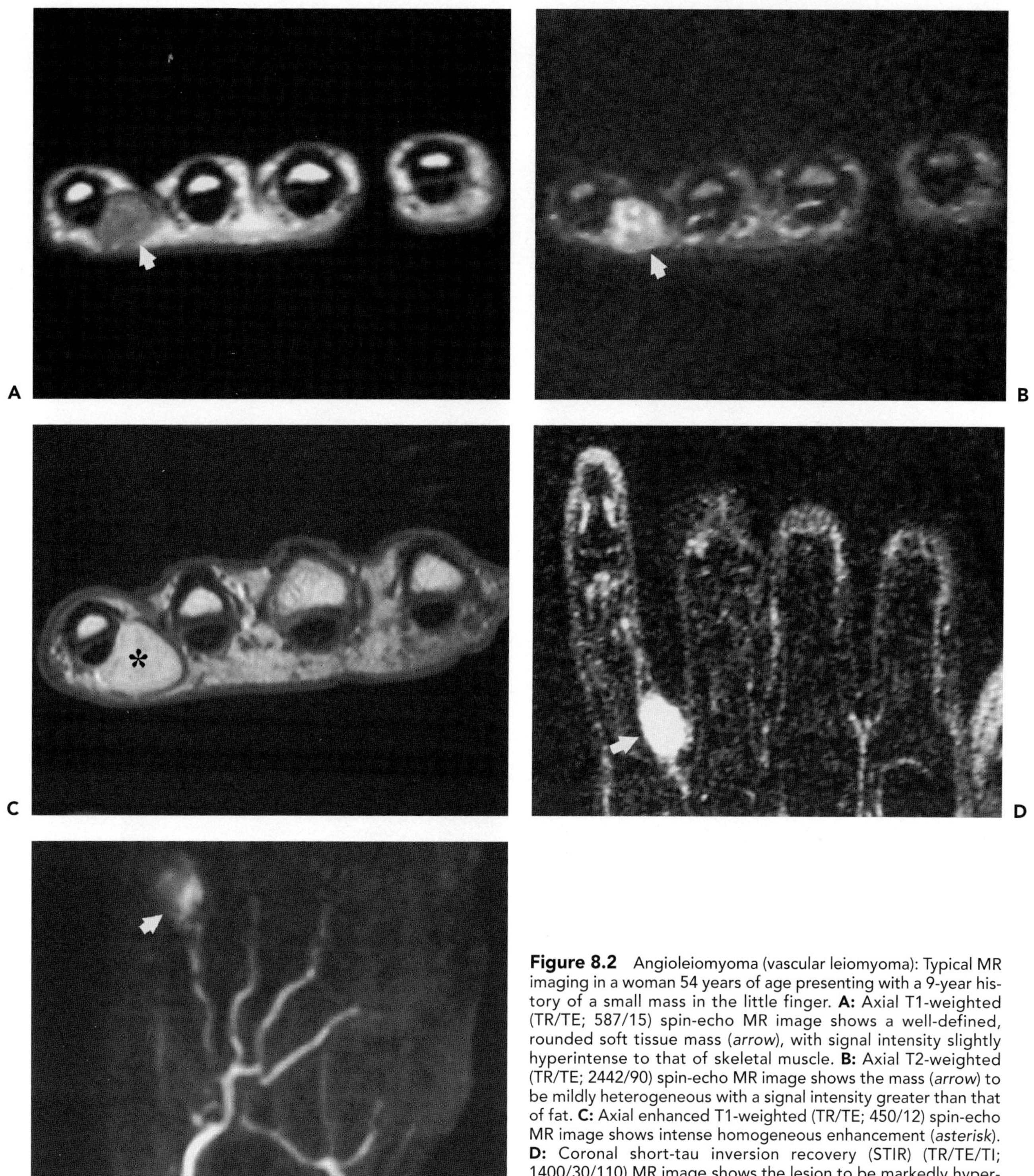

Figure 8.2 Angioleiomyoma (vascular leiomyoma): Typical MR imaging in a woman 54 years of age presenting with a 9-year history of a small mass in the little finger. **A:** Axial T1-weighted (TR/TE; 587/15) spin-echo MR image shows a well-defined, rounded soft tissue mass (*arrow*), with signal intensity slightly hyperintense to that of skeletal muscle. **B:** Axial T2-weighted (TR/TE; 2442/90) spin-echo MR image shows the mass (*arrow*) to be mildly heterogeneous with a signal intensity greater than that of fat. **C:** Axial enhanced T1-weighted (TR/TE; 450/12) spin-echo MR image shows intense homogeneous enhancement (*asterisk*). **D:** Coronal short-tau inversion recovery (STIR) (TR/TE/TI; 1400/30/110) MR image shows the lesion to be markedly hyperintense (*arrow*). **E:** Magnetic resonance angiography using enhanced 3D-volume acquisition shows the marked vascularity and early enhancement of the lesion (*arrow*).

Although radiographically detectable calcification is common in adults, it is rare in patients younger than 16 years but is reported (26,27). Extensive metaplastic ossification within the lesion is also reported (28), which is assumed to be a rare to uncommon occurrence.

On CT the lesion has soft tissue attenuation. Margins are variable, with some well-defined and others poorly delineated; the latter is more likely when the lesion arises within muscle (4,21,22). Following intravenous contrast enhancement, the lesion may show irregular or peripheral

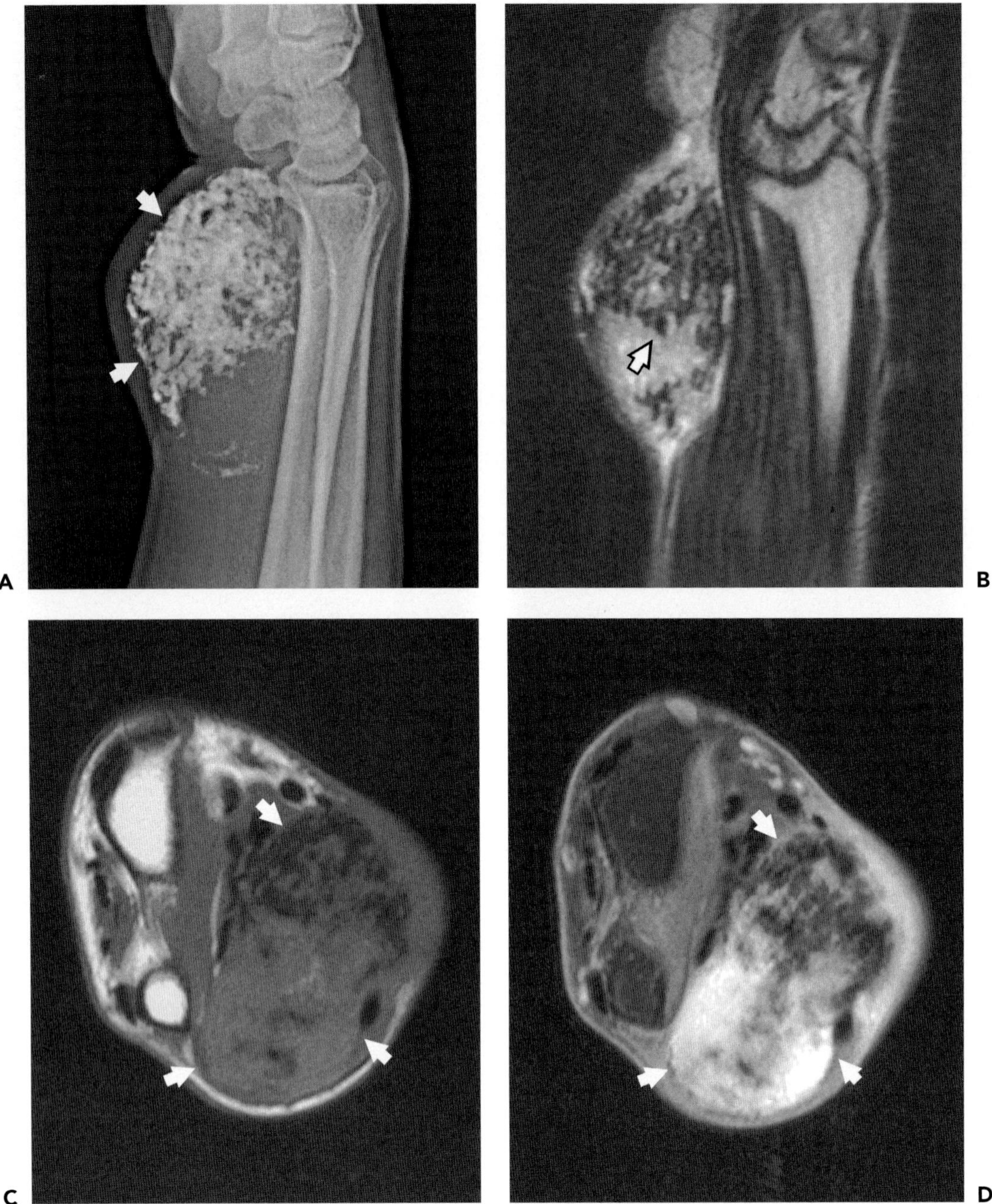

Figure 8.3 Angioleiomyoma (vascular leiomyoma): Atypical imaging in a woman 72 years of age presenting with an 8-year history of a forearm mass. **A:** Lateral radiograph of the forearm shows a densely calcified mass (*arrows*). The calcification is reminiscent of that seen in a uterine leiomyoma. **B:** Sagittal T2-weighted (TR/TE; 3500/105) fast spin-echo MR image shows multiple signal voids (*arrow*), representing areas of calcification. **C,D:** Axial T1-weighted (TR/TE; 417/14) **(C)** and enhanced fat-suppressed T1-weighted (TR/TE; 450/12) **(D)** spin-echo MR images show the subcutaneous mass (*arrows*) and intense homogeneous enhancement in the noncalcified portion of the tumor. (*continued*)

enhancement (21,22). Calcification within the lesion is well seen on CT. Large conglomerate calcifications may mimic mineralization in cartilage lesions (25).

MR experience with this lesion is extremely limited, with MR demonstrating a nonspecific, well-defined soft tissue mass. On T2-weighted sequences, a deep leiomyoma may demonstrate a variable appearance with low, intermediate, and high signal intensities noted (15,21,26,28). The lesion markedly enhances following contrast administration (21,25,28). Enhancement is usually, but not necessarily, homogeneous, and a pattern of peripheral enhancement is also reported (29). Large calcifications within the lesion

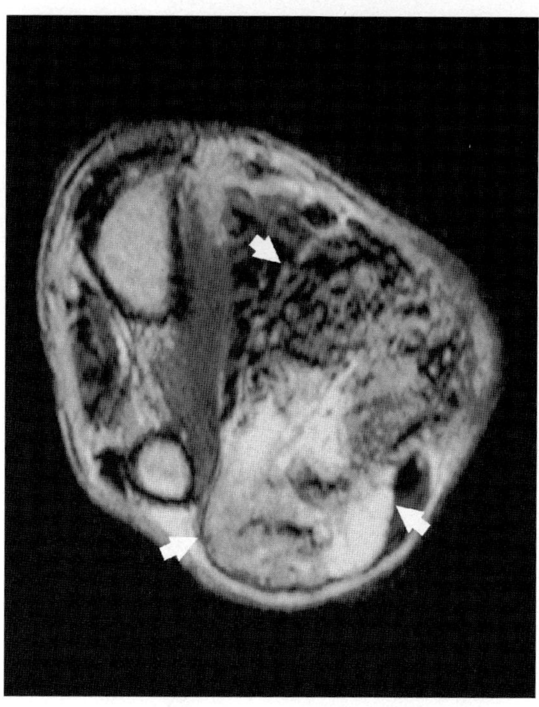

E

Figure 8.3 *(continued)* **E:** Corresponding T2-weighted (TR/TE; 4200/112) fast spin-echo MR image shows the lesion (*arrows*) to have a mixed, predominantly intermediate, signal intensity.

appear as signal voids within the mass. This great variability in MR appearances parallels that seen in uterine smooth muscle tumors (30).

Rhabdomyoma

Originally described in 1864 and termed *rhabdomyoma purum*, rhabdomyoma is a rare benign tumor composed of striated muscle cells (31,32). Although rhabdomyomas make up approximately 2% of muscle tumors (32), only 115 extracardiac rhabdomyomas were reported in the literature through 1988 (33). In a review of 18,677 benign soft tissue tumors at the AFIP, only 15 (0.1%) rhabdomyomas of soft tissue (extracardiac) were noted (1).

Classification

> **KEY CONCEPTS**
> - Rhabdomyoma is classified into cardiac and extracardiac types.
> - Extracardiac rhabdomyoma is further classified into adult, fetal, and genital types.
> - Extracardiac rhabdomyoma is not associated with tuberous sclerosis.

Rhabdomyoma is classified into cardiac and extracardiac types on the basis of location (34). More than half of those patients with cardiac rhabdomyoma have tuberous

sclerosis (35), and it is this association that suggested to some investigators that cardiac rhabdomyoma is a hamartomatous lesion (36). Unlike cardiac rhabdomyoma, extracardiac rhabdomyoma is not associated with tuberous sclerosis and likely represents a true neoplasm (34,37). Because only the extracardiac type may present as a musculoskeletal mass, cardiac lesions are not addressed here.

Extracardiac rhabdomyoma is primarily subclassified into adult and fetal types, depending on the degree of differentiation (34,38). Rarely, rhabdomyoma may occur in the genital tract (genital rhabdomyoma) (36). Although it is convenient to subclassify extracardiac rhabdomyoma, lesions may show overlapping microscopic features, suggesting they are a single group with a spectrum of rhabdomyoblastic differentiation (39).

Adult Rhabdomyoma

The adult rhabdomyoma is a benign mesenchymal tumor with mature skeletal differentiation (34). Although it may occur at any age, the tumor is found most often in middle-aged men, with a mean age in the sixth decade. The male predominance is strong at 2–5:1 (32–34,36,38,40,41). Adult-type rhabdomyoma is rare in children (42).

Adult rhabdomyomas are most commonly seen in the head and neck (90%) and may derive from the musculature of the third and fourth branchial arches (43–45) because they are reported most frequently in the larynx, pharynx, and mouth (32,46–48). Less frequent sites of involvement include the cheek, orbit, and lip (47,49,50); rare cases are reported in the somatic skeletal muscles. Rhabdomyoma may present as a circumscribed intramuscular mass of the tongue or lateral muscles of the neck (32,46), and a lesion presenting in the somatic skeletal muscle may mimic a soft tissue sarcoma. Osseous structure may be remodeled from the adjacent soft tissue mass, but osseous destruction is absent (51).

The lesion is typically a slow-growing, solitary, asymptomatic, polypoid mass. Symptoms include upper airway obstruction or mass and are often long standing, with a median duration of 2 years (34).

Multiple tumor nodules in the same anatomic site are seen in approximately 25% of cases (52); however, true multifocal lesions are unusual, representing approximately 4% of lesions (1,33,53). Bilateral pharyngeal wall lesions are reported (54). Surgery is curative (33,41), although recurrence following surgery may be caused by incomplete excision or a second lesion arising in the same location (53). Local recurrence rates as high as 42% are reported (44). There are no reported cases of malignant transformation (34,54).

Grossly, lesions are typically brown lobulated masses (55). Microscopically, lesions are composed of round to polygonal cells with abundant clear to eosinophilic cytoplasm. Adult rhabdomyomas are strongly periodic

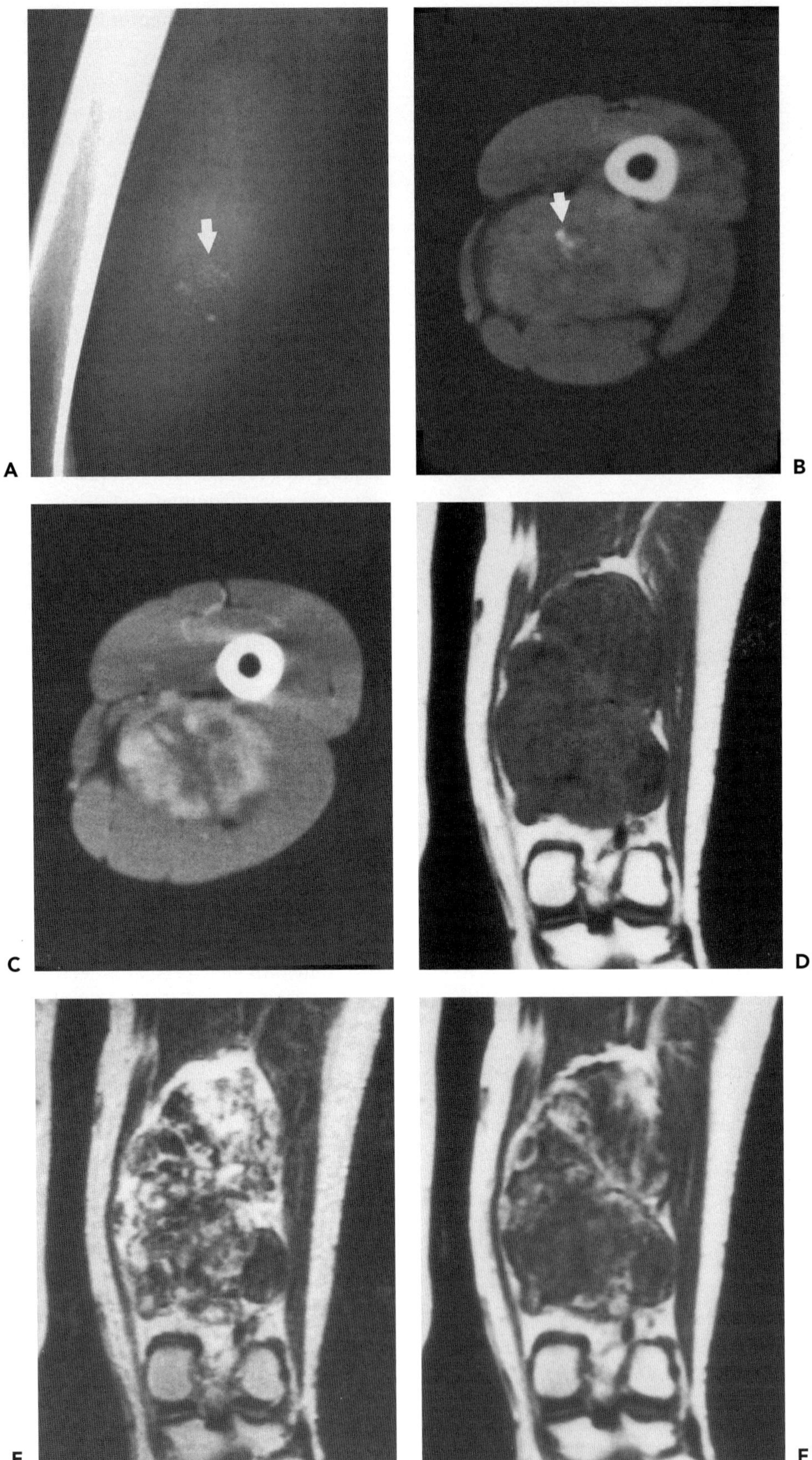

Figure 8.4 Leiomyoma of the deep soft tissue: Typical imaging features in a woman 40 years of age. **A:** Lateral radiograph shows a large soft tissue mass with prominent central mulberry-like calcifications (*arrow*), similar to that noted in uterine leiomyoma. **B:** Axial contrast-enhanced CT scan at the level of the calcifications (*arrow*) shows the mass to be well-defined with diffuse enhancement. **C:** Axial contrast-enhanced CT scan at the level superior to **(B)** shows more pronounced enhancement. **D,E:** Coronal T1-weighted (TR/TE; 410/19) **(D)** T2-weighted (TR/TE; 2100/80) **(E)** spin-echo MR images show the mass to be well-defined and markedly inhomogeneous, with prominent areas of decreased signal on all pulse sequences. **F:** Corresponding coronal T1-weighted (TR/TE; 410/19) spin-echo MR image following contrast administration shows irregular enhancement, more pronounced peripherally. (*continued*)

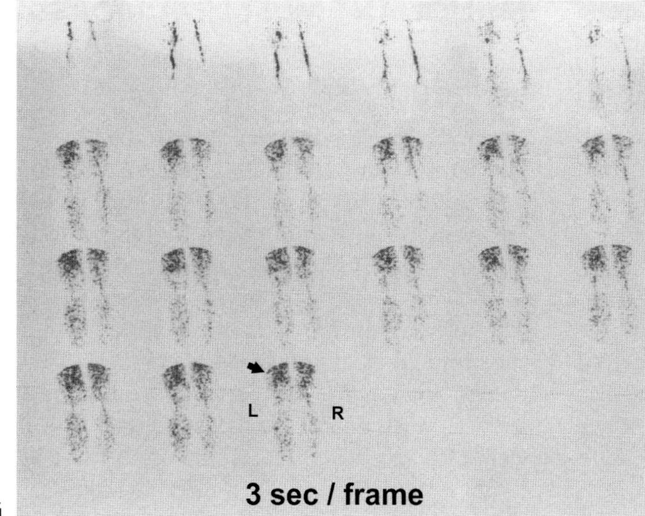
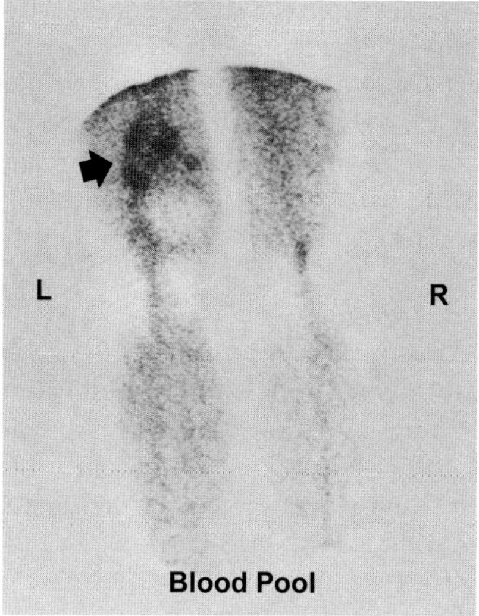

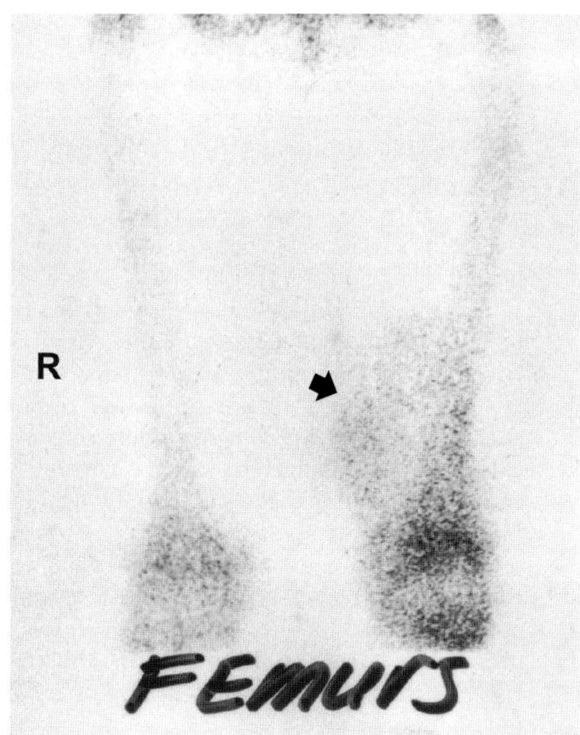

Figure 8.4 *(continued)* **G,H:** Flow **(G)** and blood pool **(H)** images from bone scintigraphy show markedly increased tracer accumulation within the mass (*arrow*). **I:** Delayed static images also show increased tracer accumulation (*arrow*).

acid-Schiff positive, reflecting a high glycogen content (55). Thin and thick filaments (myosin and actin) are dispersed randomly, and the lesions have features of disorganized skeletal muscle cells (55). Cross-striations are readily detected (5). Immunohistochemistry is useful to identify myoglobin, desmin, or both (33), with desmin the most reliable marker to identify smooth or skeletal muscle differentiation (33).

Fetal Rhabdomyoma

The fetal rhabdomyoma, less common than the adult form, is a tumor that exhibits immature skeletal muscle differentiation (32–34,39). Fetal rhabdomyoma is usually seen in children, with a median age at presentation of 4 years (32–34,39). Congenital cases are reported but rare (56). Boys are affected much more commonly than girls, approximately 2.4:1 (34,36,38,39). As is the case with adult rhabdomyoma, the lesion is most common in the head and neck, most often presenting as a well-defined, subcutaneous nodule in the posterior auricular region (39,40,57); however, it may also be located in a distribution similar to that of the adult form (40). Lesions are treated by surgical excision and local recurrence is uncommon. Metastases are not reported (34).

Fetal rhabdomyoma is usually composed of myoid tubules in a myxoid background, having a component of spindle cells (55). More differentiated cells may contain enlarged Z bands in addition to thick and thin filaments (55). Adult rhabdomyoma stains for desmin and myoglobin, but not vimentin; fetal rhabdomyoma stains for all of these markers (33).

Genital Rhabdomyoma

Genital rhabdomyoma is a rare tumor having a high degree of differentiation, with a predilection for the vagina, accruing almost exclusively in middle-aged women (32–34, 40,54). Genital rhabdomyoma may also arise from the cervix or vulva, usually presents as a polyp, and may be long standing (58). Its polypoid or cauliflower-like growth pattern may simulate sarcoma botryoids (32). Histologically, genital rhabdomyoma is similar to fetal rhabdomyoma (55) and sometimes considered to be a variant of fetal rhabdomyoma occurring in the vulvovaginal region (38,39).

Imaging of Rhabdomyoma

KEY CONCEPTS
- MR imaging shows a well-defined mass with signal intensity similar to or greater than that of skeletal muscle on T1- and T2-weighted spin-echo images.
- CT scan reveals an ill-defined lesion with attenuation similar to that of skeletal muscle.
- Homogeneous enhancement follows contrast administration.
- Hemorrhage and/or necrosis are rare.

Scant literature addresses the imaging features of extracardiac rhabdomyoma. On CT scanning, the lesion is ill-defined, demonstrating an attenuation similar to that of skeletal muscle with heterogeneous enhancement following contrast administration (38,58–60). On MR imaging, rhabdomyoma shows a relatively well-defined mass with signal intensity similar to or somewhat greater than that of skeletal muscle on T1- and T2-weighted images (38,46,50,51,58,59) and homogeneous to heterogeneous enhancement following gadolinium administration (38,46,51,59,60). Osgood et al. (50) reported a patient with a fetal rhabdomyoma in the thigh that showed signal intensities between those of skeletal muscle and fat on T1- and T2-weighted images and contained a small focus of central hemorrhagic necrosis with high signal intensity. As would be expected, the lesion demonstrates increased signal intensity on inversion recovery (fat-suppressed) imaging (45) (Figs. 8.5 and 8.6). Because rhabdomyoma is frequently found in the aerodigestive tract, it may be identified as a punctuated mass on barium studies (46).

MALIGNANT MUSCLE TUMORS

Leiomyosarcoma

Leiomyosarcoma represents approximately 9% of all classified sarcomas of soft tissue (including those located in the retroperitoneum) (2,3). It is the third most frequently encountered lesion, following undifferentiated pleomorphic sarcoma (previously classified as malignant fibrous histiocytoma [27%]) and liposarcoma (16%) (2). Although leiomyosarcoma is a relatively common soft tissue tumor, only approximately 12% to 41% of leiomyosarcomas occur in the soft tissue. In a study of 118 patients with leiomyosarcoma studied at the MD Anderson Cancer Center in Houston, Texas, between 1977 and 1983, the tumor site of origin was identified in 114 cases, of which 23 (20%) were located in the retroperitoneum and 14 (12%) were in the soft tissue (61). The remainder of these tumors were located in the alimentary and genitourinary tracts.

Radiation-induced leiomyosarcoma is reported; however, such lesions are quite rare. In a review of the literature in 2003, Demirkan et al. (62) found only 23 reported cases. Approximately a quarter of patients with radiation-induced leiomyosarcoma were treated for retinoblastoma, suggesting a relationship between leiomyosarcoma and the hereditary retinoblastoma gene, Rb1 (62).

Lesions are well-defined, with a firm, fleshy, gray to tan to white cut surface (63,64). Hemorrhage and necrosis are commonly seen in large lesions (64). Histologically, lesions are composed of intersecting, sharply marginated groups of spindle cells (64). Tumor cell nuclei are characteristically elongated and blunt ended (64). Mitotic figures are usually readily apparent. Immunohistochemistry is positive for SMA (smooth muscle actin) and desmin in the great majority of cases (64). Most karyotypes are complex and no consistent aberrations are noted (64). The number of mitotic figures varies considerably; however, 80% of retroperitoneal leiomyosarcomas average five or more mitoses/ten high-power fields (65).

In general terms, the prognosis for leiomyosarcoma is guarded. In a recent review of 1,256 malignancies, in which outcome data were available, Mankin et al. noted leiomyosarcoma had the highest death rate, at 50%, as compared to 24% for all sarcomas (66). In this report, median survival was 4.2 years (range: 1 to 11 years); with metastases at presentation being the most significant prognostic factor. In patients with metastases, the lungs are most commonly affected, seen in approximately 90% of cases. Metastases to bone (20%) and viscera and lymph nodes (17%) are much less frequent (66). Although the incidence of brain metastasis in patients with leiomyosarcoma is unknown, leiomyosarcoma is the most frequent type of soft tissue sarcoma to metastasize to the brain, representing 20% of soft tissue sarcoma brain metastases (67).

Classification

> **KEY CONCEPTS**
> - Malignant muscle tumors are classically subdivided into three groups: cutaneous, major vessel, and soft tissue.
> - Cutaneous lesions arise from the pilar structure and usually have an excellent prognosis.
> - Leiomyosarcoma in association with a major vessel is considered rare, with veins affected four to five times more frequently than arteries.
> - Soft tissue leiomyosarcoma is further divided into lesions of the somatic soft tissue and lesions of the retroperitoneum/abdomen.

Leiomyosarcoma arising in soft tissue can be divided into several subgroups: cutaneous, major vessel, and soft tissue (19,65). Cutaneous lesions arise from the pilar structures, and when limited to the dermis, they have an excellent prognosis (19). Leiomyosarcomas arising in association with major arteries and veins are rare and discussed in greater detail later. Soft tissue leiomyosarcomas make up the majority of leiomyosarcomas that come to the attention of the musculoskeletal radiologist. These soft tissue leiomyosarcomas are typically further subdivided into those arising in the peripheral or somatic soft tissues of the extremities and those arising in the retroperitoneum and abdomen (19).

Retroperitoneal/abdominal leiomyosarcomas are approximately twice as common as those arising in the somatic soft tissue. Somatic soft tissue leiomyosarcomas arise in the superficial or deep soft tissues of the extremities, where they are usually intimately associated with a small vessel (19).

Soft Tissue Leiomyosarcoma

The majority of patients presenting with soft tissue leiomyosarcoma are middle-aged to older adults, with a median age in the fifth and sixth decade (68–70), although rarely, leiomyosarcoma may present in children (17). The most common soft tissue location is the retroperitoneum, with approximately 20% to 67% of lesions occurring in this location (2,61,68–71). Leiomyosarcoma is the second most common retroperitoneal tumor in adults (72), following liposarcoma. Approximately 12% to 41% of leiomyosarcomas occur in the peripheral soft tissue (2,61,69), with the thigh the most common peripheral location (69,70).

For unknown reasons, retroperitoneal tumors occur more commonly in women, with a reported ratio ranging from 2:1 to 7:1 (19,68,69); conversely, men are more commonly affected when the lesion is in peripheral soft tissues (69). Overall, men and women are affected by leiomyosarcoma approximately equally (2). The vast majority of patients with retroperitoneal tumors present with an abdominal mass or swelling, with pain seen in only approximately 10% of patients (68). In the extremities, leiomyosarcoma typically presents as a painless, slowly growing soft tissue mass, which may appear benign clinically (70). Retroperitoneal lesions tend to be larger than those in the peripheral soft tissues, and they are generally larger than 10 cm when detected (19,68). Leiomyosarcoma of the somatic soft tissues tends to be considerably smaller than retroperitoneal leiomyosarcoma at presentation (19).

The prognosis for patients with leiomyosarcoma is guarded. The overall median 5-year survival is 35%, with a median survival of 43 months (69). The prognosis is worse for tumors larger than 5 cm and those located in the retroperitoneum (69): 80% to 95% of patients with retroperitoneal tumors die of disease within 2 to 5 years (19). Retroperitoneal tumors also metastasize more frequently than do those in the peripheral soft tissues; moreover, they generally have a poor outcome despite therapy (69). Metastases are most common to the lungs, occurring in more than half of those patients with metastatic disease (53%) (68). The liver is a close second, with 47% metastases (68). Less frequent sites of metastatic disease include the soft tissue (23%), bone, lymph nodes, and gastrointestinal tract (18% each) (68). Although mitotic rate is important in diagnosis, it does not correlate with outcome (73,74). Leiomyosarcoma lesions of the somatic soft tissue are generally smaller than retroperitoneal tumors, but they seem to have a more aggressive clinical course (19).

Leiomyosarcoma in Association with Vessels

Leiomyosarcoma may arise in association with a vessel. Such lesions were traditionally thought to be quite rare, with only limited reports in the literature. They are also quite rare at autopsy (65). Recently, it has been suggested that a vascular origin for leiomyosarcoma may be more common than previously reported; however, it is difficult to determine how frequently this occurs (65). Hashimoto et al. (75), in a review of 25 cases involving the soft tissue, noted that 6 cases (24%) demonstrated anatomic location and histologic features suggesting that the lesion arose within a venous wall. Weiss and Goldblum make a similar observation, noting that at least a third of cases arise from or involve a vessel (65). Thus, although leiomyosarcomas in association with vessels are perceived as quite rare, they may be more common than previously thought.

Venous Leiomyosarcoma. Leiomyosarcoma of the large veins is approximately four to five times more frequent than those occurring in arteries (76,77). The most common location of venous leiomyosarcoma is the inferior vena cava, accounting for approximately 50% of reported venous cases. In a report of 13 cases and review of the

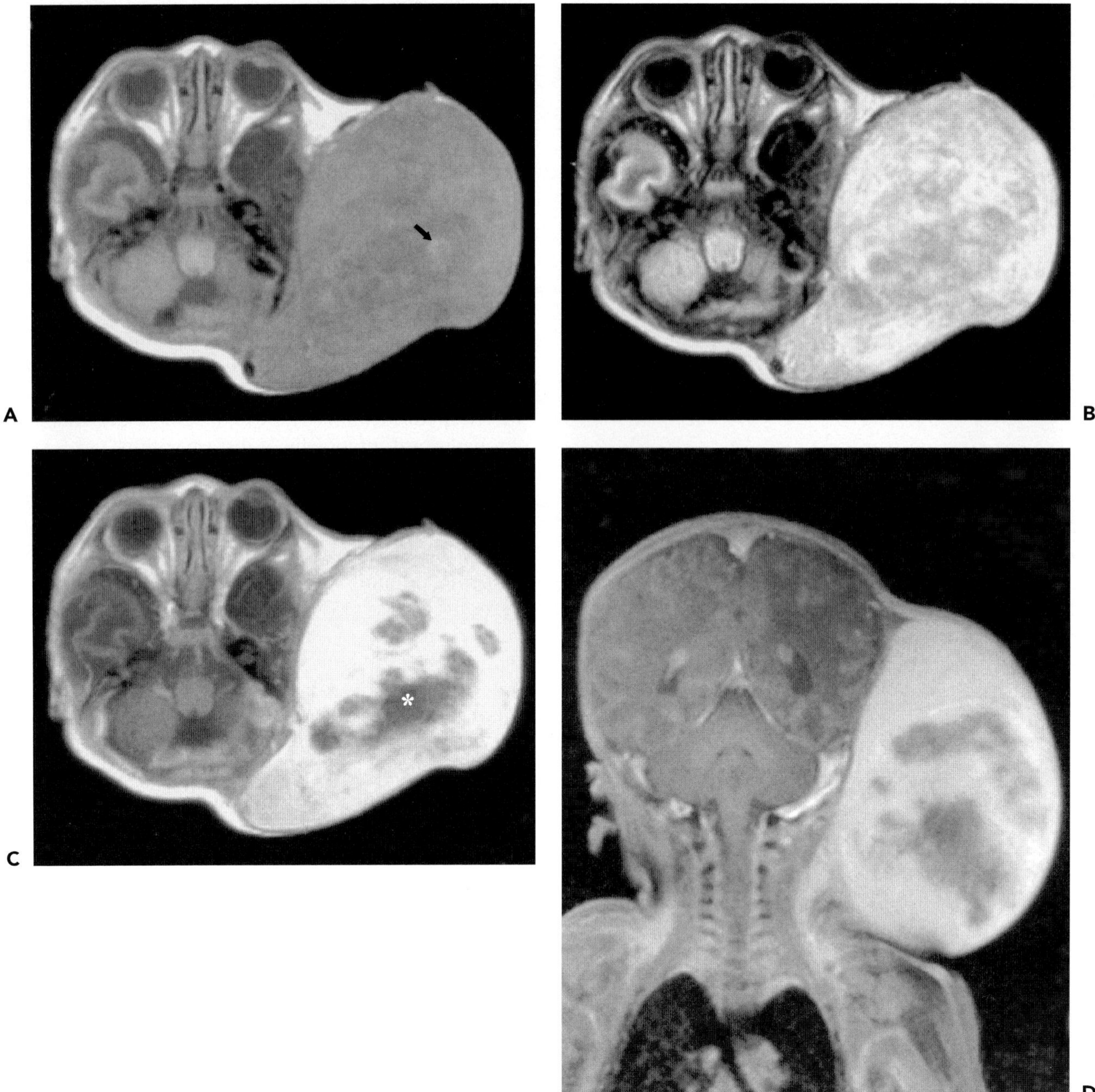

Figure 8.5 Fetal rhabdomyoma: Typical MR imaging features in a rare congenital lesion in a 1-day-old boy with a large scalp mass. **A,B:** Axial T1-weighted (TR/TE; 763/17) **(A)** spin-echo and short-tau inversion recovery (STIR) (TR/TE/TI; 7000/105/180) **(B)** MR images show a well-defined, heterogeneous, superficial mass with intermediate signal intensity on T1-weighted and high signal intensity on fluid-sensitive images. Note small area of hemorrhage (*arrow*) in **(A)**. **C,D:** Enhanced T1-weighted axial (TR/TE; 450/12) **(C)** and coronal (TR/TE; 511/17) **(D)** spin-echo MR images show intense heterogeneous enhancement with prominent central nonenhancing region (*asterisk* in **C**).

literature in 1992, Dzsinich et al. (77) found a total of 210 cases of primary venous leiomyosarcoma. Approximately a third of these cases involved the lower extremity, with only a few cases in the upper extremity. Following the vena cava, the saphenous, femoral, iliac, and popliteal veins are involved in decreasing order of frequency (78). Saphenous and femoral vein involvement occur with approximately

equal frequency and account for approximately half of all venous leiomyosarcomas not involving the vena cava (76,78). Rare lesions of the renal veins may extend into the inferior vena cava (79).

The clinical presentation of patients with venous leiomyosarcoma is quite variable. Patients may present with poorly defined pain, edema, or a mass (80). Popliteal

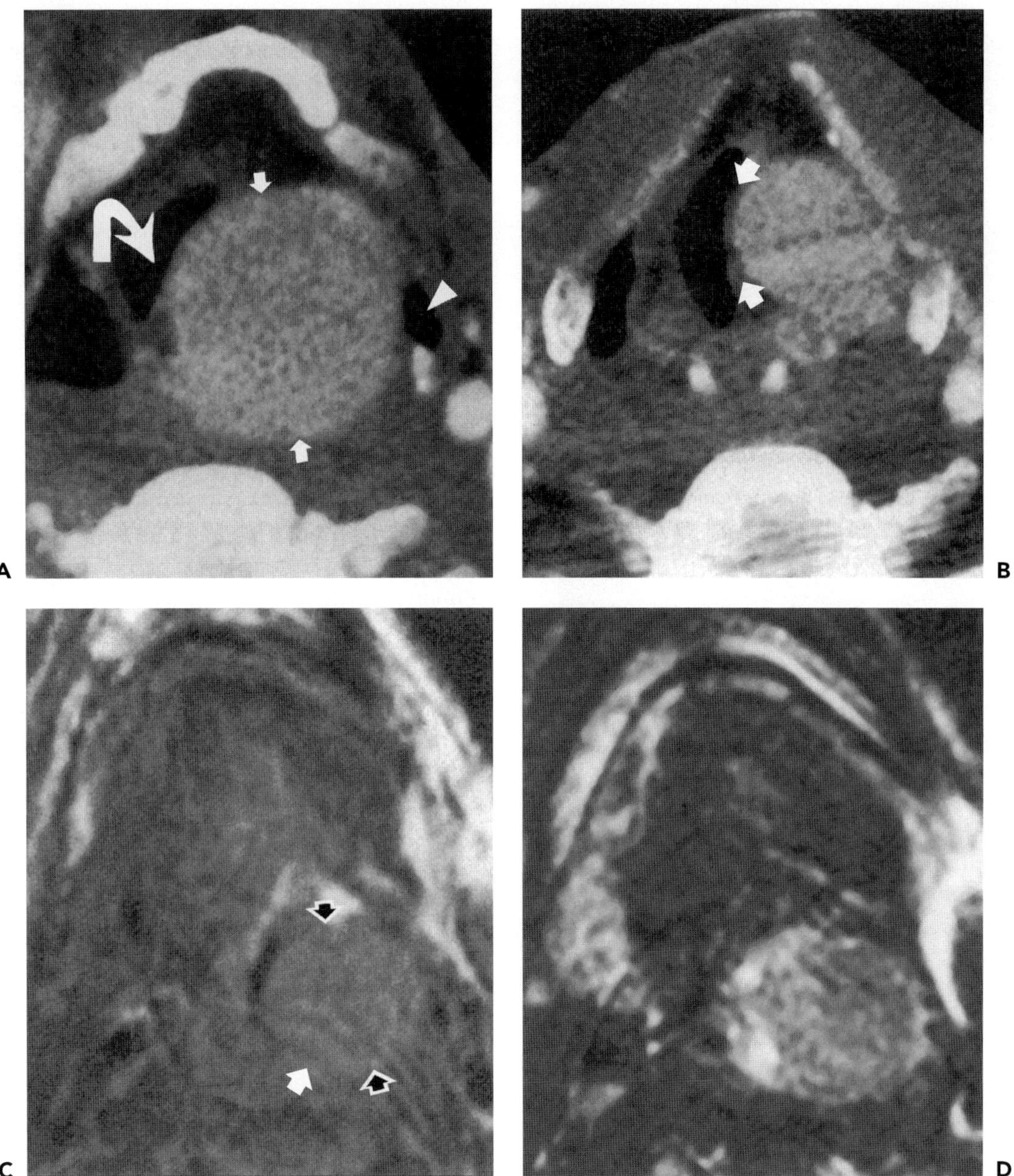

Figure 8.6 Adult rhabdomyoma: Typical CT and MR imaging features in lesion involving the paraglottic space in a man 39 years of age. **A:** Contrast-enhanced CT scan of the neck at the level of the supraglottis shows submucosal mass (*arrows*) at the level of the left aryepiglottic fold. Note airway deviation from left to right (*curved arrow*) and partial effacement of the left-sided piriform sinus (*arrowhead*). **B:** Contrast-enhanced CT scan obtained 1 cm below **(A)** shows preservation of fat plane (*arrows*), demarcating mass from mucosal surface and submucosal location. **C:** Axial T1-weighted (TR/TE; 400/9) spin-echo MR image shows submucosal mass (*black arrows*) mildly hyperintense to adjacent muscle. Indistinct margins of mass blend into adjacent prevertebral musculature (*white arrow*). **D:** Axial T2-weighted (TR/TE; 2500/90) spin-echo MR image shows the mass to be hyperintense to skeletal muscle. (*continued*)

vein leiomyosarcoma may mimic deep venous thrombosis (78). As with leiomyosarcoma elsewhere, the prognosis remains guarded, with a 5-year survival rate of 32% (78). Approximately 10% of patients have metastatic disease at the time of diagnosis, typically to the lungs or the liver (80).

Arterial Leiomyosarcoma. When leiomyosarcoma arises from the arteries, it is encountered twice as frequently in the pulmonary artery as in the major peripheral arteries (81). In a review of the literature in 2003 of nonaortic leiomyosarcoma of the peripheral arteries, Blansfield et al. (81) reported a case in the common iliac artery and

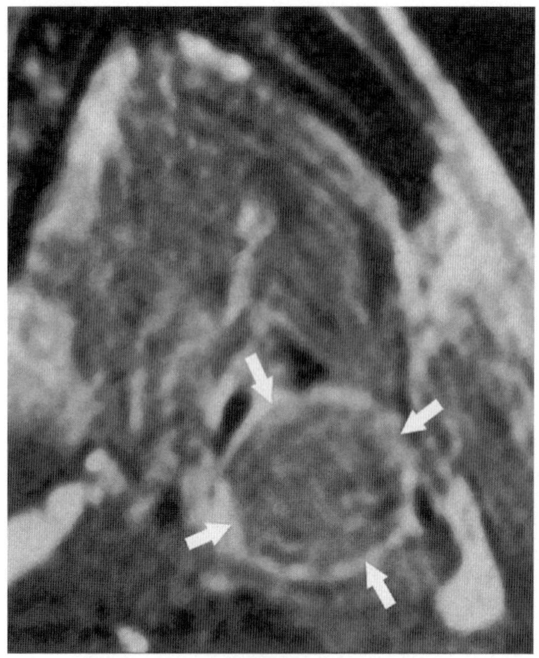

E

Figure 8.6 *(continued)* **E:** Axial enhanced T1-weighted (TR/TE; 409/9) spin-echo MR image shows mild homogeneous enhancement, with more prominent rim enhancement (*arrows*). (Case courtesy of Grace S. Liang, MD, University of Pennsylvania Medical Center; from reference 46 with permission.)

identified 18 previously reported cases of arterial leiomyosarcoma. The 19 reported patients had a mean age of 59 years (range: 33 to 79 years), with men and women affected approximately equally. The iliac artery was involved most frequently (26%), followed closely by the femoral and popliteal arteries (21% each).

Patients with leiomyosarcoma of a major peripheral artery typically present with symptoms of vascular insufficiency, pain, and mass (81). Occasionally, these tumors may be confused with pseudoaneurysms on arteriography (81). Tumor growth may be intra- or extraluminal; however, often both are present (82). In general, intraluminal growth follows the direction of blood flow (82) and associated thrombosis is common (82). Complete surgical resection is the cornerstone of treatment. Approximately half of patients develop metastatic disease, most commonly to the lungs (81). Lesions are usually large, firm, and bulky, although occasionally there are soft friable areas and even cystic areas (68). Microscopically, there are uniform, slightly tapered, eosinophilic spindle cells with elongated and blunt-ended nuclei, arranged in an interlacing fascicular pattern (68). Cell bundles occasionally are separated by myxoid or fibrous intracellular matrix, and a storiform pattern may sometimes be seen (69). Tumor necrosis is common (69). Histologic findings are not related to prognosis (69).

Superficial Leiomyosarcoma

Leiomyosarcoma accounts for approximately 2% to 6% of all sarcomas in the subcutaneous tissues (70). Superficial leiomyosarcoma affects men more commonly than women

(2–3:1) (10), arising in either the dermis or subcutis. Lesions that arise in the dermis generally present as small, firm, solitary nodules, less than 2 cm in diameter (10). Metastases to local lymph nodes may occur; however, the overall prognosis is favorable (10). Subcutaneous lesions tend to be larger and are associated with a poorer prognosis than those lesions originating in the dermis (10). Cutaneous leiomyosarcomas metastasize in 10% of cases or less; subcutaneous lesions metastasize in 30% to 40% of cases (83).

Gastrointestinal Stromal Tumor

The term *gastrointestinal stromal tumor* (GIST) is used to identify a relatively rare group of mesenchymal neoplasms that typically arise in the muscularis propria of the gastrointestinal tract wall (84). These lesions account for 0.1% to 3.0% of all gastrointestinal neoplasms and are distinct from stromal tumors of other sites (i.e., uterus, breast) (85,86). These tumors are identified immunohistochemically by the expression of c-kit proto-oncogene cell membrane protein (CD117), not seen in smooth muscle tumors (87,88). Although most GISTs are benign, tumor behavior varies with location. In the stomach, a location that accounts for 60% to 70% of all GIST tumors, the majority are benign. There is a higher percentage of malignant lesions in the small bowel, which accounts for approximately 20% to 30% of GIST tumors. The remaining 10% to 15% of lesions, found in the esophagus and colon, are usually malignant (9). Patients are typically in the sixth decade, and, unlike retroperitoneal leiomyosarcomas, which are more common in women, these tumors are more frequently encountered in men (85).

Extragastrointestinal stromal tumors are rare in comparison to their gastrointestinal counterparts (86). In a report of more than 1,000 GIST tumors, less than 7% arose outside the gastrointestinal tract, localized to the omentum, mesentery, or peritoneum (89). In a report of 116 malignant GISTs, only 3 were clearly extragastrointestinal, arising in the retroperitoneum, pelvis, and mesocolon (85).

Imaging of Leiomyosarcoma

> **KEY CONCEPTS**
> - Imaging of leiomyosarcoma is typically nonspecific.
> - Large lesions frequently demonstrate hemorrhage, necrosis, and cystic change.
> - Leiomyosarcoma in association with a major vessel shows a mass intimately associated with the vessel wall.
> - Radiographic mineralization is reported in 12% to 17% of soft tissue lesions.
> - Arteriography shows a hypervascular mass with arteriovenous shunting.

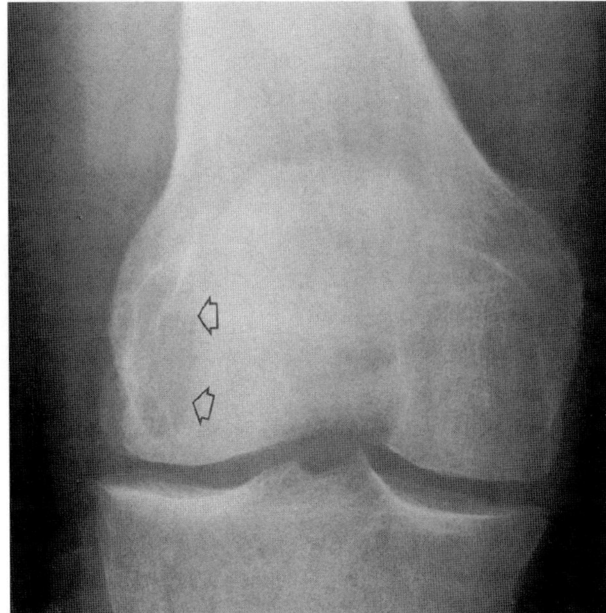

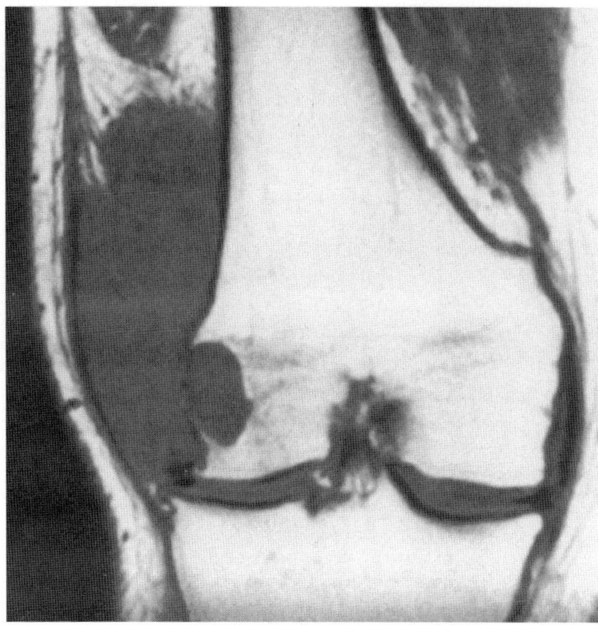

Figure 8.7   Leiomyosarcoma with bone invasion: Typical features in a man 39 years of age with a mass in the vastus lateralis muscle. **A:** Anteroposterior radiograph shows subtle area of lucency in the lateral femoral condyle (*arrows*). **B:** Corresponding coronal T1-weighted (TR/TE; 600/12) spin-echo MR image shows a nonspecific mass invading the lateral femoral condyle.

Radiographs are usually not specific, demonstrating a soft tissue mass. Calcification and invasion of the adjacent bone may be seen (Fig. 8.7). The prevalence of mineralization in leiomyosarcoma is variable and likely relatively uncommon; however, Bush et al. found mineralization in 4 (17%) of 24 cases (63). In this review, mineralization was found in 2 (12%) of 16 soft tissue lesions and in 2 (25%) of 8 osseous lesions. Mineralization in these cases ranged from faint to densely amorphous. One case was described as showing regions of ossification.

CT imaging may show a nonspecific mass (90), but especially when lesions are large, it frequently demonstrates areas of decreased attenuation corresponding to hemorrhage, necrosis, and cystic change seen grossly (Figs. 8.8 and 8.9). The CT appearance is not specific, but the diagnosis should be considered when a large mass is seen with central necrosis or liquefaction and liver metastases that also appear necrotic or cystic. Calcification is uncommonly reported (61). CT is especially useful in follow-up of patients with retroperitoneal sarcomas, assessing not only the operative bed, but also the lungs and liver. Gupta et al. (91), in a review of 33 patients with retroperitoneal sarcomas, found 25 (76%) recurred within 2 years. In this study, 4 (57%) of 7 patients with liver metastases had leiomyosarcoma.

MR imaging is typically nonspecific, reflecting a nonfatty mass (Fig. 8.10). Larger lesions are usually more heterogeneous and show necrosis (Fig. 8.11) (72). Leiomyosarcoma should be considered in the differential diagnosis for any large deep soft tissue mass with evidence of necrosis, especially those in the retroperitoneum with evidence of metastatic disease. Leiomyosarcoma typically is isointense to skeletal muscle on T1-weighted images and variably hyperintense relative to muscle on T2-weighted images, with prominent enhancement following gadolinium administration (63). Regions of mineralization show

Figure 8.8   Leiomyosarcoma: Typical CT features in a man 70 years of age with a thigh mass. Axial contrast-enhanced CT scan of the thighs shows a large inhomogeneous mass (*asterisk*) in the anterior aspect of the left thigh with large areas of hemorrhage/necrosis.

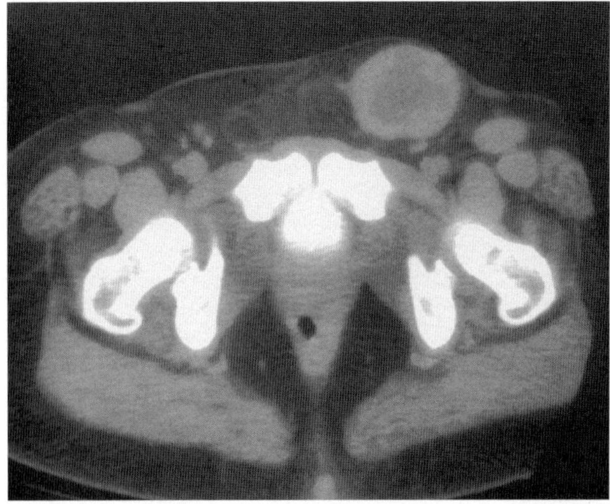

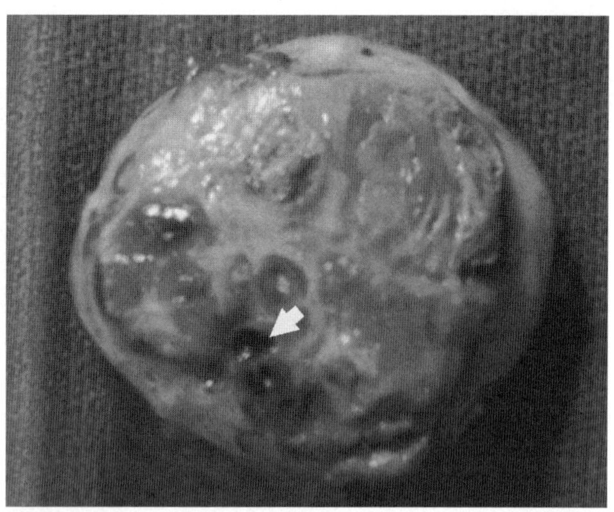

Figure 8.9 Subcutaneous leiomyosarcoma: CT features in a woman 34 years of age with a history of a mass, growing over 6 months. **A:** Axial contrast-enhanced CT scan of the thighs shows a relatively well-defined mass in the subcutaneous adipose tissue anterior to the left hip. **B:** Photograph of the bisected gross specimen shows hemorrhage and necrosis (*arrow*).

decreased signal intensity on both T1-weighted and T2-weighted images (63).

Leiomyosarcomas in association with the femoral and the greater saphenous vein are noted as well-defined masses, with a signal intensity similar to that of skeletal muscle on T1-weighted images and similar to that of fat on T2-weighted spin-echo MR images (Fig. 8.12) (82,92). Lesions may expand the lumen of the vein. Although an intermediate signal intensity is often seen, lesions may demonstrate a low to intermediate signal intensity on T1-weighted images and high signal intensity on T2-weighted images (78). If intraluminal thrombus is present, it can be distinguished from tumor when clot is subacute because of the high T1-signal intensity in subacute blood (78). Vena caval tumors may show extensive intraluminal clots (Figs. 8.13 and 8.14).

Superficial lesions are usually much smaller than deep lesions, and they may be well-defined and homogeneous; consequently, leiomyosarcoma should be included in the differential diagnosis of a nonspecific superficial mass (Fig. 8.15). Although typically small, large superficial lesions can be found, and larger lesions may demonstrate hemorrhage and necrosis usually seen in deep lesions (Fig. 8.16). Arteriography usually demonstrates a hypervascular mass (93). Arteriovenous shunting is a common finding, and intravenous tumor extension may also be seen (93).

As with other leiomyosarcomas, most GIST tumors are large at presentation, often greater than 10 cm. Extensive hemorrhage and necrosis are frequent. In general, GISTs do not exhibit lymphatic spread, and lymphadenopathy is a rare finding (88). Omental, mesenteric, or peritoneal seeding are typical in malignant disease, as are liver (50%) and lung (10%) metastases (Fig. 8.17) (88).

Rhabdomyosarcoma

Rhabdomyosarcoma is the most common childhood malignancy of soft tissue, accounting for approximately 19% of *all* childhood soft tissue sarcomas (32) and 5% to 8% of all childhood cancers (94,95). It is exceeded in number only by Wilms' tumor and neuroblastoma (96–98). Almost two-thirds of cases develop in children younger than 10 years (99). Rhabdomyosarcoma was originally thought to arise from striated muscle, but it is now regarded as a primary mesenchymal tumor in which rhabdomyoblastic differentiation has occurred (97).

Unlike tumors of adipose tissue or blood vessels, malignant tumors with skeletal muscle differentiation are much more common than benign tumors (55). The reason is unknown, as is the reason for the strong predilection for children and young adults (55). Normal myogenesis is completed by the second fetal trimester, and the association of this tumor with children suggests that intrinsic genetic and tissue factors, rather than external carcinogenic factors, are involved in its pathogenesis (55).

The vast majority of cases appear to be sporadic (99); however, an increased incidence of rhabdomyosarcoma is noted in patients with neurofibromatosis type I, with McKeen et al. (100) reporting 5 (6%) such cases among 84 patients. Rhabdomyosarcoma is also reported in association with Beckwith-Wiedemann syndrome, Li-Fraumeni syndrome, Costello syndrome, a variety of congenital anomalies, and parental use of cocaine and marijuana (99).

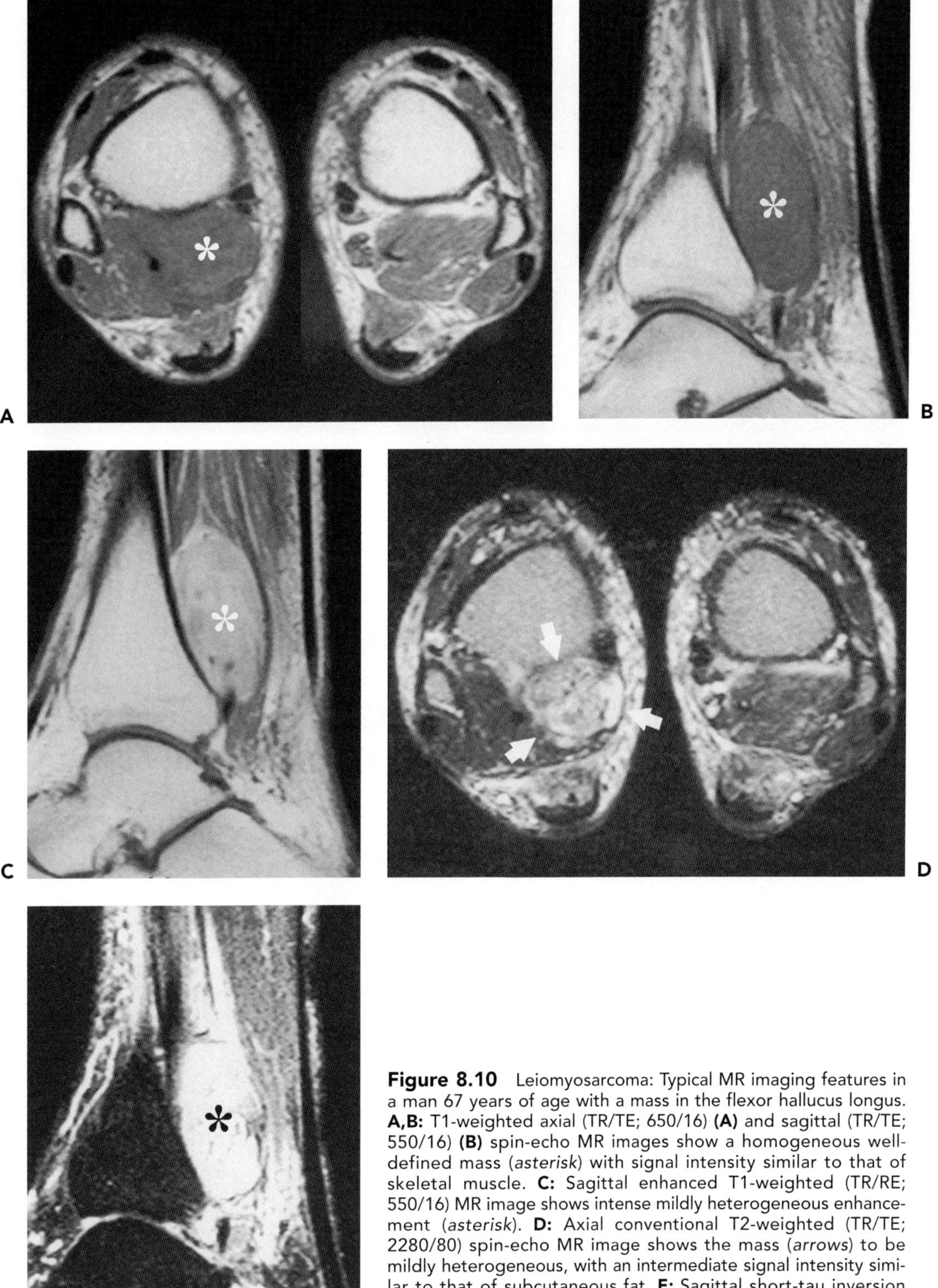

Figure 8.10 Leiomyosarcoma: Typical MR imaging features in a man 67 years of age with a mass in the flexor hallucus longus. **A,B:** T1-weighted axial (TR/TE; 650/16) **(A)** and sagittal (TR/TE; 550/16) **(B)** spin-echo MR images show a homogeneous well-defined mass (*asterisk*) with signal intensity similar to that of skeletal muscle. **C:** Sagittal enhanced T1-weighted (TR/RE; 550/16) MR image shows intense mildly heterogeneous enhancement (*asterisk*). **D:** Axial conventional T2-weighted (TR/TE; 2280/80) spin-echo MR image shows the mass (*arrows*) to be mildly heterogeneous, with an intermediate signal intensity similar to that of subcutaneous fat. **E:** Sagittal short-tau inversion recovery (STIR) (TR/TE/TI; 2117/30/130) MR image shows nonspecific increased signal intensity (*asterisk*).

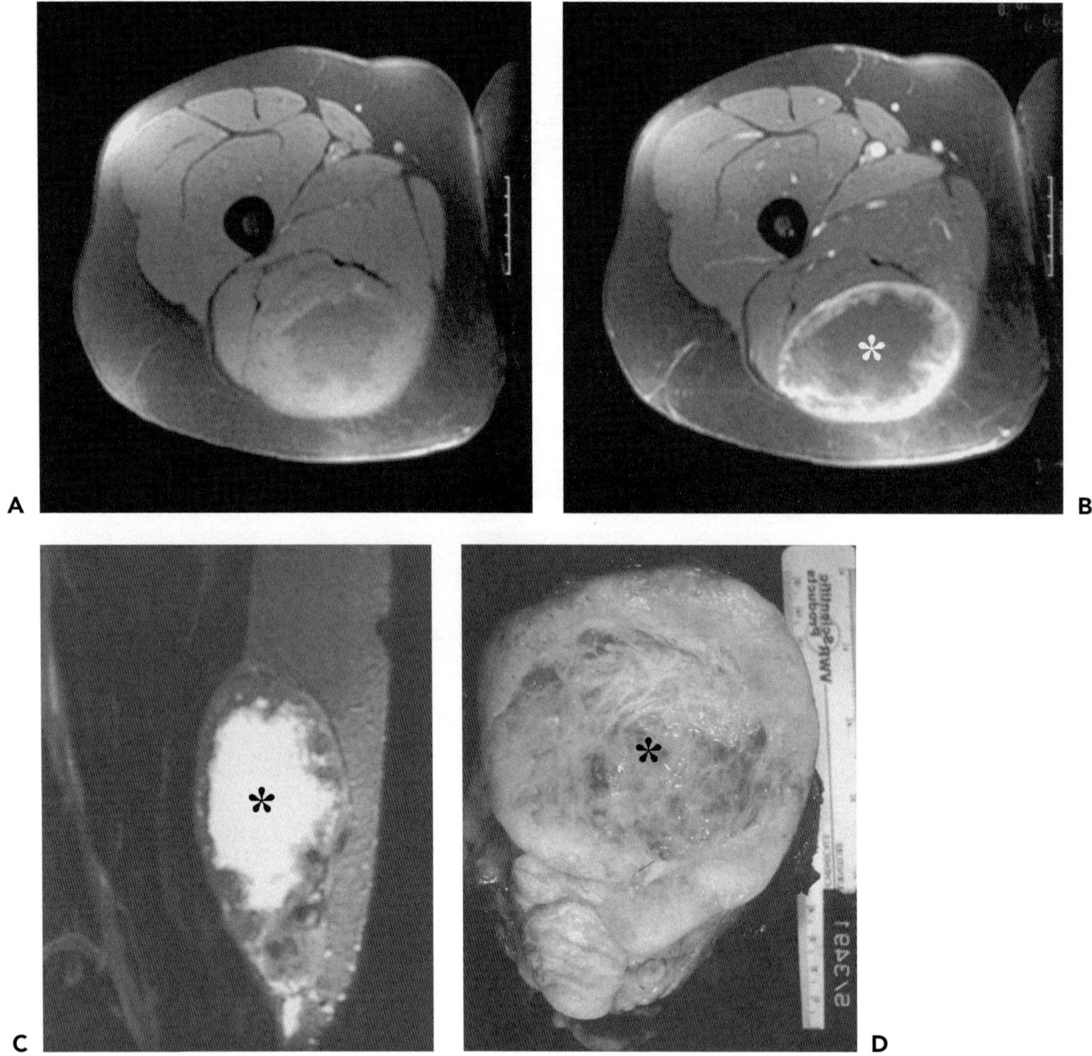

Figure 8.11 Leiomyosarcoma: Typical imaging in large intramuscular mass in the posterior compartment of the thigh of a man 41 years of age. **A,B:** Axial spoiled gradient (TR/TE/Flip; 160/4/75) MR images preceding **(A)** and following **(B)** intravenous contrast show a large mass (*asterisk*) with intense peripheral enhancement. **C:** Sagittal short-tau inversion recovery (STIR) (TR/TE/TI; 6500/77/110) MR image shows a large mass in the posterior thigh. Central high signal intensity (*asterisk*) represents central necrosis. Solid peripheral portion of the mass shows an intermediate signal intensity. **D:** Corresponding gross photograph shows central necrosis (*asterisk*) within the mass.

The most common primary sites for rhabdomyosarcoma are genitourinary (24%), parameningeal (16%), extremity (19%), orbit (9%), other head and neck (10%), and miscellaneous other sites (22%) (99). Although the lesion most typically presents as a painless mass, symptoms vary with the primary site. Genitourinary tumors may present with hematuria, whereas parameningeal lesions may demonstrate cranial nerve dysfunction (99).

There is a slight male predominance (1.67:1) (96), and whites are affected three times as frequently as blacks (32). The head and neck regions, including the orbit, maxillary antra, and nasopharynx, are most frequently involved, with approximately 60% of cases occurring in these regions (96,97). The genitourinary system accounts for approximately 14% to 25% of lesions (32,97), usually from the deep pelvic structures, in the region of the pelvic floor, bladder, and vulva and vagina (96). An estimated 15% of tumors arise in the extremities, and approximately 5% each are in the retroperitoneum and trunk (97). In a series of 558 cases reported by Enzinger and Weiss, the two most common locations were in the orbit and paratesticular region (upper pole of the testis, spermatic cord, and epididymis), each with approximately 20% of lesions (101).

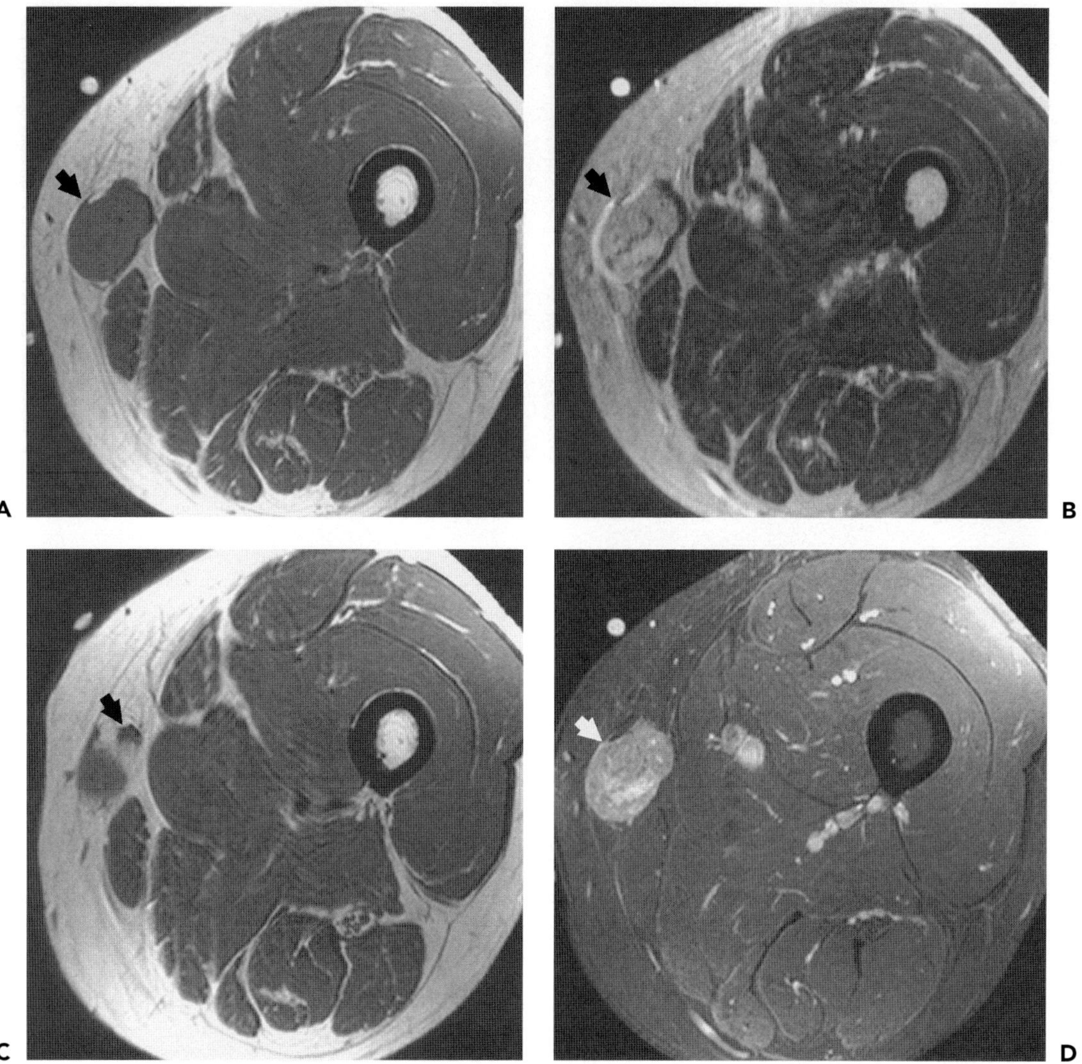

Figure 8.12   Leiomyosarcoma, saphenous vein: Typical imaging in a man 52 years of age presenting with a slowly growing thigh mass. **A,B:** Axial T1-weighted (TR/TE; 802/17) **(A)** and T2-weighted (TR/TE; 2350/80) **(B)** spin-echo MR images show a mass (*arrow*) in the subcutaneous adipose tissue of the medial thigh. The lesion shows an intermediate signal intensity on both imaging sequences. **C:** Axial T1-weighted (TR/TE; 802/17) spin-echo MR image just inferior to **(A)** at the inferior margin of the mass shows the greater saphenous vein (*arrow*) that was intimately associated with the mass. **D:** Axial fat-suppressed enhanced T1-weighted (TR/TE; 675/17) spin-echo MR image shows mildly intense heterogeneous enhancement (*arrow*). (*continued*)

Classification

> ### KEY CONCEPTS
> - Rhabdomyosarcoma is classically subdivided into three groups: embryonal, alveolar, and pleomorphic.
> - Spindle cell and botryoid rhabdomyosarcoma are variants of embryonal rhabdomyosarcoma.
> - Lesions in the head, neck, and genitourinary system are most commonly embryonal (80%).
> - Lesions in the extremities are typically alveolar (70%).

The World Health Organization (WHO) classifies rhabdomyosarcoma into three main subgroups: embryonal, alveolar, and pleomorphic. The spindle cell and botryoid rhabdomyosarcoma are considered variants of embryonal rhabdomyosarcoma (102). The botryoid and spindle cell rhabdomyosarcoma have a superior prognosis, the embryonal rhabdomyosarcoma has an intermediate prognosis, and alveolar and pleomorphic subtypes have a poor prognosis.

Embryonal Rhabdomyosarcoma

Embryonal is the most common type, accounting for approximately 55% to 70% of all rhabdomyosarcomas. It most frequently occurs in the first decade of life and is most often encountered in the orbit, head, and neck (approximately 47%) and in the genitourinary regions (approximately 28%) (3,32,39,99,102). Head and neck lesions are usually located in the soft tissues intrinsic to or

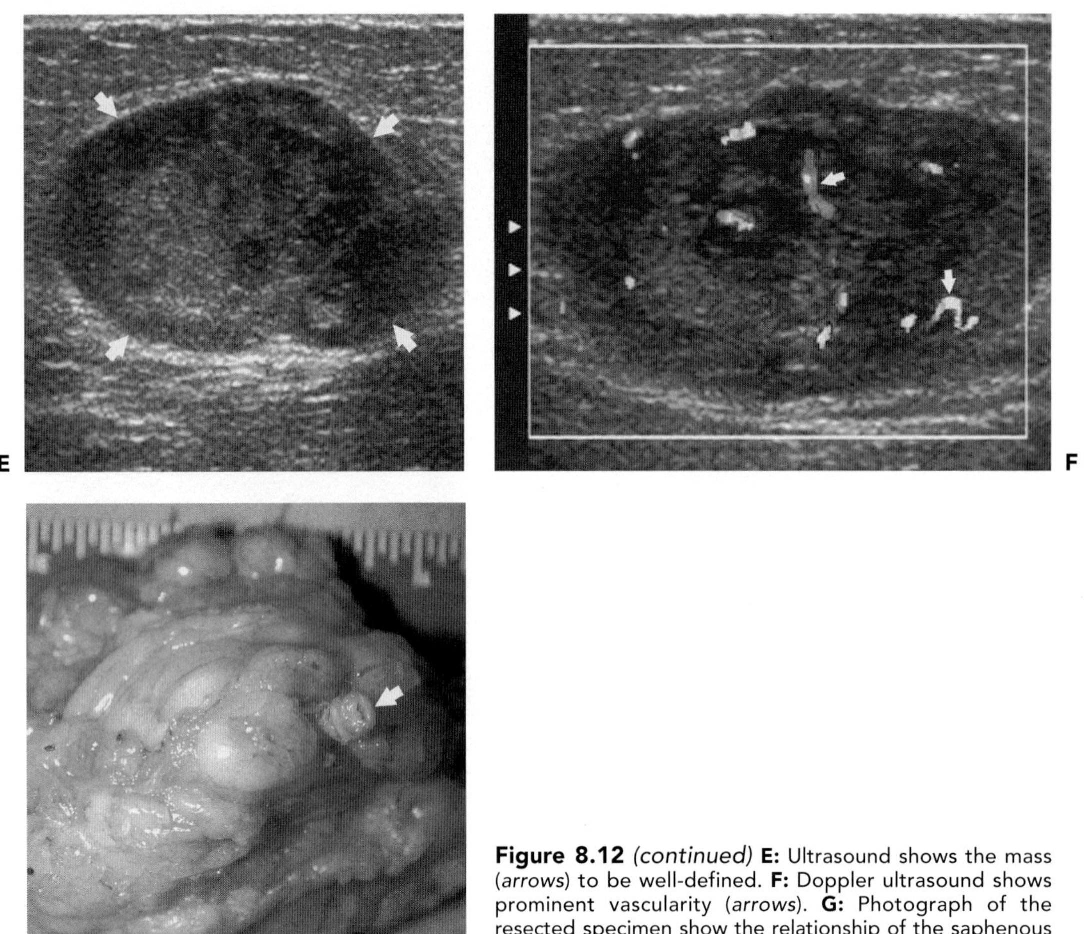

Figure 8.12 *(continued)* **E:** Ultrasound shows the mass (*arrows*) to be well-defined. **F:** Doppler ultrasound shows prominent vascularity (*arrows*). **G:** Photograph of the resected specimen show the relationship of the saphenous vein (*arrow*) to the mass.

surrounding the eyelid or orbit, oropharynx, parotid, and nasopharynx region (102).

Sarcoma botryoids is a form of embryonal rhabdomyosarcoma in which the lesion arises below the mucosa, typically in the bladder, vagina, urethra, prostate, lower rectum, or anus (97). The name *sarcoma botryoids* reflects the "bunch of grapes" appearance of the polypoid submucosal mass (97). Typically appearing in children between birth and 15 years of age, the average age at presentation is approximately 3.5 years (96,101). Embryonal rhabdomyosarcoma may occur in adults, who make up approximately 12% of patients (103); there is a slight male predominance (1.2:1) (102).

Spindle cell rhabdomyosarcoma accounts for approximately 4% of rhabdomyosarcomas and most commonly involves the scrotal soft tissue, with the remainder most frequently involving the head and neck region (102). There is a strong male predilection (101). In contrast to the typical embryonal subtype, spindle cell lesions are also found in adults, usually in nontesticular regions (102).

Embryonal rhabdomyosarcoma is most common in non-Hispanic whites, who account for 70% of the cases (102).

This compares with 14% in blacks and 10% in Hispanics (102). Embryonal rhabdomyosarcoma consists of small cells, with round to spindle-shaped hyperchromatic nuclei and varying numbers of larger cells that have eosinophilic cytoplasm characteristic of rhabdomyoblasts (3).

Alveolar Rhabdomyosarcoma

The alveolar subtype is the second most common subtype and accounts for approximately 18% to 45% of all rhabdomyosarcomas (3,39,97,99). It is more common in adolescents and young adults and is usually intramuscular (32,99). Alveolar rhabdomyosarcoma accounts for approximately 50% of all extremity lesions (104–107). In the Intergroup Rhabdomyosarcoma Study Group, the median age of affected patients was 9 years (107).

Histologically, alveolar rhabdomyosarcoma is composed of small round to oval cells forming nests, creating "alveolar" spaces separated by fibrous connective tissue (3,99). Studies demonstrate that the PAX3-FKHR and PAX7-FKHR gene fusions generated by t(2;13) and t(1;13) chromosomal translocations are specific and consistent features of alveolar rhabdomyosarcoma (99).

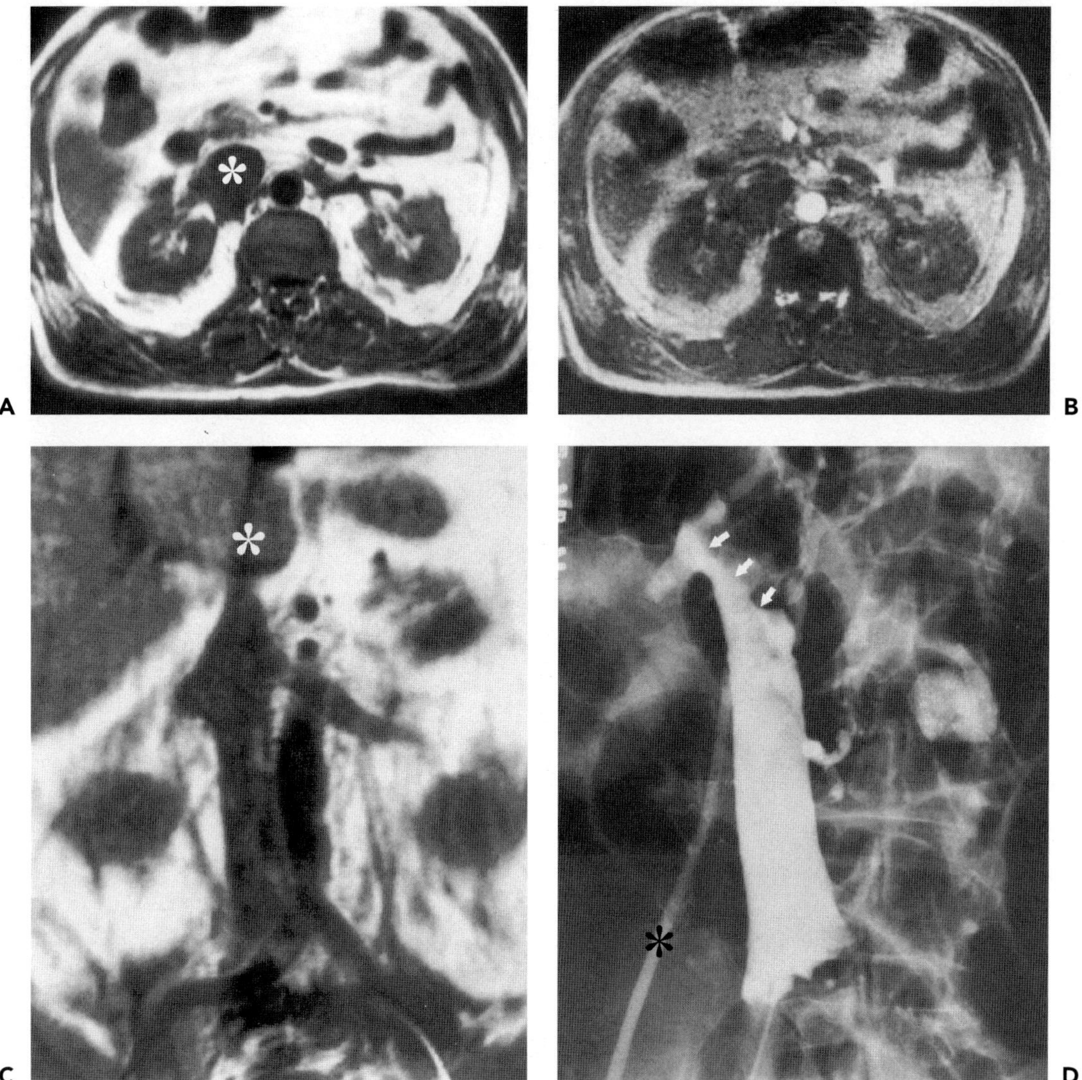

Figure 8.13   Leiomyosarcoma of the inferior vena cava: Typical imaging features in a man 62 years of age. **A:** Axial T1-weighted (TR/TE; 600/15) MR image shows a nonspecific mass in the region of the inferior vena cava (IVC) (*asterisk*). **B:** Corresponding axial gradient echo (TR/TE/Flip; 25/8/60) MR image shows no flow in the IVC. **C:** Coronal T1-weighted (TR/TE; 800/15) MR image shows a mass (*asterisk*) in the inferior vena cava with thrombus inferior to the mass. **D:** Inferior venacavagram following thrombolysis shows large filling defect (*arrows*) occluding the vena cava at the level of the renal veins with large collaterals (*asterisk*).

Pleomorphic Rhabdomyosarcoma

The pleomorphic type is a high-grade sarcoma occurring almost exclusively in adults (although it can occur rarely in children) (101,108). Affected patients are more typically men in the sixth decade (108). It is most frequently encountered in the large muscles of the extremities, especially the thigh (101). Patients usually present with a rapidly growing soft tissue mass (108).

Histologic diagnosis is difficult because of the absence of rhabdomyoblasts and the lesions' close resemblance to malignant fibrous histiocytoma (high-grade undifferenti-

ated pleomorphic sarcoma) and other pleomorphic sarcomas (101). Immunohistochemical and/or ultrastructural evaluation of sarcomatous differentiation is necessary in making the diagnosis (99). Like other rhabdomyosarcoma types, the pleomorphic subtype expresses myoglobin, desmin, MyoD1, skeletal muscle myogen, fast (skeletal muscle) myosin, and actin (101,108,109).

Staging and Prognosis

The present classification system for rhabdomyosarcoma lacks prognostic significance (32), with prognosis related to

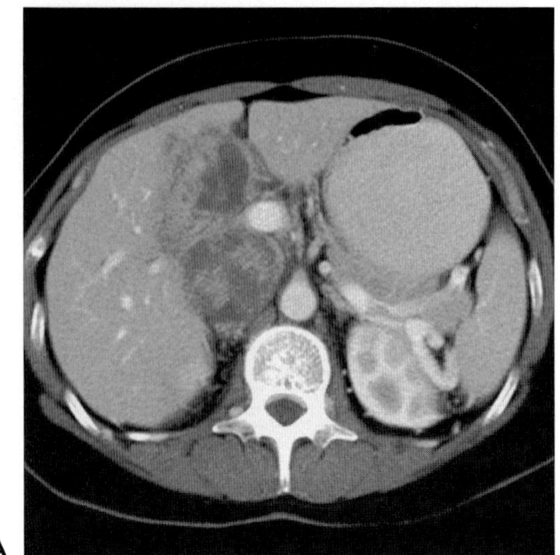
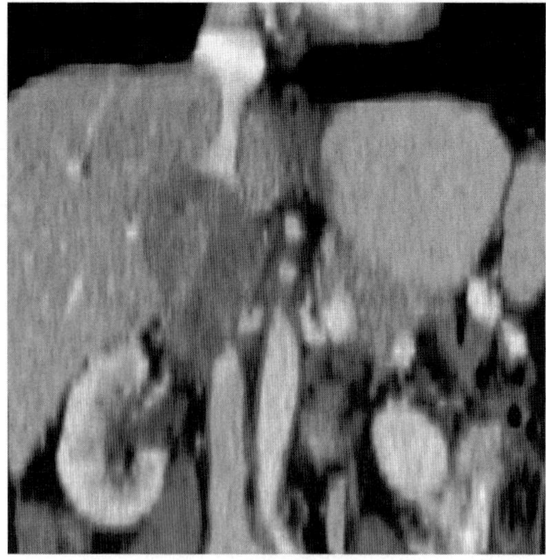

Figure 8.14 Leiomyosarcoma of the inferior vena cava: Typical CT imaging features in a woman 50 years of age. **A,B:** Axial **(A)** and reformatted coronal **(B)** enhanced CT images of the abdomen show a large heterogeneous mass arising in the inferior vena cava. The mass shows areas of decreased attenuation compatible with necrosis/hemorrhage.

stage. In general, the most favorable histologic subtype is the botryoid-embryonal type, which is rarely, if ever, found in the extremities or trunk (110). The alveolar subtype has a high rate of early regional and distant dissemination, and although it may respond initially to chemotherapy, this response is frequently short-lived (110).

Patients with rhabdomyosarcoma are classified into one of four clinical groups, based on tumor resectability, as follows: group 1, complete resection; group 2, gross resection with microscopic residual tumor or complete resection with involved nodes, extension into adjacent organs, or both; group 3, gross residual disease; and group 4, distant metastasis at diagnosis (94). Presurgical staging is based on the tumor, node, metastasis (TNM) system as described in Chapter 3.

Approximately 15% to 20% of patients with rhabdomyosarcoma have clinically detectable metastases at diagnosis; however, all patients are considered to have micrometastases at time of diagnosis (99). Hematogenous metastases are most common to lungs and pleura (96). Other sites of metastasis include bone, bone marrow, liver, and lymph nodes (96). Common sites of osseous metastases include the pelvis, long bones, spine, ribs, and skull (96,98). Bone marrow metastases at time of diagnosis are not uncommon and are seen in 6% to 16% of patients, most often in patients with alveolar rhabdomyosarcoma (104). Rarely, bone metastasis may be the initial presentation, without a clinically evident primary tumor. Shapeero

et al. (104) reported 4 (1%) such cases of 428 patients with rhabdomyosarcoma.

In general, prognosis depends on multiple factors, including tumor size, anatomic site, patient age, lesion histology, and tumor stage (95). The prognosis for this disease has improved significantly over the past 20 years, with an overall increase in survival from 25% in 1970 to 75% in 1990 (111). The results of successive treatment protocols—Intergroup Rhabdomyosarcoma Study-I (IRS-I) through IRS-IV—have now evaluated more than 4,000 patients and have seen continued improvement in the proportion of patients alive at 5 years after the start of therapy (104–106,112). Five-year survival has now increased from 55% to 75%. Of note, patients with metastatic disease at diagnosis have not benefited significantly from the more complex therapies (99).

The prognosis in adults is significantly worse than in children, with a 2-year survival of 50% in the fifth decade to 20% in the seventh decade (109,113). Such figures must be viewed with caution because adult rhabdomyosarcoma is relatively rare and studies generally reflect small patient series. Results based on a study of 82 adults at MD Anderson Cancer Center, Houston, Texas, revealed a 10-year actuarial disease-free rate of 41% and an overall survival rate of 40% (114). Patients whose disease responded to chemotherapy had a significantly better metastasis-free period (72% at 10 years) than those whose disease did not respond (19% at 10 years) (114).

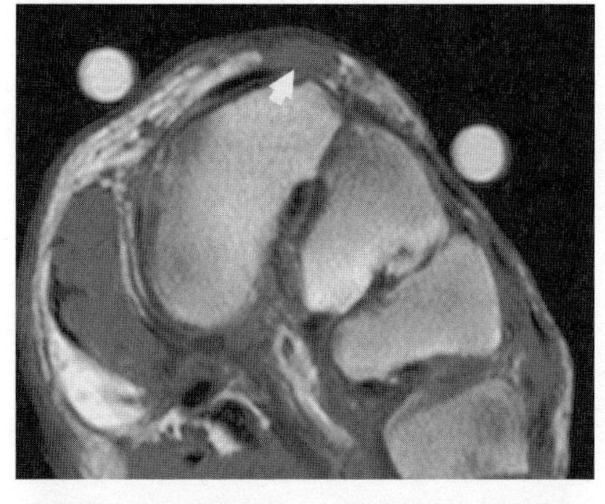
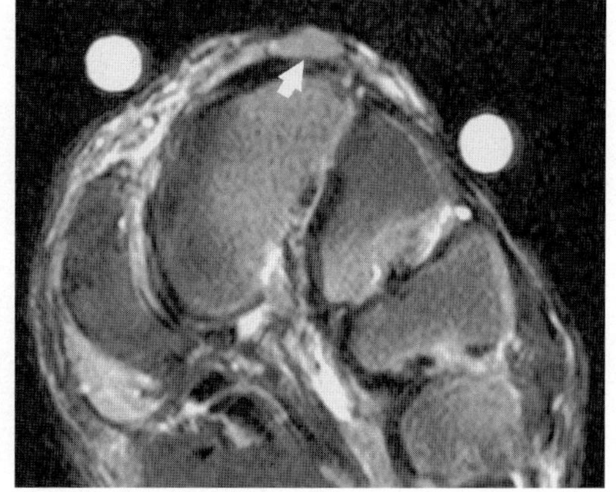
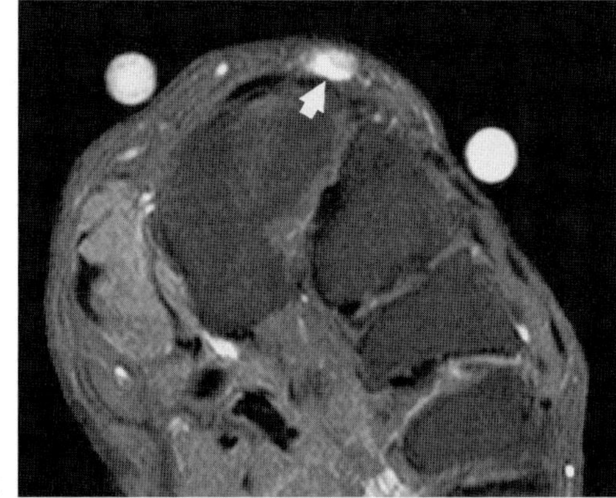

Figure 8.15 Superficial leiomyosarcoma: Typical nonspecific imaging features in a woman 68 years of age with a recurrent foot lesion. **A,B:** Coronal T1-weighted (TR/TE; 403/21) **(A)** and conventional T2-weighted (TR/TE; 2440/80) **(B)** spin-echo MR images show a small mass (*arrow*) on the dorsum of the foot with nonspecific imaging features. Note intermediate signal intensity on T2-weighted image. **C:** Coronal postcontrast T1-weighted (400/17) spin-echo MR image with fat suppression shows marked enhancement (*arrow*).

Imaging of Rhabdomyosarcoma

> **KEY CONCEPTS**
> - Local bone invasion is observed in about a quarter of cases.
> - Bone metastases are usually lytic, but mixed lesions are described.
> - MR imaging is nonspecific.
> - MR may show prominent vascularity and hemorrhage.

There are no specific radiologic features for rhabdomyosarcoma. Radiographs may reveal a nonspecific soft tissue mass (95). Local bone invasion was seen in 14 of 58 cases (24%) reported by Simmons and Tucker (96). In these cases there was a permeative pattern of bone destruction in 12 of the 14 cases, with geographic destruction, suggesting a benign process, in the remaining 2 cases. There was some degree of expansile remodeling in half the cases, and a pathologic fracture in one instance.

In the orbit, destruction of the orbital wall without enlargement of the orbit may be seen (115,116). Lesions may be associated with sclerosis and periosteal reaction, simulating neuroblastoma or Ewing sarcoma. Although not specific, such changes suggest an aggressive process, and rhabdomyosarcoma is the most frequently encountered primary malignancy of the orbit in infants and children (115).

Bone metastases are typically ill-defined lytic lesions, predominantly in the metaphysis in long bones, although there is considerable variability, mixed sclerotic and lytic lesions, and lesions with well-defined margins are noted (Fig. 8.18) (98,104). Ultrasound is a useful adjunct for the detection and evaluation of disease in the pelvis (96).

On MR imaging, the lesion has a nonspecific appearance, isointense to skeletal muscle on T1-weighted images and hyperintense on T2-weighted images (Fig. 8.19) (116). Extremity alveolar rhabdomyosarcoma, in our experience, frequently shows prominent vascularity with serpentine high-flow vessels (Fig. 8.20). Intralesional hemorrhage is also not unusual (Figs. 8.21 and 8.22). As with all MR imaging, the appearance of the lesion reflects its morphology,

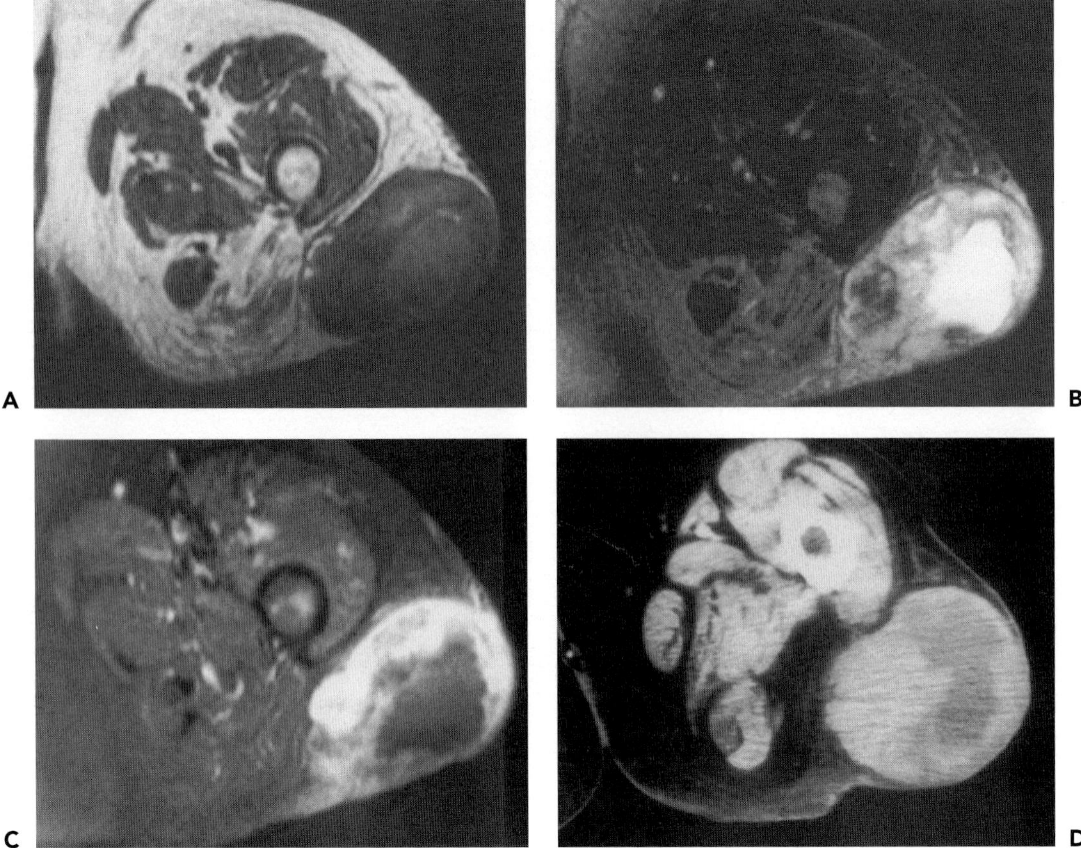

Figure 8.16 Superficial leiomyosarcoma: Imaging features similar to deep lesion in the posterior lateral aspect of the left buttocks in a woman 80 years of age. **A,B:** Axial T1-weighted (TR/TE; 600/10) **(A)** and T2-weighted (TR/TE; 4000/90) **(B)** spin-echo MR images show an inhomogeneous, well-defined mass in the left buttocks with central hemorrhage/necrosis. **C:** Corresponding axial postcontrast T1-weighted (TR/TE; 600/12) spin-echo MR image with fat suppression shows marked enhancement in the solid portions of the lesion. **D:** Axial CT scan shows decreased attenuation within the central aspect of the tumor, compatible with necrosis /hemorrhage.

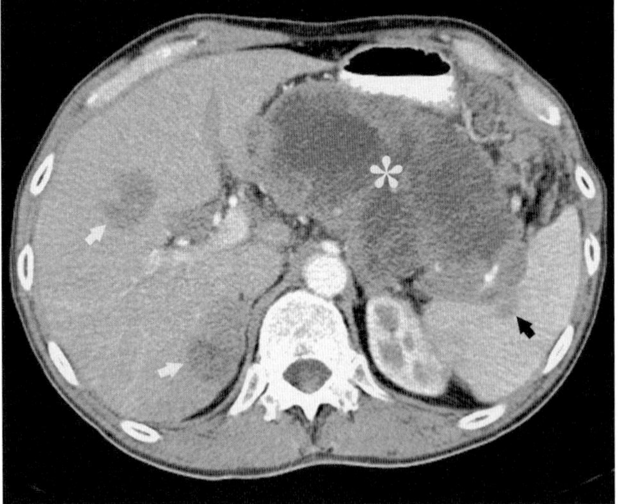

Figure 8.17 Extragastrointestinal stromal tumors: CT imaging features in a man 54 years of age. The origin of the mass (*asterisk*) was difficult to define because of its large size, but it was believed to arise from the retroperitoneum. Areas of decreased attenuation within the central aspect of the tumor are compatible with necrosis/hemorrhage. Note liver metastases (*white arrows*) and invasion of spleen (*black arrow*).

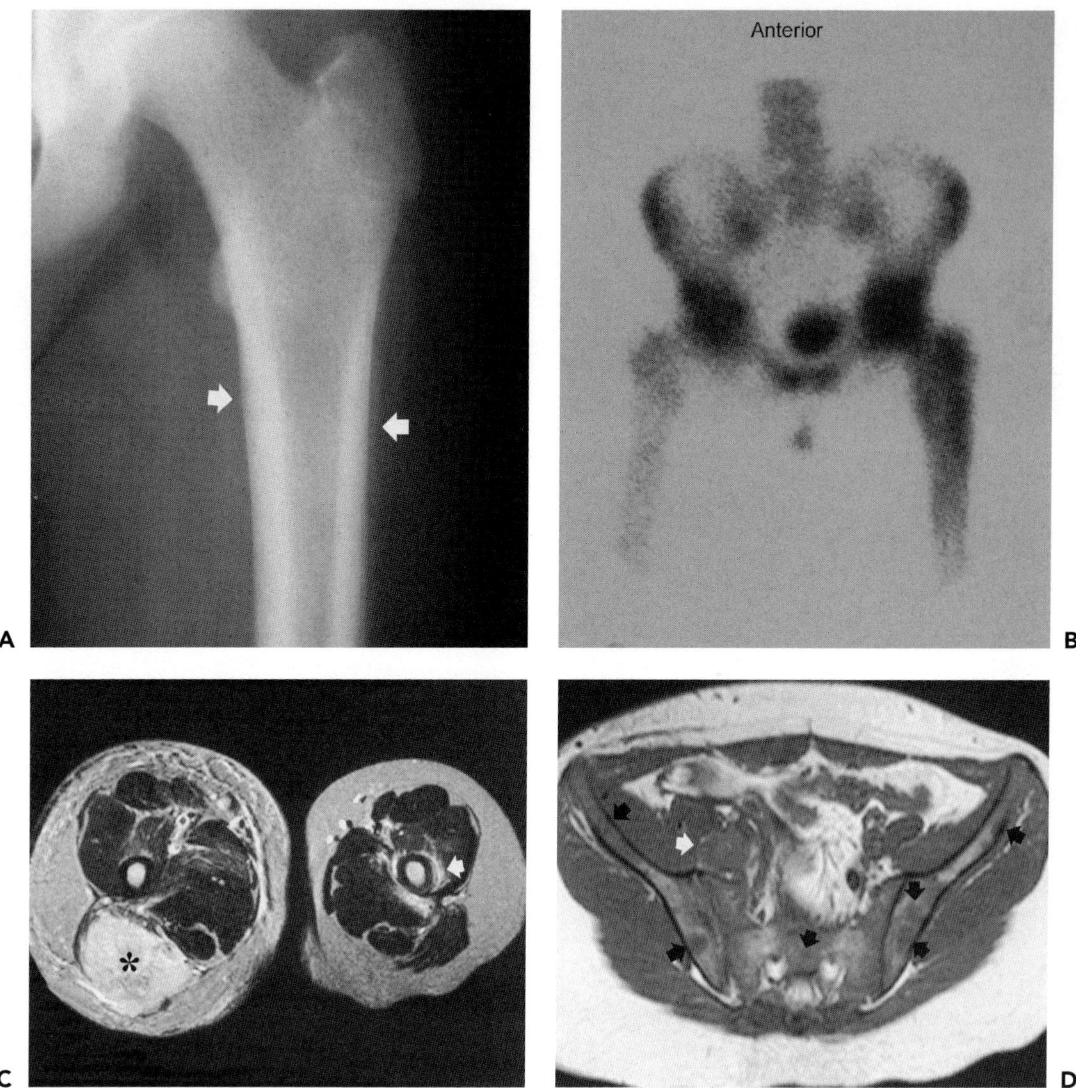

Figure 8.18   Rhabdomyosarcoma: Radiographic features in a girl 12 years of age with extensive metastatic disease. **A:** Anteroposterior radiograph of the proximal left femur shows subtle periosteal reaction (*arrows*). **B:** Anterior delayed static image MDP bone scan shows markedly increased tracer accumulation in the proximal femur. **C:** Axial T2-weighted (TR/TR; 2500/80) spin-echo MR image shows the primary mass in the right proximal thigh (*asterisk*) and left femoral metastasis (*arrow*). **D:** Axial T1-weighted (TR/TE; 700/16) spin-echo MR image of the pelvis shows numerous osseous metastases (*black arrows*) not appreciated on bone scan, as well as nodal metastasis (*white arrow*).

and decreased signal intensity on all pulse sequences, although rare in malignant lesions, is also noted (Fig. 8.23). Marked enhancement may be seen following gadolinium administration. CT imaging is also nonspecific, with areas of necrosis and hemorrhage showing a decreased attenuation on CT imaging (Fig. 8.19).

Although scant literature is available assessing the value of positron emission tomography (PET) imaging in children with sarcomas, initial reports show fluorodeoxyglucose (FDG)-PET to have a higher sensitivity than whole-body MR imaging and scintigraphy in identifying bone and bone marrow metastases (117,118).

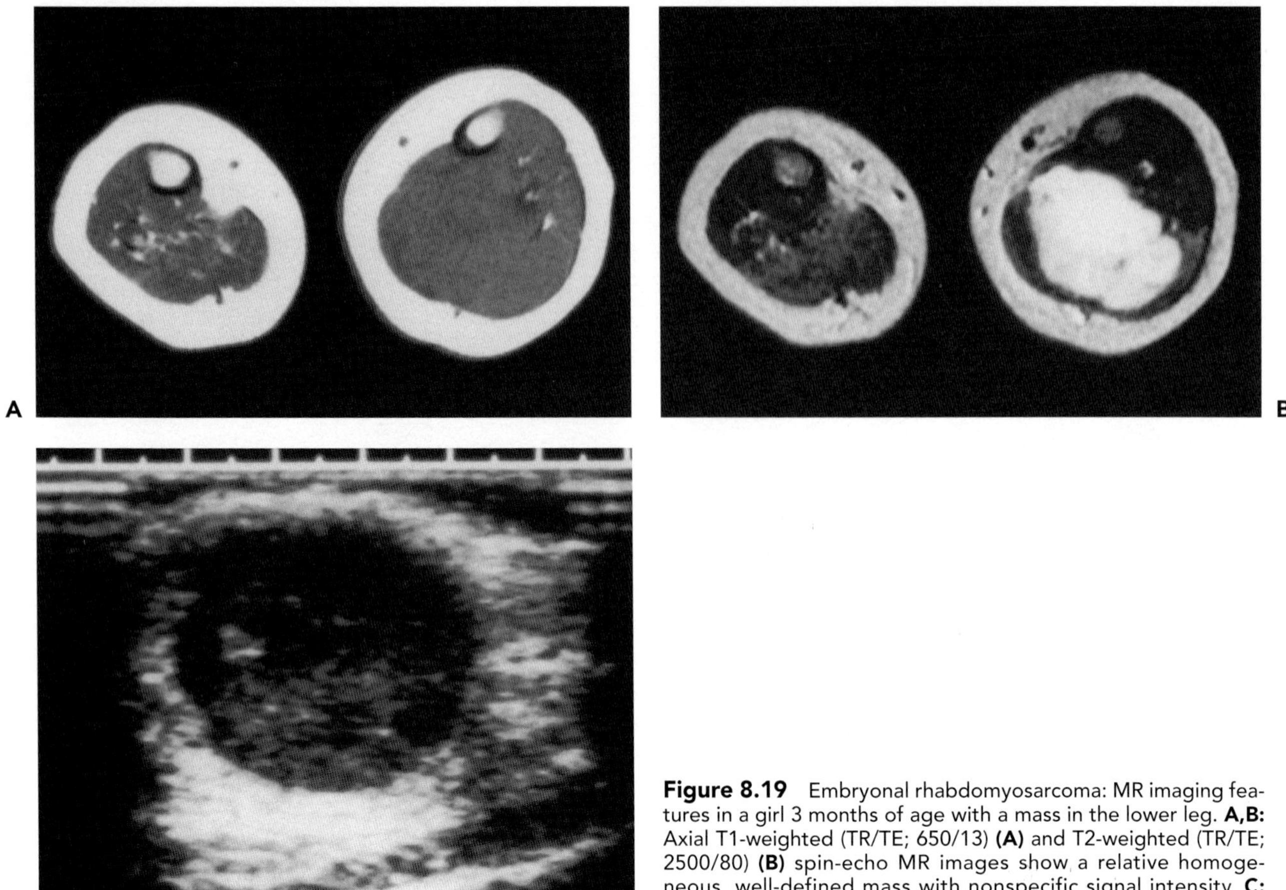

Figure 8.19 Embryonal rhabdomyosarcoma: MR imaging features in a girl 3 months of age with a mass in the lower leg. **A,B:** Axial T1-weighted (TR/TE; 650/13) **(A)** and T2-weighted (TR/TE; 2500/80) **(B)** spin-echo MR images show a relative homogeneous, well-defined mass with nonspecific signal intensity. **C:** Corresponding ultrasound shows a well-defined nonspecific soft tissue mass.

Figure 8.20 Alveolar rhabdomyosarcoma: MR imaging features in a girl 9 years of age. **A,B** Axial T1-weighted (TR/TE; 630/26) **(A)** and T2-weighted (TR/TE; 2350/80) **(B)** spin-echo MR images of the calf show a large, well-defined, heterogeneous mass. Note prominent vascularity with serpentine high-flow vessels (*arrows*). Also note bone marrow metastasis (*asterisk* in **A**).

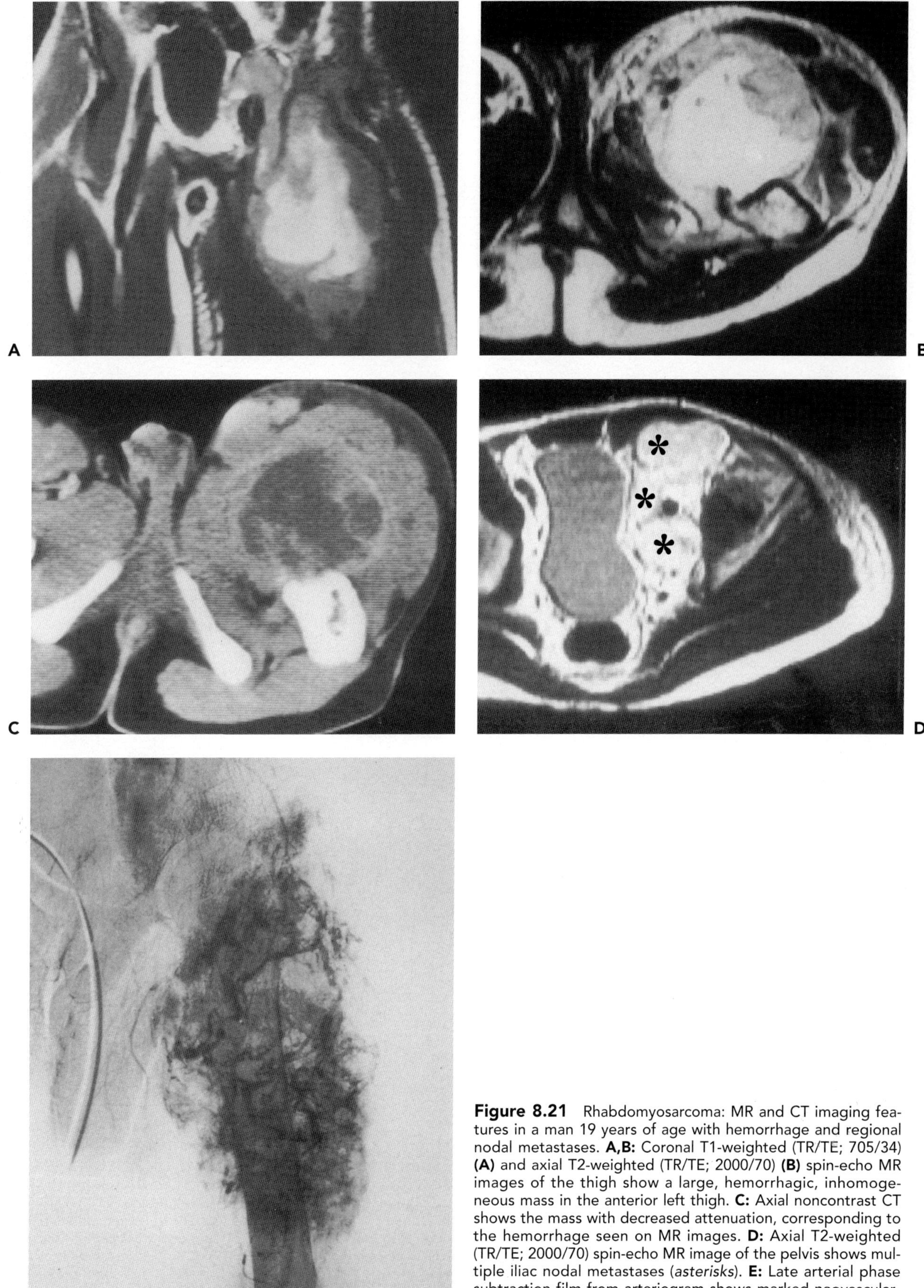

Figure 8.21 Rhabdomyosarcoma: MR and CT imaging features in a man 19 years of age with hemorrhage and regional nodal metastases. **A,B:** Coronal T1-weighted (TR/TE; 705/34) **(A)** and axial T2-weighted (TR/TE; 2000/70) **(B)** spin-echo MR images of the thigh show a large, hemorrhagic, inhomogeneous mass in the anterior left thigh. **C:** Axial noncontrast CT shows the mass with decreased attenuation, corresponding to the hemorrhage seen on MR images. **D:** Axial T2-weighted (TR/TE; 2000/70) spin-echo MR image of the pelvis shows multiple iliac nodal metastases (*asterisks*). **E:** Late arterial phase subtraction film from arteriogram shows marked neovascularity to mass.

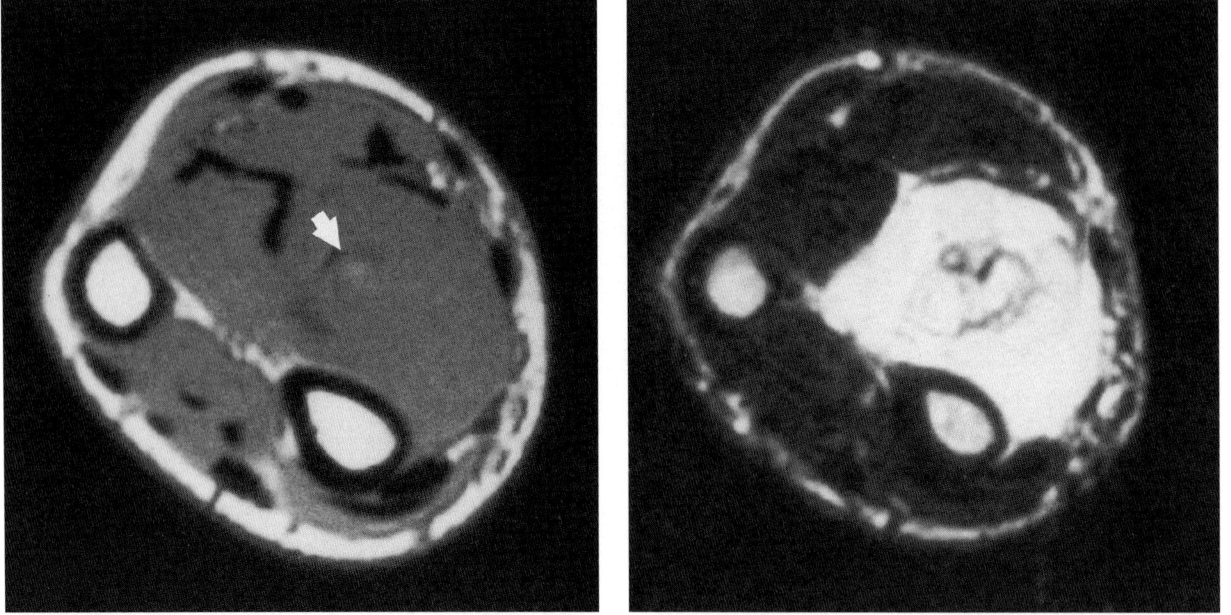

Figure 8.22   Rhabdomyosarcoma: MR imaging in a man 19 years of age with minimally hemorrhagic mass in the forearm. **A,B:** Axial T1-weighted (TR/TE; 550/12) **(A)** and T2-weighted (TE/TE; 2500/90) **(B)** spin-echo MR images show a relatively homogeneous, well-defined mass with nonspecific signal intensity. A small, poorly defined area with increased signal intensity is seen within the mass on T1-weighted image (*arrow* in **A**) compatible with a small amount of central hemorrhage.

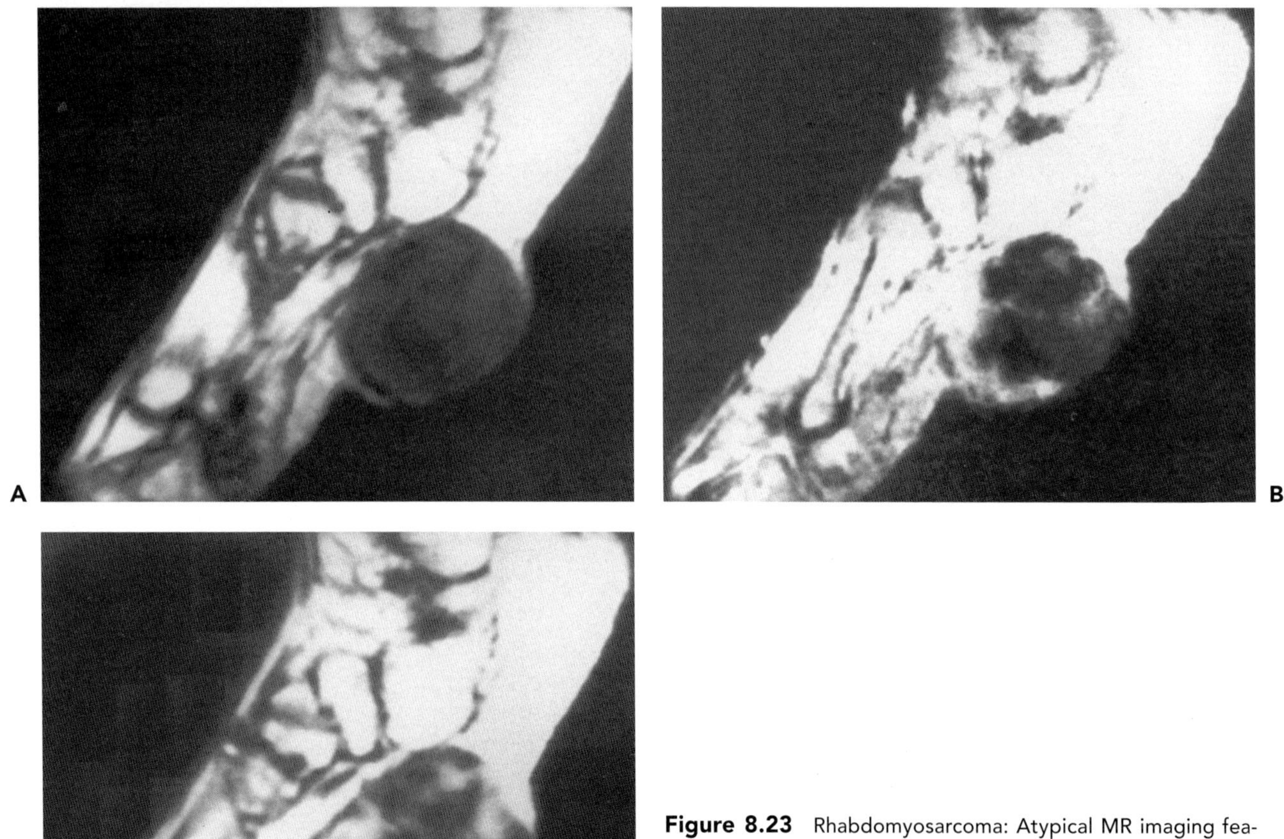

Figure 8.23   Rhabdomyosarcoma: Atypical MR imaging features in a boy 15 years of age with a foot mass. **A,B:** Sagittal T1-weighted (TR/TE; 600/20) **(A)** and T2-weighted (TR/TE; 2000/90) **(B)** spin-echo MR images of the foot show a large, well-defined mass with marked decreased signal intensity. Areas of nonspecific increased signals are seen in **B. C:** Postcontrast sagittal T1-weighted (TR/TE; 600/20) spin-echo MR image show scattered areas of intense enhancement that correspond to areas showing increased signal intensity in **B.**

REFERENCES

1. Kransdorf MJ. Benign soft-tissue tumors in a large referral population: distribution of diagnoses by age, sex and location. *AJR Am J Roentgenol.* 1995;164:395–402.

2. Kransdorf MJ. Malignant soft-tissue tumors in a large referral population: distribution of diagnoses by age, sex and location. *AJR Am J Roentgenol.* 1995;164:573–580.

3. Enjoji M, Hashimoto H. Diagnosis of soft tissue sarcomas. *Pathol Res Pract.* 1984;178:215–226.

4. Lubbers PR, Chandra R, Markle BM, et al. Case report 421. Calcified leiomyoma of the soft tissues of the right buttock. *Skeletal Radiol.* 1987; 16:252–256.

5. Lattes R. Tumors of the soft tissue. In: *Atlas of Tumor Pathology, Second Series.* Washington, DC, Armed Forces Institute of Pathology; 1982:60–65,66–69.

6. Farman AG. Benign smooth muscle tumors. *S Afr Med J.* 1975;49:1333–1340.

7. Weiss SW, Goldblum JR. Benign tumors of smooth muscle. In: *Enzinger and Weiss's Soft Tissue Tumors.* 4th ed. St. Louis: Mosby, 2001;695–726.

8. Hachisuga T, Hashimoto H, Enjoji M. Angioleiomyoma. A clinicopathologic reappraisal of 562 cases. *Cancer.* 1984;54:126–130.

9. Miettinen M. Smooth muscle tumors. In: *Diagnostic Soft Tissue Pathology.* New York: Churchill Livingstone; 2003:241–270.

10. Murphy GF, Elder DE. *Non-Melanocytic Tumors of the Skin.* Washington, DC: Armed Forces Institute of Pathology; 1991:253–256.

11. Son EJ, Oh KK, Lim EK, et al. Leiomyoma of the breast in a 50-year-old woman receiving tamoxifen. *AJR Am J Roentgenol.* 1998;171:1684–1686.

12. Freedman AM, Meland NB. Angioleiomyomas of the extremities: report of a case and review of the Mayo Clinic experience. *Plast Reconst Surg.* 1989;83:328–331.

13. Stout AP. Solitary cutaneous and subcutaneous leiomyoma. *Am J Cancer.* 1937;24:435–469.

14. Hwang JW, Ahn JM, Kang HS, et al. Vascular leiomyoma of on extremity: MR imaging-pathology correlation. *AJR Am J Roentgenol.* 1998;171:981–985.

15. Kinoshita T, Ishii K, Abe Y, et al. Angiomyoma of the lower extremity: MR findings. *Skeletal Radiol.* 1997;26:443–445.

16. Yates BJ. Angioleiomyoma: clinical presentation and surgical management. *Foot Ankle Int.* 2001;22:670–674.

17. Duchateau J, Zielonka E, Guelinckx PJ. Chronic pain: illusion or pathology? A case report of a vascular leiomyoma in the leg. *Br J Plast Surg.* 1987;40:536–537.

18. Kataoka M, Yano H, Fukunaga T, et al. Giant vascular leiomyoma in the hand. *Scand J Reconstr Hand Surg.* 1997;31:91–93.

19. Weiss SW. Smooth muscle tumors of soft tissue. *Adv Anat Pathol.* 2002;9:351–359.

20. Billings SD, Folpe AL, Weiss SW. Do leiomyomas of deep soft tissue exist? An analysis of highly differentiated smooth muscle tumors of deep soft tissue supporting two distinct subtypes. *Am J Surg Pathol.* 2001;25:1134–1142.

21. Misumi S, Irie T, Fukuda K, et al. A case of deep soft tissue leiomyoma: CT and MRI findings. *Radiat Med.* 2000;18:253– 256.

22. Herrlin K, Willén H, Rydholm A. Deep-seated soft tissue leiomyomas. Report of four patients. *Skeletal Radiol.* 1990;19:363–365.

23. Gassel F, Kraft CN, Wallny T, et al. Soft-tissue angioleiomyoma of the hand as a rare differential diagnosis of haemophilic pseudotumor. *Haemophilia.* 2001;7:528–531.

24. Ledesma-Medina J, Oh KS, Girdany BR. Calcification in childhood leiomyoma. *Radiology.* 1980;135:339–341.

25. De Mouy EH, Kaneko K, Rodriguez RP. Calcified soft tissue leiomyoma of the shoulder mimicking a chondrogenic tumor. *Clin Imaging.* 1995;19:4–7.

26. Yamato M, Nishimura G, Koguchi Y, et al. Calcified leiomyoma of deep soft tissue in a child. *Pediatr Radiol.* 1999;29:135–137.

27. López-Barea F, Rodríguez-Peralto J, Burgos E, et al. Calcified leiomyoma of deep soft tissue. Report of a case in childhood. *Virchows Archiv.* 1994;425:217–220.

28. Watson GMT, Saifuddin A, Sandison A. Deep soft tissue leiomyoma of the thigh. *Skeletal Radiol.* 1999;28:411–414.

29. Schmidt-Rohlfing B, Tietze L, Siebert CH, et al. Deep soft-tissue leiomyoma of the popliteal fossa in a 14-year-old girl. *Arch Orthop Trauma Surg.* 2001;121:604–606.

30. Siegelman ES, Outwater EK. Tissue characterization in the female pelvis by means of MR imaging. *Radiology.* 1999;212:5–18.

31. Misch KA. Rhabdomyoma purum: a benign rhabdomyoma of tongue. *J Pathol Bacteriol.* 1958;75:105–108.

32. Agamanolis DP, Dasu S, Krill CE. Tumors of skeletal muscle. *Hum Pathol.* 1986;17: 778–795.

33. Helliwell TR, Sissons MC, Stoney PJ, et al. Immunochemistry and electron microscopy of head and neck rhabdomyoma. *J Clin Pathol.* 1988;41:1058–1063.

34. Kapadia SB, Barr FG. Rhabdomyoma. In: Fletcher DM, Unni KK, Mertens F, eds. *WHO Classification of Tumors. Pathology and Genetics: Tumors of Soft Tissue and Bone.* Lyon, France: IARC Press; 2002:142–145.

35. Harding CO, Pagon RA. Incidence of tuberous sclerosis in patients with cardiac rhabdomyomas. *Am J Med Genet.* 1990;37:443–446.

36. Weiss SW, Goldblum JR. Rhabdomyoma. In: *Enzinger and Weiss's Soft Tissue Tumors.* 4th ed. St. Louis: Mosby; 2001:769–783.

37. Robbins SL, Contran RS, Kumar V. *Pathologic Basis of Disease.* 4th ed. Philadelphia: WB Saunders; 1989:1375.

38. Ho VT, Rao VM. Recurrent adult-type pharyngeal rhabdomyoma: MR appearance [Letter]. *AJR Am J Roentgenol.* 1992;159:1130–1131.

39. Dehner LP, Enzinger FM, Font RL. Fetal rhabdomyoma. An analysis of nine cases. *Cancer.* 1972;30:160–166.

40. Batsakis JG, Manning JT. Soft tissue tumors: unusual forms. *Otolaryngol Clin North Am.* 1986;19:659-683.

41. Garcia-Ruiz JA, Sanchez-Aniceto G, De La Mata-Pages R, et al. Submandibular rhabdomyoma: a case report. *Br J Oral Maxillofac Surg.* 1991;29:123–126.

42. Cacciari A, Predieri B, Mordenti M, et al. Rhabdomyoma of a rare type in a child. Case report and literature review. *Eur J Pediatr Surg.* 2001;11:66–68.

43. Blaauwgeers JL, Troost D, Dingemans KP, et al. Multifocal rhabdomyoma of the neck. Report of a case studied by fine-needle aspiration, light and electron microscopy, histochemistry, and immunohistochemistry. *Am J Surg Pathol.* 1989;13:791–799.

44. Kapadia SB, Meis JM, Frisman DM, et al. Adult rhabdomyoma of the head and neck: a clinicopathologic and immunophenotypic study. *Hum Pathol.* 1993;24:608–617.

45. Cronin CT, Keel SB, Grabbe J, et al. Adult rhabdomyoma of the extremity: a case report and review of the literature. *Hum Pathol.* 2000;31:1074–1080.

46. Liang GS, Loevner LA, Kumar P. Laryngeal rhabdomyoma involving the paraglottic space. *AJR Am J Roentgenol.* 2000;174:1285–1287.

47. Verdolini R, Goteri G, Brancorsini D, et al. Adult rhabdomyoma: report of two cases of rhabdomyoma of the lip and of the eyelid. *Am J Dermatopathol.* 2000;22:264–267.

48. Favia G, Muzio LL, Serpico R, et al. Rhabdomyoma of the head and neck: clinicopathologic features of two cases. *Head Neck.* 2003;25:700–704.

50. Ross CF. Rhabdomyoma of sternomastoid. *J Pathol Bacteriol.* 1968;95:556–558.

49. Osgood PJ, Damron TA, Rooney MT, et al. Benign fetal rhabdomyoma of the upper extremity. A case report. *Clin Orthop.* 1998;349:200–204.

51. Myung J, Kim IO, Chun JE, et al. Rhabdomyoma of the orbit: a case report. *Pediatr Radiol.* 2002;32:589–592.

52. d'more ESG, Ninfo V. Tumors of the soft tissues composed of large eosinophilic cells. *Semin Diagn Pathol.* 1999;16:178–189.

53. Schlosnagle DC, Kratochvil FJ, Weathers DR, et al. Intraoral multifocal adult rhabdomyoma. Report of a case and review of the literature. *Arch Pathol Lab Med.* 1983;107:638–642.

54. Vermeersch H, van Vugt P, Lemmerling M, et al. Bilateral recurrent adult rhabdomyoma of the pharyngeal wall. *Eur Arch Otorhinolaryngol.* 2000;257:24–26.

55. Savell VH, Parham DM. Rhabdomyomas and rhabdomyosarcomas. In: Miettinen M, ed. *Diagnostic Soft Tissue Pathology.* New York: Churchill Livingstone; 2003:287–310.

56. Smith NM, Thornton CM. Fetal rhabdomyoma: two instances of recurrence. *Pediat Pathol.* 1996;16:673–680.

57. Pradhan SA, Rajpal RM, Shrikhande SS. Extracardiac rhabdomyoma: a report of two cases. *J Surg Oncol.* 1986;33:69–71.

58. Kapadia SB, Norris HJ. Rhabdomyoma of the vagina. *Mod Pathol.* 1993;6:75A.

59. Fukuda Y, Okamura H, Nemoto T, et al. Rhabdomyoma of the base of the tongue. *J Laryngol Otol.* 2003;117:503–507.

60. Metheetrairut C, Brown DH, Cullen JB, et al. Pharyngeal rhabdomyoma: a clinico-pathological study. *J Otolaryngol.* 1992;21:257–261.

61. McLeod AJ, Zornoza J, Shirkhoda A. Leiomyosarcoma: computed tomographic findings. *Radiology.* 1984;152:133–136.

62. Demirkan F, Unal S, Cenetoglu S, et al. Radiation-induced leiomyosarcomas as second primary tumors in the head and neck region: report of 2 cases. *J Oral Maxillofac Surg.* 2003;61:259–263.

63. Bush CH, Reith JD, Spanier SS. Mineralization in musculoskeletal leiomyosarcoma: radiologic-pathologic correlation. *AJR Am J Roentgenol.* 2003;180:109–113.

64. Evans HL, Shipley J. Leiomyosarcoma. In: Fletcher DM, Unni KK, Mertens F, eds. *WHO Classification of Tumors. Pathology and Genetics: Tumors of Soft Tissue and Bone.* Lyon, France: IARC Press; 2002:131–134.

65. Weiss SW, Goldblum JR. Leiomyosarcoma. In: *Enzinger and Weiss's Soft Tissue Tumors.* 4th ed. St. Louis: Mosby; 2001:727–748.

66. Mankin HJ, Casas-Ganem J, Kim JI, et al. Leiomyosarcoma of somatic soft tissues. *Clin Orthop.* 2004;421:225–231.

67. Espat NJ, Bilsky M, Lewis JJ, et al. Soft tissue sarcoma brain metastases. Prevalence in a cohort of 3829 patients. *Cancer.* 2002;94:2706–2711.

68. Shmookler BM, Lauer DH. Retroperitoneal leiomyosarcoma. A clinicopathologic analysis of 36 cases. *Am J Surg Pathol.* 1983;7:269–280.

69. Wile AG, Evans HL, Romsdahl MM. Leiomyosarcoma of soft tissue: a clinicopathologic study. *Cancer.* 1981;48:1022–1032.

70. Brenton GE, Johnson DE, Eady JL. Leiomyosarcoma of the hand and wrist. *J Bone Joint Surg Am.* 1986;68A:139–142.

71. Hashimoto H, Daimaru Y, Tsuneyoshi M, et al. Leiomyosarcoma of the external soft tissues. *Cancer.* 1986;57:2077–2088.

72. Hartman DS, Hayes WS, Choyke PL, et al. Leiomyosarcoma of the retroperitoneum and inferior vena cava: radiologic-pathologic correlation. *Radiographics.* 1992;12:1203–1220.

73. Farshid G, Pradhan M, Goldblum J, et al. Leiomyosarcoma of somatic soft tissues: a tumor of vascular origin with multivariate analysis of outcome in 42 cases. *Am J Surg Pathol.* 2002;26:14–24.

74. Gustafson P, Willen H, Baldetorp B, et al. Soft tissue leiomyosarcoma. A population-based epidemiologic and prognostic study of 48 patients, including cellular DNA content. *Cancer.* 1992;70:114–119.

75. Hashimoto H, Daimaru Y, Tsuneyoshi M, et al. Leiomyosarcoma of the external soft tissues. A clinicopathologic, immunohistochemical, and electron microscopic study. *Cancer.* 1986;57:2077–2088.

76. Kervorkian J, Cento DP. Leiomyosarcoma of large arteries and veins. *Surgery.* 1973;73:390–400.

77. Dzsinich C, Gloviczki P, van Heerden JA, et al. Primary venous leiomyosarcoma: a rare but lethal disease. *J Vasc Surg.* 1992;15:595–603.

78. Killoran TP, Wells WA, Barth RJ, et al. Leiomyosarcoma of the popliteal vein. *Skeletal Radiol.* 2003;32:174–178.

79. Kaushik S, Neifeld JP. Leiomyosarcoma of the renal vein: imaging and surgical reconstruction. *AJR Am J Roentgenol.* 2002;179:276–277.

80. Reix T, Sevestre H, Sevestri-Pietri MA, et al. Primary malignant tumors of the venous system in the lower extremities. *Ann Vasc Surg.* 1998;12:589–596.

81. Blansfield JA, Chung H, Sullivan TR, et al. Leiomyosarcoma of the major peripheral arteries: case report and review of the literature. *Ann Vasc Surg.* 2003;17:565–570.

82. Roy C, Beaujeux R, Mutter D. Leiomyosarcoma of the femoral vein: imaging findings. *AJR Am J Roentgenol.* 1993;160:1125–1126.

83. Seynaeve PC, Mortelmans LL, DeSchepper AM. Tumors of muscular origin. In: DeSchepper AM, ed. *Imaging of Soft Tissue Tumors.* 2nd ed. Germany: Springer-Verlag; 2001:255–271.

84. Levy AD, Remotti HE, Thompson WM, et al. Anorectal gastrointestinal stromal tumors: CY and MR imaging features with clinical and pathologic correlation. *AJR Am J Roentgenol.* 2003;180:1607–1612.

85. Burkill GJ, Badran M, Al-Muderis O, et al. Malignant gastrointestinal stromal tumor: distribution, imaging features, and pattern of metastatic spread. *Radiology.* 2003;226:527–532.

86. Weiss SW, Goldblum JR. Extragastrointestinal stromal tumors. In: *Enzinger and Weiss's Soft Tissue Tumors.* 4th ed. St. Louis: Mosby; 2001:749–768.

87. Kindblom LG, Remotti HE, Aldenborg F, et al. Gastrointestinal pacemaker cell tumor (GIPACT): gastrointestinal stromal tumors show phenotypic characteristics of the interstitial cells of Cajal. *Am J Pathol.* 1998;152:1259–1269.

88. Davila RE, Faigel DO. GI stromal tumors. *Gastrointest Endosc.* 2003;58:80–88.

89. Emory TS, Sobin LH, Lukes L, et al. Prognosis of gastrointestinal smooth-muscle (stromal) tumors: dependence on anatomic site. *Am J Surg Pathol.* 1999;23:82–87.

90. Kagan AR, Steckel RJ, Mink J. Intramedullary extension of a soft-tissue neoplasm. *AJR Am J Roentgenol.* 1982;139:807–809.

91. Gupta AK, Cohan RH, Francis IR, et al. CT of recurrent retroperitoneal sarcoma. *AJR Am J Roentgenol.* 2000;174:1025–1029.

92. Stallard D, Sundaram M, Johnson FE, et al. Case report 747. Leiomyosarcoma of the great saphenous vein. *Skeletal Radiol.* 1992;21:399–401.

93. Ekelund L, Rydholm A. The value of angiography in soft tissue leiomyosarcomas of the extremities. *Skeletal Radiol.* 1983;9:201–204.

94. McCarville MB, Spunt SL, Pappo AS. Rhabdomyosarcoma in pediatric patients: the good, the bad, and the unusual. *AJR Am J Roentgenol.* 2001;176:1563–1569.

95. Herzog CE, Stewart JMM, Blakely ML. Pediatric soft tissue sarcomas. *Surg Oncol Clin North Am.* 2003;12:419–447.

96. Tannous WN, Azouz EM, Kiruluta HG, et al. CT and ultrasound imaging of pelvic rhabdomyosarcoma in children. *Pediatr Radiol.* 1989;19:530–534.

97. Dillon E, Parkin GJS. The role of diagnostic radiology in the diagnosis and management of rhabdomyosarcoma in young persons. *Clin Radiol.* 1978;29:53–59.

98. Simmons M, Tucker AK. The radiology of bone changes in rhabdomyosarcoma. *Clin Radiology.* 1978;29:47–52.

99. Meyer WH, Spunt SL. Soft tissue sarcomas of childhood. *Cancer Treat Rev.* 2004;30:269–280.

100. McKeen EA, Bodurtha J, Meadows AT, et al. Rhabdomyosarcoma complicating multiple neurofibromatosis. *J Pediatr.* 1978;93:992–993.

101. Weiss SW, Goldblum JR. Rhabdomyosarcoma. In: *Enzinger and Weiss's Soft Tissue Tumors.* 4th ed. St. Louis: Mosby; 2001:785–835.

102. Parham DM, Barr FG. Embryonal rhabdomyosarcoma. In: Fletcher DM, Unni KK, Mertens F, eds. *WHO Classification of Tumors. Pathology and Genetics: Tumors of Soft Tissue and Bone.* Lyon, France: IARC Press; 2002:146–149.

103. Lawrence W, Jegge G, Foote FW. Embryonal rhabdomyosarcoma. A clinicopathological study. *Cancer.* 1964;17:361–376.

104. Shapeero LG, Couanet D, Vanel D, et al. Bone metastases as the presenting manifestation of rhabdomyosarcoma in childhood. *Skeletal Radiol.* 1993;22:433–438.

105. Maurer HM, Gehan EA, Beltangady M, et al. The Intergroup Rhabdomyosarcoma Study-II. *Cancer.* 1993;71:1904–1922.

106. Crist W, Gehan EA, Ragab AH, et al. The Third Intergroup Rhabdomyosarcoma Study. *J Clin Oncol.* 1995;13:610–630.

107. Newton WA, Soule EH, Hamoudi AB, et al. Histopathology of childhood sarcoma, Intergroup Rhabdomyosarcoma Studies I and II: clinicopsychological correlation. *J Clin Oncol.* 1988;6:67–75.

108. Montgomery E, Barr FG. Pleomorphic rhabdomyosarcoma. In: Fletcher DM, Unni KK, Mertens F, eds. *WHO Classification of Tumors. Pathology and Genetics: Tumors of Soft Tissue and Bone.* Lyon, France: IARC Press; 2002:153–154.

109. Jones TR, Norton MS, Johnstone PAS, et al. Pleomorphic rhabdomyosarcoma in an adult forearm: a case report. *J Hand Surg.* 2002;27A:154–159.

110. Hays DM. Rhabdomyosarcoma. *Clin Orthop.* 1993;289:36–49.

111. McDowell HP. Update on childhood rhabdomyosarcoma. *Arch Dis Child*. 2003;88:354–357.
112. Crist WM, Anderson JR, Meza JL, et al. Intergroup rhabdomyosarcoma study-IV: results for patients with nonmetastatic disease. *J Clin Oncol*. 2001;19:3091–3102.
113. Lloyd RV, Hajdu SI, Knapper WH. Embryonal rhabdomyosarcoma in adults. *Cancer*. 1983;51:557–565.
114. Little DJ, Ballo MT, Kagars GK, et al. Adult rhabdomyosarcoma. *Cancer*. 2002;95:377–388.
115. Kirkpatrick JA, Capitanio MA. Radiology of the orbit in infancy and childhood. *Radiol Clin North Am*. 1972;10:143–166.
116. Judmaier W, Birbamer G, Buchberger W, et al. MR imaging of late onset orbital rhabdomyosarcoma with intracranial extension. *Magn Reson Imaging*. 1993;11:285–288.
117. Daldrup-Link HE, Franzius C, Link TM, et al. Whole-body MR imaging for detection of bone metastases in children and young adults: comparison with skeletal scintigraphy and FDG PET. *AJR Am J Roentgenol*. 2001;171:229–236.
118. Ben Arush MW, Israel O, Kedar Z, et al. Detection of isolated distant metastasis in soft tissue sarcoma by fluorodeoxyglucose positron emission tomography: case report. *Pediatr Hematol Oncol*. 2001;18:295–298.

Neurogenic Tumors

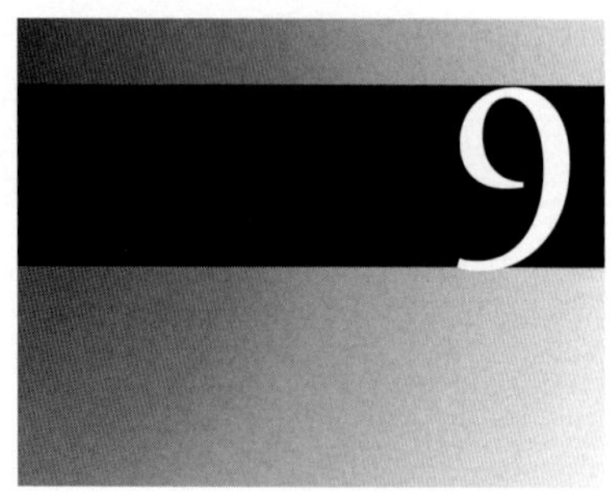

Neuromas are common, reactive, hyperplastic lesions that simulate neoplasms of nerve. True neoplasms of nerve sheath origin are not uncommon soft tissue tumors, making up approximately 12% of all benign and 7% to 8% of all malignant soft tissue neoplasms (1). Imaging characteristics often suggest a neurogenic origin for both reactive and neoplastic lesions. These distinctive features are typically related to location, such as those lesions in the region of a major nerve with an identifiable nerve entering and exiting the mass. Lesions discussed in this chapter include neuroma, schwannoma, neurofibroma, neurofibromatosis (NF), malignant peripheral nerve sheath tumor, neurothekeoma, nerve sheath myxoma, perineurioma, granular cell tumor, melanotic neuroectodermal tumor of infancy, clear cell sarcoma, paraganglioma, and primitive neural tumors.

DEVELOPMENT AND HISTOLOGIC CHARACTERISTICS OF NORMAL PERIPHERAL NERVES

We believe many of the imaging features of neurogenic tumors are a reflection of their similarity to the normal neurogenic tissue from which they are derived. Because of this relationship, an understanding of basic nerve anatomy and histologic characteristics is important.

Peripheral nerves are derived embryologically from neural crest tissue and migrating axons from the primitive neural tube (2). The two predominant supporting elements are the connective tissue stroma and Schwann cells that encase all peripheral nerve axons to varying degrees. A myelinated fiber results if only one axon is encased by one Schwann cell. Unmyelinated fibers result if a Schwann cell encases many axons.

Each peripheral nerve is surrounded by a thick connective tissue sheath called the *epineurium*. Within the nerve, groups of axons are surrounded and divided by a fibrous stroma called the *perineurium*, which creates multiple bundles of fibers or fascicles (Fig. 9.1) (2). This gross appearance of a normal nerve can be recognized at ultrasonography and MR imaging, particularly in large nerve trunks such as the

sciatic nerve, and is described as having a fascicular appearance (Fig. 9.2) (3–6). On longitudinal ultrasonography, the normal nerve texture is composed of multiple, hypoechoic parallel but discontiguous, linear bundles separated by hyperechoic bands (7,8). On MR imaging, the normal nerve is seen as multiple small circular (seen en face) or longitudinal (seen in long axis) bundles with punctate areas of higher signal intensity on T1- and T2-weighting. Vascular supply to the peripheral nerves is relatively profuse, arises from adjacent vessels, and forms longitudinally oriented channels along the nerve.

NEUROMA

Neuromas are not true soft tissue neoplasms, but represent lesions of nerve caused by reactive hyperplasia (9). Types of neuromas encountered in the soft tissue include traumatic, Morton, Pacinian, and palisaded encapsulated.

Traumatic Neuroma

> **KEY CONCEPTS**
> - Traumatic neuroma is not a true neoplasm but a reparative proliferation of an injured nerve often due to amputation.
> - The two types of traumatic neuroma are the spindle (fusiform swelling) and the lateral/terminal (bulbous termination of severed nerve) types.
> - MR and ultrasonography reveal either fusiform nerve thickening (spindle type) or entering nerve terminating in a bulbous mass (lateral/terminal type).

Traumatic neuroma is not a true neoplasm but represents an attempted, insufficient, reparative proliferation of nerve tissue to regain axonal continuity usually related to the proximal end of a severed nerve (9–16). Typically, this is associated with trauma or amputation. The incidence of traumatic neuroma is markedly reduced, and the likelihood of successful regeneration markedly improved, if the nerve ends are closely approximated following injury (13).

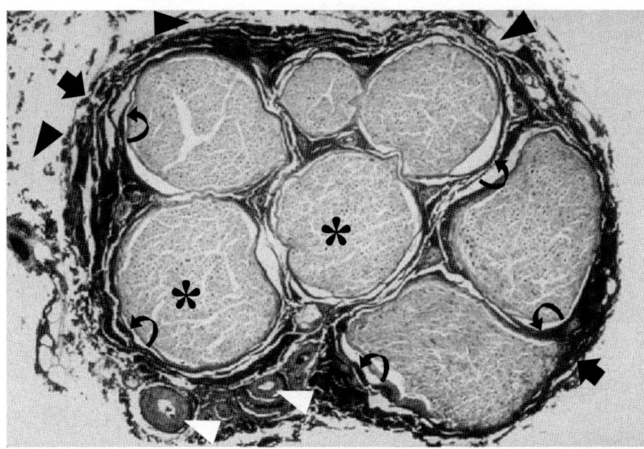

Figure 9.1 Normal nerve structure. Photomicrograph (original magnification, approximately ×20; Bielschowsky silver stain) of an axial section of normal sural nerve. Nerve is surrounded by epineurium (*straight arrows*). Bundles of nerve fibers (*asterisks*) are surrounded by perineurium (*curved arrows*), creating a fascicular appearance. Adipose tissue (*black arrowheads*) and blood vessels (*white arrowheads*) are seen about the nerve.

Clinically traumatic neuroma may be asymptomatic or painful and presents as a firm nodule at a focal pressure site. Pain may be elicited with palpation or tapping on the lesion (*Tinel sign*). The most common location for traumatic neuromas is the lower extremity, followed by the head and neck (frequently in the oral cavity; more than 50% of these lesions are related to tooth extraction) (2–5,10,12,13,16–26). Other affected sites include the radial nerve and brachial plexus (27–30).

Traumatic neuromas are divided into two major categories based on the anatomic location of the tangled, multidirectional, regenerating axonal mass with respect to the proximal nerve end (9,10). Spindle neuromas are internal,

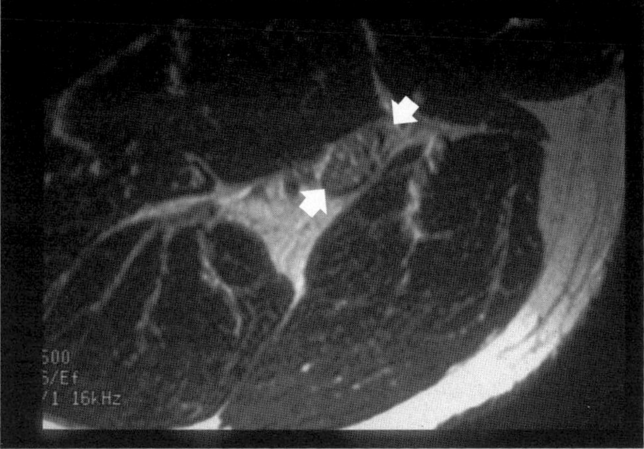

Figure 9.2 Normal nerve appearance at MR imaging. Axial T1-weighted (TR/TE; 500/20) MR image of the upper thigh shows the normal sciatic nerve (*arrows*) with small circular low-signal-intensity areas, surrounded by a background of mildly higher signal-intensity areas representing the fascicular structure of the normal nerve.

focal, fusiform swellings secondary to chronic friction or irritation to a nondisrupted, injured, but intact nerve trunk. Lateral or terminal neuromas are the result of severe trauma with partial avulsion, disruption or total transection of a nerve (9,13,16). These lesions have a bulbous-end morphology in continuity with the normal nerve proximally. They arise 1 to 12 months after transection or injury, vary in size, although they are usually less than 5 cm, with no malignant potential (9,31).

At histologic analysis, traumatic neuromas are non-neoplastic, nonencapsulated tangled masses of axons, Schwann cells, endoneurial cells, and perineurial cells, in a dense collagenous matrix with surrounding fibroblasts (9,19,26). The disorganization of the neurogenic tissue (caused by multidirectional proliferation of cells in an abortive attempt to repair the injured nerve) allows traumatic neuromas to be distinguished from neurofibroma, although discrete bundles or fascicles can be recognized.

There are only limited reports of the ultrasonographic, CT, or MR imaging appearance of traumatic neuromas (14,15,30–33). Typically, a fusiform mass or focal enlargement with an entering and exiting nerve (spindle type), or only an entering nerve terminating in a bulbous shape (lateral or terminal type), is identified (Fig. 9.3) (14,15,26,31). Ultrasonography and MR imaging are the best modalities to identify the direct relationship of the nerve to the lesion (Fig. 9.3) (34). Peer et al. reported the ability to identify injured nerves accurately by high-resolution sonography in 18 patients (35). In addition, these authors also were able to distinguish among nerve swelling (thickening but intact fascicles), compromising surrounding scar tissue (hypoechoic mass without fascicles), neuroma, and insufficient repair on high-resolution sonography. However, these authors acknowledge that difficulty may occur in distinguishing spindle cell neuromas from nerve swelling (35). Lesions of small and/or superficial nerves may not be detected radiologically or may be seen as nonspecific soft tissue masses without an entering nerve (31). Lesion margins are often well-defined, although some irregularity (likely related to multidirectional cell proliferation) is seen with ultrasonography. These imaging characteristics allow traumatic neuromas to be distinguished from other causes of amputation stump pain, including recurrent malignant tumor, phantom limb pain, bone bruise, stress fracture, lymphadenopathy, osteomyelitis, abscess, bursitis, cellulitis, hematoma, heterotopic bone, foreign bodies, atrophied stump muscles, and cicatrization or scar formation (14,26,31,36). Distinguishing lymphadenopathy from traumatic neuroma after neck dissection can be very difficult (37). Yabuuchi et al. showed that statistically significant features favoring traumatic neuroma in this situation include small short-to-long axis ratio, small short axis diameter, central hypoechoic area, less likely contact with the carotid artery, and hypointense rim on T2-weighted MR images (38).

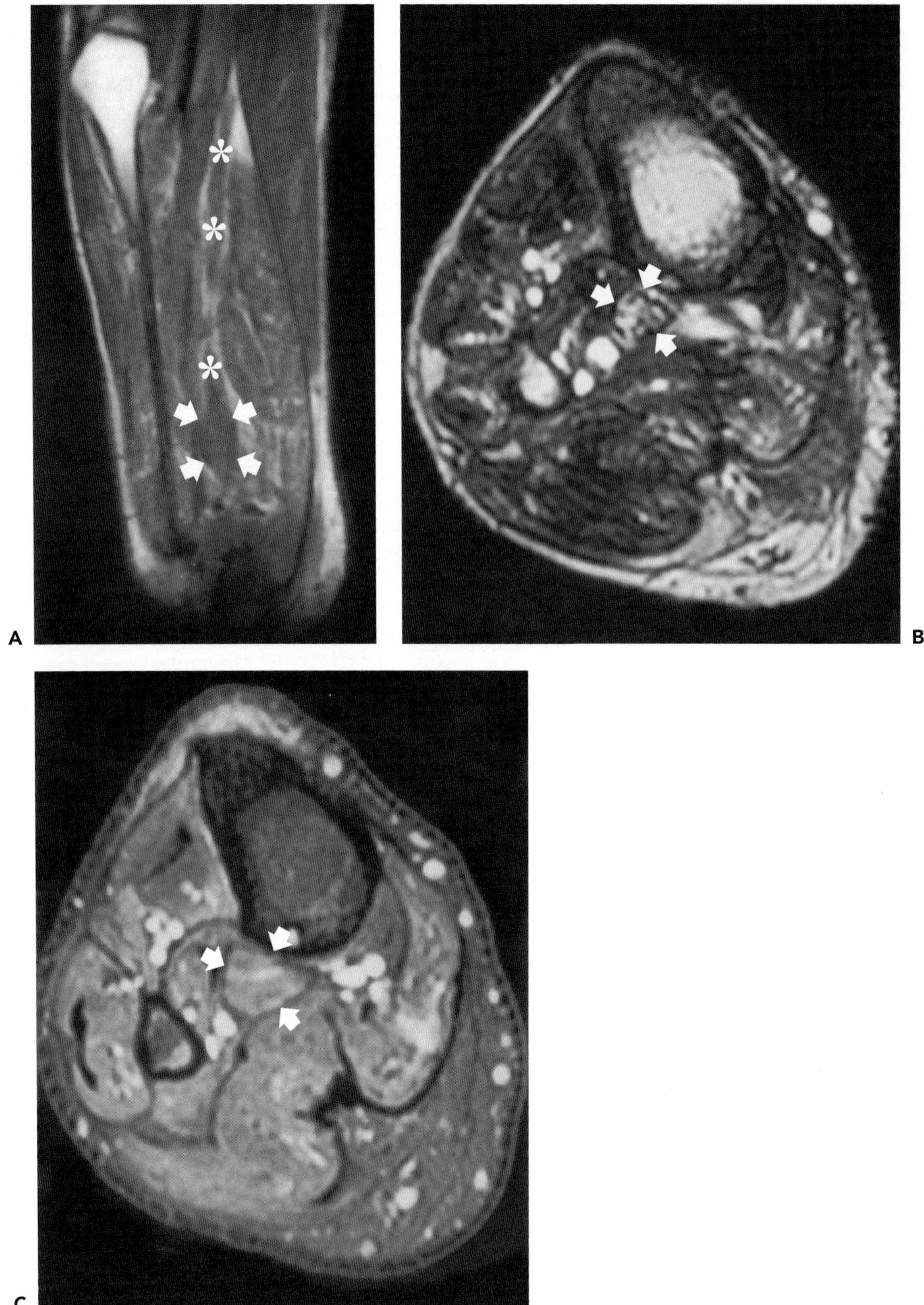

Figure 9.3   Traumatic terminal neuroma of tibial nerve in a man 33 years of age that developed after mid to distal tibial-level amputation. **A,B:** Coronal T1-weighted (TR/TE; 500/16) **(A)** and axial turbo T2-weighted (TR/TE; 4300/126) **(B)** spin-echo MR images show a mass (*arrows*) posterior to the tibia. Tubular structure (*asterisks*) represents the tibial nerve entering the mass. The axial T2-weighted MR image shows heterogeneous signal with a fascicular appearance. **C:** Axial T1-weighted (TR/TE; 600/16) spin-echo MR image following gadolinium administration shows mild enhancement (*arrows*).

Traumatic neuromas typically have intermediate signal intensity (similar to that of muscle) on T1-weighted MR images and intermediate-to-high signal intensity on T2-weighted images (26,31,32). Their signal intensity is frequently heterogeneous, with a ringlike pattern (*"fascicular sign"*), which we believe correlates with the histologic morphology of nerve fascicles and is optimally detected on T2-weighted images (Fig. 9.3) (26). Intrinsic ultrasound echogenicity (hypoechoic) and CT attenuation (similar to that of muscle) characteristics of these lesions are nonspecific (4,14,15).

Prevention of traumatic neuroma involves approximating the two severed nerve ends so that successful nerve repair and regeneration results (13,39,40). Nerve graft placement may also be performed if the nerve ends cannot be approximated. Multiple surgical techniques are available to remove the proximal nerve stump from the area of scar, which limits the potential for both traumatic neuroma development and recurrence (13,39,40). Initial conservative therapy, including acupuncture, cortisone injection (ultrasound guidance is useful), transcutaneous and direct nerve stimulation, and physical therapy is successful in up to 50% of patients (15,39–42). Surgical resection is reserved for patients in whom conservative treatment fails.

Pacinian Neuroma

Pacinian neuromas arise from hyperplasia or hypertrophy of the pacinian corpuscle. Pacinian corpuscles are mechanoreceptors and most numerous in the deep skin layers of the hands and feet, although they also occur in viscera walls, mesentery, and vessel wall adventitia. Reflecting the distribution of these normal structures, pacinian neuromas most frequently present as small superficial masses affecting the hands and feet. In the hand, lesions are most common in the index and long fingers, near the periosteum, along the lateral portion of the proximal and middle phalanges or beneath the flexor tendons at the level of the base of the proximal phalanges. The majority of pacinian neuromas are associated with a history of trauma. They are painful, and there is a female predilection (2:1 ratio). These lesions affect adults most commonly in the fifth and sixth decades of life.

At gross pathology these single or multiple lesions range from small nodules attached to interdigital nerves by a slender stalk, contiguous subepineural nodules, or simply enlargement of a pacinian corpuscle. Histologically, these lesions consist of enlarged or multiple pacinian corpuscles with fibrosis similar to that of a Morton neuroma.

Imaging of pacinian neuroma is not reported, to the best of our knowledge, although we would expect similar findings as seen in Morton neuroma (see subsequent section). Erosion of underlying bone is unusual but has been reported (9). Surgical excision with sparing of the associated nerve is curative, although symptoms occasionally persist until the pacinian corpuscle is resected.

Palisaded Encapsulated Neuroma

The palisaded encapsulated neuroma was initially described by Reed et al. in 1972 (43). Although similar to schwannoma pathologically, these lesions are clinically distinct, developing as small, asymptomatic, subcutaneous nodules affecting the face. Adults are primarily affected without a gender predilection, although some authors report a female predominance. Unlike other neuromas, these lesions are not associated with trauma and are typically encapsulated. Imaging features are not known, although we would expect a nonspecific intrinsic appearance on cross-sectional imaging. Treatment of palisaded encapsulated neuroma with surgical excision is curative.

Morton Neuroma

KEY CONCEPTS

- Morton neuroma represents perineural fibrosis about the plantar digital nerve, likely related to chronic injury, not to a neoplasm.
- It is most common in the foot, between the third and fourth or second and third metatarsal heads, with a marked female predilection.
- Morton neuroma is seen as a focal mass at the level of the metatarsal phalangeal joint, plantar to the ligament; an anatomic relationship well seen on MR and ultrasound imaging.
- T1-weighted MR images are optimal to identify a Morton neuroma. On fat-suppressed T2-weighted images the conspicuity between the fat and low-to-intermediate neuroma is reduced.
- Asymptomatic lesions are common, but are usually smaller than symptomatic lesions.

Morton neuroma is a term used to characterize a nonneoplastic lesion, originally described by Morton in 1876 as a "peculiar painful affection of the foot localized to the fourth metatarsophalangeal articulation" (44). Other terms for this lesion include *localized interdigital neuritis, plantar neuroma*, and *Morton toe* or *node*. It represents perineural fibrosis of the plantar digital nerve. The plantar digital nerve is usually affected at the level of the metatarsal head, and there is frequently an associated inflammatory response about the lesion. The nerve between the third and fourth metatarsals is most frequently involved, followed by that between the second and third metatarsals (9,44–46). Morton neuromas are uncommon between the first and second metatarsals and rare between the fourth and fifth (44,46). Similar lesions affecting the hand are described typically in males and are related to chronic occupational or recreational trauma.

Clinically, 90% of patients present with paroxysmal pain, usually elicited by exercise that may radiate into the toes or leg and is relieved by rest (44–46). Symptoms are usually present for weeks to years, and focal tenderness to palpation is frequent. Compressing the intermetatarsal space may also elicit pain (44–49). A mass is not usually palpable related to the lesion, although associated synovial cysts may be clinically evident (50). The lesions are almost invariably unilateral. Marked female predilection (as high as 18:1) has led to the suggestion that the cause is related to irritation from the wearing of high-heeled shoes, which is thought to compress the nerve against the intermetatarsal ligament. Although this pathogenesis intuitively seems correct, it has not been substantiated biomechanically, raising the question of other causes, including ischemia (51).

Asymptomatic lesions may be relatively common, with a prevalence of 30% to 33% reported in two series of 70 and 85 MR examinations, respectively (51). These asymptomatic lesions, unlike symptomatic Morton neuromas, had no significant gender predilection and were also statistically smaller than symptomatic lesions (mean transverse diameter of 4.1 to 4.5 vs. 5.3 to 5.6 mm, respectively) in several studies (51–53).

A Morton neuroma appears pathologically as a fusiform enlargement of the plantar digital nerve at its bifurcation, with thickening of the epineural fascicles, perineural fibrosis with high collagen content (*Renaut bodies*), and loss of the myelinated fibers (51,54,55). These lesions represent a primarily degenerative, rather than proliferative process.

Radiography invariably shows normal findings and is most useful for excluding other causes of pain (56,57). Ultrasonography and MR imaging are superior to CT for identifying Morton neuroma (57–62). At ultrasonography, these neuromas commonly appear as round or ovoid, well-defined, hypoechoic masses located just proximal to the metatarsal heads in the intermetatarsal space (55,56,63). Quinn et al. reported lesions to be hypoechoic in 79% of cases, mixed echotexture in 12%, and anechoic in 8% (64). Interdigital nerve continuity could be seen in only 56% of cases (64). Small lesions (<5 mm in size) can be difficult to evaluate with ultrasonography (65). In a series of 45 surgically treated patients, Kaminsky et al. reported false-negative results in two cases related to small lesion size (56). Power Doppler ultrasonography may be a valuable adjunct for identifying these lesions and often shows increased vascularity (Fig. 9.4) (66). In the study by Quinn et al., ultrasonography revealed the prospective diagnosis of Morton neuroma in 85% of 27 cases with other reports of 95% to 98% sensitivity. MR imaging had an accuracy of 90%, positive predictive value of 100%, and negative predictive value of 60% in identification of Morton neuroma in the investigation by Zanetti et al. (54). In our experience and that of others, these lesions are most evident on coronal, small field-of-view, T1-weighted images (51,54,67–70). Zanetti et al. (51) suggested three MR imaging criteria for diagnosis of Morton neuroma: (a) lesion center in the neurovascular bundle, within the intermetatarsal space, and on the plantar side of the transverse metatarsal ligament; (b) the lesion is

well-demarcated (excluding partial volume artifact from the adjacent joint capsule); and (c) the signal intensity of the lesion is similar to that of skeletal muscle on T1-weighted images and less than that of fat on T2-weighted images (likely reflecting high collagen content of fibrosis) (Figs. 9.4 and 9.5). Erikson et al. (67) reported intermetatarsal bursal fluid as an associated finding, proximal to Morton neuroma, in 67% of their cases. Zanetti et al. (51) reported a small amount of bursal fluid in the first three intermetatarsal spaces in 67% of asymptomatic patients. A large amount of intermetatarsal bursal fluid (>3 mm in transverse diameter) or fluid in the fourth intermetatarsal space should suggest an associated Morton neuroma (51).

Morton neuromas are markedly less conspicuous on T2-weighted MR images, making differentiation from surrounding muscle and fat difficult (Fig. 9.5). Use of fat-suppressed T2-weighted sequences may allow better delineation of these lesions. In our experience and that of others, the lesions often, but not invariably, enhance with intravenously administered contrast material (Fig. 9.4) (71,72). In a study of six patients with Morton neuromas, Terk et al. (69) demonstrated that fat-suppressed, contrast-enhanced MR imaging was superior for depicting lesions and detected neuromas in two patients in whom other MR imaging sequences (including fat-suppressed T2-weighted) failed to identity an abnormality. However, Williams et al. (70) reported that only 4 of 11 lesions were visible at enhanced MR imaging.

Weishaupt et al. described improved detection of Morton neuroma on MR imaging in the prone position compared to supine or upright weight-bearing positions (73,74). The supine and upright position may cause more dorsal location of the lesion, creating difficulty in detection. Quinn et al. reported 50% of lesions dorsally on sonography, which may also be a reflection of positional variation of location (73,74).

There are many cases in which metatarsal symptoms not related to Morton neuroma, had a clinical presentation suggesting that diagnosis. Zanetti et al. found that the initial clinical diagnosis of Morton neuroma was changed by MR evaluation in 28% of 54 feet (53). In 41% of cases of MR imaging, there was a significant change in location or number of neuromas, with altering of the treatment plan in 57% of cases (53). This study suggests significant implications and use for MR imaging in patients with a suspected clinical diagnosis of Morton neuroma (53).

Initial treatment of Morton neuroma is directed at modifying patient footwear. When conservative management fails, other modes of therapy are used, including neurolysis, steroid injection (ultrasound-guided), ultrasound therapy, and surgical release of the transverse metatarsal ligament for decompression (75–77). Surgical resection of the neuroma and involved nerve segment is the most successful treatment. However, the failure rate with resection is

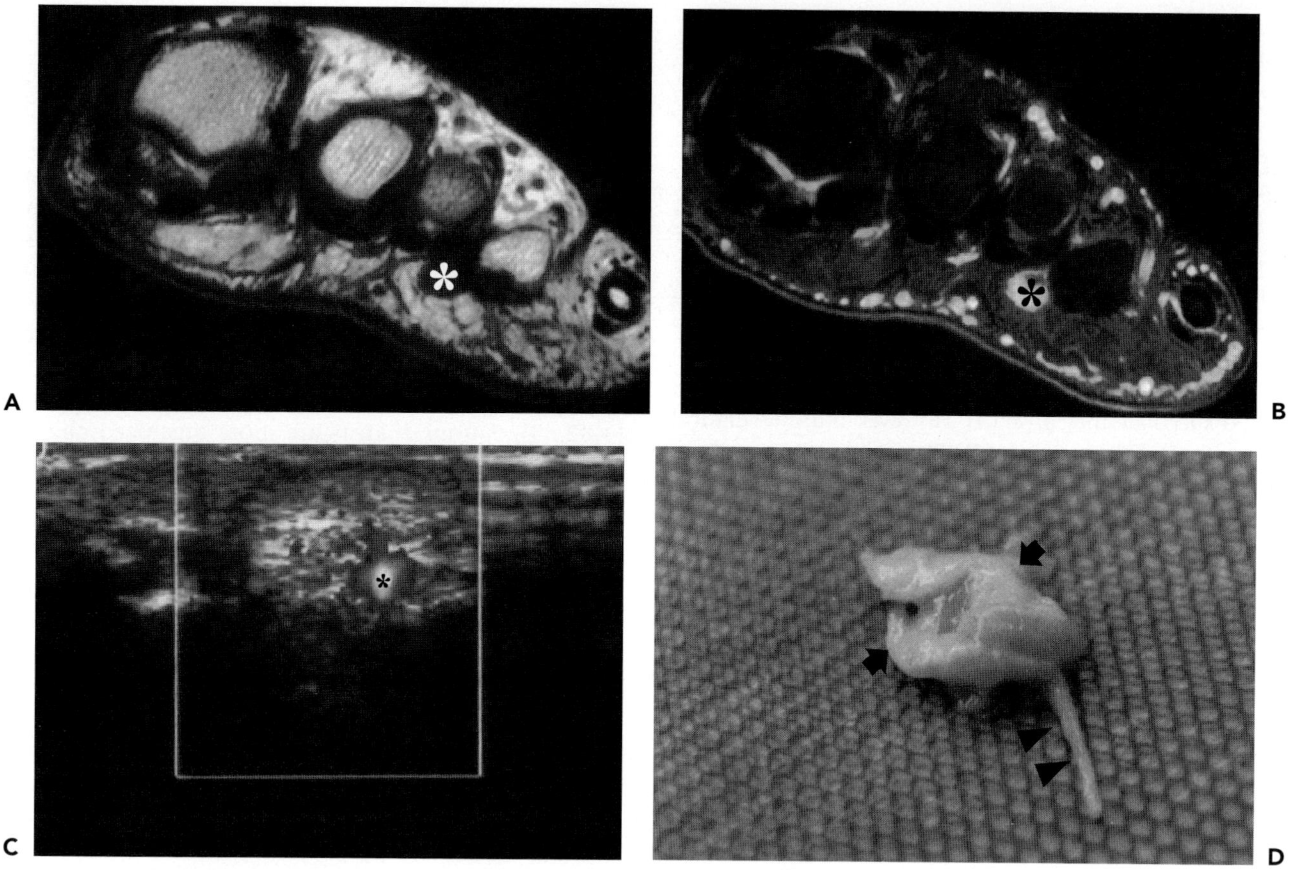

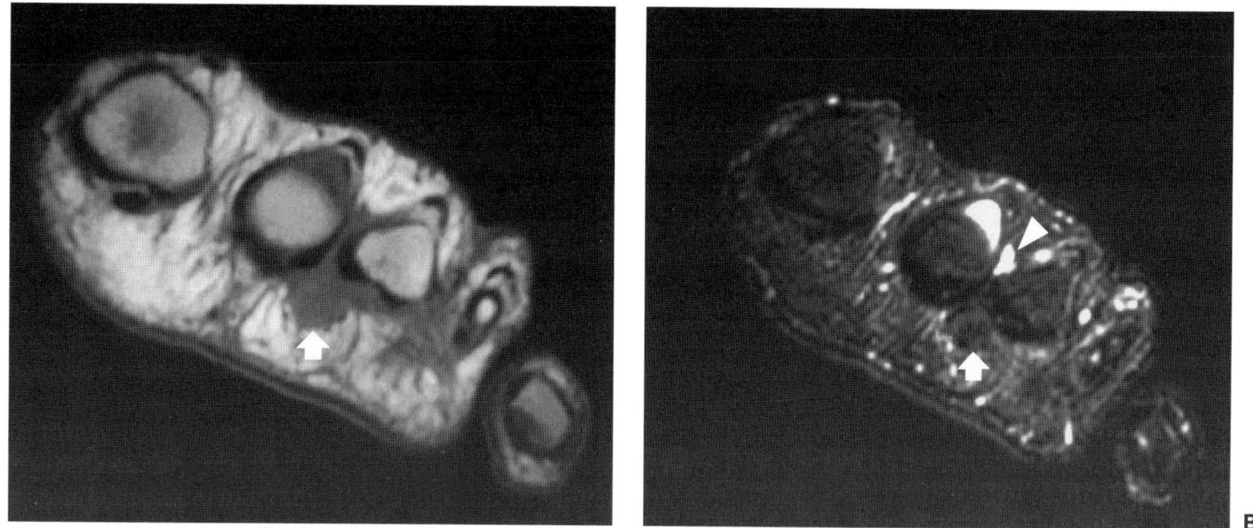

Figure 9.4 Morton neuroma in a woman 45 years of age. **A:** Short axis T1-weighted (TR/TE; 750/15) MR image shows a 6-mm mass (*asterisk*) in the interspace between the third and fourth metatarsals at the level of the metatarsal head. **B,C:** Short axis fat-suppressed contrast material–enhanced T1-weighted (TR/TE; 700/15) **(B)** MR and power Doppler ultrasound **(C)** images show marked enhancement and increased vascularity of the lesion (*asterisk*). **D:** Photograph of the resected specimen shows the entering plantar digital nerve (*arrowheads*) and the mass (*arrows*) distally representing perineural fibrosis.

Figure 9.5 Morton neuroma in a woman 39 years of age. **A,B:** Coronal T1-weighted (TR/TE; 700/15) **(A)** and T2-weighted (TR/TE; 2500/90) **(B)** spin-echo MR images show a mass (*arrow*) between the second and third metatarsal heads. The lesion has decreased signal intensity on all pulse sequences and is more difficult to detect on the long TR image. Intermetatarsal bursal fluid is also seen (*arrowhead*).

approximately 10%, likely because of development of traumatic neuroma (78).

BENIGN PERIPHERAL NERVE SHEATH TUMORS

Benign peripheral nerve sheath tumors (BPNSTs) are typically divided into two major benign groups: schwannoma (neurilemoma) and neurofibroma (79). Both the schwannoma and neurofibroma contain cells that are closely related to the normal Schwann cell, from which some would speculate they arise (9). However, multiple clinical and pathologic features usually allow distinction of these neoplasms.

Schwannoma (Neurilemoma)

KEY CONCEPTS
- Schwannomas represent 5% of all benign soft tissue tumors.
- They are also called *neurilemomas*.
- Common sites are the cutaneous tissues of the head/neck, flexor surfaces of the extremities, posterior mediastinum, and retroperitoneum.
- Affected nerve and tumor are separable within the epineurium.
- Surgical resection, with sparing of the nerve is curative.

Schwannoma is most commonly detected in patients between the ages of 20 and 50 years and occurs with equal frequency in men and women (79,80). Schwannomas are slightly less common than neurofibromas and comprise approximately 5% of all benign soft tissue tumors (81). Sites of involvement include the cutaneous nerves of the head and neck and the flexor surfaces of the extremities, particularly the peroneal and ulnar nerves. Schwannomas also show a predilection to affect sensory nerves. The posterior mediastinum and retroperitoneum are also commonly affected with deeply seated lesions. A schwannoma is almost invariably a slowly growing nonaggressive neoplasm that usually presents clinically as a painless mass, often smaller than 5 cm, without neurologic symptoms (9,82,83). Pain may be associated with large lesions, or in patients with schwannomatosis. Schwannoma is solitary in the vast majority of cases. Overall, approximately 5% of cases are plexiform or multiple and are rarely associated with von Recklinghausen disease (82,84). Schwannomas are sporadic in 90%, with 3% occurring in neurofibromatosis type 2 (NF2), 2% in patients with schwannomatosis, and 5% in association with multiple meningiomas with or without NF2 (85). Schwannomas are often mobile

in the plane transverse to the involved nerve, but movement is restricted in the longitudinal axis by nerve attachment.

At gross pathology, schwannomas are fusiform-shaped lesions, representing the mass with the entering and exiting nerve. When large nerves are affected, the mass is eccentric in relationship to the involved nerve, with nerve fibers splayed about the neoplasm. Similar to neurofibromas, schwannomas of small nerves may obliterate the nerve of origin. Both the schwannoma and the affected nerve are within a true capsule composed of the epineurium.

The histologic hallmark of schwannoma is identification of Antoni A and Antoni B regions. Lesions are also S-100 protein positive at immunohistochemical analysis (1,82,83). Antoni A areas are more organized and are hypercellular composed of spindle cells arranged in short bundles or interlacing fascicles. Antoni B regions are hypocellular, less organized, and contain more myxoid, loosely arranged tissue, with high water content. These components are intermixed within schwannomas and occur in varying amounts. Schwannomas in which Antoni A areas predominate are often called *cellular* schwannomas (86). They are more frequently located in the posterior mediastinum and retroperitoneum and constitute 25% of extremity lesions (1). Large schwannomas commonly undergo degenerative changes, including cyst formation, calcification, hemorrhage, and fibrosis and are often referred to as *ancient* schwannomas (82,83,87). Additional histologic variants of schwannoma include epithelioid and melanotic subtypes. The melanotic schwannoma deserves special mention because of several unique features. Although maintaining the basic features of schwannoma, there is often heavy pigmentation. These lesions commonly involve the spinal nerves (96%), have a mild female predilection (1.4:1 ratio), and 55% occur in association with *Carney complex* (myxomas, spotty pigmentation, and endocrine overactivity) (79,80,88,89). In addition, unlike conventional schwannoma, the melanotic variant has a significant incidence of malignant behavior with metastases reported in 13% to 26% of cases (79,80,88,89).

Schwannomas are almost universally associated with genetic aberration in chromosome 22. The specific site is frequently referred to as the NF2 gene and this encodes the Merlin protein (also termed *schwannomin*) (90). The NF2 gene is a tumor suppressor, and loss of its function is likely the initial factor in schwannoma tumorigenesis (90).

Treatment of schwannoma is usually surgical excision. The affected nerve is typically separable from the neoplasm intraoperatively after incision of the epineurium, allowing the native nerve and its function to be preserved (26). Partial resection may be performed in cases that would otherwise require nerve resection for complete removal. Recurrence is unusual, even after incomplete resection, and malignant transformation is exceedingly rare.

Neurofibroma

> **KEY CONCEPTS**
> - Neurofibromas constitute 5% of benign soft tissue tumors.
> - Three types—localized (90%), diffuse, and plexiform—are described.
> - They can involve superficial or deep nerves.
> - Neoplasm and nerve cannot be separated.
> - Complete resection requires sacrificing the nerve; thus, deep-seated lesions are often managed conservatively with observation.

Neurofibroma most commonly affects patients 20 to 30 years of age and demonstrates no sex predilection (24,79,80,83,91). These lesions constitute slightly more than 5% of all benign soft tissue tumors (1,81). Three types of neurofibromas are classically described: localized, diffuse, and plexiform (see discussion of neurofibromatosis type 1 [NF1]). The localized variety is the most common, representing approximately 90% of these lesions, and the vast majority are solitary and not associated with NF1 (1,26). Localized neurofibromas often affect superficial cutaneous nerves, although involvement of larger nerves also occurs, causing deep-seated lesions. Localized neurofibromas are slow-growing lesions, usually smaller than 5 cm at presentation and painless (1,26). The diffuse neurofibroma primarily affects children and young adults and most frequently involves the subcutaneous tissues of the head and neck. The majority of diffuse neurofibromas (90%) are isolated lesions not associated with NF1 (1,26). Diffuse neurofibromas demonstrate a plaquelike elevation of the skin with thickening of the entire subcutis.

At gross examination, localized neurofibromas show a fusiform shape, representing the mass with the entering and exiting nerve. Deep-seated lesions of large nerves (most frequently evaluated radiologically) often remain within the epineurium, and, similar to neurilemomas, they have a true capsule (3,64,65). Localized neurofibromas of small nerves commonly extend beyond the epineurium, although they often remain well-circumscribed. In contradistinction, diffuse neurofibroma is a poorly defined lesion in the subcutaneous fat that infiltrates along connective tissue septa. Unlike neurilemomas, neurofibromas are intimately intermixed and inseparable from normal nerve tissue.

At histologic analysis, a localized, solitary neurofibroma is composed of interlacing fascicles of wavy, elongated cells that often contain abundant amounts of collagen. Unlike neurilemoma, neurofibromas do not contain Antoni A and B regions (1,82,83). Myxoid areas and degenerative regions are also not as prominent as they are in neurilemoma. Diffuse neurofibroma contains very uniform, prominent fibrillary collagen. Both localized and diffuse neurofibroma are positive for S-100 protein at immunohistochemical

analysis, although generally not as extensively as schwannoma (1). Histologic variants of neurofibroma include cellular, pigmented, and epithelioid types, similar to neurilemoma. Benign neurogenic lesions composed of a mixture of neural elements, skeletal muscle, and rhabdomyomatous elements (neuromuscular hamartoma/choristoma or benign triton tumor) are also described. Genetic aberration in sporadic neurofibromas awaits confirmation, although alterations in the NF1 gene may be involved.

Treatment of localized and diffuse neurofibromas (not associated with NF1) is often surgical resection. However, in contradistinction to neurilemomas, neurofibromas cannot be separated from normal nerve, and complete excision of the neoplasm requires sacrifice of the nerve (92). Although this treatment may be acceptable in cutaneous lesions, deep-seated lesions may only be debulked or managed conservatively with observation. Surgical resection of deep-seated lesions is associated with significant patient morbidity related to nerve damage and neurologic deficits from excision (93). Local recurrence after complete excision is unusual and is more frequently associated with diffuse neurofibroma because of its infiltrative growth. Malignant transformation of these lesions, not associated with NF1, is probably rare, although the exact risk is not known.

Neurofibromatosis

> **KEY CONCEPTS**
> - Neurofibromatosis 1 (NF1) and neurofibromatosis 2 (NF2) account for 99% of cases of neurofibromatosis.
> - Musculoskeletal abnormalities predominate in NF1 versus central nervous system manifestations in NF2.
> - NF1 is a common genetic disease (1 in every 2,500 to 3,000 births).
> - New mutations cause 50% of NF1 cases.
> - The hallmark of NF1 is multiple neurofibromas, particularly plexiform lesions (essentially pathognomonic), and multiple localized neurofibromas.
> - Plexiform neurofibromas represent diffuse involvement of a long segment of the nerve and its branches (*bag of worms* appearance).
> - The incidence of malignant transformation to malignant peripheral nerve sheath tumor (MPNST) is 2% to 29%, in patients with NF1.

Several reports of neurofibromatosis predate von Recklinghausen's description in 1882 (79). However, the first association of neural and fibrous components in this disorder is attributed to von Recklinghausen (94). At least eight variations of neurofibromatosis are described, although neurofibromatosis type 1 (NF1) and neurofibromatosis type 2 (NF2) account for 99% of cases (95,96). Musculoskeletal abnormalities predominate in the most common form, NF1, as opposed to the central nervous system manifestations (bilateral acoustic neuromas, gliomas, meningiomas) of NF2 (97); therefore, we largely limit our discussion to NF1 (98–103).

NF1 is one of the most common genetic diseases, with an estimated frequency of 1 case in every 2,500 to 3,000 births (98–100,104,105). Higher frequencies are reported in Arab and Israeli subpopulations. This disease is a mesodermal dysplasia, affecting multiple organ systems, and it is inherited as an autosomal dominant trait. The penetrance of NF1 is 100%, although the expression is variable, with slightly more than 50% of patients only mildly affected (101). However, at least 50% of cases are believed to arise from new mutations, and its mutation rate (1 per 10,000 gametes per generation) is greater than that of many other common genetic disorders (98–100,104–106). Advanced paternal age (>35 years) is a predisposing factor in an estimated 80% of cases, producing a twofold increase in new mutations, although other factors are also important (9,100). The genetic abnormality is localized to the pericentromeric region of chromosome 17, which is the site of a tumor suppressor gene (9,100). This genetic focus encodes the production of the protein neurofibromin, which likely has some control in cell growth regulation.

Table 9.1 lists the clinical criteria for the diagnosis of NF1 (26), and the classic triad consists of cutaneous lesions, skeletal deformity, and mental deficiency. Café-au-lait spots are identified in approximately 90% of patients, usually within the first several years of life (9,98–100,104,105). Although café-au-lait spots are not pathognomonic of NF1 (because they are also seen in tuberous sclerosis and fibrous dysplasia), their size, distribution, and shape in NF1 aid in differentiating this condition from other diagnoses (100,104,105). Café-au-lait spots are caused by increased melanin pigment in the basal epidermal layer and represent another manifestation of the underlying neural crest abnormality. The axilla is a frequent location of café-au-lait

TABLE 9.1
CRITERIA FOR DIAGNOSIS OF NF1[a]

Six or more café-au-lait spots
Over 5 mm in greatest diameter in prepubertal patients
Over 15 mm in greatest diameter in postpubertal patients
Two or more neurofibromas (any type) or one plexiform
   neurofibroma
Axillary or inguinal freckling
Optic glioma
Two or more Lisch nodules (i.e., iris hamartomas)
Distinctive osseous lesions (e.g., sphenoid dysplasia,
   pseudarthrosis)[b]
First-degree relative with NF1, as diagnosed by preceding criteria

[a]Two or more of these criteria are required for diagnosis.
[b]See Table 9.2.
From Neurofibromatosis. Conference statement. In: National Institutes of Health Consensus Development Conference. *Arch Neurol.* 1988;575–578. Modified, with permission.

TABLE 9.2
OSSEOUS ABNORMALITIES ASSOCIATED WITH NF1

Scoliosis (short or long segment)
Kyphosis (often predominant deformity)
Facial or orbital dysplasia
Lambdoid suture defects (left-sided)
Pseudarthrosis (particularly of the tibia and congenital)
Periosteal abnormalities (reaction, cysts)
Multiple nonossifying fibromas or fibroxanthomas
Rib deformity (particularly ribbon ribs)
Posterior vertebral body scalloping (dural ectasia)

spots (9,26). Their extent often parallels disease severity. Another pigmentation abnormality seen in more than 90% of patients with NF1 (and not associated with NF2 or seen in the normal population) is the Lisch nodule, which is an asymptomatic pigmented hamartoma of the iris (98–100).

Skeletal abnormalities are common in NF1, occurring in approximately 25% to 40% of cases, again reflecting the multiorgan effects of the mesodermal dysplasia (26,100). Table 9.2 lists these osseous manifestations (Fig. 9.6) (26).

The most frequent skeletal abnormality is kyphoscoliosis. Additional features associated with NF1 include epilepsy, neuropathy, hydrocephalus (aqueductal stenosis), pseudogynecomastia in men, and fibromuscular dysplasia (renal and large cervical vessels) in women. Numerous neoplasms may also be associated with NF1 and include optic glioma, astrocytoma, glioblastoma multiforme, rhabdomyosarcoma, Triton tumor, pheochromocytoma, carcinoid tumor, nephroblastoma, gastrointestinal stromal tumor, and juvenile chronic myeloid leukemia.

The hallmark of NF1 is the neurofibroma. Neurofibromas usually occur initially in childhood or adolescence, subsequent to detection of café-au-lait spots. These lesions can occur in any location of the body, including soft tissues (superficial or deep) and viscera, and, in some reports, more commonly affect males (9). Growth of neurofibromas is usually slow; however, more rapid episodes of growth can be associated with pregnancy, puberty, or malignant transformation.

All three types of neurofibromas (localized, diffuse, and plexiform) can be associated with NF1. Localized neurofibroma is the most common type seen with NF1. However, histologically, both localized and diffuse neurofibromas are not characteristic of NF1 because most of these lesions occur in an isolated pattern which is not associated with this underlying condition. In contradistinction to localized neurofibromas in patients without any underlying disease, those associated with NF1 more frequently involve large deep nerves (particularly the sciatic nerve and brachial plexus). These neurofibromas are large in size and invariably multiple in number. Localized neurofibromas in NF1 also often affect

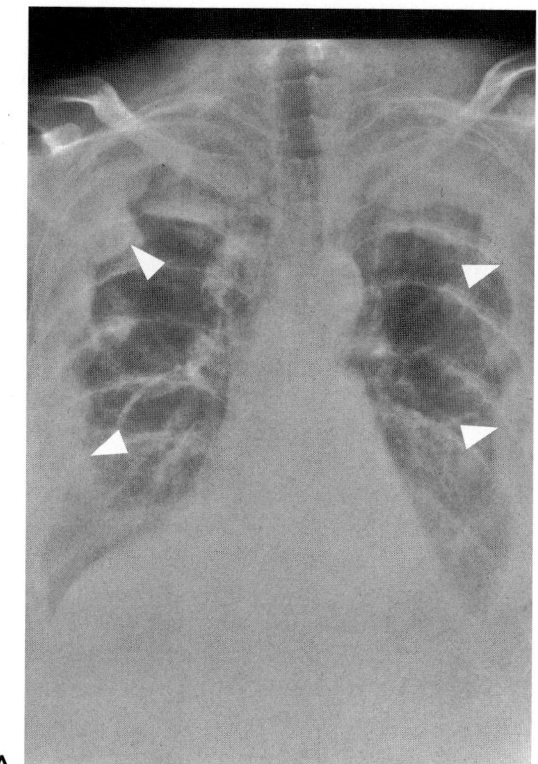
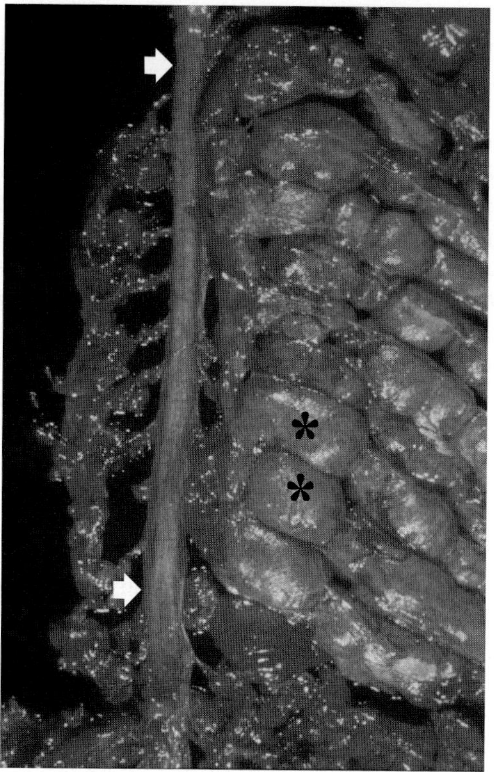

Figure 9.6 Neurofibromatosis 1 with ribbon ribs resulting from multiple plexiform neurofibromas in a 20-year-old man. **A:** Chest radiograph shows multilobulated extrapleural masses (*arrowheads*) and scalloping of all ribs with a ribbonlike appearance. **B:** Photograph of the autopsy gross specimen reveals that the rib abnormalities resulted from multiple neurofibromas of intercostal nerves (*asterisks*) arising from the spinal cord (*arrows*).

the dermis and subcutaneous tissue and are referred to as *fibroma molluscum* when pedunculated (9,26,100).

Plexiform neurofibromas are essentially pathognomonic of NF1; development of these lesions usually occurs in early childhood and precedes cutaneous neurofibromas (98–100,104,105). Pathologically, a plexiform neurofibroma represents diffuse involvement of a long nerve segment and its branches with tortuous expansion, and its gross appearance is ropelike and is described as a *bag of worms*. Because of their large size, these lesions commonly extend beyond the epineurium into the surrounding tissue. Plexiform neurofibromas may be associated with massive and disfiguring enlargement of an extremity called *elephantiasis neuromatosa*, although the segmental variant form (107–109) of NF can have a similar appearance without the other stigmata of NF1 (110–113). This condition may be accompanied by osseous hypertrophy related to chronic hyperemia.

Treatment of patients with NF1 is complicated by the multiplicity of lesions and is often nonsurgical (114). Attempts at surgical resection are usually reserved for markedly symptomatic lesions that substantially compromise function. Because of the large size of many of these lesions, surgical resection is often incomplete, leading to frequent recurrences (92). Malignant transformation to malignant peripheral nerve sheath tumor (MPNST) is the most-feared complication of NF1. The estimated prevalence

of malignant transformation varies from 2% to 29%, with an average of approximately 5% (9,26,115). The highest incidence of malignant transformation appears to be in plexiform lesions. Overall, we believe the lower figure of 2% more accurately reflects the true incidence of malignant transformation in NF1, similar to the results of the longitudinal (39-year follow-up) Danish study of 212 patients by Sorenson et al. (116).

MALIGNANT PERIPHERAL NERVE SHEATH TUMOR (MPNST)

KEY CONCEPTS

- *Malignant peripheral nerve sheath tumor* (MPNST) is the correct terminology as opposed to *malignant schwannoma* or *neurofibrosarcoma*.
- MPNST accounts for 5% to 10% of all soft tissue sarcomas.
- It affects adults 20 to 50 years of age.
- MPNST is associated with NF1 in 25% to 70% of cases.
- It usually arises in large-to-medium deep-seated nerves.
- The tumors are fusiform, a shape caused by the entering and exiting nerve.
- Treatment is wide surgical excision and adjunct therapy, although overall long-term prognosis is poor.

The World Health Organization (WHO) Committee for the Classification of Soft Tissue Tumors standardized malignant peripheral nerve sheath tumor (MPNST) as the accepted nomenclature for a spindle cell sarcoma arising from nerve, or neurofibroma, or demonstrating nerve tissue differentiation (17,80,117,118). MPNST replaces the former terminology of *malignant schwannoma, malignant neurilemoma or neurofibrosarcoma*. MPNST accounts for 5% to 10% of all soft tissue sarcomas and usually affects adult patients 20 to 50 years of age (118). Overall, there is a slight female predilection (1,17). It is estimated that these lesions are associated with NF1 in 25% to 70% of cases and that in these patients, MPNSTs occur approximately a decade earlier (28 to 40 years of age) and have a male predilection (80% of patients with MPNSTs and NF1 are male) (17). MPNSTs show a distinct propensity to affect large major or medium-sized nerves, including the sciatic nerve, brachial plexus, and sacral plexus (119). Patients present with pain and neurologic symptoms of motor weakness and sensory deficits more frequently than do patients with benign peripheral nerve sheath tumors (BPNST). In patients with NF1, sudden increase in size of a previously stable neurofibroma should be viewed with great suspicion of malignant transformation, and lead to immediate biopsy. MPNST can also be a secondary neoplasm related to previous radiation therapy. These tumors develop after a long latent period (10 to 20 years) following irradiation and account for 10% to 20% of MPNSTs, with the higher figure associated with paraspinal lesions (17,120).

MPNSTs are fusiform, a shape caused by the entering and exiting nerve, which is clearly evident at gross pathologic examination (17). The tumor frequently spreads along the entering and exiting nerve, with the epineurium and perineurium becoming thickened proximally and distally to the mass, a feature not seen in BPNSTs. The tumor cells are arranged in fascicles, resembling those seen in fibrosarcoma, and areas of hemorrhage and necrosis are frequent. Additional heterotopic regions are seen histologically in 10% to 15% of tumors, and include foci of mature cartilage and bone, rhabdomyosarcoma elements (malignant Triton tumor), angiosarcoma regions, and glandular or epithelioid components (17). MPNST with rhabdomyosarcoma, angiosarcoma, or glandular elements tend to occur in association with NF1. Epithelioid MPNST is less commonly associated with NF1 and accounts for 5% of these malignancies. Epithelioid MPNST arises in relation to a large deep nerve in 50% to 80% of cases, with the remainder in the superficial soft tissues. The majority of MPNSTs are considered to be high-grade sarcomas.

The cytogenetics of MPNST now suggest a multistep mechanism of tumorigenesis. The initial step in the process in patients with NF1 is inactivation of one or both alleles of the NF1 gene allowing neurofibroma formation (121).

Progression to MPNST is likely associated with several additional chromosomal aberrations, with particular involvement of the tumor suppression gene on chromosome 17p (122). The p53 focus is suggested as the specific culprit in allowing increased proliferation and angioinvasive capacity (122). Scientific implication of this pathway is supported by the fact that patients with MPNST show a high percentage of abnormalities at this locus, which are not seen in patients with BPNST.

Treatment of MPNST is complete surgical excision with wide resection margins. Adjuvant chemotherapy and radiation are also often employed. Radiation therapy reduces the incidence of local recurrence; however, despite this aggressive treatment, local recurrence and distant metastases are common, seen in 40% to 65% and 40% to 68% of patients, respectively (17,119). Wanebo et al. (120) reported a 5-year survival rate of only 44%. Two additional studies show 5- and 10-year survival rates ranging from 34% to 52% and 23% to 34%, respectively (120). Lesions in sites that are difficult to achieve adequate surgical margins (paraspinal, thoracic, retroperitoneal) are associated with even lower survival rates (15%). Worsened prognosis is associated with older patient age, larger tumor size (>5 cm), more central location of the tumor, high mitotic rate (>20/10 high power field [HPF]), and positive margins after resection. Although some researchers believe patients with NF1 have a significantly poorer prognosis, this contention is now somewhat controversial. Several newer reports show that all patients with MPNSTs have a similar prognosis regardless of the presence of underlying NF1 (120,123). Metastases most frequently affect the lung, bone, pleura, and retroperitoneum. Regional lymph nodes are involved in 9% of cases (17,119,120,123).

IMAGING OF SCHWANNOMA, NEUROFIBROMA, NEUROFIBROMATOSIS TYPE 1, AND MALIGNANT PERIPHERAL NERVE SHEATH TUMOR

The most common abnormality of peripheral nerve sheath tumors (PNSTs) (including BPNST, NF1, and MPNST) at radiography is a nonspecific soft tissue mass. Radiographs are also frequently normal. In rare cases, a fusiform soft tissue mass with surrounding fat may be seen. Occasionally, soft tissue and osseous overgrowth associated with elephantiasis neuromatosa and other skeletal manifestations of NF1 or the segmental variant may be recognized on radiographs (100,124). A primary osseous location for PNSTs is exceedingly rare, and bone involvement by either extrinsic erosion or invasion is unusual. Calcification (osteoid, chondroid, or amorphous) is uncommon and mild in extent when present (Fig. 9.7) (100,124). Both

KEY CONCEPTS

- Subcutaneous neurogenic neoplasms are often not imaged and have a nonspecific appearance.
- Plexiform neurofibromas have a pathognomonic imaging appearance with a serpentine morphology, representing tumor involvement of long nerve segments and their branches.
- Deep-seated neurogenic neoplasms usually have a diagnostic imaging appearance, particular on MR imaging and ultrasonography:
  - Fusiform shape with entering and exiting nerve
  - Target sign
  - Split-fat sign
  - Fascicular sign
  - Associated muscle atrophy
- Distinction of MPNST versus BPNST can be very difficult; however, imaging features favoring malignancy include size larger than 5 cm, prominent vascularity, marked heterogeneity, central necrosis, rapid growth, increased gallium uptake, and evidence of infiltrative margins in a nonplexiform lesion.

bone involvement and mineralization are more common in larger lesions and MPNST. This reflects the heterogeneity of these lesions seen pathologically.

Angiography of deep PNSTs demonstrates displacement of major vascular structures related to the site of origin of the lesion within the neurovascular bundle. The degree of increased vascularity is variable, but typically more prominent in MPNST (125–129). A characteristic at angiography that suggests a neurogenic neoplasm is the identification of corkscrew-type vessels at the upper or lower poles of the tumor. This appearance represents hypertrophy of nutrient nerve vasculature (125,127) (Fig. 9.8).

Bone scintigraphy findings of PNSTs are nonspecific and reflect the vascularity, bone involvement, or mineralization associated with the tumor. Typically, only mild uptake of radionuclide is seen on all phases of imaging, unless calcification or bone involvement is extensive. However, several reports describe gallium-67 citrate imaging as very helpful for differentiating BPNST from MPNST (126,130). Although only small numbers of patients were involved, significant uptake of gallium-67 citrate was seen in MPNST compared to minimal or no accumulation in BPNST (Figs. 9.9–9.11) (126, 130–132).

Early results with FDG-PET imaging in evaluation of neurogenic neoplasm have now reported (133). Several reports by Ahmed et al., Beaulieu et al., and Shah et al. identify marked radionuclide uptake in a significant number of patients with schwannomas (5% to 50%) with standard uptake values (SUVs) numbers greater than 2 (134–136). This limits use of FDG-PET to distinguish schwannoma from MPNST. However, Ferner et al. and Solomon et al. reported success in distinguishing plexiform neurofibromas that have undergone malignant degeneration to MPNST from benign lesions in patients with NF1 using FDG-PET (137,138).

As with other soft tissue neoplasms, these lesions are more easily characterized with cross-sectional imaging techniques (ultrasound, CT, MR) (139–145). In our opinion and experience, the most important imaging feature that should always suggest the diagnosis of neurogenic neoplasm is recognition of a fusiform mass (Figs. 9.12

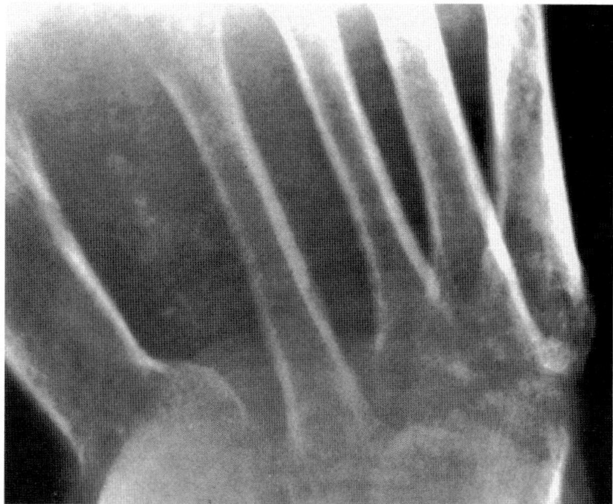
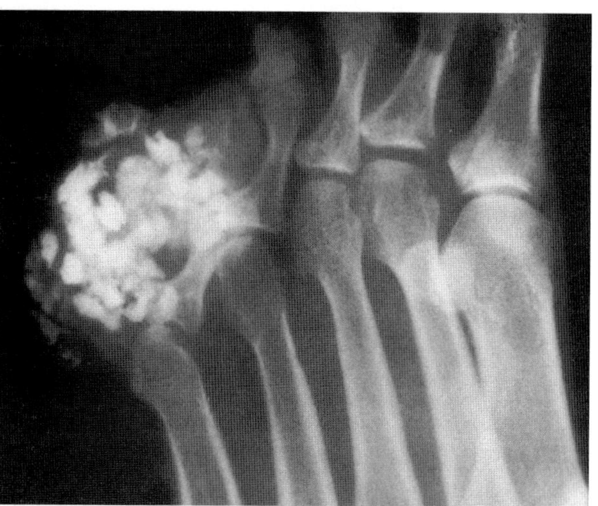

Figure 9.7 Mineralization in nerve sheath tumors in two different patients. **A:** Foot radiograph shows faint calcification between the first and second metatarsals in a patient with a malignant peripheral nerve sheath tumor. **B:** Foot radiograph shows densely mineralized neurofibroma in the fifth toe. Histology (not shown) revealed areas of chondroid and osteoid metaplasia.

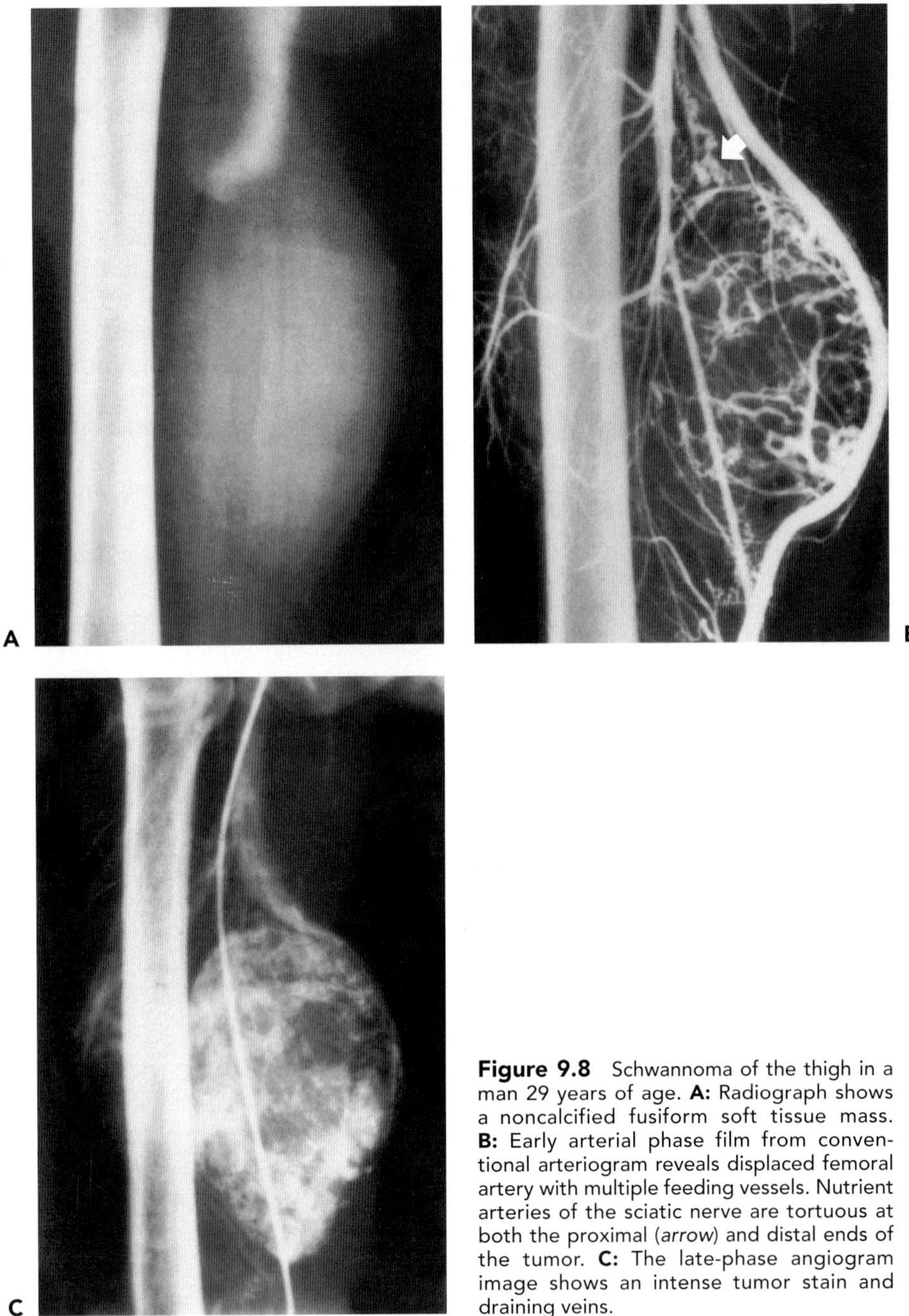

Figure 9.8 Schwannoma of the thigh in a man 29 years of age. **A:** Radiograph shows a noncalcified fusiform soft tissue mass. **B:** Early arterial phase film from conventional arteriogram reveals displaced femoral artery with multiple feeding vessels. Nutrient arteries of the sciatic nerve are tortuous at both the proximal (*arrow*) and distal ends of the tumor. **C:** The late-phase angiogram image shows an intense tumor stain and draining veins.

and 9.13) (146). This appearance is a direct reflection of the underlying gross morphology of schwannomas, localized neurofibroma, and MPNST, representing the tubular entering and exiting nerve in a typical nerve distribution. This relationship is usually easy to detect in lesions affecting large, deep nerves that are frequently imaged because the clinical presentation is that of a nonspecific soft tissue mass (Figs. 9.12 and 9.13). In contradistinction, in superficial PNSTs, it is often difficult or impossible to identify this appearance, and imaging findings are nonspecific. However, these superficial lesions, as with other cutaneous or subcutaneous lesions, often are not imaged because of the so-called ease of clinical assessment. In our experience, MR imaging and ultrasonography are superior to CT for demonstrating the virtually pathognomonic fusiform appearance of deep-seated neurilemoma, localized neurofibroma, and MPNST because of their large field of view and multiplanar capabilities (145,147,148). Cerofolini et al. (149) reported this finding in 94% of their 17 cases. PNSTs of the paraspinal region often reveal a dumbbell shape with extension into an enlarged neural foramen (150). This

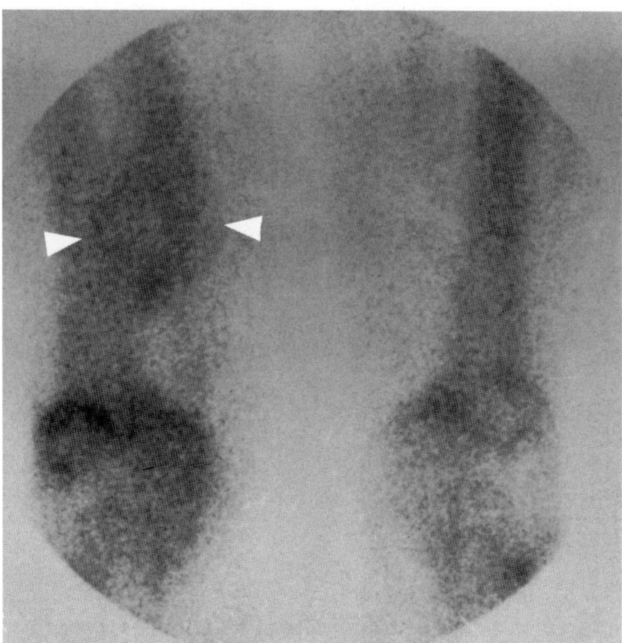

Figure 9.9 Schwannoma of the thigh in a man 61 years of age. Bone scintigraphy demonstrates mild accumulation of radionuclide (*arrowheads*).

neural foraminal component is analogous to the entering nerve seen in peripheral lesions (Fig. 9.14) (151–157). Extrinsic erosion of the posterior vertebral body and, rarely, invasion simulating a more aggressive process may also be seen (153,158). Spinal PNSTs must be differentiated from meningoceles (70% to 80% of the latter lesions occur in patients with NF1 and are often multiple) because of differences in treatment (100). Meningoceles characteristically are cystic, fill with contrast material after myelography (with or without CT), and have a posterior mediastinal location without calcification. Spinal neurofibromas in patients with NF1 are often bilateral, and a prominent disparity in size should be viewed with suspicion that the larger lesion harbors MPNST (Fig. 9.15) (151–156).

Theoretically, differentiation of deep-seated localized neurofibroma from neurilemoma should be possible because of their differences in location relative to the affected nerve. In neurilemoma, the mass is eccentric and separable from normal nerve, but in neurofibroma the two structures are intimately related, intermixed and indistinguishable. Indeed, Cerofolini et al. (149) believed they could discern this relationship in 65% of their 17 cases. In our experience, however, this distinction can be difficult because both lesions are often in deep locations within the epineurium and have similar intrinsic imaging characteristics relative to affected nerve. This similarity often precludes radiologic discrimination between these lesions in many patients, and this distinction is best accomplished in

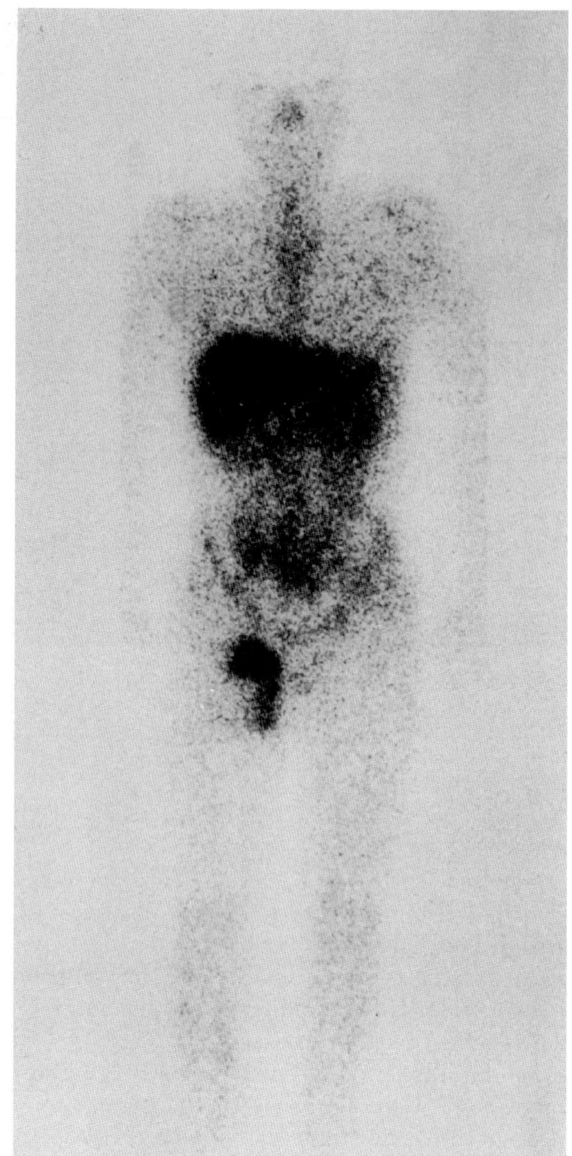

Figure 9.10 Malignant peripheral nerve sheath tumor in the left thigh of a man 22 years of age. Left thigh demonstrates intense uptake of gallium-67 5 days after injection.

neoplasms affecting large nerves such as the sciatic nerve. We believe significant eccentricity in any imaging plane of the nerve relative to the mass strongly suggests neurilemoma versus localized neurofibroma (Figs. 9.12 and 9.13) (145).

Recently, Jee et al. reported the following characteristics as statistically significant in distinguishing extra-axial localized neurofibroma (*n* = 12) from neurilemoma (*n* = 40): target sign on T2-weighted MR images (58% of neurofibromas, 65% neurilemomas); central enhancement (75% neurofibromas, 8% neurilemomas); and target sign and central enhancement (63% neurofibromas, 3% neurilemomas) (159). Features favoring extra-axial

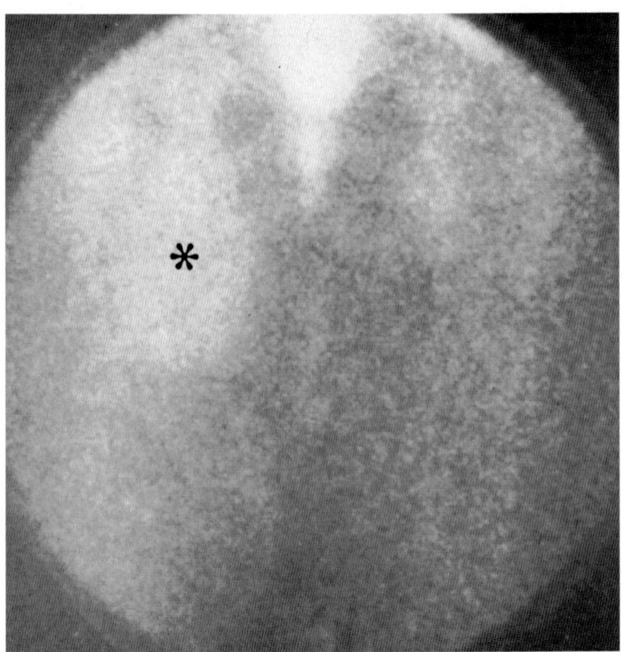

Figure 9.11 Schwannoma of the sciatic nerve in a woman 57 years of age shows relative photopenia with no significant radionuclide uptake of gallium by the tumor (*asterisk*) 2 days after injection.

TABLE 9.3

IMAGING SIGNS OF NEUROGENIC NEOPLASMS

Sign	Modality Depicting the Sign
Fusiform	MR, ultrasonography (less well-seen with CT)
Entering and exiting nerve	MR, ultrasonography (less well-seen with CT)
Low attenuation	Unenhanced CT
Target sign	T2-weighted MR (less well-seen with CT, ultrasonography)
Fascicular sign	T2- and proton density–weighted MR
Split-fat sign	T1-weighted MR (less well-seen with CT, ultrasonography)
Associated muscle atrophy	T1-weighted MR

neurilemoma versus localized neurofibroma were the fascicular appearance on T2-weighted MR images (25% neurofibromas, 63% neurilemomas); a thin hyperintense rim on T2-weighted images (8% neurofibromas, 58% neurilemomas); a combination of the above mentioned features (8% neurofibromas, 48% neurilemomas); and diffuse contrast enhancement (13% neurofibromas, 67% neurilemomas) (159). No statistically significant difference was seen between the lesions for the following features: central entering/exiting nerve (42% neurofibromas, 23% neurilemomas); peripherally entering/exiting nerve (58% neurofibromas, 77% neurilemomas); a cystic area (38% neurofibromas, 64% neurilemomas); low-signal intensity margin (100% for both lesions); peripheral contrast enhancement (13% neurofibromas, 26% neurilemomas); or target sign on contrast-enhanced MR images (11% neurofibromas, 31% neurilemomas) (159).

Plexiform neurofibromas invariably show a pathognomic imaging appearance identical to that of their gross pathologic features of diffuse nerve thickening (Figs. 9.16 and 9.17) (160–164). There is often nodularity and involvement of nerve branches that create the appearance of a serpentine "bag of worms." Patients with multiple schwannomas may reveal multiple masses (beadlike appearance) with an intrinsic appearance identical to that of other neurilemomas, usually along a single nerve distribution best seen on long axis MR images (Fig. 9.18). Unlike plexiform neurofibroma, the intervening nerve is

not typically thickened, and the nerve branches are not usually affected (Fig. 9.18) (165,166). Diffuse neurofibromas show a reticulated linear branching pattern within the subcutaneous tissue replacing the fat and creating a honeycomb appearance (Fig. 9.19) (26,167).

Table 9.3 lists the intrinsic imaging characteristics of neurogenic neoplasms. On unenhanced CT scans, PNSTs frequently have low attenuation (often as low as 5 to 25 HU) (Figs. 9.15 and 9.16) (168,169). This appearance is attributed to several factors, including high lipid content of myelin from Schwann cells, presence or entrapment of fat, endoneurial myxoid tissue with high water content (Antoni B areas in neurilemomas or myxoid areas in neurofibromas), and cystic areas (hemorrhage, necrosis or degenerated areas in ancient schwannomas) (170–175). Heterogeneity and higher attenuation may be seen in neurogenic neoplasms and is a more common feature of MPNST (128,129).

On MR images, the signal intensity of neurogenic neoplasms is relatively nonspecific and is similar to or lower than that of muscle on T1-weighted images and higher than that of fat on T2-weighted MR images. Ultrasonography typically reveals a well-defined hypoechoic mass with variable posterior acoustic enhancement (176,177). Color Doppler studies are useful to identify lesions that may simulate a ganglion on other imaging modalities with the identification of intrinsic blood flow (176). Diffuse neurofibromas often show predominant low signal intensity on T2-weighted MR images, a finding we believe is related to the high collagen content of these lesions. Heterogeneity in PNSTs is variable, although it is more prominent in MPNST (including, in uncommon cases, fluid levels and hemorrhage). Mann et al. (178) attempted to quantitate this heterogeneity in distinguishing benign PNST from MPNST by using fuzzy cluster analysis and found separation to be difficult by these characteristics alone.

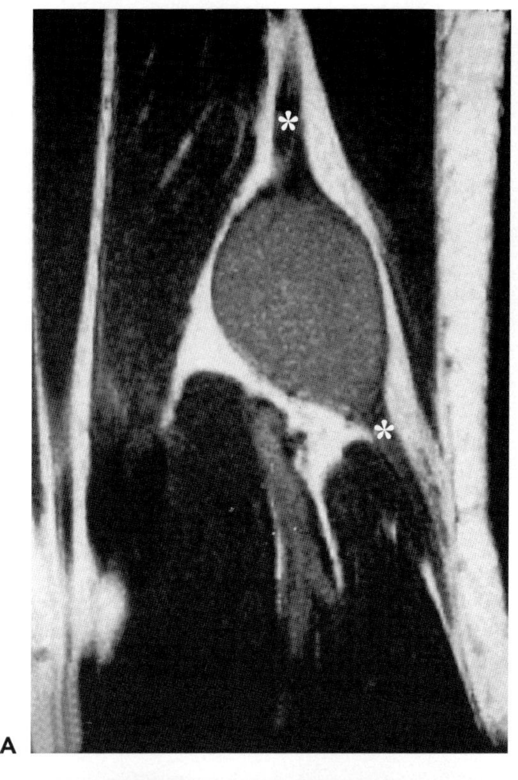

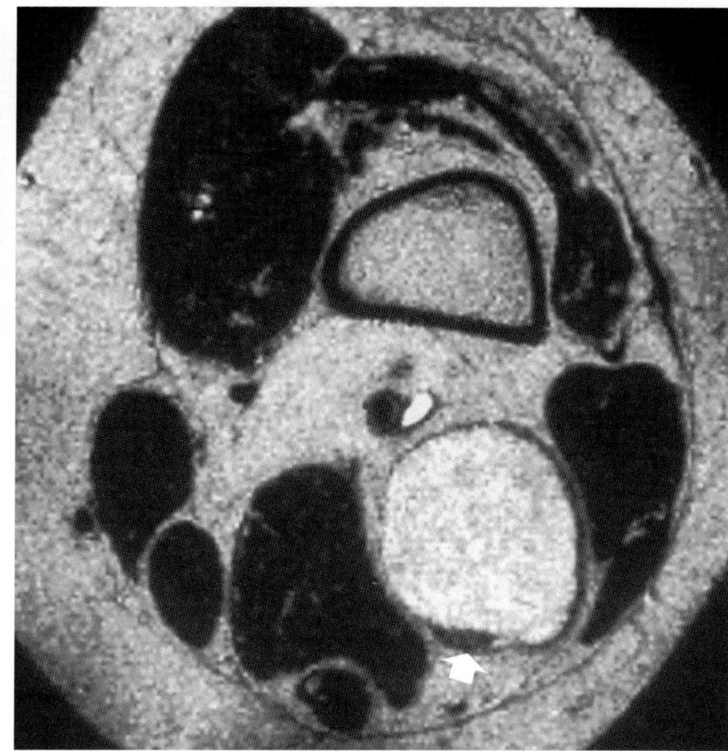

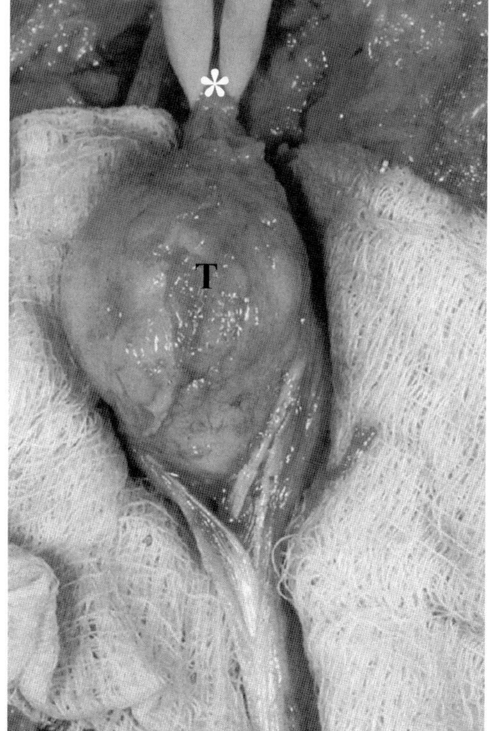

Figure 9.12 Schwannoma of the peroneal nerve in a woman 49 years of age. **A,B:** Coronal T1-weighted (TR/TE; 500/20) **(A)** and axial proton density (TR/TE; 2000/30) **(B)** spin-echo MR images reveal a fusiform intermuscular soft tissue mass with entering and exiting nerve (*asterisks*), surrounding fat is well seen in **A**, while fascicular sign is well demonstrated in **B**. The axial MR image shows the peroneal nerve in the periphery of the mass (*arrow*); the coronal image reveals mild eccentricity of the entering/exiting nerve in relationship to the mass. **C:** Intraoperative photograph shows the same relationship with the eccentric nerve (*asterisk*) easily separable from the tumor (*T*), although this was only apparent after incising of the epineurium.

The target sign is described as being nearly pathognomonic of neurofibroma on T2-weighted MR images and consists of low-to-intermediate signal intensity centrally, with a ring of high signal peripherally (Figs. 9.16 and 9.20) (151,152,155,156,179). These central areas enhance with contrast and, in the study by Lin et al.,

strongly suggested a lesion is a PNST as opposed to MPNST (141). This MR imaging finding corresponds pathologically to fibrous tissue (with high collagen content) centrally and more myxoid tissue peripherally. It is most frequent, in our experience, in plexiform neurofibroma. Suh et al. (81,156) described this finding in 70%

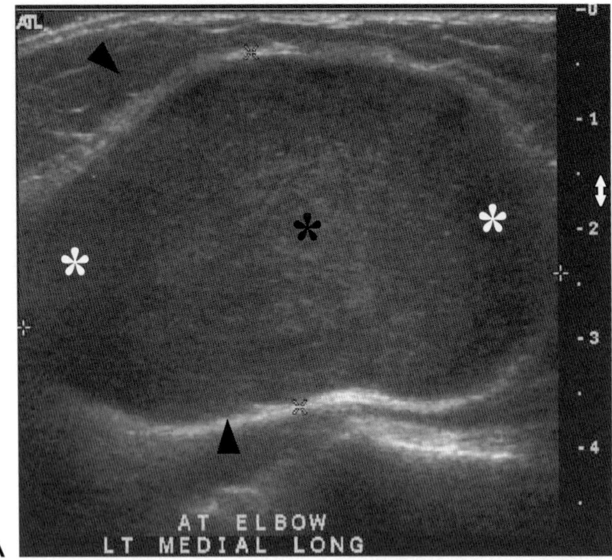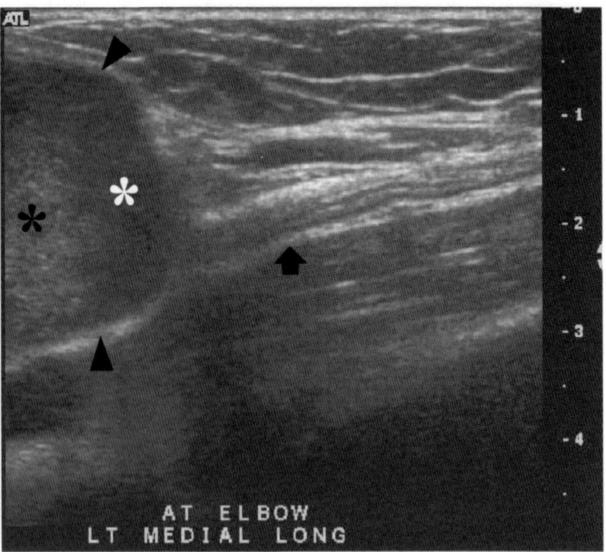

Figure 9.13 Schwannoma of the median nerve in a man 52 years of age. **A,B:** Short axis **(A)** and longitudinal sonograms **(B)** show a fusiform mass with an exiting nerve (*arrow* in **B**). The nerve is eccentric in relationship to the mass, typical of a schwannoma. Hyperechoic rim (*arrowheads*) represents the split-fat sign of an intermuscular mass, and target sign is seen with increased echogenicity centrally (*black asterisk*) and decreased echogenicity peripherally (*white asterisk*).

of 10 cases of neurofibromas. In our experience, however, this prevalence is an overestimate of the frequency of this finding, which is supported by the study of Bhargava et al. who reported this sign in 52% of 23 neurofibromas (180). We strongly agree that the MR target sign should always suggest a neurogenic neoplasm, although it can be seen less frequently in neurilemoma (Fig. 9.20) and MPNST, as well as neurofibroma (both deep-seated and superficially located lesions). The target sign was also reported in 8% of 12 MPNSTs by Bhargava et al. (180). The central areas of fibrous tissue enhance more prominently than the peripheral myxoid tissue following intravenous contrast, as reported by Ogose et al., which could also be considered a target sign (181). CT scanning can also demonstrate the target sign (peripherally low attenuation with central higher attenuation), although not as well as MR imaging, reflecting the superior contrast resolution of the latter modality (173–175). The target sign can also be identified on ultrasonography (Figs. 9.13 and 9.17) with higher echogenicity centrally, similar to CT scanning, but not as well as with MR imaging in our opinion (182).

In our experience, another intrinsic MR imaging characteristic that should suggest neurogenic neoplasm is the fascicular sign (Figs. 9.12 and 9.21) (26). This feature may be seen in both superficial and deep-seated lesions. The fascicular sign manifests as multiple, small, ringlike structures (with peripherally higher signal intensity) on either T2-weighted or proton density–weighted MR images. We believe this sign corresponds to the fascicular bundles seen pathologically in neurogenic neoplasms,

particularly in more differentiated PNSTs. This appearance recapitulates that seen in normal nerves, as described both on MR imaging and ultrasonography (4,5). The fascicular sign, as expected, is more frequent in BPNST than in MPSNT. The latter are more anaplastic neoplasms, in which this sign may be present only in small foci of the lesions.

The margins of BPNSTs are usually well-defined at ultrasonography, CT, and MR imaging (Figs. 9.12–9.14, 9.18, 9.20, and 9.21) (89,183–192). In fact, a capsule representing the epineurium (higher attenuation rim by CT, echogenic rim on ultrasonography, low signal intensity rim on all MR images) may be apparent. Unlike Beggs (32), we do not find this particularly helpful in distinguishing deep-seated localized neurofibroma from neurilemoma. The defined margin of these lesions on imaging reflects the underlying pathologic feature of both of these lesions frequently being contained within the epineurium (particularly schwannomas). Neurofibromas, although more common to extend beyond the epineurium, remain well-circumscribed in most cases, also causing a defined margin on imaging. However, indistinct margins are far more frequent in MPNSTs as a result of more infiltrative growth (Figs. 9.22 and 9.23). We believe any ill-defined margin, particularly on MR imaging (T2-weighted, short-tau inversion recovery [STIR], or postcontrast), of a deep-seated nonplexiform PNST strongly suggests MPNST. Plexiform neurofibromas may also show ill-defined margins, and diffuse neurofibromas always appear indistinct and infiltrative because of their subcutaneous spread along connective tissue septae (26,160).

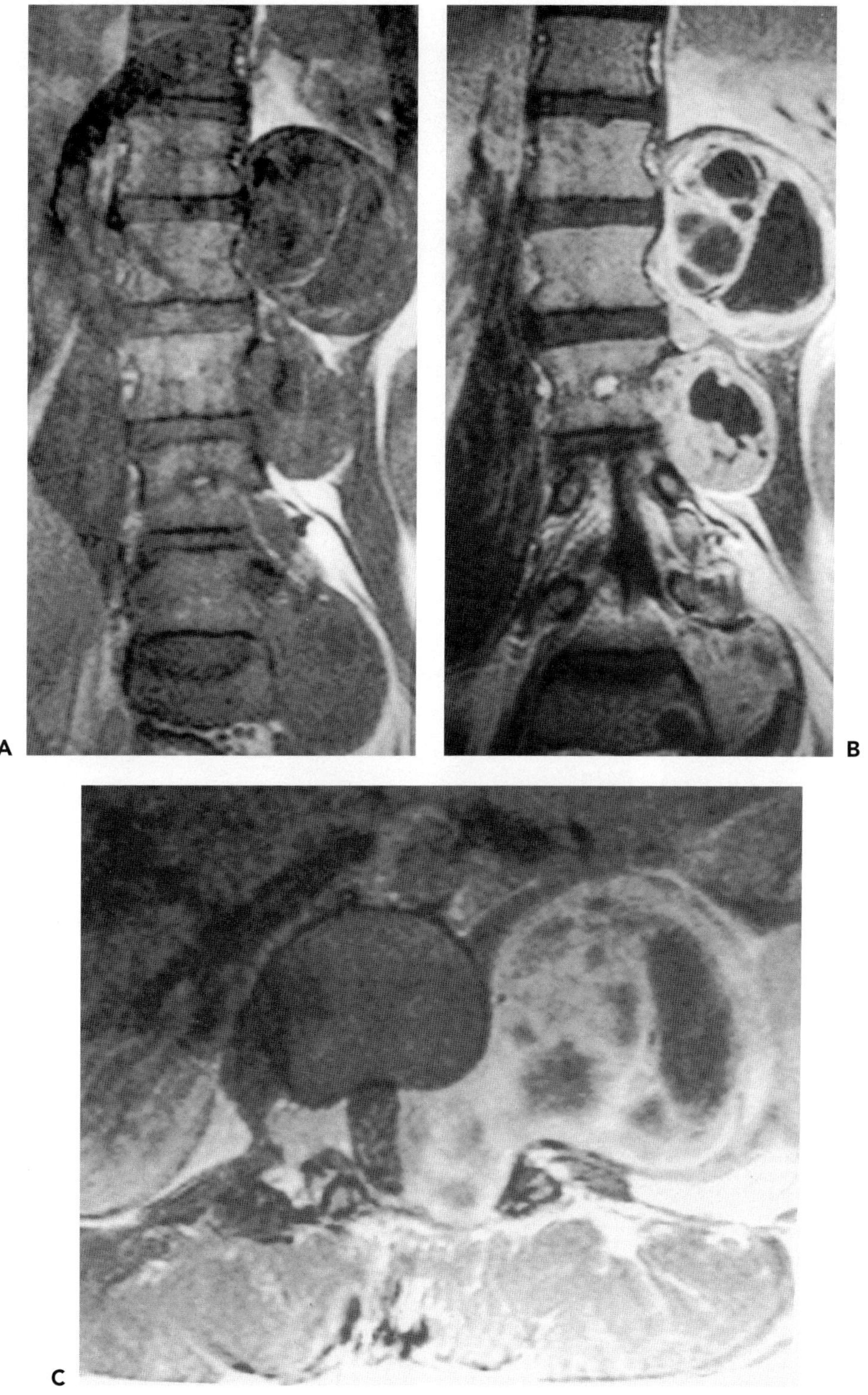

Figure 9.14   Multiple spinal neurofibromas in a woman 38 years of age with neurofibromatosis 1. **A,B:** Coronal T1-weighted (TR/TE; 500/16) spin-echo MR images of the lumbar spine preceding **(A)** and following **(B)** gadolinium administration show multiple paraspinal masses. Nonenhancing areas represent central hemorrhage or necrosis. **C:** Axial T1-weighted (TR/TE; 717/16) spin-echo MR image following gadolinium shows the dumbbell shape to better advantage, representing the entering nerve extending into the neural foramina. Note small contralateral lesion.

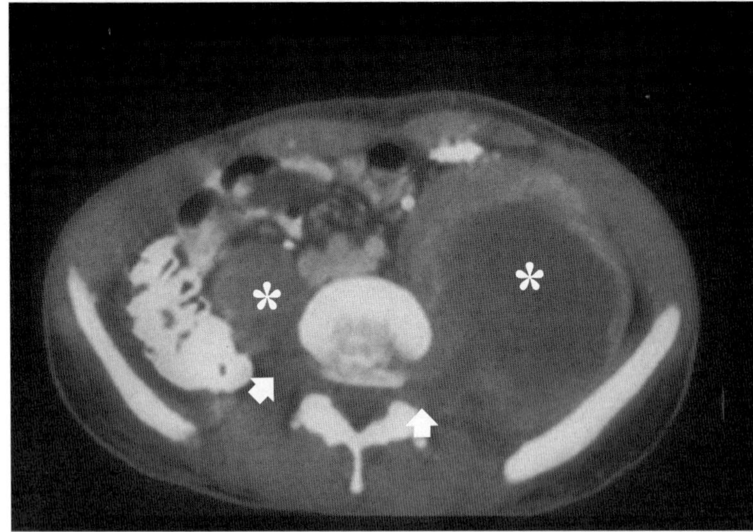

Figure 9.15 Multiple spinal neurofibromas in a man 40 years of age with neurofibromatosis 1. Axial CT shows low attenuation paraspinal lesions (*asterisks*) with extension into the neural foramina (*arrows*). The much larger lesion on the left proved to be a malignant peripheral nerve sheath tumor.

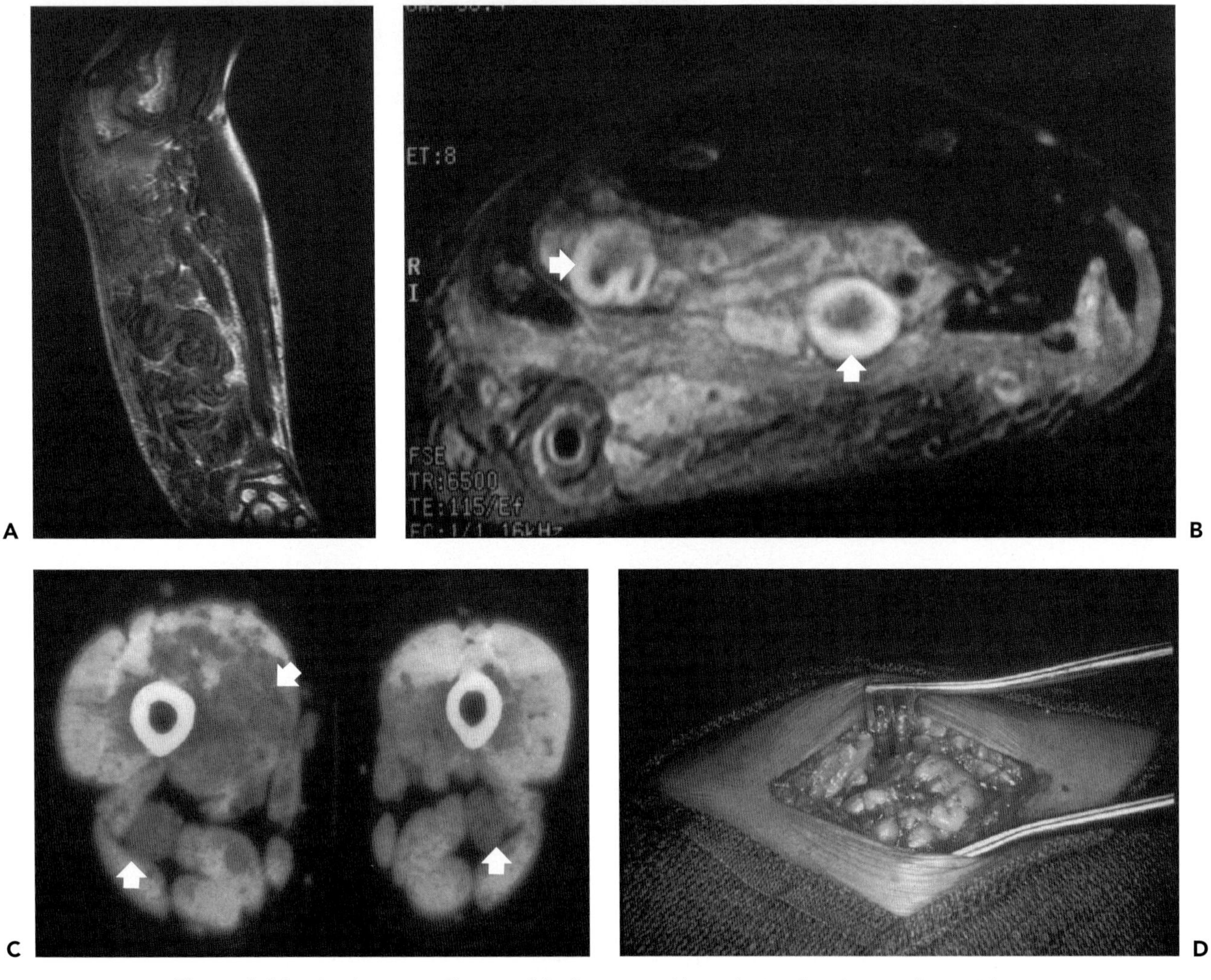

Figure 9.16 Plexiform neurofibroma of the forearm and lower leg in a boy 8 years of age with neurofibromatosis 1. **A,B:** Coronal T1-weighted (TR/TE; 500/20) **(A)** and axial turbo spin-echo T2-weighted (TR/TE; 6500/115) **(B)** MR images show serpentine plexiform neurofibroma with a "bag of worms" appearance. The target sign with high signal intensity peripherally and low signal centrally (*arrows*) is seen in several lesions on the axial T2-weighted image. **C:** CT of lower leg reveals multiple low attenuation neurofibromas (*arrows*). **D:** Intraoperative photograph also shows serpentine "bag of worms" appearance.

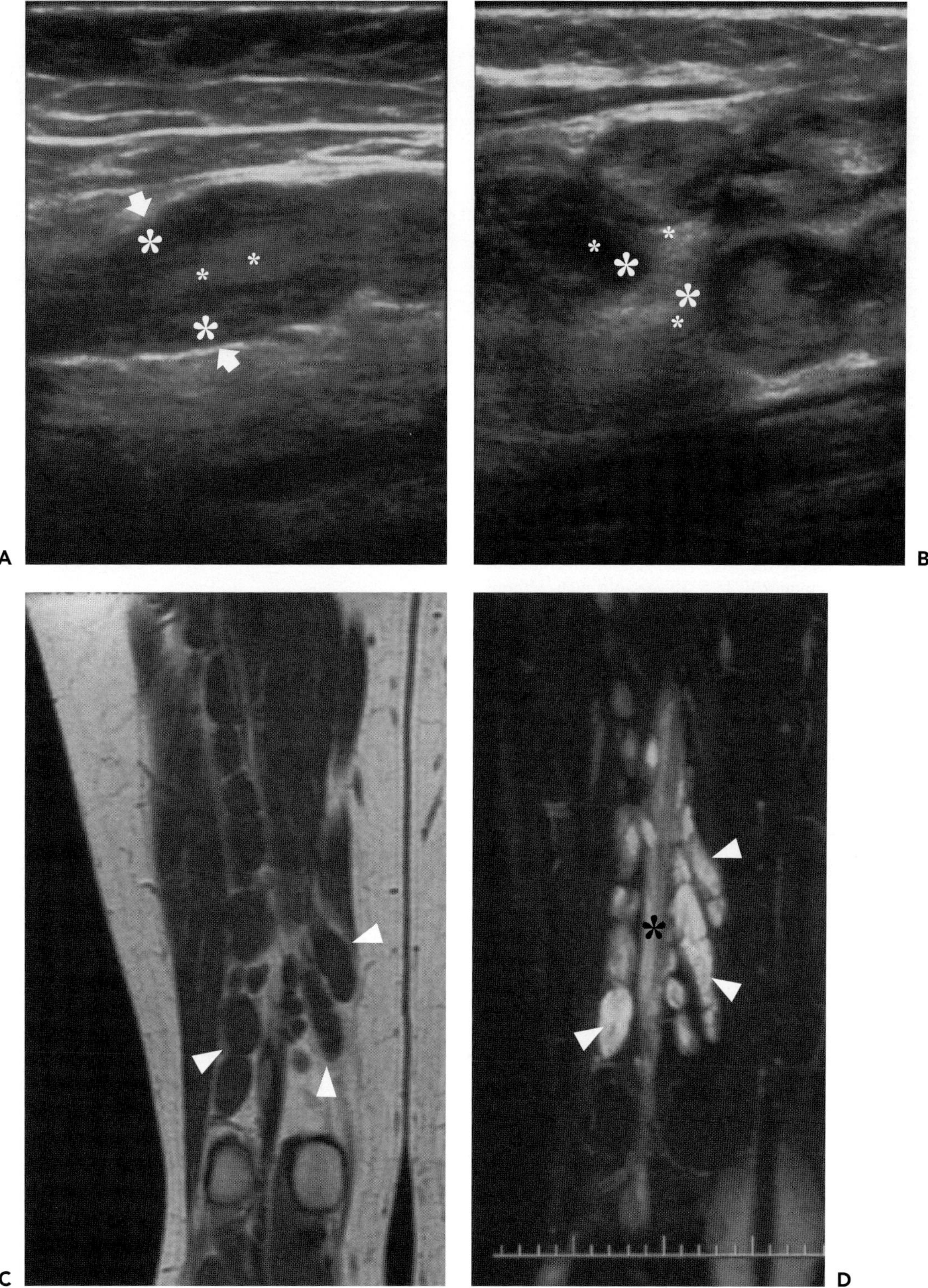

Figure 9.17 Plexiform neurofibroma in a woman 33 years of age with neurofibromatosis 1. **A,B:** Long **(A)** and short **(B)** axis sonograms show plexiform morphology with diffusely thickened nerve (*arrows*), with higher echogenicity centrally (*smaller asterisks*), and lower echogenicity peripherally (*larger asterisks*). **C,D:** Coronal T1-weighted (TR/TE; 500/15) **(C)** and fat-suppressed T2-weighted (TR/TE; 3000/50) **(D)** MR images reveal the diffusely thickened and nodular sciatic nerve (*black asterisk*) and involvement to the nerve branches (*arrowheads*).

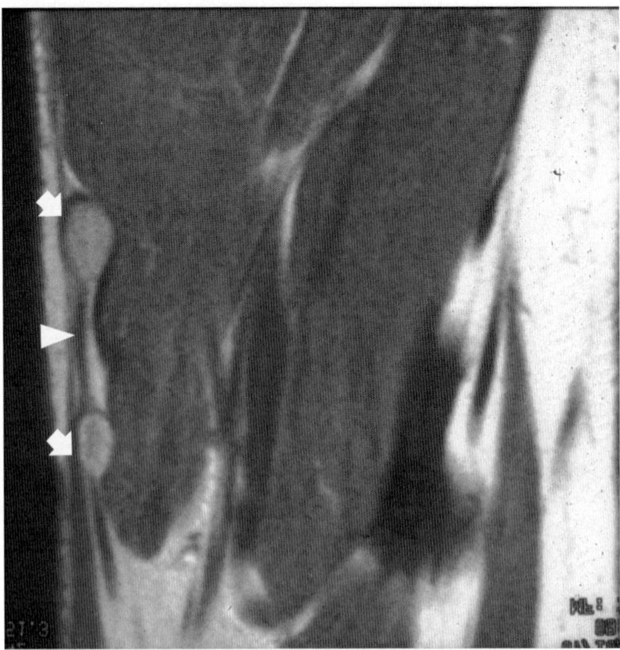

Figure 9.18 Schwannomatosis in a 35-year-old man without neurofibromatosis. Coronal proton density MR image (TR/TE; 2500/30) shows two schwannomas (*arrows*) with normal thickness intervening peroneal nerve (*arrowhead*).

TABLE 9.4

DIFFERENTIATING BENIGN AND MALIGNANT PERIPHERAL NEUROECTODERMAL TUMORS

	BPNST[a]	MPNST[b]
Fusiform shape	Common	Common
Entering/exiting nerve	Common	Common
Target sign	Common	Uncommon
Fasicular sign	Common, diffuse	Uncommon, focal
Split-fat sign	Common, complete	Common (may be incomplete)
Size	<5 cm	>5 cm
Margins	Defined	Ill-defined
Central necrosis	Uncommon	Common
Gallium uptake	No	Yes
FDG-PET uptake	Variable	Yes
Rapid growth	No	Yes
Vascularity	Variable	Prominent

[a]Benign peripheral nerve sheath tumor
[b]Malignant peripheral nerve sheath tumor

A rim of fat (split-fat sign) is often present about deep-seated neurogenic neoplasms and has been described previously on CT scans, although is much easier to appreciate on T1-weighted MR imaging (Figs. 9.12 and 9.17) (170). The split-fat sign can also be seen on ultrasonography as a hyperechoic rim about the mass, as well as the entering and exiting nerve (Figs. 9.13 and 9.21). Because the neurovascular bundle is surrounded by fat, masses arising in this site maintain a rim of fat about them as they slowly enlarge. Although not a specific sign for PNST, this finding suggests tumor origin in the intermuscular space about the neurovascular bundle of which neurogenic neoplasms are the most frequent cause. Intramuscular masses do not demonstrate this feature unless they involve the entire muscle compartment extending to the fat in the intermuscular septae. The split-fat sign is more common in BPNST and lesions of large nerves. MPNST less frequently demonstrates a complete fat rim, reflecting its more infiltrative growth pattern.

Muscle atrophy with striated increased fat content and/or decreased size is associated with PNST and reported by Stull et al. (191) to occur in 23% of cases. Muscle atrophy is not commonly seen with other soft tissue masses. This finding can be quite subtle in muscle supplied by the affected nerve, may require comparison to the normal side, and is best seen on T1-weighted MR imaging (Fig. 9.24).

Contrast enhancement on CT or MR imaging, similar to angiography appearances, is variable in both BPNST and MPNST. Generally, more contrast enhancement is apparent in MPNST (26,193). The pattern of enhancement is also variable, commonly either heterogeneous and diffuse or peripheral (Fig. 9.21) (194). However, as described previously, lesions demonstrating the target sign typically enhance more prominently centrally (Fig. 9.25) (195). In addition, Lee and Boles reported a case of schwannoma with no enhancement (196,197). Irregular nodular peripheral enhancement with central necrosis is typical of MPNST. However, central necrosis can also be seen in ancient schwannomas (Figs. 9.14 and 9.26) (198–200). Ancient schwannoma is one of few benign lesions that can demonstrate this feature, and it represents an important exception to the general rule that central necrosis implies malignancy (Figs. 9.14 and 9.26) (201,202). Contrast-enhanced MR images (and T2-weighted sequences) may demonstrate growth of neurogenic neoplasm into the entering and exiting nerve and surrounding soft tissues. This imaging appearance is an ominous sign of MPNST as opposed to BPNST in nonplexiform lesions, and reflects the growth seen pathologically (Figs. 9.22 and 9.23) (132).

Differentiation of BPNST from MPNST is also often very difficult. Imaging features suggestive of malignancy include large size (>5 cm), prominent vascularity or enhancement, infiltrative margins, marked heterogeneity with central necrosis, rapid growth, and increased uptake of gallium-67 citrate (Figs. 9.10, 9.13, 9.20–9.23) (Table 9.4). Recognition of these imaging features is important for prospective diagnosis and to help guide therapy in the clinical management of these patients.

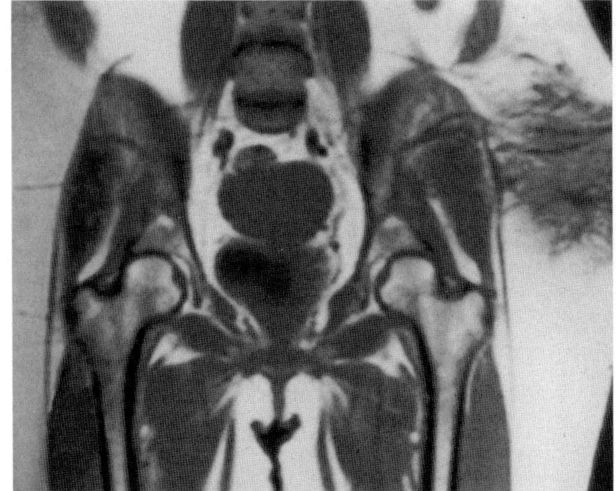

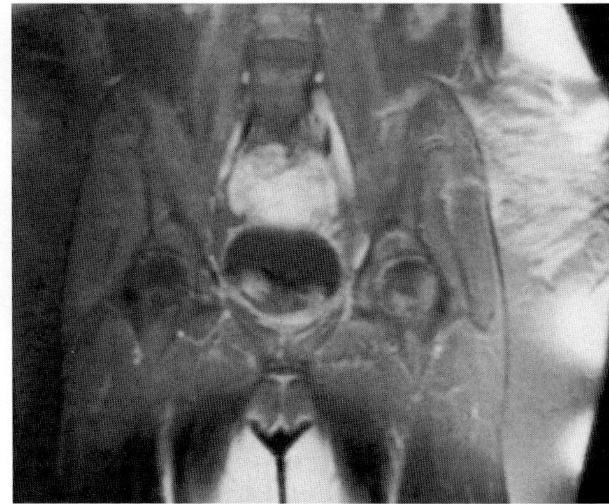

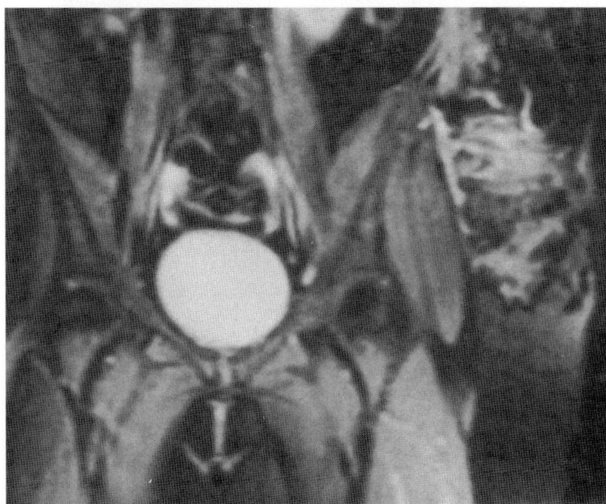

Figure 9.19 Diffuse neurofibroma of the buttock in a woman 31 years of age without neurofibromatosis. **A,B:** Coronal T1-weighted spin-echo MR images **(A)** before and corresponding fat-suppressed postcontrast T1-weighted image **(B)** show an infiltrative mass in the subcutaneous fat, with linear branching components. There is significant enhancement after contrast injection. **C:** Coronal proton density spin-echo MR image reveals heterogeneous high signal intensity.

NEUROTHEKEOMA AND NERVE SHEATH MYXOMA

Neurothekeoma and nerve sheath myxoma were previously thought to represent variations of the same lesion, but they are now considered to be distinct lesions based on histologic differences. Nerve sheath myxomas reveal schwannian features, whereas neurothekeoma shows fibroblastic or myofibroblastic derivation. However, both lesions typically involve the superficial tissues of the head, face, neck, or shoulders and show a female predilection (2:1 ratio). Deep-seated lesions are very rare (Fig. 9.27). Nerve sheath myxoma affects adults in the third to fifth decade, whereas neurothekeoma involves primarily children and young adults.

Similar to other subcutaneous lesions, these tumors are rarely subject to radiologic evaluation. We would expect that both lesions would demonstrate nonspecific features of a subcutaneous mass, but that imaging would reflect the high water content of nerve sheath myxoma (Fig. 9.27).

These benign lesions have no malignant potential, and complete excision is curative.

PERINEURIOMA

> **KEY CONCEPTS**
> - Perineurioma is a rare neoplasm of cells surrounding nerves.
> - There are two types: intraneural and extraneural (soft tissue).
> - Intraneural perineurioma shows diffuse thickening of a relatively long nerve segment, both pathologically and radiologically.
> - Imaging of intraneural lesions, particularly MR, is pathognomonic and may obviate the need for biopsy.
> - Soft tissue perineurioma has nonspecific imaging features and is usually subcutaneous.
> - Treatment is usually observation of intraneural perineurioma, and surgical resection of soft tissue perineurioma.

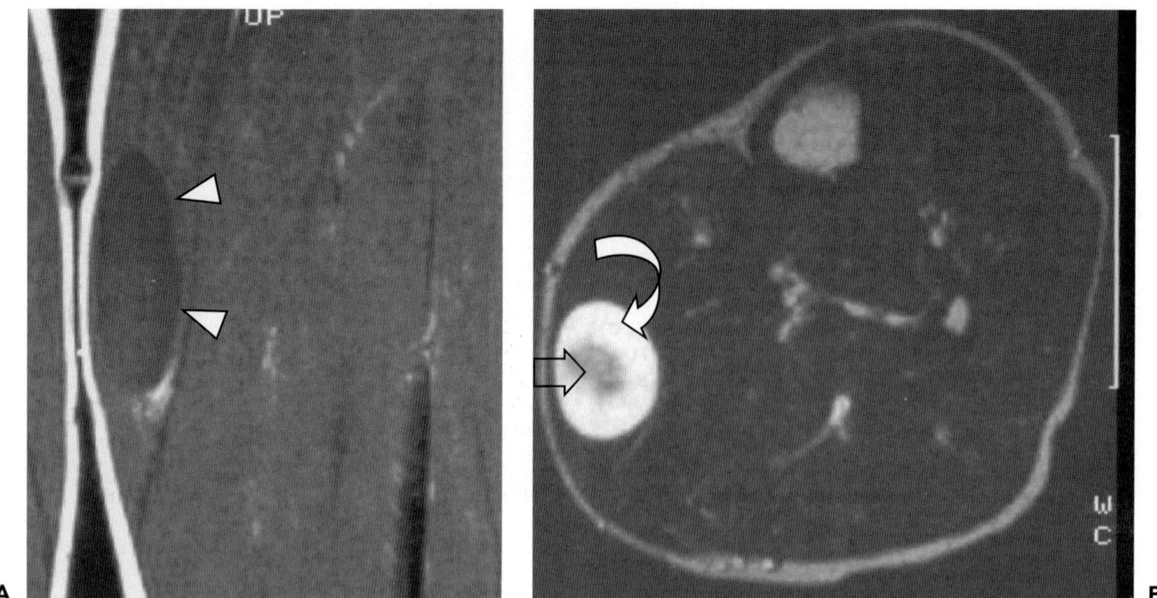

Figure 9.20 Neurilemoma in a man 35 years of age with a palpable soft tissue mass in the calf. **A:** Coronal T1-weighted (TR/TE; 500/20) MR image shows an elongated, low-signal-intensity mass (*arrowheads*). **B:** On the axial T2-weighted (TR/TE; 2000/90) MR image, the mass has peripheral high signal intensity (*white arrow*) with low signal intensity centrally (*black arrow*), representing the target sign. No entering or exiting nerve is seen because the affected nerve is a small gastrocnemius intramuscular branch.

Perineurial cells form the outer lining of peripheral nerve fascicles, analogous to the meningeal cells in the pia-arachnoid membrane. Perineurioma, described in 1978 by Lazarus and Trombetta, represents a rare soft tissue tumor composed of cells resembling normal perineurium without Schwann cell components (203). These lesions are rare and represent less than 1% of soft tissue neoplasms. There are two distinct types of these lesions: the intraneural perineurioma and the extraneural, or soft tissue, perineurioma. More than 30 cases of intraneural perineurioma have been reported to date (204). These lesions were formerly diagnosed as hypertrophic neuropathy and considered to be reactive lesions. However, further pathologic evaluation with clonal abnormalities (monosomy) related to chromosome 22 now provides proof of their neoplastic nature. Adolescents or young adults are usually affected with an equal sex distribution. The most common symptom is muscle weakness, and atrophy may be apparent. Nerves of the upper extremity are most commonly involved, followed by those of the lower extremity. Only one nerve is typically affected, with a single case of adjacent spinal nerve involvement reported (204). At gross pathologic examination there is symmetric tubular enlargement of the affected nerve (from 2 cm to 10 cm), without involvement of its branches. Histologically, ropelike bundles of perineurial cells surround indistinct nerve fibers.

Soft tissue perineuriomas are most common in the subcutaneous tissues of the hand, affect adults of all ages, and have a female predominance (4:1) except for the sclerosing subtype (male predilection). These lesions are solitary, well-circumscribed, but nonencapsulated masses of perineurial cells, but unlike their intraneural counterpart, they do not surround a nerve. Soft tissue perineuriomas demonstrate the same cytogenetic abnormality as intraneural lesions.

Radiologic evaluation of these lesions is only rarely reported. In our experience, intraneural perineuriomas have a distinctive, pathognomic appearance, particularly on MR imaging. The affected nerve is diffusely thickened for a long extent with high signal intensity on T2-weighting and enhancement following intravenous contrast (Fig. 9.28). Similar morphologic features would be expected on CT scanning or sonography and reflect the underlying pathology. In contradistinction to plexiform neurofibroma or an infectious neuritis (such as that seen in leprosy), the nerve branches are not involved (no "bag of worms" appearance), and no surrounding inflammation is identified. The imaging appearance of soft tissue perineurioma is not described, to the best of our knowledge, but we would expect nonspecific characteristics with detection of a soft tissue mass.

These lesions are benign, with only rare and controversial description of a malignant variant. Surgical excision of soft tissue perineurioma is curative and there have been no reports of recurrence. Intraneural perineurioma demonstrates neither risk of recurrence nor metastases on long-term follow-up, and thus biopsy alone is considered sufficient for diagnosis. Biopsy should be directed to fascicles that are nonfunctional by direct nerve stimulation. We would suggest that imaging alone is diagnostic and may supplant the need for biopsy. Surgical resection of intraneural perineurioma is to be avoided to retain nerve function even if only partial. Resection, even though curative, of nonfunctional, localized,

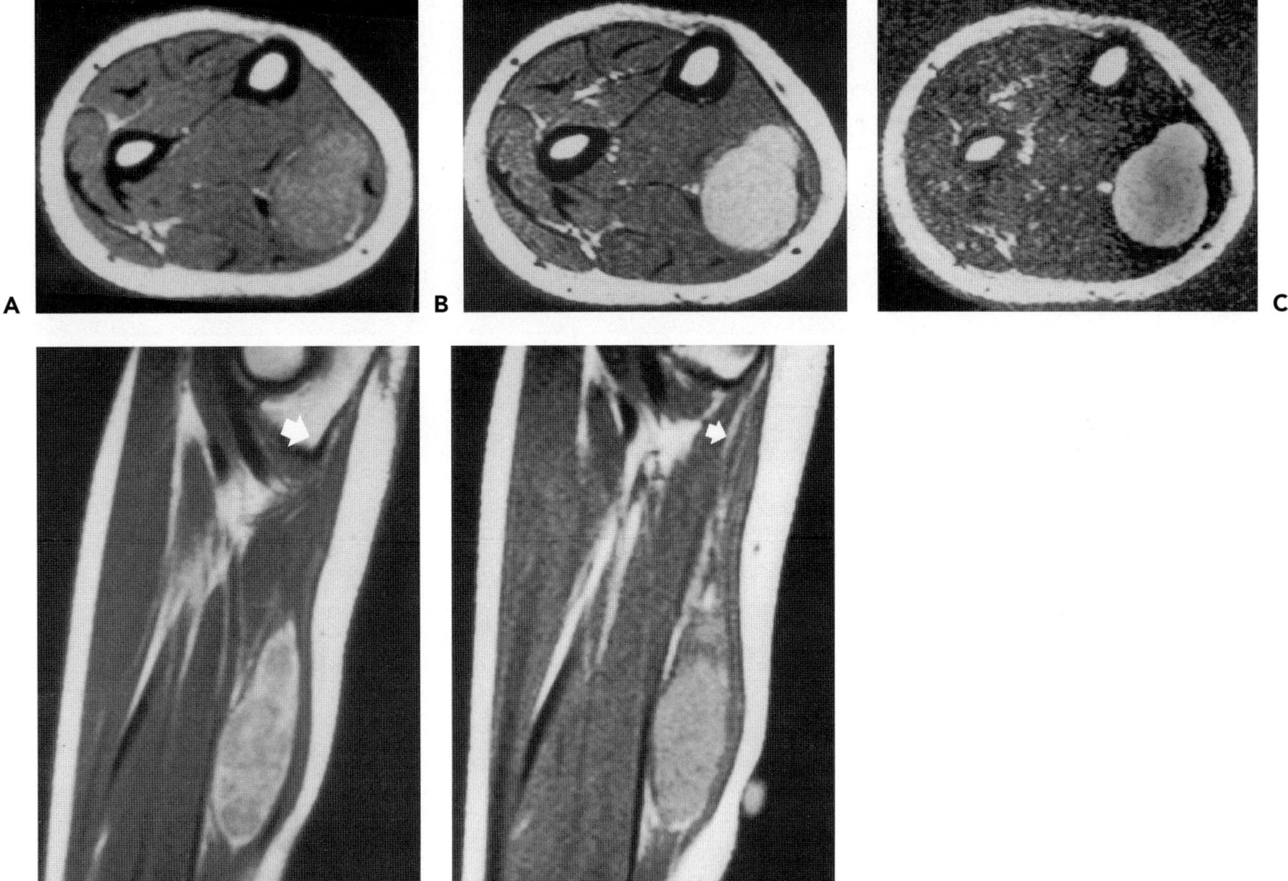

Figure 9.21 Schwannoma of the forearm (ulnar nerve) in a 15-year-old girl. **A–C:** Axial T1-weighted (TR/TE; 616/25) **(A)**, proton density (TR/TE; 2000/25) **(B)** and T2-weighted (TR/TE; 2000/90) **(C)** spin-echo MR images show a well-defined mass with fascicular sign (best seen on long TR images). The relationship of the ulnar nerve to the mass (schwannoma versus neurofibroma) is difficult to distinguish. **D,E:** Sagittal T1-weighted (TR/TE; 578/16) **(D)** spin-echo MR image preceding intravenous gadolinium, and corresponding T1-weighted (TR/TE; 600/15) **(E)** image following contrast reveal a fusiform mass. Nerve is seen proximally (*arrow* in **D**). Note surrounding rim of fat (split-fat sign) and mild peripheral enhancement.

affected nerve with graft placement and reconstruction, may not be associated with recovery of function.

GRANULAR CELL TUMOR

> ### KEY CONCEPTS
> - Granular cell tumor is a relatively common lesion of nerve origin affecting medium- to small-sized nerves.
> - It is most common in the head/neck (particularly related to the tongue), chest, breast, and upper extremity.
> - MR imaging features commonly reported are relatively low-to-intermediate signal intensity centrally and high signal intensity peripherally on long TR images.
> - Lesion margins may be irregular.
> - The vast majority of these tumors are benign, with surgical resection curative.

Initially the granular cell tumor was believed to be of muscle origin, and the term *granular myoblastoma* was used. Evidence now strongly suggests that this lesion is of nerve origin. Other former terms for this neoplasm included *granular cell neurogenic tumor, granular cell neuroma, granular cell neurofibroma,* and *granular cell schwannoma* (9). Granular cell tumors are relatively common lesions. They occur most frequently in the fourth to sixth decade, are twice as common in women, and have a predilection for blacks. Lesions are often in the skin or subcutaneous tissue, although a deep intramuscular location (205) can also occur and usually develops in close association to small-to-medium-sized nerves. The most common location is the head and neck (particularly the tongue) (Fig. 9.29), followed by the chest wall, breast, and arm (9,206–209). These lesions most frequently present as small painless masses, and approximately 10% to 15% occur at multiple

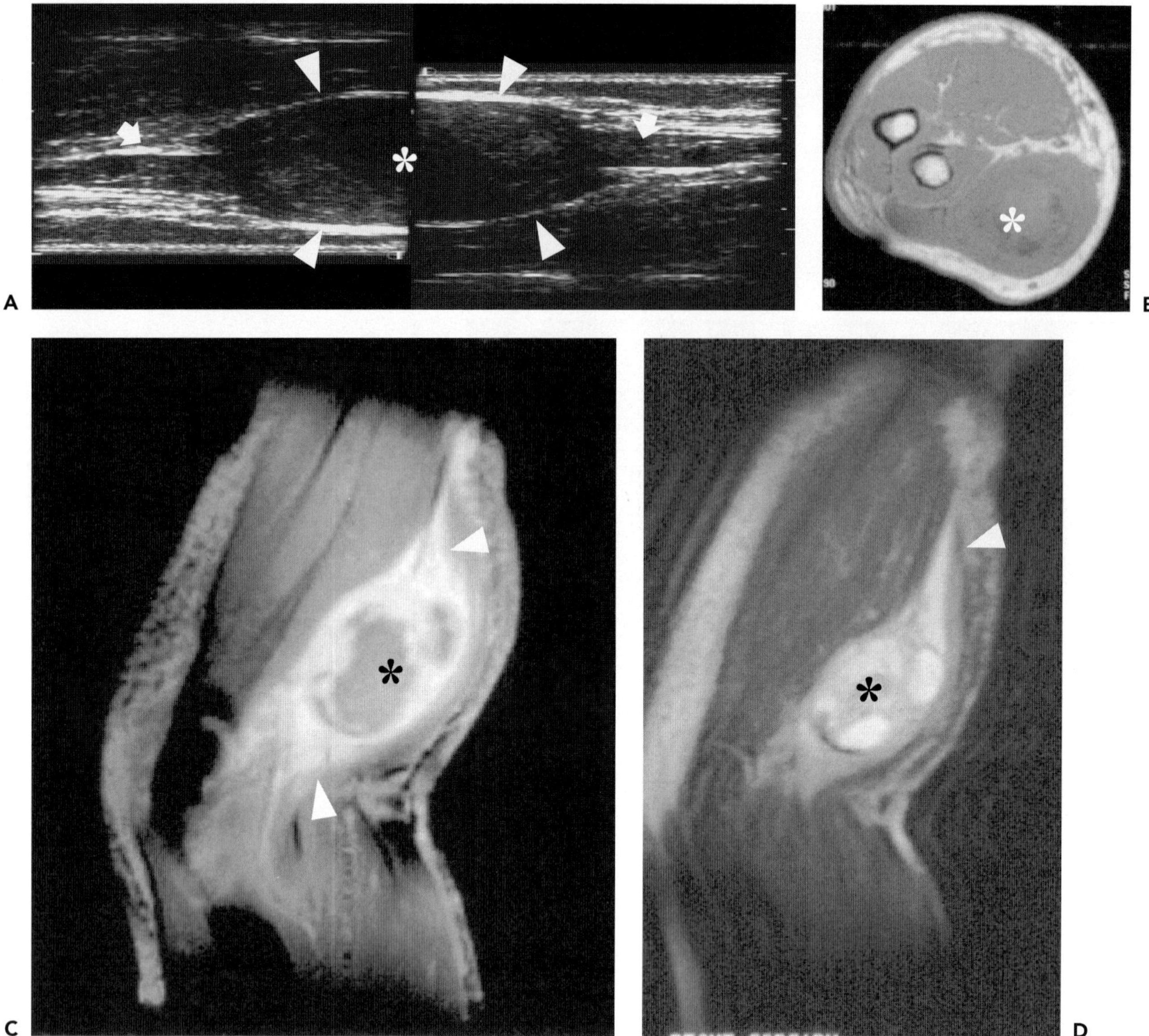

Figure 9.22   Malignant peripheral nerve sheath tumor of the radial nerve in a man 24 years of age with neurofibromatosis 1 and clinical rapid enlargement of a forearm mass. **A:** Spliced long axis sonogram shows the mass (*asterisk*) with entering and exiting nerve (*arrows*) and split-fat sign (*arrowheads*). **B–D:** Multiple MR images including axial T1-weighting (TR/TE; 500/20) **(B)**, sagittal enhanced, fat-suppressed T1-weighted (TR/TE; 500/20) **(C)** and sagittal T2-weighted (TR/TE; 3000/115) **(D)**, reveal a large (>5 cm) necrotic forearm mass (*asterisk*) with irregular margins and extension along the entering and exiting nerves (*arrowheads*).

locations, with as many as 50 sites reported in some cases. Multiple lesions may be metachronous or synchronous in occurrence.

Pathologically, the vast majority of lesions are benign, with only 1% to 2% being malignant and showing metastatic potential (9,210). Lesions are often closely associated with or replace adjacent peripheral nerves (9,206,207). Benign granular cell tumor is usually smaller than 3 cm as opposed to the malignant variety, which is typically larger than 4 cm. Malignant granular cell tumor should demonstrate three or more of the following histologic features: necrosis, spindling, vesicular nuclei with prominent nucleoli, increased mitotic activity (>2 mitoses/HPF), high nucleocytoplasmic ratio, or pleomorphism. Histologically, the lesions are nonencapsulated and are composed of cells with prominent granular eosinophilic cytoplasm.

Imaging of these lesions has only been recently reported, again related to the fact that superficial lesions are often not evaluated radiologically (3,208,209,211–213). The largest series are by Blacksin et al. and Elkousy et al. of 5 and 10 patients, respectively (214,215). These neoplasms are seen as subcutaneous nodular masses. Deep-seated lesions may show an intimate relationship to a nerve

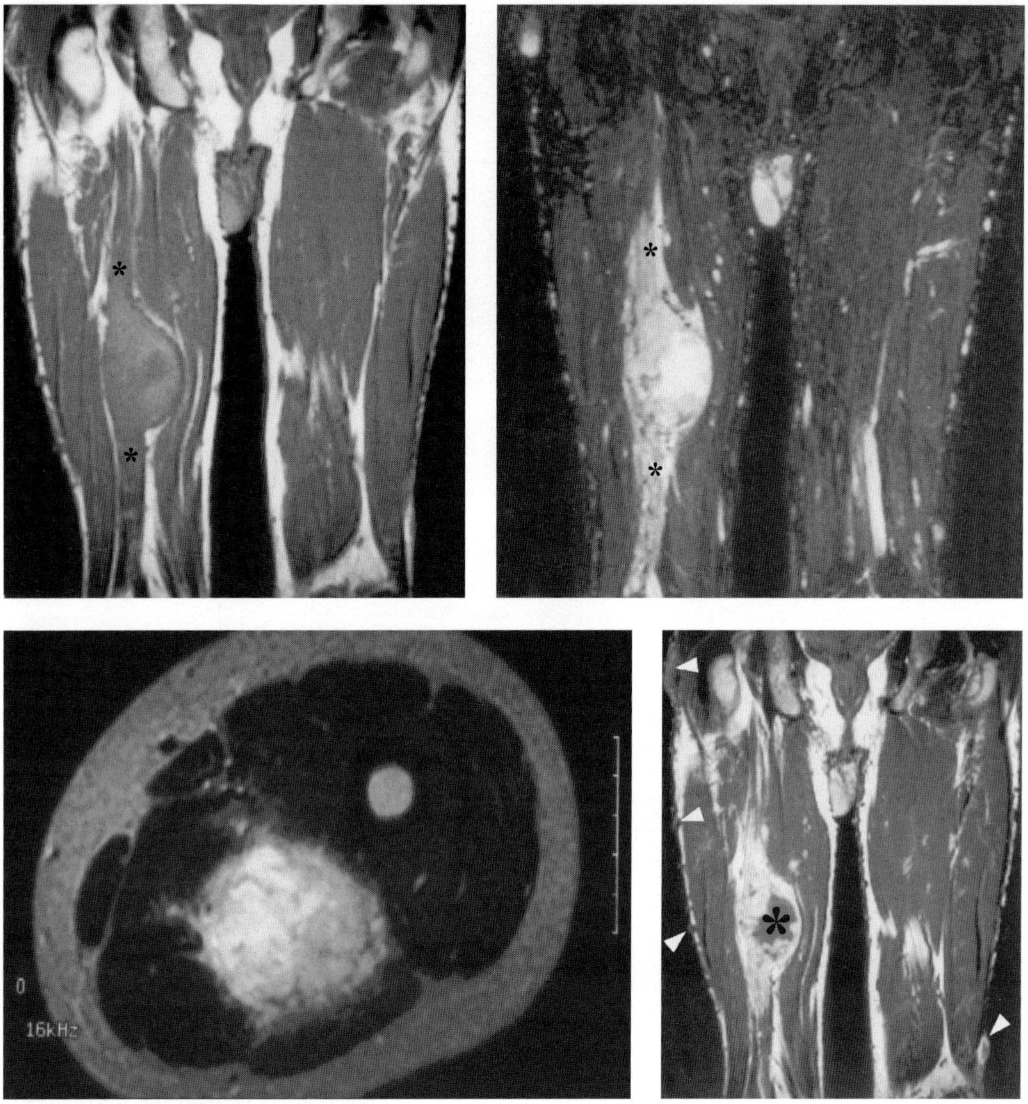

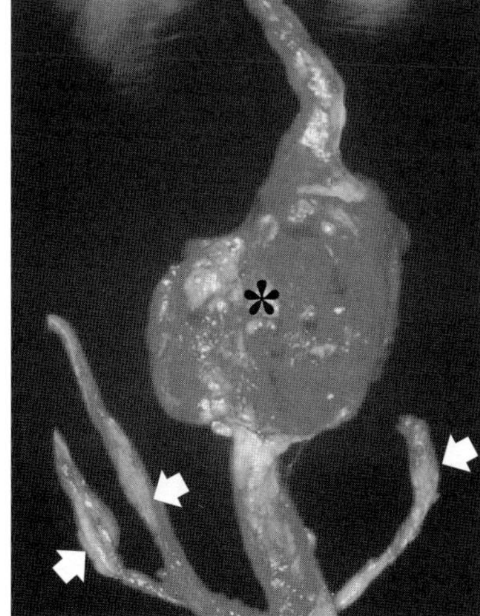

Figure 9.23 Malignant peripheral nerve sheath tumor (MPNST) in the thigh of a man 42 years of age with neurofibromatosis 1 (NF1). **A–C:** Coronal T1-weighted (TR/TE; 634/18) **(A)** spin-echo, coronal short-tau inversion recovery (STIR) (TR/TE/TI; 3000/60/160) **(B)** and axial T2-weighted (TR/TE; 2500/100) **(C)** MR images show a large fusiform mass in the mid-right thigh. Thickened sciatic nerve (*asterisks*) is seen entering and exiting the mass, and mild irregular margins are demonstrated on the axial image. **D:** Coronal T1-weighted (TR/TE; 634/18) spin-echo MR image following intravenous gadolinium shows extensive peripheral enhancement and tumor extending along thickened entering and exiting sciatic nerve. Nonenhancing central necrosis (*asterisk*) has low signal on T1-weighting and high signal on T2-weighting. Numerous superficial neurofibromas are also seen (*several are marked with arrowheads*), suggesting NF1. Large tumor size (>5 cm), irregular margins, and extension along the nerve all suggest MPNST as opposed to benign neurofibroma. **E:** Photograph of gross specimen shows multinodular thickening of a plexiform neurofibroma of both sciatic nerve and its branches (*white arrows*) and the necrotic MPNST (*asterisk*).

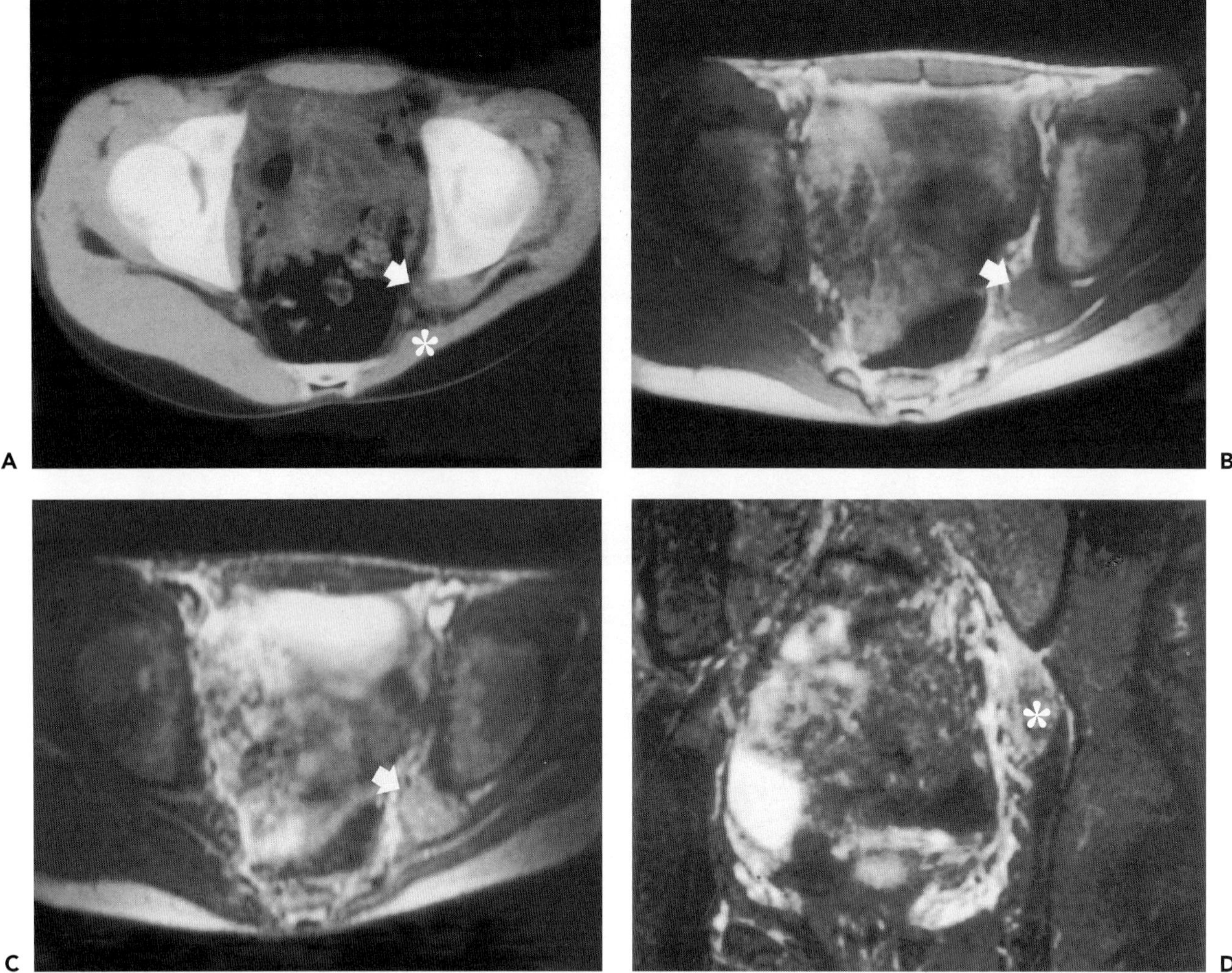

Figure 9.24   Malignant peripheral nerve sheath tumor in a girl 12 years of age without neurofibromatosis. **A:** Noncontrast axial CT shows a mass (*arrow*) related to the sciatic nerve, with marked atrophy of gluteal musculature (*asterisk*). **B,C:** Axial T1-weighted (TR/TE; 600/24) **(B)** and T2-weighted (TR/TE; 2000/90) **(C)** spin-echo MR images reveal a relatively well-defined mass (*arrow*). The fascicular pattern is best seen on axial T2-weighted image. Left gluteal muscle atrophy is again noted. **D:** Coronal turbo T2-weighted (TR/TE; 4000/108) spin-echo MR image shows the sciatic nerve entering the mass (*asterisk*).

(212). Low signal intensity on T2-weighted MR images, with a peripheral rim of high signal intensity that may reveal infiltrative margins has also been described as a suggestive feature of this diagnosis (Fig. 9.30) (216). Lesions larger than 4 cm with invasion of adjacent structures, including bone, should raise suspicion of a malignant granular cell tumor.

Surgical resection is usually curative for benign granular cell tumors. Malignant granular cell tumors demonstrate significant metastatic potential with a 40% risk of mortality. Metastases in malignant granular cell tumors (50% of patients) usually require several years to occur following excision of the original lesion, and usually follow local recurrence. Metastases most frequently affect the lymph nodes, lung, liver, and bone. Reports of small numbers of patients suggest that adjuvant radiation therapy and chemotherapy are not effective in treatment of malignant lesions.

MELANOTIC NEUROECTODERMAL TUMOR OF INFANCY

The original description of the melanotic neuroectodermal tumor of infancy was by Krompecher in 1918, and approximately 150 to 200 cases have been reported to date (217). The vast majority of evidence suggests a neural crest origin. Additional terms for this lesion include *congenital*

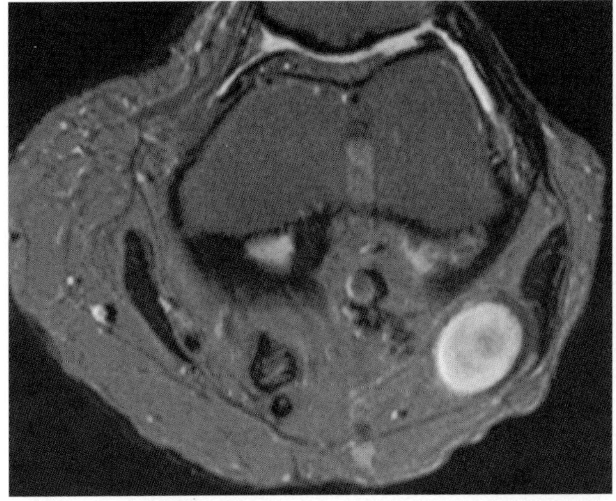

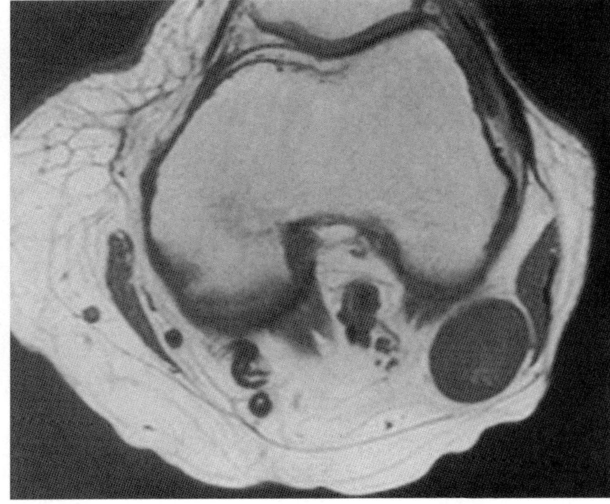

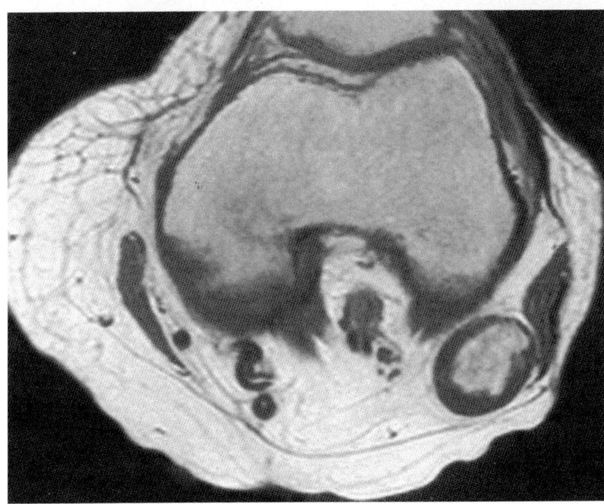

Figure 9.25 Neurofibroma of the peroneal nerve in a woman 77 years of age. **A:** Axial T2-weighted (TR/TE; 2200/80) spin-echo MR image shows a characteristic target appearance, with a central zone of low signal intensity and a peripheral zone of higher signal intensity. **B,C:** Axial T1-weighted (TR/TE; 577/16) spin-echo MR images before **(B)** and after **(C)** gadolinium administration show enhancement of the central area that corresponds to a solid central, tightly packed, cellular portion with fibrous tissue and xanthomatous areas. The peripheral nonenhancing region corresponds to loosely arranged myxoid stroma.

> **KEY CONCEPTS**
> - Melanotic neuroectodermal tumors of infancy are rare lesions involving the mandible, maxilla, or calvarium in an infant younger than 5 months of age.
> - They can appear quite aggressive, with both bone and soft tissue involvement.
> - These tumors tend to have prominent low-to-intermediate signal intensity on T2-weighted MR images.
> - Association of patient age, lesion location, and MR appearance is distinctive.

melanocarcinoma, melanotic adamantinoma, retinal anlage tumor, pigmented epulis of infancy, and *melanotic progonoma* (217–221). This tumor usually develops in patients younger than 6 months of age, but is only occasionally identified at birth. Rapid enlargement causing facial disfigurement and a protuberant blue-black mass (related to melanin) arising from the mandible, maxilla, or calvarium, is usually seen at presentation. Other rare reported locations include the epididymis, mediastinum, uterus, and shoulder. Multicentric melanotic neuroectodermal tumors of infancy are also rarely reported.

A neural crest origin of this tumor is supported pathologically by the ultrastructure identification of neurofilaments and neurosecretory granules. Variable amounts of melanin pigment are also present. Elevated levels of vanillylmandelic acid (VMA) are also rarely associated with this tumor.

Treatment primarily involves surgical resection; however, recurrence is seen in nearly 50% of patients (9,217–221). In addition, although melanotic neuroectodermal tumor of infancy is generally considered to be a benign lesion, metastases are reported in 2% to 10% of cases (9). Sporadic reports of the use of adjuvant chemotherapy are also available.

Imaging of this tumor is not extensively reported, reflecting its rare occurrence, with the largest series consisting of five patients reported by Mirich et al. in 1991

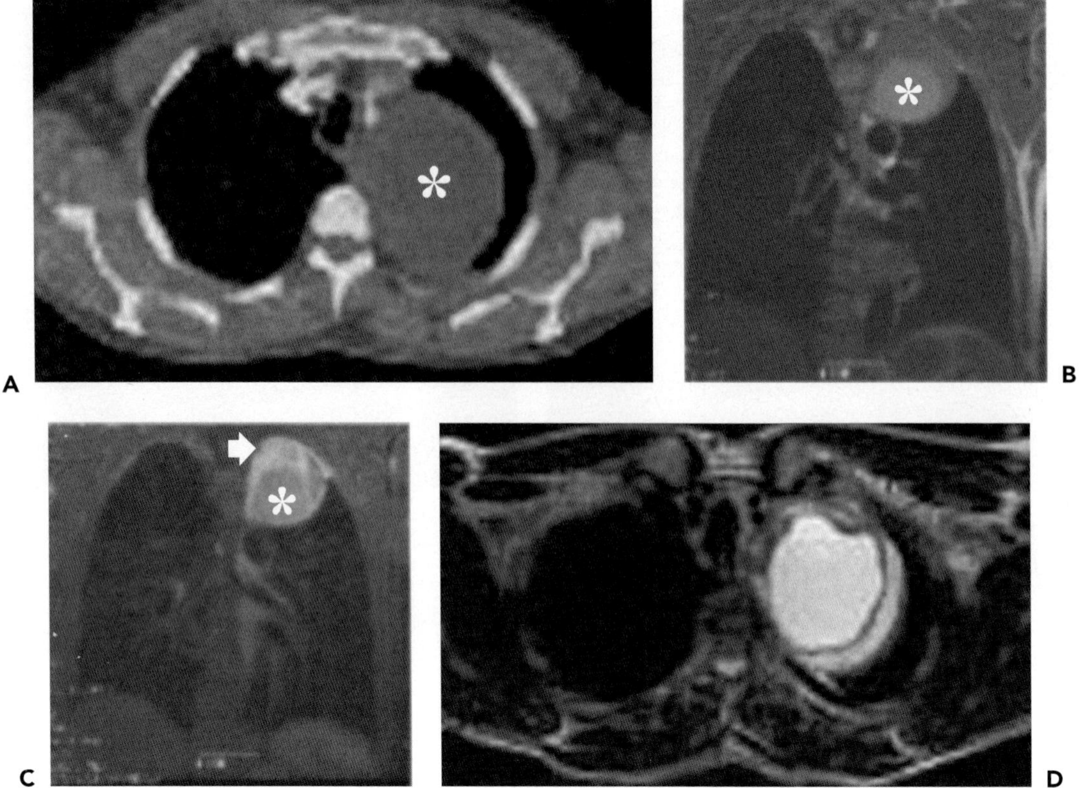

Figure 9.26 Ancient schwannoma in a man 51 years of age without neurofibromatosis. **A:** Axial CT shows low attenuation mass (*asterisk*) in the superior mediastinum. **B,C:** Fat-suppressed coronal T1-weighted (TR/TE; 500/20) MR images preceding **(B)** and following **(C)** contrast show a mass in the left upper chest with a large focus of nonenhancing hemorrhage inferiorly (*asterisk*). More solid tumor superiorly shows diffuse enhancement (*arrow* in **C**). **D:** Axial T2-weighted (TR/TE; 3500/110) MR image shows high signal intensity from both hemorrhagic and nonhemorrhagic areas.

(217–221). The lesion typically involves both bone and soft tissue, with lytic destruction and expansile remodeling of the mandible, maxilla, or skull. Reactive hyperostosis and osteogenesis may also be present. CT generally reveals relatively homogeneous replacement of bone with an associated soft tissue mass. CT after contrast typically reveals uniform enhancement (220,221). MR imaging with its multiplanar imaging capability is optimal to delineate lesion extent and involvement of surrounding structures prior to surgical resection (Fig. 9.31) (218,221). Mirich et al. reported intermediate signal intensity on T1-weighted and slightly hyperintense signal intensity with heterogenicity on T2-weighted MR images (221). In the case report by Atkinson et al., low intensity was present, presumably reflecting the paramagnetic properties of melanin (218). Our experience with this lesion on MR imaging is that the T2-weighted images show heterogeneity with prominent low-to-intermediate signal intensity, and these tumors mildly enhance following intravenous contrast administration (Fig. 9.31). Homogeneous stain during the venous phase of angiography has also been reported (220). We believe that patient age, lesion location, and MR features are distinctive of this lesion.

CLEAR CELL SARCOMA

KEY CONCEPTS
- Clear cell sarcoma is a rare neoplasm, also referred to as *melanoma of soft parts*, but melanin is microscopic.
- Young adults (20 to 40 years of age) are affected most commonly.
- The lower extremity accounts for 25% of cases, with 43% in the foot and ankle.
- Suggestive feature of diagnosis, best seen on MR imaging, is a mass having components not only surrounding, but also within a tendon, ligament, or aponeurosis.
- Theoretic effects of melanin (high signal on T1-weighting, low signal on T2-weighting) are not prominent because of the minute amount present.
- Prognosis is poor despite aggressive therapy.

Clear cell sarcoma is a rare neoplasm accounting for 1% of all soft tissue sarcomas. It was originally described by Enzinger in 1965 and is also referred to as *malignant melanoma of soft parts* (222). Young adults between 20 and

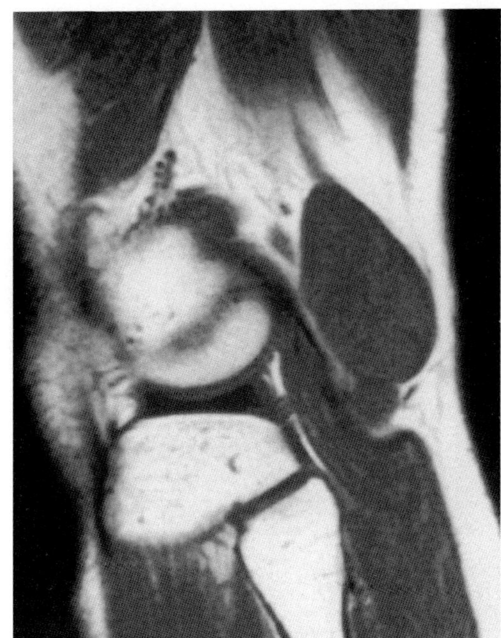
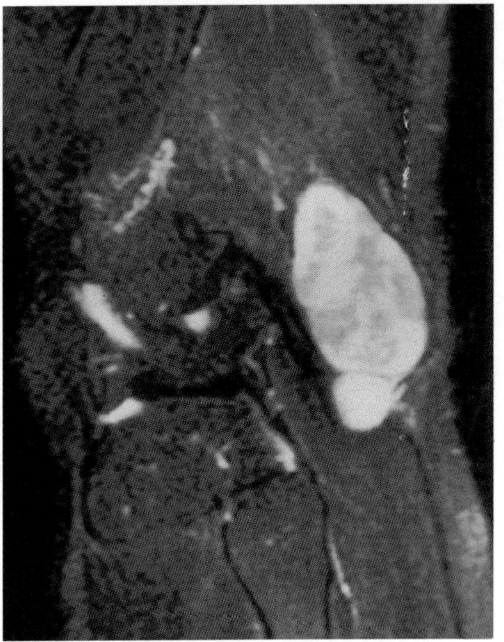

Figure 9.27 Neurothekeoma of the popliteal fossa in a 35 year old woman. **A,B:** Sagittal T1-weighted **(A)** and T2-weighted **(B)** spin-echo MR images show a lobular mass in the popliteal fossa. The mass reveals low-to-intermediate signal intensity on the short TR image and areas of marked high intensity on the long TR image. (Case courtesy of Martha C. Nelson, MD.)

40 years of age are most commonly involved. Women are affected slightly more frequently than men (3:2 ratio) (223–225). Clear cell sarcoma is a lesion intimately associated with or in a tendon, ligament, or aponeurosis. The lower extremity is involved in 75% of cases, with a particular predilection for the foot/ankle (43% of cases) followed by the knee and thigh (222–231). Other less commonly affected sites include the upper extremity (22% to 25%), trunk (2%), and head/neck (1%) (17,232). In the upper extremity, involvement of the hand and wrist is most common, paralleling the distribution in the lower extremity.

Pathologically, clear cell sarcoma encompasses nearby tendon, ligament, or aponeurosis and is composed of nests or fascicles of cells with clear abundant cytoplasm (222,223,227,229). Intracellular melanin and premelanosome granules can be identified in 72% of cases (222,223). Small amounts of iron are also seen in many patients. Immunohistochemical stains suggest neural crest origin and associated melanin production (S-100 protein, neuron-specific enolase homatropine methylbromide [HMB45]). Unlike malignant melanomas, cytogenetic abnormalities are reported in patients with this lesion, particularly translocation of the long arms of chromosomes 12 and 22 (17,227,233,234).

Treatment usually involves aggressive resection or amputation and adjuvant chemotherapy and radiation therapy (228,229). Unfortunately, prognosis in these patients is poor, with frequent local recurrence and metastases. Mortality rates range from 37% to 59% in the largest series (17,228,229). Survival at 5, 10, and 20 years was 67%, 33%, and 10%, respectively, in series at the Mayo Clinic (224,225). Multiple local recurrences are not uncommon and often precede development of distant metastases. Regional lymph node involvement develops in up to 50% of patients. In fact, regional lymph node dissection is often part of the initial treatment because of this common route of extension. Unfavorable prognostic factors include tumor size greater than 5 cm, necrosis, and local recurrence.

Radiographs in cases of clear cell sarcoma are often nonspecific with evidence of a soft tissue mass, although small lesions may not be detected. Associated bone involvement, by direct extension, has been considered rare in previous reports. However, we reviewed our cases at the Armed Forces Institute of Pathology (AFIP) and osseous invasion was seen in 5 of 14 patients (Fig. 9.32) (36%). The osseous involvement had an aggressive lytic appearance on radiographs, except in one case, where periosteal reaction alone was present. This frequency of osseous involvement should perhaps not be surprising, considering the primary tumor focus is within tendon or aponeurosis immediately adjacent to bone. Not unexpectedly, bone scans in patients with osseous extension show increased uptake of radionuclide. Calcification is only rarely reported in clear cell sarcoma (17).

Cross-sectional imaging of clear cell sarcoma by sonography, CT, or MR imaging more clearly suggests primary

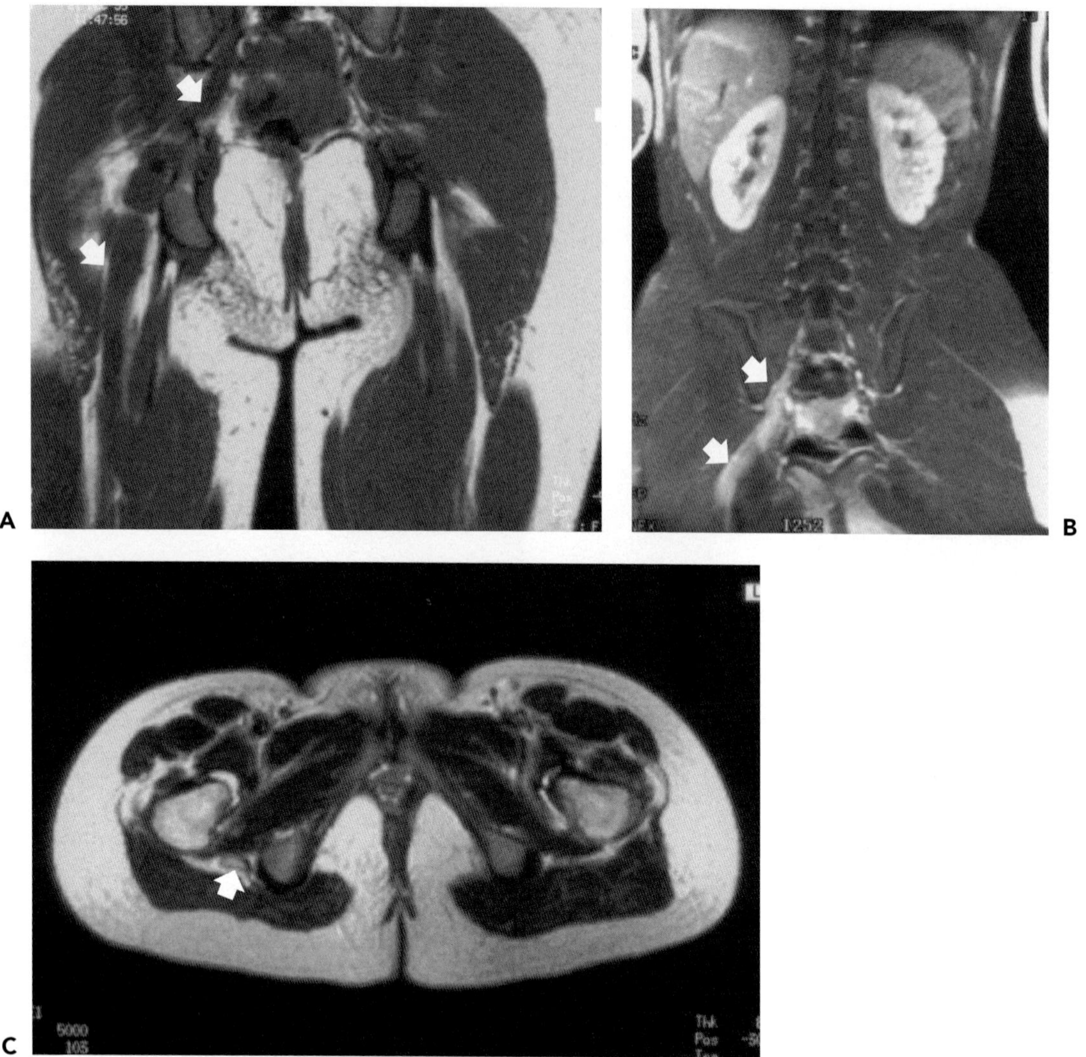

Figure 9.28 Perineurioma in a girl 13 years of age with right lower extremity neurologic symptoms. **A–C:** Coronal T1-weighted (TR/TE; 420/22) **(A)**, enhanced fat-suppressed T1-weighted (TR/TE; 500/16) **(B)**, and axial T2-weighted (TR/TE; 5000/106) **(C)** MR images show diffuse thickening of the sciatic nerve (*arrows*) with intermediate-to-high signal intensity on the long TR image and enhancement. Only the sciatic nerve is involved and not its branches, and no surrounding inflammation is seen.

involvement of the tendon, ligament, or aponeurosis. It is this location that should strongly suggest the diagnosis, and this anatomic relationship is best evaluated by MR imaging. CT scanning generally shows a soft tissue mass with attenuation equal to that of muscle. The lesion margins are often indistinct without evidence of a pseudocapsule. Because masses are often large at presentation and engulf multiple surrounding structures, it can be difficult to determine mass origin to a single tendon, ligament, or aponeurosis on axial CT images. Reports of sonographic evaluation of clear cell sarcoma are limited, but we would expect the lesion to appear as an aggressive infiltrating solid mass.

The largest imaging series of 21 patients, reported by De Beuckeleer et al., noted a slightly higher signal intensity than that of muscle on T1-weighted MR images in 52% of patients as a helpful finding suggesting clear cell sarcoma (235). Although we have also observed this imaging appearance, in our experience, this is not uncommon in other neoplasms, and it is so mild that we do not find it useful as a distinguishing feature. MR imaging typically reveals relatively homogeneous signal intensity on T1-weighting with more heterogeneity on T2-weighting. In our 10 cases with MR imaging, 70% had overall higher signal intensity than that of fat, and only 30% showed low-to-intermediate signal intensity (lower than that of fat) on T2-weighted images (Figs. 9.32 and 9.33). Low signal intensity on long TR MR images and high signal on T1-weighting in clear cell sarcoma is attributed to the effects of melanin (paramagnetic relaxation enhancement of surrounding tissues) (Fig. 9.32). Low signal intensity on long TR images was reported in 50% of lesions in the study by Wetzel et al.

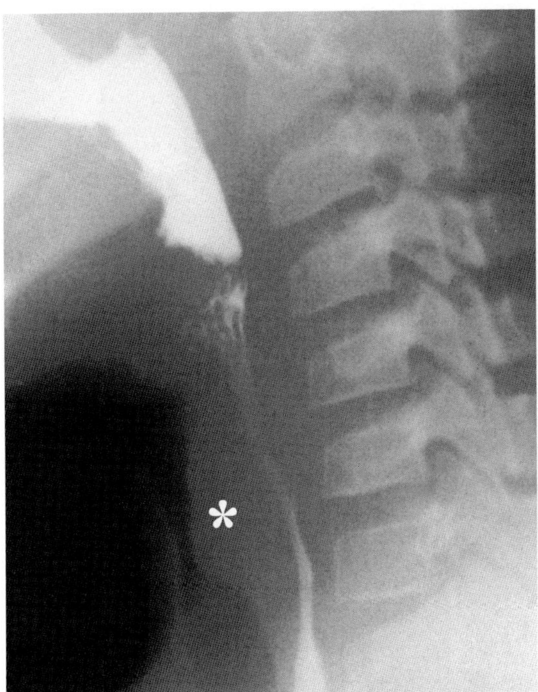
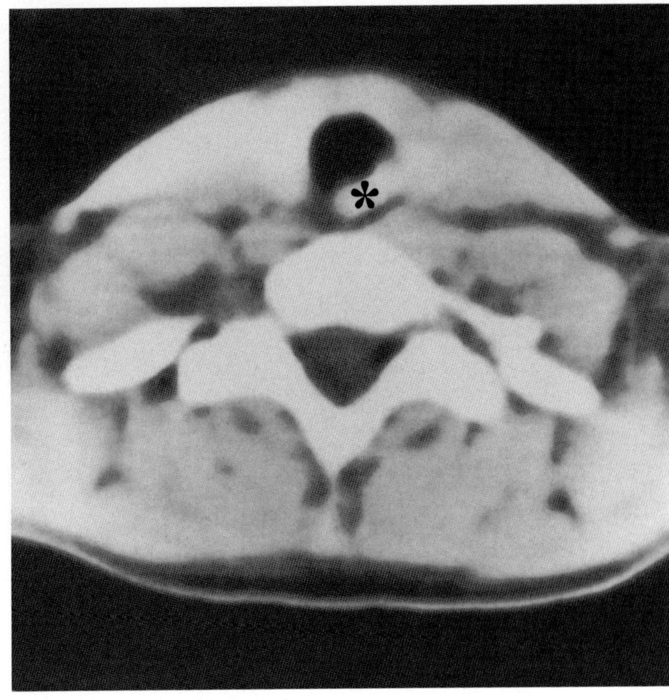

Figure 9.29 Granular cell tumor of subglottic region in a girl 8 years of age. **A:** Lateral radiograph after barium ingestion shows subglottic mass (*asterisk*). **B:** Axial noncontrast CT reveals a postero-lateral mass (*asterisk*).

(231). They suggested this finding may be related to lesions with a large amount of melanin (231). Others have questioned this effect of melanin, and additional causes of low MR signal intensity include hemosiderin and fibrous content (236). However, the majority of cases of clear cell sarcomas, in our experience, do not show low signal intensity on T2-weighted MR images, but reveal nonspecific intermediate-to-high signal intensity. Prominent enhancement after intravenous contrast administration is often apparent on CT or MR imaging (237).

We do not believe the minute amounts of melanin in these lesions are likely to cause significant or characteristic signal intensity in agreement with studies that suggest up to 23% melanin is required to increase the T1-weighted signal. The most distinctive feature of clear cell sarcoma on MR imaging is its primary involvement of a tendon, ligament, or aponeurosis with fusiform growth proximally and distally along and within this affected fibrous structure (Figs. 9.32 and 9.33). This manifestation is particularly well-shown on long axis MR images. This intimate relationship of tumor to ligament, tendon, or aponeurosis is best appreciated in lesions that involve large tendons or are imaged early in their course, prior to extensive invasion of surrounding structures. Clear cell sarcomas that do not demonstrate this relationship to tendons have a nonspecific cross-sectional imaging appearance (Fig. 9.34). Involvement of subcutaneous tissues and dermis with ulceration is not infrequent in cases of clear cell sarcoma.

PARAGANGLIOMA

KEY CONCEPTS

- Paragangliomas are rare neoplasms in extra-adrenal sites.
- They are most common about the carotid body (chemodectoma) and jugulotympanic region (glomus jugulare tumor).
- Multiple extra-adrenal paragangliomas appear in up to 20% of patients.
- The marked vascularity of these lesions is reflected on ultrasonography, CT, and MR imaging with serpentine high- and low-flow components.
- Indium-111 octreotide scanning has high sensitivity in detecting lesions larger than 1.5 cm.
- Treatment is complete surgical excision if possible; malignant paragangliomas account for 6% to 9% of lesions.

Paragangliomas are rare neuroendocrine neoplasms accounting for 0.03% of all neoplasms and 0.6% of all head and neck neoplasms (238–240). These tumors arise from the paraganglia, which represent neural crest cells associated with autonomic ganglia distributed from the skull base to the pelvic floor (241). Paragangliomas may be functional (producing catecholamines) or nonfunctional (not producing catecholamines-nonchromaffin). The World Health Organization subdivides these lesions into

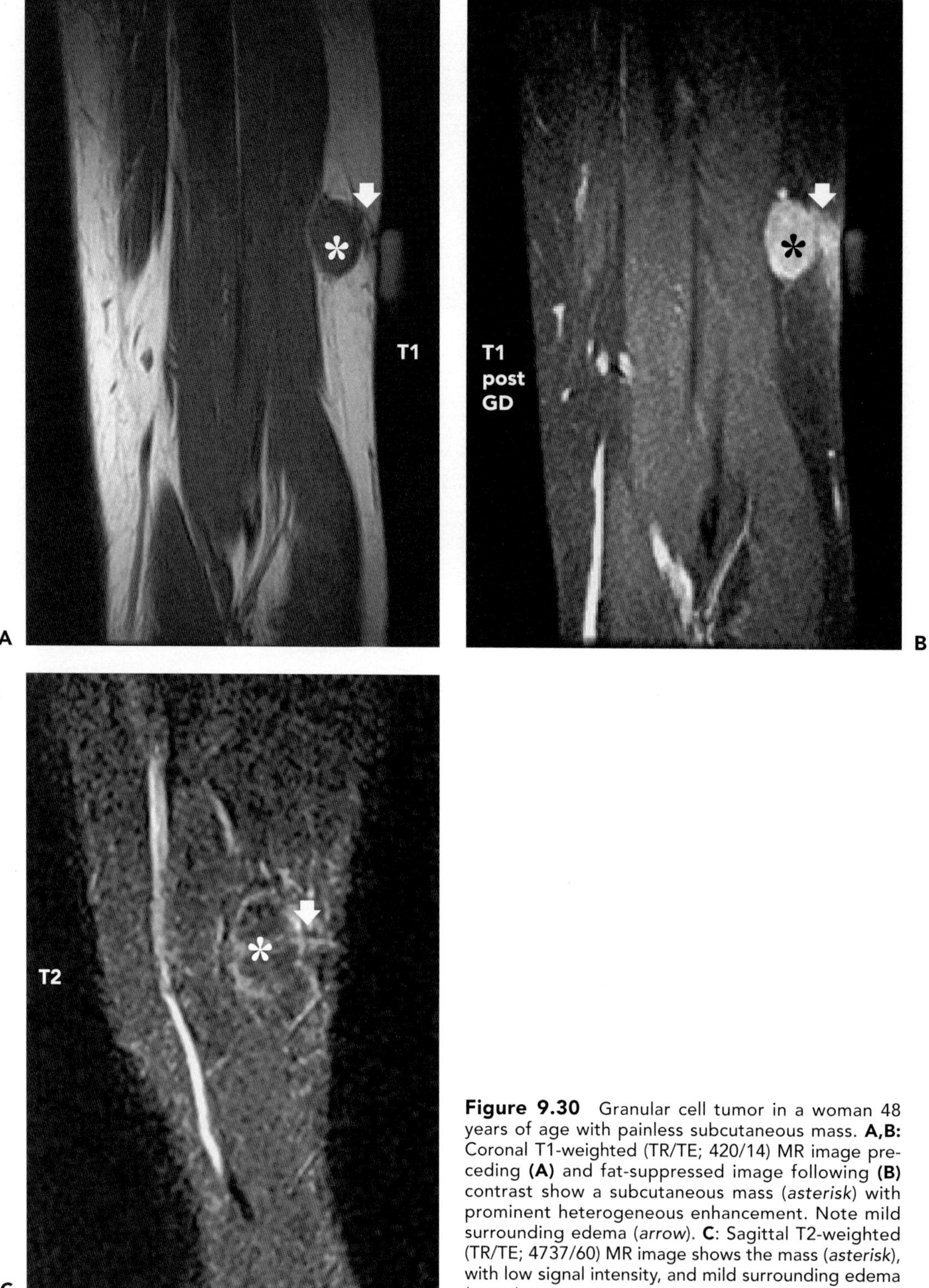

Figure 9.30 Granular cell tumor in a woman 48 years of age with painless subcutaneous mass. **A,B:** Coronal T1-weighted (TR/TE; 420/14) MR image preceding **(A)** and fat-suppressed image following **(B)** contrast show a subcutaneous mass (*asterisk*) with prominent heterogeneous enhancement. Note mild surrounding edema (*arrow*). **C:** Sagittal T2-weighted (TR/TE; 4737/60) MR image shows the mass (*asterisk*), with low signal intensity, and mild surrounding edema (*arrow*).

four types, including: (a) those arising from the adrenal medulla (pheochromocytoma; not further discussed); (b) aorticosympathetic, related to the sympathetic chain and retroperitoneal ganglia; (c) parasympathetic, associated with the carotid, vagal, and visceral autonomic ganglia; and (d) other paragangliomas. Common sites of extra-adrenal paragangliomas include those of the carotid body (Fig. 9.35), jugulotympanic region, vagal body (Fig. 9.36), mediastinum (aortic body), and retroperitoneum, although numerous unusual foci are also described (242, 243). Paragangliomas of either the carotid body or glomus jugulare account for 80% of all lesions.

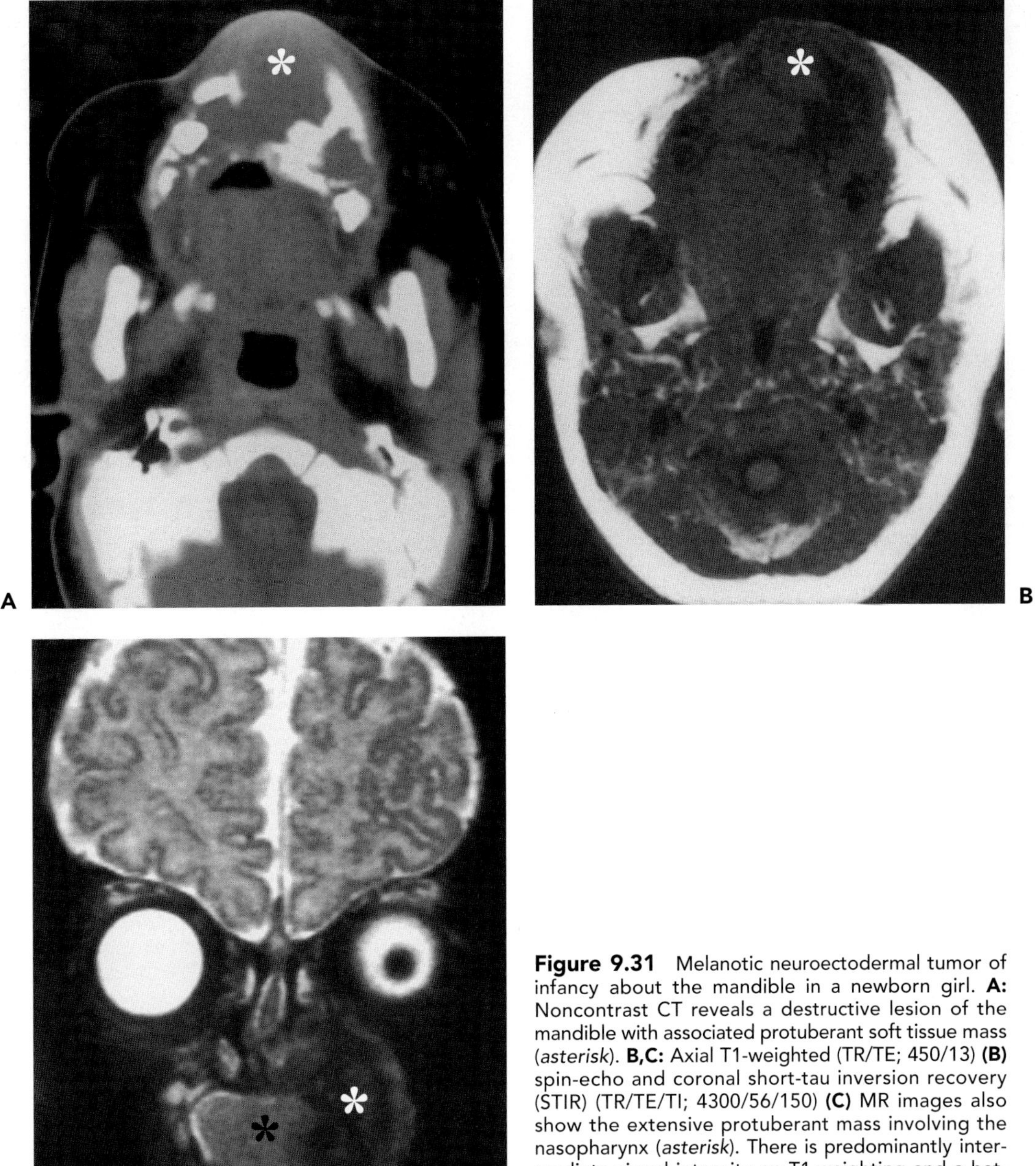

Figure 9.31 Melanotic neuroectodermal tumor of infancy about the mandible in a newborn girl. **A:** Noncontrast CT reveals a destructive lesion of the mandible with associated protuberant soft tissue mass (*asterisk*). **B,C:** Axial T1-weighted (TR/TE; 450/13) **(B)** spin-echo and coronal short-tau inversion recovery (STIR) (TR/TE/TI; 4300/56/150) **(C)** MR images also show the extensive protuberant mass involving the nasopharynx (*asterisk*). There is predominantly intermediate signal intensity on T1-weighting and a heterogeneous pattern on the long TR image with areas of intermediate signal intensity (*black asterisk*) and other regions with low signal intensity (*white asterisk*).

Carotid body paragangliomas are commonly referred to as *chemodectomas,* a term proposed by Mulligan in 1950. Reports conflict on whether carotid body or glomus jugulare lesion is the most frequent extra-adrenal paraganglioma. However, many reports suggest carotid body lesions are most common and account for 60% of all head/neck paragangliomas. These paragangliomas are generally nonfunctional and arise from the carotid body (chemoreceptor to monitor arterial oxygen levels and blood pH) along the posterior aspect of the common carotid artery bifurcation (239). Chemodectomas are more frequent in high-altitude regions and in patients with chronic obstructive pulmonary disease, perhaps related to chronic hypoxia-induced hyperplasia. Patients are typically affected in the fifth to seventh decades (peak prevalence: 45 to 50 years of age), and the sex distribution is equal, except for lesions associated with high altitude where women predominate (241). Patients usually present with a slowly growing (5 mm per year) painless mass. Bruit may be apparent, and pressure applied to the mass may initiate symptoms of increased heart rate (carotid sinus syndrome). Other symptoms include hoarseness, stridor, vertigo, dysphasia, and tongue paresis. Treatment is usually surgical, which is curative in

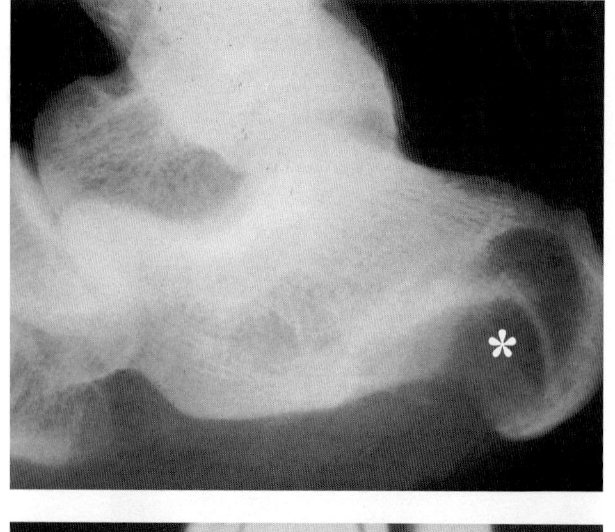

A

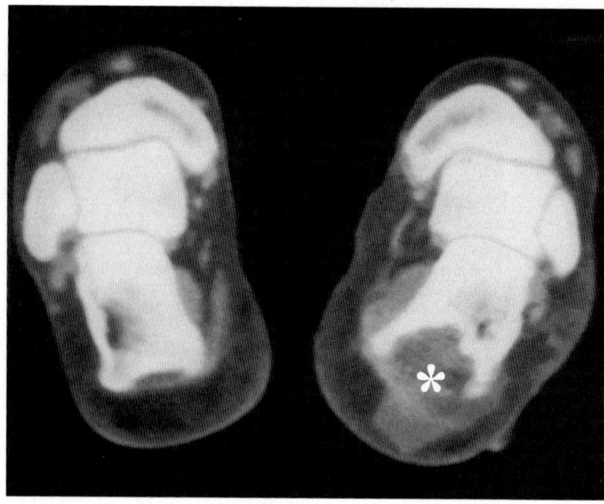

B

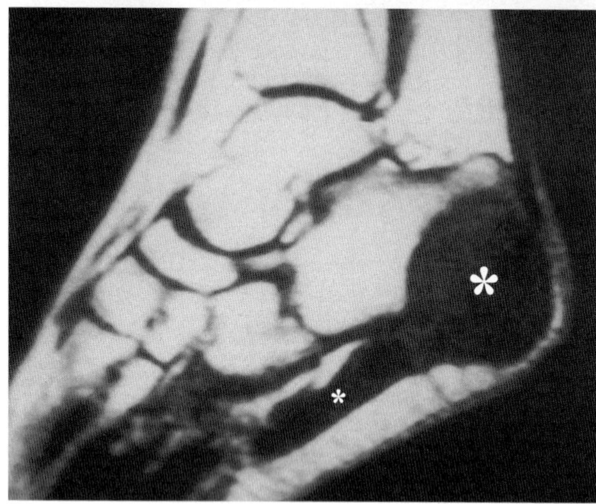

C

Figure 9.32 Clear cell sarcoma of the foot in a woman 28 years of age. **A:** Lateral radiograph shows a large plantar mass with associated destruction of the calcaneus (*asterisk*). **B:** Noncontrast oblique coronal CT demonstrates the mass (*asterisk*) to be heterogeneous with an attenuation similar to that of muscle, extending into the calcaneus. **C:** Sagittal T2-weighted spin-echo MR image (TR/TE; 2000/90) reveals a large mass (*large asterisk*) involving the calcaneus, and extending into the plantar aponeurosis (*small asterisk*). Note low signal intensity of mass.

most cases if the resection is complete (244). The metastases of malignant chemodectoma (6% to 9% of patients) most frequently affect regional lymph nodes (50% of metastases), lung, and bone (241,245–247). All large benign unresectable and malignant paragangliomas are radiosensitive.

Multiple paragangliomas are present in up to 20% of patients, either synchronously or metachronously (248). This is particularly common in familial cases (10% of chemodectomas), 90% of which arise in the carotid body and show an autosomal dominant inheritance pattern (249). Familial paragangliomas occur at a younger age and reveal cytogenetic aberrations with evidence of linkage to 11q22.3-q23.2. Chemodectomas are bilateral in 2% to 7% of patients, and in patients with a familial lesion, the incidence of bilaterality increases to 31% (250–252). Paragangliomas may also be associated with multiple endocrine neoplasia (MEN), neuroectodermal syndromes (neurofibromatosis), and rarely, von Hippel-Lindau disease.

The second most common extra-adrenal paraganglioma in most series, is the jugulotympanic lesion, referred to as *glomus jugulare tumor*. These paragangliomas arise from the auricular branch of the vagus nerve, the tympanic branch of the glossopharyngeal nerve, or the jugular vein bulb (253–256). They are the most frequent neoplasms of the middle ear, and the vast majority are nonfunctional (241,256). Women are affected far more frequently than men (4–6:1 ratio), with the highest incidence in the fifth decade of life. Clinical symptoms are common, including pulsatile tinnitus, conductive hearing loss, and other cranial nerve palsies (40% of patients). Multiple staging systems accurately depict the clinical course of these lesions. Lesions that are amenable to complete surgical resection rarely recur. The incidence of malignant lesions with metastases (similar sites as seen with chemodectoma) is estimated at 1% to 4% (239).

Vagal paraganglioma was first described by Stout in 1935 and is the third most common extra-adrenal

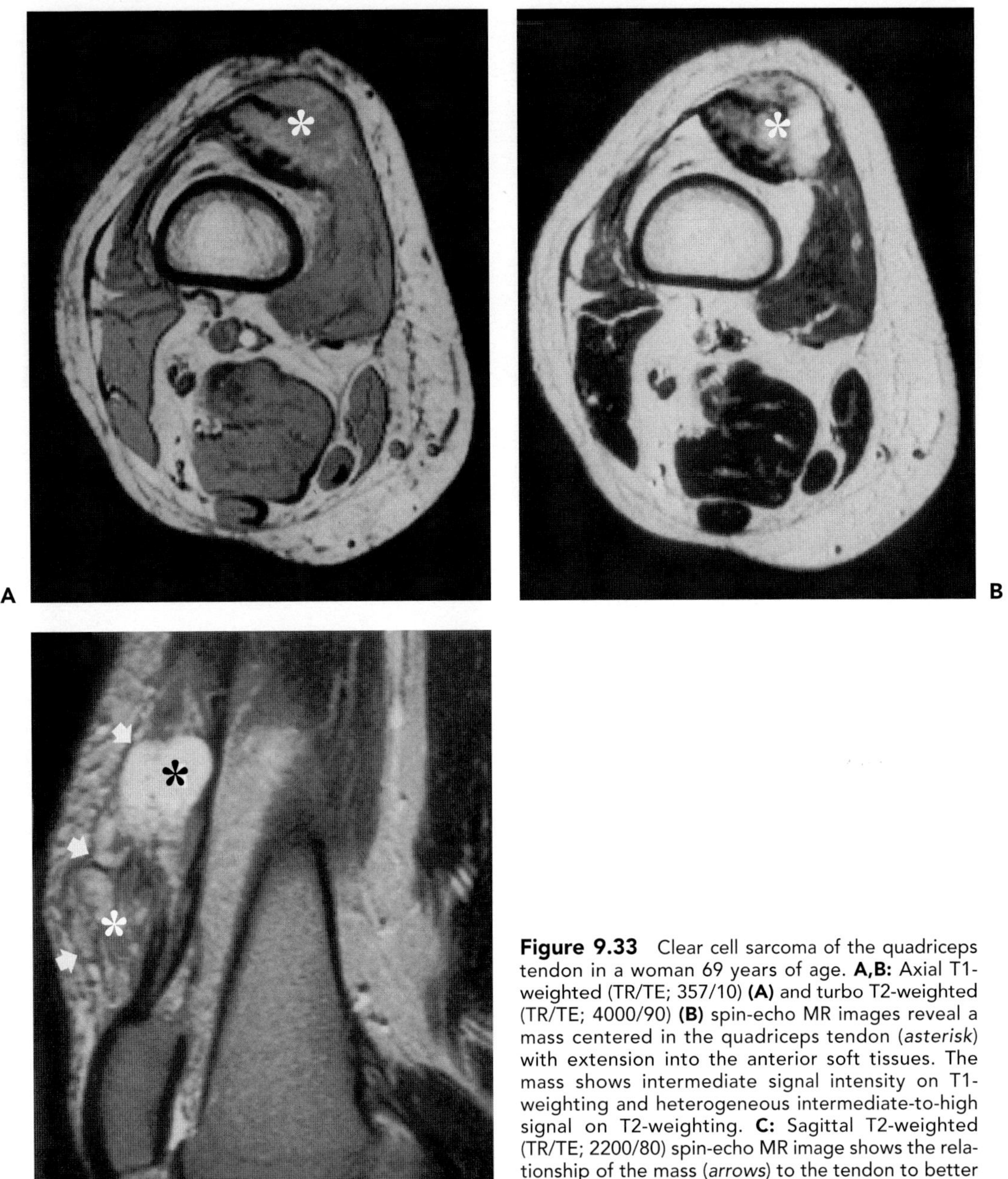

Figure 9.33 Clear cell sarcoma of the quadriceps tendon in a woman 69 years of age. **A,B:** Axial T1-weighted (TR/TE; 357/10) **(A)** and turbo T2-weighted (TR/TE; 4000/90) **(B)** spin-echo MR images reveal a mass centered in the quadriceps tendon (*asterisk*) with extension into the anterior soft tissues. The mass shows intermediate signal intensity on T1-weighting and heterogeneous intermediate-to-high signal on T2-weighting. **C:** Sagittal T2-weighted (TR/TE; 2200/80) spin-echo MR image shows the relationship of the mass (*arrows*) to the tendon to better advantage, as well as the high (*black asterisk*) and intermediate (*white asterisk*) signal intensity areas.

paraganglioma, accounting for 5% of lesions (239). These lesions most commonly arise behind the angle of the mandible (83% of cases) (257). Vagal paragangliomas usually extend along the perineurium, as opposed to a focal mass, and they are slowly growing and painless. There is a female-to-male ratio of 2.7:1, and 10% to 15% of cases have multiple lesions (257). Surgical resection is difficult without sacrificing the vagus nerve. Malignancy with metastases occurs in 10% to 20% of lesions (239).

Other extra-adrenal paragangliomas arise related to the aortic body, within the posterior mediastinum or in the retroperitoneum along the periaortic sympathetic chain (including the organs of Zuckerkandl). The vast majority of these lesions are nonfunctional, except retroperitoneal lesions that produce norepinephrine in 25% to 60% of cases (258–260). Clinical symptoms are usually related to the mass and involvement of adjacent structures, although functional lesions may produce systemic signs such as hypertension, headaches, and palpitations with norepinephrine production as opposed to hypotension and cardiac arrhythmias in epinephrine-producing lesions. The incidence of malignant paragangliomas with metastases from these primary sites ranges from 2% to 16% (241). Metastatic foci usually involve regional lymph nodes, bone, liver, and lung.

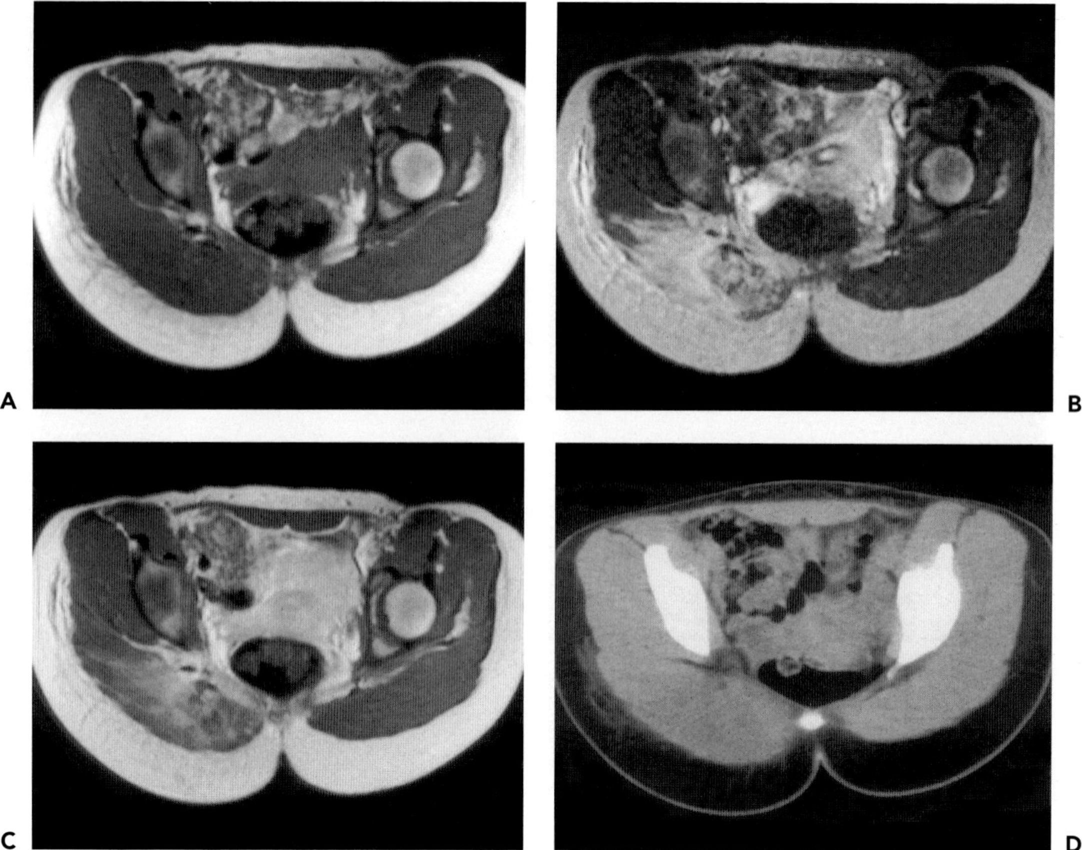

Figure 9.34 Clear cell sarcoma of the buttocks in a girl 15 years of age with a nonspecific appearance. **A,B:** Axial T1-weighted (TR/TE; 700/15) **(A)** and T2-weighted (TR/TE; 2100/80) **(B)** spin-echo MR images reveal a mass in the gluteus maximus. The mass shows an intermediate signal intensity on T2-weighted images. There is marked associated edema. **C:** Axial T1-weighted image following gadolinium administration shows mild enhancement of the mass, with diffuse enhancement of the surrounding edema. **D:** The lesion is poorly delineated on corresponding noncontrast CT.

Pathologically, extra-adrenal paragangliomas are most commonly solid, defined masses. When bisected, a fibrous pseudocapsule and multiple blood vessels are well seen on the cut surface. Histologically, these lesions are composed of chief cells and sustentacular cells, with a surrounding fibrovascular stroma. The chief cells are arranged in compact nests (termed *zellballen ball of cells*).

Paragangliomas are richly vascular tumors, and radiologic imaging reflects this characteristic. Most masses are not apparent on radiographs, although larger lesions, particularly in a mediastinal location, may be apparent on chest radiographs. Ultrasonography of carotid body tumors is reported by Derchi et al. to reveal solid heterogeneous (1.2 cm to 5.0 cm) masses within the carotid bifurcation in 22 of 23 cases (261). Lesions are often heterogeneously hypoechoic, and Doppler analysis typically detects low-resistance arterial blood flow (Fig. 9.35) (262,263). CT and MR imaging also detect these masses and involvement of surrounding structures. Splaying of the common carotid bifurcation is a common manifestation of chemodectoma on ultrasound, CT, or MR imaging (264). CT

reveals a soft tissue mass with marked postcontrast enhancement (Fig. 9.35) (265). Areas of osseous destruction and expansion are not uncommon with paragangliomas of the skull base and middle ear; these manifestations are best depicted by CT (256). MR imaging appearance has been described by Olsen et al. with demonstration of serpentine areas of signal void representing high vascular flow (12 of 15 cases), similar to arteriovenous hemangioma (Figs. 9.35 and 9.36) (246). Lesions are generally low-to-intermediate intensity on T1-weighted MR images and intermediate-to-very-high signal on T2-weighting (Figs. 9.35 and 9.36). Lesions were heterogeneous on all pulse sequences, creating a "salt and pepper" appearance on long TR sequences (Figs. 9.35 and 9.36) (246). The "salt" represents high signal intensity in slow-flow vascular components or hemorrhage, and the "pepper" represents areas of signal void from high-flow regions. The salt and pepper appearance occurs in lesions larger than 1 cm, but is not considered pathognomonic because it may occur in other hypervascular neoplasms (particularly renal or thyroid metastases). Similar to that seen on CT, an

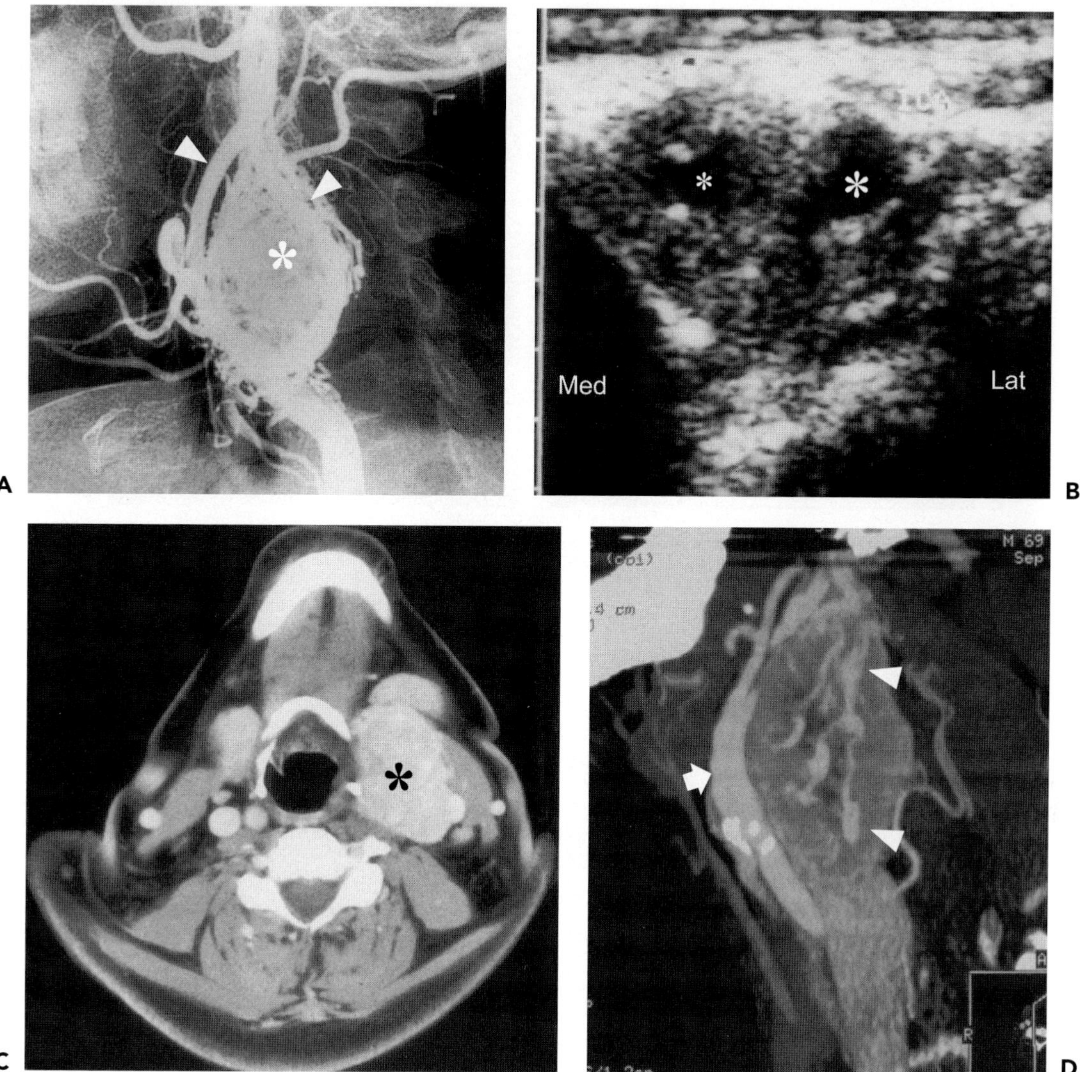

Figure 9.35   Paraganglioma of the carotid body in several different patients. **A:** Angiogram shows intense staining in the chemodectoma (*asterisks*) with splaying of carotid vessels (*arrows*). **B:** Sonogram shows heterogeneous solid mass. Internal (*large asterisk*) and external (*small asterisk*) carotid arteries are well-seen. **C,D:** Contrast-enhanced axial CT **(C)** and sagittal reconstruction **(D)** show marked tumor enhancement (*asterisk*), splaying of carotid vessels (*arrow*), and high-flow serpentine internal vascularity (*arrowheads*). (*continued*)

intense pattern of enhancement occurs following intravenous contrast administration. Paragangliomas may reveal the so-called dropout phenomenon with MR angiography (266). Standard doses of gadolinium show a progressive increase in signal intensity caused by T1-shortening. However, with higher doses of contrast, magnetic susceptibility leads to a transient decreased signal intensity (T2-shortening) 24 to 42 seconds after injection, followed by progressive increased signal intensity (267,268).

Angiography of paragangliomas usually reveals profuse vascularity with large serpentine nutrient vessels, heterogeneous dense capillary stain, and early draining veins (Fig. 9.35) (250,252,269). In evaluation of chemodec-

tomas, the contralateral carotid artery should also be studied to evaluate for a second tumor as well as to assess adequacy of cross filling, in case major vessels must be sacrificed at surgical resection (250,252). Preoperative embolization may be performed to lessen blood loss during surgery.

Scintigraphy with I-131 (or I-123) metaiodobenzylguanidine (MIBG), a structural analogue of norepinephrine, is also used to detect functional paragangliomas with a high degree of accuracy (242,270–273). In the study by von Gils et al., MIBG demonstrated 88% of extra-adrenal functioning paragangliomas as focal areas of marked radionuclide uptake (242). MIBG scanning is

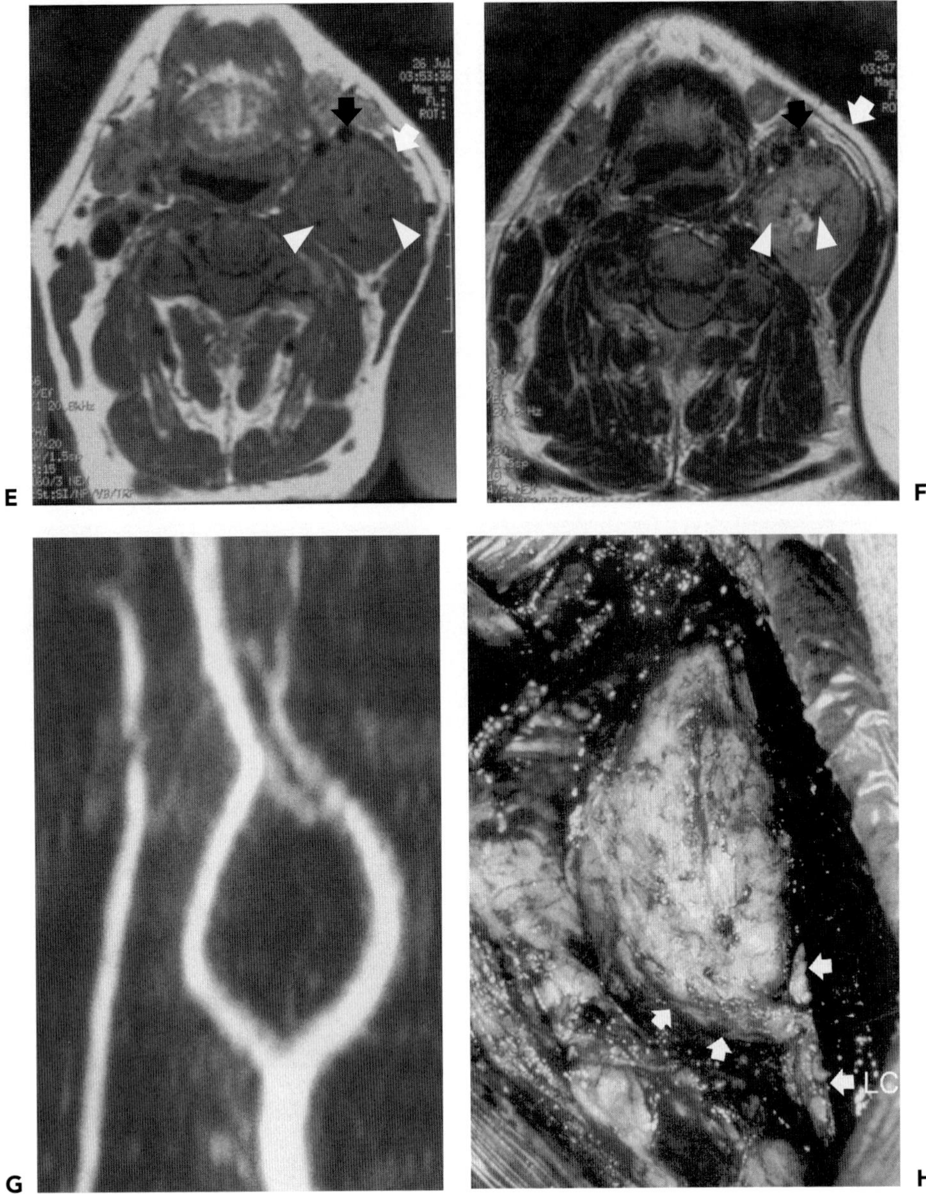

Figure 9.35 *(continued)* **E,F:** Axial T1-weighted (TR/TE; 366/22) **(E)** and T2-weighted (TR/TE; 4066/122) **(F)** spin-echo MR images show the mass (*white arrow*) to have well-defined margins, with heterogeneous, but predominantly intermediate signal intensity on long TR images. Low signal intensity flow voids (*arrowheads*) results from rapid blood flow, and the carotid vessels are displaced (*black arrows*). **G:** MR angiography study also shows splaying of carotid vessels by tumor. **H:** Intraoperative photograph demonstrate mass with splaying of carotid vessels (*arrows*).

reported to detect tumors as small as 0.2 grams and is also very useful to identify local recurrence and metastatic disease (242,271). However, false positives can occur associated with other neural crest tumors (neuroblastoma, schwannoma, medullary carcinoma of thyroid) and false negatives with certain medications (insulin, antidepressants, cocaine, amphetamines). In addition, spatial resolution limitations of scintigraphy usually require evaluation by CT or MR imaging as well, prior to surgical resection. Currently indium-111 octreotide is the agent of choice for nuclear medicine detection of paragangliomas (274–276). Octreotide imaging shows high sensitivity in detecting paragangliomas larger than 1.5 cm, but it is insensitive for lesions smaller than 1 cm (274–276). Octreotide is more sensitive than MIBG for identifying lesions, primarily because of its ability to detect both functional and nonfunctional paragangliomas (274–276). Octreotide is particularly useful in demonstrating multiple lesions, metastases, local recurrence, and in differentiating neurogenic tumors.

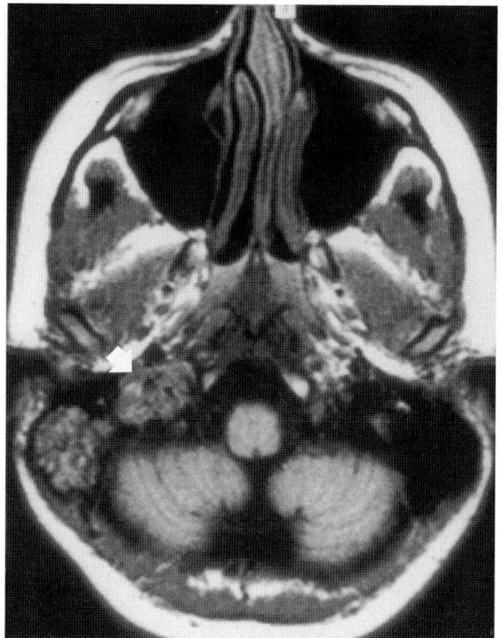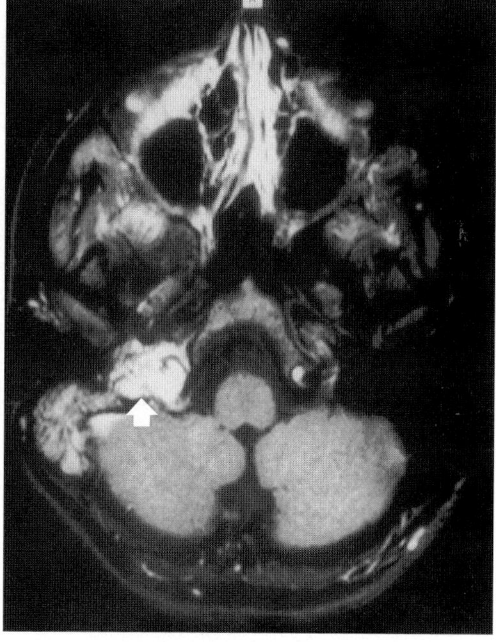

Figure 9.36   Paragangliomas (glomus jugulare and glomus tympanicum) in a woman 18 years of age complaining of pulsatile tinnitus. **A,B:** Axial T1-weighted (TR/TE; 600/15) **(A)** and fat-suppressed enhanced T1-weighted (TR/TE; 750/20) **(B)** spin-echo MR images show paragangliomas with prominent enhancement (*arrow*). Signal voids are indicative of the high degree of tumor vascularity. The patient had an additional paraganglioma with a small lesion about the ipsilateral carotid (not shown).

PRIMITIVE NEURAL TUMORS

Neuroblastoma/Ganglioneuroblastoma/Ganglioneuroma

> ### KEY CONCEPTS
> - Primitive neural tumors are neoplasms that include neuroblastoma, ganglioneuroblastoma, and ganglioneuroma; they represent lesions of varying degrees of differentiation.
> - These lesions frequently involve young patients and common extra-adrenal locations include the abdomen, retroperitoneum, posterior mediastinum, and pelvis.
> - Treatment and prognosis depend on the clinical stage of the lesion.
> - Intrinsic imaging characteristics are typically nonspecific, and calcification is frequently observed on CT.

Primitive neural tumors arise from neural crest origin and thus, they occur along the sympathetic ganglia and within the adrenal medulla (not discussed further). In order of least to most differentiated, neuroblastoma is composed of primitive neuroblasts (resembling the fetal adrenal and representing a small, round, blue cell tumor), ganglioneuroblastoma contains both primitive neuroblast and maturing ganglion cells, and finally, the

ganglioneuroma is made up of mature Schwann cells and ganglion cells (Figs. 9.37–9.39) (277–279). As expected, the malignant potential and behavior is directly related to the degree of differentiation. Clinically, patients usually present with evidence of a soft tissue mass or the secondary effects of the lesion on surrounding structures. Neuroblastoma patients frequently (80% to 90%) demonstrate elevated amounts of catecholamines and their byproducts, with resulting clinical symptoms (277). Ganglioneuroblastoma and ganglioneuroma less commonly manifest elevated catecholamine levels. Ganglioneuromas, even if large, are often asymptomatic. Numerous cytogenetic abnormalities are detected, with the most common related to the short arm of chromosome 1 (described in up to 70% of patients with neuroblastoma) (277).

Neuroblastoma is the third most common malignant tumor in childhood (1 per 10,000 live births), following leukemia and brain tumors, and it causes 15% of cancer deaths in children (277,278,280–284). The vast majority of these lesions occur sporadically, with a small number following an autosomal dominant pattern of inheritance. Neuroblastoma represents the most frequent solid neoplasm arising outside the central nervous system in infants and children. This tumor is significantly less common in blacks. Neuroblastoma and ganglioneuroblastoma are generally seen in young patients. In fact, 50% of neuroblastomas are found before the age of 2 years (25% congenital

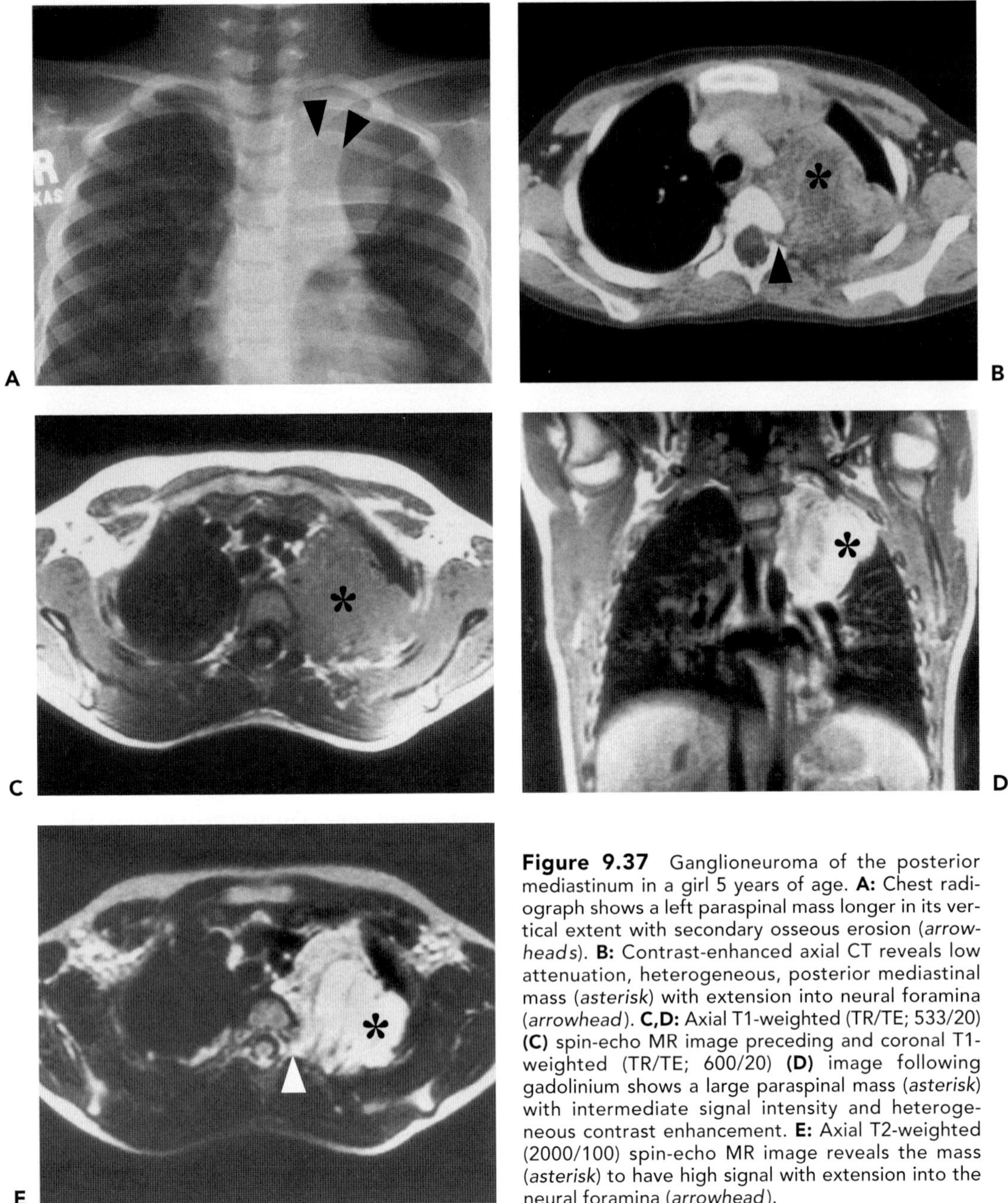

Figure 9.37 Ganglioneuroma of the posterior mediastinum in a girl 5 years of age. **A:** Chest radiograph shows a left paraspinal mass longer in its vertical extent with secondary osseous erosion (*arrowheads*). **B:** Contrast-enhanced axial CT reveals low attenuation, heterogeneous, posterior mediastinal mass (*asterisk*) with extension into neural foramina (*arrowhead*). **C,D:** Axial T1-weighted (TR/TE; 533/20) **(C)** spin-echo MR image preceding and coronal T1-weighted (TR/TE; 600/20) **(D)** image following gadolinium shows a large paraspinal mass (*asterisk*) with intermediate signal intensity and heterogeneous contrast enhancement. **E:** Axial T2-weighted (2000/100) spin-echo MR image reveals the mass (*asterisk*) to have high signal with extension into the neural foramina (*arrowhead*).

and most of these are adrenal), 90% by 5 years of age, 96% in the first decade of life, and 3.5% in the second decade (277,278,281,285). The peak age of presentation of neuroblastoma is 18 months. Ganglioneuromas, in contrast, are usually diagnosed after the age of 10 years (277,285).

Neuroblastomas and ganglioneuroblastoma are located in a paramidline position from the skull base to the lower pelvis, with the adrenal (not discussed further) being the single most frequent site. Extra-adrenal neuroblastoma locations include the abdomen (63%), most of which are retroperitoneal (Fig. 9.39), posterior mediastinum (14%), neck (5%), pelvis (5%), and brain (2%) (281,286).

Ganglioneuroblastomas most frequently affect the abdomen, followed by the mediastinum, neck, and lower extremity (Fig. 9.38). Ganglioneuromas are most common in the posterior mediastinum (39% to 43%) and the retroperitoneum (32% to 52%) (277,285) (Fig. 9.37). Neural immunohistochemical markers are usually positive but are nonspecific.

Treatment of these lesions is usually complete surgical removal, except in neuroblastoma patients with stage 4 disease. The most important prognostic factor for neuroblastoma is the clinical stage according to the International Neuroblastoma Staging System (Table 9.5) (284).

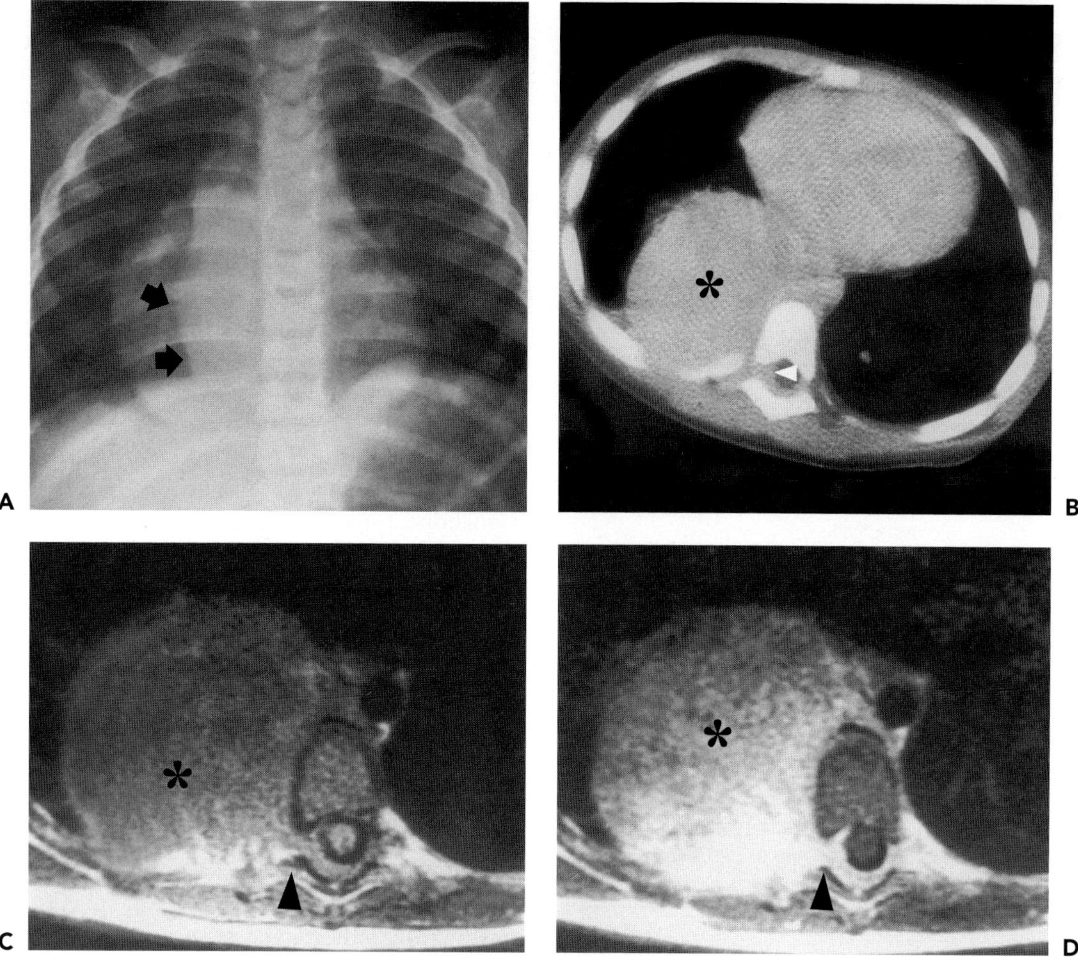

Figure 9.38 Ganglioneuroblastoma of the posterior mediastinum in a girl 2 years of age. **A:** Chest radiograph reveals a right posterior mediastinal mass (*arrows*). **B:** Noncontrast axial CT shows the large soft tissue mass (*asterisk*) with extension into a neural foramen (*arrowhead*). **C,D:** Axial T1-weighted spin-echo (TR/TE; 500/20) MR image preceding **(C)** and following **(D)** gadolinium administration show diffuse heterogeneous enhancement and extension into neural canal. (*arrowhead by the mass*).

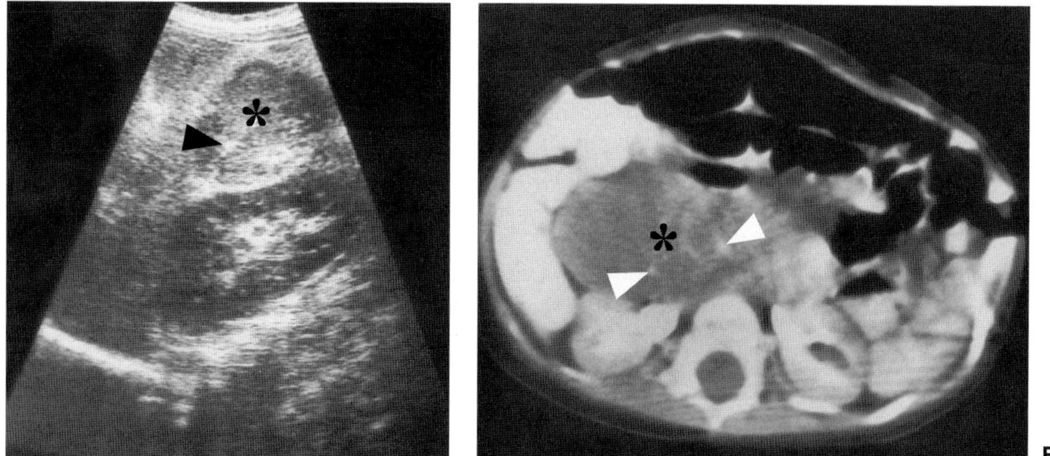

Figure 9.39 Neuroblastoma of the retroperitoneum in a boy 18 months of age. Laboratory tests demonstrated elevated catecholamines. **A:** Abdominal sonogram shows an echogenic mass (*asterisk*) anterior to the kidney. Small echogenic focus with shadowing (*arrowhead*) resulting from calcification is seen. **B:** Contrast-enhanced axial CT reveals the mass (*asterisk*) containing small calcifications (*arrowheads*). Calcifications were not well-seen on radiographs (not shown).

TABLE 9.5

INTERNATIONAL NEUROBLASTOMA STAGING SYSTEM

Stage	Definition
1	Localized tumor confined to area of origin; complete gross excision, with or without microscopic residual disease; representative ipsilateral lymph nodes negative for tumor.
2A	Localized tumor with incomplete gross excision; representative ipsilateral nonadherent lymph nodes negative for tumor microscopically.
2B	Localized tumor with or without complete gross excision, with ipsilateral nonadherent lymph nodes positive for tumor. Enlarged contralateral lymph nodes must be negative for tumor microscopically.
3	Unresectable unilateral tumor infiltrating across the midline, with or without regional lymph node involvement; or localized unilateral tumor with contralateral regional lymph node involvement; or midline tumor with bilateral extension by infiltration (unresectable) or by lymph node involvement.
4	Any primary tumor with dissemination to distant lymph nodes, bone, bone marrow, liver, skin, and/or other organs (except as defined for stage 4S).
4S	Localized primary tumor (as defined for stage 1, 2A, or 2B), with dissemination limited to skin, liver, and/or bone marrow.

Children with stage 1 and 2 disease have a 3-year survival rate of 90%; stage 4S, 80%; stage 3 and 4, 30%. The overall 3-year survival rate is 50% (277,284). Diagnosis of neuroblastoma at a younger age (particularly less than 1 year) also improves survival rates (77% vs. 38% for those with diagnosis at ages greater than 2 years) (284). Metastatic disease is present in nearly 70% of neuroblastoma patients at presentation, with bone, lymph node, liver, and skin the most frequent sites (281). Metastasis to bone (60% of cases) is a particularly ominous finding almost invariably associated with a fatal outcome (281). Spontaneous regression or maturation of neuroblastoma or ganglioneuroblastoma is reported in 1% to 2% of patients, usually in children younger than 1 year and in patients with stage 4S disease (277,281,284). Additional favorable prognostic factors include histologic tumor type and some laboratory and genetic markers (low serum ferritin, neuron-specific enolase, hyperdiploidy, lack of N-myc amplification gene sequence sites, high expression of TrkA [tyrosine kinase receptor A] nerve growth factor), and no allelic loss of 1p (277). Patients with neuroblastoma located in the retroperitoneum or adrenal have a worse prognosis that those with lesions in the pelvic or paraspinal (cervical/thoracic) regions.

Histologic features are also used to divide patients into those with and without differentiated stroma, with prognostic implications. These various factors can be used to divide patients into three risk groups: low, intermediate, and high. Low-risk patients are usually adequately managed with surgery alone. Intermediate-risk patients usually require chemotherapy and second-look surgery. High-risk patients receive dose-intensive chemotherapy; bone marrow and blood stem cell transplantation are also used. Patients with 4S disease are individualized for treatment depending on age (older or younger than 4 weeks) and for those older than 4 weeks of age, the presence of unfavorable biologic markers. Patients with stage 4 disease may be treated with radiation and chemotherapy as opposed to surgical excision (281). Ganglioneuroblastomas generally have a less malignant clinical course than neuroblastoma. Ganglioneuroma, in contrast, is almost invariably a benign tumor and surgical resection is curative. Ganglioneuromas only rarely undergo malignant transformation; this association has been reported in a patient with HIV.

Imaging of these neoplasms in extra-adrenal locations is often nonspecific. Location of the lesion along the sympathetic chain is important for diagnosis. Paraspinal lesions may extend into the spinal canal (Figs. 9.37 and 9.38). Calcification is seen in approximately 55% of retroperitoneal neuroblastomas on radiographs (85% by CT) (Fig. 9.39) and in 20% to 30% of ganglioneuromas (281,287). CT and MR imaging are best to evaluate and stage disease extent of the soft tissue mass (280–285). CT is superior to detect the presence of calcification (Figs. 9.37–9.39). Dietrich et al. suggested that MR imaging is superior to CT in determining tumor extent because of its multiplanar capabilities and superior contrast resolution (282). The MR imaging signal intensity of neuroblastoma is generally nonspecific with low-to-intermediate intensity on T1-weighting and intermediate-to-high signal on T2-weighting. Similarly, CT reveals a nonspecific soft tissue attenuation mass. Higher signal intensity on T2-weighted images likely corresponds to increased myxoid tissue and is more common in ganglioneuroma (Fig. 9.37) (288). Curvilinear bands of low signal intensity on long TR images causing a whorled appearance have been described in ganglioneuroma (289,290). Amundson et al., in reporting the ultrasound results in 10 cases, noted focal areas or lobules of increased echogenicity within 4 (40%) of ganglioneuroblastomas neuroblastomas in their series, and they believe this finding is characteristic because it was not seen in 43 other abdominal neoplasms (280,291, 292). Ganglioneuromas tend to surround adjacent major vascular structures partially or completely without compromising blood flow. CT scanning of ganglioneuroma may show gradual delayed heterogeneous contrast enhancement. We are not aware of any radiologic findings that distinguish neuroblastoma, ganglioneuroblastoma, or ganglioneuroma. Paraspinal ganglioneuroblastoma and ganglioneuroma typically are long, vertical, posterior mediastinal tumors (285,293,294). Radioiodine MIBG scintigraphy may demonstrate radionuclide uptake within both primary and metastatic primitive neuroectodermal neoplasms (295,296).

Primitive Neuroectodermal Tumor (PNET)/ Extraskeletal Ewing Sarcoma

---

KEY CONCEPTS

- Primitive neuroectodermal tumor (PNET) and extraskeletal Ewing sarcoma were previously considered to be distinct malignant lesions, but may represent a single entity.
- These lesions frequently affect young patients (10 to 30 years of age) with common locations including the paravertebral region, chest wall (Askin tumor), retroperitoneum, and lower extremities.
- Clinical history is often of a rapidly enlarging mass.
- Treatment is surgical resection and adjuvant chemotherapy.
- Imaging frequently reveals only a nonspecific mass, although high-flow vascular channels are often identified within the lesion.

Extraskeletal Ewing sarcoma and primitive neuroectodermal tumor (PNET) are similar soft tissue sarcomas likely derived from neuroectodermal origin (279,297). Ewing sarcoma was originally described in 1921; PNET was reported 3 years earlier by Stout (298,299). Synonyms for PNET include *peripheral neuroepithelioma* and *peripheral neuroblastoma*. Extraskeletal Ewing sarcoma and PNET can occur in bone or soft tissue, although our discussion is limited to soft tissue lesions. These neoplasms previously were considered to be distinct lesions because of purported differences in clinical behavior and pathologic appearance (300). Although still controversial, newer studies suggest a common genetic abnormality and clinical behavior, and these lesions may well represent a single entity; therefore, it may be preferable to consider these lesions together in the same family of tumors (300).

Both extraskeletal Ewing sarcoma and PNET usually affect young patients between 10 and 30 years of age (277,301). However, in review of some studies, the age range of patients was reported to be wider in PNET: from birth to 81 years (301–306). Males are affected slightly more commonly than females. Extraskeletal Ewing sarcoma is rarely seen in blacks. The most frequently involved locations include the paravertebral region, chest wall (PNET Askin tumor; see later discussion), retroperitoneum, and lower extremities. Clinical presentation is usually that of a rapidly growing soft tissue mass, often 5 cm to 10 cm in size at diagnosis. No elevation of catecholamine levels is seen, unlike neuroblastoma. Interestingly, 90% to 95% of patients show a reciprocal translocation of the long arm of chromosomes 11 and 22 (q24;q12) with both extraskeletal Ewing sarcoma and PNET (307).

Pathologically, these lesions are small, round, blue cell neoplasms, usually rich in glycogen. Previous distinction of PNET from extraskeletal Ewing sarcoma required detection of rosette formation in the former. In addition, electron microscopy revealed filaments and microtubules, and immunohistochemical stains should be positive for neuron-specific enolase and at least one other neural marker in PNET, although this distinction has become obscured over time (277,301–308). Both lesions express the product of the MIC2 gene in up to 95% of cases, providing further credence to a histogenetic linkage.

Treatment usually involves chemotherapy followed by surgical resection, and prognosis has progressively improved (309,310). Radiation therapy may also be used in some cases as an adjunct. Several studies have shown that the overall prognosis of PNET is worse than that of extraskeletal Ewing sarcoma (311). Schmidt et al. reported a disease-free survival rate of only 45% with PNET versus 60% for extraskeletal Ewing sarcoma (311). Other reports suggest a survival rate of only 30% for PNET and 65% to 70% for extraskeletal Ewing sarcoma (3-year survival rate of 80% for smaller tumors vs. 32% for larger lesions) (277,303,306). However, other studies do not confirm this disparity in prognosis, with 5-year survival rates in PNET ranging from 56% to 68% (312). Factors that worsen prognosis are large tumor size at diagnosis and evidence of extensive necrosis. Metastases and local recurrence are usually seen in the first 2 years after diagnosis. Sites of metastatic involvement are most commonly lung and bone.

Imaging appearance of these lesions has not been extensively evaluated (309,313–315). Findings are usually nonspecific, and to the best of our knowledge, no imaging features are described to allow distinction of extraskeletal Ewing sarcoma from PNET. O'Keeffe et al. reported that most frequently the lesions are hypoechoic on ultrasound and low attenuation on CT (314). However, in our experience, CT scanning shows attenuation similar to that of muscle without evidence of calcification. MR imaging also reveals nonspecific features with low-to-intermediate signal intensity on T1-weighting and generally intermediate-to-high signal intensity on T2-weighting (Fig. 9.40). The high cellularity of these lesions likely accounts for the common appearance of intermediate signal intensity on long TR images. Areas of hemorrhage, with high signal on all MR imaging pulse sequences, are not infrequent. Neoplasm margins may be relatively well-defined with a pseudocapsule, or may appear infiltrative.

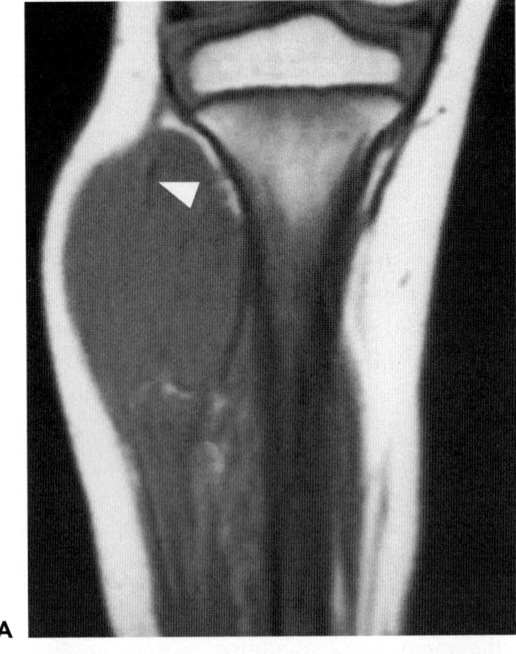

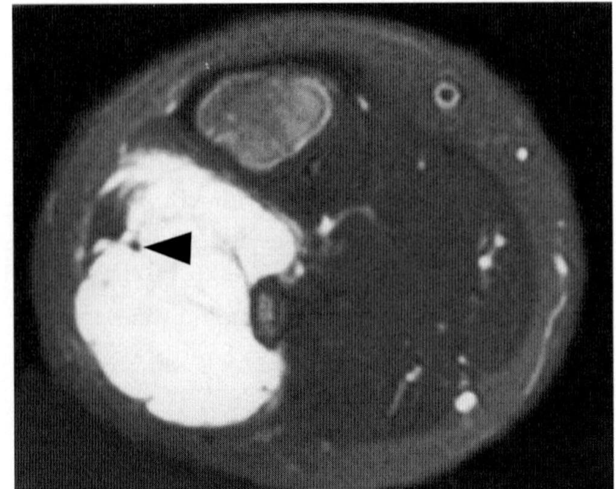

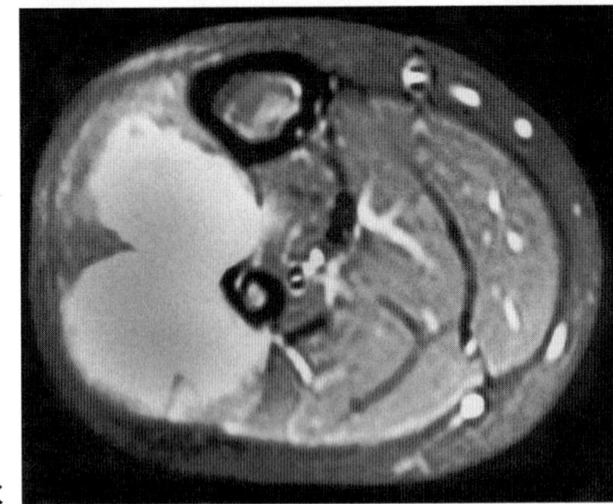

Figure 9.40 Extraskeletal Ewing sarcoma of the calf in a girl 5 years of age. **A,B:** Coronal T1-weighted (TR/TE; 633/16) **(A)** and axial turbo T2-weighted (TR/TE; 3000/102) **(B)** spin-echo MR images show a large soft tissue mass in the lateral aspect of the lower leg. The mass is relatively well-defined and homogeneous with nonspecific signal intensity. Flow voids (*arrowhead*) represent rapidly flowing blood in small peripheral vascular channels are also seen. **C:** Axial T1-weighted (TR/TE; 800/16) spin-echo MR image with fat suppression following contrast administration shows striking contrast enhancement, reflecting the lesion's marked vascularity.

The angiographic appearance is described as hypervascular, although this is not an invariable finding. MR imaging frequently reveals definable high-flow (low intensity on all MR imaging pulse sequences) vascular channels within the mass, often more prominent peripherally (Fig. 9.40). This is not a unique feature of PNET or extraskeletal Ewing sarcoma, since it can also be seen with vascular neoplasms (hemangiopericytoma, hemangioendothelioma, and angiosarcoma), alveolar soft part sarcoma, and alveolar rhabdomyosarcoma. Prominent contrast enhancement is also a feature of these lesions, in our experience, on CT or MR imaging, although O'Keeffe et al. only reported enhancement in 4 of 11 patients on CT (314). Associated involvement of bone is unusual, and bone scintigraphy is usually normal.

Askin Tumor

Extraskeletal Ewing sarcoma/PNET occurring in the chest wall was formerly referred to as *Askin tumor,* and this term is often retained for lesions in the thoracopulmonary region (316). In 1979, Askin et al. described a small cell malignant tumor of the thoracopulmonary region in children and adolescents that is now generally believed to be equivalent to other extraskeletal Ewing sarcoma/PNET (316). These lesions are usually large and seen in young adults and children. A chest wall mass is the typical clinical presentation with or without pain. Lesions are most common in young females (3:1), and are almost exclusively unilateral (277,316). Associated rib destruction is common and seen in more than 50% of cases (317). There is typically a large associated pleural effusion, which may be loculated or form pseudotumors. Constitutional symptoms, including fever, anorexia, and weight loss, may also be present.

Grossly, the lesions are multilobulated, gray-white masses, with foci of hemorrhage and necrosis. The tumor is usually circumscribed but not encapsulated. On microscopy, the tumor is composed of small round cells with an identical appearance, as previously described, for extraskeletal Ewing sarcoma/PNET.

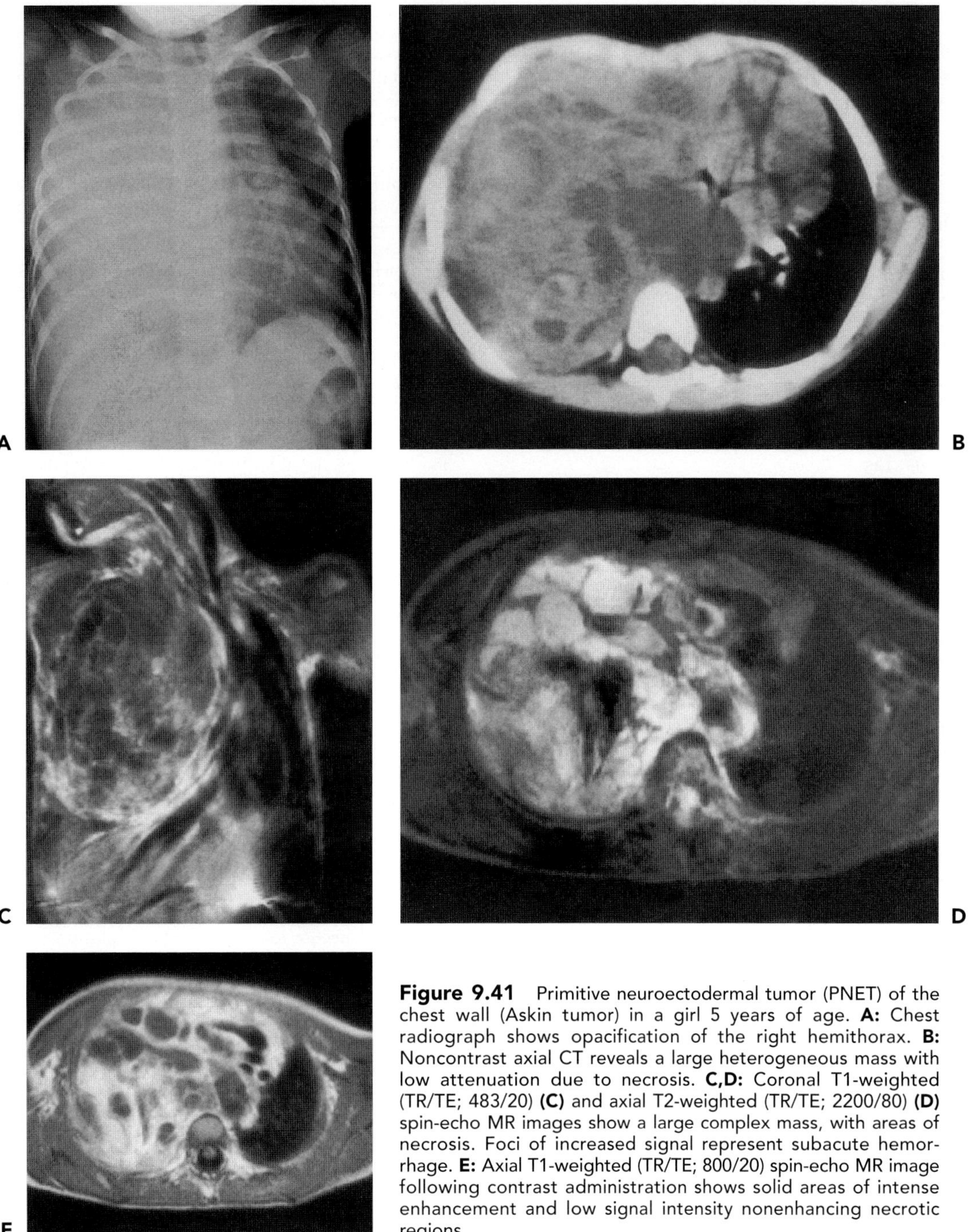

Figure 9.41 Primitive neuroectodermal tumor (PNET) of the chest wall (Askin tumor) in a girl 5 years of age. **A:** Chest radiograph shows opacification of the right hemithorax. **B:** Noncontrast axial CT reveals a large heterogeneous mass with low attenuation due to necrosis. **C,D:** Coronal T1-weighted (TR/TE; 483/20) **(C)** and axial T2-weighted (TR/TE; 2200/80) **(D)** spin-echo MR images show a large complex mass, with areas of necrosis. Foci of increased signal represent subacute hemorrhage. **E:** Axial T1-weighted (TR/TE; 800/20) spin-echo MR image following contrast administration shows solid areas of intense enhancement and low signal intensity nonenhancing necrotic regions.

Chest radiographs reveal a large pleural mass, which is usually a combination of pleural mass and fluid. Associated parenchymal disease is seen in approximately 25% of cases (Fig. 9.41) (318,319). Calcification is seen on radiographs in 10% of cases (318,319). Ipsilateral hilar and mediastinal adenopathy, as well as pneumothorax may also be present.

On CT scans, the lesion appears as a unilateral heterogeneous mass of mixed attenuation, often with associated rib destruction (25% to 63% of cases) and pleural fluid (318–320). In the study by Winer-Muram et al, lesions were commonly heterogeneous with signal intensity greater than that of muscle on T1-weighting (88%) (Fig. 9.41) (320). On T2-weighted MR images, high signal intensity was seen in all cases (Fig. 9.41) (320). Prominent contrast enhancement has been reported, reflecting the rich vascularity of these lesions on MR imaging (319–321).

Metastases are seen at presentation in 10% to 38% of patients (277). Recurrent thoracic disease is seen in more than 50% of patients, either with local recurrent disease, mediastinal nodes, or pulmonary nodules. Bone metastases develop in approximately 25% of patients, and lesions may be osteoblastic (277,316). The prognosis is poor; the median survival in Askin's original 20 patients was only 8 months (316).

REFERENCES

1. Kransdorf MJ. Malignant soft-tissue tumors in a large referral population: distribution of diagnoses by age, sex, and location. *AJR Am J Roentgenol.* 1995;164:129–134.
2. Damjanov I. Anderson's pathology. In: Kissane J, ed. *Peripheral Nervous System.* 10th ed. St. Louis: Mosby; 1996:2799–2803.
3. Fornage BD. Peripheral nerves of the extremities: imaging with US. *Radiology.* 1988;167:179–182.
4. Graif M, Seton A, Nerubai J, et al. Sciatic nerve: sonographic evaluation and anatomic-pathologic considerations. *Radiology.* 1991;181:405–408.
5. Ikeda K, Haughton VM, Ho KC, et al. Correlative MR-anatomic study of the median nerve. *AJR Am J Roentgenol.* 1996;167:1233–1236.
6. Filler AG, Howe FA, Hayes CE, et al. Magnetic resonance neurography. *Lancet.* 1993;341:659–661.
7. Martinoli C, Bianchi S, Derchi LE. Tendon and nerve sonography. *Radiol Clin North Am.* 1999;37:691–711, viii.
8. Silvestri E, Martinoli C, Derchi LE, et al. Echotexture of peripheral nerves: correlation between US and histologic findings and criteria to differentiate tendons. *Radiology.* 1995;197:291–296.
9. Enzinger F, Weiss SW. Benign tumors of peripheral nerves. In: Weiss SW, Goldblum JR, eds. *Soft Tissue Tumors.* 3rd ed. St. Louis: Mosby; 1995:821–888.
10. Das Gupta TK, Brasfield RD. Amputation neuromas in cancer patients. *N Y State J Med.* 1969;69:2129–2132.
11. Donnal JF, Blinder RA, Coblentz CL, et al. MR imaging of stump neuroma. *J Comput Assist Tomogr.* 1990;14:656–657.
12. Fisher GT, Boswick JA Jr. Neuroma formation following digital amputations. *J Trauma.* 1983;23:136–142.
13. Huber G, Lewis D. Amputation neuromas: their development and prevention. *Arch Surg.* 1920;1:85–113.
14. Singson RD, Feldman F, Slipman CW, et al. Postamputation neuromas and other symptomatic stump abnormalities: detection with CT. *Radiology.* 1987;162:743–745.
15. Singson RD, Feldman F, Staron R, et al. MRI of postamputation neuromas. *Skeletal Radiol.* 1990;19:259–262.
16. Spencer PS. The traumatic neuroma and proximal stump. *Bull Hosp Joint Dis.* 1974;35:85–102.
17. Enzinger F, Weiss SW. Malignant tumors of Peripheral Nerves. In: *Soft Tissue Tumors.* 3rd ed. St. Louis: Mosby; 1995:889–928.
18. Lee SH, Jung HG, Park YC, et al. Results of neurilemoma treatment: a review of 78 cases. *Orthopedics.* 2001;24:977–980.
19. Appiah-Anane S. Amputation neuroma: a late complication following sagittal split osteotomy of the mandible. *J Oral Maxillofac Surg.* 1991;49:1218–1220.
20. Detenbeck LC. Infrapatellar traumatic neuroma resulting from dashboard injury. *J Bone Joint Surg Am.* 1972;54:170–172.
21. Feller SR, Evans RD. Proper digital neuroma of the fifth toe. *J Am Podiatr Med Assoc.* 1996;86:187–188.
22. Gregg JM. Studies of traumatic neuralgias in the maxillofacial region: surgical pathology and neural mechanisms. *J Oral Maxillofac Surg.* 1990;48:228–237; discussion 238–239.
23. Peszkowski MJ, Larsson A. Extraosseous and intraosseous oral traumatic neuromas and their association with tooth extraction. *J Oral Maxillofac Surg.* 1990;48:963–967.
24. Rodeo SA, Sobel M, Weiland AJ. Deep peroneal-nerve injury as a result of arthroscopic meniscectomy. A case report and review of the literature. *J Bone Joint Surg Am.* 1993;75:1221–1224.
25. Sist TC Jr, Greene GW. Traumatic neuroma of the oral cavity. Report of thirty-one new cases and review of the literature. *Oral Surg Oral Med Oral Pathol Oral Radiol Endod.* 1981;51:394–402.
26. Kransdorf MJ, Murphey M. Neurogenic tumors. In: *Imaging of Soft Tissue Tumors.* Philadelphia: WB Saunders; 1997:235–273.
27. Attarian DE. Neuromas of the superficial radial nerve. *Mil Med.* 1988;153:393–394.
28. Kneeland JB, Kellman GM, Middleton WD, et al. Diagnosis of diseases of the supraclavicular region by use of MR imaging. *AJR Am J Roentgenol.* 1987;148:1149–1151.
29. Stahl S, Kaufman T, Ben-David B. Neuroma of the superficial branch of the radial nerve after intravenous cannulation. *Anesth Analg.* 1996;83:180–182.
30. Gupta RK, Mehta VS, Banerji AK, et al. MR evaluation of brachial plexus injuries. *Neuroradiology.* 1989;31:377–381.
31. Boutin RD, Pathria MN, Resnick D. Disorders in the stumps of amputee patients: MR imaging. *AJR Am J Roentgenol.* 1998;171:497–501.
32. Beggs I. Pictorial review: imaging of peripheral nerve tumours. *Clin Radiol.* 1997;52:8–17.
33. Bodner G, Huber B, Schwabegger A, et al. Sonographic detection of radial nerve entrapment within a humerus fracture. *J Ultrasound Med.* 1999;18:703–706.
34. Provost N, Bonaldi VM, Sarazin L, et al. Amputation stump neuroma: ultrasound features. *J Clin Ultrasound.* 1997;25:85–89.
35. Peer S, Bodner G, Meirer R, et al. Examination of postoperative peripheral nerve lesions with high-resolution sonography. *AJR Am J Roentgenol.* 2001;177:415–419.
36. Henrot P, Stines J, Walter F, et al. Imaging of the painful lower limb stump. *Radiographics.* 2000;20(special issue):S219–S235.
37. Huang LF, Weissman JL, Fan C. Traumatic neuroma after neck dissection: CT characteristics in four cases. *AJNR Am J Neuroradiol.* 2000;21:1676–1680.
38. Yabuuchi H, Kuroiwa T, Fukuya T, et al. Traumatic neuroma and recurrent lymphadenopathy after neck dissection: comparison of radiologic features. *Radiology.* 2004;233:523–529.
39. Burchiel KJ, Johans TJ, Ochoa J. The surgical treatment of painful traumatic neuromas. *J Neurosurg.* 1993;78:714–719.
40. Tada K, Nakashima H, Yoshida T, et al. A new treatment of painful amputation neuroma: a preliminary report. *J Hand Surg [Br].* 1987;12:273–276.
41. Ernberg LA, Adler RS, Lane J. Ultrasound in the detection and treatment of a painful stump neuroma. *Skeletal Radiol.* 2003;32:306–309.
42. Thomas AJ, Bull MJ, Howard AC, et al. Peri operative ultrasound guided needle localisation of amputation stump neuroma. *Injury.* 1999;30:689–691.
43. Reed RJ, Bliss BO. Morton's neuroma. Regressive and productive intermetatarsal elastofibrosis. *Arch Pathol.* 1973;95:123–129.
44. Morton T. A peculiar and painful affection of the fourth metatarsophalangeal articulation. *Am J Med Sci.* 1876;71:37–45.
45. Alexander IJ, Johnson KA, Parr JW. Morton's neuroma: a review of recent concepts. *Orthopedics.* 1987;10:103–106.
46. Mann RA, Reynolds JC. Interdigital neuroma—a critical clinical analysis. *Foot Ankle.* 1983;3:238–243.
47. Lassmann G. Morton's toe: clinical, light and electron microscopic investigations in 133 cases. *Clin Orthop.* 1979;142:73–84.
48. Mulder JD. The causative mechanism in Morton's metatarsalgia. *J Bone Joint Surg Br.* 1951;33-B:94–95.
49. Torriani M, Kattapuram SV. Technical innovation. Dynamic sonography of the forefoot: The sonographic Mulder sign. *AJR Am J Roentgenol.* 2003;180:1121–1123.
50. Bossley CJ, Cairney PC. The intermetatarsophalangeal bursa—its significance in Morton's metatarsalgia. *J Bone Joint Surg Br.* 1980;62-B:184–187.
51. Zanetti M, Strehle JK, Zollinger H, et al. Morton neuroma and fluid in the intermetatarsal bursae on MR images of 70 asymptomatic volunteers. *Radiology.* 1997;203:516–520.
52. Bencardino J, Rosenberg ZS, Beltran J, et al. Morton's neuroma: is it always symptomatic? *AJR Am J Roentgenol.* 2000;175:649–653.
53. Zanetti M, Strehle JK, Kundert HP, et al. Morton neuroma: effect of MR imaging findings on diagnostic thinking and therapeutic decisions. *Radiology.* 1999;213:583–588.
54. Zanetti M, Ledermann T, Zollinger H, et al. Efficacy of MR imaging in patients suspected of having Morton's neuroma. *AJR Am J Roentgenol.* 1997;168:529–532.

55. Redd RA, Peters VJ, Emery SF, et al. Morton neuroma: sonographic evaluation. *Radiology.* 1989;171:415–417.

56. Kaminsky S, Griffin L, Milsap J, et al. Is ultrasonography a reliable way to confirm the diagnosis of Morton's neuroma? *Orthopedics.* 1997;20:37–39.

57. Turan I, Lindgren U, Sahlstedt T. Computed tomography for diagnosis of Morton's neuroma. *J Foot Surg.* 1991;30:244–245.

58. Mendicino SS, Rockett MS. Morton's neuroma. Update on diagnosis and imaging. *Clin Podiatr Med Surg.* 1997;14:303–311.

59. Resch S, Stenstrom A, Jonsson A, et al. The diagnostic efficacy of magnetic resonance imaging and ultrasonography in Morton's neuroma: a radiological-surgical correlation. *Foot Ankle Int.* 1994;15:88–92.

60. Sartoris DJ, Brozinsky S, Resnick D. Magnetic resonance images. Interdigital or Morton's neuroma. *J Foot Surg.* 1989;28:78–82.

61. Shapiro PP, Shapiro SL. Sonographic evaluation of interdigital neuromas. *Foot Ankle Int.* 1995;16:604–606.

62. Sobiesk GA, Wertheimer SJ, Schulz R, et al. Sonographic evaluation of interdigital neuromas. *J Foot Ankle Surg.* 1997;36:364–366.

63. Oliver TB, Beggs I. Ultrasound in the assessment of metatarsalgia: a surgical and histological correlation. *Clin Radiol.* 1998;53:287–289.

64. Quinn TJ, Jacobson JA, Craig JG, et al. Sonography of Morton's neuromas. *AJR Am J Roentgenol.* 2000;174:1723–1728.

65. Pollak RA, Bellacosa RA, Dornbluth NC, et al. Sonographic analysis of Morton's neuroma. *J Foot Surg.* 1992;31:534–537.

66. Read JW, Noakes JB, Kerr D, et al. Morton's metatarsalgia: sonographic findings and correlated histopathology. *Foot Ankle Int.* 1999;20:153–161.

67. Erickson SJ, Canale PB, Carrera GF, et al. Interdigital (Morton) neuroma: high-resolution MR imaging with a solenoid coil. *Radiology.* 1991;181:833–836.

68. Hoskins CL, Sartoris DJ, Resnick D. Magnetic resonance imaging of foot neuromas. *J Foot Surg.* 1992;31:10–16.

69. Terk MR, Kwong PK, Suthar M, et al. Morton neuroma: evaluation with MR imaging performed with contrast enhancement and fat suppression. *Radiology.* 1993;189:239–241.

70. Williams JW, Meaney J, Whitehouse GH, et al. MRI in the investigation of Morton's neuroma: which sequences? *Clin Radiol.* 1997;52:46–49.

71. Theodoresco B, Lalande G. Magnetic resonance and Morton's neuroma [in French]. *Rev Chir Orthop Reparatrice Appar Mot.* 1991;77:273–275.

72. Unger HR Jr, Mattoso PQ, Drusen MJ, et al. Gadopentetate-enhanced magnetic resonance imaging with fat saturation in the evaluation of Morton's neuroma. *J Foot Surg.* 1992;31:244–246.

73. Weishaupt D, Treiber K, Jacob HA, et al. MR imaging of the forefoot under weight-bearing conditions: position-related changes of the neurovascular bundles and the metatarsal heads in asymptomatic volunteers. *J Magn Reson Imaging.* 2002;16:75–84.

74. Weishaupt D, Treiber K, Kundert HP, et al. Morton neuroma: MR imaging in prone, supine, and upright weight-bearing body positions. *Radiology.* 2003;226:849–856.

75. Beskin J. Primary and salvage procedures for Morton's interdigital neuroma. In: Myerson M, ed. *Current Therapy in Foot and Ankle Surgery.* St. Louis: Mosby-Yearbook; 1994:183–187.

76. Biasca N, Zanetti M, Zollinger H. Outcomes after partial neurectomy of Morton's neuroma related to preoperative case histories, clinical findings, and findings on magnetic resonance imaging scans. *Foot Ankle Int.* 1999;20:568–575.

77. Wu J, Chiu DT. Painful neuromas: a review of treatment modalities. *Ann Plast Surg.* 1999;43:661–667.

78. Ruuskanen MM, Niinimaki T, Jalovaara P. Results of the surgical treatment of Morton's neuralgia in 58 operated intermetatarsal spaces followed over 6 (2–12) years. *Arch Orthop Trauma Surg.* 1994;113:78–80.

79. Weiss S, Goldblum J. Benign tumors of peripheral nerves. In: Weiss SW, Goldblum JR, eds. *Enzinger and Weiss's Soft Tissue Tumors.* 4th ed. St. Louis: Mosby; 2001:1111–1207.

80. Miettinen M. Nerve sheath tumors. In: *Diagnostic Soft Tissue Pathology.* New York: Churchill Livingstone; 2003:343–378.

81. Kransdorf MJ. Benign soft-tissue tumors in a large referral population: distribution of specific diagnoses by age, sex, and location. *AJR Am J Roentgenol.* 1995;164:395–402.

82. Scheithauer BW, Woodruff JM, Erlandson RA. Tumors of peripheral nervous system. In: Rosai J, Sobin LH, eds. *Atlas of Tumor Pathology.* Washington, DC: Armed Forces Institute of Pathology; 1999;1–415.

83. Stout A. The peripheral manifestations of the specific nerve sheath tumor (neurilemmoma). *Am J Cancer.* 1935;24:751–796.

84. Sheikh S, Gomes M, Montgomery E. Multiple plexiform schwannomas in a patient with neurofibromatosis. *J Thorac Cardiovasc Surg.* 1998;115:240–242.

85. Ogose A, Hotta T, Morita T, et al. Multiple schwannomas in the peripheral nerves. *J Bone Joint Surg Br.* 1998;80:657–661.

86. Alberghini M, Zanella L, Bacchini P, et al. Cellular schwannoma: a benign neoplasm sometimes overdiagnosed as sarcoma. *Skeletal Radiol.* 2001;30:350–353.

87. Russell D, Rubinstein L. *Pathology of Tumors of the Nervous System.* Baltimore: William and Wilkins; 1989.

88. Scheithauer B, Woodruff JM, Erlandson RA. *Atlas of Tumor Pathology: Tumors of the Peripheral Nervous System.* Bethesda, MD: Armed Forces Institute of Pathology; 1999.

89. Walker CW, Adams BD, Barnes CL, et al. Case report 667. Fibrolipomatous hamartoma of the median nerve. *Skeletal Radiol.* 1991;20:237–239.

90. Shaw RJ, Paez JG, Curto M, et al. The Nf2 tumor suppressor, Merlin, functions in Rac-dependent signaling. *Dev Cell.* 2001;1:63–72.

91. Ferner RE, O'Doherty MJ. Neurofibroma and schwannoma. *Curr Opin Neurol.* 2002;15:679–684.

92. Kehoe NJ, Reid RP, Semple JC. Solitary benign peripheral-nerve tumours. Review of 32 years' experience. *J Bone Joint Surg Br.* 1995;77:497–500.

93. Donner TR, Voorhies RM, Kline DG. Neural sheath tumors of major nerves. *J Neurosurg.* 1994;81:362–373.

94. von Recklinghausen F. Ueber die multiplen Fibrome der Haut und igre Beziehung zu den multiplen Neuromen. Berlin: August Hirschwald; 1882.

95. Cnossen MH, de Goede-Bolder A, van den Broek KM, et al. A prospective 10 year follow up study of patients with neurofibromatosis type 1. *Arch Dis Child.* 1998;78:408–412.

96. Friedman DP. Segmental neurofibromatosis (NF-5): a rare form of neurofibromatosis. *AJNR Am J Neuroradiol.* 1991;12: 971–972.

97. Evans DG, Huson SM, Donnai D, et al. A genetic study of type 2 neurofibromatosis in the United Kingdom. I. Prevalence, mutation rate, fitness, and confirmation of maternal transmission effect on severity. *J Med Genet.* 1992;29:841–846.

98. Neurofibromatosis. Conference statement. In: National Institutes of Health Consensus Development Conference. *Arch Neurol.* 1988;575–578.

99. Neurofibromatosis 1 (Recklinghausen disease) and neurofibromatosis 2 (bilateral acoustic neurofibromatosis). An update. In: ed. National Institutes of Health Conference. *Ann Intern Med.* 1990;39–52.

100. Feldman F. Tuberous sclerosis, neurofibromatosis, and fibrous dysplasia. In: *Diagnosis of Bone and Joint Disorders.* 3rd ed. Philadelphia: WB Saunders; 1995:4361–4379.

101. Gutmann DH, Aylsworth A, Carey JC, et al. The diagnostic evaluation and multidisciplinary management of neurofibromatosis 1 and neurofibromatosis 2. *JAMA.* 1997;278:51–57.

102. Huson SM, Hughes RAC. Neurofibromatosis 1: a clinical and genetic overview. In: SM H, RAC H, eds. *The Neurofibromatoses: A Pathogenetic and Clinical Overview.* Cambridge: Cambridge University Press; 1994;60–203.

103. Mulvihill JJ, Parry DM, Sherman JL, et al. NIH conference. Neurofibromatosis 1 (Recklinghausen disease) and neurofibromatosis 2 (bilateral acoustic neurofibromatosis). An update. *Ann Intern Med.* 1990;113:39–52.

104. Holt JF. 1977 Edward B. D. Neuhauser lecture: neurofibromatosis in children. *AJR Am J Roentgenol.* 1978;130:615–639.

105. Riccardi VM. Von Recklinghausen neurofibromatosis. *N Engl J Med.* 1981;305:1617–1627.

106. Ruggieri M, Huson SM. The clinical and diagnostic implications of mosaicism in the neurofibromatoses. *Neurology.* 2001;56: 1433–1443.

107. Ingordo V, D'Andria G, Mendicini S, et al. Segmental neurofibromatosis: is it uncommon or underdiagnosed? *Arch Dermatol.* 1995;131:959–960.

108. Ogose A, Hotta T, Imaizumi S, et al. Deep-seated segmental neurofibromatosis without cafe au lait spots. *Skeletal Radiol.* 2000;29:543–547.

109. Sieb JP, Schultheiss R. Segmental neurofibromatosis of the sciatic nerve: case report. *Neurosurgery.* 1992;31:1122–1125; discussion 1125.

110. Harris WC Jr, Alpert WJ, Marcinko DE. Elephantiasis neuromatosa in von Recklinghausen's disease. A review and case report. *J Am Podiatry Assoc.* 1982;72:70–72.

111. Hertzanu Y, Hirsch M, Peiser J, et al. Computed tomography of elephantiasis neuromatosa. *J Comput Assist Tomogr.* 1989;13:156–158.

112. Roy SM, Ghosh AK. Elephantiasis neuromatosa: a clinicopathologic study of four cases. *J Indian Med Assoc.* 1992;90:185–187.

113. Stevens KJ, Ludman CN, Sully L, et al. Magnetic resonance imaging of elephantiasis neuromatosa. *Skeletal Radiol.* 1998;27:696–701.

114. Packer RJ, Gutmann DH, Rubenstein A, et al. Plexiform neurofibromas in NF1: toward biologic-based therapy. *Neurology.* 2002;58:1461–1470.

115. Evans DG, Baser ME, McGaughran J, et al. Malignant peripheral nerve sheath tumours in neurofibromatosis 1. *J Med Genet.* 2002;39:311–314.

116. Sorensen SA, Mulvihill JJ, Nielsen A. Long-term follow-up of von Recklinghausen neurofibromatosis. Survival and malignant neoplasms. *N Engl J Med.* 1986;314:1010–1015.

117. Kleihues P, Cavenee W. World Health Organization Classification of Tumors. In: Fletcher CDM, Unni KK, Mertens F, eds. *Pathology and Genetics Tumors of the Nervous System.* Lyon, France: IARC Press; 2000.

118. Weiss S, Goldblum J. Malignant tumors of the peripheral nerves. In: Weiss SW, Goldblum JR, eds. *Enzinger and Weiss's Soft Tissue Tumors.* 4th ed. St. Louis: Mosby; 2001:1209–1263.

119. Ducatman BS, Scheithauer BW, Piepgras DG, et al. Malignant peripheral nerve sheath tumors. A clinicopathologic study of 120 cases. *Cancer.* 1986;57:2006–2021.

120. Wanebo JE, Malik JM, VandenBerg SR, et al. Malignant peripheral nerve sheath tumors. A clinicopathologic study of 28 cases. *Cancer.* 1993;71:1247–1253.

121. Kourea HP, Cordon-Cardo C, Dudas M, et al. Expression of p27(kip) and other cell cycle regulators in malignant peripheral nerve sheath tumors and neurofibromas: the emerging role of p27(kip) in malignant transformation of neurofibromas. *Am J Pathol.* 1999;155:1885–1891.

122. Nielsen GP, Stemmer-Rachamimov AO, Ino Y, et al. Malignant transformation of neurofibromas in neurofibromatosis 1 is associated with CDKN2A/p16 inactivation. *Am J Pathol.* 1999;155:1879–1884.

123. Hruban RH, Shiu MH, Senie RT, et al. Malignant peripheral nerve sheath tumors of the buttock and lower extremity. A study of 43 cases. *Cancer.* 1990;66:1253–1265.

124. Biondetti PR, Vigo M, Fiore D, et al. CT appearance of generalized von Recklinghausen neurofibromatosis. *J Comput Assist Tomogr.* 1983;7:866–869.

125. Berlin O, Stener B, Lindahl S, et al. Vascularization of peripheral neurilemomas: angiographic, computed tomographic, and histologic studies. *Skeletal Radiol.* 1986;15:275–283.

126. Levine E, Huntrakoon M, Wetzel LH. Malignant nerve-sheath neoplasms in neurofibromatosis: distinction from benign tumors by using imaging techniques. *AJR Am J Roentgenol.* 1987;149:1059–1064.

127. Stener B, Angervall L, Nilsson L, et al. Angiographic and histologic studies of the vascularization of peripheral nerve tumors. *Clin Orthop.* 1969;66:113–124.

128. Littlewood AH, Stilwell JH. The vascular features of plexiform neurofibroma with some observations on the importance of pre-operative angiography and the value of pre-operative intra-arterial embolisation. *Br J Plast Surg.* 1983;36:501–506.

129. Patel YD, Morehouse HT. Neurofibrosarcomas in neurofibromatosis: role of CT scanning and angiography. *Clin Radiol.* 1982;33:555–560.

130. Hammond JA, Driedger AA. Detection of malignant change in neurofibromatosis (von Recklinghausen's disease) by gallium-67 scanning. *Can Med Assoc J.* 1978;119:352–353.

131. Kaplan IL, Swayne LC, Baydin JA. Uptake of Ga-67 citrate in a benign neurofibroma. *Clin Nucl Med.* 1989;14:224.

132. Kobayashi H, Kotoura Y, Sakahara H, et al. Schwannoma of the extremities: comparison of MRI and pentavalent technetium-99m-dimercaptosuccinic acid and gallium-67-citrate scintigraphy. *J Nucl Med.* 1994;35:1174–1178.

133. Eary JF, Conrad EU. Positron emission tomography in grading soft tissue sarcomas. *Semin Musculoskelet Radiol.* 1999;3:135–138.

134. Ahmed AR, Watanabe H, Aoki J, et al. Schwannoma of the extremities: the role of PET in preoperative planning. *Eur J Nucl Med.* 2001;28:1541–1551.

135. Beaulieu S, Rubin B, Djang D, Conrad E, et al. Positron emission tomography of schwannomas: emphasizing its potential in preoperative planning. *AJR Am J Roentgenol.* 2004;182:971–974.

136. Shah N, Sibtain A, Saunders MI, et al. High FDG uptake in a schwannoma: a PET study. *J Comput Assist Tomogr.* 2000;24:55–56.

137. Ferner RE, Lucas JD, O'Doherty MJ, et al. Evaluation of (18)fluorodeoxyglucose positron emission tomography ((18)FDG PET) in the detection of malignant peripheral nerve sheath tumours arising from within plexiform neurofibromas in neurofibromatosis 1. *J Neurol Neurosurg Psychiatry.* 2000;68:353–357.

138. Solomon SB, Semih Dogan A, Nicol TL, et al. Positron emission tomography in the detection and management of sarcomatous transformation in neurofibromatosis. *Clin Nucl Med.* 2001;26:525–528.

139. Hems TE, Burge PD, Wilson DJ. The role of magnetic resonance imaging in the management of peripheral nerve tumours. *J Hand Surg [Br].* 1997;22:57–60.

140. Kransdorf MJ, Jelinek JS, Moser RP Jr, et al. Soft-tissue masses: diagnosis using MR imaging. *AJR Am J Roentgenol.* 1989;153:541–547.

141. Lin J, Martel W. Cross-sectional imaging of peripheral nerve sheath tumors: characteristic signs on CT, MR imaging, and sonography. *AJR Am J Roentgenol.* 2001;176:75–82.

142. Soderlund V, Goranson H, Bauer HC. MR imaging of benign peripheral nerve sheath tumors. *Acta Radiol.* 1994;35:282–286.

143. Kilcoyne RF, Richardson ML, Porter BA, et al. Magnetic resonance imaging of soft tissue masses. *Clin Orthop.* 1988;228:13–19.

144. Sundaram M, McGuire MH, Herbold DR. Magnetic resonance imaging of soft tissue masses: an evaluation of fifty-three histologically proven tumors. *Magn Reson Imaging.* 1988;6:237–248.

145. Murphey MD, Smith WS, Smith SE, et al. From the archives of the AFIP. Imaging of musculoskeletal neurogenic tumors: radiologic-pathologic correlation. *Radiographics.* 1999;19:1253–1280.

146. Beaman FD, Kransdorf MJ, Menke DM. Schwannoma: radiologic-pathologic correlation. *Radiographics.* 2004;24:1477–1481.

147. Hoddick WK, Callen PW, Filly RA, et al. Ultrasound evaluation of benign sciatic nerve sheath tumors. *J Ultrasound Med.* 1984;3:505–507.

148. King AD, Ahuja AT, King W, et al. Sonography of peripheral nerve tumors of the neck. *AJR Am J Roentgenol.* 1997;169:1695–1698.

149. Cerofolini E, Landi A, DeSantis G, et al. MR of benign peripheral nerve sheath tumors. *J Comput Assist Tomogr.* 1991;15:593–597.

150. Li MH, Holtas S. MR imaging of spinal neurofibromatosis. *Acta Radiol.* 1991;32:279–285.

151. Bass JC, Korobkin M, Francis IR, et al. Retroperitoneal plexiform neurofibromas: CT findings. *AJR Am J Roentgenol.* 1994;163:617–620.

152. Burk DL Jr, Brunberg JA, Kanal E, et al. Spinal and paraspinal neurofibromatosis: surface coil MR imaging at 1.5 T1. *Radiology.* 1987;162:797–801.

153. Demachi H, Takashima T, Kadoya M, et al. MR imaging of spinal neurinomas with pathological correlation. *J Comput Assist Tomogr.* 1990;14:250–254.

154. Hu HP, Huang QL. Signal intensity correlation of MRI with pathological findings in spinal neurinomas. *Neuroradiology.* 1992;34:98–102.

155. Lewis TT, Kingsley DP. Magnetic resonance imaging of multiple spinal neurofibromata-neurofibromatosis. *Neuroradiology.* 1987;29:562–564.

156. Suh JS, Abenoza P, Galloway HR, et al. Peripheral (extracranial) nerve tumors: correlation of MR imaging and histologic findings. *Radiology.* 1992;183:341–346.

157. Khong PL, Goh WH, Wong VC, et al. MR imaging of spinal tumors in children with neurofibromatosis 1. *AJR Am J Roentgenol.* 2003;180:413–417.
158. Inaoka T, Takahashi K, Hanaoka H, et al. Paravertebral neurinoma associated with aggressive intravertebral extension. *Skeletal Radiol.* 2001;30:286–289.
159. Jee WH, Oh SN, McCauley T, et al. Extraaxial neurofibromas versus neurilemmomas: discrimination with MRI. *AJR Am J Roentgenol.* 2004;183:629–633.
160. Sullivan TP, Seeger LL, Doberneck SA, et al. Case report 828: plexiform neurofibroma of the tibial nerve invading the medial and lateral gastrocnemius muscles and plantaris muscle. *Skeletal Radiol.* 1994;23:149–152.
161. Gossios KJ, Guy RL. Case report: imaging of widespread plexiform neurofibromatosis. *Clin Radiol.* 1993;47:211–213.
162. Stull MA, Kransdorf MJ, Devaney KO. Langerhans cell histiocytosis of bone. *Radiographics.* 1992;12:801–823.
163. Hallisey MJ, Nelson MC, Muraki A, et al. Case report 547: plexiform neurofibroma involving a dorsal root ganglion. *Skeletal Radiol.* 1989;18:314–317.
164. Poussaint TY, Jaramillo D, Chang Y, et al. Interobserver reproducibility of volumetric MR imaging measurements of plexiform neurofibromas. *AJR Am J Roentgenol.* 2003;180:419–423.
165. Katsumi K, Ogose A, Hotta T, et al. Plexiform schwannoma of the forearm. *Skeletal Radiol.* 2003;32:719–723.
166. Yamamoto T, Maruyama S, Mizuno K. Schwannomatosis of the sciatic nerve. *Skeletal Radiol.* 2001;30:109–113.
167. Peh WC, Shek TW, Yip DK. Magnetic resonance imaging of subcutaneous diffuse neurofibroma. *Br J Radiol.* 1997;70:1180–1183.
168. Fortman BJ, Kuszyk BS, Urban BA, et al. Neurofibromatosis type 1: a diagnostic mimicker at CT. *Radiographics.* 2001;21:601–612.
169. Reinbold WD, Wimmer B, Adler CP, et al. Radiologic findings in peripheral neurilemoma. *Eur J Radiol.* 1987;7:268–273.
170. Cohen LM, Schwartz AM, Rockoff SD. Benign schwannomas: pathologic basis for CT inhomogeneities. *AJR Am J Roentgenol.* 1986;147:141–143.
171. Feyerabend T, Schmitt R, Lanz U, et al. CT morphology of benign median nerve tumors. Report of three cases and a review. *Acta Radiol.* 1990;31:23–25.
172. Kumar AJ, Kuhajda FP, Martinez CR, et al. Computed tomography of extracranial nerve sheath tumors with pathological correlation. *J Comput Assist Tomogr.* 1983;7:857–865.
173. Pierallini A, Bastianello S, Antonini G, et al. CT findings in peripheral mononeuropathies. *Zentralbl Neurochir.* 1993;54:66–71.
174. Thiebot J, Laissy JP, Delangre T, et al. Benign solitary neurinomas of the sciatic popliteal nerves CT study. *Neuroradiology.* 1991;33:186–188.
175. Zingale A, Consoli V, Tigano G, et al. CT morphology of a median nerve neurilemmoma at the arm. Case report and review. *J Neurosurg Sci.* 1993;37:57–59.
176. Beggs I. Sonographic appearances of nerve tumors. *J Clin Ultrasound.* 1999;27:363–368.
177. Reynolds DL Jr, Jacobson JA, Inampudi P, et al. Sonographic characteristics of peripheral nerve sheath tumors. *AJR Am J Roentgenol.* 2004;182:741–744.
178. Mann FA, Murphy WA, Totty WG, et al. Magnetic resonance imaging of peripheral nerve sheath tumors. Assessment by numerical visual fuzzy cluster analysis. *Invest Radiol.* 1990;25:1238–1245.
179. Banks KP. The target sign: extremity. *Radiology.* 2005;234:899–900.
180. Bhargava R, Parham DM, Lasater OE, et al. MR imaging differentiation of benign and malignant peripheral nerve sheath tumors: use of the target sign. *Pediatr Radiol.* 1997;27:124–129.
181. Ogose A, Hotta T, Morita T, et al. Tumors of peripheral nerves: correlation of symptoms, clinical signs, imaging features, and histologic diagnosis. *Skeletal Radiol.* 1999;28:183–188.
182. Stuart RM, Koh ES, Breidahl WH. Sonography of peripheral nerve pathology. *AJR Am J Roentgenol.* 2004;182:123–129.
183. Chui MC, Bird BL, Rogers J. Extracranial and extraspinal nerve sheath tumors: computed tomographic evaluation. *Neuroradiology.* 1988;30:47–53.
184. Damascelli B, Landoni L, Spreafico C. Magnetic resonance imaging of extracranial neurogenic tumors. *J Med Imaging.* 1987;1:27–37.
185. Declercq H, De Man R, Van Herck G, et al. Case report 814: fibrolipoma of the median nerve. *Skeletal Radiol.* 1993;22:610–613.
186. Glasier CM, Williamson MR, Lange TA. MRI of peripheral neurofibromas in children. *Orthopedics.* 1989;12:269–272.
187. Nichols J, Tehranzadeh J. Benign neurilemmoma in the posterior soft tissues of the right thigh. Case report 325. *Skeletal Radiol.* 1985;14:136–140.
188. Petasnick JP, Turner DA, Charters JR, et al. Soft-tissue masses of the locomotor system: comparison of MR imaging with CT. *Radiology.* 1986;160:125–133.
189. Roberts CS, Fetto JF, Fay CM. Neurilemoma in the distal part of the thigh. A case report. *J Bone Joint Surg Am.* 1989;71:1082–1083.
190. Santi MD, Mitsunaga MM, Lockett JL. Total sacrectomy for a giant sacral schwannoma. A case report. *Clin Orthop.* 1993;294:285–289.
191. Stull MA, Moser RP Jr, Kransdorf MJ, et al. Magnetic resonance appearance of peripheral nerve sheath tumors. *Skeletal Radiol.* 1991;20:9–14.
192. Varma DG, Moulopoulos A, Sara AS, et al. MR imaging of extracranial nerve sheath tumors. *J Comput Assist Tomogr.* 1992;16:448–453.
193. Moon WK, Im JG, Han MC. Malignant schwannomas of the thorax: CT findings. *J Comput Assist Tomogr.* 1993;17:274–276.
194. Friedman DP, Tartaglino LM, Flanders AE. Intradural schwannomas of the spine: MR findings with emphasis on contrast-enhancement characteristics. *AJR Am J Roentgenol.* 1992;158:1347–1350.
195. Gouliamos AD, Kontogiannis DS, Androulidakis J, et al. Spinal neurilemmomas and neurofibromas: central dot sign in postgadolinium MRI. *J Comput Assist Tomogr.* 1993;17:446–448.
196. Lee JA, Boles CA. Peripheral schwannoma lacking enhancement on MRI. *AJR Am J Roentgenol.* 2004;182:534–535.
197. Nemeth A, Patel S. Peripheral schwannoma lacking enhancement on MRI [Letter to Editor]. *AJR Am J Roentgenol.* 2004;182:534–535.
198. Graviet S, Sinclair G, Kajani N. Ancient schwannoma of the foot. *J Foot Ankle Surg.* 1995;34:46–50.
199. Hide IG, Baudouin CJ, Murray SA, et al. Giant ancient schwannoma of the pelvis. *Skeletal Radiol.* 2000;29:538–542.
200. Loke TK, Yuen NW, Lo KK, et al. Retroperitoneal ancient schwannoma: review of clinico-radiological features. *Australas Radiol.* 1998;42:136–138.
201. Isobe K, Shimizu T, Akahane T, et al. Imaging of ancient schwannoma. *AJR Am J Roentgenol.* 2004;183:331–336.
202. Schultz E, Sapan MR, McHeffey-Atkinson B, et al. Case report 872. "Ancient" schwannoma (degenerated neurilemoma). *Skeletal Radiol.* 1994;23:593–595.
203. Lazarus SS, Trombetta LD. Ultrastructural identification of a benign perineurial cell tumor. *Cancer.* 1978;41:1823–1829.
204. Heilbrun ME, Tsuruda JS, Townsend JJ, et al. Intraneural perineurioma of the common peroneal nerve. Case report and review of the literature. *J Neurosurg.* 2001;94:811–815.
205. Aaron AD, Nelson MC, Azumi N, et al. Case report 820: Granular cell tumor of striated muscle. *Skeletal Radiol.* 1994;23:63–66.
206. Hurrell MA, McLean C, Desmond P, et al. Malignant granular cell tumour of the sciatic nerve. *Australas Radiol.* 1995;39:86–89.
207. Mukherji SK, Castillo M, Rao V, et al. Granular cell tumors of the subglottic region of the larynx: CT and MR findings. *AJR Am J Roentgenol.* 1995;164:1492–1494.
208. Reuter KL, Raptopoulos V, DeGirolami U, et al. Ultrasonography of a plexiform neurofibroma of the popliteal fossa. *J Ultrasound Med.* 1982;1:209–211.
209. Shimamura K, Osamura RY, Ueyama Y, et al. Malignant granular cell tumor of the right sciatic nerve. Report of an autopsy case with electron microscopic, immunohistochemical, and enzyme histochemical studies. *Cancer.* 1984;53:524–529.
210. Fanburg-Smith JC, Meis-Kindblom JM, Fante R, et al. Malignant granular cell tumor of soft tissue: diagnostic criteria and clinicopathologic correlation. *Am J Surg Pathol.* 1998;22:779–794.

211. Chinn DH, Filly RA, Callen PW. Unusual ultrasonographic appearance of a solid schwannoma. *J Clin Ultrasound.* 1982;10:243–245.

212. Hughes DG, Wilson DJ. Ultrasound appearances of peripheral nerve tumours. *Br J Radiol.* 1986;59:1041–1043.

213. Kudawara I, Ueda T, Yoshikawa H. Granular cell tumor of the subcutis: CT and MRI findings. A report of three cases. *Skeletal Radiol.* 1999;28:96–99.

214. Blacksin MF, White LM, Hameed M, et al. Granular cell tumor of the extremity: magnetic resonance imaging characteristics with pathologic correlation. *Skeletal Radiol.* 2005;34:625–631.

215. Elkousy H, Harrelson J, Dodd L, et al. Granular cell tumors of the extremities. *Clin Orthop.* 2000;380:191–198.

216. Tsuchida T, Okada K, Itoi E, et al. Intramuscular malignant granular cell tumor. *Skeletal Radiol.* 1997;26:116–121.

217. Krompecher E. Zur histogenese und morphologie der adamantinome und sonstiger kiefergeschwulste. *Pathol Res Pract.* 1918;64:169–197.

218. Atkinson GO Jr, Davis PC, Patrick LE, et al. Melanotic neuroectodermal tumor of infancy. MR findings and a review of the literature. *Pediatr Radiol.* 1989;20:20–22.

219. Cutler LS, Chaudhry AP, Topazian R. Melanotic neuroectodermal tumor of infancy: an ultrastructural study, literature review, and reevaluation. *Cancer.* 1981;48:257–270.

220. Kozlowski K, Masel J, Sprague P, et al. Mandibular and paramandibular tumors in children. Report of 16 cases. *Pediatr Radiol.* 1981;11:183–192.

221. Mirich DR, Blaser SI, Harwood-Nash DC, et al. Melanotic neuroectodermal tumor of infancy: clinical, radiologic, and pathologic findings in five cases. *AJNR Am J Neuroradiol.* 1991;12:689–697.

222. Enzinger FM. Clear-cell sarcoma of tendons and aponeuroses. An analysis of 21 cases. *Cancer.* 1965;18:1163–1174.

223. Chung EB, Enzinger FM. Malignant melanoma of soft parts. A reassessment of clear cell sarcoma. *Am J Surg Pathol.* 1983;7:405–413.

224. Eckardt JJ, Pritchard DJ, Soule EH. Clear cell sarcoma. A clinicopathologic study of 27 cases. *Cancer.* 1983;52:1482–1488.

225. Lucas DR, Nascimento AG, Sim FH. Clear cell sarcoma of soft tissues. Mayo Clinic experience with 35 cases. *Am J Surg Pathol.* 1992;16:1197–1204.

226. Andrew TA. Clear cell sarcoma of the hand. *Hand.* 1982;14:200–203.

227. Limon J, Debiec-Rychter M, Nedoszytko B, et al. Aberrations of chromosome 22 and polysomy of chromosome 8 as non-random changes in clear cell sarcoma. *Cancer Genet Cytogenet.* 1994;72:141–145.

228. Morishita S, Onomura T, Yamamoto S, et al. Clear cell sarcoma of tendons and aponeuroses (malignant melanoma of soft parts) with unusual roentgenologic findings. Case report. *Clin Orthop.* 1987;216:276–279.

229. Raynor AC, Vargas-Cortes F, Alexander RW, et al. Clear-cell sarcoma with melanin pigment: a possible soft-tissue variant of malignant melanoma. Case report. *J Bone Joint Surg Am.* 1979;61:276–280.

230. Sartoris DJ, Haghighi P, Resnick D. Case report 423: clear-cell sarcoma plantar aspect of right foot. *Skeletal Radiol.* 1987;16:325–332.

231. Wetzel LH, Levine E. Soft-tissue tumors of the foot: value of MR imaging for specific diagnosis. *AJR Am J Roentgenol.* 1990;155:1025–1030.

232. Deenik W, Mooi WJ, Rutgers EJ, et al. Clear cell sarcoma (malignant melanoma) of soft parts: a clinicopathologic study of 30 cases. *Cancer.* 1999;86:969–975.

233. Graadt van Roggen JF, Mooi WJ, Hogendoorn PC. Clear cell sarcoma of tendons and aponeuroses (malignant melanoma of soft parts) and cutaneous melanoma: exploring the histogenetic relationship between these two clinicopathological entities. *J Pathol.* 1998;186:3–7.

234. Speleman F, Delattre O, Peter M, et al. Malignant melanoma of the soft parts (clear-cell sarcoma): confirmation of EWS and ATF-1 gene fusion caused by a t(12;22) translocation. *Mod Pathol.* 1997;10:496–499.

235. De Beuckeleer LH, De Schepper AM, Vandevenne JE, et al. MR imaging of clear cell sarcoma (malignant melanoma of the soft parts): a multicenter correlative MRI-pathology study of 21 cases and literature review. *Skeletal Radiol.* 2000;29:187–195.

236. Gomori JM, Grossman RI, Shields JA, et al. Choroidal melanomas: correlation of NMR spectroscopy and MR imaging. *Radiology.* 1986;158:443–445.

237. Schnarkowski P, Peterfy CG, Johnston JO, et al. Clear cell sarcoma mimicking peripheral nerve sheath tumor. *Skeletal Radiol.* 1996;25:197–200.

238. Bishop GB Jr, Urist MM, el Gammal T, et al. Paragangliomas of the neck. *Arch Surg.* 1992;127:1441–1445.

239. Rao AB, Koeller KK, Adair CF. From the archives of the AFIP. Paragangliomas of the head and neck: radiologic-pathologic correlation. Armed Forces Institute of Pathology. *Radiographics.* 1999;19:1605–1632.

240. Weiss S, Goldblum J. Paraganglioma. In: Weiss SW, Goldblum JR, eds. *Enzinger and Weiss's Soft Tissue Tumors.* 4th ed. St. Louis: Mosby; 2001:1323–1360.

241. Enzinger F, Weiss SW. Paraganglioma. In: Weiss SW, Goldblum JR, eds. *Soft Tissue Tumors.* 3rd ed. St. Louis: Mosby; 1995:965–990.

242. van Gils AP, Falke TH, van Erkel AR, et al. MR imaging and MIBG scintigraphy of pheochromocytomas and extraadrenal functioning paragangliomas. *Radiographics.* 1991;11:37–57.

243. Williams E, Siebenmann R, Sobin L. Histological typing of endocrine tumors. In: Fletcher CDM, Unni KK, Mertens F, eds. *WHO International Histological Classification of Tumors.* Geneva: World Health Organization; 1980:33–39.

244. Leonetti JP, Donzelli JJ, Littooy FN, et al. Perioperative strategies in the management of carotid body tumors. *Otolaryngol Head Neck Surg.* 1997;117:111–115.

245. Duncan AW, Lack EE, Deck MF. Radiological evaluation of paragangliomas of the head and neck. *Radiology.* 1979;132: 99–105.

246. Olsen WL, Dillon WP, Kelly WM, et al. MR imaging of paragangliomas. *AJR Am J Roentgenol.* 1987;148:201–204.

247. Kawai A, Healey JH, Wilson SC, et al. Carotid body paraganglioma metastatic to bone: report of two cases. *Skeletal Radiol.* 1998;27:103–107.

248. Grimley P. Multicentric paragangliomas and associated neuroendocrine tumors. In: Brunson K, ed. *Local Invasion and Spread of Cancer.* Dordrecht, The Netherlands: Kluwer Academic; 1989:49–61.

249. Zaslav AL, Myssiorek D, Mucia C, et al. Cytogenetic analysis of tissues from patients with familial paragangliomas of the head and neck. *Head Neck.* 1995;17:102–107.

250. Bosniak MA, Seidenberg B, Rubin IC, et al. Angiographic demonstration of bilateral carotid body tumors. *Am J Roentgenol Radium Ther Nucl Med.* 1964;92:850–854.

251. Farr HW. Carotid body tumors. A thirty year experience at Memorial Hospital. *Am J Surg.* 1967;114:614–619.

252. Jacobs JB, Chretien PB, Sugarbaker E, et al. Arteriographic discovery of a small contralateral carotid body tumor. *Radiology.* 1969;93:837–838.

253. Lack EE, Cubilla AL, Woodruff JM, et al. Paragangliomas of the head and neck region: a clinical study of 69 patients. *Cancer.* 1977;39:397–409.

254. Oberman HA, Holtz F, Sheffer LA, et al. Chemodectomas (nonchromaffin paragangliomas) of the head and neck. A clinicopathologic study. *Cancer.* 1968;21:838–851.

255. Rice RP, Holman CB. Roentgenographic manifestations of tumors of the glomus jugulare (chemodectoma). *Am J Roentgenol Radium Ther Nucl Med.* 1963;89:1201–1208.

256. Shugar MA, Mafee MF. Diagnosis of carotid body tumors by dynamic computerized tomography. *Head Neck Surg.* 1982;4:518–521.

257. Weissman JL. Case 21: glomus vagale tumor. *Radiology.* 2000;215:237–242.

258. Falke TH, van Gils AP, van Seters AP, et al. Magnetic resonance imaging of functioning paragangliomas. *Magn Reson Q.* 1990;6:35–64.

259. Schmedtje JF Jr, Sax S, Pool JL, et al. Localization of ectopic pheochromocytomas by magnetic resonance imaging. *Am J Med.* 1987;83:770–772.

260. Velchik MG, Alavi A, Kressel HY, et al. Localization of pheochromocytoma: MIBG [correction of MIGB], CT, and MRI correlation. *J Nucl Med.* 1989;30:328–336.

261. Derchi LE, Serafini G, Rabbia C, et al. Carotid body tumors: US evaluation. *Radiology.* 1992;182:457–459.

262. Jansen JC, Baatenburg de Jong RJ, Schipper J, et al. Color Doppler imaging of paragangliomas in the neck. *J Clin Ultrasound.* 1997;25:481–485.

263. Makarainen H, Paivansalo M, Hyrynkangas K, et al. Sonographic patterns of carotid body tumors. *J Clin Ultrasound.* 1986;14:373–375.

264. Mukherji SK, Kasper ME, Tart RP, et al. Irradiated paragangliomas of the head and neck: CT and MR appearance. *AJNR Am J Neuroradiol.* 1994;15:357–363.

265. Som PM, Braun IF, Shapiro MD, et al. Tumors of the parapharyngeal space and upper neck: MR imaging characteristics. *Radiology.* 1987;164:823–829.

266. van den Berg R, van Gils AP, Wasser MN. Imaging of head and neck paragangliomas with three-dimensional time-of-flight MR angiography. *AJR Am J Roentgenol.* 1999;172:1667–1673.

267. Vogl T, Bruning R, Schedel H, et al. Paragangliomas of the jugular bulb and carotid body: MR imaging with short sequences and Gd-DTPA enhancement. *AJR Am J Roentgenol.* 1989;153:583–587.

268. Vogl TJ, Juergens M, Balzer JO, et al. Glomus tumors of the skull base: combined use of MR angiography and spin-echo imaging. *Radiology.* 1994;192:103–110.

269. Idbohrn H. Angiographical diagnosis of carotid body tumours. *Acta Radiol.* 1951;35:115–123.

270. Chatal JF, Charbonnel B. Comparison of iodobenzylguanidine imaging with computed tomography in locating pheochromocytoma. *J Clin Endocrinol Metab.* 1985;61:769–772.

271. Quint LE, Glazer GM, Francis IR, et al. Pheochromocytoma and paraganglioma: comparison of MR imaging with CT and I-131 MIBG scintigraphy. *Radiology.* 1987;165:89–93.

272. van Gils AP, van der Mey AG, Hoogma RP, et al. Iodine-123-metaiodobenzylguanidine scintigraphy in patients with chemodectomas of the head and neck region. *J Nucl Med.* 1990;31:1147–1155.

273. Welch TJ, Sheedy PF II, van Heerden JA, et al. Pheochromocytoma: value of computed tomography. *Radiology.* 1983;148:501–503.

274. Krenning EP, Kwekkeboom DJ, Bakker WH, et al. Somatostatin receptor scintigraphy with [111In-DTPA-D-Phe1]- and [123I-Tyr3]-octreotide: the Rotterdam experience with more than 1000 patients. *Eur J Nucl Med.* 1993;20:716–731.

275. Kwekkeboom DJ, van Urk H, Pauw BK, et al. Octreotide scintigraphy for the detection of paragangliomas. *J Nucl Med.* 1993;34:873–878.

276. Myssiorek D, Palestro CJ. 111 Indium pentetreotide scan detection of familial paragangliomas. *Laryngoscope.* 1998;108:228–231.

277. Enzinger F, Weiss SW. Primitive neuroectodermal tumors and related lesions. In: Weiss SW, Goldblum JR, eds. *Soft Tissue Tumors.* 3rd ed. St. Louis: Mosby; 1995:929–964.

278. Stout A. Ganglioneuroma of the sympathetic nervous system. *Surg Gynecol Obstet.* 1947;84:101–110.

279. Miettinen M. Neuroectodermal and neural tumors. In: *Diagnostic Soft Tissue Pathology.* New York: Churchill Livingstone; 2003:379–401.

280. Amundson GM, Trevenen CL, Mueller DL, et al. Neuroblastoma: a specific sonographic tissue pattern. *AJR Am J Roentgenol.* 1987;148:943–945.

281. David R, Lamki N, Fan S, et al. The many faces of neuroblastoma. *Radiographics.* 1989;9:859–882.

282. Dietrich RB, Kangarloo H, Lenarsky C, et al. Neuroblastoma: the role of MR imaging. *AJR Am J Roentgenol.* 1987;148:937–942.

283. Evans AE. Staging and treatment of neuroblastoma. *Cancer.* 1980;45:1799–1802.

284. Stark DD, Moss AA, Brasch RC, et al. Neuroblastoma: diagnostic imaging and staging. *Radiology.* 1983;148:101–105.

285. Armstrong EA, Harwood-Nash DC, Ritz CR, et al. CT of neuroblastomas and ganglioneuromas in children. *AJR Am J Roentgenol.* 1982;139:571–576.

286. Page D, DeLellis R, Hough A. Tumors of the adrenal. In: *Atlas of Tumor Pathology,* 2nd Series, Fascicle 23. Washington, DC: Armed Forces Institute of Pathology; 1985.

287. Rha SE, Byun JY, Jung SE, et al. Neurogenic tumors in the abdomen: tumor types and imaging characteristics. *Radiographics.* 2003;23:29–43.

288. Ichikawa T, Koyama A, Fujimoto H, et al. Retroperitoneal ganglioneuroma extending across the midline: MR features. *Clin Imaging.* 1993;17:19–21.

289. Ichikawa T, Ohtomo K, Araki T, et al. Ganglioneuroma: computed tomography and magnetic resonance features. *Br J Radiol.* 1996;69:114–121.

290. Zhang Y, Nishimura H, Kato S, et al. MRI of ganglioneuroma: histologic correlation study. *J Comput Assist Tomogr.* 2001;25:617–623.

291. Jasinski RW, Samuels BI, Silver TM. Sonographic features of retroperitoneal ganglioneuroma. *J Ultrasound Med.* 1984;3:413–415.

292. White SJ, Stuck KJ, Blane CE, et al. Sonography of neuroblastoma. *AJR Am J Roentgenol.* 1983;141:465–468.

293. Otal P, Mezghani S, Hassissene S, et al. Imaging of retroperitoneal ganglioneuroma. *Eur Radiol.* 2001;11:940–945.

294. Radin R, David CL, Goldfarb H, et al. Adrenal and extra-adrenal retroperitoneal ganglioneuroma: imaging findings in 13 adults. *Radiology.* 1997;202:703–707.

295. Harbert JC, Robertson JS, Held KD. Meta (131) iodobenzylguanidine therapy of malignant pheochromocytomas and other neuroendocrine lesions. In: *Nuclear Medicine Therapy.* New York: Thieme; 1987:99–108.

296. Munkner T. 131I-meta-iodobenzylguanidine scintigraphy of neuroblastomas. *Semin Nucl Med.* 1985;15:154–160.

297. Weiss S, Goldblum J. Primitive neuroectodermal tumors and related lesions. In: Weiss SW, Goldblum JR, eds. *Enzinger and Weiss's Soft Tissue Tumors.* 4th ed. St. Louis: Mosby; 2001:1265–1321.

298. Ewing J. Diffuse endothelioma of bone. *Proc NY Soc Pathol.* 1921;21:17–24.

299. Stout A. A tumor of the ulnar nerve. *Proc NY Soc Pathol.* 1918;12:2–12.

300. Parham DM, Hijazi Y, Steinberg SM, et al. Neuroectodermal differentiation in Ewing's sarcoma family of tumors does not predict tumor behavior. *Hum Pathol.* 1999;30:911–918.

301. Dehner LP. Primitive neuroectodermal tumor and Ewing's sarcoma. *Am J Surg Pathol.* 1993;17:1–13.

302. Cavazzana AO, Ninfo V, Roberts J, et al. Peripheral neuroepithelioma: a light microscopic, immunocytochemical, and ultrastructural study. *Mod Pathol.* 1992;5:71–78.

303. Gillespie JJ, Roth LM, Wills ER, et al. Extraskeletal Ewing's sarcoma. Histologic and ultrastructural observations in three cases. *Am J Surg Pathol.* 1979;3:99–108.

304. Hashimoto H, Enjoji M, Nakajima T, et al. Malignant neuroepithelioma (peripheral neuroblastoma). A clinicopathologic study of 15 cases. *Am J Surg Pathol.* 1983;7:309–318.

305. Kushner BH, Hajdu SI, Gulati SC, et al. Extracranial primitive neuroectodermal tumors. The Memorial Sloan-Kettering Cancer Center experience. *Cancer.* 1991;67:1825–1829.

306. Shimada H, Newton WA Jr, Soule EH, et al. Pathologic features of extraosseous Ewing's sarcoma: a report from the Intergroup Rhabdomyosarcoma Study. *Hum Pathol.* 1988;19:442–453.

307. Turc-Carel C, Aurias A, Mugneret F, et al. Chromosomes in Ewing's sarcoma. I. An evaluation of 85 cases of remarkable consistency of t(11;22)(q24;q12). *Cancer Genet Cytogenet.* 1988;32:229–238.

308. Meister P, Gokel JM. Extraskeletal Ewing's sarcoma. *Virchows Arch.* 1978;378:173–179.

309. Hoffer FA, Gianturco LE, Fletcher JA, et al. Percutaneous biopsy of peripheral primitive neuroectodermal tumors and Ewing's sarcomas for cytogenetic analysis. *AJR Am J Roentgenol.* 1994;162:1141–1142.

310. Marina NM, Etcubanas E, Parham DM, et al. Peripheral primitive neuroectodermal tumor (peripheral neuroepithelioma) in children. A review of the St. Jude experience and controversies in diagnosis and management. *Cancer.* 1989;64:1952–1960.

311. Schmidt D, Herrmann C, Jurgens H, Harms D. Malignant peripheral neuroectodermal tumor and its necessary distinction from Ewing's sarcoma. A report from the Kiel Pediatric Tumor Registry. *Cancer.* 1991;68:2251–2259.

312. Jurgens H, Exner U, Gadner H, et al. Multidisciplinary treatment of primary Ewing's sarcoma of bone. A 6-year experience of a European Cooperative Trial. *Cancer.* 1988;61:23–32.

313. Allam K, Sze G. MR of primary extraosseous Ewing sarcoma. *AJNR Am J Neuroradiol.* 1994;15:305–307.

314. O'Keeffe F, Lorigan JG, Wallace S. Radiological features of extraskeletal Ewing sarcoma. *Br J Radiol.* 1990;63:456–460.

315. Rose JS, Hermann G, Mendelson DS, et al. Extraskeletal Ewing sarcoma with computed tomography correlation. *Skeletal Radiol.* 1983;9:234–237.

316. Askin FB, Rosai J, Sibley RK, et al. Malignant small cell tumor of the thoracopulmonary region in childhood: a distinctive clinicopathologic entity of uncertain histogenesis. *Cancer.* 1979;43: 2438–2451.

317. Faubert C, Inniger R. MRI and pathological findings in two cases of Askin tumors. *Neuroradiology.* 1991;33:277–281.

318. Fink IJ, Kurtz DW, Cazenave L, et al. Malignant thoracopulmonary small-cell ("Askin") tumor. *AJR Am J Roentgenol.* 1985; 145:517–520.

319. Saifuddin A, Robertson RJ, Smith SE. The radiology of Askin tumours. *Clin Radiol.* 1991;43:19–23.

320. Winer-Muram HT, Kauffman WM, Gronemeyer SA, et al. Primitive neuroectodermal tumors of the chest wall (Askin tumors): CT and MR findings. *AJR Am J Roentgenol.* 1993;161: 265–268.

321. Burge HJ, Novotny DB, Schiebler ML, et al. MRI of Askin's tumor. Case report at 1.5 T. *Chest.* 1990;97:1252–1254.

Synovial Tumors

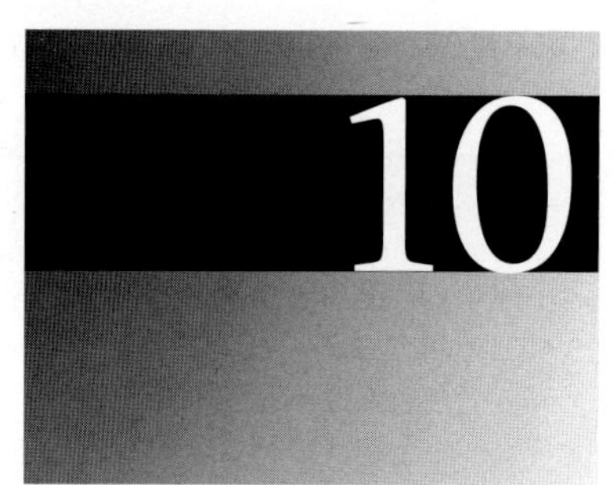

In this chapter we review those lesions that are usually found in and around joints. These lesions are commonly encountered in clinical practice, and although it is useful to consider these as a group for purposes of diagnosis and differential, it is important to remember that they have a diverse origin. The World Health Organization (WHO) does not include a classification category for synovial lesions; however, synovial lesions that are categorized by the WHO are included as *tumors of uncertain differentiation* and *so-called fibrohistiocytic tumors* (1). The former group includes synovial sarcoma; the latter includes the spectrum of benign proliferative disorders of the synovium (giant cell tumor of tendon sheath and pigmented villonodular synovitis). Synovial cyst and ganglion are also included in this chapter, as is synovial chondromatosis. Synovial hemangioma and synovial lipoma are discussed in the chapters on vascular and fatty tumors, respectively.

BENIGN LESIONS

Benign synovial lesions frequently present as juxta-articular masses, and in clinical practice these lesions are especially prevalent. This section discusses the spectrum of benign synovial lesions, beginning with proliferative disorders of the synovium. We have included many tumorlike lesions such as *ganglion*, which is a myxoid lesion and is best considered a pseudotumor, and *synovial chondromatosis*, which evidence now suggests is a benign neoplasm.

Benign Synovial Proliferative Lesions

Benign proliferative lesions of the synovium of the joint, bursa and tendon sheath represent a family of abnormalities (1,2). The most common of these is the localized *giant cell tumor of tendon sheath*, which represents the localized form of this spectrum of synovial proliferations, which, when diffuse and intra-articular, is termed *pigmented villonodular synovitis* (PVNS) (2,3). In general, lesion extent and growth is influenced by anatomic location (2). The true nature of these lesions has long been debated; however, newer

evidence suggests they are neoplastic rather than reactive (2,4). Synonyms for giant cell tumor of tendon sheath include *tenosynovial giant cell tumor* and *nodular tenosynovitis*.

Classification

> **KEY CONCEPTS**
> - The two main forms of benign synovial proliferative lesions are the localized form (giant cell tumor of tendon sheath) and the diffuse intra-articular form (PVNS).
> - Giant cell tumor of tendon sheath is further subdivided into localized type (also known as *nodular tenosynovitis*) and diffuse type (considered to be *extra-articular* PVNS).
> - *Nodular synovitis* is the term applied to focal intra-articular lesions.

Although the nomenclature describing benign synovial proliferative lesions is often confusing, it is useful to remember that it describes multiple manifestations of a single disease state arising from the synovium of the joint, bursae, and tendon sheath (5). Currently, these lesions are usually divided according to their site (intra- or extra-articular) and pattern of growth (localized or diffuse) (6).

The localized form of giant cell tumor of tendon sheath or nodular tenosynovitis usually presents as a nodular or polypoid mass, most commonly in the hand and wrist. In its diffuse form, giant cell tumor of tendon sheath is less well-defined and typically occurs adjacent to the large is often joints. Diffuse giant cell tumor of tendon sheath is often considered to be the soft tissue or extra-articular counterpart of PVNS. As PVNS can occasionally occur outside the joint, localized giant cell tumor of tendon sheath can occasionally occur within a joint. Such intra-articular cases of giant cell tumors of tendon sheath are termed *nodular synovitis* in order to distinguish them from those arising from the tendon sheath. Finally, current usage applies the term PVNS to cases in which there is diffuse involvement of a joint.

Giant Cell Tumor of Tendon Sheath

> ### KEY CONCEPTS
> - Localized giant cell tumor of tendon sheath is approximately seven times more common than PVNS.
> - Typically seen in adults, the peak incidence occurs in the third to fifth decade.
> - This mass is one of the most common soft tissue masses of the hand, second only to ganglion.
> - Patients present with a slowly growing mass; recurrence following surgery is not uncommon.
> - The diffuse type of giant cell tumor of tendon sheath shows a skeletal distribution similar to that of PVNS, but has a more aggressive behavior and higher rate of recurrence than the localized form.
> - Intra-articular giant cell tumor of tendon sheath is termed *nodular synovitis.*

As noted, the giant cell tumor of tendon sheath occurs in either a localized or diffuse form (2). The localized form usually presents as an encapsulated, well-defined nodular or polypoid mass, most commonly in the hand or wrist (Fig. 10.1). In its diffuse form, the lesion is less well-defined and grossly characterized by shaggy, beardlike projections (representing hypertrophic synovial villi) (4). Clearly, the distinction between the localized and diffuse form is on occasion blurred and a function of its gross, as well as its microscopic, appearance. The diffuse form of giant cell tumor of tendon sheath is rare and usually occurs adjacent to large weight-bearing joints and in most, although not all, cases represents extra-articular extension of PVNS (2). Ushijima et al., in reporting a 20-year experience with 208 cases, found tenosynovial giant cell tumor (localized form) to be more than seven times more common than PVNS (diffuse intra-articular form).

Localized Giant Cell Tumor of Tendon Sheath

Localized giant cell tumor of tendon sheath, also termed *nodular tenosynovitis* or *tenosynovial giant cell tumor*, is one of the most common soft tissue masses of the hand (8,9), second in frequency only to ganglion. Patients are typically adults, with a peak incidence in the third to fifth decades (7,8,10), with a slight female predominance (1.5–2.1:1) (7,8,10,11). The overwhelming majority of lesions arise in the hand and wrist, with this location accounting for 65% to 89% of lesions (6,7,11,12). In the hand, the lesion more commonly affects the volar aspect of the digits than the dorsal surface, although lesions may be lateral or circumferential (7,8,11). Involvement is most commonly seen in the first three fingers (7,8,11). The foot and ankle account for approximately 5% to 15% of lesions, with these most often in the first two toes (7,8,11,12).

Most patients present with soft tissue swelling or a slowly enlarging, painless, soft tissue mass, which is freely mobile under the skin but attached to deeper structures (7,8,11,12). Pain is not uncommon and may be aggravated by activity (10). Lesions may progress slowly or remain stable for many years. Multiple lesions are quite unusual but are reported (7), and in our experience they are usually seen with recurrent tumors. Local recurrence is not uncommon and may be seen in approximately 7% to 44% of cases (7,8,13,14), although it is much less frequent than in the diffuse form of the disease.

The lesion is typically a small, rubbery, well-encapsulated, multinodular mass, tan to brown to yellow in color (7,8). The gross color of the lesion varies with the amount of foam cells and hemosiderin deposition within the tumor (7). Lesions are usually smaller than 2 to 4 cm (7,8,13). On microscopic evaluation there is synovial proliferation with scattered multinucleated giant cells, macrophages, fibroblasts, and xanthoma cells. Varying amounts of hemosiderin may be seen (7,8). In general, the diffuse form is larger than the localized form (13).

Nodular Synovitis

Uncommonly, a giant cell tumor of tendon sheath can occur within a joint. Such lesions may be termed *nodular synovitis*. An intra-articular lesion is considered to be nodular synovitis (as opposed to PVNS) only when it is a well-defined, solitary nodule, with no associated hemorrhagic or xanthochromic effusion (13). Although unusual, nodular synovitis is typically within the knee, with two-thirds of cases occurring within the infrapatellar fat pad (15). Other less common locations include the suprapatellar pouch, intercondylar notch, and posterior cruciate ligament (15). It is difficult to estimate the prevalence of nodular synovitis, but in series evaluating knee lesions, PVNS is approximately four times more common than nodular synovitis (16).

Clinical symptoms are nonspecific but are similar to those of mechanical derangement and include pain, swelling, fullness, joint line tenderness, palpable mass, and locking (15,17,18). Nodular synovitis is histologically similar to PVNS, but it has a different natural history with a relatively limited risk of local recurrence, in stark contrast to that of PVNS (16).

Diffuse Giant Cell Tumor of Tendon Sheath

The diffuse form of giant cell tumor of tendon sheath, also termed *florid synovitis*, *proliferative synovitis*, or *extra-articular PVNS*, is much less common and is considered the soft tissue counterpart of diffuse PVNS of the joint (2,4). It shows a skeletal distribution similar to that of PVNS and generally develops completely or predominantly outside a large joint. In most, although not all, cases it is thought to represent extra-articular extension of PVNS (2). The diffuse form of giant cell tumor of tendon sheath is more aggressive than the

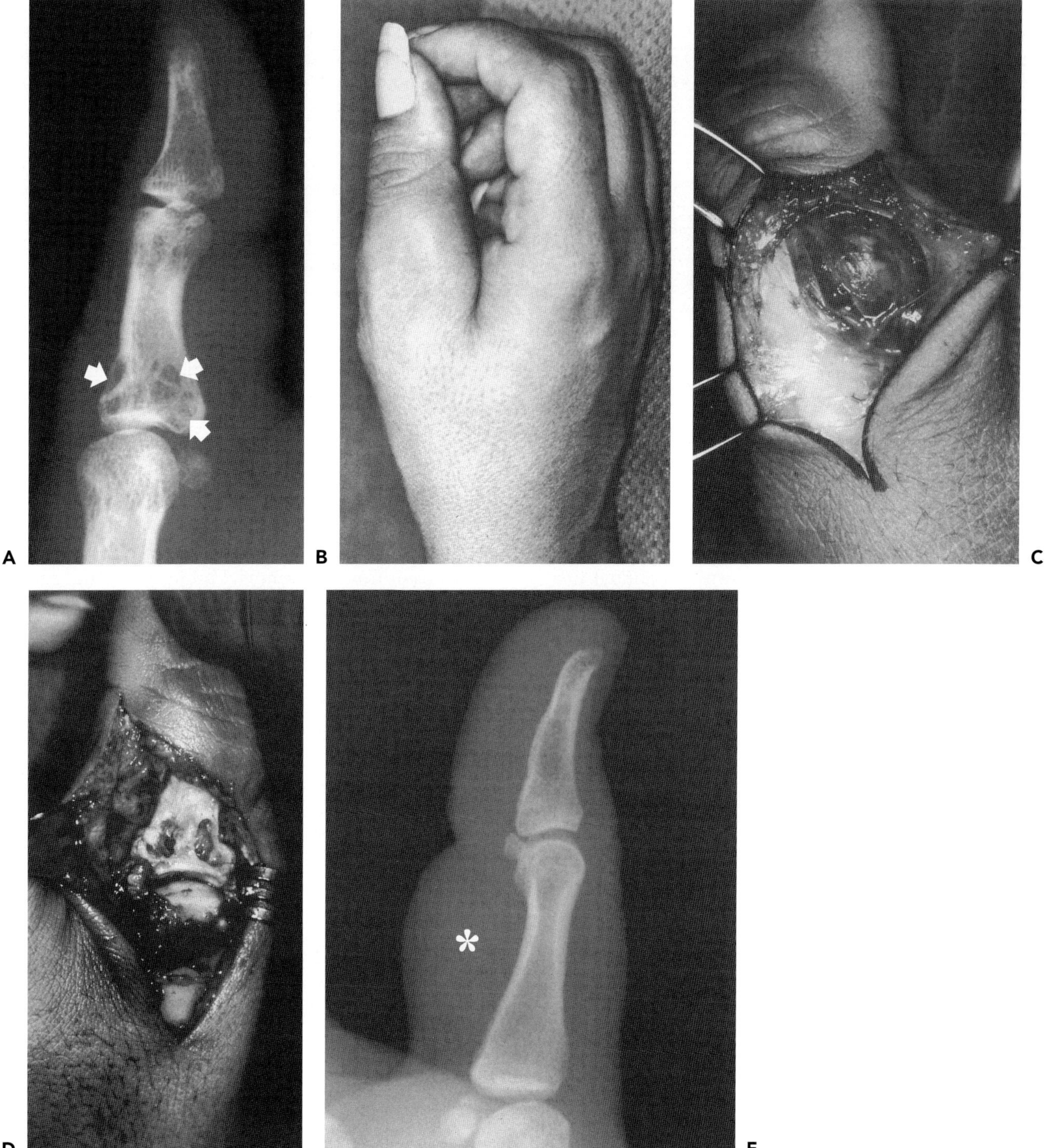

Figure 10.1 Giant cell tumor of tendon sheath (nodular tenosynovitis): Typical radiographic features in two patients. **A:** Radiograph of the thumb in a woman 26 years of age shows multiple, well-defined, geographic lesions with sclerotic margins (*arrows*), most prominent in the base of the proximal phalanx. **B:** Preoperative clinical photograph of the thumb shows marked fusiform enlargement. **C:** The nodular character of the mass is apparent grossly at surgery. **D:** Intraoperative photograph shows the well-defined lesions in the base of the proximal phalanx, corresponding to erosions seen on radiograph. **E:** Radiograph of a second patient shows a soft tissue mass (*asterisk*) adjacent to the flexor tendon of the thumb.

localized form, and it has an increased incidence of local recurrence that may be as high as 40% to 50%, considerably higher than that of the localized form (13). Calcification is reported in diffuse giant cell tumor of tendon sheath (19).

Pigmented Villonodular Synovitis

> **KEY CONCEPTS**
> - Pigmented villonodular synovitis most commonly involves the large joints: 75% to 80% occur in the knee.
> - Other joints affected, in order of decreasing frequency, include the hip, ankle, shoulder, and elbow.
> - Grossly, the lesion is likened to a "shaggy red beard"; reddish color is the result of iron pigment.
> - Patients present with a slowly growing mass; recurrence following surgery is not uncommon.
> - The lesion is typically associated with serosanguineous or xanthochromic joint effusion.

Pigmented villonodular synovitis (PVNS) is most common in the third and fourth decades of life (20). It occurs equally in both men and women, with an annual incidence of approximately 1.8 to 2.0 per million persons (20). It most commonly involves the large joints, with approximately 75% to 80% of cases occurring in the knee (6,21). Other large joints affected, in order of decreasing frequency, include the hip, ankle, shoulder, and elbow (6,21,22). Involvement of more than one joint is distinctly unusual (23); however, Cotten et al. (24) noted probable bilateral involvement in 2 (3%) of 58 patients with PVNS of the hip. In addition to the hips, bilateral involvement is reported in the shoulders and wrists (25,26). Patients usu-

ally complain of mechanical pain, which increases with motion and is improved by rest (24). Swelling and decreased range of motion may also be seen. The time interval from onset of symptoms to clinical presentation varies from months to years (21,27). Patients are usually adults (28), although it is reported in children as young as 4.5 years (29). Childhood PVNS may be a different lesion and is reported in conjunction with synovial hemangioma. Recurrent hemorrhage within the hemangioma is suggested as an etiology (30).

Synovectomy remains the preferred treatment. Both traditional and arthroscopic synovectomy are used. In patients with PVNS, the recurrence rate is lower and clinical results better in patients treated with extended synovectomy (16). Recurrence rates are typically quite high, approaching 50% (31). Total joint replacement relieves pain and restores function in selected patients and is recommended for those with significant cartilage loss and secondary osteoarthritis (21,32).

Lesions are usually much larger and more irregular in shape than those seen in nodular tenosynovitis. Grossly, the lesion is likened to a "shaggy red beard" to emphasize the villous or frondlike synovial projections. The reddish or rust color is the result of iron pigment (hemosiderin) within the lesion (27,33). Pathologically, PVNS is characterized by synovial hyperplasia with multinucleated giant cells and a characteristic pigmentation caused by both intra- and extracellular hemosiderin (Fig. 10.2) (21,34). Early lesions demonstrate large villi projecting into the joint space, and with time, these become adherent (Fig. 10.2). Long-standing lesions can show fibrosis and hyalinization (34). Foam or xanthoma cells may also be seen in mature lesions (35). There is typically an associated joint

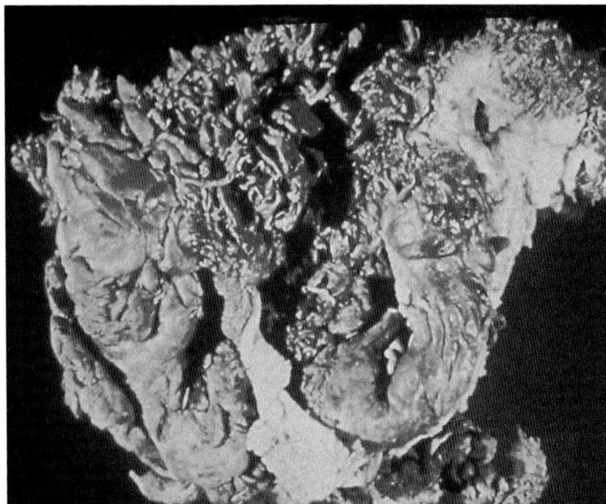

A

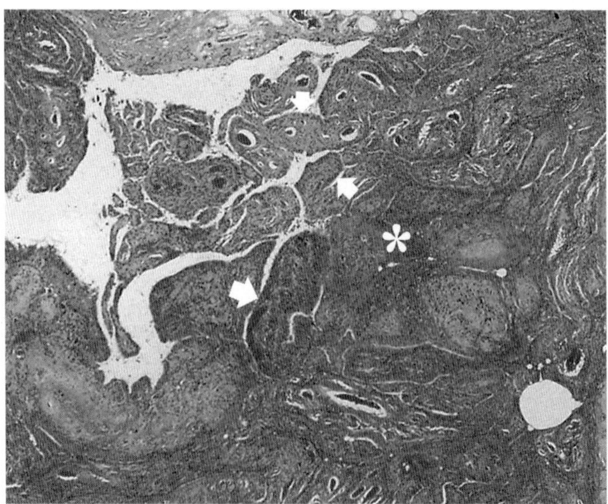

B

Figure 10.2 Pigmented villonodular synovitis: Typical gross and histologic features. **A:** Gross photograph shows multiple villous or frondlike projections. Lesions are typically reddish or rust color as a result of hemosiderin deposition within the tumor. **B:** Low-power photomicrograph shows frondlike growth pattern (*arrows*) and hemosiderin deposition (*asterisk*).

effusion with serosanguineous or xanthochromic fluid (21,27).

Malignant Pigmented Villonodular Synovitis

> **KEY CONCEPTS**
> - Malignant PVNS is quite rare.
> - It may occur with long-standing disease and multiple recurrences or at initial presentation.
> - Recent studies of malignant PVNS indicate that it is a distinct entity.
> - Limited experience shows an imaging appearance similar to that of a conventional lesion.

Rare cases of PVNS and giant cell tumors of tendon sheath (malignant tenosynovial giant cell tumor) with metastases are reported (2,36–40). Such tumors are quite unusual and are reported in patients with long-standing disease who have had multiple recurrences, as well as in patients at the time of initial presentation (40). Malignant PVNS and giant cell tumor of tendon sheath are defined as lesions in which benign tumors coexist with frankly malignant areas or, alternatively, in cases in which frankly malignant areas are present in recurrent lesions (2,4,37,38). Newer studies of malignant PVNS suggest that it is a distinct entity with a histologic architecture similar to that of conventional PVNS (40). This concept is supported by identification of consistent trisomies in chromosome 5 and 7 (39). Our limited experience with the imaging appearance of malignant PVNS is that it shows an appearance similar to that of conventional lesions.

Imaging of Benign Proliferative Lesions

Giant Cell Tumor of Tendon Sheath

Radiographs of patients with giant cell tumor of tendon sheath (tenosynovial giant cell tumor; nodular tenosynovitis) most commonly demonstrate a soft tissue mass (8,10). Pressure erosions of bone are seen in about 15% of cases overall (7,11). Radiographs are entirely normal in approximately 20% of cases (Fig. 10.1) (11). In a large review, Ushijima et al. (7) reviewed the radiographs of 56

> **KEY CONCEPTS**
> - Radiographs are normal in 20% of cases; pressure erosions appear in 15% to 20%.
> - MR imaging usually shows a well-defined mass intimately associated with the tendon.
> - Lesions are intermediate on T1 with a signal intensity equal to or less than that of skeletal muscle.
> - T2 imaging shows a signal intensity equal to or less than that of fat.
> - Lesions typically show intense gadolinium enhancement.

patients with giant cell tumor of tendon sheath and found osseous abnormalities in 18 (32%), including pressure erosions in 12 (21%), cystic change in 4 (7%), and degenerative change in 4 (7%). Karasick and Karasick (11) reported the radiographic findings in 36 patients and noted periosteal reaction in 3 (8%), calcifications in 2 (6%), and intraosseous invasion in 1 (3%). The intralesional calcifications may mimic those of synovial chondromatosis, periosteal chondroma, or calcific tendonitis (11). Although unusual, both dystrophic calcification and cartilaginous metaplasia may be seen (11). Lesions in the feet and ankles are more likely to produce pressure erosions in the adjacent bone, secondary to the dense ligaments and the propensity of these to prevent outward growth (7).

Because the diagnosis is usually suggested clinically, CT and MR are not commonly used; therefore, experience with this lesion is limited. MR typically demonstrates a nonspecific, well-defined mass adjacent to a tendon. Lesions are hypointense on T1-weighted spin-echo images with signal intensity approximately equal to that of skeletal muscle. Signal intensities greater and less than that of skeletal muscle are reported (13,14). On T2-weighted images, lesions are more heterogeneous with decreased signal intensity, typically equal to or less than that of fat (Fig. 10.3) (13,28). This variable signal on T2-weighted images reflects the lesion's morphology and hemosiderin content. Intense enhancement following gadolinium administration is seen in the vast majority of cases (14). MR imaging readily identifies osseous erosions (Fig. 10.4). The MR imaging features of tenosynovial giant cell tumor are relatively constant and allow a successful diagnosis even in atypical locations (Fig. 10.5). Rarely, multifocal local recurrence may be seen (Fig. 10.6).

Technetium-99m methylene diphosphonate bone scintigraphy is rarely used in the diagnosis of tenosynovial giant cell tumor. Osseous erosions may produce increased tracer accumulation, but such findings are uncommon and seen in only a minority of cases. Thallium (T1-201) scintigraphic features are reported (41) and discussed later.

Nodular Synovitis

> **KEY CONCEPTS**
> - MR imaging shows a well-defined, pedunculated, small nodular or polypoid intra-articular soft tissue mass.
> - T1-weighted images show a signal intensity similar to that of skeletal muscle.
> - T2-weighted signal intensity is variable, usually equal to or less than that of fat.
> - Rounded or curvilinear regions of low signal intensity may be seen, representing hemosiderin-laden areas.

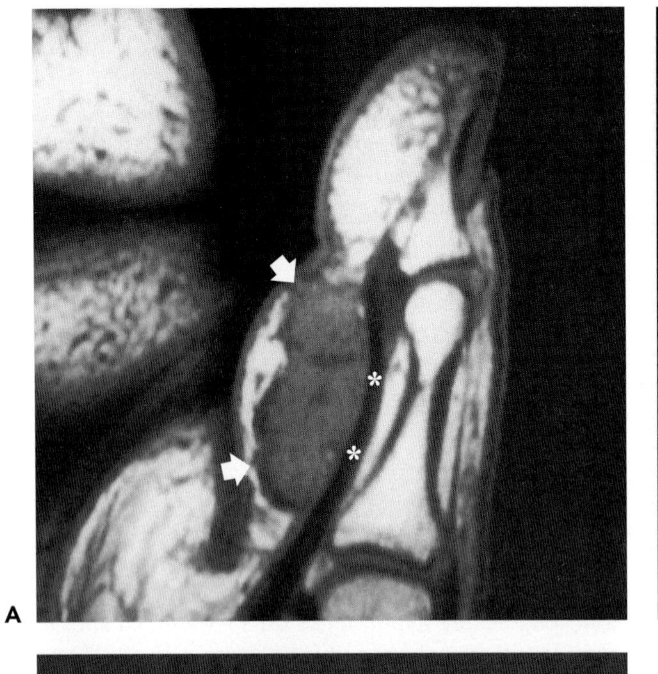

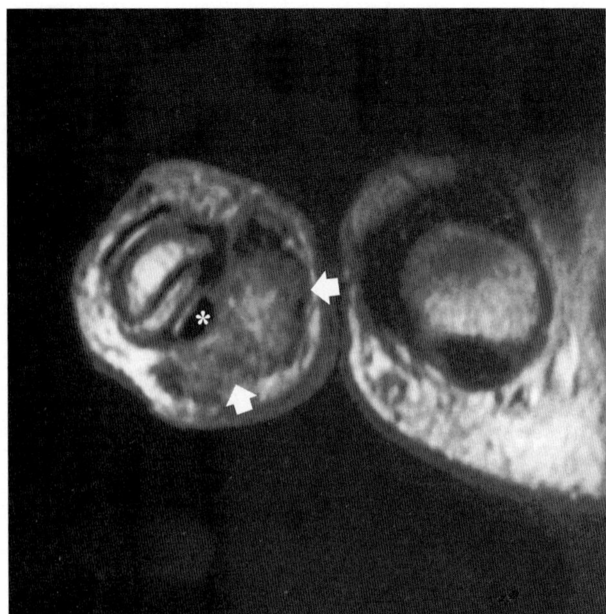

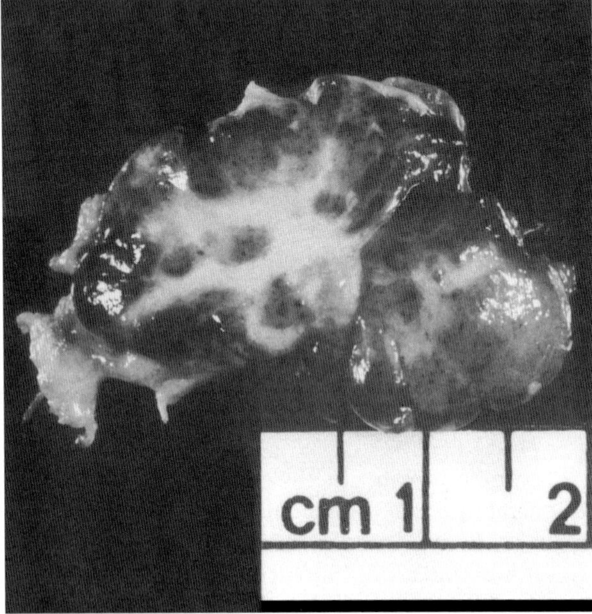

Figure 10.3 Giant cell tumor of tendon sheath (nodular tenosynovitis): Typical MR imaging findings in a woman 32 years of age presenting with a slightly painful thumb mass, increasing in size over the previous 14 months. **A,B:** Sagittal T1-weighted (TR/TE; 300/25) **(A)** and axial T2-weighted (TR/TE; 2000/80) **(B)** spin-echo MR images of the thumb show a well-defined, lobulated mass (*arrows*) arising adjacent to the flexor pollicis longus tendon (*asterisks*) of the thumb. **C:** Gross photograph of the resected specimen shows nodular character of the lesion, as well as areas of dense fibrosis.

The MR imaging of nodular synovitis is typically that of a well-defined small, nodular or polypoid intra-articular soft tissue mass. The lesion usually shows a signal intensity similar to that of skeletal muscle on T1-weighted images and a variable signal intensity on T2-weighted images (15) (Fig. 10.7). In our experience, the T2-weighted signal intensity is usually equal to or less than that of fat. Rounded or curvilinear regions of low signal intensity may be identified within the mass, representing hemosiderin-laden areas (15,18). These regions demonstrate "blooming" on gradient images typical of hemosiderin-laden tissue. Huang et al. (15) noted linear or cleftlike high signal intensity areas within lesions on T2-weighted images in 7 (33%) of 21 cases, speculating that the high signal intensity area represented necrosis.

Prominent contrast enhancement is typically seen. Caution must be used when fat-suppressed, fluid-sensitive images are viewed because these sequences often do not demonstrate the typical decreased-to-intermediate signal intensity seen on non-fat-suppressed T2-weighted images. Radiographs are typically unremarkable, although longstanding lesions may cause pressure erosions on the adjacent joints (Fig. 10.8).

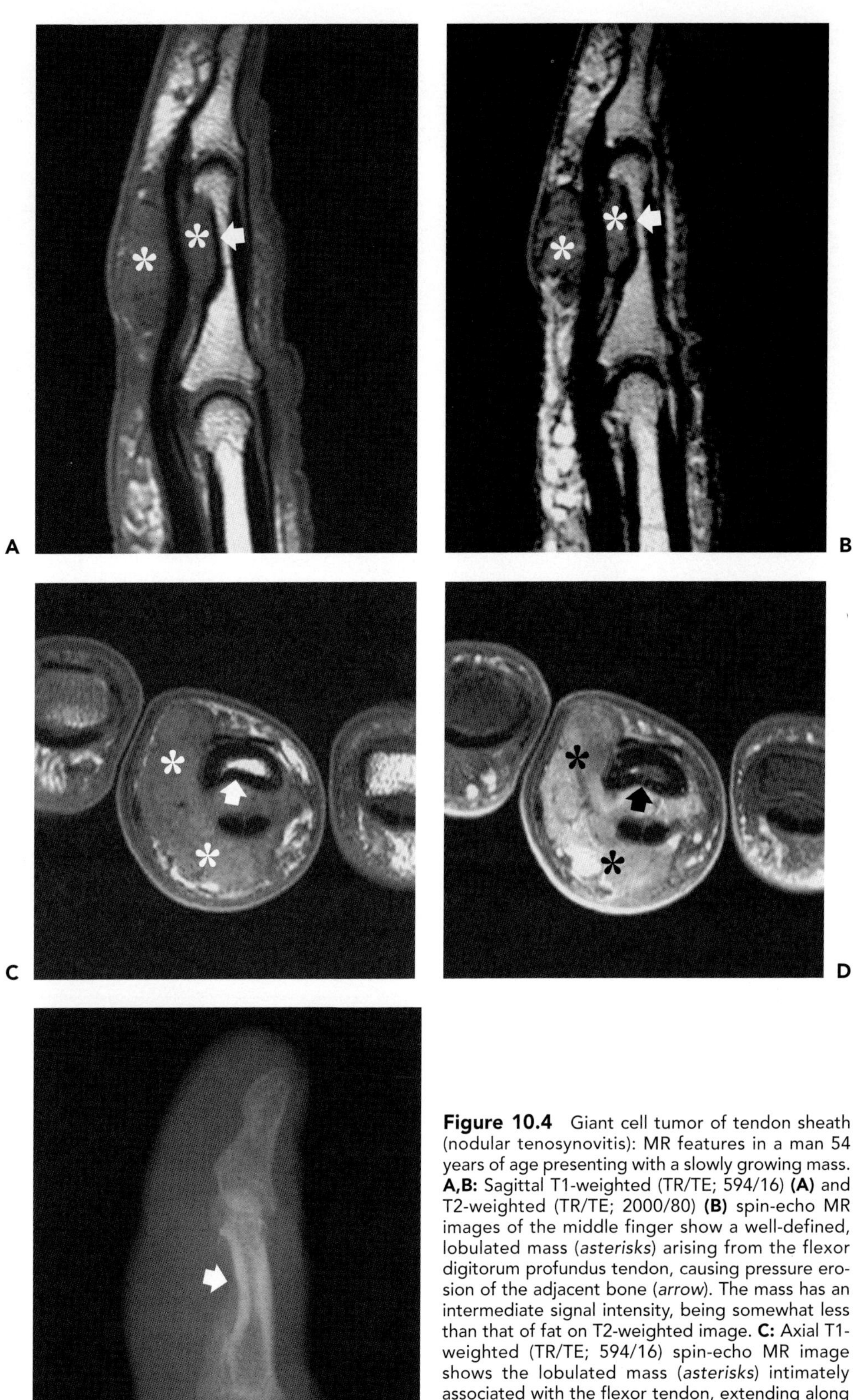

Figure 10.4 Giant cell tumor of tendon sheath (nodular tenosynovitis): MR features in a man 54 years of age presenting with a slowly growing mass. **A,B:** Sagittal T1-weighted (TR/TE; 594/16) **(A)** and T2-weighted (TR/TE; 2000/80) **(B)** spin-echo MR images of the middle finger show a well-defined, lobulated mass (*asterisks*) arising from the flexor digitorum profundus tendon, causing pressure erosion of the adjacent bone (*arrow*). The mass has an intermediate signal intensity, being somewhat less than that of fat on T2-weighted image. **C:** Axial T1-weighted (TR/TE; 594/16) spin-echo MR image shows the lobulated mass (*asterisks*) intimately associated with the flexor tendon, extending along the radial aspect of the finger. Note osseous erosion (*arrow*). **D:** Axial enhanced fat-suppressed T1-weighted (TR/TE; 594/16) spin-echo MR image shows prominent enhancement of the mass (*asterisks*). Osseous erosion (*arrow*) is again seen. **E:** Lateral radiograph of the middle finger shows the extrinsic pressure osseous erosion (*arrow*).

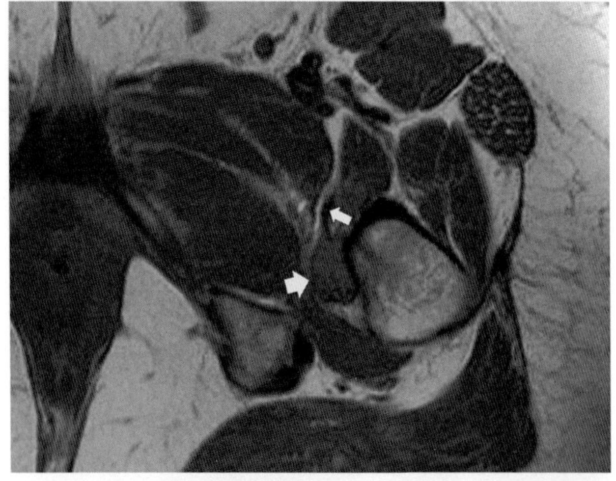

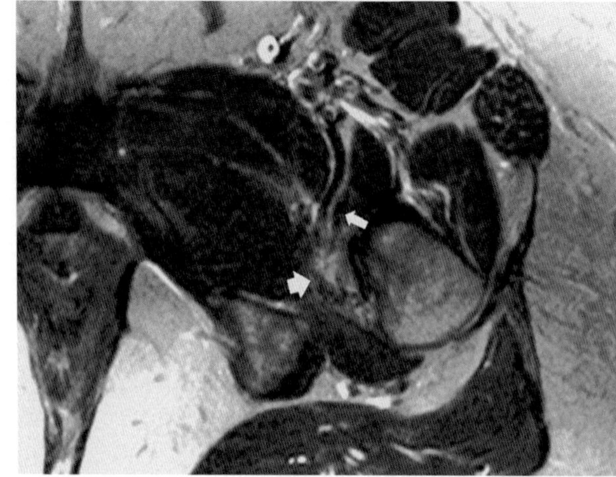

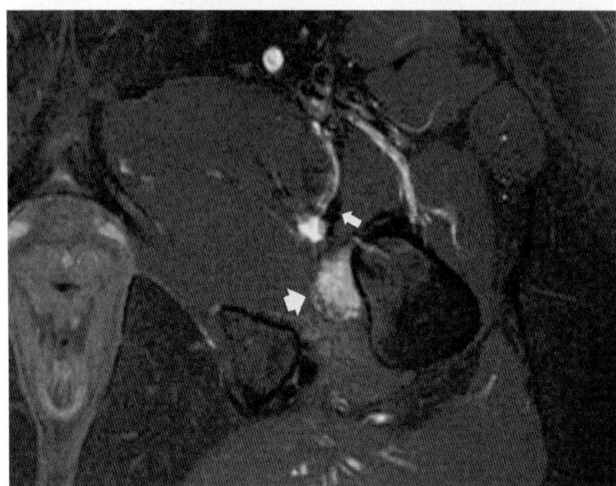

Figure 10.5 Giant cell tumor of tendon sheath (nodular tenosynovitis): Typical MR features in an unusual location, in a woman 50 years of age presenting with hip pain. **A,B:** Corresponding axial T1-weighted (TR/TE; 683/17) **(A)** and T2-weighted (TR/TE; 2640/80) **(B)** spin-echo MR images of the hip show a mass (*small arrow*) intimately associated with the iliopsoas tendon (*large arrow*). The mass has a signal intensity similar to that of muscle in **(A)** and similar to that of fat in **(B)**. **C:** Axial enhanced fat-suppressed T1-weighted (TR/TE; 400/17) spin-echo MR image shows prominent enhancement of the mass (*small arrow*). Note iliopsoas tendon (*large arrow*).

Diffuse Giant Cell Tumor of Tendon Sheath

> ### KEY CONCEPTS
> - Diffuse form of giant cell tumor of tendon sheath shows a nodular to multinodular mass adjacent to a large joint.
> - Signal intensity is similar to that of PVNS.

The diffuse form of giant cell tumor of tendon sheath shows imaging features that have characteristics of both giant cell tumor of tendon sheath and PVNS. The lesion tends to grow as a multinodular juxta-articular mass, with a growth pattern similar to that of giant cell tumor of tendon sheath and a signal intensity and vascularity more akin to that of PVNS (Figs. 10.9 and 10.10).

Pigmented Villonodular Synovitis

Radiographs may be normal and show a noncalcified soft tissue mass, joint effusion, or bone erosions (Fig. 10.11) (21,42). Erosive bone lesions are seen in approxi-

> ### KEY CONCEPTS
> - In PVNS, radiographs may show a noncalcified mass; 50% of joints show bone erosions.
> - Erosions are most common in joints with tight capsules, such as the hip (93%) and shoulder (75%).
> - Erosions are most characteristic when on both sides of a joint.
> - MR imaging typically shows a diffuse, multinodular intra-articular mass with decreased signal on T1/T2.
> - Gradient images show "blooming" caused by hemosiderin deposition within the mass.

mately 50% of all cases (21), most commonly in joints with tight capsules, such as the hip (93%) and shoulder (75%), and least commonly in the knee (26%) (21). These erosive changes are usually geographic lytic lesions, with well-defined, thinly sclerotic margins. They are most characteristic when multiple and on both sides of the joint (Fig. 10.12). The joint space is usually

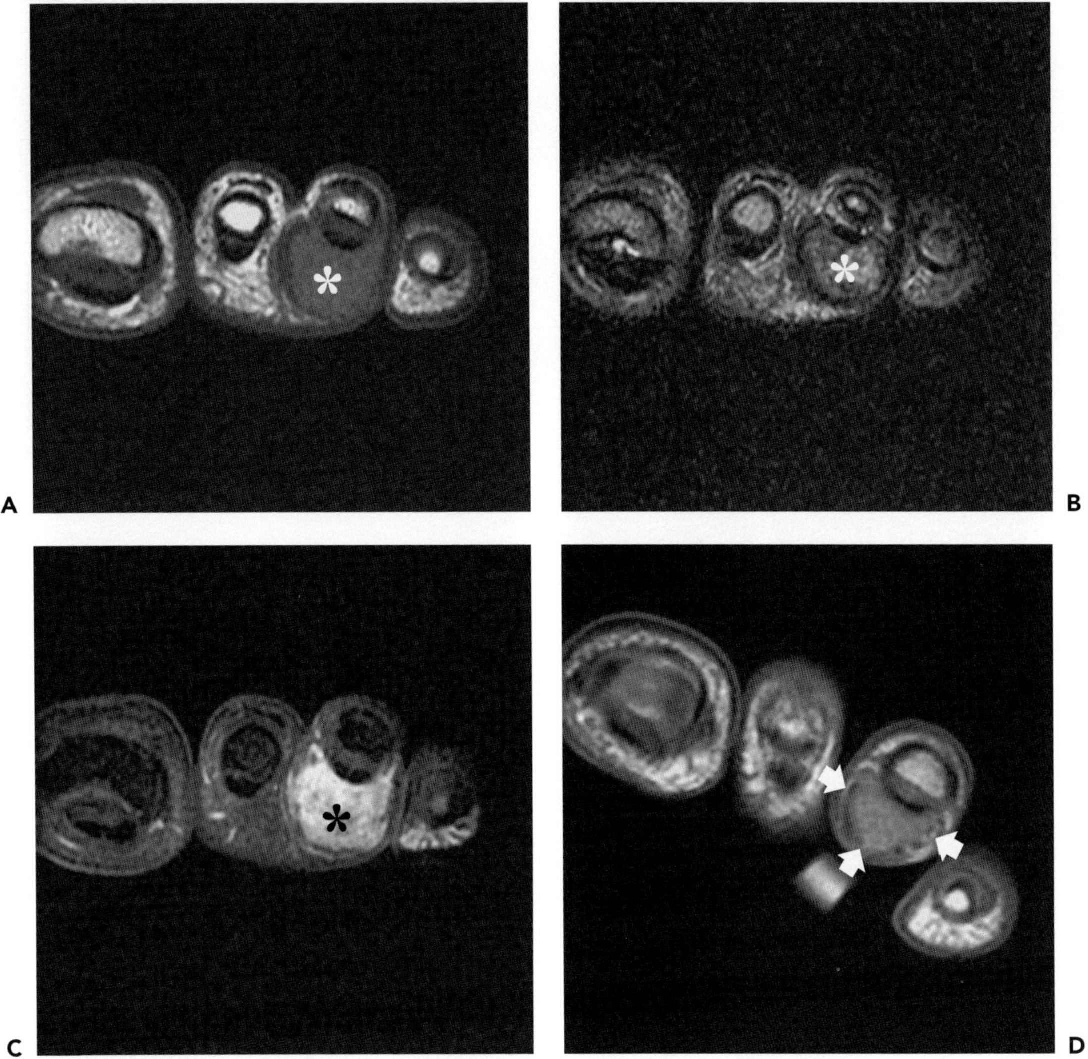

Figure 10.6 Recurrent giant cell tumor of tendon sheath (nodular tenosynovitis): Multifocal recurrence in a man 19 years of age. **A,B:** Coronal T1-weighted (TR/TE; 467/17) **(A)** and T2-weighted (TR/TE; 2000/80) **(B)** spin-echo MR images of the third toe show an intermediate signal intensity mass (*asterisks*) associated with the flexor tendon. **C:** Corresponding enhanced coronal T1-weighted (TR/TE; 467/17) spin-echo MR image of the third toe show extensive heterogeneous enhancement. **D:** Four years following resection, the patient noted a recurrent mass. Coronal T1-weighted (TR/TE; 400/14) spin-echo MR image of the third toe shows a mass (*arrows*), with signal intensity similar to that of the original lesion. (*continued*)

preserved, as is bone mineralization (21). Uncommonly, radiographic features may mimic those of arthritis with localized loss of joint space, osteosclerosis, osteophytosis, and subchondral cyst formation or uniform joint space loss, osteoporosis, and cortical erosions (Fig. 10.13) (24). Radiologic calcification within the mass is reported (43), but it is rare and should suggest an alternative diagnosis.

Three-phase bone scintigraphy demonstrates increased tracer accumulation on flow and blood-pool images. Patients with erosive bone changes have increased bone uptake of the radionuclide on delayed images in the region of those defects (Fig. 10.14) (42). Thallium (Tl-201) imaging shows significant uptake on early images and retention on delayed images. In PVNS, thallium demonstrates a diffuse, nodular, juxta-articular pattern. In contrast, the uptake in tenosynovial giant cell tumor is more focal (41). PVNS also demonstrates hypermetabolic activity on 18-fluorine fluorodeoxyglucose positron emission tomography (PET) imaging (44).

Limited experience with ultrasonography shows a complex echogenic mass within an enlarged bursa that contains fluid and septations (42). Arthrography demonstrates a lobulated intra-articular mass. The joint capacity is normal

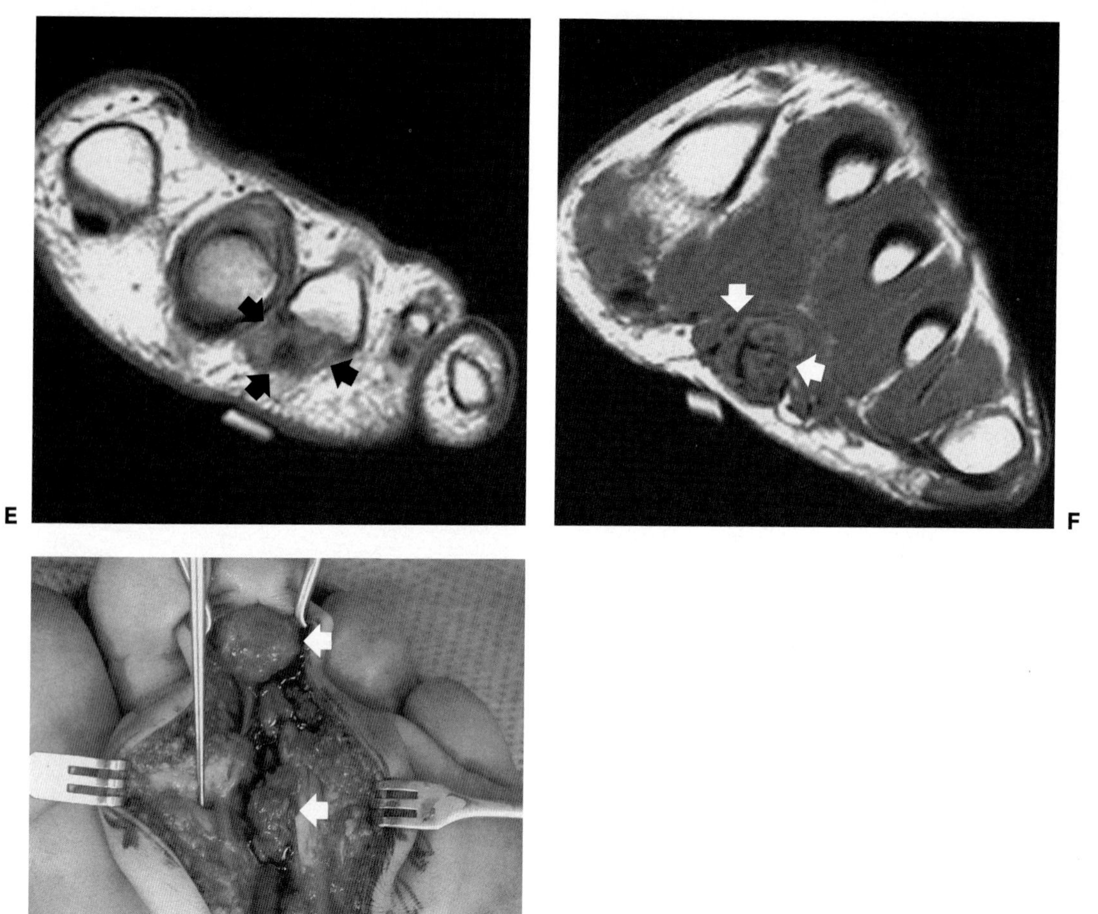

Figure 10.6 *(continued)*   **E,F:** Coronal T1-weighted (TR/TE; 400/14) spin-echo imaging more proximally shows two additional masses (*arrows*), adjacent to the metatarsal head **(E)** and in the midfoot **(F)**. **G:** Intraoperative photo shows the three masses (*arrows*) along the flexor tendon. Note nodular morphology of the masses.

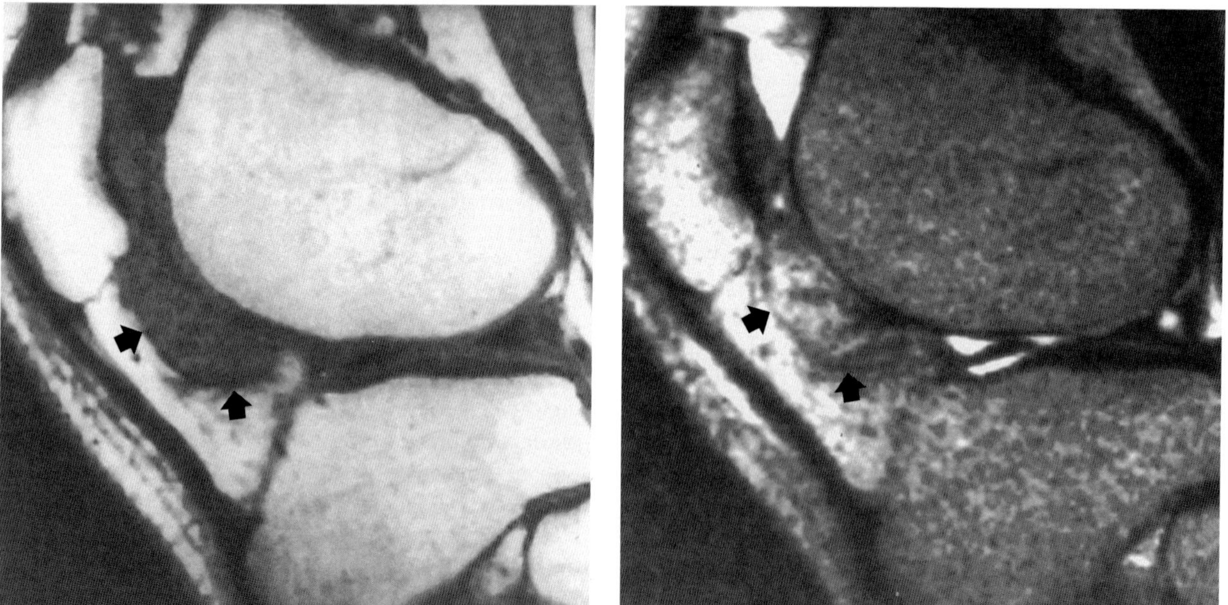

Figure 10.7   Nodular synovitis: MR features in a man 24 years of age, presenting with an 8-month history of knee pain. **A,B:** Sagittal T1-weighted (TR/TE; 500/17) **(A)** and T2-weighted (TR/TE; 2500/84) **(B)** spin-echo MR images of the knee show a well-defined mass (*arrows*) within the knee joint with intermediate signal intensity.

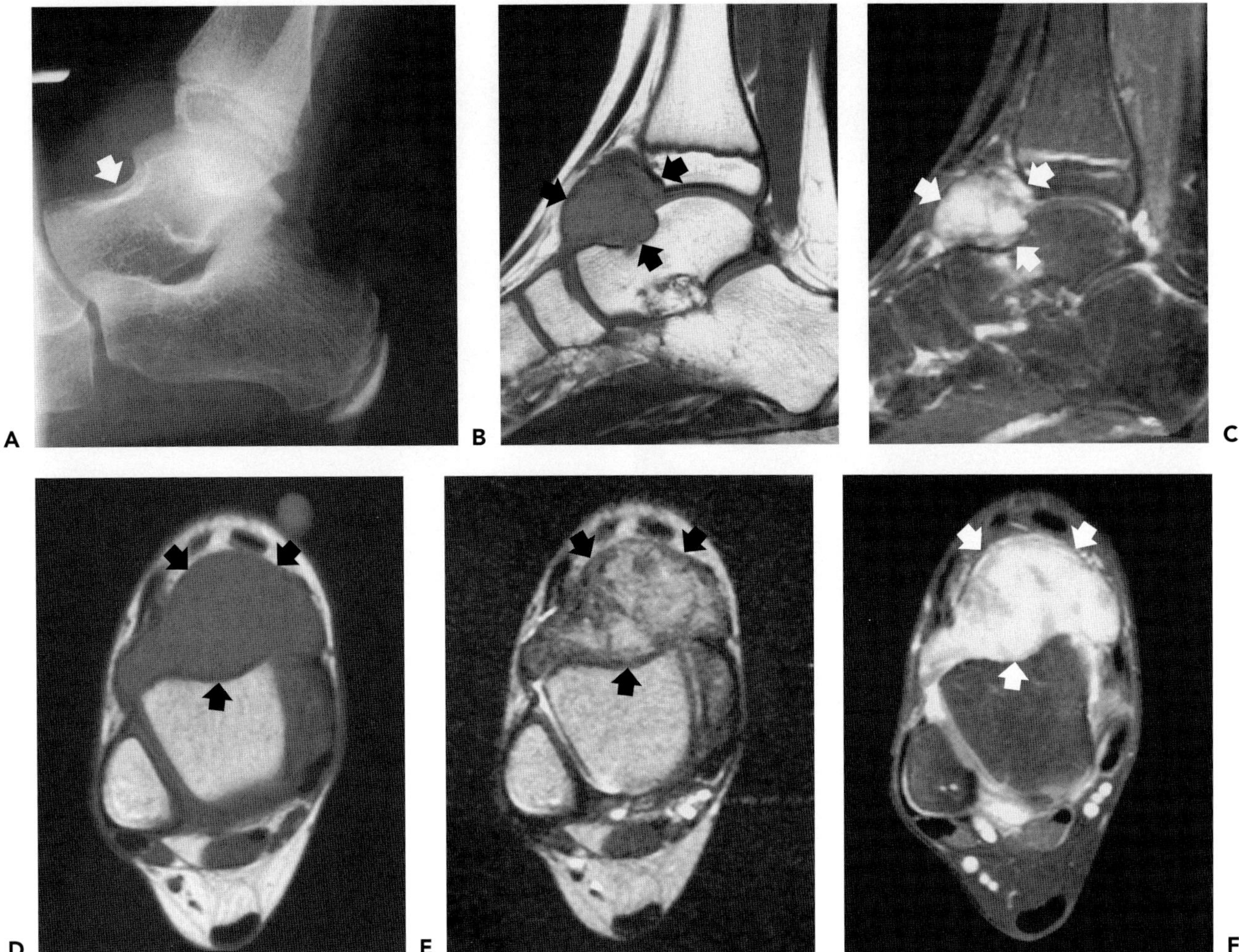

Figure 10.8 Nodular synovitis: Typical radiographic and MR imaging features in a girl 8 years of age presenting with an ankle mass. **A:** Lateral radiograph of the ankle shows well-defined pressure erosion (*arrow*) in the neck of the talus. Note adjacent soft tissue mass. **B,C:** Corresponding sagittal T1-weighted (TR/TE; 575/20) **(B)** spin-echo and short-tau inversion recovery (STIR) (TR/TE/TI; 4700/30/150) **(C)** MR images of the ankle show the mass (*arrows*) anterior to the ankle joint. Note increased signal intensity of the mass on STIR image. **D,E:** Corresponding axial T1-weighted (TR/TE; 450/12) **(D)** and conventional T2-weighted (TR/TE; 2000/80) **(E)** spin-echo MR images of the ankle show a typical intermediate signal intensity mass (*arrows*). **F:** Corresponding enhanced fat-suppressed axial T1-weighted (TR/TE; 850/12) spin-echo MR shows extensive relatively homogeneous enhancement throughout the mass (*arrows*).

and the aspirated fluid is usually serosanguineous (21,42). Arteriography is nonspecific and may reveal a vascular mass that is indistinguishable from a malignant neoplasm, with numerous irregular vessels, "tumor blush," and arteriovenous shunting (Figs. 10.10 and 10.12) (21,16,42,45). Rare, mature, hyalinized lesions may be radiographically avascular (34).

On CT scanning, the erosive lesions are sharply defined with sclerotic margins (42). Subtle erosions, not visible on radiographs, may also be identified. CT demonstrates a soft tissue mass, which may show an increased attenuation relative to that of muscle on noncontrast examination, caused by hemosiderin deposition within the lesion

(20,33,42,46). A joint effusion may also be seen (Figs. 10.12 and 10.13) (42).

The MR appearance of PVNS is typically characteristic, demonstrating a heterogeneous synovial-based mass. The mass may extend along the synovial surface (Fig. 10.15) or may be associated with marked thickening of the synovium (Fig. 10.16). As the lesion increases in size, it extends away from the joint space (Fig. 10.12) (42). The mass is usually well-defined, but margins may be obscure and difficult to separate from adjacent muscle. Large lesions may be subdivided by septae, likely representing the edges of the individual nodules comprising the lesion (47). On T1-weighted spin-echo images, the

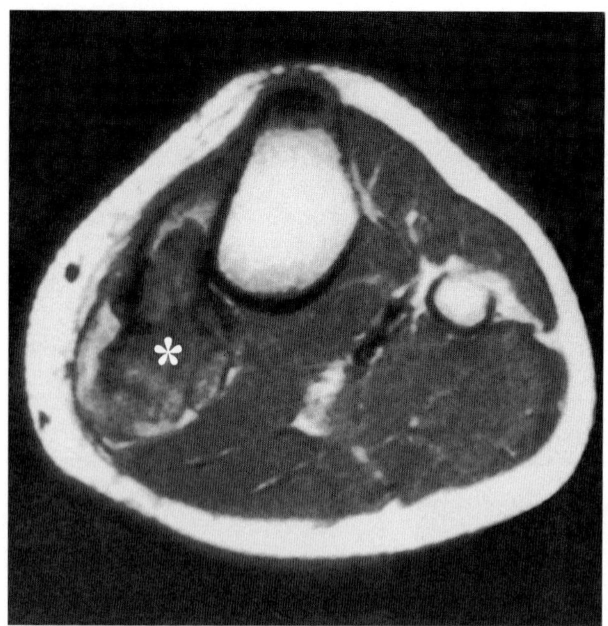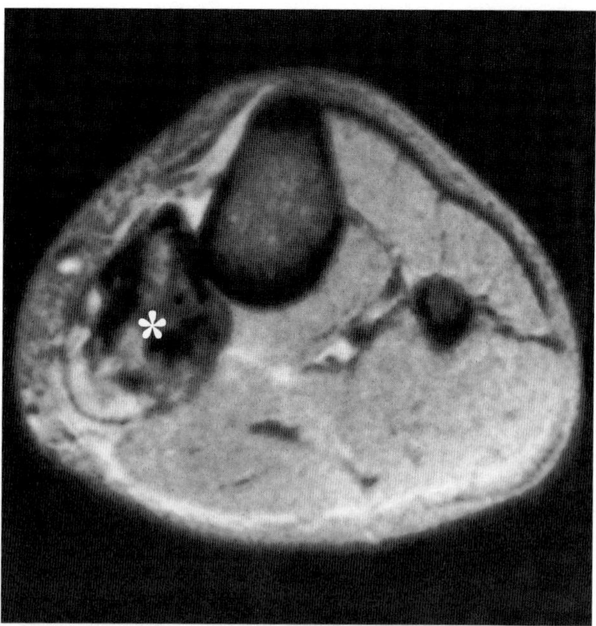

Figure 10.9 Diffuse giant cell tumor of tendon sheath: MR imaging features in a girl 16 years of age with a mass adjacent to the knee. **A,B:** Axial T1-weighted (TR/TE; 400/19) **(A)** spin-echo and gradient-echo (TR/TE; 317/10/15) MR images of the knee show a lobulated mass (*asterisk*) adjacent to the medial aspect of the knee. **(B)** The mass shows increased susceptibility on gradient-echo image, compatible with hemosiderin deposition within the mass. Note associated edema extending along fascial planes. Edema was felt to be caused by infarction within the mass.

overall signal intensity of the mass is similar to that, or less than that, of skeletal muscle. A similar pattern is seen on T2-weighted images, although scattered areas of high signal may be present (20,42,47,48). The decreased signal intensity is usually more pronounced on long TR/TE images because of the preferential shortening of T2 relaxation times caused by hemosiderin (Figs. 10.13, 10.15–10.17) (20,27,46,49). This decreased signal intensity is more pronounced at high field strengths (27,48,50); therefore, this feature is useful in distinguishing PVNS from synovitis with rice body formation, which does not show susceptibility artifact on gradient-echo sequences (51). Intense contrast enhancement is typically seen; however, enhancement is variable and a function of the degree of fibrosis and the amount of hemosiderin within the tumor (26,52).

Collections of lipid-laden macrophages (foam cells) may appear as focal areas of increased signal intensity on T1-weighted and intermediate signal intensity on T2-weighted images (47). PVNS shows significant enhancement following gadolinium administration (47). Predominantly cystic lesions are described; however, these are relatively uncommon and represent less than 10% of cases (47). Associated edema was noted in the bone adjacent to an erosion, or in the nearby soft tissues, in 6 (23%) of 26 patients reported by Hughes et al. (47). All 6 patients had either prominent erosions, subchondral synovial tissue, or cysts.

The lytic bone lesions seen on radiographs and CT are typically well seen on MR (42). Coexistent joint effusions and focal fluid collections are present in more than 50% of cases, appearing as areas of low signal on T1-weighted images, with marked hyperintensity on T2-weighted images (42). These joint effusions are usually surrounded by low signal intensity, hemosiderin-laden synovial tissue. Joint fluid is most common in the knee but is less common in those joints with tight capsules (47).

Although PVNS is most common in the large joints, it may arise in association with bursae. It is described in the pes anserinus bursa, subacromial bursa, and many juxta-articular bursae (Fig. 10.18) (53). The appearance of malignant PVNS is similar to that of conventional PVNS (Fig. 10.19).

Synovial Cyst

The term *synovial cyst* is used loosely for any synovial-lined juxta-articular fluid collection. A synovial cyst usually represents an extension of the joint fluid and typically is the result of chronic effusion from mechanical internal derangement or arthropathy (54).

Classification

Although there is no uniformly accepted classification for synovial cysts, the term *popliteal cyst* is used for synovial cysts that form in the normally occurring gastrocnemius-semimembranosus bursa. Synovial cysts are distinguished from other juxta-articular fluid collections in that they are lined by synovium.

KEY CONCEPTS

- *Synovial cyst* is a term loosely used for any synovial-lined juxta-articular fluid collection.
- The *popliteal cyst* is the most common synovial cyst, representing fluid accumulation in the normally occurring gastrocnemius-semimembranosus bursa.

Popliteal Cyst

The most frequently encountered synovial cyst is the popliteal cyst, which occurs in the medial posterior aspect of the knee and is the result of a slit-shaped communication of the knee joint with the normally occurring gastrocnemius-semimembranosus bursa (55). This communication is more common in older individuals because of degeneration and reduced elasticity of the joint capsule (55,56). The incidence of popliteal cyst increases with age (56,57), demonstrated arthrographically in 16% of patients in the second decade of life, 36% in the third decade, increasing to 54% beyond the fifth decade (56). In a study of adult cadavers, a communication between the knee joint and the gastrocnemius-semimembranosus bursa was found in more than half the cases (58). The term

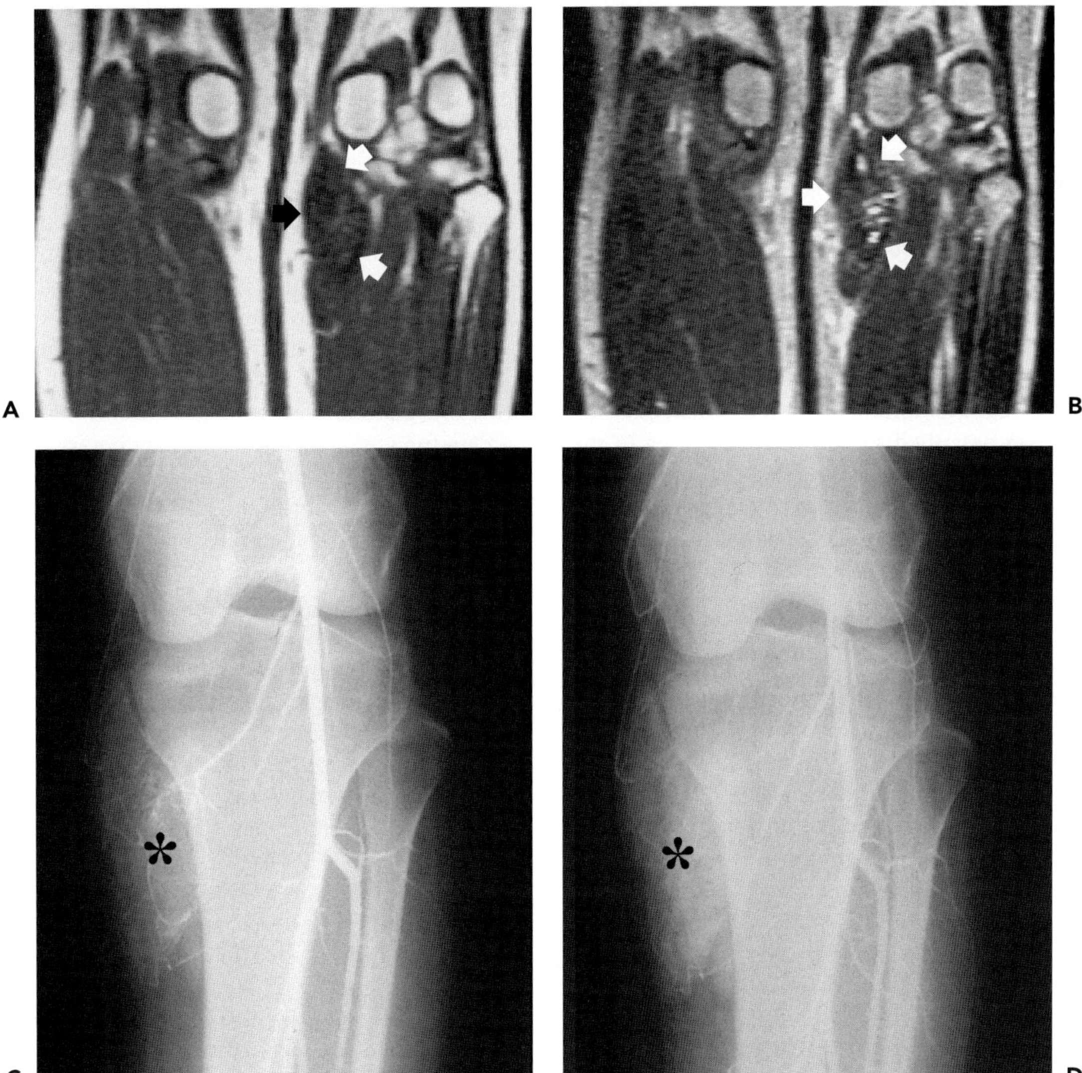

Figure 10.10 Diffuse giant cell tumor of tendon sheath: MR imaging features in a woman 26 years of age. **A,B:** Coronal T1-weighted (TR/TE; 480/22) **(A)** and T2-weighted (TR/TE; 2000/80) **(B)** spin-echo MR images of the knee show a lobulated mass (*arrows*) adjacent to the medial aspect of the knee. The mass shows markedly decreased signal intensity compatible with that of a hemosiderin-laden mass. **C,D:** Early **(C)** and late **(D)** arterial images from a conventional arteriogram show the mass (*asterisk*) with prominent hypervascularity.

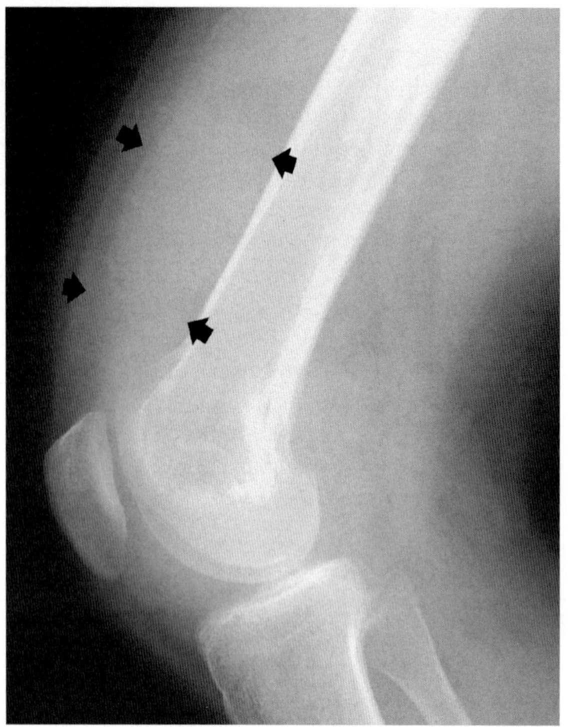

Figure 10.11 Pigmented villonodular synovitis: Radiographic features in a woman 36 years of age. Lateral radiograph shows a large joint effusion. No osseous erosions are seen.

Baker cyst is usually reserved for those cases in which this gastrocnemius-semimembranosus bursa is distended by fluid (55). Baker described eight cases of swelling in the popliteal region in 1877, concluding that the swelling was the result of "fluid which had escaped from the interior knee-joint." On the basis of his original observations and six additional cases in other joints, he hypothesized that these synovial cysts were the result of synovial membrane herniation and cyst formation caused by osteoarthritis (55,59,60).

The gastrocnemius-semimembranosus bursa is a composite of two parts: the gastrocnemius bursa and the semimembranosus bursa (61). There is often a central septum between these parts, which may be incomplete or complete, and depending on this division, one or both may distend (61). The semimembranosus bursa is larger and medial to the gastrocnemius portion. Each of these individual bursea can be further subdivided into an anterior and posterior horn. Although popliteal cysts may extend in any direction, they most commonly extend inferomedially (62). Less commonly they extend laterally or proximally (62). Rarely, popliteal cysts may dissect into the adjacent vastus medialis muscle, medial head of the gastrocnemius muscle (62), or semimembranosus muscle.

The relationship between popliteal cysts and meniscal injury was previously emphasized with approximately 80% to 90% of popliteal cysts associated with a meniscal tear (56,57). The meniscal tear is usually in the posterior horn of the medial meniscus, although 10% to 15% are lateral by arthrography and 38% are lateral by MR imaging (57). There is also an association with previous meniscectomy, collateral and cruciate ligament injury, articular cartilage damage (chondromalacia patella and degenerative arthritis), intra-articular osteochondral bodies, rheumatoid arthritis, and other arthritides (56,57,63,64). Wolfe and Colloff suggested that it is the presence of an effusion-producing intra-articular lesion rather than the specific injury that is important in the production of a popliteal cyst (56). In general, cysts in younger patients tend to be small and not associated with intra-articular pathology (56,65). It is suspected that the initial insult is relatively minor, with enlargement resulting from subsequent injury. This may help explain the increase in cyst size and number with age (56). Popliteal cysts are frequently seen in children with juvenile rheumatoid arthritis (65).

The actual incidence of popliteal cyst is difficult to establish, and it is likely to be age-related. In a recent study of the MR imaging examinations of 1,113 patients referred for evaluation of internal derangement of the knee, the incidence of popliteal cyst was 5% (57). The incidence of popliteal cyst demonstrated by arthrography ranges between 7% to 42% (56,57,66–68). This higher incidence is probably caused by the distension of the normally collapsed bursa during arthrography (57). Similar results were reported in a comparison between the results of sonography (15%) and arthrography (42%) (63).

Patients with popliteal cyst may be asymptomatic or may present with pain or signs and symptoms suggesting internal derangement of the knee, and only uncommonly do they present for the evaluation of a mass (56,64,66). Bierbaum (66) noted that a popliteal cyst was clinically evident in only 2 of 33 patients identified as having them on arthrography, and at best, less than half of those lesions noted on arthrography were detectable on clinical examination (69,70). Popliteal cysts may also be confused with proliferation of adipose tissue, tortuosity, or aneurysmal dilation of the popliteal artery, thrombosed vessel, or tumor (63). Cysts may dissect into the calf or rupture, causing symptoms that may clinically simulate thrombophlebitis (71,72). Rarely, dissecting popliteal cyst and thrombophlebitis may coexist (73,74). Mink and Deutsch suggested the term *pseudo-pseudo thrombophlebitis syndrome* to describe a deep venous thrombosis (DVT) occurring secondary to a ruptured popliteal cyst (73,74). Because popliteal cysts are lined by synovium, they are subject to synovial processes such as PVNS and synovial chondromatosis (65).

Other Synovial Cysts

Although the popliteal cyst is the prototypical example, it represents only one specific type of synovial cyst. In the knee, synovial cysts may extend anteriorly, laterally, or

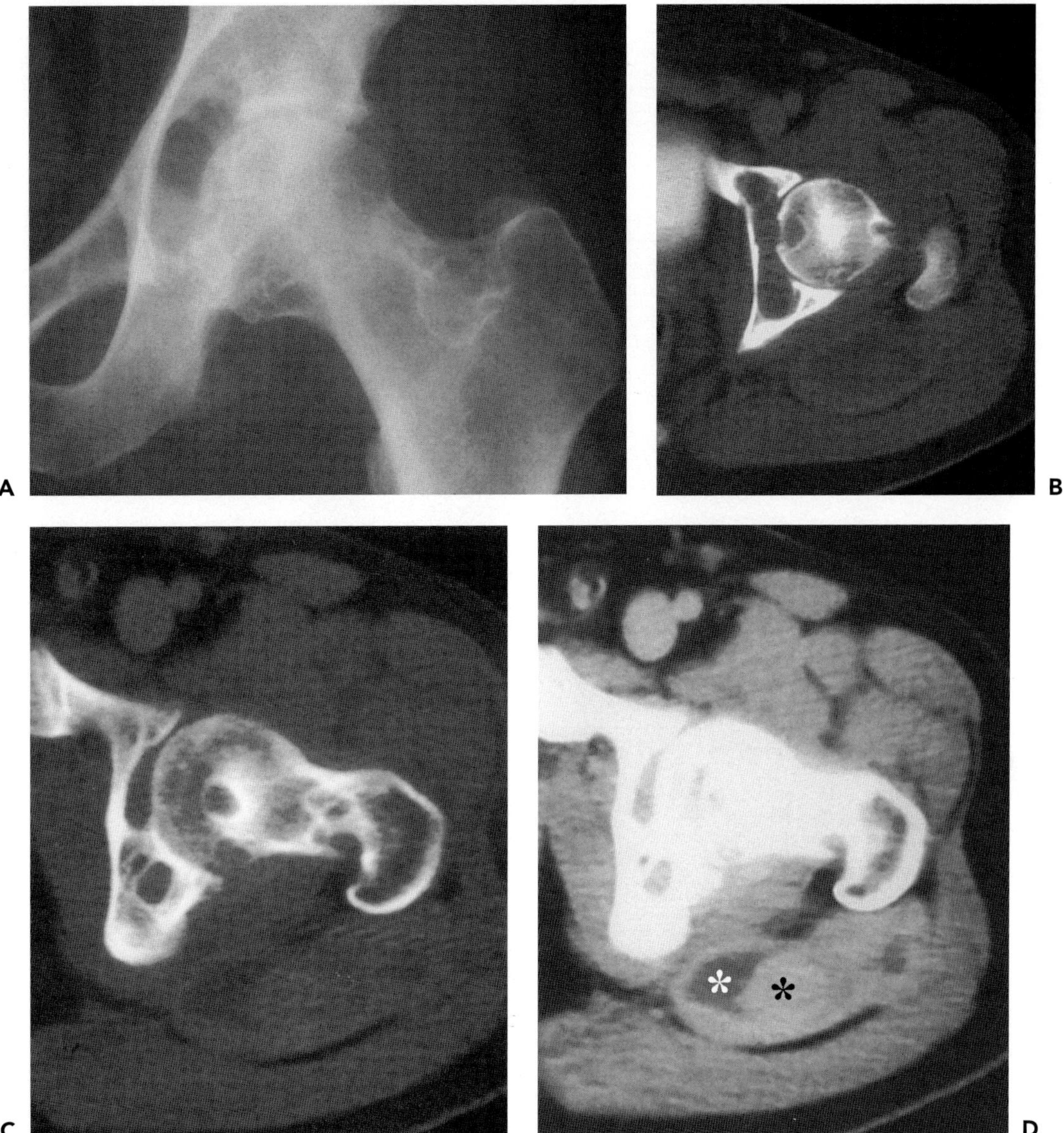

Figure 10.12 Pigmented villonodular synovitis: Radiographic and imaging features in a man 41 years of age. **A:** Anteroposterior radiograph shows multiple, well-defined, geographic, lytic lesions with sclerotic margins on both sides of the joint, with preservation on the joint space. **B:** Axial enhanced CT scan at the level of the hip joint displayed on bone window shows multiple well-defined erosions with sclerotic margins in both the femur and acetabulum. **C:** Axial enhanced CT scan at the level of the midneck, just distal to **B**, displayed on bone window, shows multiple, smaller, well-defined lesions. **D:** Axial enhanced CT scan at the level of the midneck displayed on soft tissue window shows increased attenuation to the juxta-articular mass (*black asterisk*) with associated joint effusion (*white asterisk*). (*continued*)

medially from the joint or be associated with the popliteal tendon or the proximal tibiofibular joint (75–78). Synovial cysts may be bursal in origin, not communicating with the knee joint (75–78). Seidl et al. (79) identified 5 (3.8%) cysts, originating at the apex of the suprapatellar pouch extending in a cranial direction, in 132 knee arthrograms from patients with rheumatoid arthritis. Interestingly, popliteal cysts were found in 75 (57%) of these cases.

The knee joint communicates with the proximal tibiofibular joint in approximately 10% of adults, and tibiofibular cysts are more common in patients with joint effusions (65). Synovial cysts from the tibiofibular joints may be associated with pain that radiates down the calf and may be exacerbated by squatting (65). Tibiofibular joint cysts may also be associated with peroneal nerve dysfunction. Synovial cysts from the hip joint are a rare cause of lower extremity DVT (80).

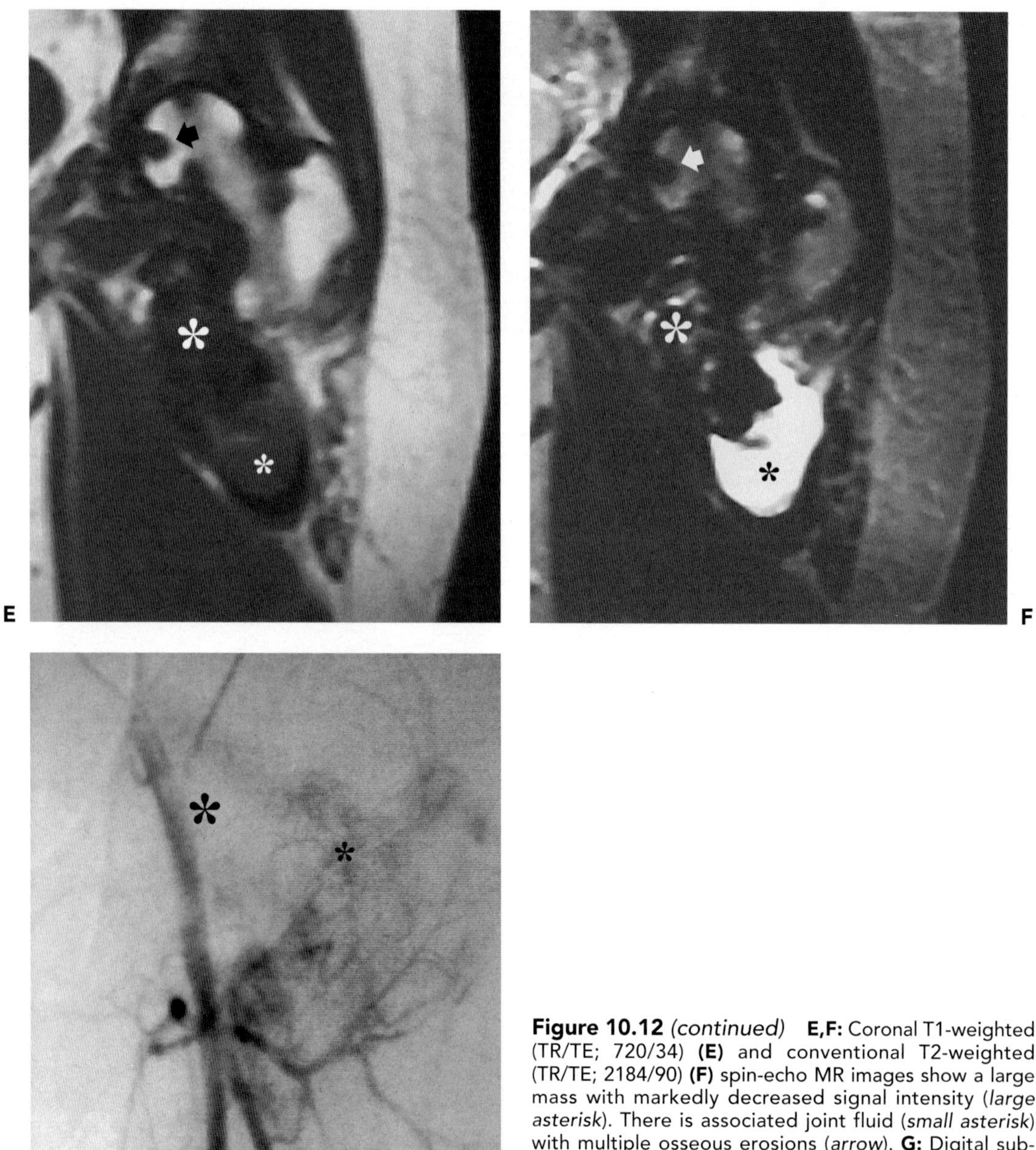

Figure 10.12 *(continued)* **E,F:** Coronal T1-weighted (TR/TE; 720/34) **(E)** and conventional T2-weighted (TR/TE; 2184/90) **(F)** spin-echo MR images show a large mass with markedly decreased signal intensity (*large asterisk*). There is associated joint fluid (*small asterisk*) with multiple osseous erosions (*arrow*). **G:** Digital subtraction image from arteriogram shows "tumor blush" around the acetabulum, femoral head, neck, and intertrochanteric region. The large asterisk marks the center of the femoral head; the small asterisk marks the well-defined lesion at the base of the femoral neck.

Giant synovial cysts, defined as large well-defined cavities filled with synovial fluid and lined by synoviumlike tissue, are also reported in association with rheumatoid arthritis and, less often, trauma, osteoarthritis, gout, systemic lupus erythematosus, and juvenile rheumatoid arthritis (81). These cysts typically involve the large joints, such as the knee, shoulder, and elbow, but they also are seen in the wrist, hand, foot, and ankle (81). Giant synovial cysts are also reported in pseudarthroses; they are thought to be caused by synovial proliferation with secondary formation of a fluid-filled, synovial-lined cavity (82). They occur most frequently following trauma to the femur, tibia, clavicle, metatarsal, ulna, and radius (83).

Bursae

Bursae are synovial-lined structures usually located between osseous surfaces, ligaments, or tendons (65,84). Because they normally contain only limited fluid, bursae are usually not readily identified on imaging studies. Superficial bursae do not communicate with the joint space (85).

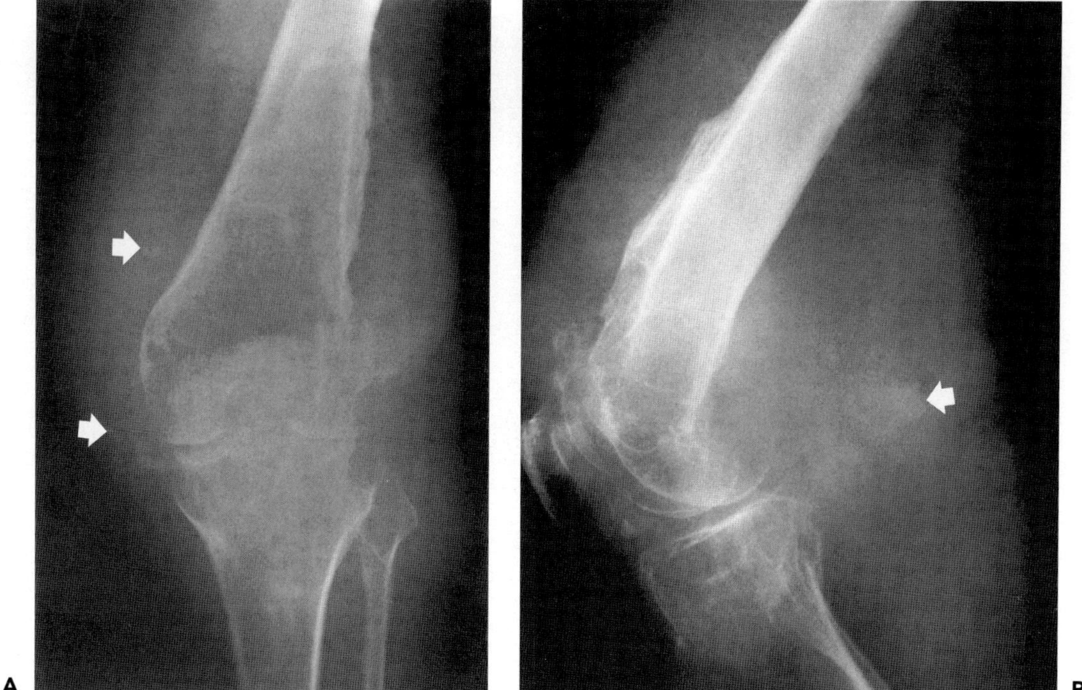

Figure 10.13 Pigmented villonodular synovitis: Unusual radiographic features in a man 41 years of age. **A,B:** Anteroposterior **(A)** and lateral **(B)** radiographs of the knee show extensive destructive change with a large associated soft tissue mass. Subtle calcification/ossification (*arrows*) is seen posteriorly and medially.

Inflammation from a variety of processes, such as overuse, trauma, infection, hemorrhage, or internal derangement, causes thickening of the synovial membrane and fluid accumulation within bursae (65). Fibrous adhesions may also be seen with long-standing bursitis (85). When bursitis is chronic, it may be complicated by hemorrhage and calcification; consequently it may mimic a soft tissue sarcoma (84).

Imaging of Synovial Cysts

A popliteal cyst is located between the tendons of the medial head of the gastrocnemius and semimembranosus muscles; hence this anatomic relationship defines the lesion (62). A small communication to the knee joint

often is observed on imaging studies (Fig. 10.20). MR imaging typically demonstrates a mass with low signal on T1-weighted and high signal on T2-weighted spin-echo MR images (86,87). Septations may be identified within the lesion (Fig. 10.21). The gastrocnemius-semimembranosus bursa is located superficial to the medial head of the gastrocnemius muscle (65). Fluid within it can be seen wrapping around the medial gastrocnemius tendon on transaxial images, concave toward the midline (65). Not uncommonly, a popliteal cyst may extend anterolaterally, communicating with the subgastrocnemius bursa (65). Unbending adherence to the anatomic requirements for the diagnosis of a popliteal cyst minimizes interpretive errors (Fig. 10.22).

The fluid from a ruptured popliteal cyst typically dissects along the medial aspect of the medial gastrocnemius muscle (Figs. 10.23 and 10.24). The protein-containing synovial fluid within the cyst may result in an increased signal intensity on T1-weighted images (88). Sundaram et al. (86) also reported a case in which the lesion appeared as intense as fat on T1-weighted images. Blood products within the cyst, from subclinical hemorrhage, may also be responsible for increased signal on T1-weighted images (Fig. 10.25) (82). Contrast enhancement may be seen in the cyst wall on both CT and MR imaging (Fig. 10.21) (89). Imaging features on CT mirror those on MR imag-

---

KEY CONCEPTS

- Uncomplicated cysts image as homogeneous fluid-filled masses.
- A popliteal cyst is located between the tendons of the medial head of the gastrocnemius and the semimembranosus muscles; this anatomic relationship defines this lesion.
- Any synovial cyst may be complicated by processes such as inflammation or hemorrhage.

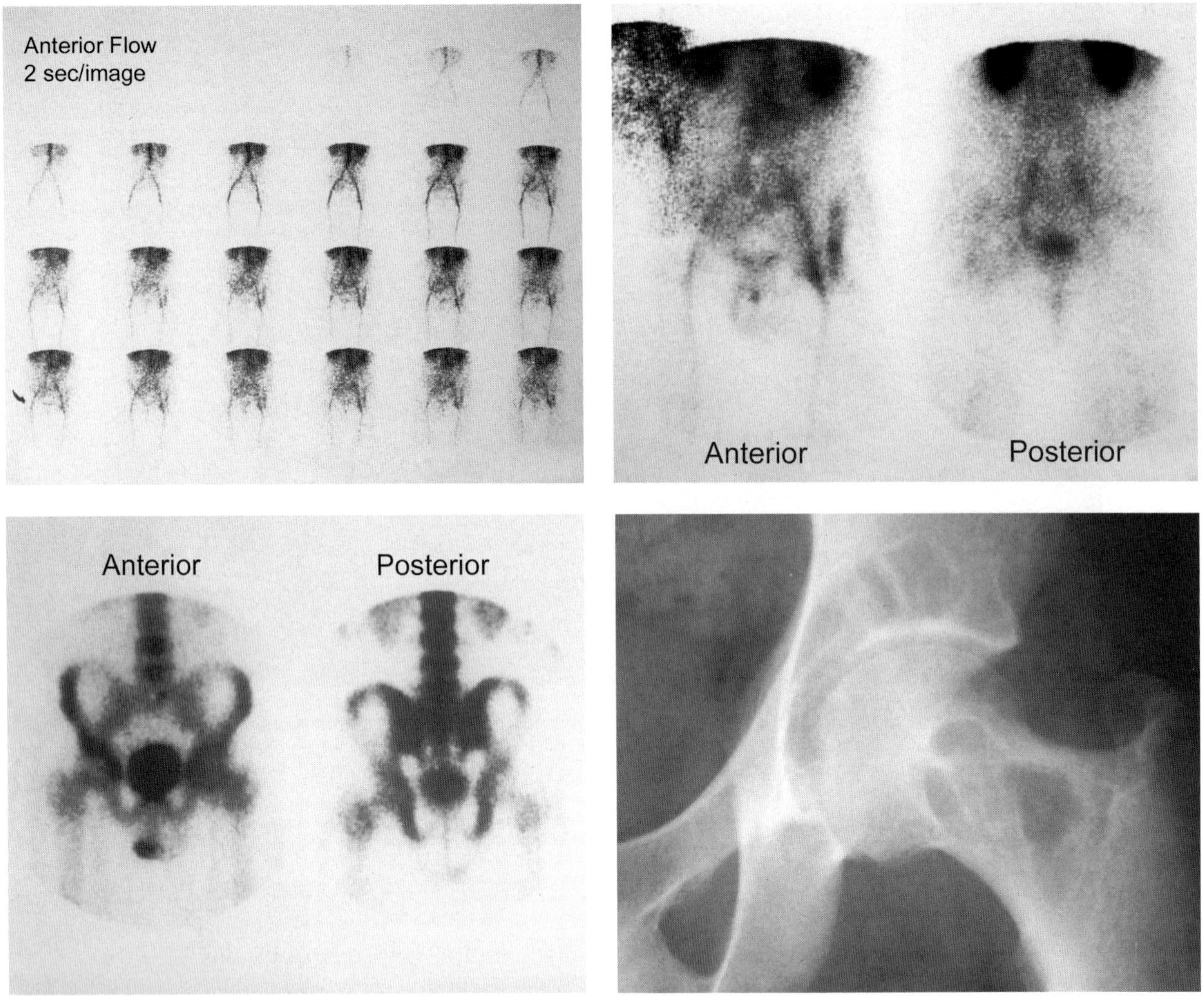

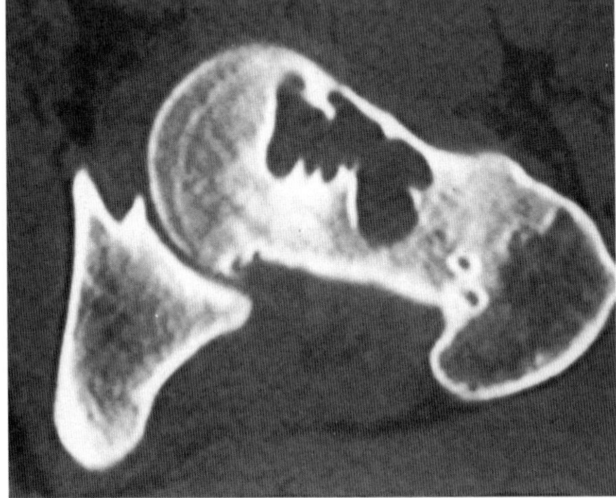

Figure 10.14 Pigmented villonodular synovitis: Technetium-99m methylene diphosphonate bone scan features in a man 32 years of age. **A,B:** Flow **(A)** and blood-pool **(B)** images show increased tracer accumulation in the soft tissues adjacent to the hip. Area of increased uptake in the left upper aspect of image **B** is an artifact from flow study. **C:** Delayed static images also show increased tracer accumulation within the acetabulum and femoral head and neck. **D:** Corresponding radiograph shows well-defined, geographic, lytic lesions with sclerotic margins on both sides of the joint, with preservation on the joint space. **E:** Axial noncontrast CT scan at the level of the midfemoral neck, displayed on bone window, shows the extent of intraosseous involvement in the femoral neck.

ing, demonstrating a homogeneous mass of approximately water density (89), usually with an associated joint effusion.

Arthrography, with lateral films of a flexed knee, may confuse a popliteal cyst with a bulging posterior knee capsule (81). A synovial cyst must be seen while the knee is in an extended position (81). Sonography reliably detects clinically significant popliteal cysts as hypoechoic fluid collections in the popliteal fossa (64,81). Sonography may also detect dissection into the calf or up into the thigh, as a

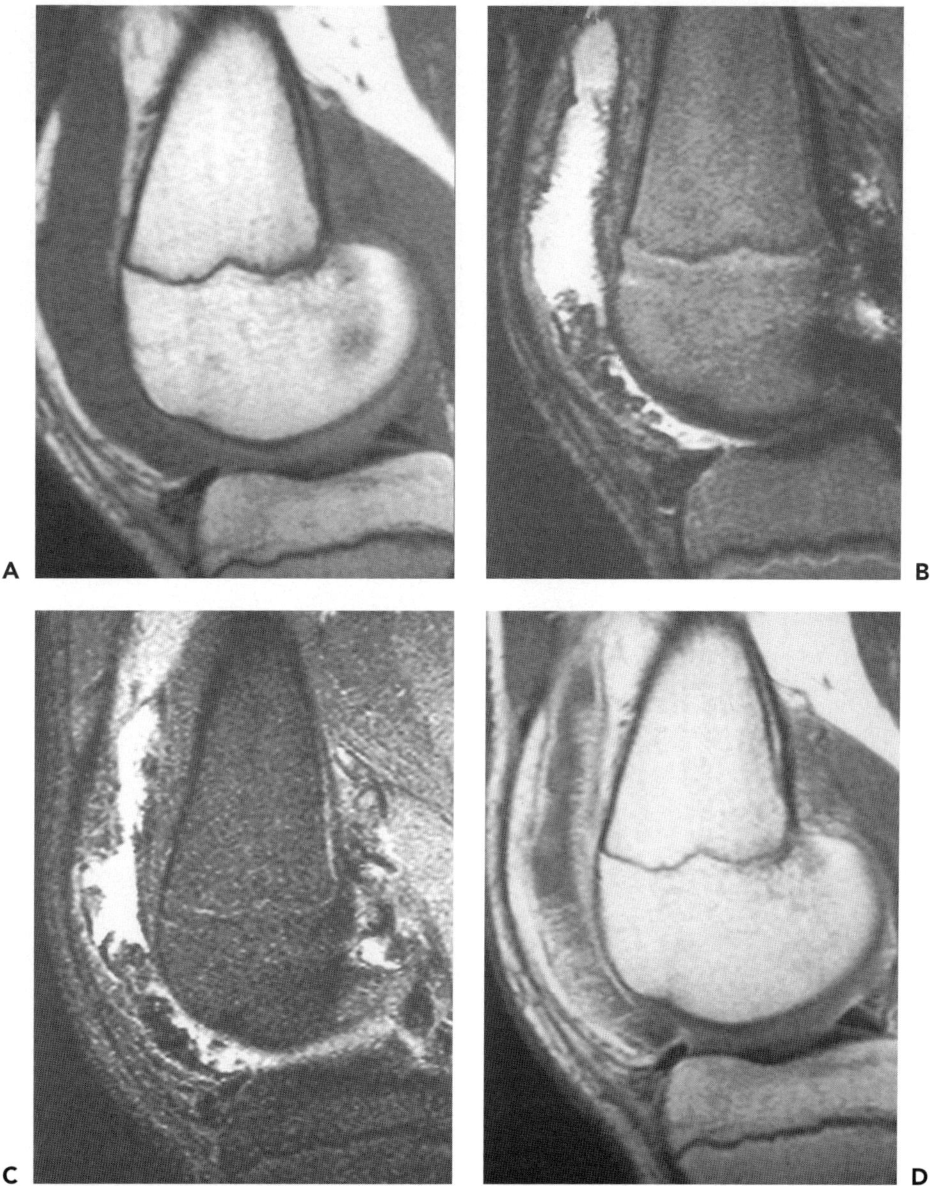

Figure 10.15 Pigmented villonodular synovitis: Typical MR imaging features in the knee of a boy 15 years of age presenting with a nontraumatic bloody knee joint effusion. **A,B:** Sagittal T1-weighted (TR/TE; 700/16) **(A)** and conventional T2-weighted (TR/TE; 2500/80) **(B)** spin-echo MR images show numerous irregular masses extending from the synovial surface. The lesions show more pronounced signal loss in **B. C:** Corresponding gradient-echo (TR/TE; 800/13) MR image shows "blooming," indicative of hemosiderin-laden tissue. **D:** Postcontrast T1-weighted (TR/TE; 700/16) spin-echo MR image shows extensive enhancement.

result of rupture (64). The popliteal artery is readily visualized with sonography; therefore, differentiation of a synovial cyst from a popliteal artery aneurysm is usually not difficult (64). Homogeneous hypoechoic neoplasms may mimic a popliteal cyst.

Synovial cysts image as simple homogeneous fluid collections. Often, a communicating neck may be seen from the originating structure, such as the proximal tibiofibular or hip joint (Fig. 10.26) (80). Uncomplicated bursitis also typically images as simple fluid collections on imaging

studies (Fig. 10.27). The imaging appearance of complicated bursitis is far more varied. Hemorrhagic bursitis shows imaging characteristics reflecting constituent blood and blood products, pannus, fluid, hemosiderin, and inflammation (84). These complicating factors typically result in a heterogeneous mass on imaging studies (Fig. 10.28). Dystrophic calcification, which may be more apparent on radiographs, contributes to the complex appearance by producing areas of decreased signal intensity on MR imaging (84).

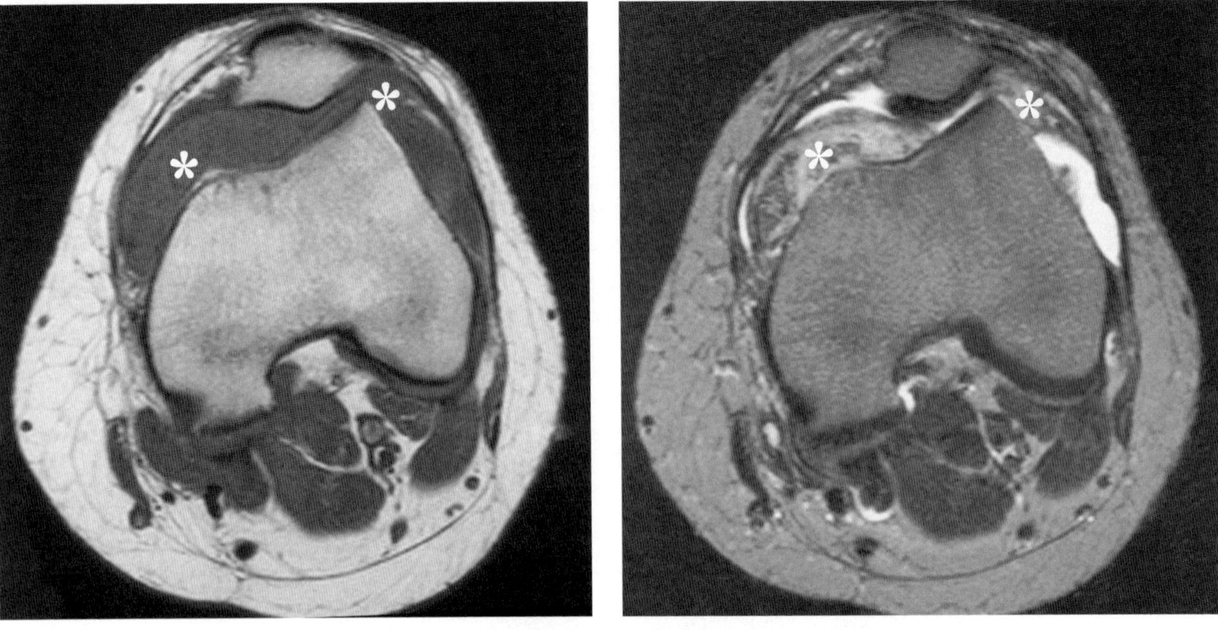

Figure 10.16 Pigmented villonodular synovitis: Typical MR imaging features in the knee of a woman 38 years of age. **A,B:** Axial T1-weighted (TR/TE; 650/15) **(A)** and conventional T2-weighted (TR/TE; 2500/80) **(B)** spin-echo MR images show a large multifocal, synovial-based mass (*asterisks*) with intermediate-to-decreased signal intensity.

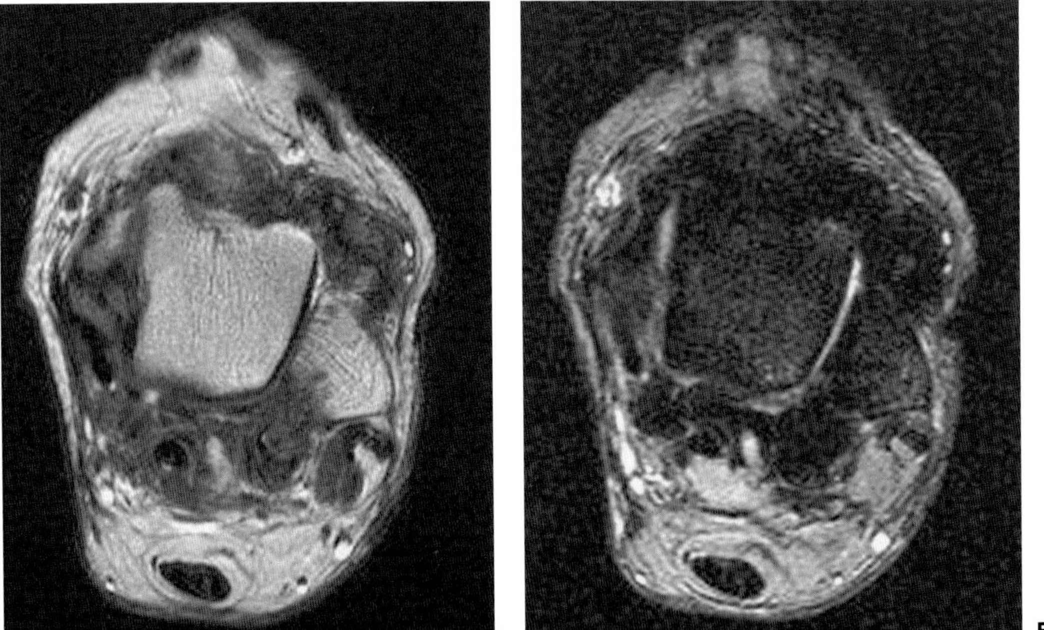

Figure 10.17 Pigmented villonodular synovitis: Typical "blooming" effects of hemosiderin in a woman 60 years of age with involvement of the ankle. **A,B:** Axial fast spin-echo T2-weighted (TR/TE; 4570/80) **(A)** and gradient-echo (TR/TE; 785/20) **(B)** MR images show a mass surrounding the ankle joint with marked loss of signal from the mass on gradient image **B.**

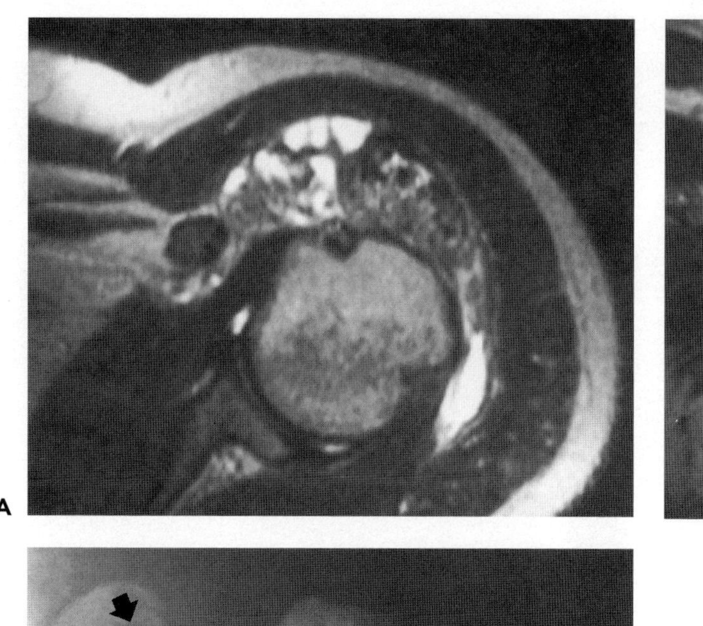

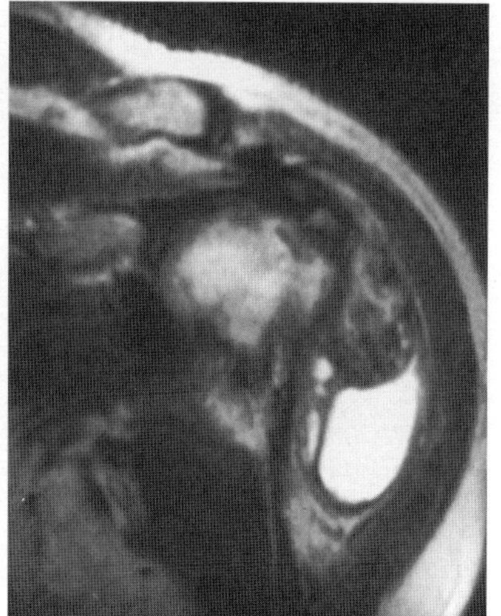

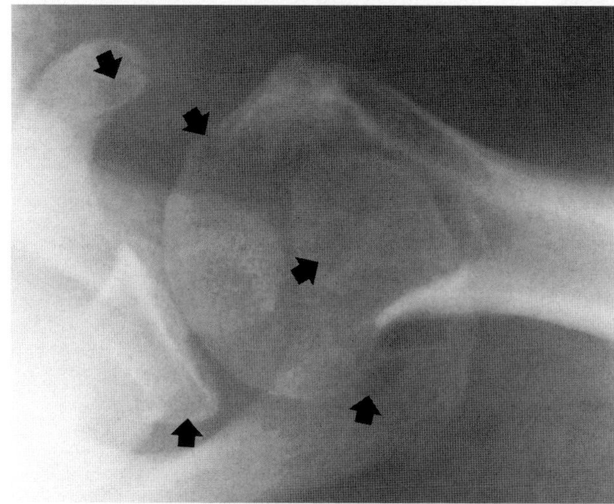

Figure 10.18 Bursal pigmented villo-nodular synovitis: Typical features in the sub-acromial/subdeltoid bursa of the shoulder in a woman 40 years of age. **A,B:** Axial T2-weighted (TR/TE; 2300/80) **(A)** and coronal T2-weighted (TR/TE; 2500/80) **(B)** spin-echo MR images of the shoulder show a mass in the subacromial/subdeltoid bursa with typical imaging features of PVNS. Note decreased signal intensity and associated effusion. **C:** Axillary radiograph of the shoulder shows well-defined erosions in the acromion, coracoid, glenoid, and humerus (*arrows*).

Ganglion

Classification

> ### KEY CONCEPTS
> - A ganglion is a tumorlike lesion of unknown origin that typically arises in the juxta-articular soft tissue.
> - No definitive classification system is available.
> - Ganglia can be conveniently divided into *juxta-articular*, *intra-articular*, and *periosteal* types.

A ganglion is a tumorlike lesion of unknown origin that arises in the juxta-articular soft tissue. Ganglia have been recognized since antiquity and were described by Hippocrates as a "knot of tissue containing mucoid flesh" (90,91). Synovial herniation and tissue degeneration, as well as repeated trauma, are suggested as causes (2,92).

Although their histogenesis is in question, they are classified as myxoid lesions and are presumably caused by a coalescence of small cysts formed by the myxomatous degeneration of periarticular connective tissue (2,93). Although the juxta-articular location of ganglia suggests they are the result of synovial herniation through a defect in the joint capsule or tendon sheath, communication between ganglia and the adjacent joint or tendon sheath is uncommon (65,94). When such a communication is present, it is difficult, if not impossible, to determine if such a communication is secondary or primary.

Because ganglia are not tumors, they are not addressed by the World Health Organization; therefore, there is no rigid classification. We find it convenient to separate them into three broad types: conventional *juxta-articular* ganglia (typical lesions arising in the juxta-articular region); *intra-articular* ganglia (those arising within a joint, usually associated with cruciate ligaments); and *periosteal* ganglia (those associated with the periosteum).

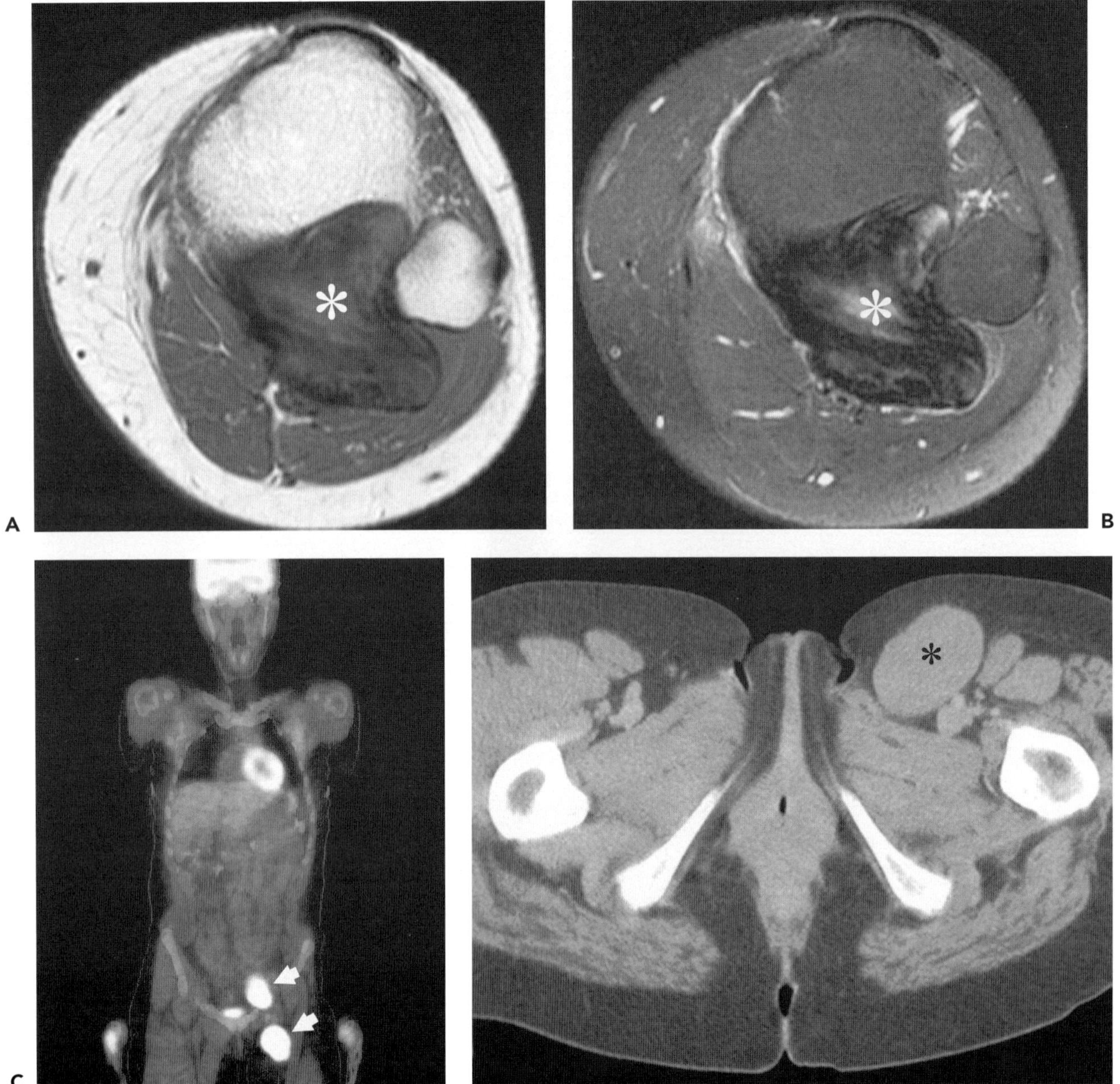

Figure 10.19 Malignant pigmented villonodular synovitis: Imaging features in a woman 35 years of age with a long history of PVNS. The patient's initial lesion in the left knee was treated by synovectomy more than 20 years ago and she has had multiple local recurrences. **A,B:** Axial T1-weighted (TR/TE; 608/14) **(A)** and fat-suppressed T2-weighted (TR/TE; 3800/77) **(B)** spin-echo MR images of the knee show a mass with decreased signal intensity and typical imaging features of PVNS. **C:** Positron emission tomography (PET)/CT shows two hypermetabolic foci in the left groin (*arrows*). **D:** Axial enhanced CT scan of the groin shows enlarged inguinal node (*asterisk*) corresponding to hypermetabolic focus seen on PET/CT. (*continued*)

Juxta-Articular Ganglion

Juxta-articular ganglia are quite common, and approximately 70% of ganglia are located around the wrist. Ganglia account for 50% to 70% of all soft tissue masses of the wrist (95,96). In a review of 625 wrist MR imaging examinations, el-Noueam et al. (97) found ganglia in 120 patients (19%); 80% were on the radial side, 18% on the ulna side, and 2% in the lunotriquetral articulation. In that study, volar lesions outnumbered dorsal lesions 1.6:1. Less commonly, ganglia arise in the foot, although ganglia may develop adjacent to any joint or tendon sheath (98,99). Typically presenting in young adults (25 to 45 years of age), there is female predominance (2,92,96). Patients may note a palpable mass (Fig. 10.29), although lesions are often asymptomatic. About half the cases are associated with tenderness, mild pain, or functional impairment (2,92). Ganglia may grow, diminish in size, or resolve spontaneously (90). In some cases they may compress adjacent structures and be the cause of nerve palsy (100). Fritz et al. (101) reported 27 patients with entrapment of the suprascapular nerve, noting ganglion as the cause in 21 (78%) cases. Ganglia may also extend from the joint into the adjacent muscle. Bianchi et al. (102) reported six ganglia extending from the proximal tibiofibular joint.

Most ganglia are small, measuring 1.5 to 2.5 cm. Lesions may be unilocular or multilocular, are typically rounded to lobular in shape, and are adjacent to joint capsules or tendon sheaths (90). Microscopically, thick-walled cystic spaces are seen in association with myxoid areas, which may be outside the cystic spaces (2). The lesion is surrounded by dense connective tissue and filled with viscous, gelatinous fluid that is rich in hyaluronic acid and other mucopolysaccharides (103). There is no discernible internal lining cell type (Fig. 10.29) (93).

Intra-Articular Ganglion

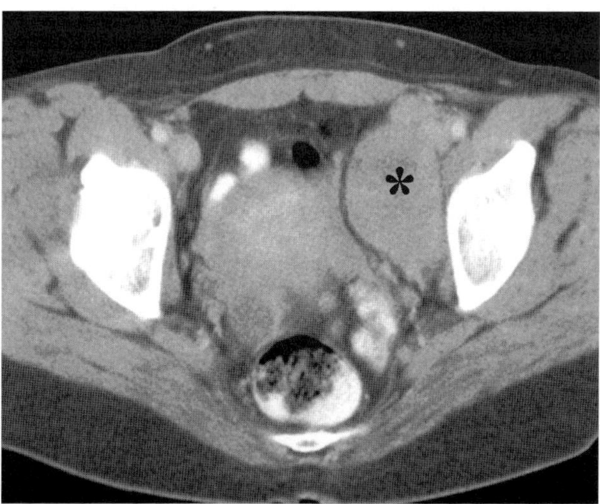

E

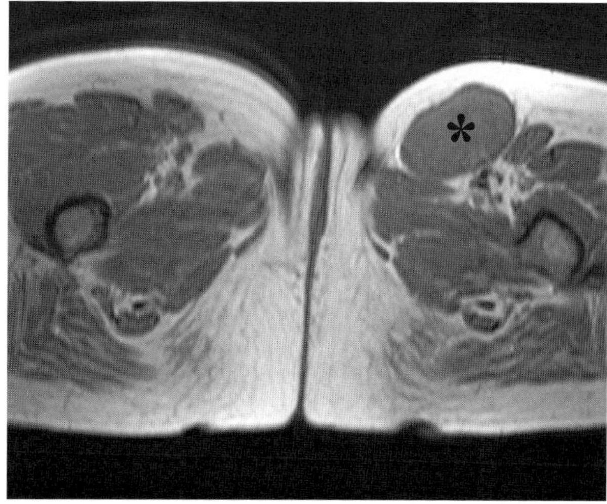

F

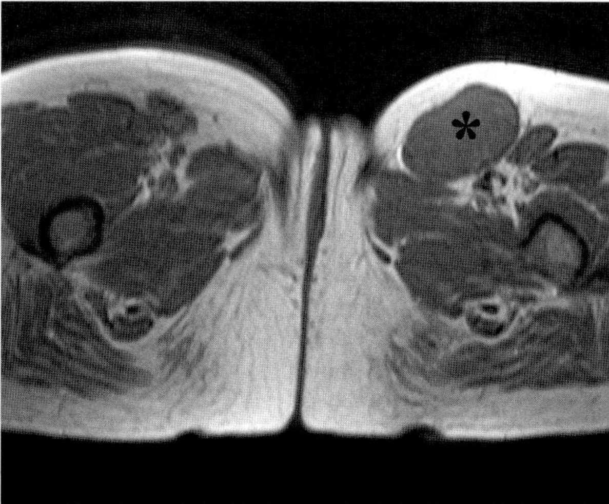

G

Figure 10.19 *(continued)* **E:** Axial enhanced CT scan of the pelvis shows external iliac node (*asterisk*) corresponding to PET/CT abnormality. **F,G:** Axial T1-weighted (TR/TE; 723/15) **(F)** and T2-weighted (TR/TE; 3530/69) **(G)** spin-echo MR images of the groin show the inguinal node (*asterisk*).

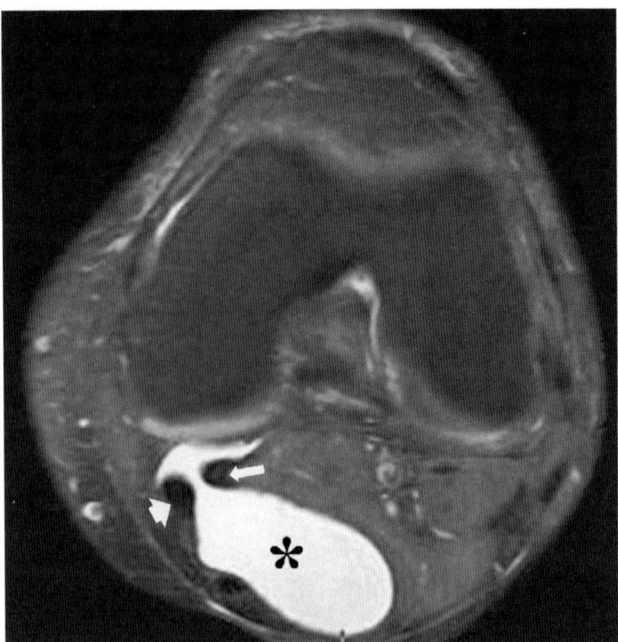

Figure 10.20 Popliteal cyst: Typical MR imaging appearance. Axial fat-suppressed fast spin-echo proton density (TR/TE; 4000/24) MR image shows fluid in a distended gastrocnemius-semimembranosus bursa (*asterisk*), communicating with the knee joint. The bursa lies between the tendons of the medial head of the gastrocnemius muscles (*long arrow*) and semimembranosus (*short arrow*).

Intra-articular ganglia are relatively rare lesions that were initially identified in association with the anterior cruciate ligament at autopsy by Caan in 1924 (104). Reported with an incidence on MR imaging of 0.9 to 1.3% (105,106), intra-articular ganglia may be within or adjacent to the cruciate ligaments (107–109). The incidence on MR imaging correlates well with a 0.8% incidence found on arthroscopy (110). Cruciate ganglia are classified by their origin into three types: type 1, located anterior to the anterior cruciate ligament; type 2, located between the anterior and posterior cruciate ligament; and type 3, posterior to the posterior cruciate ligament (107). At arthroscopy, nearly two-thirds of ganglia originate from the anterior cruciate ligament, most frequently from the tibial insertion (110). Although the cause of cruciate ganglia is unknown, they are presumed to arise from mucinous degeneration of connective tissue, a mechanism similar to that of other ganglia (111). Other theories of pathogenesis suggest origin from herniation of synovial tissue through a capsular defect, similar to the mechanism suggested for wrist ganglia (105). In contrast to juxta-articular ganglia, which show a recurrence rate of approximately 20%, the recurrence rate for intra-articular ganglia is extremely low (108). This difference in natural history suggests these lesions may have distinct underlying causes (108).

Cruciate ganglia may coexist with mucoid degeneration of the cruciate ligament (108). In a study of 74 patients with ganglion-like abnormalities of the anterior cruciate ligament, Bergin et al. (111) found that 56

patients (76%) had discrete ganglia, 18 patients (24%) had mucoid degeneration, and 26 patients (35%) had features of both. Intraosseous abnormalities frequently coexist with cruciate ligament ganglia, and MRI-diagnosed intraosseous abnormalities are found in two-thirds of patients with anterior cruciate ligament ganglia and three-quarters of patients with mucoid degeneration (108).

Clinical symptoms are variable, but patients are usually asymptomatic, with approximately 90% of lesions believed to be incidental findings at arthroscopy (110). When present, symptoms include pain, mechanical locking, clicking, and limitation of motion (109,111). Cysts anterior to the anterior cruciate ligament tend to limit extension; those behind the posterior cruciate ligament limit flexion (110). A variety of treatments are used, including arthroscopic aspiration, arthroscopic excision, surgical excision, and ultrasound-guided aspiration (112).

Periosteal Ganglion

KEY CONCEPTS

- The periosteal ganglion is a rare lesion; the majority are found in the region of the pes anserinus.
- Presenting symptoms include swelling and mild tenderness.
- Occasionally, periosteal ganglion presentation may mimic that of internal derangement of the knee.
- Most patients are adults in the fourth and fifth decades.

Periosteal ganglion is a rare lesion. Okada et al. (113) reported three cases and found 17 previous cases in their 1996 review of the medical literature. Periosteal ganglia are more common in men (approximately 70% of cases) (114). The majority of lesions are found in the region of the pes anserinus (113,114). The remaining lesions mainly affect the ends of long tubular bones, including the distal shafts of the ulna, radius, femur, and medial malleolus (114–117). Patients usually present with swelling and mild tenderness. When the knee is involved, symptoms may mimic those associated with internal derangement (114). Most patients are adults in the fourth or fifth decade, although the lesions have been reported in children (113,115). While the cause is unknown, periosteal ganglia are thought to derive from mucinous degeneration of the periosteum (115,118). Other theories speculate that periosteal ganglia develop when fluid migrates from a distended joint into the periarticular soft tissue (119). De Maeseneer et al. (119) reported a case in which a tibial periosteal ganglion filled following injection of contrast into the knee joint.

Treatment options include excision, puncture, and aspiration, with or without injection of corticosteroids (115,119). If a communication with the adjacent joint exists, this should also be excised. In the knee, the lesion is

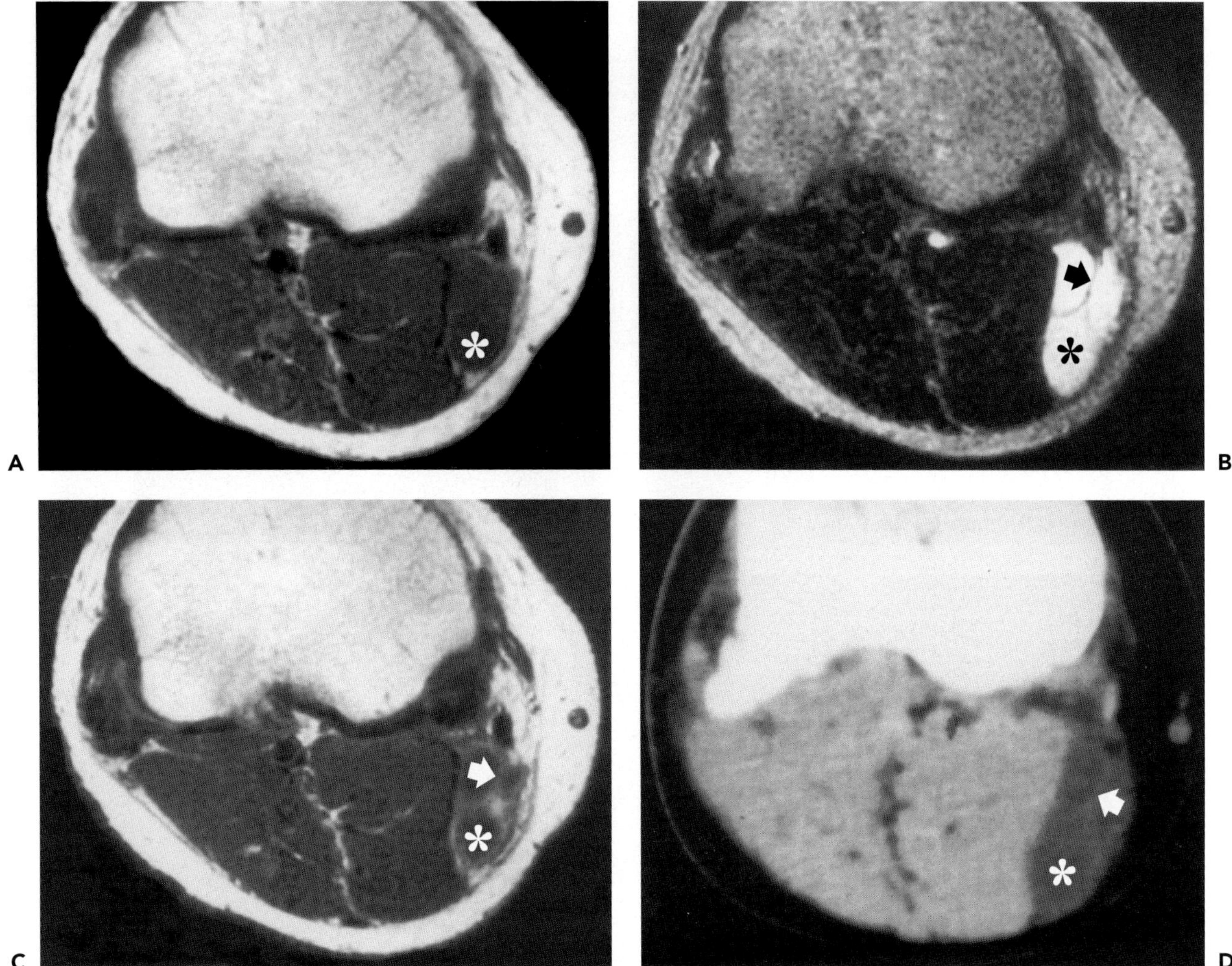

Figure 10.21 Popliteal cyst: Septated appearance in a man 22 years of age. **A,B:** Axial T1-weighted (TR/TE; 733/16) **(A)** and T2-weighted (TR/TE; 1800/80) **(B)** spin-echo MR images show a fluid collection located between the tendons of the medial head of the gastrocnemius and semimembranosus muscles (*asterisk*). Subtle thin septations are seen within the cyst (*arrow*) in **B. C:** Axial T1-weighted (TR/TE; 567/20) spin-echo MR image following contrast administration shows enhancement at the periphery of the lesion (*asterisk*), as well as around septations (*arrow*) within the lesion. **D:** Corresponding axial CT scan, displayed on soft tissue window, shows the cystic nature of the lesion (*asterisk*), as well as the septations (*arrow*) within it.

readily differentiated from pes anserine bursitis, which is characterized on MR imaging by the presence of fluid beneath the tendons of the pes anserinus at the medial aspect of the tibia near the joint line (120). As with periosteal ganglia, patients with pes anserine bursitis may present with signs and symptoms mimicking those of internal derangement.

Imaging of Ganglia

Radiographs in patients with juxta-articular ganglia may be normal or may reveal a soft tissue mass. The adjacent bone occasionally demonstrates evidence of bone resorption caused by pressure remodeling or periosteal new bone (2). Ultrasound and MR imaging are both effective in detecting ganglia; however, the lower cost of ultrasound makes it use-

> ### KEY CONCEPTS
> - Uncomplicated ganglia image as multilobulated cystlike lesions.
> - Lesions are typically well-defined, often with a corrugated appearance.
> - MR imaging may show peripheral enhancement and, rarely, central enhancement.
> - Ultrasound is useful as the initial imaging modality.
> - Periosteal ganglia may show cortical scalloping caused by extrinsic pressure remodeling.

ful as the first imaging modality of choice (96). Ultrasound readily detects even small ganglia, which may be identified as small fluid collections, appearing as well-defined

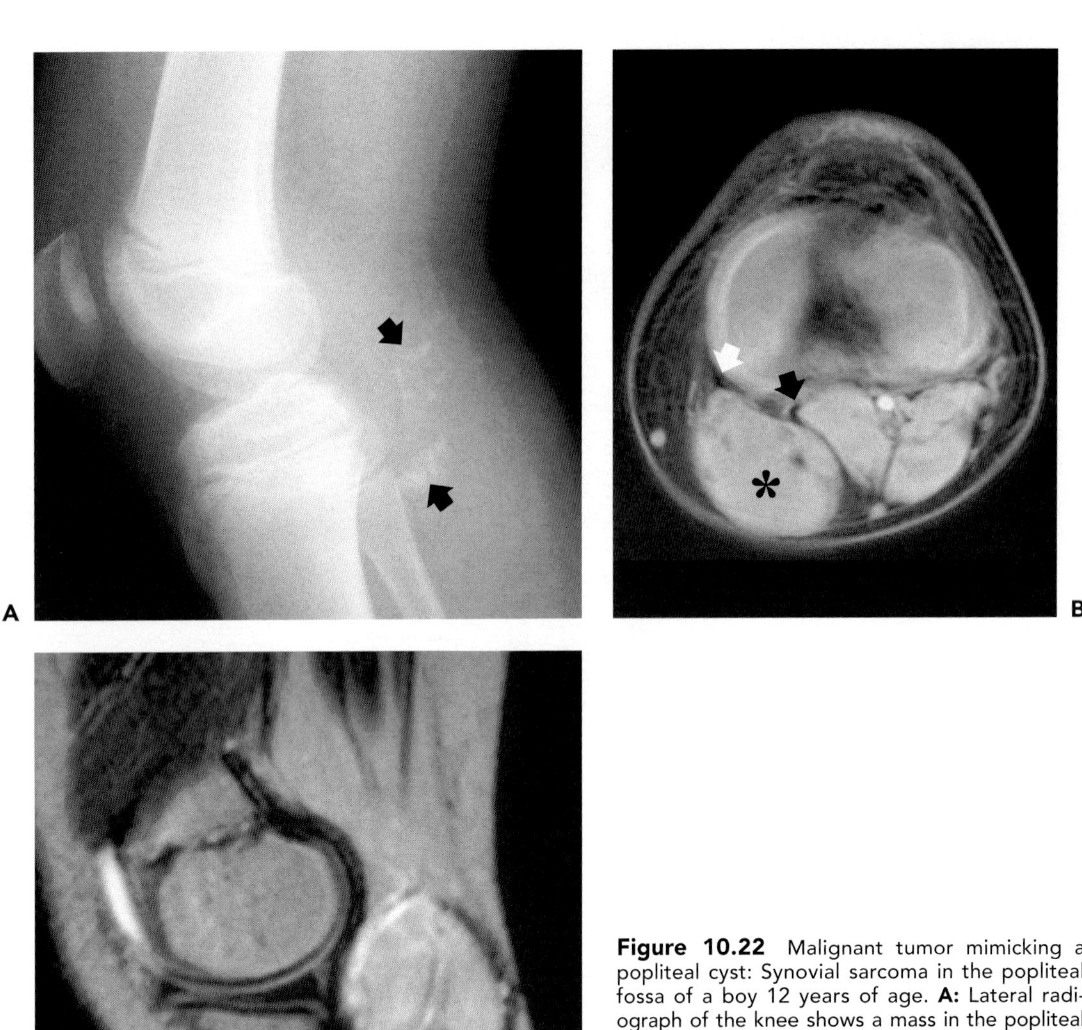

Figure 10.22 Malignant tumor mimicking a popliteal cyst: Synovial sarcoma in the popliteal fossa of a boy 12 years of age. **A:** Lateral radiograph of the knee shows a mass in the popliteal fossa with multiple small calcifications (*arrows*). **B:** Axial gradient-echo (TR/TE/Flip angle; 20/9/25 degrees) MR image shows rounded mass (*asterisk*) along the medial aspect of the knee. The mass does not communicate with the knee joint, nor is it located between the tendons of the medial head of the gastrocnemius (*black arrow*) and semimembranosus (*white arrow*) muscles. **C:** Sagittal fast spin-echo T2-weighted (TR/TE; 2873/85) MR image shows a well-defined, intermediate signal intensity mass adjacent to the gastrocnemius muscle. Note focus of decreased signal intensity (*arrow*) from calcification. (Courtesy of H. Thomas Temple, MD, University of Miami.)

homogeneously anechoic masses (96,97,100,121,122). Occasionally, septations may be present (96). Long-standing lesions may demonstrate a more complex cystic appearance, especially if complicated by hemorrhage or infection. Following aspiration, ganglia may demonstrate internal echoes mimicking those of a solid tumor (95,122). Occasionally, a communication to the joint may be demonstrated (94), or "pseudopodia" may be seen extending toward the joint (96).

A ganglion typically appears as a multilobulated cyst-like mass on MR imaging with low signal intensity on T1-weighted images and high signal intensity on T2-weighted or fluid-sensitive images (Fig. 10.30) (100,101,103,107,123). Uncommonly, it may be isointense or slightly hyperintense to muscle on T1-weighted spin-echo images (90), with the increased signal intensity on T1-weighted images caused by a high protein content within the lesion. This may also create an attenuation higher than that of simple fluid on CT scanning. Rim enhancement may be seen following gadolinium administration, although less commonly, more extensive enhancement may be noted (Figs. 10.30 and 10.31) (101,122). Feldman et al. (90) noted sharply defined, delicate internal septa, creating a characteristic corrugated or

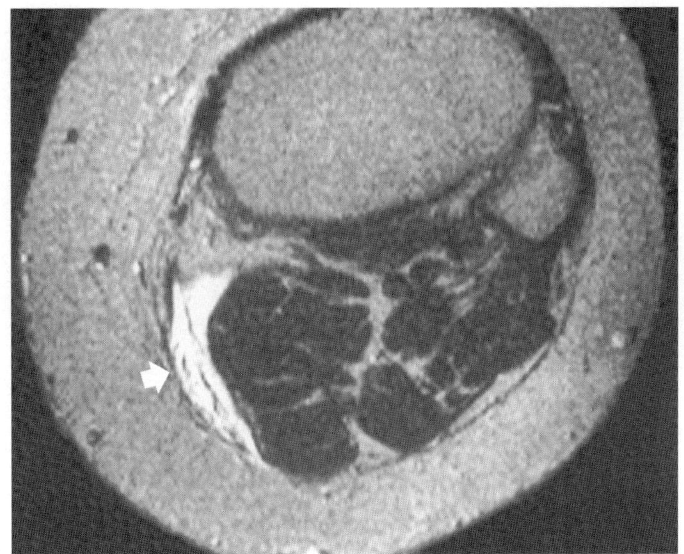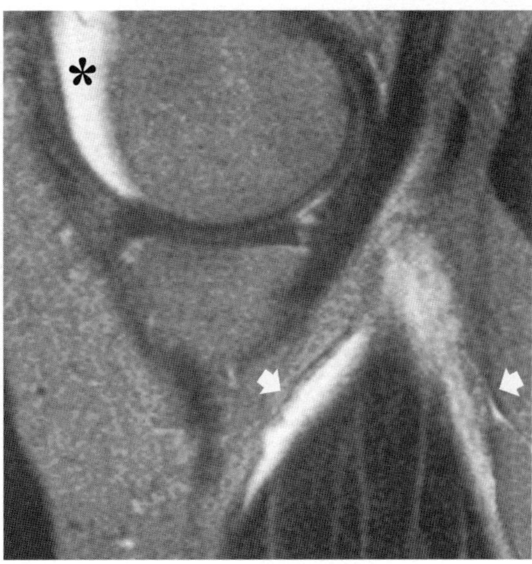

Figure 10.23 Dissecting popliteal cyst: Typical MR imaging features in a woman 46 years of age. **A,B:** Axial **(A)** and sagittal **(B)** T2-weighted (TR/TE; 2500/90) spin-echo MR images of the knee show a fluid collection along the medial aspect of the medial head of the gastrocnemius muscle (*arrows*). Note associated joint effusion (*asterisk*) in **B.**

compartmentalized MR imaging appearance in 13 of 17 cases, as well as small fluid-filled pseudopodia in 11 of 17 cases. MR imaging not only localizes the lesion, but it identifies its relationship to adjacent structures, including vessels, tendons, and nerves (123). The relationship to adjacent joints, capsules, and tendons is best demonstrated on long TR/TE or gradient imaging sequences (90). Ganglia may be associated with major vessels in 10% to 20% of cases, making aspiration difficult (Fig. 10.31) (123,124). When adjacent nerves are compressed (compressive neuropathy), MR imaging may reveal abnormalities in the corresponding muscle groups, including atrophy, fat infiltration, and increased signal intensity on T2-weighted images (Fig. 10.32).

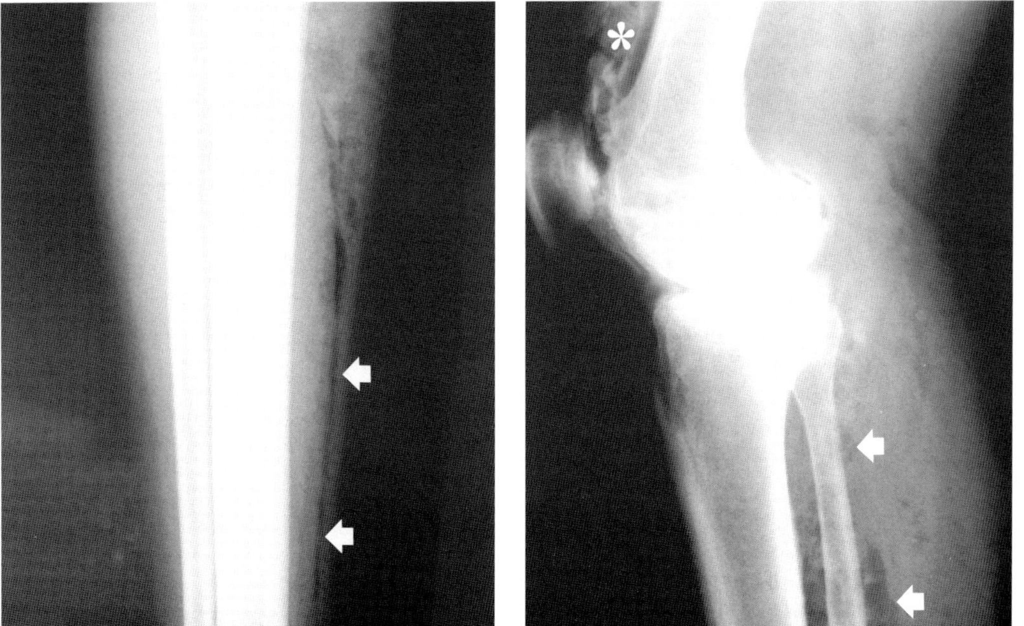

Figure 10.24 Dissecting popliteal cyst: Arthrographic features in a woman 56 years of age. **A,B:** Anteroposterior **(A)** and lateral radiographs **(B)** of the lower leg following arthrogram show contrast and air dissecting into the lower leg along the medial head of the gastrocnemius muscle (*arrows*). Note contrast in joint on lateral radiograph (*asterisk*) from double-contrast arthrogram in **B.**

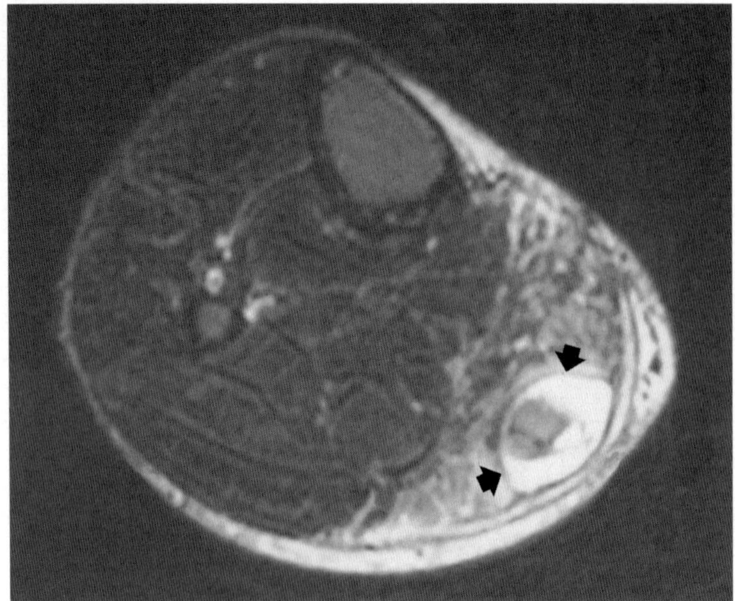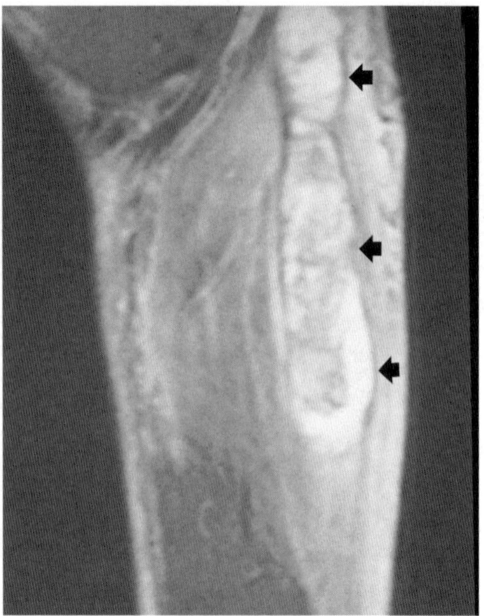

Figure 10.25 Hemorrhagic dissecting popliteal cyst: Imaging features in a woman 59 years of age. **A,B:** Axial fast spin-echo inversion recovery (TR/TE; 6000/85) **(A)** and sagittal T2-weighted (TR/TE; 2000/68) **(B)** spin-echo MR images of the knee show a complex fluid collection along the medial aspect of the medial head of the gastrocnemius muscle (*arrows*). Note associated edema and inflammatory change.

The MR imaging appearance of intra-articular cruciate ganglia is also quite characteristic. Recht et al. (109) reported the MR imaging features in 16 cases and noted that those associated with the posterior cruciate ligament typically appeared as well-defined, multiloculated cysts along the surface of the ligament, and those associated with the anterior cruciate ligament typically had a fusiform appearance along the course of and interspersed within the fibers of the ligament (Fig. 10.33). MR imaging criteria for anterior cruciate ganglia include fluid signal in the substance of the ligament, mass effect on the cruciate ligament fibers, lobulated margins, and anterior cruciate ligament fluid disproportionate to joint fluid (Fig. 10.34) (111). MR imaging criteria for mucoid degeneration of the anterior cruciate ligament are poor delineation of the anterior cruciate ligament fibers on T1-weighted or proton density sequences, with delineation on T2-weighted sequences (111). As with juxta-articular ganglia, the signal intensity of the ganglia on T2-weighted images may be complex.

Periosteal ganglia may also show a characteristic imaging appearance. The hallmark of radiographic diagnosis is cortical scalloping, caused by extrinsic pressure remodeling (113–117,119). Thick spicules of reactive periosteal new bone may extend from the scalloped area (114,116,117,119). The periosteal spicules may be oriented perpendicular to the underlying cortex and appear thick and well-defined (119). CT demonstrates a well-defined soft tissue mass adjacent to cortical bone, with an attenuation equal to that of fluid (114,119). MR imaging shows a homogeneous, well-

defined juxtacortical mass with signal intensity approximately equal to that of skeletal muscle on T1-weighted images and brighter than that of fat on T2-weighted spin-echo MR images (Fig. 10.35) (114,116,117,119). Peripheral enhancement can be seen following gadopentetate administration, although the cyst itself should not enhance (119). Sonography demonstrates a hypoechoic, juxtacortical collection, with interspersed hyperechoic linear lines corresponding to the areas on new bone formation (119).

Juxta-Articular Myxoma

KEY CONCEPTS

- Juxta-articular myxoma is a rare myxoid lesion closely resembling ganglion and intramuscular myxoma.
- Patients typically present with an enlarging juxta-articular mass.
- The lesion is usually seen in the third to fifth decade, and is three times more common in men.
- Approximately 85% of cases occur around the knee.
- Juxta-articular myxoma is likely related to meniscal cyst.

The juxta-articular myxoma is a rare myxoid tumor that bears a close histological resemblance to intramuscular myxoma (125). The histological similarity of these two lesions suggests a common pathogenesis; however, recent genetic studies indicate that juxta-articular and intramus-

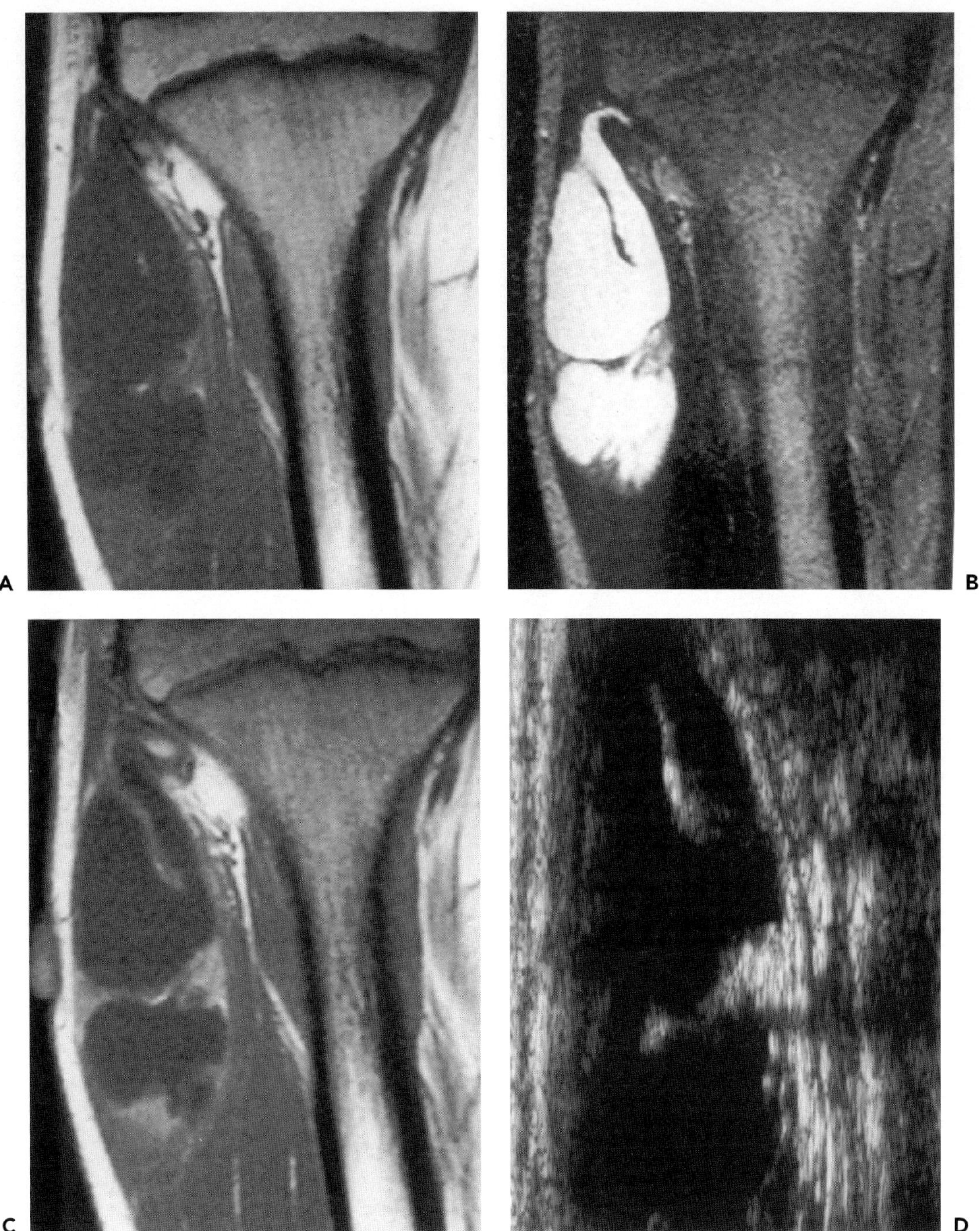

Figure 10.26 Synovial cyst: Typical imaging features in a boy 12 years of age with an enlarging calf mass for 11 months. **A,B:** Coronal T1-weighted (TR/TE; 567/20) **(A)** and T2-weighted (TR/TE; 1800/80) **(B)** spin-echo MR images of the knee show a well-defined mass adjacent to the proximal tibiofibular joint. The mass originates from the joint and has a signal intensity compatible with that of fluid. **C:** Coronal T1-weighted (TR/TE; 567/20) spin-echo MR image following gadolinium administration shows peripheral enhancement. **D:** Corresponding ultrasound shows the mass is fluid-filled. At surgery, the lesion was fluid-filled and lined by synovium.

cular myoma represent distinct entities with different underlying molecular mechanisms (125). Juxta-articular myxoma, also known as *periarticular myxoma*, usually occurs around large joints, particularly the knee (2,126). Although juxta-articular myxoma has histological features similar to those of a myxoma, it is frequently associated with cystic change that closely resembles a ganglion (2,126). The origin of the cystic change is uncertain but is suspected to be the result of motion, friction, or torsion affecting certain joints and adjacent structures (126). The

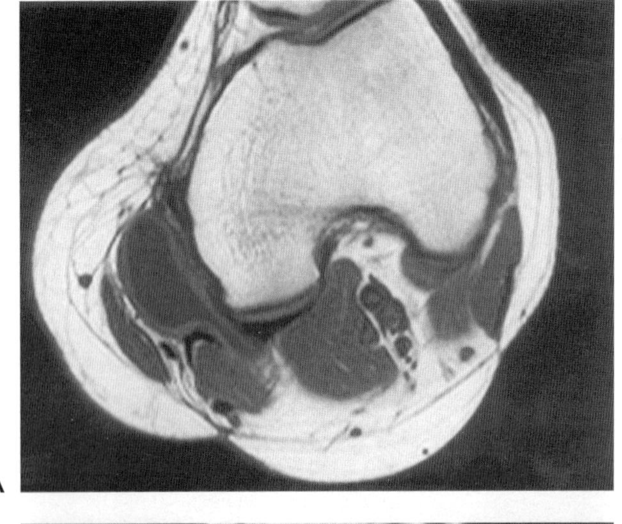

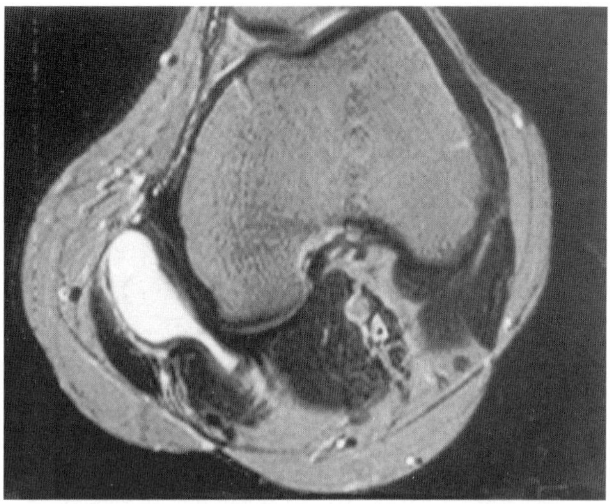

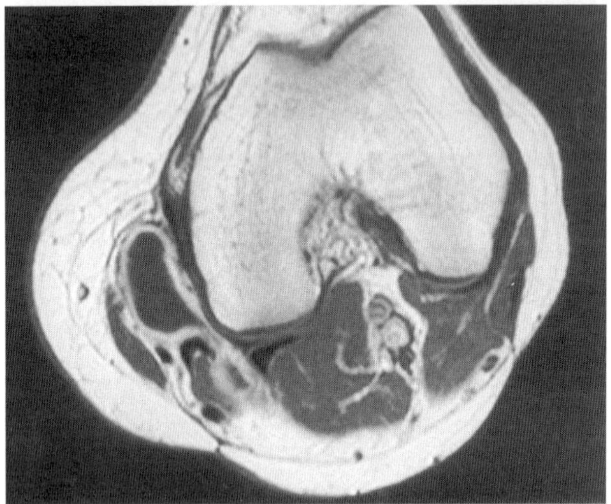

Figure 10.27 Uncomplicated bursitis: Typical imaging appearance in a woman 51 years of age. **A,B:** Axial T1-weighted (TR/TE; 700/16) **(A)** and conventional T2-weighted (TR/TE; 2000/80) **(B)** spin-echo MR images show a mass in the medial aspect of the right knee, with signal intensity compatible with that of fluid. Note inflammatory rind with slight increased signal intensity in **(A)**. **C:** Axial T1-weighted (TR/TE; 700/16) spin-echo MR image following contrast administration shows peripheral enhancement, likely caused by inflammation and fibrovascular connective tissue in the wall.

role of trauma in the development of juxta-articular myxoma is uncertain; however, trauma may explain its predilection for the knee and frequent association with degenerative joint disease (126).

Most patients present with an enlarging, painful mass (126–129), usually in the third to fifth decade of life, although children may also be affected (126,127). Juxta-articular myxoma is more common in males by almost 3:1 (125,126,128). Approximately 85% of lesions occur around the knee, a quarter of which involve the meniscus (126,128). Other reported joints include the shoulder, elbow, hip, ankle, and foot (129,130). The lesion has a tendency to recur locally, with a recurrence rate as high as 34% (126).

Grossly, the lesion tends to be small, usually 3 cm to 4 cm, but it may be considerably larger. The vast majority (90%) contain multiple cystic spaces and may resemble a ganglion grossly and microscopically; however, the latter have a much less-developed myxoid component (126).

Juxta-articular myxoma is characterized by large amounts of myxoid material and a paucity of cells, with a poorly developed vascular pattern (2). The lesion is rich in hyaluronic acid and glycosaminoglycans (2). In long-standing cases, there may be calcification of the myxoid material (131). Recurrence following surgery is not uncommon, occurring in approximately a third of cases (126).

Juxta-articular myxoma may be distinguished clinically from ganglion in that the latter occurs predominantly in the hand and wrist of young women, is associated with the tendon or joint capsule, and is usually much smaller (126). The relationship between meniscal cyst and juxta-articular myxoma is more complex. Both are seen predominantly in middle-aged men. Meis and Enzinger (126) noted 14 patients with meniscal involvement in their report of 65 cases of juxta-articular myxoma, 9 (64%) of which involved the lateral meniscus. In five cases, a meniscal tear was identified. The similarity in clinical presentation

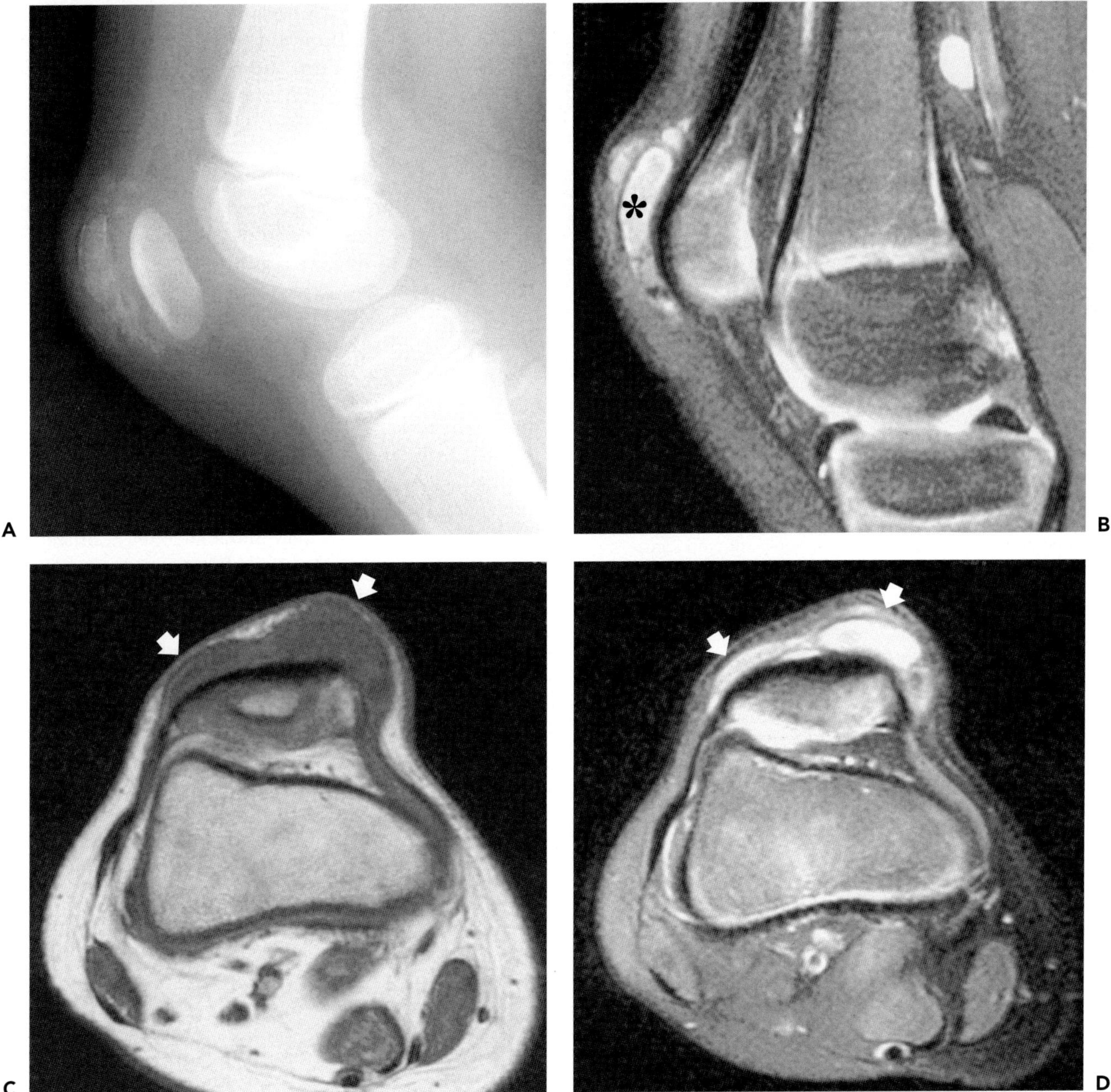

Figure 10.28 Calcific prepatellar bursitis: Imaging appearance in a girl 6 years of age presenting with a prepatellar mass. **A:** Lateral radiograph shows a lobulated, calcified, prepatellar mass. **B:** Sagittal, fat-suppressed, fast proton density (TR/TE; 3250/51) spin-echo MR image shows a lobulated prepatellar mass (*asterisk*). Note small reactive node in the popliteal fossa. **C,D:** Axial T1-weighted (TR/TE; 600/12) **(C)** and fat-suppressed fast proton density (TR/TE; 3850/52) **(D)** spin-echo MR images show a lobulated prepatellar mass (*arrows*). The mass has a fluidlike signal intensity. The decreased signal intensity from the mineralization seen on radiograph is not well appreciated.

and skeletal distribution suggests that these lesions are likely related.

Imaging of Juxta-Articular Myxoma

There is scant literature on the radiologic appearance of juxta-articular myxoma; however, lesions image similar to ganglion and myxoma, demonstrating a signal intensity less than that of skeletal muscle on T1-weighted images and brighter than that of fat on T2-weighted spin-echo MR images (Figs. 10.36 and 10.37) (131). Inhomogeneous enhancement is seen following gadopentetate administration (131). Clearly, the full spectrum of the radiologic appearance is unknown, and cases in which the lesion demonstrated an inhomogeneous intermediate signal intensity (similar to that of fat) on T2-weighted images are described (129,131).

> ### KEY CONCEPTS
> - Limited reports of imaging features are available.
> - MR imaging features are similar to those of a ganglion, with fluidlike signal intensity.
> - Lesions with intermediate signal intensity on T2-weighted MR images are reported.
> - Inhomogeneous enhancement is observed following gadopentetate.

Synovial Chondromatosis

> ### KEY CONCEPTS
> - Synovial chondromatosis is a benign lesion characterized by the formation of multiple cartilaginous nodules in the synovium.
> - It occurs most commonly in synovium of joints, but also occurs in tendons and bursae.
> - The knee is by far the most commonly affected joint, involved in more than 50% of cases.
> - It most commonly affects patients in the third through fifth decades of life.
> - Men are affected approximately two to four times more frequently than women.

Synovial chondromatosis is a benign lesion characterized by the formation of multiple cartilaginous nodules in the synovium of the joints, tendons, and bursae (132,133). Synovial chondromatosis was traditionally considered to be a self-limiting, proliferative, metaplastic process, rather than a true tumor (132); however, newer reports note abnormal cytogenetic findings, suggesting that synovial chondromatosis is a neoplastic process, with chromosome 6 losses described in a majority of cases (133,134).

Whatever its true nature, synovial chondromatosis is the result of the formation of intrasynovial cartilaginous or osteocartilaginous nodules (132). It is included in this discussion as a tumorlike process. Milgram identified three distinct phases of synovial chondromatosis. In the earliest phase, there is active intrasynovial disease with the formation of cartilaginous masses within the synovium, but no loose bodies. In phase 2, there are osteochondral nodules in the synovium, as well as osteochondral bodies lying free within the joint cavity. In the final phase, there are free osteochondral bodies without synovial-based disease (132). Once formed, the loose bodies may remain free floating, conglomerate with other loose bodies into a large mass, or reattach themselves to the synovium and subsequently be resorbed or continue to grow (Fig. 10.38) (132,133,135–139). This entity is also referred to as *synovial osteochondromatosis*; however, ossification may not be present and the term *synovial chondromatosis* is therefore preferred.

Synovial chondromatosis usually occurs within a joint, although it may occur in a tendon sheath (tenosynovial chondromatosis), usually in the hand or foot (140) or, as rarely reported, in a popliteal cyst (141) or an extra-articular bursa (140,142,143). Synovial chondromatosis should not

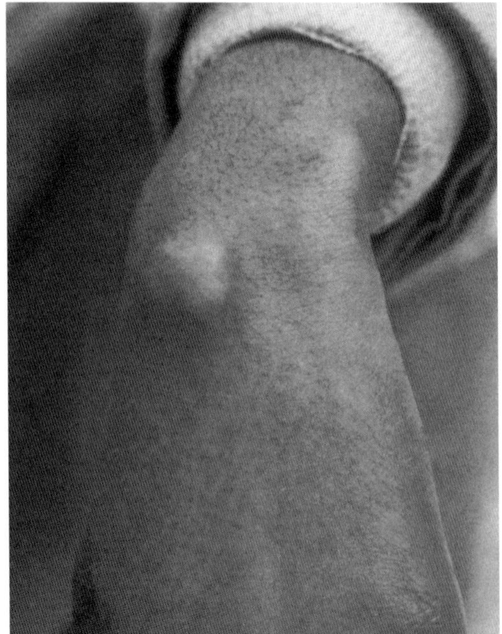
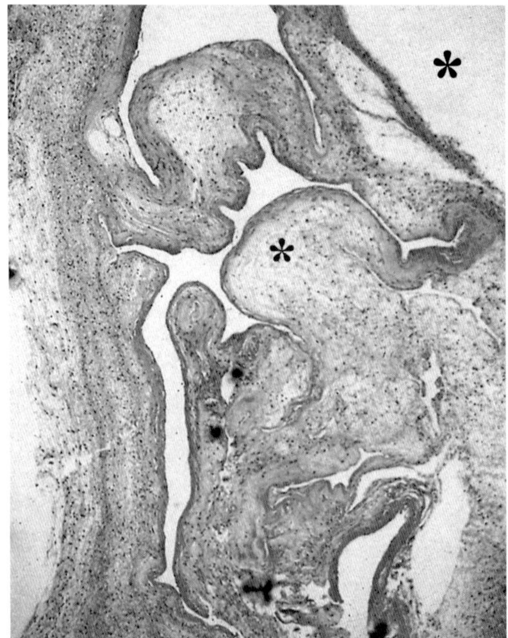

Figure 10.29 Juxta-articular ganglion: Clinical and microscopic appearance. **A:** Dorsal ganglion of the wrist in a woman 21 years of age. Clinical photo shows a prominent soft tissue mass. **B:** Low-power photomicrograph of a typical ganglion shows thick-walled cystic spaces in association with myxoid areas within the walls (*small asterisk*). The lesion is filled with viscous, gelatinous fluid (*large asterisk*) that is rich in hyaluronic acid and other mucopolysaccharides. There is no discernible internal lining cell type.

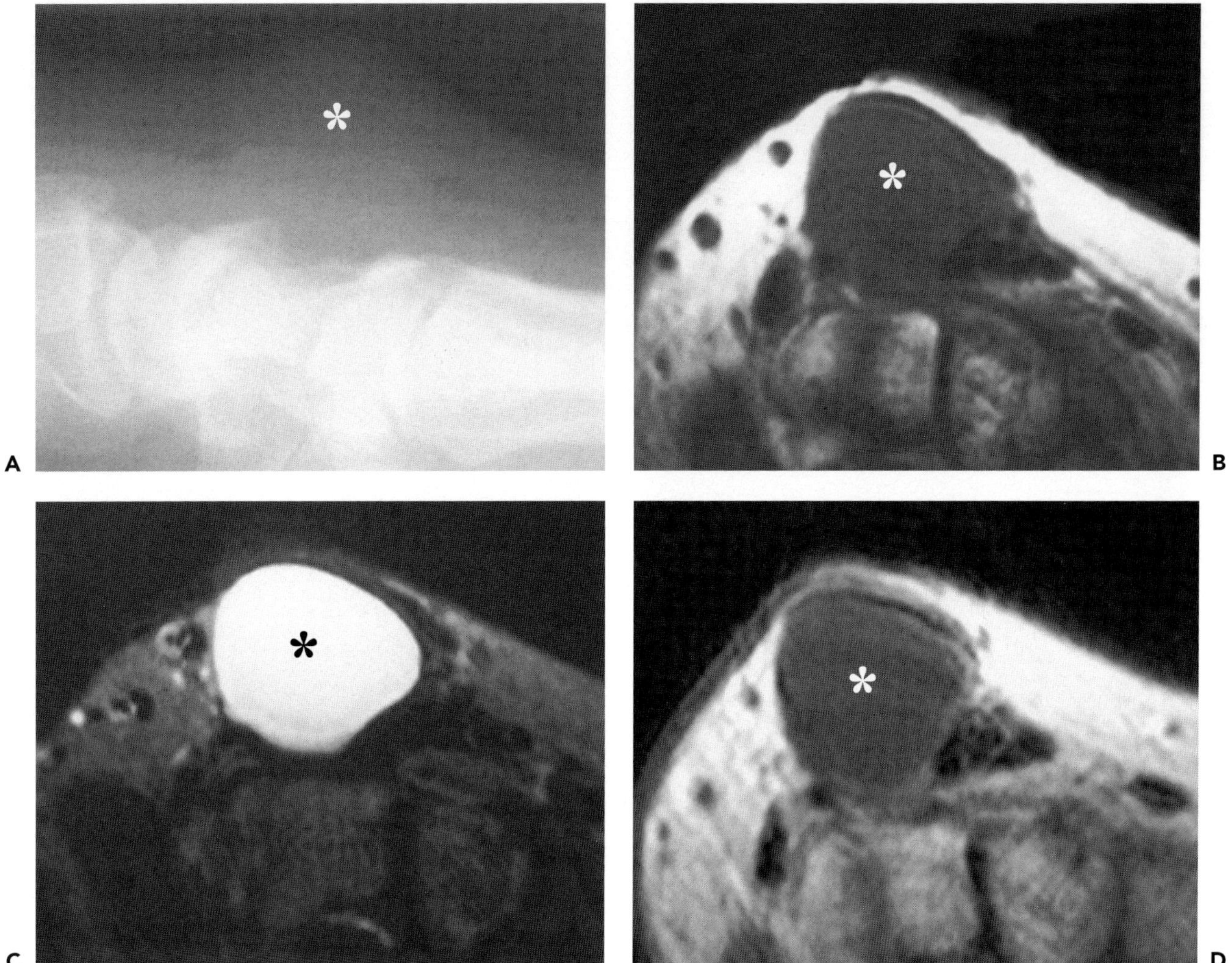

Figure 10.30   Ganglion: Typical MR imaging features in a woman 49 years of age with an enlarging dorsal wrist mass. **A:** Lateral radiograph of the wrist shows a noncalcified mass (*asterisk*) on the dorsal aspect of the wrist. **B,C:** Axial T1-weighted (TR/TE; 700/20) **(B)** and conventional T2-weighted (TR/TE; 2000/90) **(C)** spin-echo MR images of the wrist show a well-defined mass (*asterisk*) on the dorsum of the wrist. The mass originates from the dorsum of the wrist joint and has a signal intensity compatible with that of fluid. **D:** Axial enhanced T1-weighted (TR/TE; 700/20) spin-echo MR image of the mass (*asterisk*) following gadolinium administration shows faint peripheral enhancement.

be confused with other causes of intra-articular osteocartilaginous bodies (secondary chondromatosis), which may be the result of trauma, osteoarthritis, osteonecrosis, neuropathic arthropathy, rheumatoid arthritis, or osteochondritis desiccans (140,143–145).

The knee, by far the most commonly affected joint, is involved in more than 50% of cases, approximately 10% of which are bilateral (132,140,142). Other commonly affected joints (in order of decreasing frequency) include the elbow, hip, and shoulder. Virtually any joint may be affected, however, including the temporomandibular, interphalangeal, and vertebral facet joints (132,146–150). Symptoms, including swelling and stiffness, may be associated with pain and locking (143,151,152).

True extra-articular spread is rarely reported, and is most common in the knee, with extension into a popliteal bursa (135). In the hip, extra-articular spread is into the iliopsoas bursa, which normally communicates with the hip joint in 10% to 15% of patients (135). Extra-articular spread from the hip may also extend into the obturator externus bursa (135). Compressive nerve palsy secondary to bursal distension is reported (151). Symptoms are often insidious and the disease progresses slowly (132).

Synovial chondromatosis is most common in the third to fifth decades, although it may affect individuals of all ages. Men are affected approximately two to four times more frequently than women (143,147,152). The disease process tends to be progressive, and osteoarthritis is a frequent complication (153–156). Treatment usually consists of removal of the intra-articular bodies. The process may stabilize over time, and the affected synovium is removed only when the disease is active (142). Local

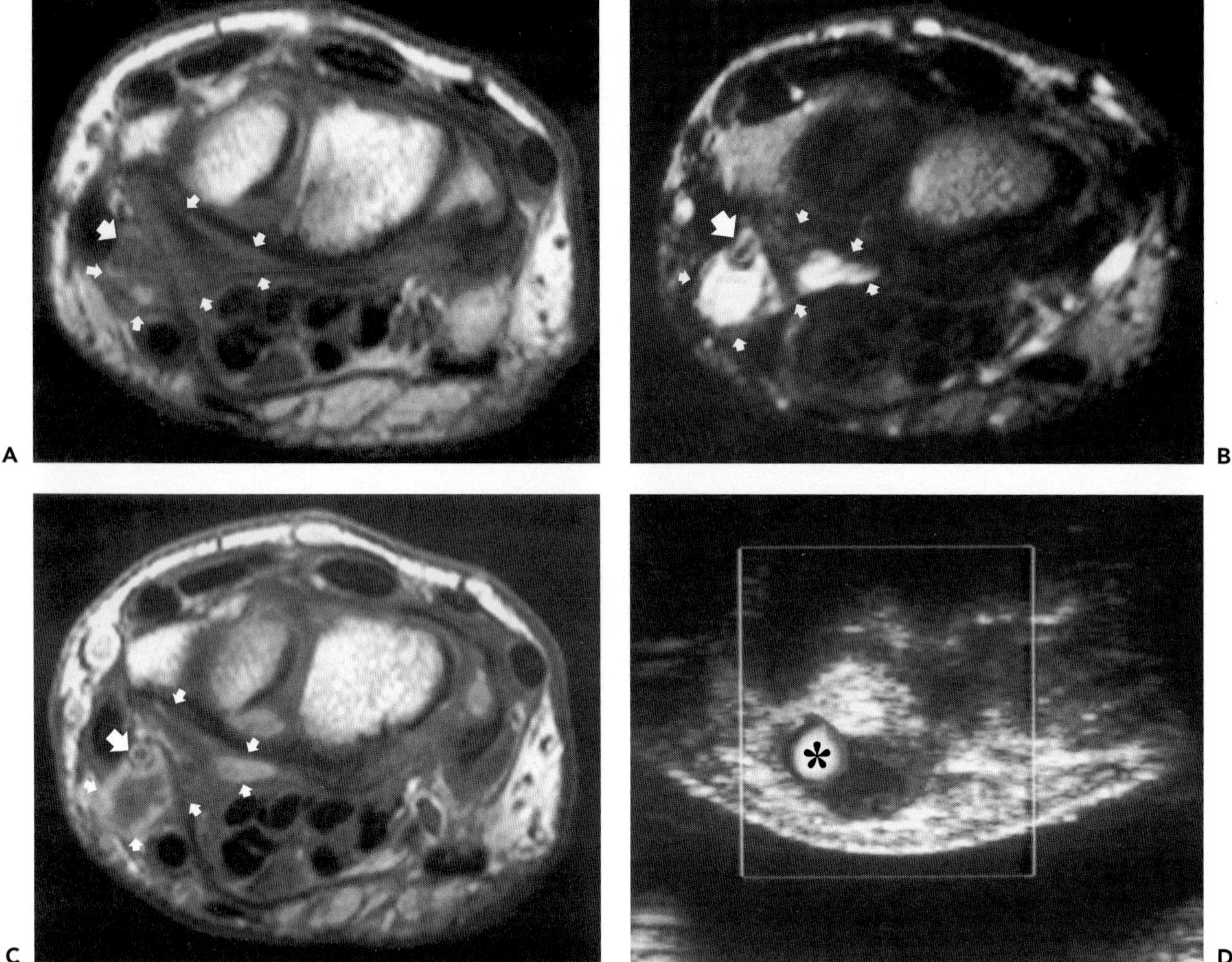

Figure 10.31 Ganglion: Atypical MR imaging features in a woman 49 years of age with a recurring wrist mass. **A,B:** Axial T1-weighted (TR/TE; 600/20) **(A)** and conventional T2-weighted (TR/TE; 2000/90) **(B)** spin-echo MR images show a mass (*small arrows*) adjacent to the volar aspect of the radiocarpal joint. Note the position of the ulnar artery (*large arrow*). The mass is relatively well-defined, with heterogeneous signal intensity. **C:** Corresponding axial T1-weighted (TR/TE; 600/20) spin-echo MR image following contrast administration shows significant heterogeneous contrast enhancement, more pronounced peripherally. **D:** Power Doppler ultrasound shows the complex cystic nature of the mass and better delineates its relationship to the ulnar artery (*asterisk*).

recurrence is common, with recurrence rates more than 25% (137,145).

Lesions consist of white-gray translucent nodules of hyaline cartilage attached to the synovium. These may be separate or coalescent, forming a conglomerate mass. These conglomerate masses are sometimes referred to as giant synovial chondroma and may measure up to 20 cm. Giant synovial chondroma may also form by the continued growth of a solitary synovial chondroma (98). Giant synovial chondromas may coexist with classic synovial chondromatosis (152).

Synovial chondromatosis is reported in association with multiple *rice bodies* (157). Rice bodies, which are small, are composed of tissue resembling coarse collagenous fiber,

reticulin, and elastin (158), and are named for their resemblance to small grains of polished rice (157–159). They are usually seen in patients with chronic arthritis, most commonly rheumatoid arthritis; however, they may occur in association with seronegative arthropathies and chronic, low-grade, synovial infections such as *Mycobacterium marinum* (159).

Histologic examination of synovial chondromatosis demonstrates foci of hyaline cartilage beneath the synovial surface and within the subsynovial connective tissue (Fig. 10.39) (138). The cartilaginous nodules frequently calcify, and they may establish an intact blood supply and undergo enchondral ossification (155). Ossified nodules can develop a fatty marrow (Fig. 10.40) (155). The hypercellularity and

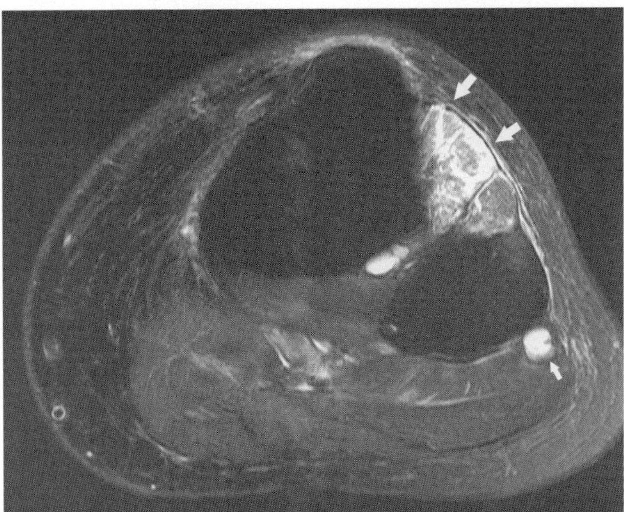

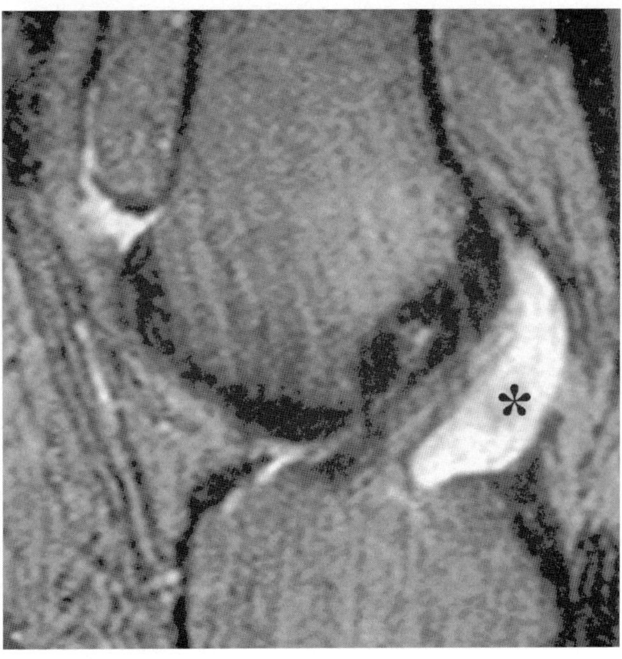

Figure 10.32 Ganglion causing compressive neuropathy: MR imaging feature. Transverse fat-suppressed fast T2-weighted MR image (TR/TE; 4390/80) shows a small ganglion adjacent to the fibular head, compressing the peroneal nerve (*small arrow*). The ganglion continued along the course of the nerve and compressed the deep branch of the peroneal nerve, causing denervation changes in the anterior compartment (*arrows*).

Figure 10.33 Cruciate ganglion: Typical MR imaging features in a woman 34 years of age. Sagittal conventional T2-weighted (TR/TE; 2200/80) spin-echo MR image shows the lesion associated with the anterior cruciate ligament, with signal intensity similar to that of fluid.

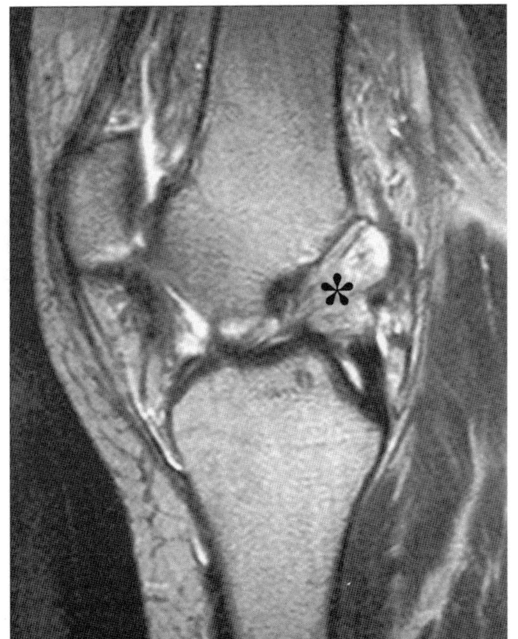

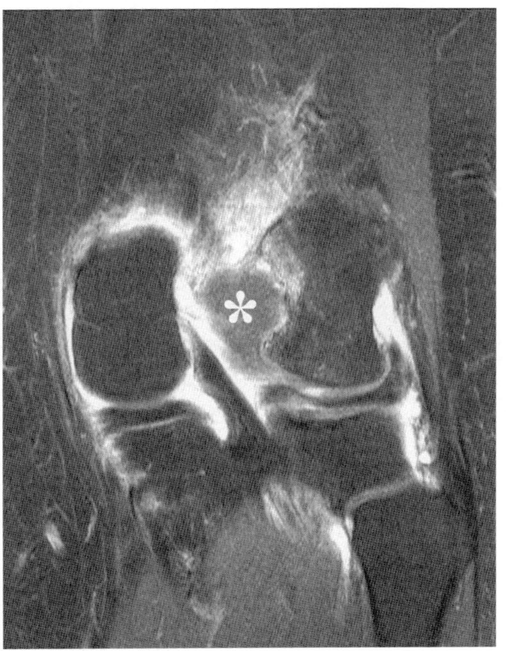

A

B

Figure 10.34 Anterior cruciate ganglion: MR imaging appearance in a woman 48 years of age. **A:** Conventional T2-weighted (TR/TE; 2000/80) spin-echo MR image shows a mass (*asterisk*) within the anterior cruciate ligament. **B:** Coronal, fat-saturated T1-weighted (TR/TE; 644/14) spin-echo MR image following contrast administration shows no significant enhancement (*asterisk*). Note mild erosion of the lateral femoral condyle.

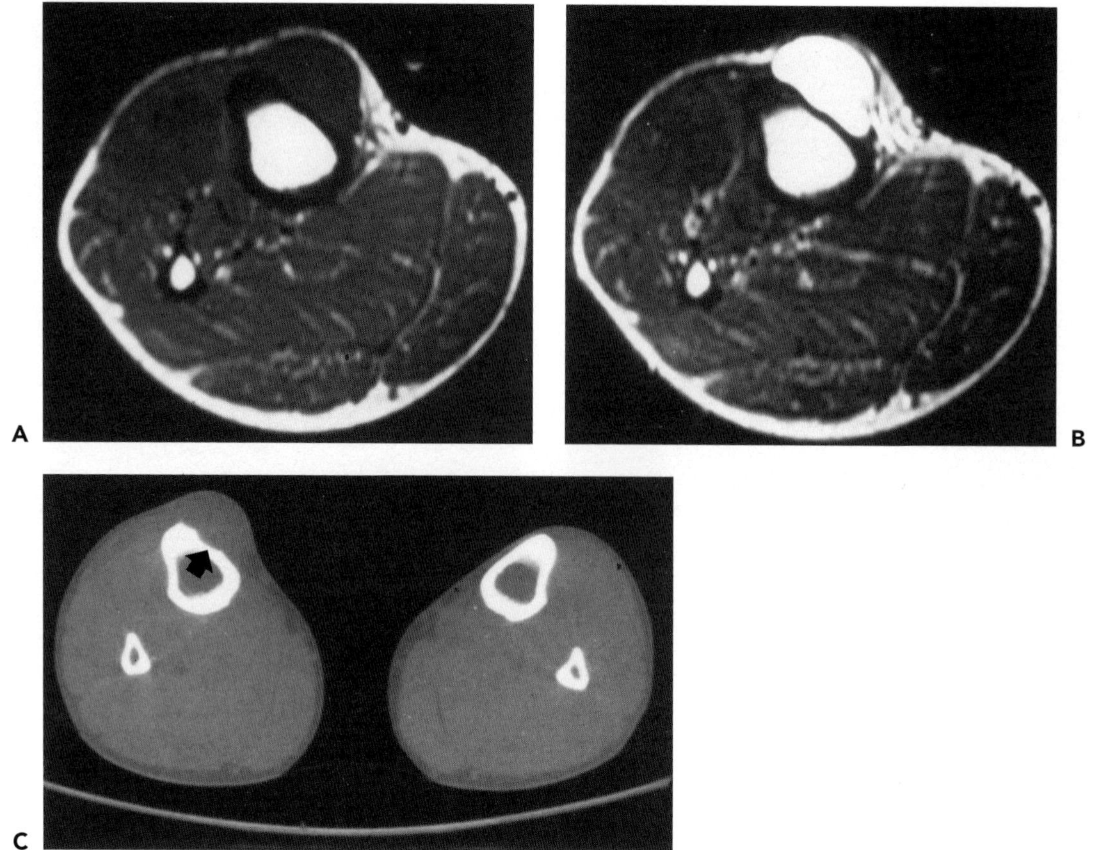

Figure 10.35   Periosteal ganglion: Typical imaging features in a man 45 years of age with a 10-year history of a soft tissue mass. **A,B:** Axial T1-weighted (TR/TE; 600/20) **(A)** and conventional T2-weighted (TR/TE; 1800/80) **(B)** spin-echo MR images show a well-defined, cystlike, lobulated mass adjacent to and scalloping the anterior medial tibia. **C:** Corresponding axial CT displayed on bone window shows the cortical remodeling (*arrow*) to better advantage.

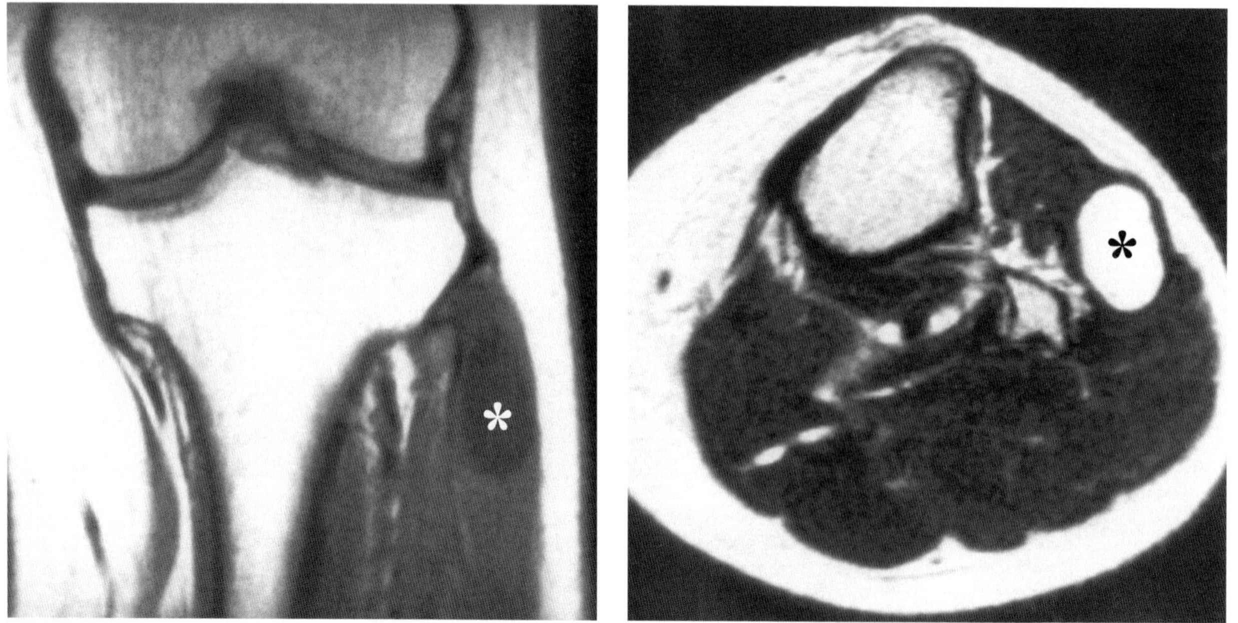

Figure 10.36   Juxta-articular myxoma: MR imaging features in a woman 48 years of age. **A,B:** Coronal T1-weighted (TR/TE; 600/30) **(A)** and axial T2-weighted (TR/TE; 2000/75) **(B)** spin-echo MR images show a lobulated mass (*asterisk*), which images similar to fluid, adjacent to the lateral aspect of the knee.

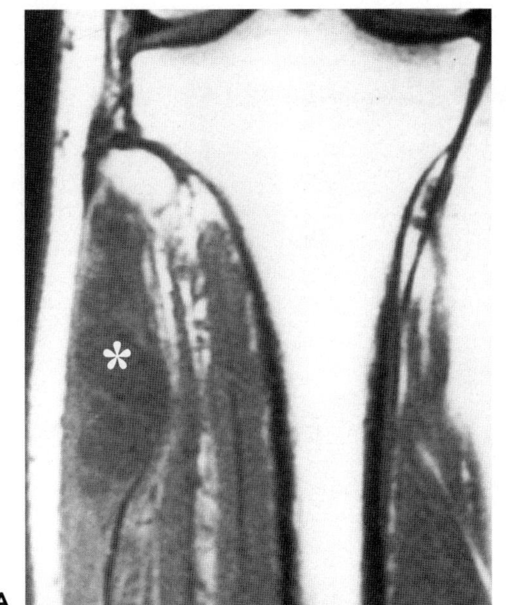

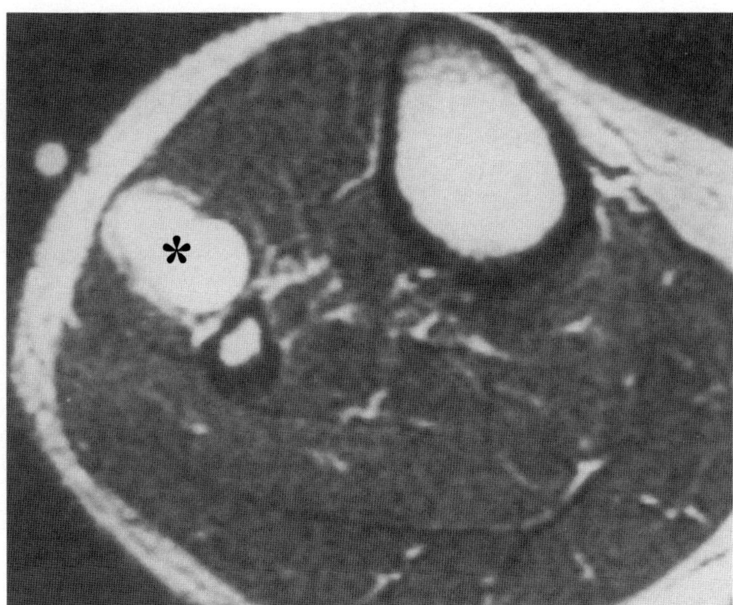

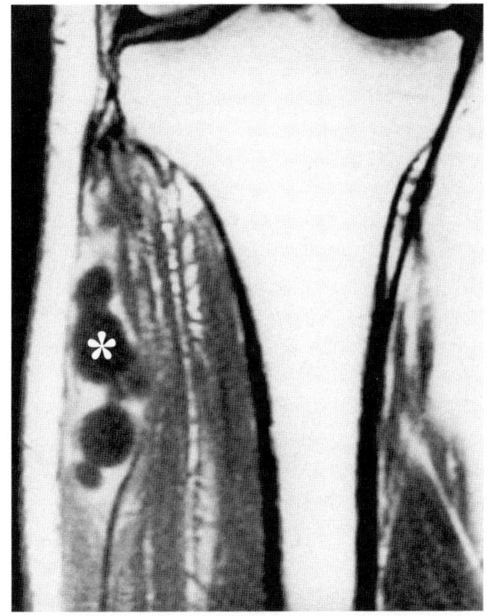

Figure 10.37 Juxta-articular myxoma: MR imaging features in a woman 49 years of age. **A,B:** Coronal T1-weighted (TR/TE; 550/20) **(A)** and axial T2-weighted (TR/TE; 2350/70) **(B)** spin-echo MR images show a mass (*asterisk*) that images similar to that of fluid. **C:** Coronal T1-weighted (TR/TE; 550/20) SE MR image shows marked enhancement in portions of the mass (*asterisk*).

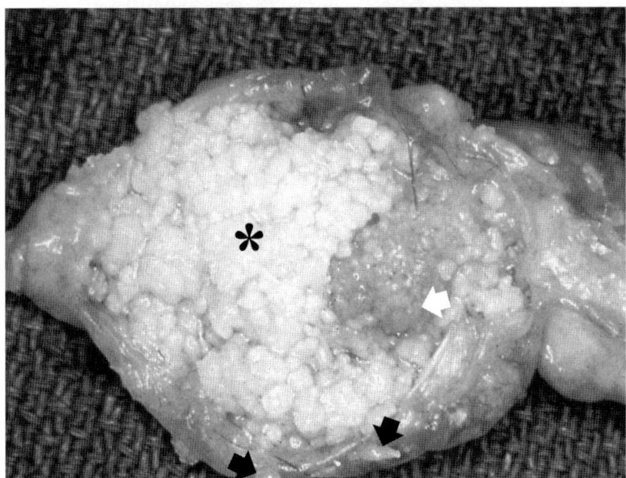

Figure 10.38 Synovial osteochondromatosis: Gross features. Photograph of surgical specimen of synovium shows multiple cartilaginous loose bodes on the synovial surface (*asterisk* and *black arrows*). Note nodularity of the synovial surface (*white arrow*) caused by intrasynovial cartilaginous nodules.

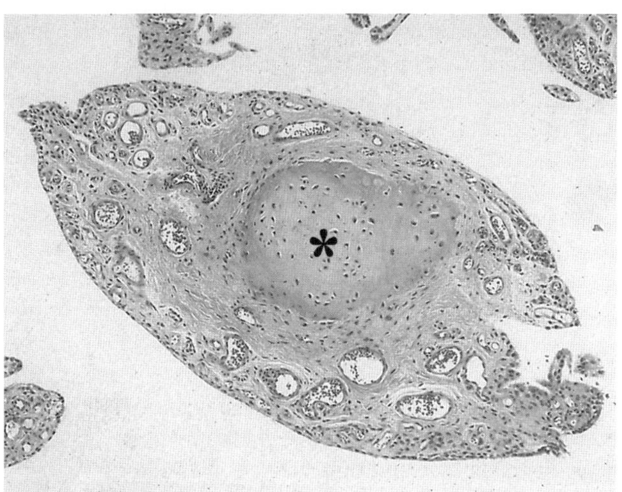

Figure 10.39 Synovial osteochondromatosis: Microscopic features. High-power photomicrograph shows foci of hyaline cartilage (*asterisk*) surrounded by synovium.

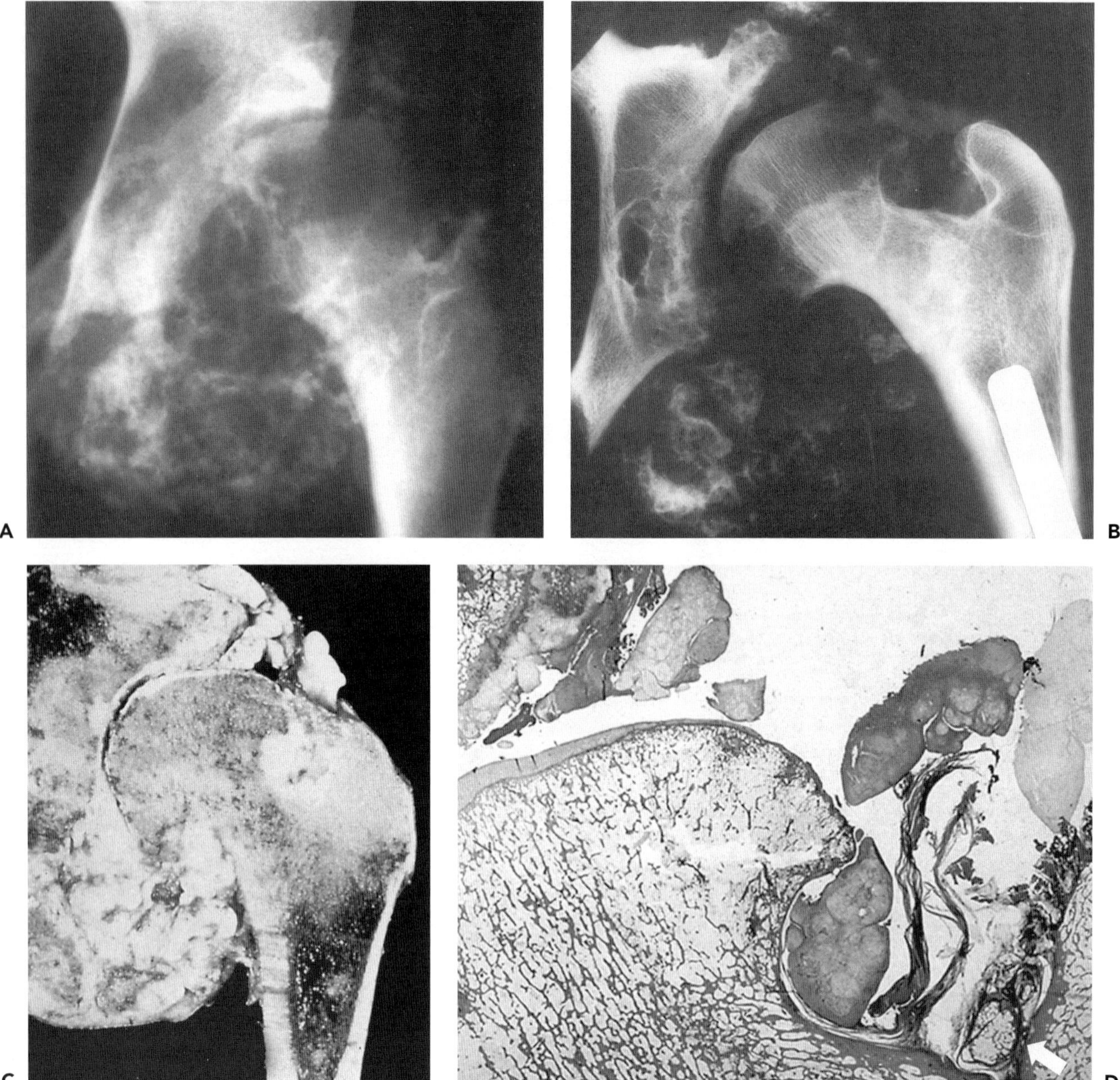

Figure 10.40 Synovial chondromatosis: Radiographic features in long-standing involvement of the hip in a man 29 years of age. **A:** Anteroposterior radiograph of the hip shows a large mineralized juxta-articular mass. **B:** Specimen radiograph shows portions of the mineralized mass, as well as secondary degenerative change and osseous remodeling. **C:** Photograph of the resected specimen show the extensive synovial chondromatosis and secondary degenerative change. **D:** Macrosection of the hip joint shows numerous synovial chondromas. Note small synovial osteochondroma with central marrow (*arrow*). Note also the secondary degeneration that includes thinning and irregularity of the articular surface and osseous remodeling.

nuclear atypia of these extraskeletal cartilaginous lesions may suggest malignancy (138); however, the absence of an aggressive clinical course and documented metastases in patients with synovial chondromatosis indicates they are not malignant. The criteria necessary to establish malignancy in extraskeletal cartilaginous lesions differ from those of bone (138). Chondrosarcoma arising in association with synovial

chondromatosis is extremely rare, with only a small number of cases reported (138,160–162). This entity is discussed more fully later in this chapter.

Imaging of Synovial Chondromatosis
Radiographs may be unremarkable or show evidence of a synovial-based, intra-articular, soft tissue mass, with or

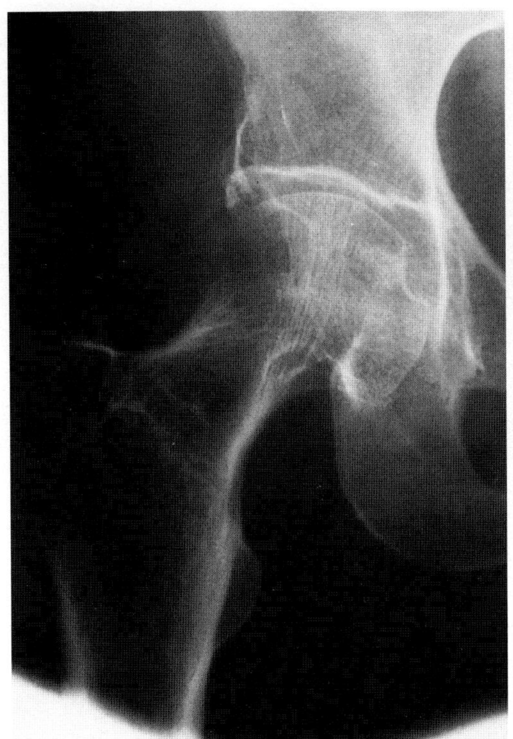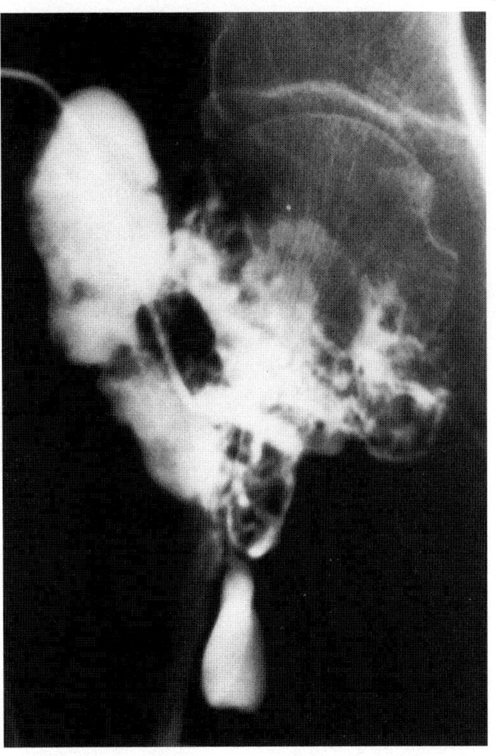

Figure 10.41 Synovial chondromatosis: "Apple core" circumferential erosions of the hip in a woman 73 years of age with a 20-year history of hip pain. **A:** Anteroposterior radiograph of the hip shows a vague mass with multiple circumferential erosions of the femoral neck, resembling an apple core. **B:** Arthrogram shows multiple intra-articular filling defects representing multiple nonmineralized synovial chondromas.

without calcification. The pattern of mineralization varies greatly with the calcification or ossification of the cartilaginous nodules, and the size of the mass or masses ranges from a few millimeters to several centimeters (143). Calcification is present in approximately two-thirds of patients (137,144,152). An osseous shell of remodeled

> ## KEY CONCEPTS
> - Radiographs may be unremarkable or show evidence of a synovial-based, intra-articular soft tissue mass.
> - Calcification occurs in approximately two-thirds of patients.
> - There are three distinct patterns on MR imaging:
>   - Most common pattern: lobulated intra-articular nodules showing intermediate signal intensity on T1-weighted images and high signal intensity on T2-weighted images, with focal signal voids.
>   - Lobulated homogeneous intra-articular nodules with intermediate signal intensity on T1-weighted images and high signal intensity on T2-weighted images, without focal signal voids.
>   - Ring-like signal voids surrounding central areas with imaging characteristics similar to that of fat.

lamellar bone may occasionally be seen (153). There may be associated degenerative joint disease (osteoarthritis), with narrowing of the joint space (154,163) and well-defined osseous erosions on both sides of the joint. Osseous erosion is more likely to be seen in joints with a tight capsule, such as the hip, rather than in the more capacious joint capsules, such as the knee (Fig. 10.40) (34). It is difficult to accurately estimate the percentage of patients with osseous involvement. Norman and Steiner (164) reported 30 lesions in 28 patients, noting intra-articular erosions in 9 (30%): 7 involving the hip and 2 affecting the shoulder. Erosions were either small defects involving the cortex or large circumferential, erosive lesions resembling an apple core (Fig. 10.41). Ill-defined erosive change is also reported (165). The joint may be widened because of the accumulation of chondral bodies within the joint space (Fig. 10.42). Osteoporosis is typically absent (154). Rarely, osseous erosions may be extensive enough to cause a pathologic fracture (164). When radiographs demonstrate erosion of bone on both sides of a synovial joint, the differential diagnosis should include synovial processes such as rheumatoid arthritis, pigmented villonodular synovitis, amyloid arthropathy, and degenerative joint disease (osteoarthritis) (154,163).

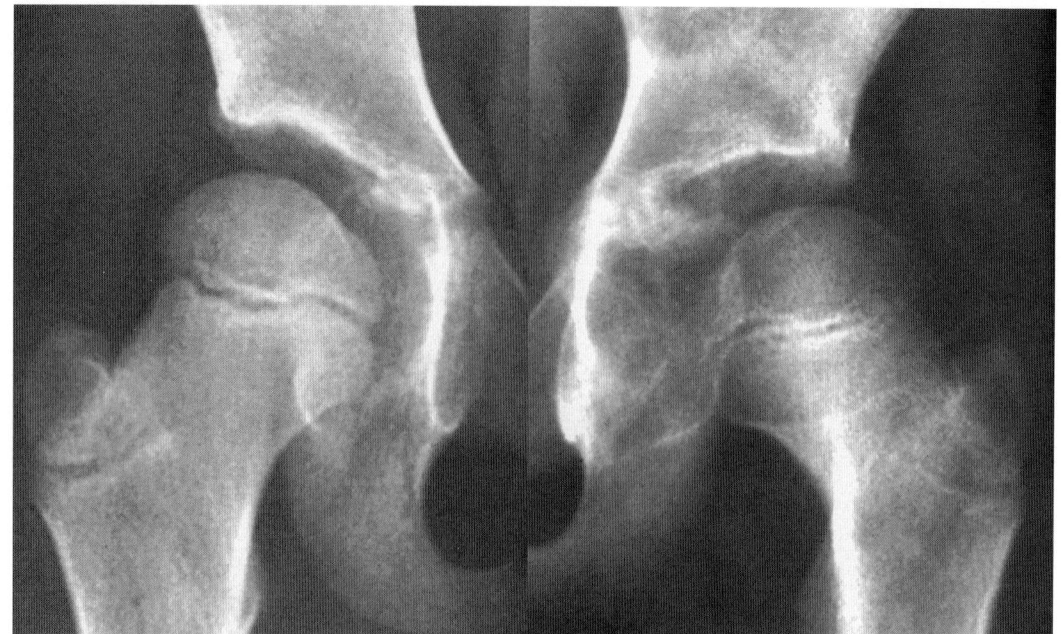

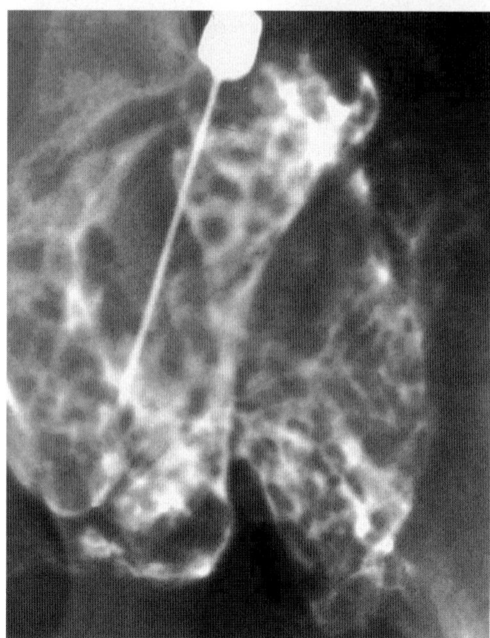

Figure 10.42 Synovial chondromatosis: Radiographic features in a girl 9 years of age presenting with left hip pain. **A:** Anteroposterior radiograph of the hips show widening of the left hip joint caused by nonmineralized, intra-articular synovial chondromatosis. **B:** Arthrogram shows multiple intra-articular filling defects representing multiple nonmineralized synovial chondromas.

CT may demonstrate a joint effusion with multiple, calcified intra-articular bodies (Fig. 10.43) (142). CT, as well as MR imaging, may be extremely useful to confirm the extraosseous origin of the lesion when radiographs are equivocal (166). Arthrography shows multiple filling defects and is especially useful in identifying nonmineralized intra-articular loose bodies (150,163). Arthrography is also useful in evaluating the joint space (163). Sonography may be useful in selected cases. It is probably of limited value for heavily calcified lesions in that the intense calcification obscures the more characteristic lobulated architecture seen in more modestly mineralized lesions (167).

Kramer et al. (155) described three distinct patterns on MR imaging in patients with synovial chondromatosis. The most common pattern, seen in more than three-quarters of patients, is characterized by lobulated, homogeneous, intra-articular nodules with intermediate signal intensity on T1-weighted images and high signal intensity on T2-weighted images (similar to fluid), with focal areas of signal void on all pulse sequences (Fig. 10.44). The focal areas of signal void correspond to foci of calcification. The remaining cases had a similar appearance but with no signal voids (Fig. 10.45) or signal voids surrounding central areas with imaging characteristics similar to

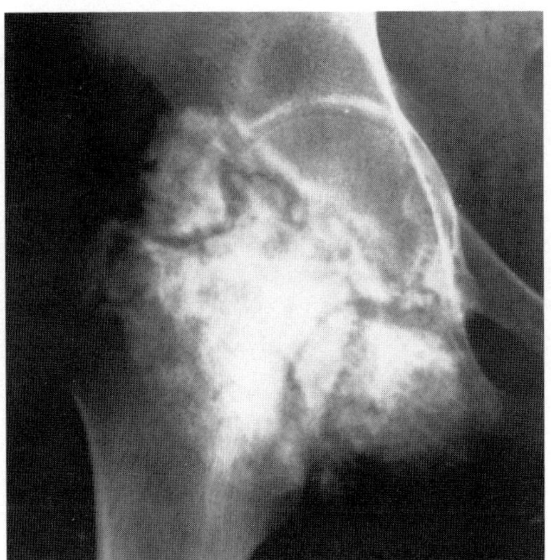
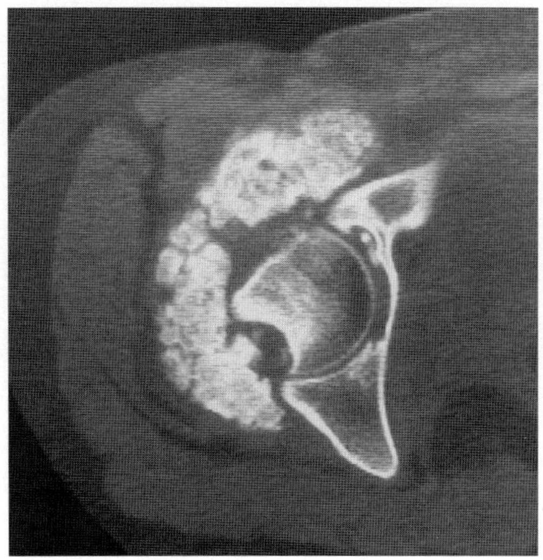

Figure 10.43 Synovial chondromatosis: Radiographic and CT imaging features in extensively mineralized lesions of the hip in a 21-year-old woman with hip pain for 3 years. **A:** Anteroposterior radiograph of the hip shows marked calcification around the hip joint. **B:** Noncontrast axial CT through the femoral head shows extensive juxta-articular calcification. Erosions are seen in the acetabulum and femoral head suggesting a synovial-based process. Erosions were not appreciated on radiographs.

that of fat (Fig. 10.46). These correspond, respectively, to cases in which there are no chondroid calcifications and cases in which a fatty marrow has developed within the osteocartilaginous bodies. These patterns are in keeping with previously reported cases (157–159,168–172). The lobular configuration with homogeneous high signal intensity on long TR/TE images typically associated with hyaline cartilage lesions may be absent, perhaps secondary to the cellularity of the lesions and enchondral bone formation (170). Conglomerate masses of synovial chondromatosis, especially when not significantly mineralized, may have a nonspecific appearance and mimic a sarcoma. Careful attention to the growth pattern of the lesion as originating from the joint may be helpful in suggesting a synovial origin (Fig. 10.47).

The imaging appearance of lesions originating outside a joint in a tendon sheath (Fig. 10.48) or bursa (Fig. 10.49) is similar. The origin of large lesions may be difficult to determine, and the pattern of hyaline cartilage enhancement may simulate an abscess (Fig. 10.50). Synovial chondromatosis may also arise in the bursa, overlying an osteochondroma (171). Such cases may present as an enlarging, painful soft tissue mass and may suggest malignant transformation (156).

Synovial chondromatosis may occur in association with multiple rice bodies (157). When synovial chondromatosis is mineralized, the distinction is readily made. In those cases in which there is no mineralization, the distinction is considerably more difficult. Although rice bodies demonstrate a morphologic appearance simulating that of synovial chondromatosis on MR imaging, the

entities can be distinguished because rice bodies typically show a signal intensity relatively similar to that of muscle on T1- and T2-weighted images (Fig. 10.51) (157,159,172), whereas synovial chondromatosis demonstrates an intermediate to high signal intensity on T2-weighted images.

MALIGNANT LESIONS

Synovial Chondrosarcoma

Synovial chondrosarcoma is a rare neoplasm. Although its origin is controversial, it is now accepted that synovial chondrosarcoma may arise de novo or from preexisting synovial chondromatosis (136,138,160–162,173–176). Patients with synovial chondrosarcoma present with complaints of pain, swelling, and decreased range of motion (174). These symptoms are often long standing; moreover,

---

KEY CONCEPTS

- Synovial chondrosarcoma is a rare neoplasm.
- It may arise de novo or from preexisting synovial chondromatosis.
- The vast majority of cases occur in the knee joint (75%), followed by the hip (15%), and ankle and elbow (5% each).
- Clinical and radiographic features mimic those of synovial chondromatosis; however, a permeative pattern of osseous destruction and sudden exacerbation of symptoms suggests malignant transformation.

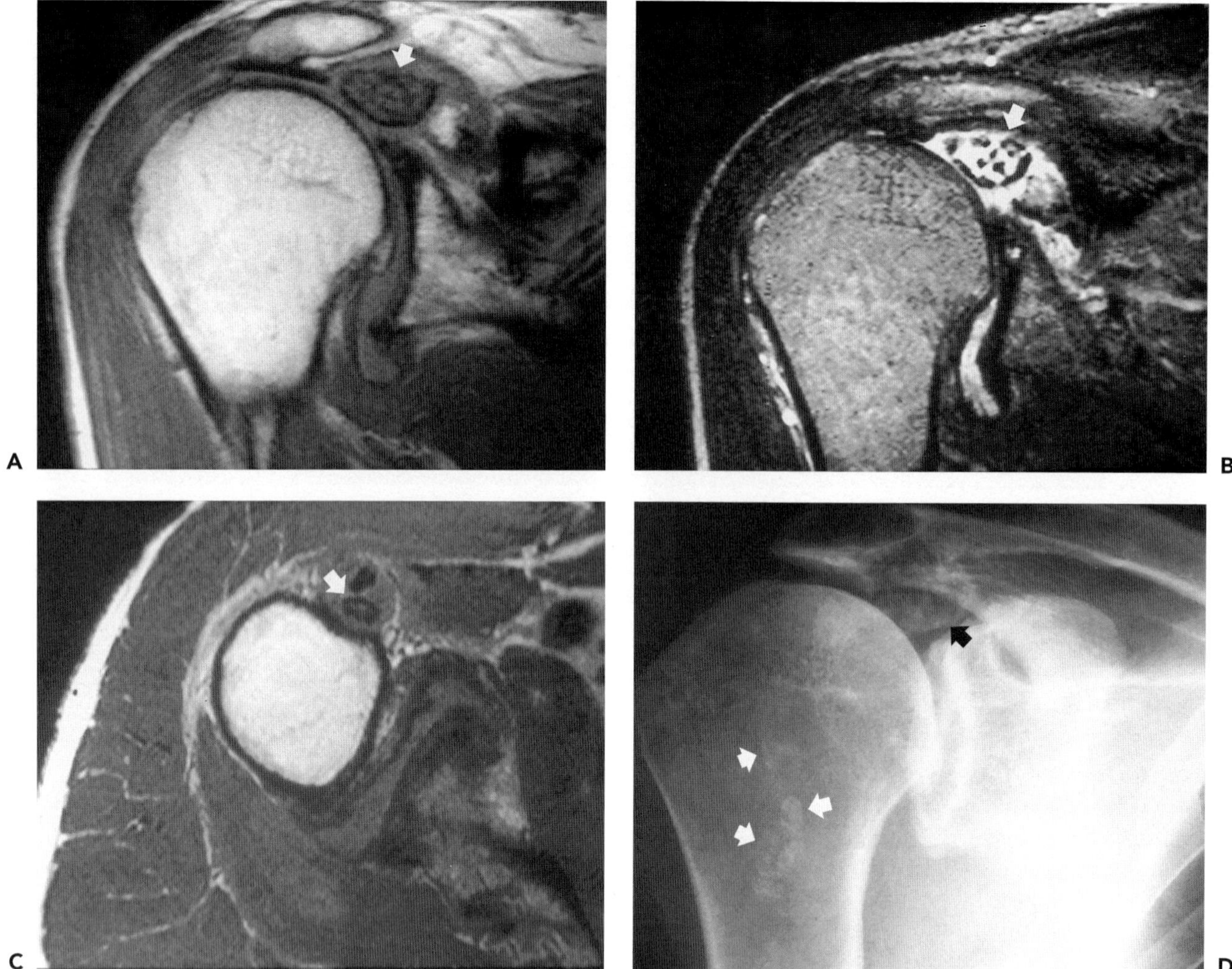

Figure 10.44 Synovial chondromatosis: Typical MR imaging features in a man 70 years of age with shoulder pain. **A,B:** Coronal T1-weighted (TR/TE; 650/20) **(A)** and conventional T2-weighted (TR/TE; 2500/80) **(B)** spin-echo MR images show a joint effusion with lobulated, intra-articular loose bodies (*arrow*) show an intermediate signal intensity on T1-weighted images and high signal intensity on T2-weighted images. Note focal areas of signal void on all pulse sequences. **C:** Axial T1-weighted (TR/TE; 620/20) spin-echo MR image shows loose body in biceps tendon sheath (*arrow*). **D:** Anteroposterior radiograph of the shoulder shows multiple mineralized loose bodies (*arrows*) corresponding to the focal signal voids.

the clinical and radiographic features of synovial chondromatosis and synovial chondrosarcoma are typically similar (137,173,174,176,177). The distinction between these lesions on a histologic basis is also difficult and misdiagnosis of synovial chondromatosis as synovial chondrosarcoma is a well-known pitfall in orthopedic pathology (177).

Kenan et al. (173) in 1993 reported a case of synovial chondrosarcoma, reviewed the literature, and found 19 previously reported cases arising in synovial chondromatosis. Patients ranged from 33 to 72 years of age, with males affected almost twice as frequently as females. All patients had synovial chondromatosis, with symptoms present from 1 to 26 years. The vast majority of cases (75%) occurred in

the knee joint, followed by the hip (15%), and ankle and elbow (5% each). Only seven patients developed pulmonary metastases, and ultimately, the development of pulmonary metastases may be the only absolute way to distinguish this entity from synovial chondromatosis.

Bertoni et al. (178) reported 10 cases of synovial chondrosarcoma; two were considered to be primary. In five cases there was evidence of preexisting synovial chondromatosis, and in the remaining three, there was a suggestion of preexisting disease. Although these authors were unable to distinguish synovial chondrosarcoma from synovial chondromatosis clinically or radiographically, they suggested differentiation on a histologic basis, by identifying the loss of the "clustering" growth pattern that is typical of synovial

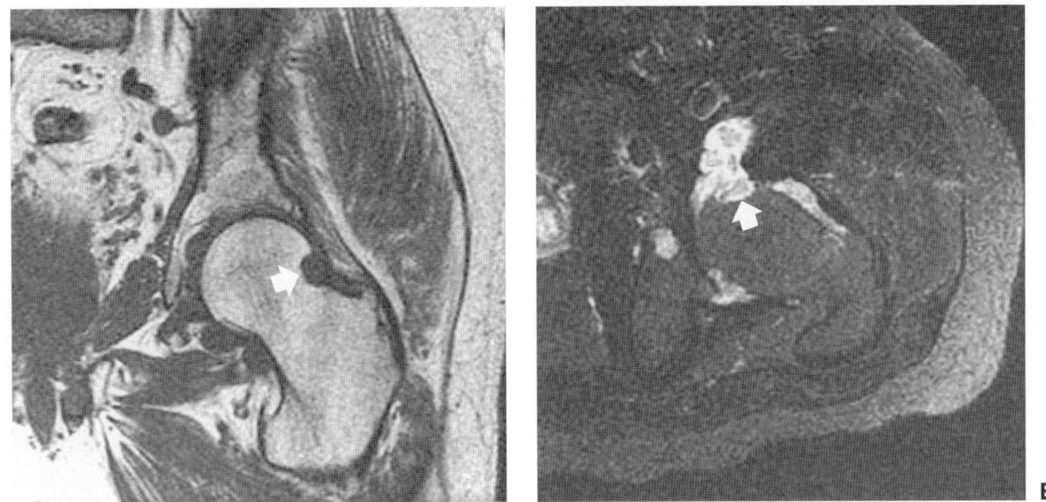

Figure 10.45 Synovial chondromatosis: Less common MR imaging features in a man 75 years of age. **A,B:** Coronal T1-weighted (TR/TE; 633/17) **(A)** and axial fat-suppressed fast spin-echo T2-weighted (TR/TE; 4000/91) **(B)** MR images show a heterogeneous joint effusion with lobulated intra-articular bodies. Note osseous erosions (*arrow*).

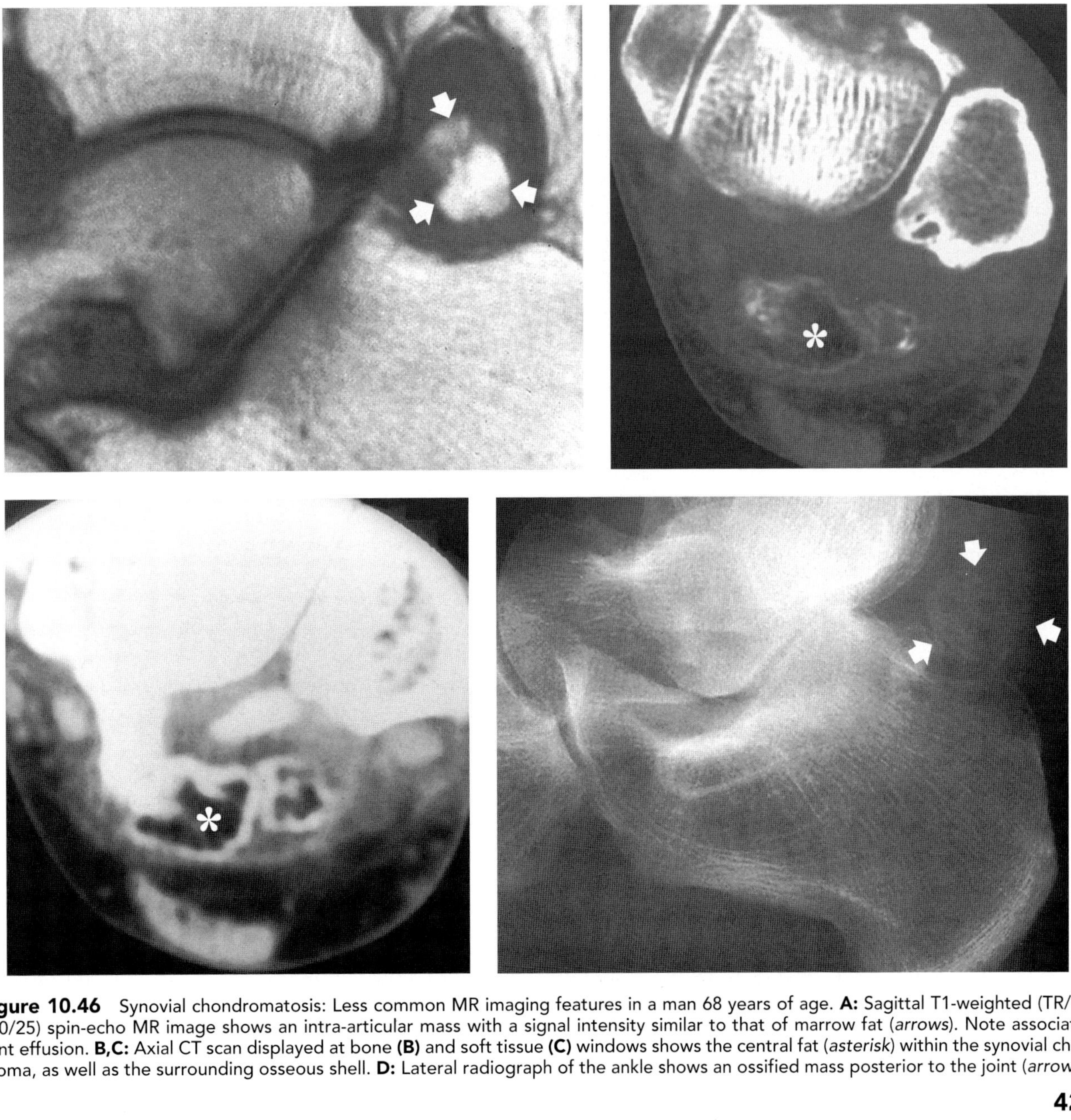

Figure 10.46 Synovial chondromatosis: Less common MR imaging features in a man 68 years of age. **A:** Sagittal T1-weighted (TR/TE; 600/25) spin-echo MR image shows an intra-articular mass with a signal intensity similar to that of marrow fat (*arrows*). Note associated joint effusion. **B,C:** Axial CT scan displayed at bone **(B)** and soft tissue **(C)** windows shows the central fat (*asterisk*) within the synovial chondroma, as well as the surrounding osseous shell. **D:** Lateral radiograph of the ankle shows an ossified mass posterior to the joint (*arrows*).

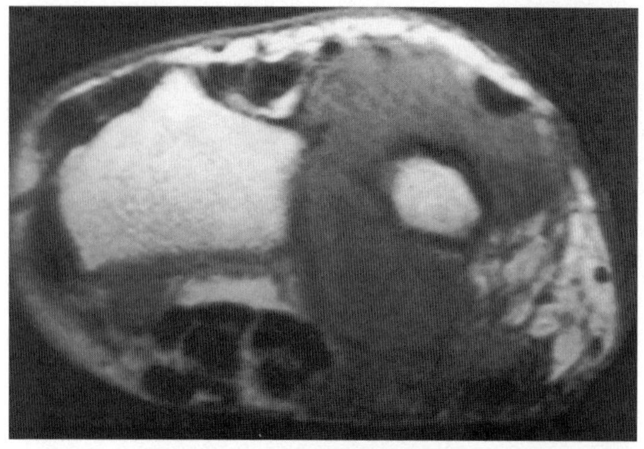

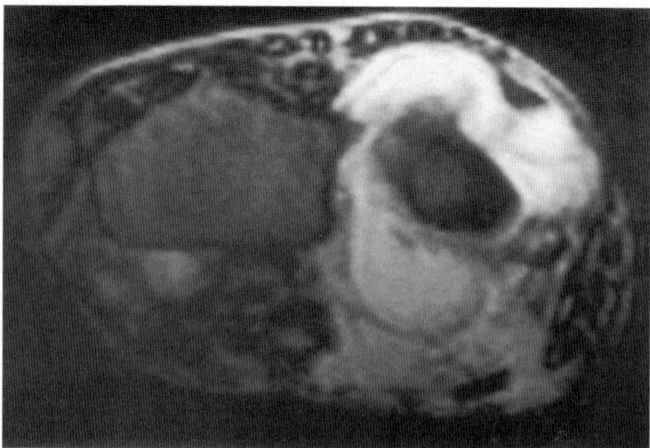

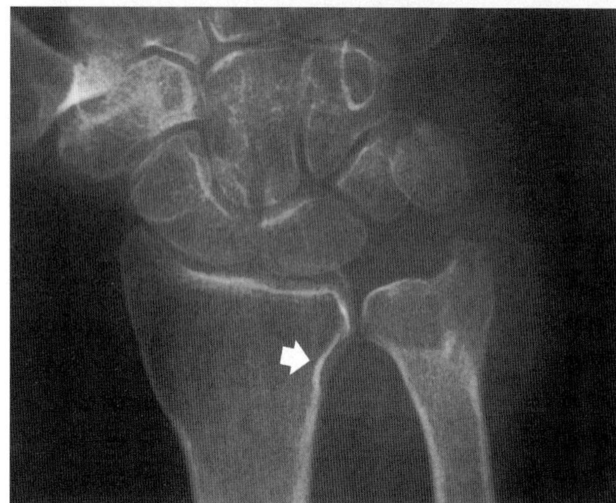

Figure 10.47 Synovial chondromatosis: Conglomerate mass in the wrist of a woman 77 years of age. **A,B:** Axial T1-weighted (TR/TE; 617/20) **(A)** and T2-weighted (TR/TE; 2000/90) **(B)** spin-echo MR images of the wrist show a mass surrounding the distal ulna, centered on the distal radioulnar joint. **C:** Anteroposterior radiograph of the wrist shows a large mass in the region of the distal radioulnar joint. Note subtle osseous erosion (*arrow*). The pattern of circumferential growth of the mass would be quite unusual for a tumor.

chondromatosis, myxoid change in the matrix, areas of necrosis, and spindling at the periphery of chondroid lobules.

Although the radiographic features of synovial chondromatosis and synovial chondrosarcoma may be identical, Wuisman et al. (179) have suggested CT and MR imaging features may be useful in distinguishing these lesions. In synovial chondrosarcoma, the more rapid and aggressive growth of the lesion leads to a permeative pattern of osseous destruction, rather than the pressure erosions seen with synovial chondromatosis (Fig. 10.52) (179). Additionally, a sudden exacerbation of symptoms may also suggest malignant transformation (180).

Synovial Sarcoma

Synovial sarcoma is a well-recognized soft tissue malignancy that typically arises in young adults between 15 and 35 years of age. First reported in 1893, it is a relatively common primary soft tissue sarcoma, accounting for approximately 5% to 10% of all malignant mesenchymal neoplasms (2,181). The term *synovial sarcoma* is a misnomer, in that the lesion does not arise from or differentiate toward the synovium (182,183) and its origin is likely from undifferentiated mesenchymal tissue (2,184). The lesion typically demonstrates epithelial features; con-

KEY CONCEPTS

- Synovial sarcoma represents approximately 5% to 10% of all sarcomas; patients are usually between 15 and 35 years of age.
- The most common malignancy of the foot, ankle, and lower extremity in patients between 6 and 35 years of age.
- True intra-articular lesions are quite rare.
- Metastases or local recurrence is seen in approximately 80% of patients.
- Metastases are present at the time of initial diagnosis in about 16% to 25% of cases.
- The prognosis is guarded.

sequently, it is proposed that synovial sarcoma be renamed *carcinosarcoma* or *spindle cell carcinoma of soft tissue* (183).

Clinically, presentation spans a wide range in age, although synovial sarcoma is most prevalent between 15 and 35 years of age (2). It is reported in children and is sometimes noted at birth (185). In a report of 672 cases seen in consultation over a 10-year period by the Department of Soft Tissue Pathology at the Armed Forces Institute of Pathology, the mean patient age was 32 years,

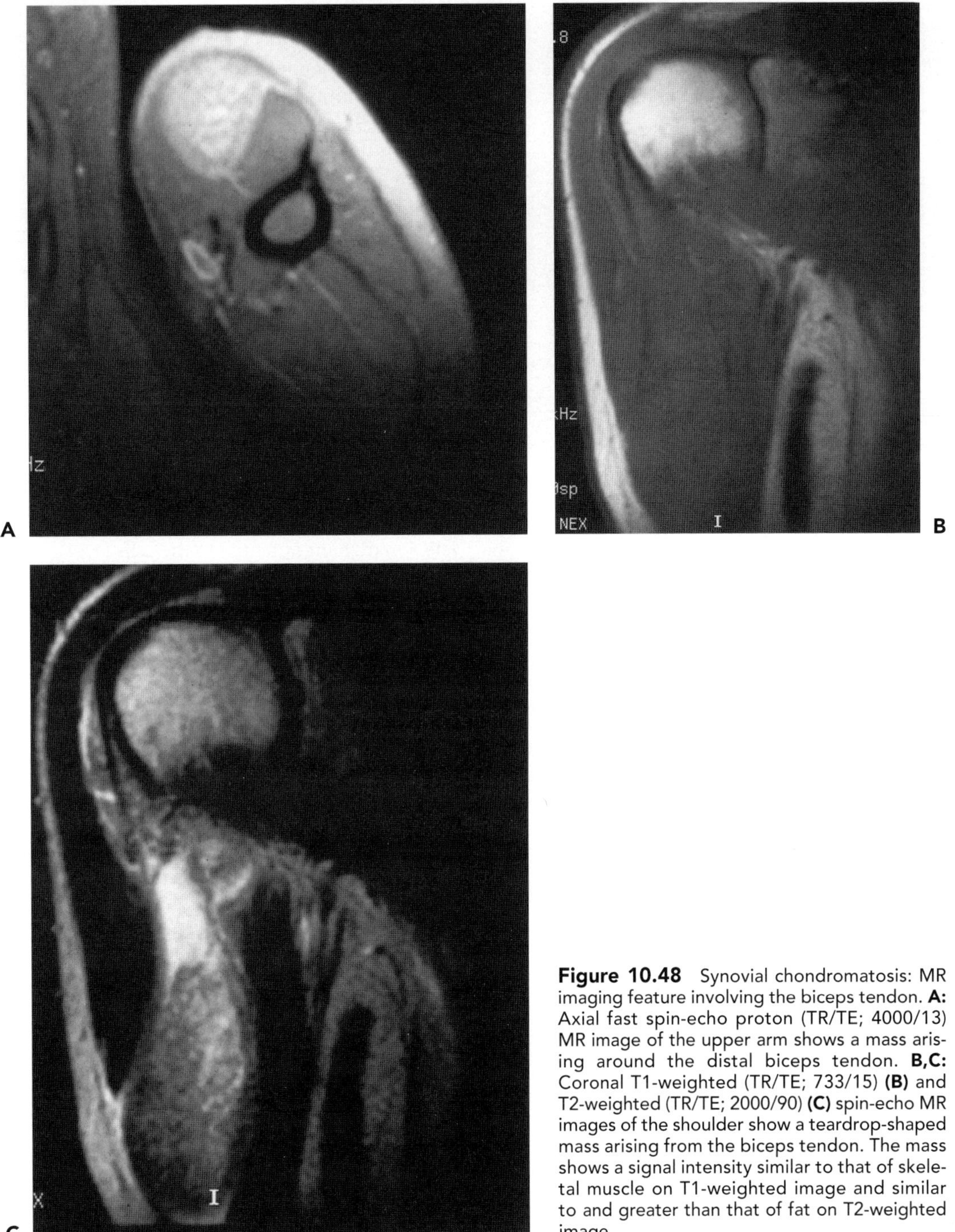

Figure 10.48 Synovial chondromatosis: MR imaging feature involving the biceps tendon. **A:** Axial fast spin-echo proton (TR/TE; 4000/13) MR image of the upper arm shows a mass arising around the distal biceps tendon. **B,C:** Coronal T1-weighted (TR/TE; 733/15) **(B)** and T2-weighted (TR/TE; 2000/90) **(C)** spin-echo MR images of the shoulder show a teardrop-shaped mass arising from the biceps tendon. The mass shows a signal intensity similar to that of skeletal muscle on T1-weighted image and similar to and greater than that of fat on T2-weighted image.

with 80% of patients between 14 and 58 years of age, and males and females affected equally (181).

Patients with synovial sarcoma generally present with a palpable soft tissue mass, which may be quite slow-growing and may clinically simulate a benign process (186). Pain is often present, and additional complaints include sensory and/or motor dysfunction distal to the lesion. The duration of symptoms is quite variable and may be present for days to weeks, or as long as 20 years prior to initial diagnosis (187).

The majority (80% to 95%) of synovial sarcomas occur in the extremities, with approximately 60% to 70% located in the lower limbs (2,187,188). It is the most common malignancy of the foot and ankle in patients between 6 and 45 years of age, and the most common malignancy of the lower extremity in patients between 6 and 35 years of age (181). Fewer than 10% of cases are intra-articular. This figure must be viewed with caution because many lesions that involve the joint do so by extension from an extra-articular

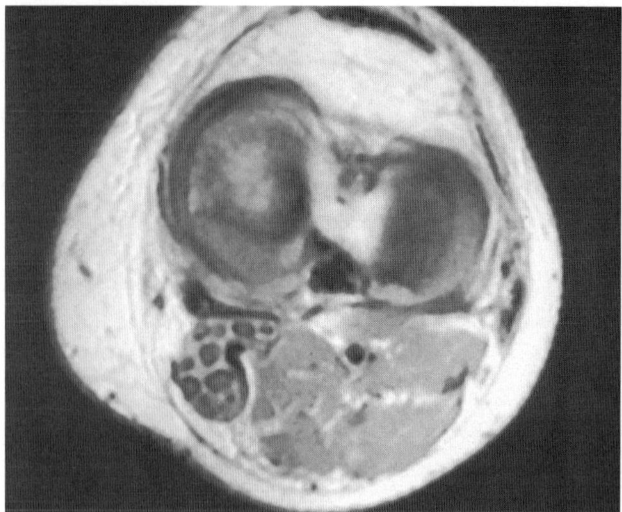

Figure 10.49 Synovial chondromatosis: MR imaging features involving the gastrocnemius-semimembranosus bursa. Axial fast spin-echo proton MR image shows multiple loose bodies in a popliteal cyst.

origin. In our experience, true intra-articular lesions are quite rare. Other rare sites of involvement include the neck, pharynx, larynx, precoccygeal and paravertebral regions, thoracic and abdominal wall, and heart (2,189–194).

Metastases or local recurrence is seen in approximately 80% of patients (195). Metastases are present at the time of initial diagnosis in approximately 16% to 25% of patients (195,196), but are reported as long as 35 years following initial diagnosis (197). Pulmonary foci account for approximately 59% to 94% of metastatic lesions (188,195,198). After the lungs, metastases to lymph nodes (4% to 18%) and bone (8% to 11%) are most common, although multiple sites may be affected (187,195,198–201). Soft tissue metastases are also reported (202). Local recurrence is frequent, seen in approximately 20% to 26% of patients, occurring in the excision scar or the amputation stump, often within 2 years of initial presentation (188,193,198,200).

The prognosis remains guarded, although the biologic activity of the tumor is variable. The median survival after diagnosis is 32 to 33 months, with the 5-year survival rate approximately 27% to 61% (188,198,203,204). Median survival following first recurrence is less than half that at diagnosis (198). Lesions that demonstrate extensive calcification have a more favorable prognosis (205), as do younger patients, those with tumors smaller than 5 cm, and those lesions located in the extremities (188). The size of the tumor is the most important variable in determining prognosis (188). Multivariate analysis has shown that sizes greater than 10 cm and sizes 5 to 10 cm are associated with an 18-fold and a 3.1-fold increased risk of death, respectively, as compared with tumors smaller than 5 cm (203). In analyses of tumor location, Deshmukh et al. (203) noted that patients with distal extremity lesions had a 10-year survival of 65%. Survival dropped to 48% for proxi-

mal extremity lesions, and there were no 10-year survivors with truncal tumors. Rare truly intra-articular lesions often have a much better prognosis in that they present earlier when the tumor is small.

Histologically, synovial sarcoma is biphasic, composed of both epithelial and spindle cell components. Diagnosis is usually based on the presence of both of these cellular elements in at least a portion of the tumor, although monophasic variants have been described (Fig. 10.53) (2). In these cases, immunocytochemical markers are used to demonstrate the presence of both vimentin (a mesenchymal intermediate filament) and cytokeratin (an epithelial intermediate filament) within the tumor. In general, patients with biphasic histology demonstrate a better overall survival. Synovial sarcoma cells are characterized by the presence of a translocation involving chromosomes X and 18 [t(X,18)(p11,q11)] (184,206) occurring in more than 90% of cases (183). Genetic studies show that this translocation fuses two normal genes to form an abnormal fusion protein that confers a malignant potential to the cells (184).

In most patients, lesions are relatively deep; however, superficial subcutaneous lesions may be seen (207). There is no agreement on the significance of microscopic subtype on prognosis, but in general, monophasic synovial sarcomas behave more aggressively and metastasize earlier than biphasic lesions (2,208,209). No imaging differences are reported between the monophasic and biphasic variants (210). Calcification is generally localized to areas of hyalinization within the spindle cell component of the tumor (2). Chondroid and osseous metaplasia may also be found and is rarely extensive (211).

Imaging of Synovial Sarcoma

Routine radiographs may be interpreted as normal in approximately half of patients (188). When a lesion is identified, it is most commonly a well-defined, round or lobulated, soft tissue mass (2,212). As many as a third of cases demonstrate calcification (less commonly ossification), often in the periphery of the tumor (Fig. 10.54) (2,137,184,187). In rare cases of intra-articular synovial

---

KEY CONCEPTS

- Radiographs are normal in approximately half of cases; a third demonstrate calcification.
- Adjacent bone involvement (periosteal reaction, osseous remodeling, or frank bony invasion) is seen in 11% to 20% of cases.
- MR imaging usually shows a nonspecific inhomogeneous mass.
- Change compatible with previous hemorrhage may be seen in more than 40% of patients, with fluid-fluid levels in 10% to 25% of lesions on MR imaging.
- T2-weighted MR images may show a "triple" signal intensity caused by a mixture of cystic (hemorrhagic and necrotic) and solid elements.

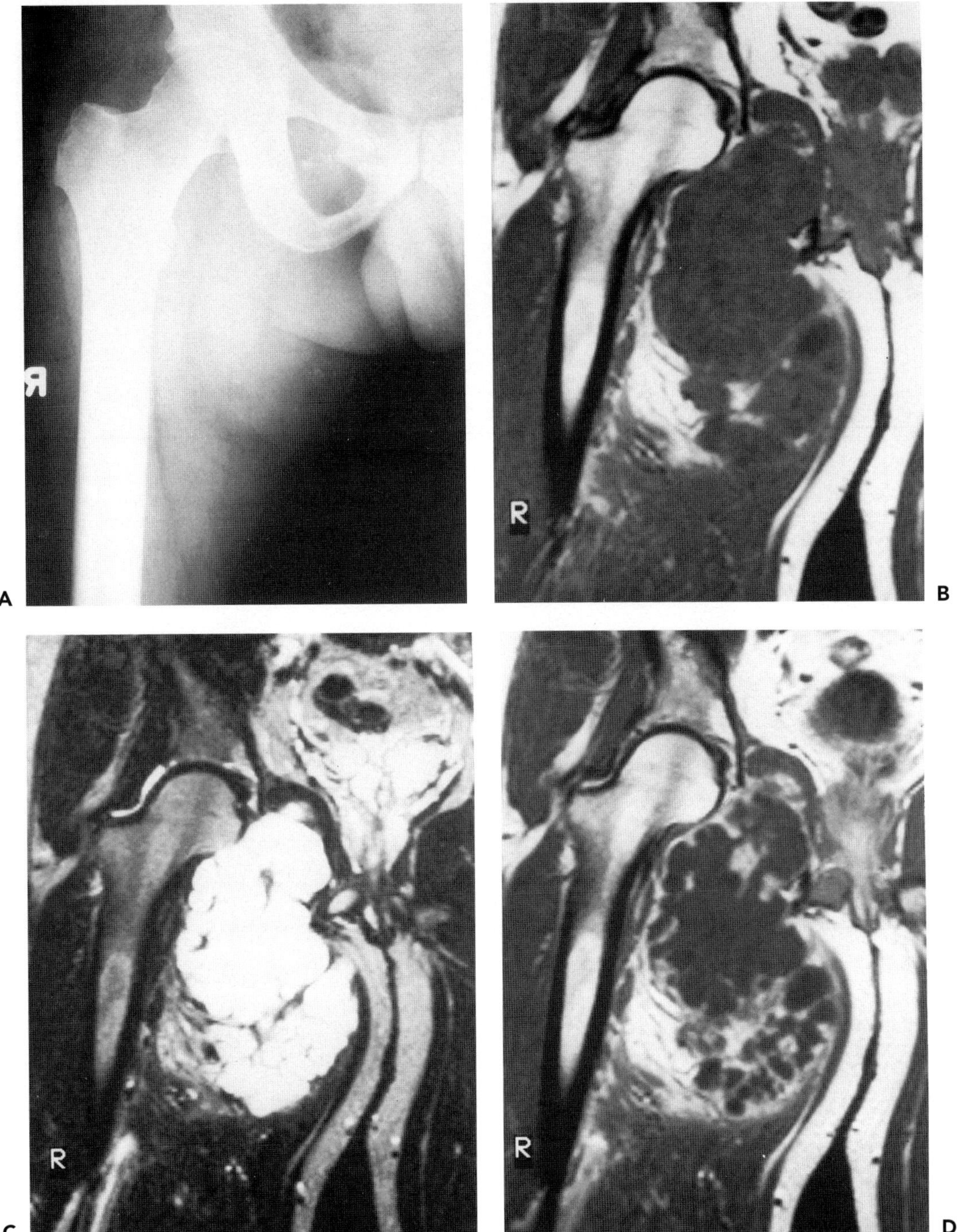

Figure 10.50 Extra-articular synovial chondromatosis: Lesion arising in the region of the hip. **A:** Anteroposterior radiograph of the hip shows a large mass with minimal calcification. **B,C:** Coronal T1-weighted (TR/TE; 761/18) **(B)** and T2-weighted (TR/TE; 2912/80) **(C)** spin-echo MR images show a well-defined, lobulated mass. The signal intensity is similar to that of skeletal muscle on T1-weighted image and greater than that of fat on T2-weighted image, suggesting fluid. **D:** Coronal T1-weighted (TR/TE; 761/18) spin-echo MR image following contrast administration shows peripheral enhancement, also suggesting fluid. Nonenhancing areas correspond to conglomerate, lobular hyaline cartilaginous mass.

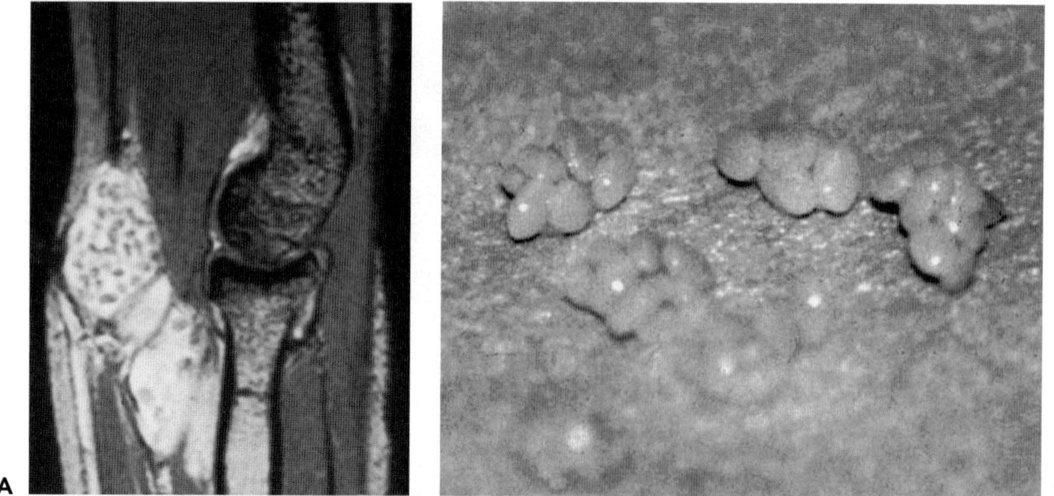

Figure 10.51   Multiple rice bodies: Imaging feature mimicking synovial chondromatosis in a woman with rheumatoid arthritis affecting the elbow. **A:** Sagittal T2-weighted spin-echo MR image shows multiple small intra-articular lesions with signal intensity similar to that of muscle. **B:** Gross photograph of portion of the resected material shows the lesions, resemblance to "grains of rice."

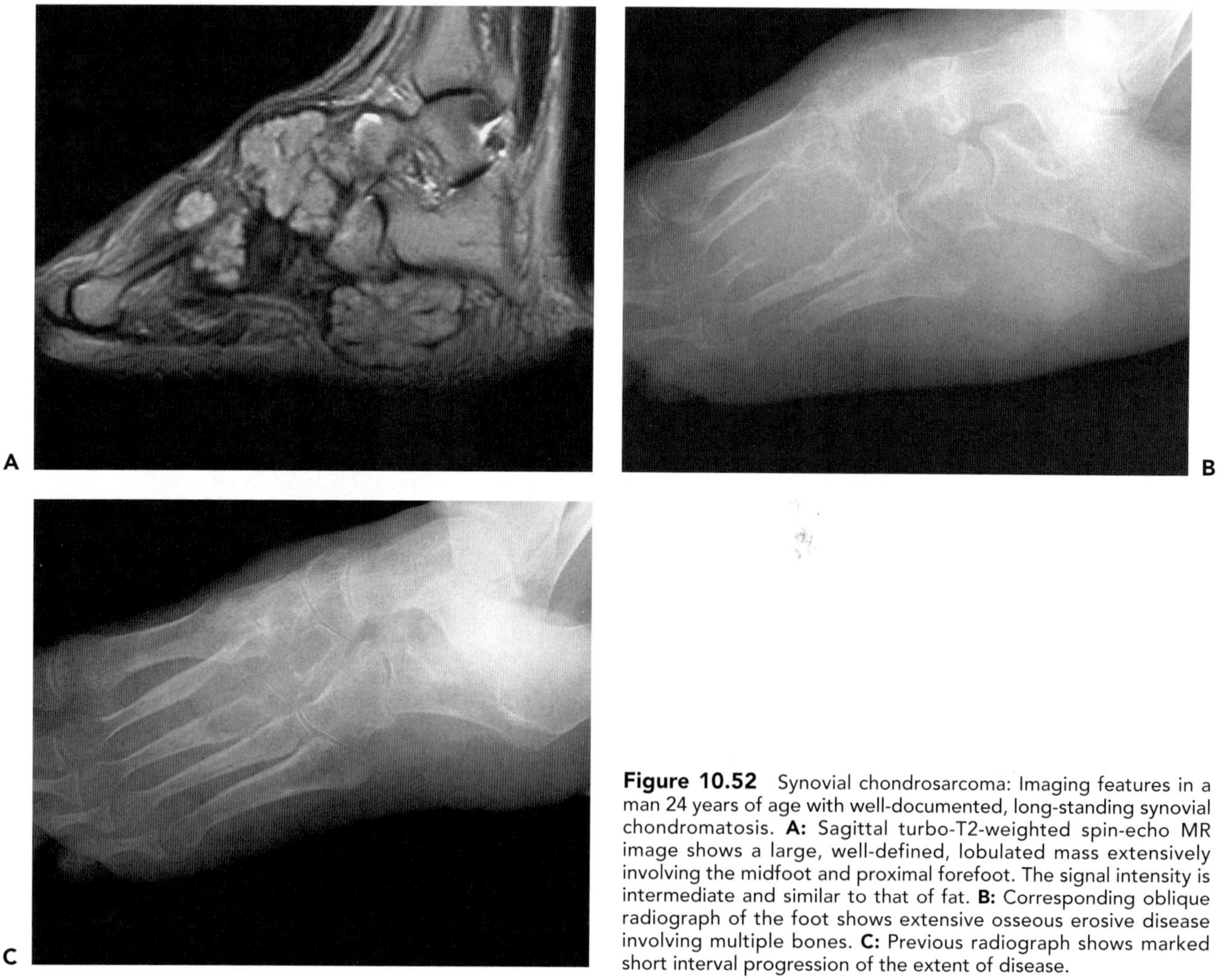

Figure 10.52   Synovial chondrosarcoma: Imaging features in a man 24 years of age with well-documented, long-standing synovial chondromatosis. **A:** Sagittal turbo-T2-weighted spin-echo MR image shows a large, well-defined, lobulated mass extensively involving the midfoot and proximal forefoot. The signal intensity is intermediate and similar to that of fat. **B:** Corresponding oblique radiograph of the foot shows extensive osseous erosive disease involving multiple bones. **C:** Previous radiograph shows marked short interval progression of the extent of disease.

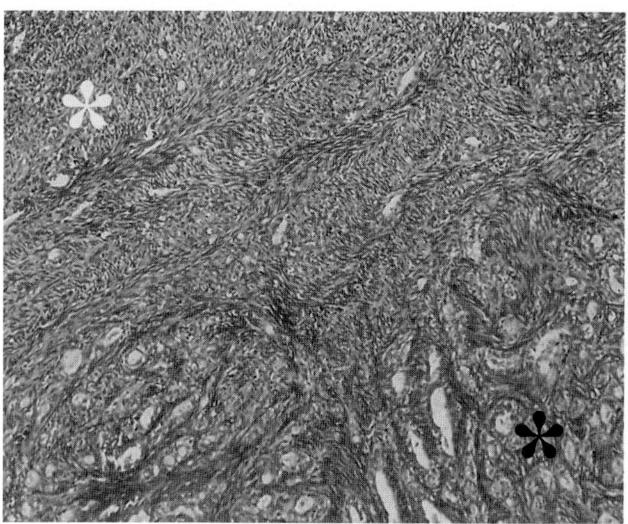

Figure 10.53 Synovial sarcoma: Histology. Low-power photomicrograph shows biphasic tumor with epithelial (*black asterisk*) and spindle cell (*white asterisk*) components.

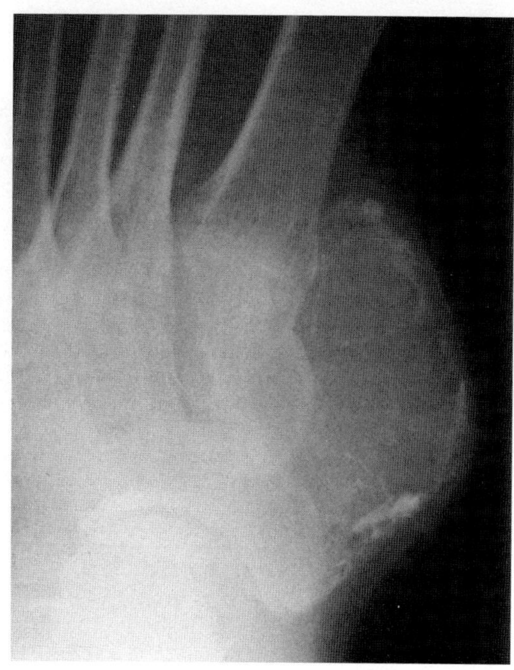

Figure 10.54 Synovial sarcoma: Radiographic features in a woman 17 years of age with a slow-growing soft tissue mass. The lesion shows moderate mineralization, which is predominantly peripheral.

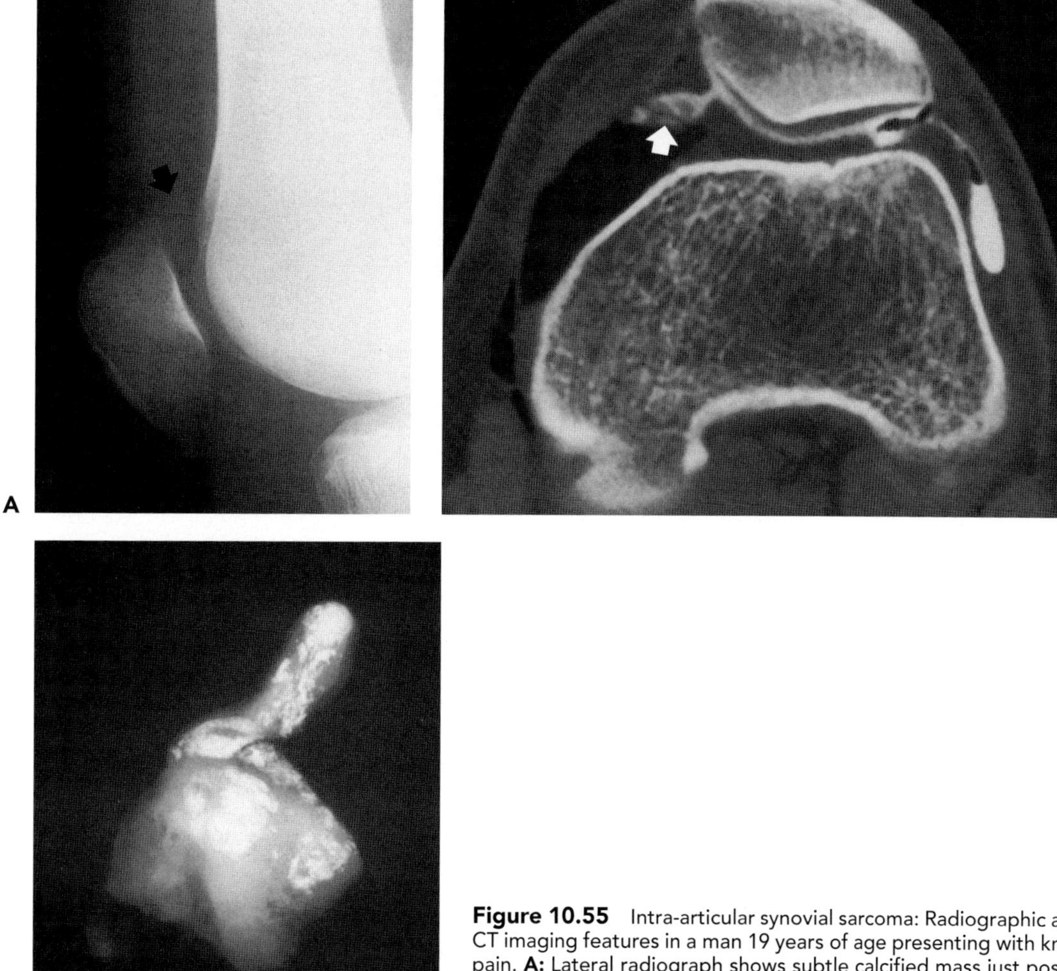

Figure 10.55 Intra-articular synovial sarcoma: Radiographic and CT imaging features in a man 19 years of age presenting with knee pain. **A:** Lateral radiograph shows subtle calcified mass just posterior to the superior pole of the patella (*arrow*). **B:** Axial CT scan from following arthrogram shows subtle mineralized mass (*arrow*) just medial to the patella. **C:** Specimen radiograph shows the lesion to be extensively mineralized.

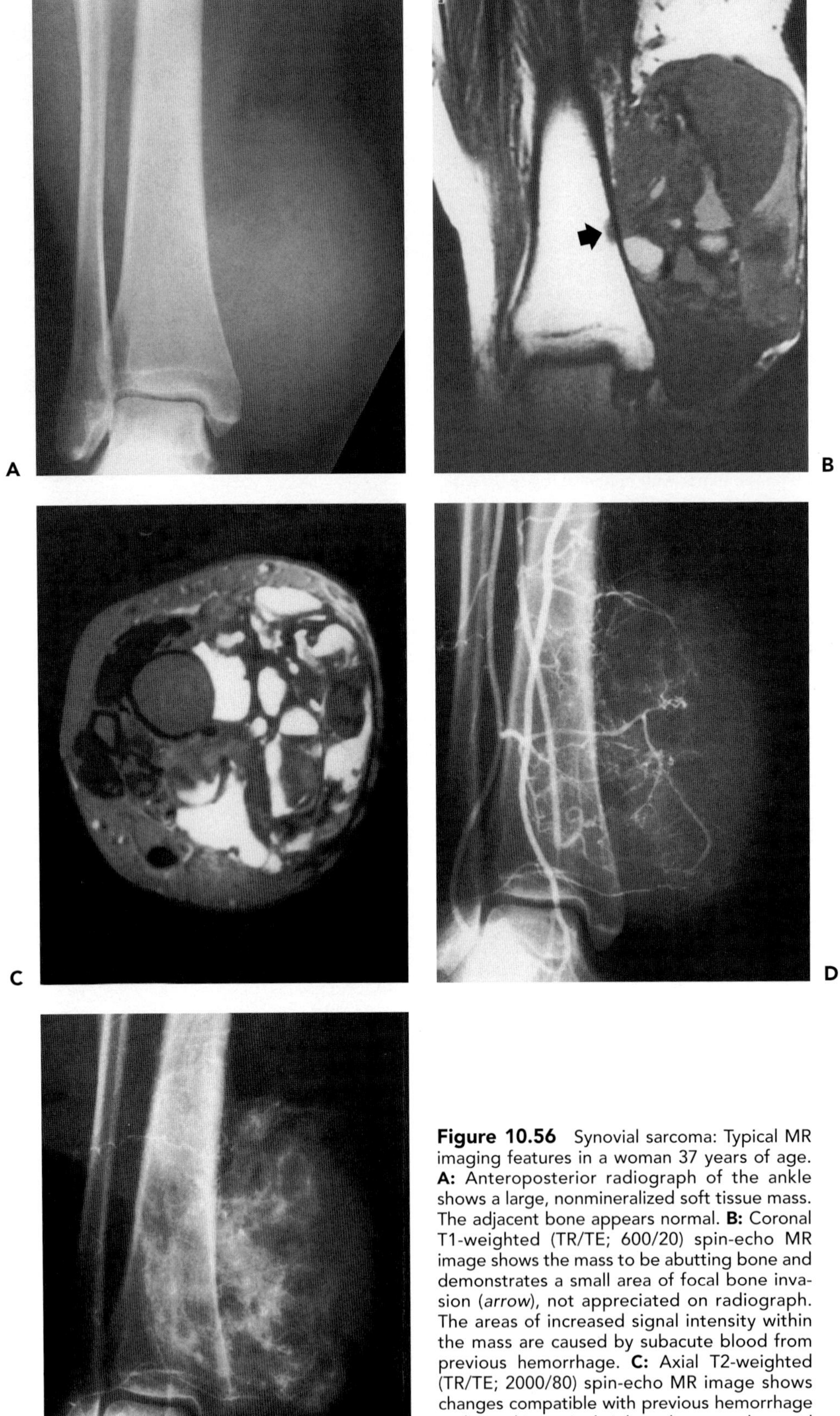

Figure 10.56 Synovial sarcoma: Typical MR imaging features in a woman 37 years of age. **A:** Anteroposterior radiograph of the ankle shows a large, nonmineralized soft tissue mass. The adjacent bone appears normal. **B:** Coronal T1-weighted (TR/TE; 600/20) spin-echo MR image shows the mass to be abutting bone and demonstrates a small area of focal bone invasion (*arrow*), not appreciated on radiograph. The areas of increased signal intensity within the mass are caused by subacute blood from previous hemorrhage. **C:** Axial T2-weighted (TR/TE; 2000/80) spin-echo MR image shows changes compatible with previous hemorrhage and signal intensity brighter than, equal to, and less than that of fat. **D,E:** Late arterial phase (**D**) and capillary phase (**E**) films from arteriogram shows marked vascularity to the mass.

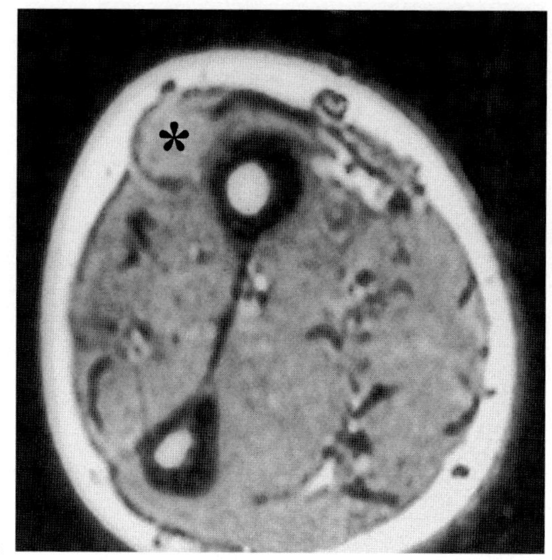
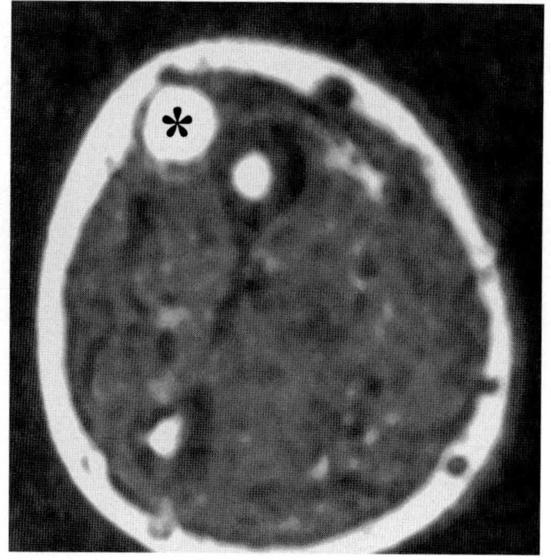

Figure 10.57 Synovial sarcoma: MR imaging appearance in the forearm of a boy 9 years of age. **A,B:** Axial T1-weighted (TR/TE; 600/16) **(A)** and T2-weighted (TR/TE; 2500/70) **(B)** spin-echo MR images show an innocent-appearing, well-defined, intramuscular nodule (*asterisk*) in the forearm. No calcification was identified on radiographs (not shown).

sarcoma, lesion mineralization may suggest synovial chondromatosis or loose body (Fig. 10.55) (182). Coexistent adjacent bone involvement, manifested by periosteal reaction, osseous remodeling (caused by pressure from the adjacent tumor), or frank bony invasion, is seen in 11% to 20% of cases (2,187,188,212). Lamellated periosteal reaction is reported, but it is rare (213). Although CT scanning is frequently viewed as superior to MR imaging in the identification of cortical invasion, osseous invasion is well-demonstrated on MR imaging, with reported sensitivity and specificity of 100% and 93%, respectively (214).

CT is particularly useful to identify soft tissue calcifications (193), especially those that are subtle or in areas where the osseous anatomy is complex, such as in the pelvis or shoulder. CT scan may also show areas of hemorrhage, necrosis, or cyst formation within the tumor (185). CT defines the mass and readily confirms bone involvement (185,193). Scans with intravenous contrast may be helpful in differentiating the mass from the adjacent muscle and the neurovascular bundle (185,193), although clearly this is better assessed with MR imaging. CT remains the modality of choice for evaluation of the chest to exclude metastatic disease. Calcification may be identified in pulmonary metastases (211).

On MR imaging the lesion is usually a nonspecific, inhomogeneous mass, with signal intensity approximately equal to that of skeletal muscle on T1-weighted and equal to and/or higher than that of subcutaneous fat on T2-weighted spin-echo MR images (207,215). The lesion may demonstrate a multiloculated configuration with internal septation (215). Marked inhomogeneity is typically present on T2-weighted images, although small lesions are more likely to be homogeneous (210). Change

compatible with previous hemorrhage may be seen in more than 40% of patients (210) and may suggest a cyst-like appearance to portions of the lesion (216). Fluid-fluid levels are reported in 10% to 25% of lesions on MR imaging (207,210,215). Jones et al. (210) reported the MR imaging findings of synovial sarcoma in 34 patients, noting 12 (35%) had areas that were hyperintense, isointense, and hypointense to fat on T2-weighted images (Fig. 10.56). This heterogeneous "triple" signal intensity was caused by a mixture of cystic (hemorrhage and necrosis) and solid elements. Although not pathognomonic for synovial sarcoma, this finding in conjunction with evidence of hemorrhage and fluid-fluid levels in a deep mass in the appropriate age individual should suggest the diagnosis. Imaging features associated with a poorer prognosis include proximal location, size greater than 5 cm, absence of calcification, presence of hemorrhage, and presence of triple signal pattern (204).

Margins are variable but are typically well-defined, although less commonly, portions of the margins may be poorly defined or infiltrating (210,215,217). Well-defined homogeneous lesions with nonspecific signal intensity may appear to be deceptively innocent (Fig. 10.57). Signal intensity similar to that of skeletal muscle on both T1- and T2-weighted images have also reported (215). The soft tissue calcifications frequently seen on radiographs may not be detected on MR imaging (207,215), although larger calcifications may be identified as areas of decreased signal intensity on all pulse sequences (Fig. 10.58).

Scintigraphy may be normal or show significantly increased uptake of technetium-99m MDP caused by mineralization within the tumor, which may not be apparent on radiographs (218,219). Flow and blood-pool images may

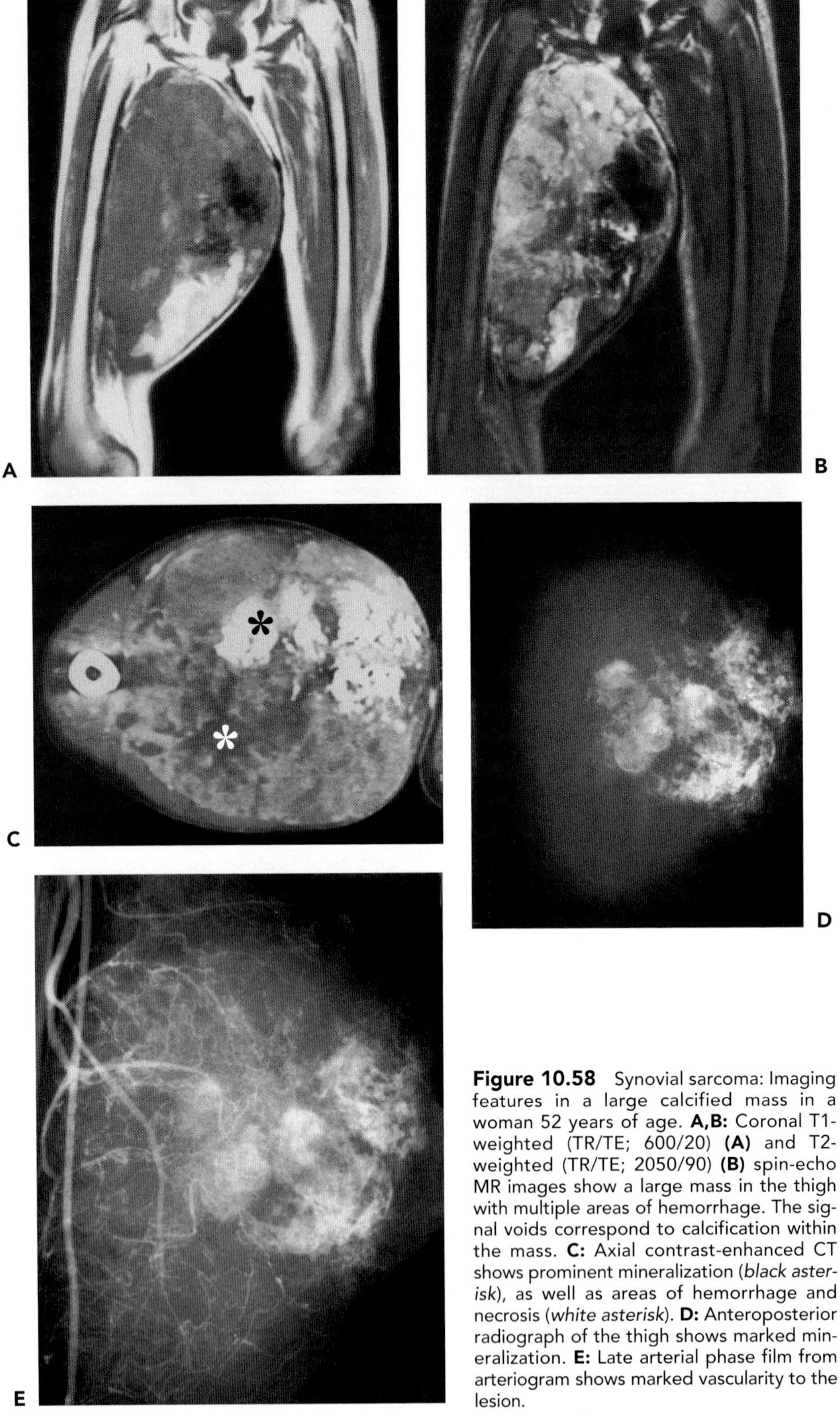

Figure 10.58 Synovial sarcoma: Imaging features in a large calcified mass in a woman 52 years of age. **A,B:** Coronal T1-weighted (TR/TE; 600/20) **(A)** and T2-weighted (TR/TE; 2050/90) **(B)** spin-echo MR images show a large mass in the thigh with multiple areas of hemorrhage. The signal voids correspond to calcification within the mass. **C:** Axial contrast-enhanced CT shows prominent mineralization (*black asterisk*), as well as areas of hemorrhage and necrosis (*white asterisk*). **D:** Anteroposterior radiograph of the thigh shows marked mineralization. **E:** Late arterial phase film from arteriogram shows marked vascularity to the lesion.

show marked focal tracer accumulation, reflecting the vascularity of the lesion, with decreased tracer accumulation in areas of hematoma formation (218,219). Arteriography will reflect this, demonstrating hypervascularity (Fig. 10.56).

REFERENCES

1. Fletcher CDM, Unni KK, Mertens F. *WHO Classification of tumors. Pathology and Genetics: Tumors of Soft Tissue and Bone.* Lyon, France: IARC Press; 2002.
2. Weiss SW, Goldblum JR. Benign tumors and tumor-like lesions of synovial tissue. In: *Enzinger and Weiss's Soft Tissue Tumors.* 4th ed. St. Louis: Mosby; 2001:1037–1062.
3. Jaffe HL, Lichtenstein L, Sutro CJ. Pigmented villonodular synovitis, bursitis and tenosynovitis. *Arch Pathol Lab Med.* 1941;31: 731–765.
4. Ferrer J, Namiq A, Carda C, et al. Diffuse type of giant-cell tumor of tendon sheath: an ultrastructural study of two cases with cytogenetic support. *Ultrastruct Pathol.* 2002;26:15–21.
5. Granowitz SP, D'Antonio J, Mankin HL. The pathogenesis and long-term end results of pigmented villonodular synovitis. *Clin Orthop.* 1976;114:335–351.
6. de St Aubain Somerhausen N, Cal Cin P. Giant cell tumor of tendon sheath. In: Fletcher DM, Unni KK, Mertens F, eds. *WHO Classification of Tumors. Pathology and Genetics: Tumors of Soft Tissue and Bone.* Lyon, France: IARC Press; 2002:110–111.
7. Ushijma M, Hashimoto H, Tsuneyoshi M, et al. Giant cell tumor of the tendon sheath (nodular tenosynovitis). A study of 207 cases to compare the large joint group with the common digit group. *Cancer.* 1986;57:875–884.
8. Savage RC, Mustafa ED. Giant cell tumor of tendon sheath (localized nodular tenosynovitis). *Plastic Surg.* 1984;13:205–210.
9. Bogumill GP, Sullivan DJ, Baker GI. Tumors of the hand. *Clin Orthop.* 1975;108:214–222.
10. Oyemade GA-A, Abioye A-A. A clinicopathologic review of benign giant cell tumors of tendon sheaths in Ibadan, Nigeria. *Am J Surg.* 1977;134:392–395.
11. Karasick D, Karasick S. Giant cell tumor of tendon sheath: spectrum of radiologic findings. *Skeletal Radiol.* 1992;21:219–224.
12. Kransdorf MJ. Benign soft-tissue tumors in a large referral population: distribution of diagnoses by age, sex and location. *AJR Am J Roentgenol.* 1995;164:395–402.
13. Jelinek JS, Kransdorf MJ, Shmookler BM, et al. Giant cell tumor of tendon sheath: MR imaging in nine cases. *AJR Am J Roentgenol.* 1994;162:919–922.
14. Kitagawa Y, Ito H, Amano Y, et al. MR imaging for preoperative diagnosis and assessment of local tumor extent on localized giant cell tumor of tendon sheath. *Skeletal Radiol.* 2003;32:633–638.
15. Huang GS, Lee CH, Chan WP, et al. Localized nodular synovitis of the knee: MR imaging appearance and clinical correlates in 21 patients. *AJR Am J Roentgenol.* 2003;181:539–543.
16. De Ponti A, Sansone V, Malchere M. Result of arthroscopic treatment of pigmented villonodular synovitis of the knee. *Arthroscopy.* 2003;19:602–607.
17. Dunstan E, Freeman R, Dowd G. Two contrasting presentations of localised pigmented villonodular synovitis of the knee. *Knee Surg Sports Traumatol Arthrosc.* 2002;10:352–354.
18. Kim RS, Lee JY, Lee KY. Localized pigmented villonodular synovitis attached to the posterior cruciate ligament of the knee. *Arthroscopy.* 2003;19:e37–e40.
19. Sundaram M, McGuire MH, Fletcher J, et al. Magnetic resonance imaging of lesions of synovial origin. *Skeletal Radiol.* 1986;15: 110–116.
20. Al-Nakshabandi NA, Ryan AG, Choudur H, et al. Pigmented villonodular synovitis. *Clin Radiol.* 2004;59:414–420.
21. Dorwart RH, Genant HK, Johnston WH, et al. Pigmented villonodular synovitis of synovial joints: clinical, pathologic and radiologic features. *AJR Am J Roentgenol.* 1984;143:877–885.
22. Dorwart RH, Genant HK, Johnston WH, et al. Pigmented villonodular synovitis of the shoulder: radiologic-pathologic assessment. *AJR Am J Roentgenol.* 1984;143:886–888.
23. Wagner ML, Spjut HJ, Dutton RV, et al. Polyarticular pigmented villonodular synovitis. *AJR Am J Roentgenol.* 1981;136: 821–823.
24. Cotten A, Flipo RM, Chastanet P, et al. Pigmented villonodular synovitis of the hip: review of radiographic features in 58 patients. *Skeletal Radiol.* 1995;24:1–6.
25. Patkar D, Prasad S, Shah J, et al. Pigmented villonodular synovitis: magnetic resonance features of an unusual case of bilateral hip joint involvement. *Australas Radiol.* 2000;44:458–459.
26. Jamieson TW, Curran JJ, Desmet A-A, et al. Bilateral pigmented villonodular synovitis of the wrists. *Orthop Rev.* 1990;19: 432–436.
27. Spritzer CE, Dalinka MK, Kressel HY. Magnetic resonance imaging of pigmented villonodular synovitis: a report of two cases. *Skeletal Radiol.* 1987;16:316–319.
28. Balsara ZN, Stainken BF, Martinez AJ. Case report. MR imaging of localized giant cell tumor of the tendon sheath involving the knee. *J Comput Assist Tomgr.* 1989;13:159–162.
29. Sundaram M, Chalk D, Merenda J, et al. Case report 563. Pigmented villonodular synovitis (PVNS) of knee. *Skeletal Radiol.* 1989;18:463–465.
30. Bobechko WP, Kostiuk JP. Childhood villonodular synovitis. *Can J Surg.* 1968;1:480–486.
31. Byers PD, Cotton RE, Deacon OW, et al. The diagnosis and treatment of pigmented villonodular synovitis. *J Bone Joint Surg.* 1868;50B:290–305.
32. Gonzalez Della Valle A, Piccaluga F, Potter HG, et al. Pigmented villonodular synovitis of the hip: 2- to 23-year followup study. *Clin Orthop.* 2001;388:187–199.
33. Rosenthal DI, Aronow S, Murray WT. Iron content of pigmented villonodular synovitis detected by computed tomography. *Radiology.* 1979;133:409–411.
34. Rosenthal DI, Coleman PK, Schiller AL. Pigmented villonodular synovitis: correlation of angiographic and histologic findings. *AJR Am J Roentgenol.* 1980;135:581–585.
35. Jaffe HL, Lichtenstein L, Sutro CJ. Pigmented villonodular synovitis, bursitis and tenosynovitis. *Arch Pathol Lab Med.* 1941;31:731–765.
36. Carstens PHB, Howell RS. Case report. Malignant giant cell tumor of tendon sheath. *Virchows Arch.* 1979;382:237–243.
37. Wu NL, Hsiao PF, Chen BF, et al. Malignant giant cell tumor of the tendon sheath. *Int J Dermatol.* 2004;43:54–57.
38. de St Aubain Somerhausen N, Cal Cin P. Diffuse-type giant cell tumor. In: Fletcher DM, Unni KK, Mertens F, eds. *WHO Classification of Tumors. Pathology and Genetics: Tumors of Soft Tissue and Bone.* Lyon, France: IARC Press; 2002:112–114.
39. Layfield LJ, Meloni-Ehrig A, Liu K, et al. Malignant giant cell tumor of synovium (malignant pigmented villonodular synovitis). *Arch Pathol Lab Med.* 2000;124:1636–1641.
40. Bertoni F, Unni KK, Beabout JW, et al. Malignant giant cell tumor of the tendon sheaths and joints (malignant pigmented villonodular synovitis). *Am J Surg Pathol.* 1997;21:153–163.
41. Mackie GC. Pigmented villonodular synovitis and giant cell tumor of the tendon sheath: scintigraphic findings in 10 cases. *Clin Nucl Med.* 2003;28:881–885.
42. Jelinek JS, Kransdorf MJ, Utz JA, et al. Imaging of pigmented villonodular synovitis with emphasis on magnetic resonance imaging. *AJR Am J Roentgenol.* 1989;152:337–342.
43. Linderbaum BL, Hunt T. An unusual presentation of pigmented villonodular synovitis. *Clin Orthop.* 1977;122:263–267.
44. Kitapci MT, Coleman RE. Incidental detection of pigmented villonodular synovitis on FDG PET. *Clin Nucl Med.* 2003;28: 668–669.
45. Weisz GM, Gal A, Kitchener PN. Magnetic resonance imaging in the diagnosis of aggressive villonodular synovitis. *Clin Orthop.* 1988;236:303–305.
46. Mohana-Borges AVR, Chung CB, Resnick D. Monoarticular arthritis. *Radiol Clin North Am.* 2004;42:135–149.
47. Hughes TH, Sartoris DJ, Schweitzer ME, et al. Pigmented villonodular synovitis: MRI characteristics. *Skeletal Radiol.* 1995;24: 7–12.
48. Kottal RA, Vogler JB, Matamoros A, et al. Pigmented villonodular synovitis: a report of MR imaging in two cases. *Radiology.* 1987;163:551–553.
49. Cotton A, Flipo RM, Mestdagh H, et al. Diffuse pigmented villonodular synovitis of the shoulder. *Skeletal Radiol.* 1995;24: 311–313.
50. Stark DD, Mosley ME, Brown BR, et al. Magnetic resonance imaging and spectroscopy of hepatic iron overload. *Radiology.* 1985;154:137–142.

51. Spence LD, Adams J, Gibbons D, et al. Rice body formation in bicipito-radial bursitis: ultrasound, CT, and MRI findings. *Skeletal Radiol.* 1998;27:30–32.

52. Dale K, Smith HJ, Paus AC, et al. Dynamic MR-imaging in the diagnosis of pigmented villonodular synovitis of the knee. *Scand J Rheumatol.* 2000;29:336–339.

53. Abdelwahab IF, Kenan S, Steiner GC, et al. True bursal pigmented villonodular synovitis. *Skeletal Radiol.* 2002;31:354–358.

54. Murphey MD, Kransdorf MJ. Radiologic evaluation of soft tissue tumors. In: Miettinen M, ed, *Diagnostic Soft Tissue Pathology.* New York: Churchill Livingstone; 2003:13–39.

55. Lindgren PG, Willén R. Gastrocnemio-semimembranosus bursa and its relation to the knee joint. Anatomy and histology. *Acta Radiologica.* 1977;18:497–512.

56. Wolfe RD, Colloff B. Popliteal cysts. An arthrographic study and review of the literature. *J Bone Joint Surg.* 1972;54A: 1057–1063.

57. Fielding JR, Franklin PD, Kustan J. Popliteal cysts: a reassessment using magnetic resonance imaging. *Skeletal Radiol.* 1991;20: 433–435.

58. Wilson PD, Eyre-Brook AL, Francis JD. A clinical and anatomic study of the semimembranosus bursa in relation to popliteal cyst. *J Bone Joint Surg.* 1938;20:963–984.

59. Baker WM. On the formation of synovial cysts in the leg in connection with disease of the knee-joint. *St Bartholomews Hosp Rep.* 1877;13:245–261.

60. Baker WM. The formation of abnormal synovial cysts in connection with the joints (second communication). St Bartholomews Hosp Rep 1885;21:177–190.

61. Lee KR, Cox GG, Neff JR, et al. Cystic masses of the knee: arthrographic and CT evaluation. *AJR Am J Roentgenol.* 1987;148: 329–334.

62. Fang CS, McCarthy CL, McNally EG. Intramuscular dissection of Baker's cysts: report on three cases. *Skeletal Radiol.* 2004;33: 367–371.

63. Hermann G, Yeh HC, Lehr-Janus C, et al. Diagnosis of popliteal cyst: double-contrast arthrography and sonography. *AJR Am J Roentgenol.* 1981;137:369–372.

64. Richardson ML, Selby B, Montana MA, et al. Ultrasonography of the knee. *Radiol Clin North Am.* 1988;26:63–75.

65. McCarthy CL, McNally EG. The MRI appearance of cystic lesions around the knee. *Skeletal Radiol.* 2004;33:187–209.

66. Bierbaum BE. Double contrast knee arthrography. A safe and reliable aid to diagnosis of "internal derangement." *J Trauma.* 1968; 8:165–176.

67. Butt WP, McIntyre JL. Double-contrast arthrography of the knee. *Radiology.* 1969;92:487–499.

68. Nicholas JA, Freiberger RH, Killoran PJ. Double-contrast arthrography of the knee. *J Bone Joint Surg.* 1970;52A:203–220.

69. Genovese GR, Joyson MIV, Dixon ASJ. Protective value of synovial cysts in rheumatoid arthritis. *Ann Rheum Dis.* 1972;31: 179–182.

70. Moore CP, Sarti DA, Louie JS. Ultrasonic demonstration of popliteal cysts in rheumatoid arthritis. *Arthritis Rheum.* 1975; 18:577–580.

71. McDonald DG, Leopold GR. Ultrasound B-scanning in the differentiation of Baker's cyst and thrombophlebitis. *Br J Radiol.* 1972;45:729–732.

72. Good AE. Rheumatoid arthritis, Baker's cyst and "thrombophlebitis." *Arthritis Rheum.* 1964;7:56–64.

73. Lazarus ML, Ray CE, Maniquis CG. MRI findings on concurrent acute DVT and dissecting popliteal cyst. *Magn Reson Imaging.* 1994;12:155–158.

74. Mink JH, Deutsch AL. *MRI of the Musculoskeletal System: A Teaching File.* New York: Raven Press; 1990.

75. Shepherd JR, Helms CA. Atypical popliteal cyst due to lateral synovial herniation. *Radiology.* 1981;140:66.

76. Corbetti F, Schiavon F, Fiocco U, et al. Unusual antefemoral dissecting cyst. *Br J Radiol.* 1985;58:675–677.

77. Palmer DG. Antero-medial synovial cysts at the knee joint in rheumatoid disease. *Australas Radiol.* 1972;16:79–83.

78. O'Dell JR, Anderson PA, Hollister JR, et al. Anterior tibial mass: an unusual complication of popliteal cyst. *Arthritis Rheum.* 1984;27:113–115.

79. Seidl G, Scherak O, Hofner W. Antefemoral dissecting cysts in rheumatoid arthritis. *Radiology.* 1979;133:343–347.

80. Sugiura M, Komiyama T, Akagi D, et al. Compression of the iliac vein by a synovial cyst. *Ann Vasc Surg.* 2004;18:369–371.

81. Fedullo LM, Bonakdarpour A, Moyer RA, et al. Giant synovial cysts. *Skeletal Radiol.* 1984;12:90–96.

82. Morris CS, Beltran JL. Giant synovial cyst associated with a pseudarthrosis of a rib: MR appearance. *AJR Am J Roentgenol.* 1990;155:337–338.

83. Heppenstall RB, Brighton CT, Esterhai JL, et al. Synovial pseudarthrosis: a clinical, roentgenographic-scintigraphic, and pathologic study. *J Trauma.* 1987;27:463–470.

84. Stahnke M, Mangham DC, Davies AM. Calcific haemorrhagic bursitis anterior to the knee mimicking a soft tissue sarcoma: report of two cases. *Skeletal Radiol.* 2004;33:363–366.

85. Friedman L, Finlay K, Jurria-ans E. Ultrasound of the knee. *Skeletal Radiol.* 2001;30:361–377.

86. Sundaram M, McGuire MH, Fletcher J, et al. Magnetic resonance imaging of lesions of synovial origin. *Skeletal Radiol.* 1986;15: 110–116.

87. Langer JE, Meyer SJF, Dalinka MK. Imaging of the knee. *Radiol Clin North Am.* 1990;28:975–990.

88. Hartzman S, Reicher MA, Bassett LW, et al. MR imaging of the knee. Part II. Chronic disorders. *Radiology.* 1987;162: 553–557.

89. Schwimmer M, Edelstein G, Heiken JP, et al. Synovial cysts of the knee: CT evaluation. *Radiology.* 1985;154:175–177.

90. Feldman F, Singson RD, Staron RB. Magnetic resonance imaging of para-articular and ectopic ganglia. *Skeletal Radiol.* 1989;18: 353–358.

91. Hippocrates. *On Joints.* Withington ET, trans. London: W. Heinemann; 1927:277.

92. Conrad EU, Enneking WF. Common soft tissue tumors. *Clin Symp.* 1990;42:21.

93. Butt WP, McIntyre JL. Double-contrast arthrography of the knee. *Radiology.* 1969;92:487–499.

94. DeFlaviis L, Nessi R, Del Bo P, et al. High-resolution ultrasonography of wrist ganglia. *J Clin Ultrasound.* 1987;15:17–22.

95. Haller J, Resnick D, Greenway G, et al. Juxta-acetabular ganglionic (or synovial) cysts: CT and MR features. *J Comput Assist Tomogr.* 1989;13:976–983.

96. Cardinal E, Buckwalter KA, Braunstein EM, et al. Occult dorsal carpal ganglion: comparison of US and MR imaging. *Radiology.* 1994;193:259–262.

97. el-Noueam KI, Schweitzer ME, Blasbalg R, et al. Is a subset of wrist ganglia the sequela of internal derangements of the wrist joint? MR imaging findings. *Radiology.* 1999;212:537–540.

98. Kirby EJ, Shereff MJ, Lewis MM. Soft-tissue tumors and tumor-like lesions of the foot. *J Bone Joint Surg.* 1989;71A:621–626.

99. Fornage BD, Rifkin MD. Ultrasound examination of the hand and foot. *Radiol Clin North Am.* 1988;26:109–129.

100. Ogino T, Minami A, Kato H. Diagnosis of radial nerve palsy caused by ganglion with use of different imaging techniques. *J Hand Surg.* 1991;16A:230–235.

101. Fritz RC, Helms CA, Steinbach LS, et al. Suprascapular nerve entrapment: evaluation with MR imaging. *Radiology.* 1992;182: 437–444.

102. Bianchi S, Abdelwahab IF, Kenan S, et al. Intramuscular ganglia arising from the superior tibiofibular joint: CT and MR evaluation. *Skeletal Radiol.* 1995;24:253–256.

103. Tom BM, Rao VM, Farole A. Bilateral temporomandibular joint ganglion cysts: CT and MR characteristics. *AJNR Am J Neuroradiol.* 1990;11:746–748.

104. Caan P. Zystenbildung im ligamentum cruciatum ant genus. *Deutsch Z Chir.* 1924;186:403–408.

105. Angelides AC, Wallace PF. The dorsal ganglion of the wrist: its pathogenesis, gross and microscopic anatomy, and surgical treatment. *J Hand Surg [Am].* 1976;1:228–235.

106. McLaren DB, Buckwalter KA, Vahey TN. The prevalence and significance of cyst-like changes at the cruciate ligament attachments in the knee. *Skeletal Radiol.* 1992;21:365–369.

107. Zantop T, Rusch A, Hassenpflug J, et al. Intra-articular ganglion cysts of the cruciate ligaments: case report and review of the literature. *Arch Orthop Trauma Surg.* 2003;123:195–198.

108. Kakutani K, Yoshiya S, Matsui N, et al. An intraligamentous ganglion cyst of the anterior cruciate ligament after a traumatic event. *Arthroscopy.* 2003;19:1019–1022.

109. Recht MP, Applegate G, Kaplan P, et al. The MR appearance of cruciate ganglion cysts: a report of 16 cases. *Skeletal Radiol.* 1994;23:597–600.

110. Krudwig WK, Schulte KK, Heinemann C. Intra-articular ganglion cysts of the knee joint: a report of 85 cases and review of the literature. *Knee Surg Sports Traumatol Arthrosc.* 2004;12:123–129.

111. Bergin D, Morrison WB, Carrino JA, et al. Anterior cruciate ligament ganglia and mucoid degeneration: coexistence and clinical correlation. *AJR Am J Roentgenol.* 2004;182:1283–1287.

112. DeFriend DE, Schranz PJ, Silver DA. Ultrasound-guided aspiration of posterior cruciate ligament ganglion cysts. *Skeletal Radiol.* 2001;30:411–414.

113. Okada K, Unoki E, Kubota H, et al. Periosteal ganglion: a report of three new cases including MRI findings and a review of the literature. *Skeletal Radiol.* 1996;25:153–157.

114. Abdelwahab IF, Kenan S, Hermann G, et al. Periosteal ganglia: CT and MR imaging features. *Radiology.* 1993;188:245–248.

115. Blanco JF, De Pedro JA, Paniagua JC. Periosteal ganglion in a child. *Arch Orthop Trauma Surg.* 2003;123:115–117.

116. Chiba T, Hatori M, Abe Y, et al. Periosteal ganglion of the radius: a case report. *Tohoku J Exp Med.* 1998;185:71–78.

117. Valls R, Melloni P, Darnell A, et al. Diagnostic imaging of tibial periosteal ganglion. *Eur Radiol.* 1997;7:70–72.

118. McCarthy EF, Maltz S, Steiner GC, et al. Periosteal ganglion: a cause of cortical bone erosion. *Skeletal Radiol.* 1983;10:243–246.

119. De Maeseneer M, De Boeck H, Shahabpour M, et al. Subperiosteal ganglion cyst of the tibia. A communication with the knee demonstrated by delayed arthrography. *J Bone Joint Surg Br.* 1999;81:643–646.

120. Forbes JR, Helms CA, Janzen DL. Acute pes anserine bursitis: MR imaging. *Radiology.* 1995;194:525–527.

121. Fornage BD, Schernberg FL, Rifkin MD. Ultrasound examination of the hand. *Radiology.* 1985;155:785–788.

122. Hashimoto BE, Hayes AS, Ager JD. Sonographic diagnosis and treatment of ganglion cysts causing suprascapular nerve entrapment. *J Ultrasound Med.* 1994;13:671–674.

123. Weiss KL, Beltran J, Lubbers LM. High-field MR surface-coil imaging of the hand and wrist. Part II. Pathologic correlation and clinical relevance. *Radiology.* 1986;160:147–152.

124. Johnson J, Kilgore E, Newmeyer W. Tumorous lesions of the hand. *J Hand Surg.* 1985;10:284–286.

125. Okamoto S, Hisaoka M, Meis-Kindblom JM, et al. Juxta-articular myxoma and intramuscular myxoma are two distinct entities. Activating Gs alpha mutation at Arg 201 codon does not occur in juxta-articular myxoma. *Virchows Arch.* 2002;440:12–15.

126. Meis JM, Enzinger FM. Juxta-articular myxoma: a clinical and pathologic study of 65 cases. *Hum Pathol.* 1992;23:639–646.

127. Daluiski A, Seeger LL, Doberneck SA, et al. A case of juxta-articular myxoma of the knee. *Skeletal Radiol.* 1995;24:389–391.

128. Ozcanli H, Ozenci AM, Gurer EI, et al. Juxta-articular myxoma of the wrist: a case report. *J Hand Surg [Am].* 2005;30:165–167.

129. Minkoff J, Stecker S, Irizarry J, et al. Juxta-articular myxoma: a rare cause of painful restricted motion of the knee. *Arthroscopy.* 2003;19:e143–e150.

130. Echols PG, Omer GE Jr, Crawford MK. Juxta-articular myxoma of the shoulder presenting as a cyst of the acromioclavicular joint: a case report. *J Shoulder Elbow Surg.* 2000;9:157–159.

131. King DG, Saifuddin A, Preston HV, et al. Magnetic resonance imaging of juxta-articular myxoma. *Skeletal Radiol.* 1995;24:145–147.

132. Milgram JW. Synovial osteochondromatosis. A histopathological study of thirty cases. *J Bone Joint Surg Am* 1977;59A:792–801.

133. Buddingh EP, Krallman P, Neff JR, et al. Chromosome 6 abnormalities are recurrent in synovial chondromatosis. *Cancer Genet Cytogenet.* 2003;140:18–22.

134. Sandberg A-A. Genetics of chondrosarcoma and related tumors. *Curr Opin Oncol.* 2004;16:342–354.

135. Robinson P, White LM, Kandel R, et al. Primary synovial osteochondromatosis of the hip: extracapsular patterns of spread. *Skeletal Radiol.* 2004;33:210–215.

136. Wenger DE, Sundaram M, Unni KK, et al. Acral synovial chondrosarcoma. *Skeletal Radiol.* 2002;31:125–129.

137. Sheldon PJ, Forrester DM, Learch TJ. Imaging of intra-articular masses. *Radiographics.* 2005;25:105–119.

138. Chung EB, Enzinger FM. Extraskeletal osteosarcoma. *Cancer.* 1987;60:1132–1142.

139. Milgram JW. The development of loose bodies in human joints. *Clin Orthop.* 1977;124:292–303.

140. Sim FH, Dahlin DC, Ivins JC. Extra-articular synovial chondromatosis. *J Bone Joint Surg.* 1977;59A:492–495.

141. Abu-Yousef MM, El-Khoury GY. Case report 307. Synovial osteochondromatosis limited to a popliteal cyst. *Skeletal Radiol.* 1985;13:234–238.

142. Milgram JW, Hadesman WM. Synovial osteochondromatosis in the subacromial bursa. *Clin Orthop.* 1988;236:154–159.

143. Pope TL, Keats TE, de Lange EE, et al. Idiopathic synovial chondromatosis in two unusual sites: inferior radioulnar joint and ischial bursa. *Skeletal Radiol.* 1987;16:205–208.

144. Murphy FP, Dahlin DC, Sullivan CR. Articular synovial chondromatosis. *J Bone Joint Surg.* 1962;44A:77–86.

145. Villacin AB, Brigham LN, Bullough PG. Primary and secondary synovial chondrometaplasia. Histologic and clinicoradiologic differences. *Human Pathol.* 1979;10:439–451.

146. Coscia MF, Edmonson AS, Pitcock JA. Paravertebral synovial osteochondromatosis. A case report. *Spine.* 1986;11:82–87.

147. Giustra PE, Furman RS, Roberts L, et al. Synovial osteochondromatosis involving the elbow. *AJR Am J Roentgenol.* 1976;127:347–348.

148. Silver CM, Simon SD, Litchman HM, et al. Synovial chondromatosis of the temporomandibular joint: a case report. *J Bone Joint Surg.* 1971;53A:777–780.

149. Akhtar M, Mahajan S, Kott E. Synovial chondromatosis of the temporomandibular joint: a case report. *J Bone Joint Surg.* 1977;59A:266–267.

150. Bloom R, Pattinson JN. Osteochondromatosis of the hip joint. *J Bone Joint Surg.* 1951;33B:80–84.

151. Fahmy NRM, Noble J. Ulnar palsy as a complication of synovial osteochondromatosis of the elbow. *Hand.* 1981;13:308–310.

152. Edeiken J, Edeiken BS, Ayala AG, et al. Giant solitary synovial chondromatosis. *Skeletal Radiol.* 1994;23:23–29.

153. Lagier R. Case report 451. Primary synovial osteochondromatosis of the knee with extensive bone formation observed over a period of 13 years. *Skeletal Radiol.* 1987;16:660–665.

154. Friedman B, Nerubay J, Blankstein A, et al. Case report 439. Synovial chondromatosis (osteochondromatosis) of the right hip: "hidden" radiologic manifestations. *Skeletal Radiol.* 1987;16:504–508.

155. Kramer J, Recht M, Deely DM, et al. MR appearance of idiopathic synovial osteochondromatosis. *J Comput Assist Tomogr.* 1993;17:772–776.

156. Schofield TD, Pitcher JD, Youngberg R. Synovial chondromatosis simulating neoplastic degeneration of osteochondromatosis: findings on MRI and CT. *Skeletal Radiol.* 1994;23:99–102.

157. Tan CHA, Rai SB, Chandy J. MRI appearances of multiple rice body formation in chronic subacromial and subdeltoid bursitis, in association with synovial chondromatosis. *Clin Radiol.* 2004;59:753–757.

158. Resnick D. Rheumatoid arthritis and the seronegative spondyloarthropathies: radiographic and pathologic concepts. In: Resnick D, ed, *Diagnosis of Bone and Joint Disorders.* 4th ed. Philadelphia: WB Saunders; 2002:837–987.

159. Lee EY, Rubin DA, Brown DM. Recurrent *Mycobacterium marinum* tenosynovitis of the wrist mimicking extra-articular synovial chondromatosis on MR images. *Skeletal Radiol.* 2004;33:405–408.

160. Milgram JW, Addison RG. Synovial osteochondromatosis of the knee. Chondromatous recurrence with possible chondrosarcomatous degeneration. *J Bone Joint Surg.* 1976;58A:264–266.

161. Goldman RL, Lichtenstein L. Synovial chondrosarcoma. *Cancer.* 1964;17:1233–1240.

162. King JW, Spjut HJ, Fechner RE, et al. Synovial chondromatosis of the knee joint. *J Bone Joint Surg.* 1967;49A:1389–1396.

163. Goldberg RP, Weissman BN, Naimark A, et al. Femoral neck erosions: sign of hip joint synovial disease. *AJR J Roentgenol.* 1983;141:107–111.

164. Norman A, Steiner GC. Bone erosion in synovial chondromatosis. *Radiology.* 1986;161:749–752.

165. Hermann G, Abdelwahab IF, Klein M, et al. Synovial chondromatosis. *Skeletal Radiol.* 1995;24:298–300.

166. Sundaram M, McGuire MH, Fletcher J, et al. Magnetic resonance imaging of lesions of synovial origin. *Skeletal Radiol.* 1986;15:110–116.

167. Roberts D, Miller TT, Erlanger SM. Sonographic appearance of primary synovial chondromatosis of the knee. *J Ultrasound Med.* 2004;23:707–709.

168. Tuckerman G, Wirth CZ. Case report. Synovial osteochondromatosis of the shoulder: MR findings. *J Comput Assist Tomogr.* 1989;13:360–361.

169. Blandino A, Salvi L, Chirico G, et al. Synovial chondromatosis of the ankle: MR findings. *Clin Imaging.* 1992;16:34–36.

170. Cohen EK, Kressel HY, Frank TS, et al. Hyaline cartilage-origin bone and soft-tissue neoplasms: MR appearance and histologic correlation. *Radiology.* 1988;167:477–481.

171. Erickson SJ, Fitzgerald SW, Quinn SF, et al. Long head tendon of the shoulder: normal anatomy and pathologic findings on MR imaging. *AJR Am J Roentgenol.* 1992;158:1091–1096.

172. Chen A, Wong LY, Sheu CY, et al. Distinguishing multiple rice body formation in chronic subacromial-subdeltoid bursitis from synovial chondromatosis. *Skeletal Radiol.* 2002;31:119–121.

173. Kenan S, Abdelwahab IF, Klein MJ, et al. Case report 817. Synovial chondrosarcoma secondary to synovial chondromatosis. *Skeletal Radiol.* 1993;22:623–626.

174. Taconis WK, van der Heul RO, Taminiau AM. Synovial chondrosarcoma: report of a case and review of the literature. *Skeletal Radiol.* 1997;26:682–685.

175. Hermann G, Klein MJ, Abdelwahab IF, et al. Synovial chondrosarcoma arising in synovial chondromatosis of the right hip. *Skeletal Radiol.* 1997;26:366–369.

176. Ontell FR, Greenspan A. Chondrosarcoma complicating synovial chondromatosis: findings with magnetic resonance imaging. *Can Assoc Radiol.* 1994;45:318–323.

177. Blokx WA, Rasing LA, Veth RP, et al. Late malignant transformation of biopsy proven benign synovial chondromatosis: an unexpected pitfall. *Histopathology.* 2000;36:564–566.

178. Bertoni F, Unni KK, Beabout JW, et al. Chondrosarcomas of the synovium. *Cancer.* 1991;67:155–162.

179. Wuisman PI, Noorda RJ, Jutte PC. Chondrosarcoma secondary to synovial chondromatosis. Report of two cases and a review of the literature. *Arch Orthop Trauma Surg.* 1997;116:307–311.

180. Hallam P, Ashwood N, Cobb J, et al. Malignant transformation in synovial chondromatosis of the knee? *Knee.* 2001;8:239–342.

181. Kransdorf MJ. Malignant soft-tissue tumors in a large referral population: distribution of diagnoses by age, sex and location. *AJR Am J Roentgenol.* 1995;164:129–134.

182. Ishida T, Iijima T, Moriyama S, et al. Intra-articular calcifying synovial sarcoma mimicking synovial chondromatosis. *Skeletal Radiol.* 1996;25:766–769.

183. Fisher C, de Bruijm DRH, Geurts van Kessel A. Synovial sarcoma. In: Fletcher DM, Unni KK, Mertens F, eds. *WHO Classification of Tumors. Pathology and Genetics: Tumors of Soft Tissue and Bone.* Lyon, France: IARC Press; 2002:200–204.

184. McCarville MB, Spunt SL, Skapek SX, et al. Synovial sarcoma in pediatric patients. *AJR Am J Roentgenol.* 2002;179:797–801.

185. Israels SJ, Chan HSL, Daneman A, et al. Synovial sarcoma in childhood. *AJR Am J Roentgenol.* 1983;142:803–806.

186. Bogumill GP, Bruna PD, Barrick EF. Malignant lesions masquerading as a popliteal cyst. *J Bone Joint Surg.* 1981;63-A:474–477.

187. Cadman NL, Soule EH, Kelley PJ. Synovial sarcoma: an analysis of 134 tumors. *Cancer.* 1965;18:613–627.

188. Wright PH, Sim FH, Soule EH, Taylor WF. Synovial sarcoma. *J Bone Joint Surg.* 1982;64A:112–122.

189. Genest P, Kim TH, Katsarkas A, et al. Calcified synovial sarcoma of the oropharynx. *Br J Radiol.* 1983;56:580–582.

190. Batsakis JG, Nishiyama RH, Sullinger GD. Synovial sarcoma of the neck. *Arch Otolaryngol.* 1961;85:327–331.

191. Roth JA, Enzinger FM, Tannenbaum MT. Synovial sarcoma of the neck: a follow up study of 24 cases. *Cancer.* 1975;35:1243–1253.

192. Shmookler BM, Enzinger FM, Brannon RB. Orofacial synovial sarcoma: a clinicopathologic study of 11 new cases and review of the literature. *Cancer.* 1982;50:269–276.

193. Treu EBWM, de Slegte RGM, Golding RP, et al. CT findings in paravertebral synovial sarcoma. *J Comput Assist Tomogr.* 1986;10:460–462.

194. Tahir T, Sanjiv G. Synovial sarcoma of the right ventricle. *Am Heart J.* 1991;121:933–938.

195. Ryan JR, Baker LH, Benjamin RS. The natural history of metastatic synovial sarcoma. The experience of the Southwest Oncology Group. *Clin Orthop.* 1982;164:257–260.

196. Paulino AC. Synovial sarcoma prognostic factors and patterns of failure. *Am J Clin Oncol.* 2004;27:122–127.

197. Sutro J. Synovial sarcoma of the soft parts in the first toe: recurrence after thirty-five year interval. *Bull Hosp Jt Dis.* 1976;37:105–109.

198. Vezeridis MP, Moore R, Karakousis CP. Metastatic patterns in soft tissue sarcomas. *Arch Surg.* 1983;118:915–918.

199. Mazeron JJ, Suit HD. Lymph nodes as sites of metastases from sarcomas of soft tissue. *Cancer.* 1987;60:1800–1808.

200. Pack GT, Ariel IM. Treatment of cancer and allied diseases. In: Pack GT, Ariel IM, eds. *Tumors of the Soft Somatic Tissues and Bone.* Vol 8. New York: Harper & Row; 1965;8–39.

201. Ariel IM. Incidence of metastases to lymph nodes from soft-tissue sarcomas. *Semin Surg Oncol.* 1988;4:27–29.

202. Meyer CA, Kransdorf MJ, Jelinek JS, et al. Case report 716. Soft tissue metastasis in synovial sarcoma. *Skeletal Radiol.* 1992;21:128–131.

203. Deshmukh R, Mankin HJ, Singer S. Synovial sarcoma: the importance of size and location for survival. *Clin Orthop.* 2004;419:155–161.

204. Tateishi U, Hasegawa T, Beppu Y, et al. Synovial sarcoma of the soft tissues: prognostic significance of imaging features. *J Comput Assist Tomogr.* 2004;28:140–148.

205. Varela-Duran J, Enzinger FM. Calcifying synovial sarcoma. *Cancer.* 1982;50:345–352.

206. Oliveria AM, Fletcher CDM. Molecular prognostication for soft tissue sarcomas: are we ready yet? *J Clin Oncol.* 2004;22:4031–4034.

207. Mahajan H, Lorigan JG, Shirkhoda A. Synovial sarcoma: MR imaging. *Magn Res Imaging.* 1989;7:211–216.

208. Evans HL. Synovial sarcoma. A study of 23 biphasic and 17 probable monophasic examples. *Pathol Annu.* 1980;15:309–331.

209. Hajdu SI, Shiu MH, Fortner JG. Tenosynovial sarcoma: a clinicopathological study of 136 cases. *Cancer.* 1977;39:1201–1217.

210. Jones BC, Sundaram M, Kransdorf MJ. Synovial sarcoma: MR imaging findings in 34 patients. *AJR Am J Roentgenol.* 1993;161:827–830.

211. Maxwell JR, Yao L, Eckardt JJ, et al. Case report 878. Densely calcifying synovial sarcoma of the hip metastatic to the lungs. *Skeletal Radiol.* 1994;23:673–675.

212. Horowitz AL, Resnick D, Watson RC. The roentgen features of synovial sarcoma. *Clin Radiol.* 1973;24:481–484.

213. Blacksin M, Adesoksan A, Benevenia J. Case report 871. Synovial sarcoma, monophasic type. *Skeletal Radiol.* 1994;23:589–591.

214. Elias DA, White LM, Simpson DJ, et al. Osseous invasion by soft-tissue sarcoma: assessment with MR imaging. *Radiology.* 2003;229:145–152.

215. Morton MJ, Berquist TH, McLeod RA, et al. MR imaging of synovial sarcoma. *AJR Am J Roentgenol.* 1990;156:337–340.

216. Nakanishi H, Araki N, Sawai Y, et al. Cystic synovial sarcomas: imaging features with clinical and histopathologic correlation. *Skeletal Radiol.* 2003;32:701–707.

217. DeCoster TA, Kamps BS, Craven JP. Magnetic resonance imaging of a foot synovial sarcoma. *Orthopedics.* 1991;14:169–171.

218. Braeuning MP, Park HE. Three-phase Tc-99m MDP scan findings of a soft tissue sarcoma. *Clin Nucl Med.* 1990;15:572–573.

219. Rice S, Stewart CA. Synovial sarcoma seen on bone scan. *Clin Nucl Med.* 1990;15:445–446.

Extraskeletal Osseous and Cartilaginous Tumors

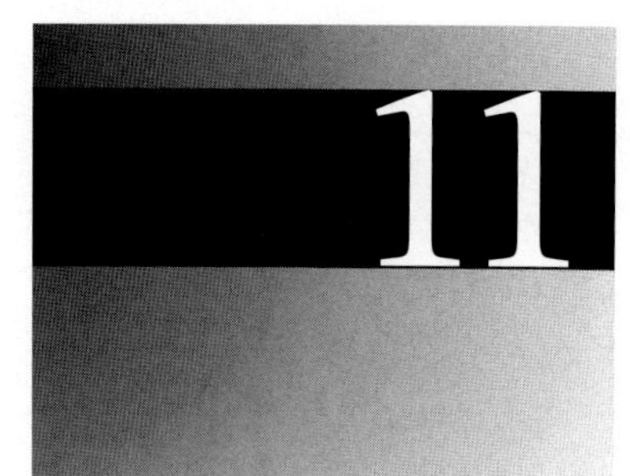

The radiologic images of extraskeletal osseous and cartilaginous tumors of the extremities are often sufficiently characteristic to suggest a specific diagnosis. This is particularly true with regard to myositis ossificans and fibrodysplasia ossificans progressiva, as well as selected instances of soft tissue chondroma and extraskeletal osteosarcoma.

The World Health Organization (WHO) currently classifies only soft tissue chondroma and extraskeletal osteosarcoma as chondro-osseous tumors (1). Myositis ossificans and fibro-osseous pseudotumor of the digits are currently classified as fibroblastic/myofibroblastic tumors. Extraskeletal myxoid chondrosarcoma is classified as a tumor of uncertain differentiation. Rather than limit this chapter to those lesions strictly defined as chondro-osseous tumors, we have chosen to demonstrate the radiologic spectrum of extraskeletal osseous and cartilaginous tumors and tumorlike conditions. Such lesions are not uncommon in clinical practice, and although it is useful to group these lesions together for purposes of differential diagnosis, they have diverse origins.

With the exception of bizarre parosteal osteochondromatous proliferation (BPOP), lesions of the periosteum and juxtacortical regions are not considered to be soft tissue and not addressed here. Several soft tissue tumors, such as lipoma, liposarcoma, peripheral nerve sheath tumor, and so on, may contain metaplastic bone and/or cartilage; however, they are not considered to be osseous or cartilaginous tumors.

BENIGN LESIONS

Benign Osseous Lesions

> **KEY CONCEPTS**
> - Myositis ossificans is the most common benign bone-forming lesion.
> - It is termed *panniculitis ossificans* when it arises in the subcutis.
> - It is termed *fasciitis ossificans* when it arises in the fascia.
> - It is termed *florid reactive periostitis* or *fibro-osseous pseudotumor* when it arises in the periosteum.

Benign osseous lesions are relatively uncommon, accounting for less than 1% of all benign soft tissue masses undergoing biopsy (2). The actual prevalence is difficult to ascertain with certainty because the radiographic features are often characteristic, and many lesions are not excised or biopsied. The most common benign bone-forming lesion is myositis ossificans. Variants of this lesion located in the subcutis are termed *panniculitis ossificans*, and those in the fascia are referred to as *fasciitis ossificans* (3,4). When the lesion arises in the periosteum, it is typically located in the hand (and less commonly in the foot), and is known as *florid reactive periostitis of the tubular bones of the hands and feet* or *fibro-osseous pseudotumor of the digits* (4).

Myositis Ossificans

> ### KEY CONCEPTS
> - Myositis ossificans is a benign, solitary, self-limiting, ossifying soft tissue mass.
> - A history of trauma is often absent.
> - The most frequent symptoms are pain, tenderness, and soft tissue mass.
> - The lesion may be an incidental finding.
> - Patients are usually young adults with a mean age in the third decade; myositis ossificans is quite rare in children.
> - Approximately 80% of cases arise in the large muscles of the extremities, with the thigh the most common location.
> - A distinct zoning pattern is present microscopically in which lesional maturation progresses from an immature, central, nonossified cellular focus to a peripheral rim of mature lamellar bone.

Myositis ossificans is a benign, solitary, self-limiting, ossifying soft-tissue mass typically occurring within skeletal muscle. A history of trauma is often absent; no distinction is made between lesions of atraumatic and traumatic origin. The pathogenesis of myositis ossificans is unknown and the term *myositis* is a misnomer because no primary inflammation of skeletal muscle is associated with the process (4,5). Synonyms include *pseudomalignant osseous tumor of soft tissue, extraosseous localized nonneoplastic bone and cartilage formation, myositis ossificans circumscripta, pseudomalignant myositis ossificans,* and *heterotopic ossification* (5–8).

The most frequent symptoms are pain, tenderness, and a soft tissue mass; however, the lesion may be an incidental finding. Uncommonly, patients may be febrile, with an elevated erythrocyte sedimentation rate (9). Although many cases may be related to a single traumatic event or repeated minor trauma, no history of injury is found in approximately 25% to 40% of patients (9–11). The incidence of myositis ossificans following a direct muscle injury is reported to be between 9% and 17% of cases (12). It is also suggested that lesions may be a reaction to infection (10).

Patients are usually young adults with a mean age in the third decade (13); myositis ossificans is quite rare in children (9). Heifetz et al. estimate that only 1% of myositis ossificans occurs in the first decade (14). Approximately 80% of cases arise in the large muscles of the extremities (15), with the thigh the most common location. Myositis ossificans is not a premalignant lesion and in most reported cases of malignant transformation, the presence of preexisting myositis ossificans is poorly documented (4). Consequently, true malignant transformation is likely to be extremely rare. Local excision is generally curative. A case report documented marked clinical improvement in a mineralized lesion adjacent to the knee, following 6

months of alendronate (Fosamax) therapy, obviating the need for surgery (16). Spontaneous lesion regression and resolution are reported (17).

Lesions are typically well-circumscribed and rimmed by compressed fibrous connective tissue, which is frequently surrounded by or contains atrophic skeletal muscle. Typically, a distinct zoning pattern is present, in which lesional maturation progresses from an immature, central, nonossified cellular focus to osteoid, and finally to a peripheral rim of mature lamellar bone (Fig. 11.1). Central nodular fasciitis-like areas and chondro-osseous nodules may also be seen. As lesions mature, the nodular fasciitis-like areas in the intratrabecular spaces become areas of delicate fibrosis, containing thin-walled, ectatic, vascular channels that eventually become replaced by both adipose tissue and mature bone in the oldest lesions.

Imaging of Myositis Ossificans

> ### KEY CONCEPTS
> - Radiographs show:
>   - Faint calcification within 2 to 6 weeks.
>   - A sharply circumscribed osseous mass within 6 to 8 weeks.
>   - Smaller, mature mass by 5 to 6 months.
> - Bone technetium-99m diphosphonate scintigraphy demonstrates intense focal tracer accumulation.
> - MR imaging features vary with lesion age:
>   - Early lesions demonstrate a high signal intensity on T2-weighted images with associated edema.
>   - Intermediate lesions are similar but demonstrate a rim of curvilinear decreased signal intensity corresponding to the lesions' peripheral ossification.
>   - Mature (late) lesions are well-defined, inhomogeneous masses with a signal intensity equal to or less than that of fat on all pulse sequences.
>   - Active lesions demonstrate enhancement following intravenous gadolinium administration.

Radiographs of myositis ossificans show faint calcification within 2 to 6 weeks of onset of symptoms (5,9). A sharply circumscribed, osseous mass is usually apparent by 6 to 8 weeks (although it may be seen much earlier), becoming smaller and mature by 5 to 6 months (11,18–20). Lesions are often deep and may be associated with the periosteum, but they are usually separated from it by a radiolucent zone (Figs. 11.2 and 11.3) (20). Recognition of the pattern of mineralization with peripheral mature ossification is essential in establishing the radiologic diagnosis and allows differentiation from other mineralized lesions, especially extraskeletal and juxtacortical osteosarcoma. Short interval follow-up (3 to 4 weeks) may be invaluable in confirming the diagnosis (Fig. 11.4). It has been our experience that mature lesions

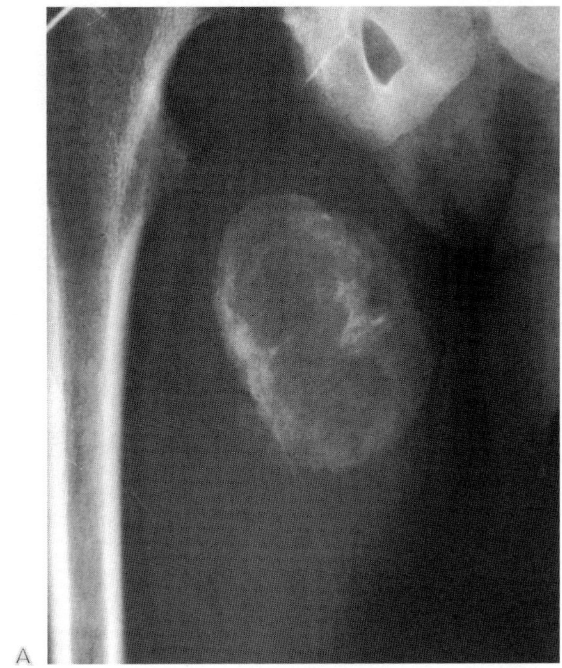
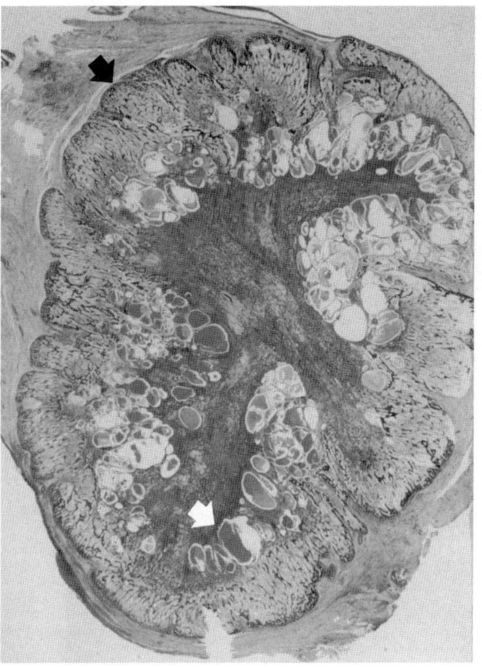

Figure 11.1 Myositis ossificans: Macroscopic section of a lesion in the thigh of a girl 11 years of age. **A:** Anteroposterior radiograph of the thigh shows a well-defined mass with a distinct osseous character, more mature peripherally. **B:** Low-power photomicrograph shows the zoning phenomenon of myositis ossificans with a peripheral rim of mature bone (*black arrow*) and a central cellular area composed of fibroblasts. Note prominent central hemorrhagic cystic spaces (*white arrow*). Original magnification ×1, trichrome stain.

are often densely mineralized, making it more difficult to appreciate the zoning pattern of maturation (Fig. 11.5).

Bone technetium-99m diphosphonate scintigraphy demonstrates intense focal tracer accumulation on all phases, including flow and blood-pool images (Figs. 11.2, 11.3, 11.5, and 11.6). Early in the course, delayed static images show only mild increased tracer accumulation in the soft tissues, although this rapidly progresses to markedly increased focal tracer accumulation (21). Serial scintigraphy is used to evaluate the activity and maturity of heterotopic ossification in paraplegics (22). In such cases, when activity is reduced, the ossification is judged to be mature, and surgery may be performed with little risk of recurrence (22).

Ultrasound shows an oval, hypoechoic mass with a central reflective core, which corresponds to the lesion zonal architecture seen pathologically (9). The zonal pattern may not be appreciated in early lesions (9). With maturity, increased hyperechogenicity is noted in the peripheral rind of mineralization (9).

The CT appearance of myositis ossificans is well-described and varies with the age of the lesion (18,23–25). CT scanning of early lesions, within the first 2 weeks, shows a relatively low attenuation mass without mineralization (9). A rim of mineralization around lesions is usually well-seen after 4 to 6 weeks (Figs. 11.4 and 11.6). The center of the mass may have decreased CT tissue attenuation (18,23), again reflecting its similarity to

nodular fasciitis (26). Mature lesions may show diffuse ossification (Fig. 11.5). Surrounding edema may be seen on CT but is better appreciated on MR imaging (Figs. 11.6 and 11.7) (9,27).

In the early active phase of myositis ossificans, arteriography shows a diffuse tumor blush and fine neovascularity (28); consequently, it may mimic a neoplasm. Mature lesions are avascular (27,28).

The MR appearance of myositis ossificans changes with the lesion's age, reflecting the evolving histology. Early lesions, prior to radiographically visible mineralization, demonstrate a signal intensity greater than that of fat on T2-weighted spin-echo MR images. The lesions are moderately inhomogeneous with diffuse surrounding soft tissue edema (27,29). On corresponding T1-weighted images, the lesion is usually isointense to skeletal muscle. Margins are poorly defined and may be recognized only secondarily by mass effect and displacement of fascial planes (Fig. 11.2) (27,29). Curvilinear areas of decreased signal intensity may be seen within lesions, corresponding to peripheral mineralization (Fig. 11.4). Intermediate lesions are similar but typically demonstrate a rim of curvilinear decreased signal intensity corresponding to the lesions' peripheral ossification. Irregular areas of decreased signal intensity may be seen coursing through lesions as well, again corresponding to areas of mineralization. As expected, these areas of mineralization are often best appreciated retrospectively and are far more apparent on CT.

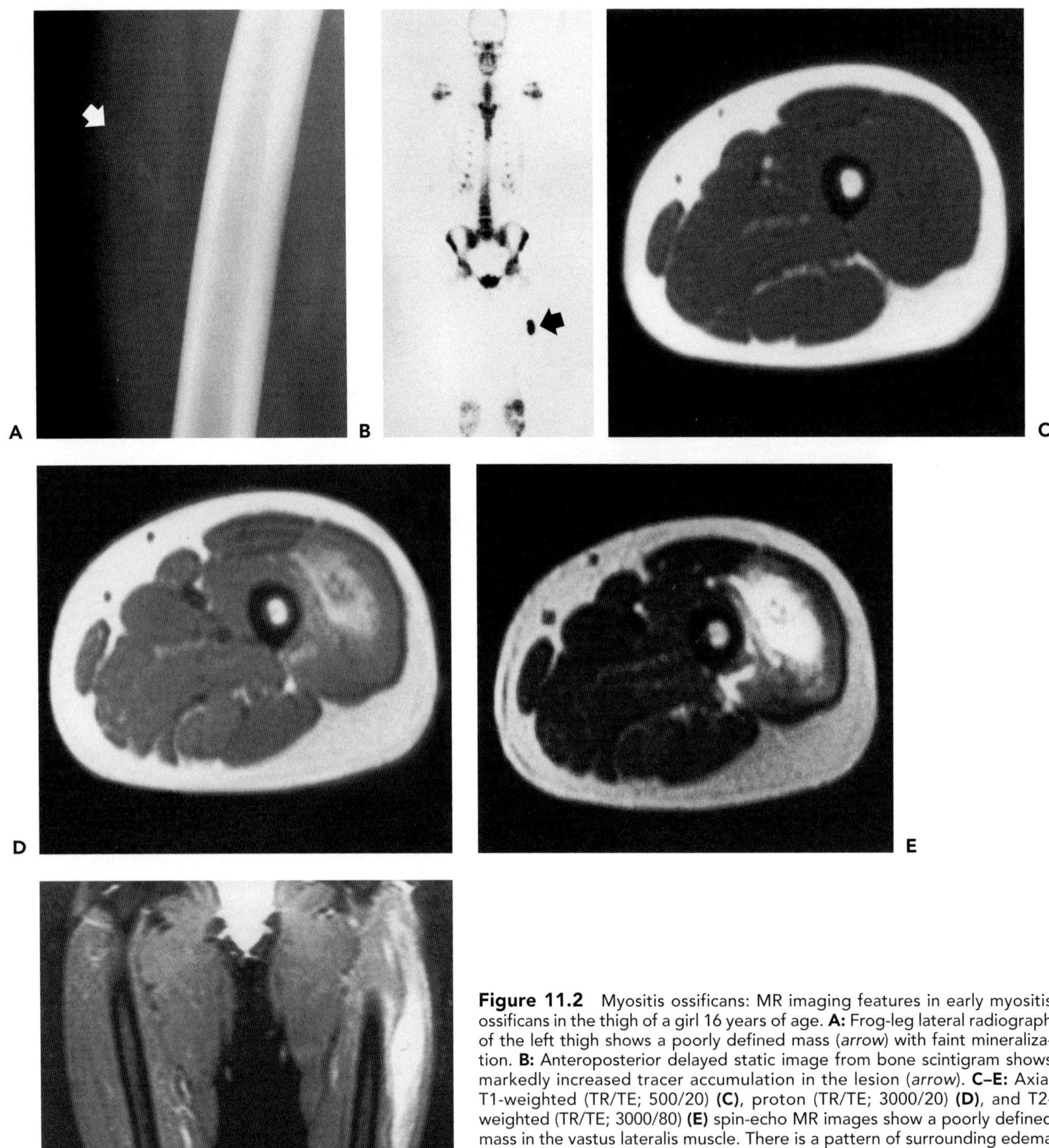

Figure 11.2 Myositis ossificans: MR imaging features in early myositis ossificans in the thigh of a girl 16 years of age. **A:** Frog-leg lateral radiograph of the left thigh shows a poorly defined mass (*arrow*) with faint mineralization. **B:** Anteroposterior delayed static image from bone scintigram shows markedly increased tracer accumulation in the lesion (*arrow*). **C–E:** Axial T1-weighted (TR/TE; 500/20) **(C)**, proton (TR/TE; 3000/20) **(D)**, and T2-weighted (TR/TE; 3000/80) **(E)** spin-echo MR images show a poorly defined mass in the vastus lateralis muscle. There is a pattern of surrounding edema extending into adjacent muscles. The areas of decreased signal within the lesion in **D** and **E** correspond to the areas of vague mineralization seen on radiograph. **F:** Coronal short-tau inversion recovery (STIR) (TR/TE/TI; 300/25/170) MR image shows the extent of associated edema.

Infrequently, fluid-fluid levels may be detected and are consistent with previous hemorrhage (30). This is not an uncommon histologic finding in the inner, most immature, portion of the lesion (Fig. 11.4). Fluid-fluid levels are a nonspecific finding and are reported in other soft tissue lesions including synovial sarcoma and hemangioma (30). MR signal changes compatible with edema in the adjacent bone marrow (poorly defined areas of increased signal intensity on T2-weighted and decreased signal on T1-weighted spin-echo MR images) are also noted infrequently (6).

Mature (late) lesions are well-defined heterogeneous masses with a signal intensity approximating that of fat on all pulse sequences, with a surrounding rind of absent/decreased signal. Absent/decreased signal is also seen

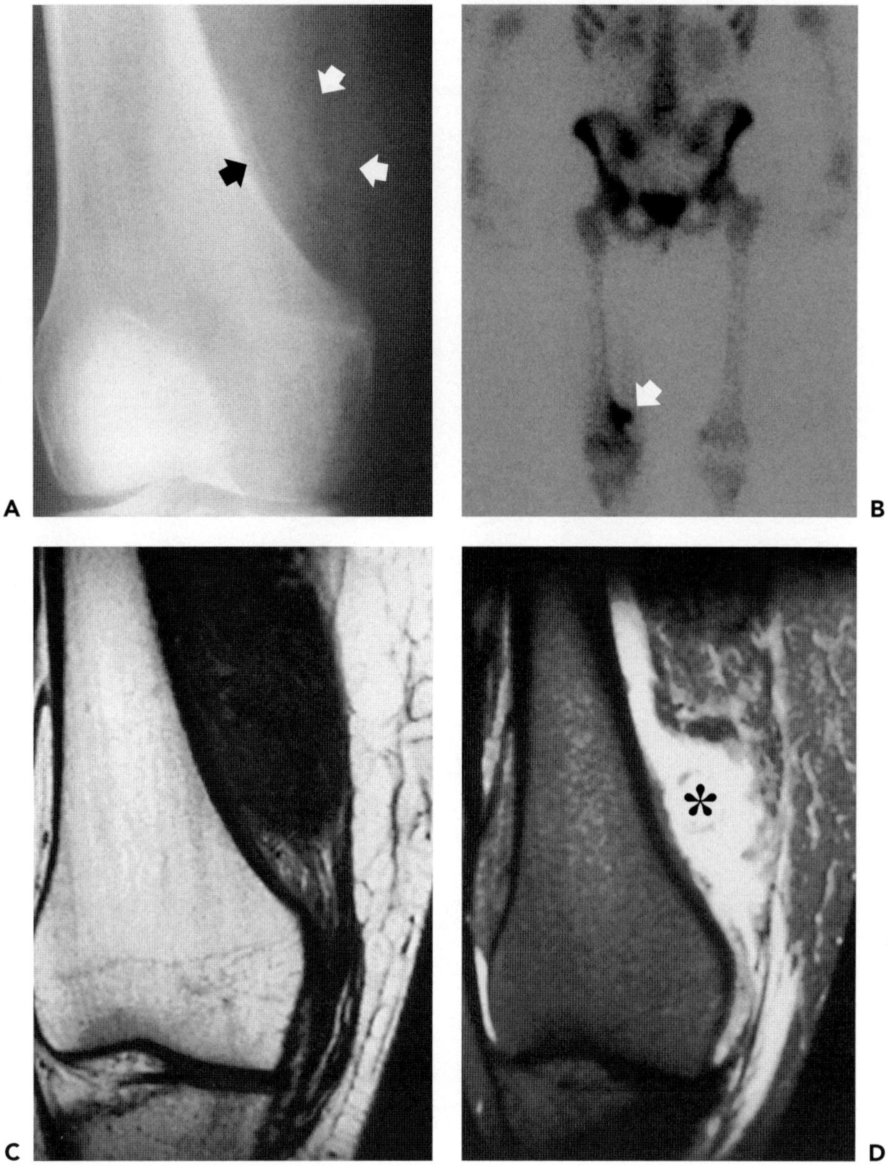

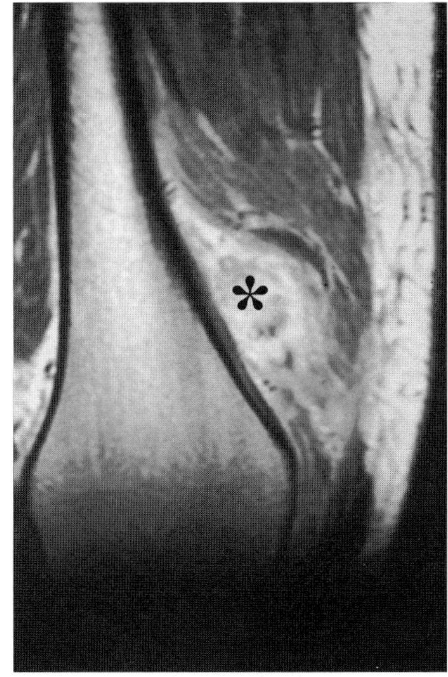

Figure 11.3 Myositis ossificans: MR imaging features in early myositis ossificans in the distal thigh of a boy 15 years of age. **A:** Anteroposterior radiograph of the left thigh shows a poorly defined mass with minimal mineralization (*white arrows*), as well as lamellated periosteal new bone on the adjacent femur (*black arrow*). **B:** Static delayed image from bone scintigram shows markedly increased tracer accumulation in the lesion and the associated periosteal reaction (*arrow*). **C:** Coronal T1-weighted (TR/TE; 300/16) spin-echo MR image shows the lesion to be mildly inhomogeneous with a signal intensity similar to that of skeletal muscle. The lesion is not delineated from the surrounding muscle. **D:** Corresponding coronal T2-weighted (TR/TE; 2300/90) spin-echo MR image shows the lesion (*asterisk*) to be poorly defined and not well-delineated from the surrounding edema. **E:** Coronal postcontrast T1-weighted (TR/TE; 500/17) spin-echo MR image shows marked enhancement in the lesion (*asterisk*) and associated edema. (Case courtesy of B.J. Manaster, MD, PhD.)

441

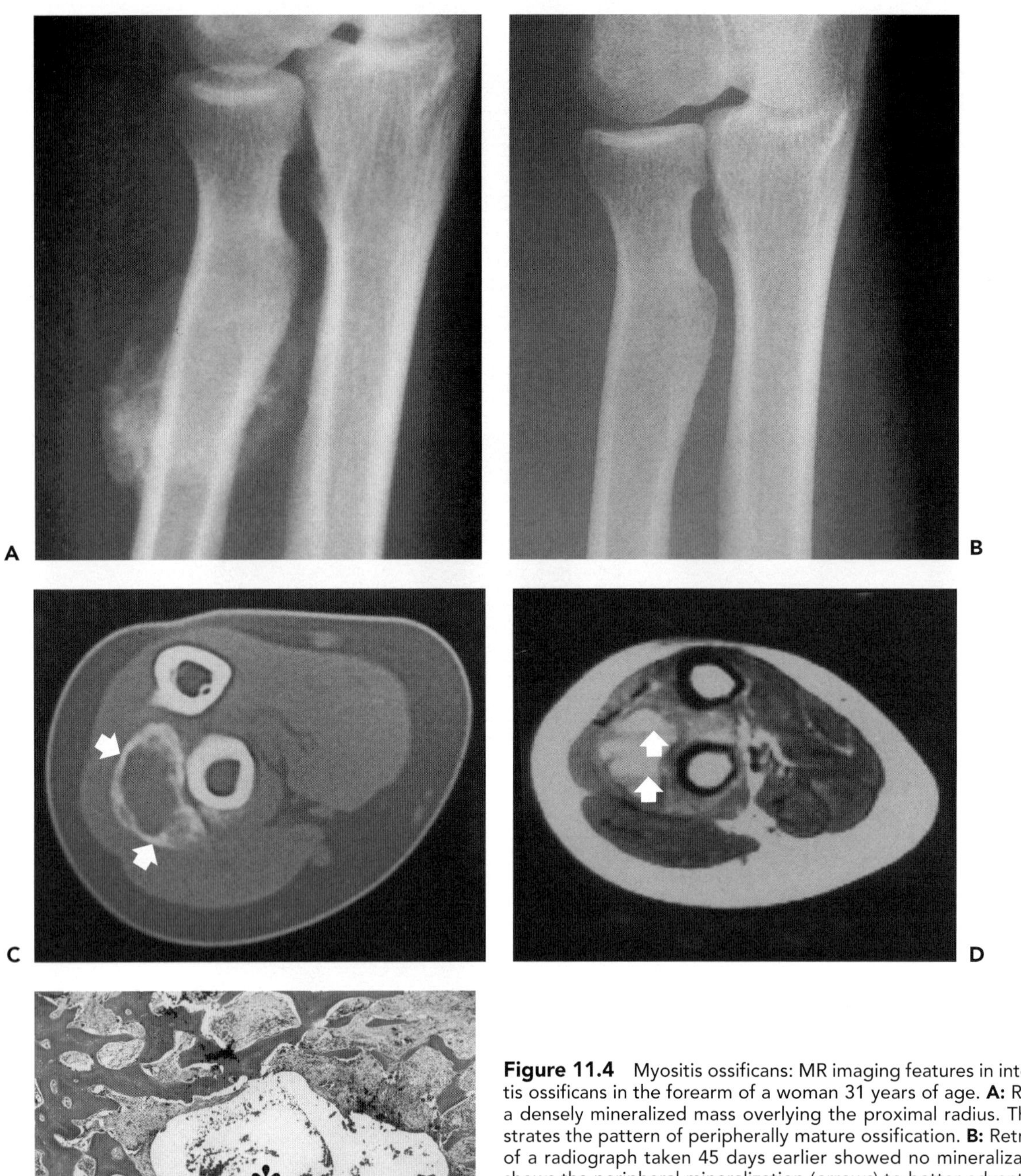

Figure 11.4 Myositis ossificans: MR imaging features in intermediate myositis ossificans in the forearm of a woman 31 years of age. **A:** Radiograph shows a densely mineralized mass overlying the proximal radius. The lesion demonstrates the pattern of peripherally mature ossification. **B:** Retrospective review of a radiograph taken 45 days earlier showed no mineralization. **C:** Axial CT shows the peripheral mineralization (*arrows*) to better advantage. **D:** Axial T1-weighted (TR/TE; 500/40) spin-echo MR image shows the lesion with fluid-fluid levels (*arrows*) adjacent to proximal radius. The areas of increased signal intensity adjacent to the lesion may be related to hemorrhage. The dense peripheral mineralization is not readily apparent on MR imaging. **E:** Photomicrograph shows mature lamellar bone surrounding hemorrhagic cysts (*asterisks*). Regions between trabeculae consist of densely packed fibroblasts and myofibroblasts with occasional multinucleated giant cells. Cellularity simulates a sarcoma. (Original magnification ×30, hematoxylin and eosin.)

within the lesion, secondary to dense ossification and fibrosis (Fig. 11.5) (27,29).

The areas of increased signal intensity seen centrally within early lesions on T2-weighted images are probably related to the extremely cellular central areas of proliferating fibroblasts and myofibroblasts within a myxoid stroma or extracellular matrix. These areas are histologically and radiologically similar in appearance to nodular fasciitis (26). Areas of hyaline cartilage may also contribute to this appearance. The inhomogeneous areas of intermediate signal seen within late myositis ossificans on T2-weighted images reflect areas of mature fat between bone trabeculae of the lesion. These same areas have a high signal intensity on T1-weighted images. The areas of decreased signal

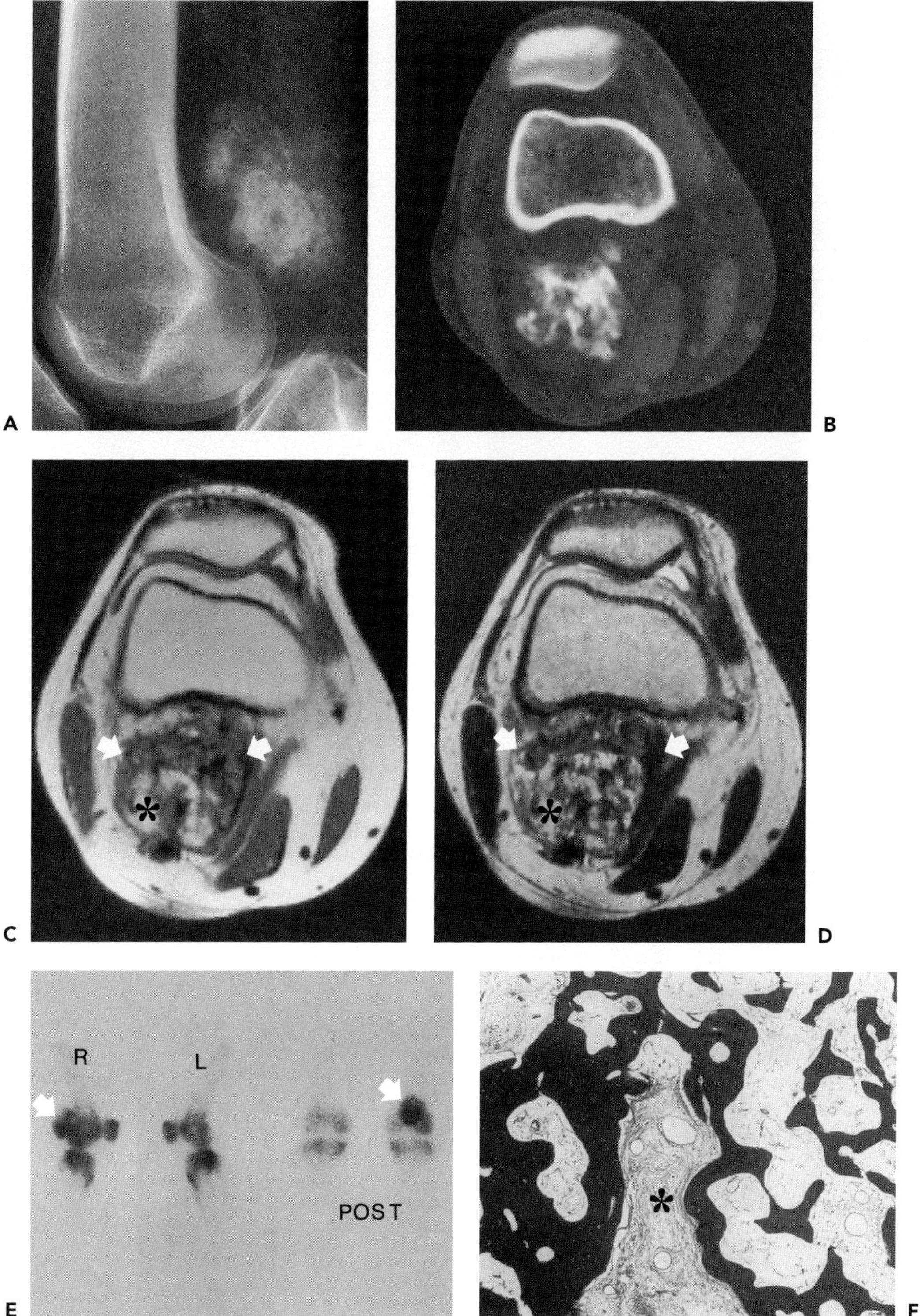

Figure 11.5 Mature myositis: Imaging features in mature (late) myositis ossificans in popliteal fossa of a man 35 years of age. **A:** Radiograph shows a densely mineralized mass in the popliteal fossa. **B:** Axial CT scan displayed at bone window shows irregular diffuse mineralization throughout the mass. The attenuation coefficient of the nonmineralized area is difficult to assess, but areas imaging similar to fat can be seen. **C,D:** Axial T1-weighted (TR/TE; 500/30) **(C)** and T2-weighted (TR/TE; 2500/80) **(D)** spin-echo MR images show a well-defined mass (*arrows*) in the popliteal fossa. Areas of increased signal within mass (*asterisk*) have a signal intensity similar to that of subcutaneous fat. **E:** Lateral and posterior delayed static image from bone scintigram shows markedly increased tracer accumulation in the lesion (*arrows*). **F:** Photomicrograph shows mature lamellar bone corresponding to the densely mineralized portions of the mass. Regions between trabeculae (*asterisk*) consist of adipose tissue and delicate fibrous connective tissue. (Original magnification ×30, hematoxylin and eosin.)

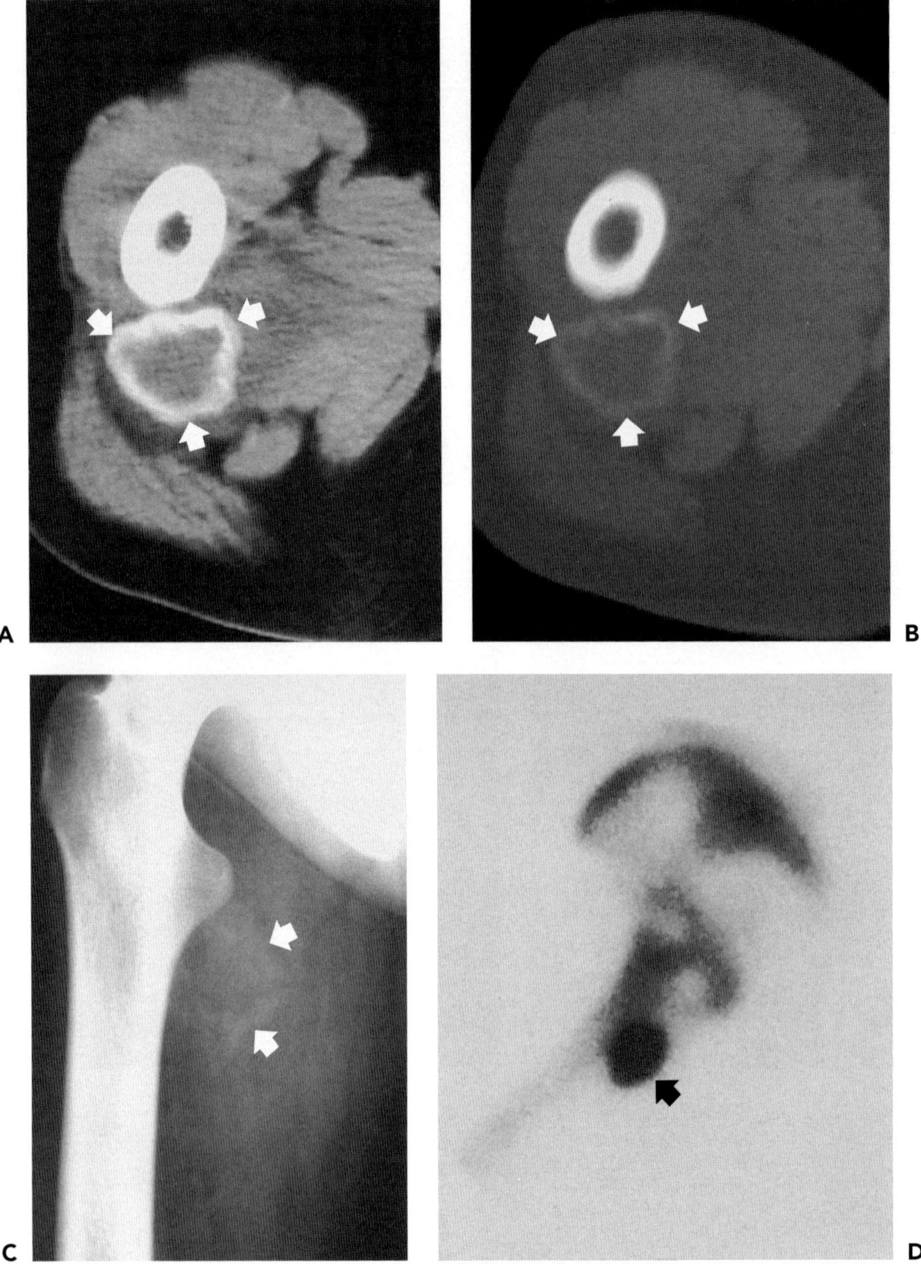

Figure 11.6 Myositis ossificans: Imaging features in intermediate myositis ossificans in a woman 20 years of age presenting with a 6-week history of a lump in the thigh. There was no history of previous injury. **A,B:** Axial CT scans displayed at soft tissue **(A)** and bone **(B)** windows show the peripheral mineralization to better advantage, as well as decreased attenuation in the surrounding soft tissue caused by edema. **C:** Corresponding radiograph shows faint peripheral mineralization (*arrows*). **D:** Delayed image from bone scintigram shows markedly increased tracer accumulation in the lesion (*arrow*). (*continued*)

intensity on both pulse sequences represent the bone trabeculae of the lesion. Areas of hemosiderin deposition from previous hemorrhage and fibrosis may also contribute to areas of decreased signal intensity on both pulse sequences.

Active lesions demonstrate enhancement following intravenous contrast administration (27,31). Although understanding of enhancement is incomplete, the vascularity seen arteriographically is likely responsible, at least in part, for the contrast enhancement seen on MR imaging (32). Surrounding enhancement reflects associated edema (23). The use of gadolinium-enhanced imaging does not facilitate diagnosis (31).

Soft Tissue Aneurysmal Bone Cyst

The soft tissue aneurysmal bone cyst is an extremely rare lesion that is histologically indistinguishable from its

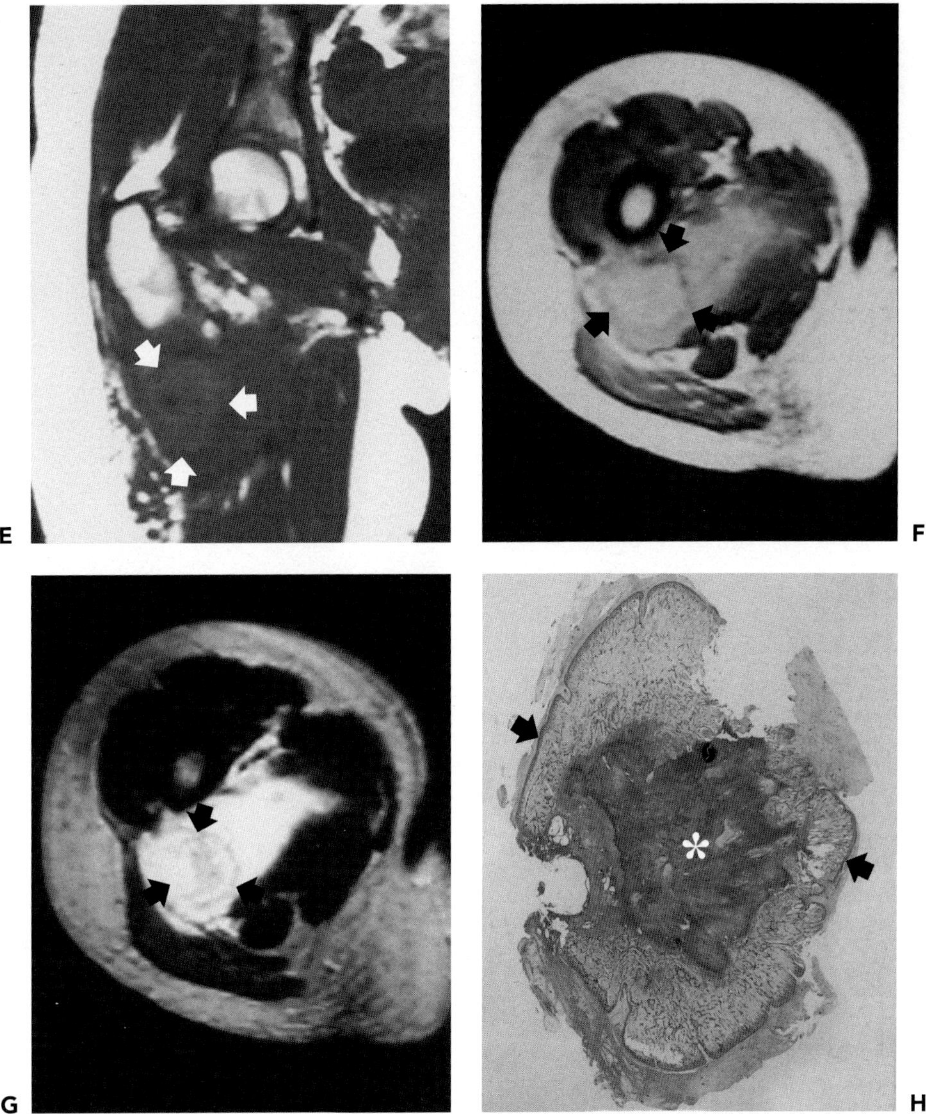

Figure 11.6 *(continued)*   **E:** Coronal T1-weighted (TR/TE; 750/20) spin-echo MR image shows the lesion (*arrows*) to be mildly inhomogeneous with a signal intensity slightly greater than that of skeletal muscle. **F,G:** Axial proton (TR/TE; 2200/20) **(F)** and T2-weighted (TR/TE; 2200/70) **(G)** spin-echo MR images show the lesion as a nonspecific area of increased signal. The decreased signal correlates to the mineralized portion of the mass (*arrows*), which is less well-seen on T2-weighted image. This is likely because of the window and level of the image, with the lesion not delineated from the surrounding edema. **H:** Low-power photomicrograph of the lesion shows the zoning phenomenon of myositis ossificans with a peripheral rim of mature lamellar bone (*arrows*) surrounding a central cellular area composed of immature bone and fibroblasts (*asterisk*).

intraosseous counterpart (34). In a report of a case in 2004, Wang et al. (35) noted only 12 previously reported cases. The cause of soft tissue aneurysmal bone cyst remains uncertain; however, it does show overlapping morphologic features with those of myositis ossificans (Fig. 11.4) (34). Although it is suggested that both myositis ossificans and soft tissue aneurysmal bone cyst may represent responses to injury, soft tissue aneurysmal bone cyst may be a distinct clinicopathologic entity (34,36).

On radiographs and CT scanning, soft tissue aneurysmal bone cyst demonstrates a well-organized peripherally mineralized mass, resembling myositis ossificans (35). MR imaging reveals a hemorrhagic lesion with multiple fluid-fluid levels and no solid component except for thin intralesional septa (35).

Myositis Ossificans Variants

Lesions with a histologic appearance similar to that of myositis ossificans, but which are located in the subcutis, are termed *panniculitis ossificans*. Panniculitis ossificans is seen most commonly in the subcutaneous tissues of the upper extremities in women (37). These lesions demonstrate a

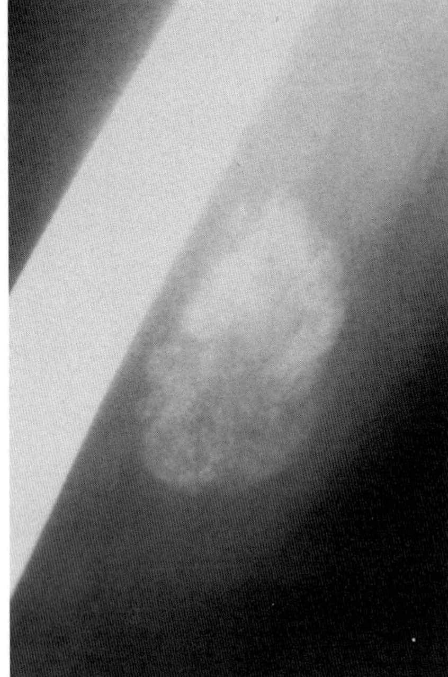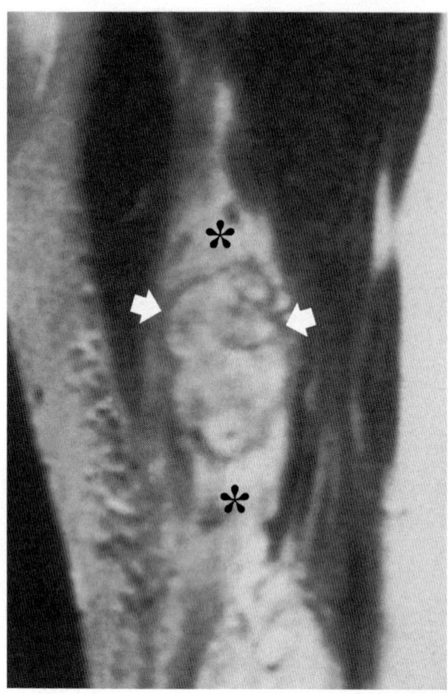

Figure 11.7 Myositis ossificans: MR imaging features in intermediate myositis ossificans in a woman 24 years of age. **A:** Lateral radiograph shows a well-mineralized mass in the posterior thigh. **B:** Coronal T2-weighted (TR/TE; 2200/80) spin-echo MR image shows the mass to have a rind of decreased signal (*arrows*) corresponding to the peripheral mineralization, as well as surrounding edema (*asterisks*).

> ### KEY CONCEPTS
> - Panniculitis ossificans is seen most commonly in the sub-cutaneous tissues of the upper extremities in women.
> - Fibro-osseous pseudotumor is typically located in the hand.
>   - Lesions are most often in the index finger, followed by the middle and little fingers.
>   - Patients with fibro-osseous pseudotumor of the digits are usually young, with a mean age of 30 years of age.
>   - Males and females are affected equally.

less-prominent zoning phenomenon. When the lesion occurs in the fascia, it is termed *fasciitis ossificans* (4,37). Although these lesions are not specifically addressed in the imaging literature, their radiologic appearance is similar to that described for myositis ossificans.

The term *fibro-osseous pseudotumor of the digits* is used for a variant of myositis ossificans occurring predominantly in the fingers, and occasionally in the toes, of young adults (38). Also known as *florid reactive periostitis of the tubular bones of the hands and feet* (39), this lesion arises in association with the periosteum. It typically is located in the hand, and as with the other myositis ossificans variants, this lesion typically lacks the well-defined zoning phenomenon seen in conventional myositis ossificans. Lesions are found most often in the index finger, followed by the middle and little fingers, although they may be seen in any of

the digits (38). Digital lesions are found most commonly in the proximal phalanx, followed by the distal and middle phalanx (38). Patients usually present with fusiform swelling or mass.

Patients with fibro-osseous pseudotumor of the digits are usually young, with a mean age of about 30 years. Lesions are relatively uncommon, and in a 10-year review of soft tissue tumors seen by the Department of Soft Tissue Pathology at the Armed Forces Institute of Pathology (AFIP), only 12 cases of fibro-osseous pseudotumor were diagnosed. The average patient age was 32 years (range 4 to 64 years); females were affected twice as often as males (2). Other series note patients with fibro-osseous pseudotumor are on average more than a decade older than those with myositis ossificans; and males and females are affected equally (13).

Myositis ossificans and fibro-osseous pseudotumor represent the same pathological process; minor histological differences are believed to be related to the different site of involvement (13). When these diagnoses are suspected clinically and radiologically, this information should be shared with the pathologist. In a review of 50 cases of myositis ossificans and 14 cases of fibro-osseous pseudotumor by de Silva and Reid, a malignant diagnosis was suggested by the referring pathologist in 23% of the cases of myositis ossificans and 9% of the cases of fibro-osseous pseudotumor (13). It is also suggested that florid reactive periostosis is related to bizarre parosteal osteochondromatous proliferation (BPOP) (40). The nature of the relationship is discussed more fully in the section on BPOP.

Imaging of Myositis Ossifican Variants

> ### KEY CONCEPTS
> - The image appearances of paniculitis ossificans and fasciitis ossificans are likely similar to myositis ossificans.
> - Fibro-osseous pseudotumor of the digits will show a mass on radiographs; half will have visible calcification and a similar number will have periosteal thickening.
> - Fibro-osseous pseudotumor may not demonstrate the peripherally mature pattern of ossification seen in myositis ossificans.

The appearances of panniculitis ossificans and fasciitis ossificans are not specifically addressed in the imaging literature. Our limited experience with these lesions suggests that their imaging appearance is similar to that described for myositis ossificans (Fig. 11.8).

Radiographs of patients with fibro-osseous pseudotumor of the digits (florid reactive periostitis of the tubular bones of the hands and feet) demonstrate a soft tissue mass. Approximately half have visible calcification and a similar number have focal periosteal thickening (38,41). A lucent band typically is present between the density and the normal cortex (Figs. 11.9–11.11) (41). The lesion, especially in its early phase, may mimic a juxtacortical osteosarcoma, although such lesions are quite rare in the digits. The lesion may not demonstrate the peripherally mature pattern seen in myositis ossificans (38). Cortical erosion may occasionally be seen (Fig. 11.12) (38). The radiographic differential also often includes periosteal chondroma and chondroma of soft parts. Noncalcified lesions may mimic a giant cell tumor of tendon sheath.

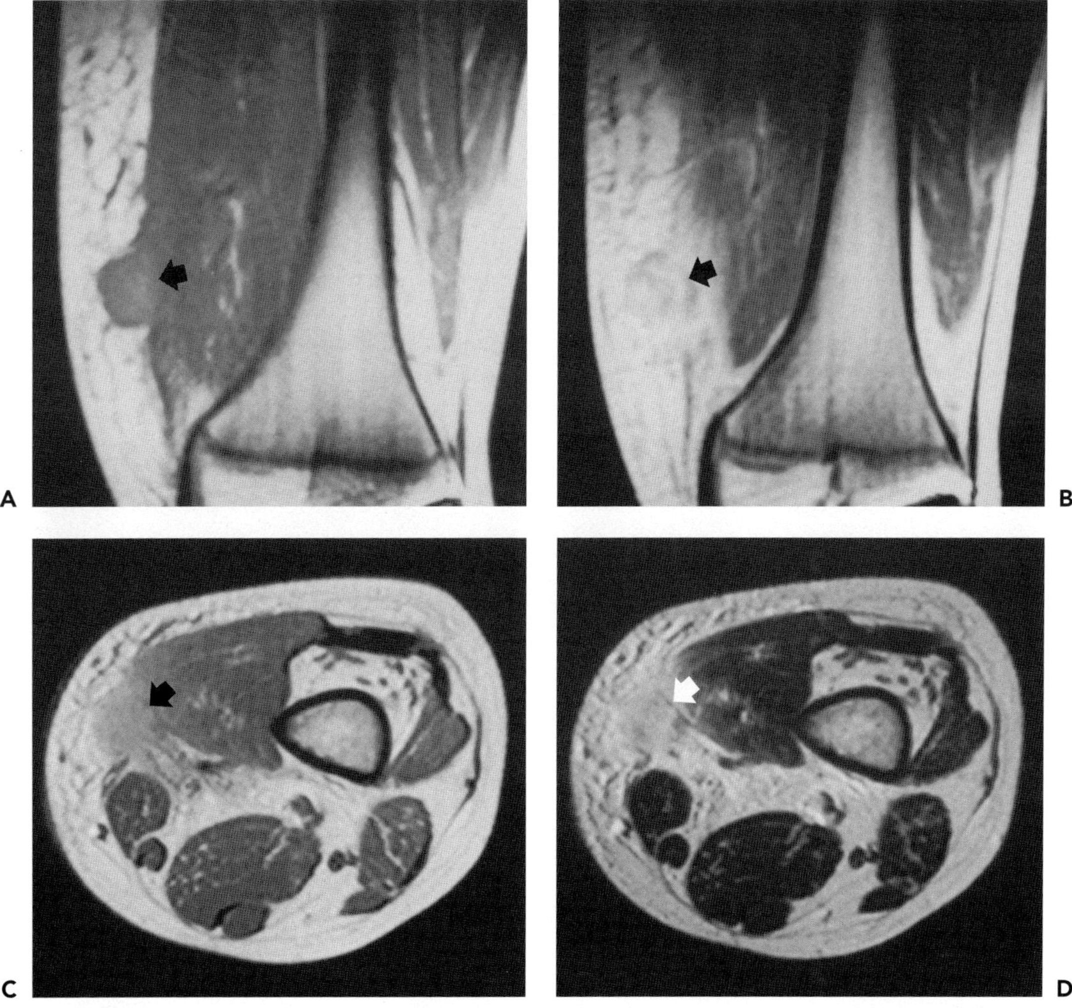

Figure 11.8 Panniculitis ossificans: MR imaging features in early panniculitis ossificans in a boy 9 years of age. **A,B:** Coronal T1-weighted (TR/TE; 600/20) spin-echo MR images preceding **(A)** and following **(B)** contrast show a small, rounded lesion (*arrow*) in the subcutaneous adipose tissue, immediately adjacent to the vastus medialis muscle. Note extensive enhancement and surrounding enhancing edema. **C,D:** Axial proton (TR/TE; 1800/20) **(C)** and T2-weighted (TR/TE; 1800/80) **(D)** spin-echo MR images show the lesion (*arrow*) with edema in the adjacent fat and muscle.

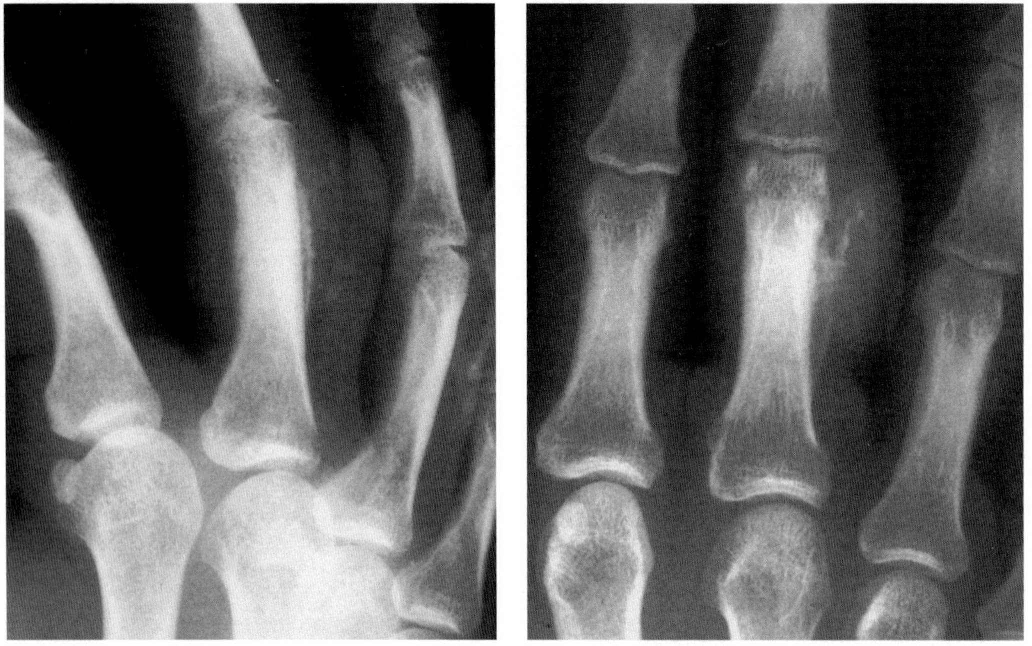

Figure 11.9   Fibro-osseous pseudotumor of the digits: Radiographic features in the middle finger of a man 29 years of age. **A,B:** Oblique **(A)** and anteroposterior **(B)** radiographs show a prominent soft tissue mass with associated bone production and extensive periosteal new bone.

Shigeru et al. (42) reported the imaging findings in two cases. CT scan in one case, with the lesion between the bases of the first and second metacarpals, showed a soft tissue mass having rimlike mineralization at the periphery with associated periosteal new bone. MR imaging in this case showed a poorly defined high signal intensity mass on T2-weighted images, with a thin peripheral rim of decreased signal corresponding to the calcification identified on CT. MR imaging in a second case involving the ring finger also showed a lobulated mass around the base of the finger, with relatively decreased signal intensity on both T1- and T2-weighted images. A thin rim of markedly decreased signal was also seen, although it was not correlated. Associated marrow edema was also noted (Fig. 11.12).

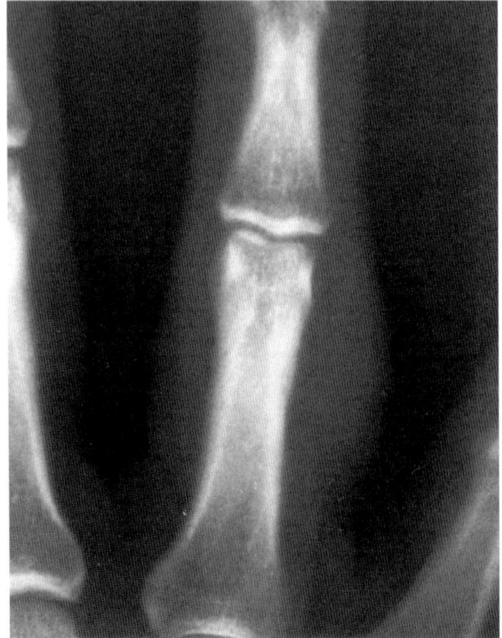
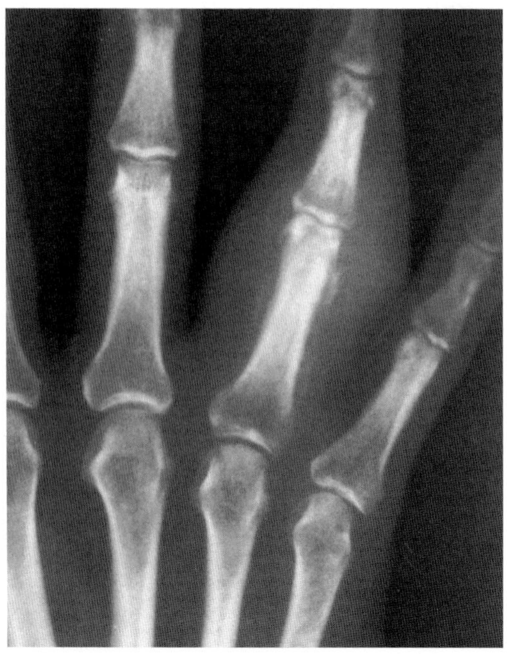

Figure 11.10   Fibro-osseous pseudotumor of the digits: Radiographic features in the ring finger of a man 40 years of age. **A:** Initial radiograph shows soft tissue swelling, without identifiable bone formation. **B:** Follow-up radiograph 6 weeks later shows extensive associated periosteal new bone. Such cases exemplify the name florid reactive periostitis of the tubular bones of the hands and feet.

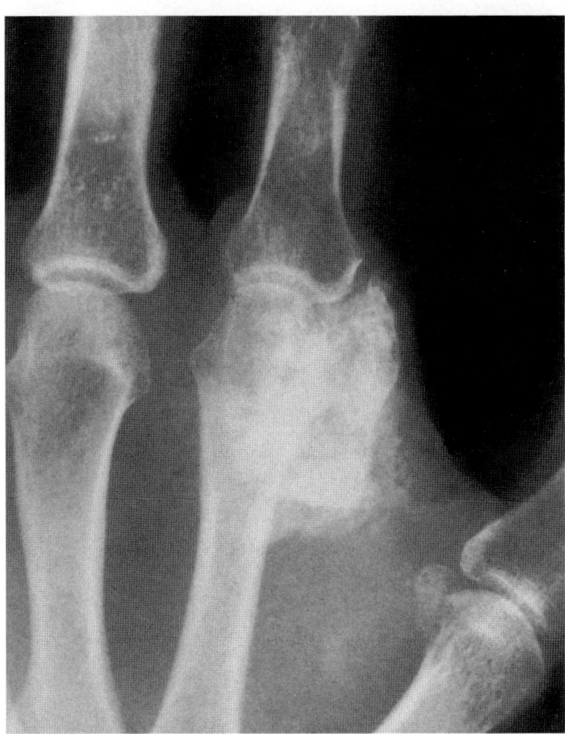

Figure 11.11 Fibro-osseous pseudotumor of the digits: Radiographic features. Radiograph shows densely mineralized mass in the index finger.

Bizarre Parosteal Osteochondromatous Proliferation (BPOP)

> ### KEY CONCEPTS
> - Patients with BPOP are typically adults, with the mean patient age in the fourth decade.
> - It occurs most frequently in the hands (55%), feet (15%), and long bones (27%).
> - Trauma is implicated as a cause.
> - Symptoms are usually related to the size of the lesion.
> - Excision is curative and the usual treatment.
> - Local recurrence is common (35% to 58%).

Bizarre parosteal osteochondromatous proliferation (BPOP) is a histologically and radiologically distinct lesion initially described by Nora in 1983, in a report of 35 cases affecting the tubular bones of the hands and feet (43). Subsequent reports documented that although most cases involve the small tubular bones, long bone involvement may be seen (44–49). The lesion arises from the surface of bone on the outer aspect of the periosteum and appears as a calcified mass broadly attached to the cortex (45).

Patients are typically adults, with the mean patient age in the fourth decade, although BPOP is reported in children and older adults (43,46–49). Overall, males and females are affected equally, although this varies somewhat between reported series.

BPOP was initially described in the hands and feet, with these anatomic areas representing 55% and 15%,

respectively, of all cases (43,46). Long bone lesions are present in about 27% of cases (46). Although none of the patients in the original report had a history of trauma, previous injury was associated with the lesion in a number of subsequent reports: Smith et al. reported a history of trauma in 5 (71%) of 7 cases (43,44,46,47,49). BPOP is also reported adjacent to post-traumatic myositis ossificans (44).

Patient symptoms are usually related to the size of the lesion. Excision is curative and the usual treatment. Local recurrence following primary excision is common, with local recurrence rates of 35% to 58% (43,46,49). Subsequent recurrence is reported in about a quarter of patients (43,46). Although most cases are treated surgically, those followed with serial radiographs show slow progressive growth (47,49).

Histologically, the lesion is a disordered mass of bone, cartilage, and fibrous tissue that has a broad-based attachment to the underlying cortex and a gross appearance similar to that of a small osteochondroma. The lesion shows hypercellularity with marked proliferative activity, irregular bony-cartilaginous interfaces, and enlarged, bizarre, and binucleate chondrocytes (43,47). The histologic appearance may mimic that of a chondrosarcoma (43). The fibrocartilagenous and myxoid tissue may be abundant in some cases (49). Early lesions usually show an absence of bone attachment, with a solid attachment developing over time (49). In spite of the high rate of recurrence and the disturbing histologic appearance of these lesions, malignant transformation and metastases are not reported.

It is suggested that florid reactive periostosis and BPOP represent different ends of a spectrum of lesions, and a case of florid reactive periostosis developing into BPOP has been reported (40). Probably common to these lesions is an initial traumatic insult (50). If this reaction remains contained within the periosteum, florid reactive periostosis develops. If the periosteum is violated, a reactive process develops and extends from the cortex to the adjacent areolar tissue (50). In the latter case, the blood supply is more limited, causing the lesion to have a proliferative appearance. Despite the proposed relationship between these lesions, it is of interest that there are virtually no recurrences with florid reactive periostosis, whereas the recurrence rate of BPOP may be greater than 50% (40).

Imaging of Bizarre Parosteal Osteochondromatous Proliferation

> ### KEY CONCEPTS
> - Radiographs reveal a well-defined, pedunculated or sessile mass.
> - Lesions arise from the cortical surface without altering bone architecture.
> - A cleavage plane between the mass and the cortex may be seen.
> - MR imaging is nonspecific.

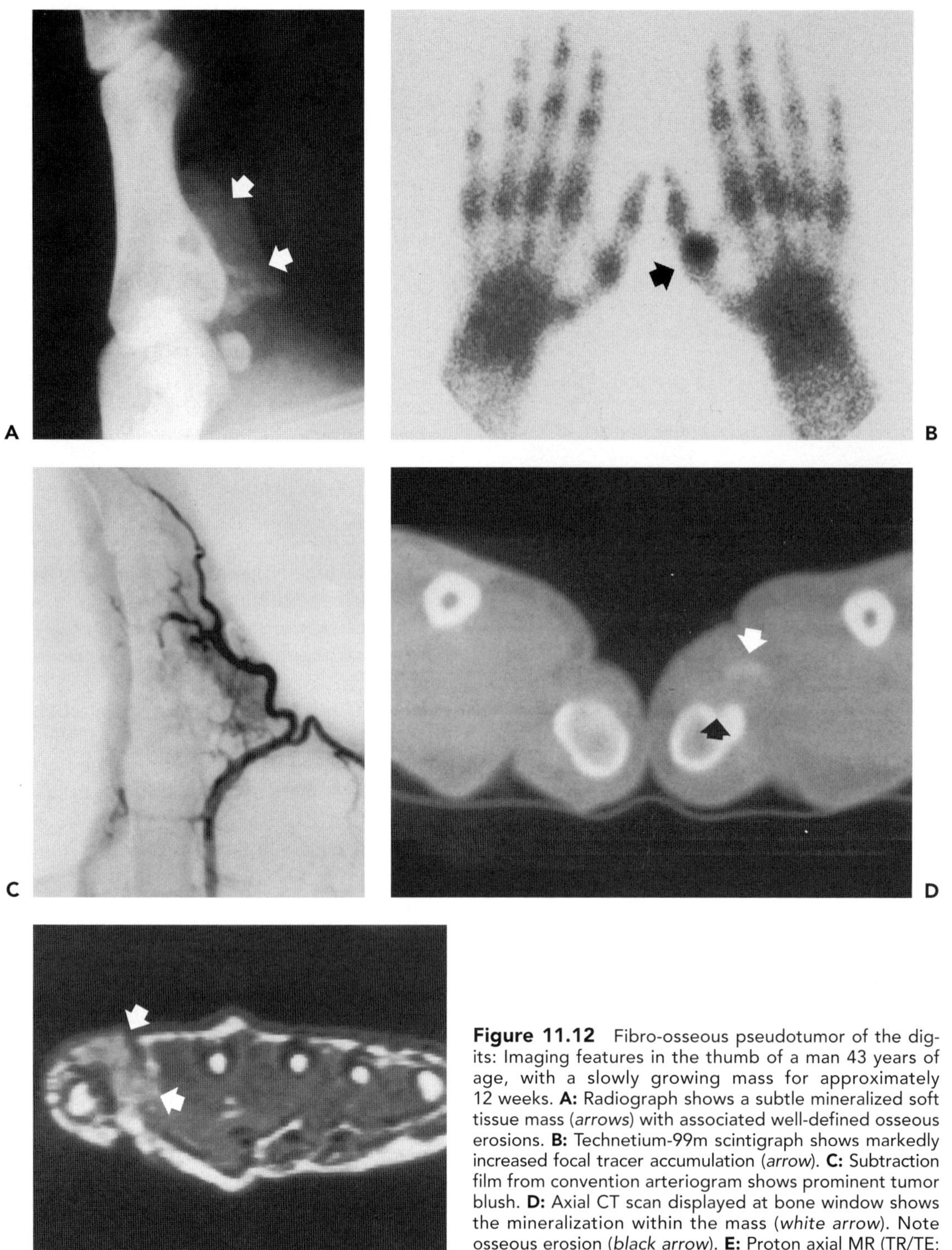

Figure 11.12 Fibro-osseous pseudotumor of the digits: Imaging features in the thumb of a man 43 years of age, with a slowly growing mass for approximately 12 weeks. **A:** Radiograph shows a subtle mineralized soft tissue mass (*arrows*) with associated well-defined osseous erosions. **B:** Technetium-99m scintigraph shows markedly increased focal tracer accumulation (*arrow*). **C:** Subtraction film from convention arteriogram shows prominent tumor blush. **D:** Axial CT scan displayed at bone window shows the mineralization within the mass (*white arrow*). Note osseous erosion (*black arrow*). **E:** Proton axial MR (TR/TE; 2000/40) shows a poorly defined soft tissue mass (*arrows*).

Radiographs reveal a well-defined, pedunculated or sessile mass arising from the cortical surface of bone without alteration of the architecture of the underlying cortex (Figs. 11.13 and 11.14) (47). The osteochondromatous excrescence typically shows prominent mineralization and a broad base attachment to the underlying cortex and lacks the cortical and medullary continuity seen in an osteochondroma (47,49). A cleavage plane between the mass

and the cortex may be observed in some cases (49). Periosteal reaction is not seen (47).

CT scan shows a normal contour to the native cortex, as well as a lack of cortical and medullary continuity (Figs. 11.13 and 11.14). Helliwell et al. (45) described a case in the radius with focal cortical invasion. MR imaging is nonspecific, with mildly heterogeneous enhancement (45). Recurrent lesions show similar radiologic features (Fig. 11.14).

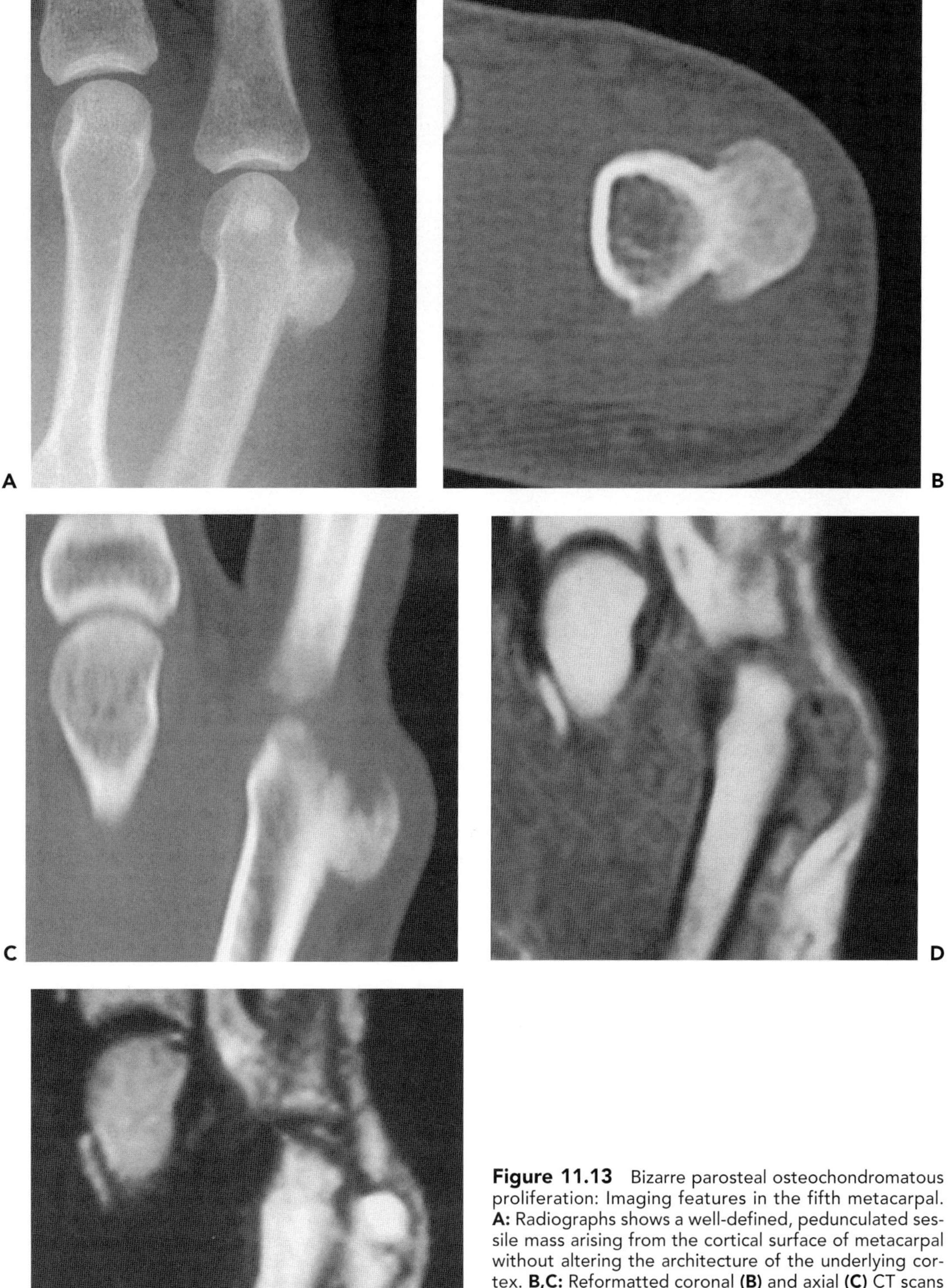

Figure 11.13 Bizarre parosteal osteochondromatous proliferation: Imaging features in the fifth metacarpal. **A:** Radiographs shows a well-defined, pedunculated sessile mass arising from the cortical surface of metacarpal without altering the architecture of the underlying cortex. **B,C:** Reformatted coronal **(B)** and axial **(C)** CT scans show the densely mineralized mass and its broad-based attachment to the adjacent cortex. The lesion lacks the cortical and medullary continuity seen in osteochondroma. **D,E:** Coronal T1-weighted (TR/TE; 300/18) **(D)** and turbo T2-weighted (TR/TE; 4100/125) **(E)** spin-echo MR images show the mass originating from the surface of the bone without medullary involvement.

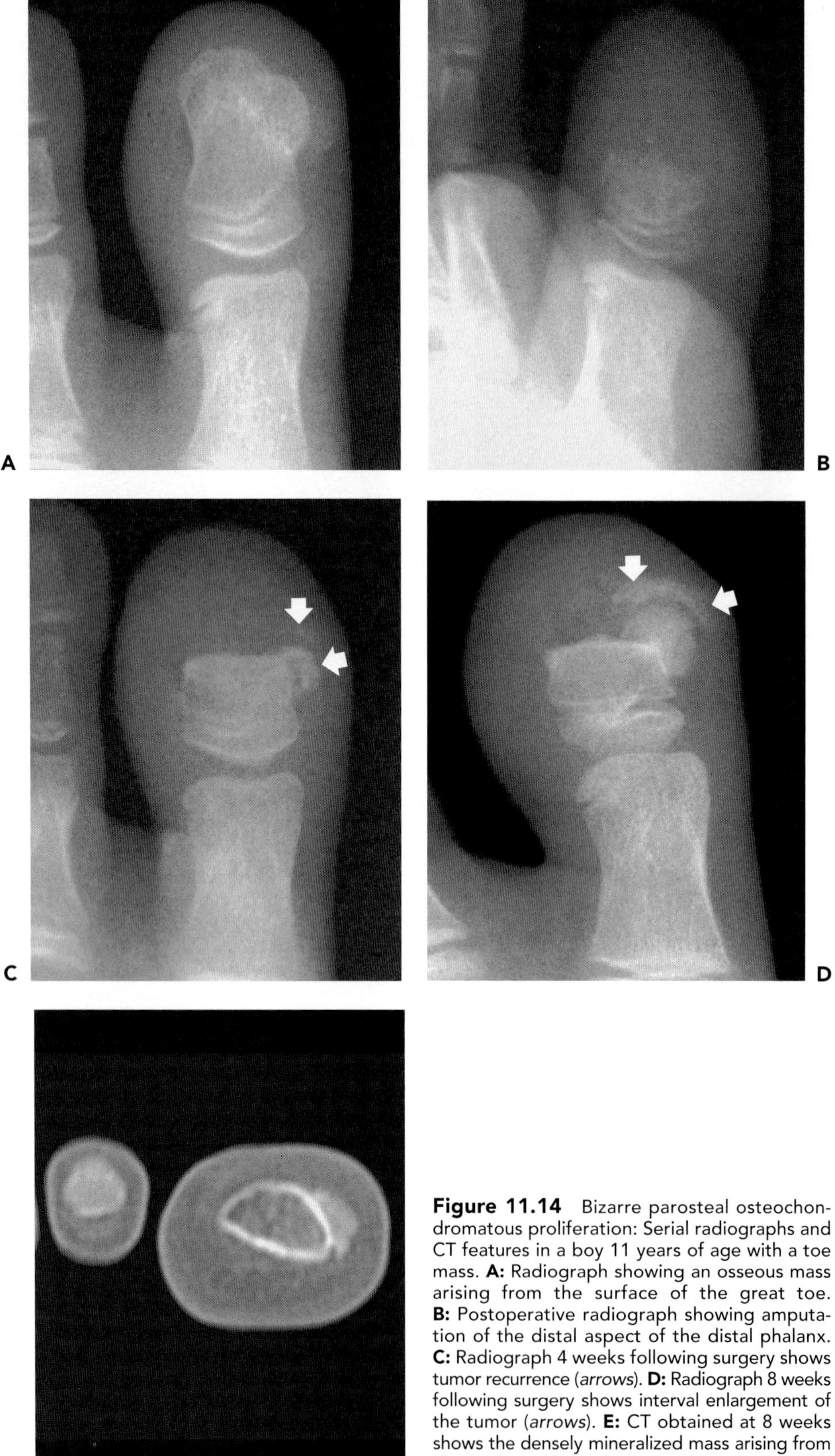

Figure 11.14 Bizarre parosteal osteochondromatous proliferation: Serial radiographs and CT features in a boy 11 years of age with a toe mass. **A:** Radiograph showing an osseous mass arising from the surface of the great toe. **B:** Postoperative radiograph showing amputation of the distal aspect of the distal phalanx. **C:** Radiograph 4 weeks following surgery shows tumor recurrence (*arrows*). **D:** Radiograph 8 weeks following surgery shows interval enlargement of the tumor (*arrows*). **E:** CT obtained at 8 weeks shows the densely mineralized mass arising from the surface of the bone without altering the cortex.

Fibrodysplasia Ossificans Progressiva

> ### KEY CONCEPTS
> - Fibrodysplasia ossificans progressiva is a rare, progressive disorder characterized by fibroblastic proliferation, calcification, and ossification of subcutaneous fat, tendons, aponeuroses, ligaments, and skeletal muscle.
> - It is usually sporadic and may be an autosomal dominant trait with variable penetrance.
> - The average age of onset of ossification is 5 years; by 15 years of age, severely restricted upper limb mobility is seen in 95% of patients.
> - Heart, diaphragm, larynx, tongue, and sphincter muscles are spared, as are all smooth muscle structures.
> - Diagnosis is based on characteristic skeletal deformities and soft tissue ossifications:
>   - Most characteristic skeletal malformation is symmetric hypoplasia of the great toes.
>   - Similar abnormalities may be seen in the thumbs.
>   - Less common deformities include vertebral hypoplasia and short, broad femoral necks.

Fibrodysplasia ossificans progressiva (FOP), is a rare, slowly progressive disorder characterized by fibroblastic proliferation, subsequent calcification, and ossification of subcutaneous fat, tendons, aponeuroses, ligaments, and skeletal muscle. It is usually associated with symmetric malformation of the digits, especially the great toes and thumbs; short broad femoral necks; and vertebral anomalies. The bone-forming lesions in FOP are typically precipitated by local trauma, underscoring the previous designation of myositis ossificans progressiva; however, this designation is a misnomer and is no longer used. FOP is a disease that affects primarily connective tissue; changes in muscle are secondary (51).

The disease is usually sporadic but may be inherited as an autosomal dominant trait with variable penetrance (52,53). FOP is quite rare, with an estimated prevalence of 0.6 per million persons (54). Patients are usually children, with about half presenting by 2 years of age (51,54). Patients usually present with localized soft tissue swelling, which may be accompanied by pain, edema, and a low-grade fever (51). These early lesions are typically in the neck or paraspinal region (55). Appendicular and distal lesions usually appear later (56).

Previous trauma is inconsistently identified as a cause of the soft tissue lesions (54). In time, the soft tissue swelling resolves and the soft tissue masses coalesce, fibrose, and calcify, leading to the formation of "bony bridges" that cause restriction of respiration and ambulation and skeletal contractures. The ossification process may occur quickly, with doughy nodules progressing to well-

defined ossified lesions within weeks (57), although ossification is usually not identified until 4 to 6 months following the appearance of a mass (58). The average age of onset of ossification is 5 years (58); most affected individuals have soft tissue heterotopic bone formation by 10 years of age (54,56). By 15 years of age, 95% of patients have severely restricted upper limb mobility, and patients are usually wheelchair-bound by the third decade (59).

Although the ectopic ossification is independent of skeletal maturation, maturing ectopic ossification forms rigid synostoses between the normal skeletal structures (56). The rigid synostoses bridge and immobilize joints, markedly restricting motion (Figs. 11.15 and 11.16) (56). The heart, diaphragm, larynx, tongue, and sphincter muscles are spared, as are all smooth muscle structures (59).

The diagnosis is usually made on the basis of the characteristic skeletal deformities and soft tissue ossifications (55). The most characteristic skeletal malformation is seen in the great toe, with shortening of the first metatarsal and proximal phalanx (56). This anomaly is present at birth and is usually associated with a monophalangic first toe (fused phalanges) (56). Similar abnormalities may be seen in the thumbs (56). Hand abnormalities are never present as an isolated finding (56). Less common skeletal deformities include vertebral hypoplasia, variable degrees of vertebral fusion, and short, broad femoral necks (56). Ossification of ligamentous insertions may produce exostosislike abnormalities (56). Kyphoscoliosis is a common finding and is the result of asymmetric, heterotopic ossification involving the rib cage and paraspinal regions (56). The temporomandibular joint is involved in almost three-quarters of patients and is often the last joint affected (60). Delayed diagnosis is not uncommon, even after the onset of ectopic ossification (55); Connor and Evans (58) report an average delay of greater than 3 years in such patients.

The disease course is characterized by remissions and exacerbations. Local trauma, including surgery and intramuscular injections, are implicated in disease progression (51,57,61,62); however, most often the cause of disease exacerbations is unknown (63). Influenzalike viral illnesses are linked to disease flare-ups, which may be the result of previously unrecognized viral muscle injury (61). Some patients succumb to the disease at an early age. Long-term survival is not uncommon; however, most patients do not have a normal life span (54).

Various treatments are used for FOP, including steroids, mineral-binding agents, and calcium-blocking agents; although, no effective long-term treatment has been found (52,54,64,65). Newer evidence suggests that 13-cis-retinoic acid (Accutane) may reduce the rate of involvement of previously unaffected joints (63).

Lymphocytes in patients with FOP produce excess levels of bone morphogenic protein-4 (BMP4) (67). This protein is involved in the development of FOP, and genetically

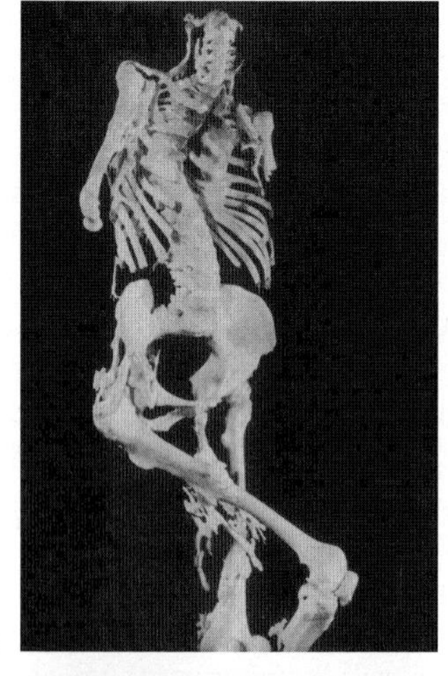

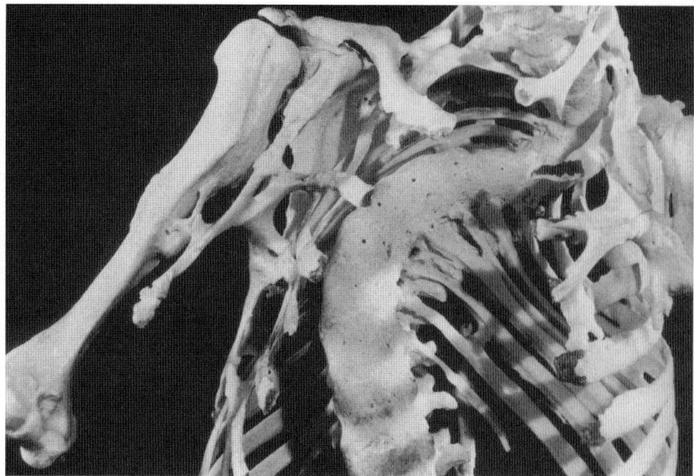

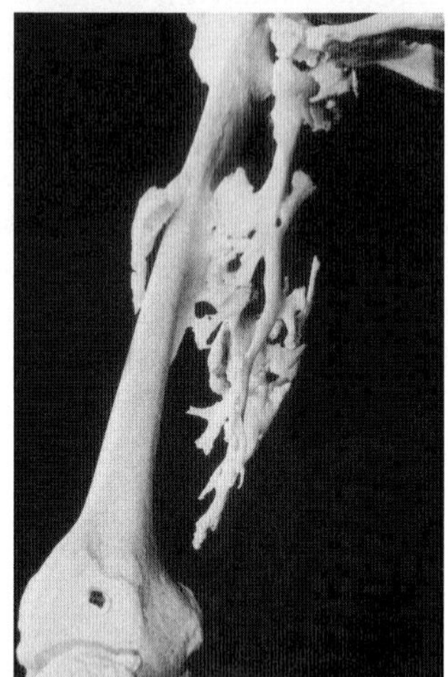

Figure 11.15 Fibrodysplasia ossificans progressiva: Skeletal remains of a woman 44 years of age. **A:** Photograph of skeletal remains shows extensive involvement with numerous bony bridges fixing the extremities and neck. **B,C:** Detailed examination of the right humerus **(B)** and right femur **(C)** shows the bridging bone to better advantage. (Case courtesy of Dr. Donald J. Ortner, Smithsonian Institution.)

altered mice that overexpress NMP4 develop an FOP-like phenotype (67). Microscopic evaluation of the active fibroproliferative lesions in FOP show that they form within muscle and other soft connective tissues, eventually developing enchondral bone formation (52,67). Genetic mutations are reported on chromosome 17 (17q21–22) and chromosome 4 (4q21–31) (52,55).

Imaging of Fibrodysplasia Ossificans Progressiva

KEY CONCEPTS

- Radiographic features are most diagnostic and include:
  - Microdactyly of the great toes and thumbs.
  - Short, broad femoral neck.
  - Narrowed anteroposterior dimension to the cervical and lumbar vertebral bodies.
  - Osseous excrescences at ligamentous attachments.
- Scintigraphy is useful in determining extent of involvement.
- CT is useful in detecting early soft tissue abnormalities and early ossification.
- MR imaging features are nonspecific.

The major radiographic features of FOP were well-described and categorized by Thickman et al. (51); they include ectopic ossification, short bone abnormalities, and vertebral abnormalities. In addition, there may be epiphyseal changes, calcaneal spurs, high patella, hallux valgus, and cortical thickening of the tibia (51).

Ectopic ossification usually begins in the neck and paravertebral region and progresses to ossified bars and bony bridges throughout the soft tissue (51). Virtually all patients have microdactyly of the great toes, and there is a high association with other congenital anomalies, including macrodactyly of the thumbs, shortening of the middle phalanx of the little finger, and a short, broad femoral neck (51,56,57). The vertebral bodies in the cervical and lumbar regions have a narrowed anteroposterior dimension, and there may be fusion of the posterior arches in the cervical spine (Figs. 11.17 and 11.18) (51). Osseous excrescences may be seen at ligamentous attachments and may simulate small osteochondromas or osteochondromatosis (Fig. 11.19). Because of the characteristic skeletal deformities, radiographs remain the most useful modality for diagnosis (56).

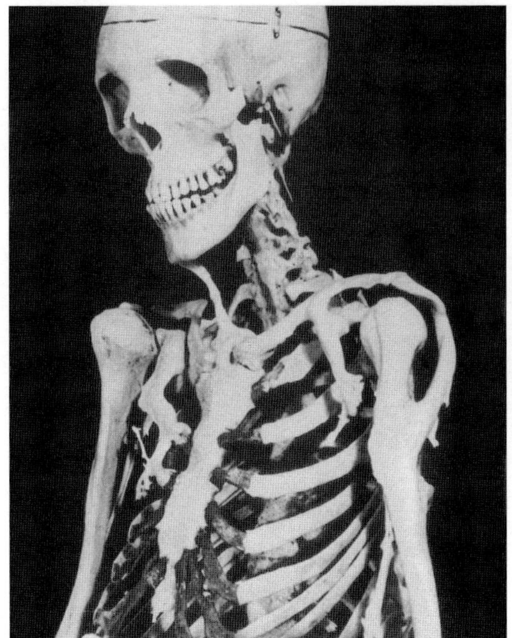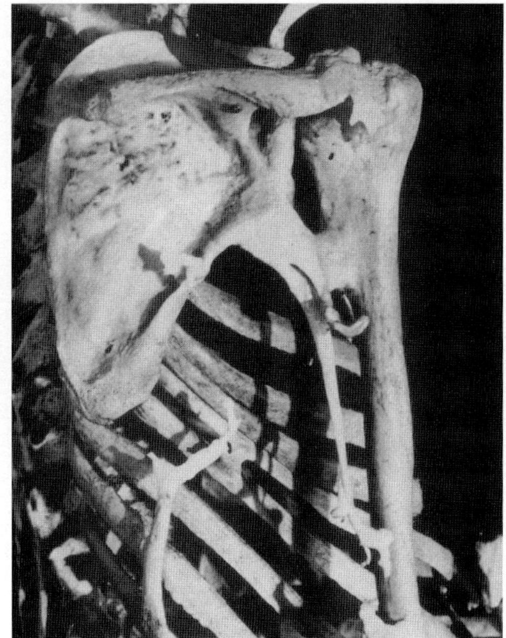

Figure 11.16 Fibrodysplasia ossificans progressiva: Skeletal remains in a woman 48 years of age. **A:** Skeletal remains show extensive involvement with numerous bony bridges fixing the upper body and neck. **B:** Posterior view of the left shoulder shows bridging of bone between the scapula, humerus, and ribs. (Case courtesy of Dr. Donald J. Ortner, Smithsonian Institution.)

Bone scintigraphy demonstrates increased tracer accumulation and detects sites of ectopic ossification before they are noted on radiographs (56,69,70). Scintigraphy may be useful in determining extent of involvement as well as identifying areas of new involvement (69).

CT is useful in detecting early soft tissue abnormalities and early ossification before they are apparent on radiographs (57). In this early phase, CT demonstrates swelling of fascial planes and edematous muscle, without evidence of ectopic ossification (Fig. 11.19) (55,57). CT also demonstrates that ossification occurs at random points within the fascia and not as an advancing sheet, developing adjacent to, and extending around muscle (57). This tends to confirm the impression that the initial focus of the process is within the connective tissue (57).

There is scant literature documenting the MR appearance of FOP. In a case reported by Caron et al. (62) in which there was involvement of the chest wall, MR images showed a nonspecific soft tissue mass with prolonged T1- and T2-relaxation times (Fig. 11.19). Follow-up scanning 1 year later demonstrated a decrease in the size of the mass, as well as a decrease in the signal intensity on T2-weighted spin-echo MR images and a small focal area of relatively absent signal intensity on all pulse sequences. The latter was not correlated with radiographs but was believed to represent calcification, ossification, or dense fibrous tissue (62). In this case, MR was also useful in demonstrating a new area of chest wall involvement.

Similar MR imaging features were noted by Hagiwara et al. (55), in a report of a case in a boy 21 months of age. In that case involving preosseous lesions of the chest and shoulders, the authors noted the lesion had a nonspecific signal intensity, similar to that of skeletal muscle on T1-weighted and a high signal intensity on T2-weighted MR images. Following intravenous gadolinium administration, the lesion showed marked homogeneous enhancement, likely reflecting the high vascularity of the fibrovascular tissue seen in early lesions (55).

The lesions of FOP predominantly spread along the fascial planes as an interstratified sheetlike mass between muscular bundles (55). Adjacent muscle may show abnormal signal and marginal enhancement; however, the disease affects the connective tissue between the muscles predominantly, and changes in the muscle are secondary (55).

Osteoma

KEY CONCEPTS
- Osteoma is an extremely rare tumor.
- Almost all cases are reported in the posterior tongue or in the skin.
- Patients present with a slow-growing, hard, palpable mass.
- Simple excision is curative.

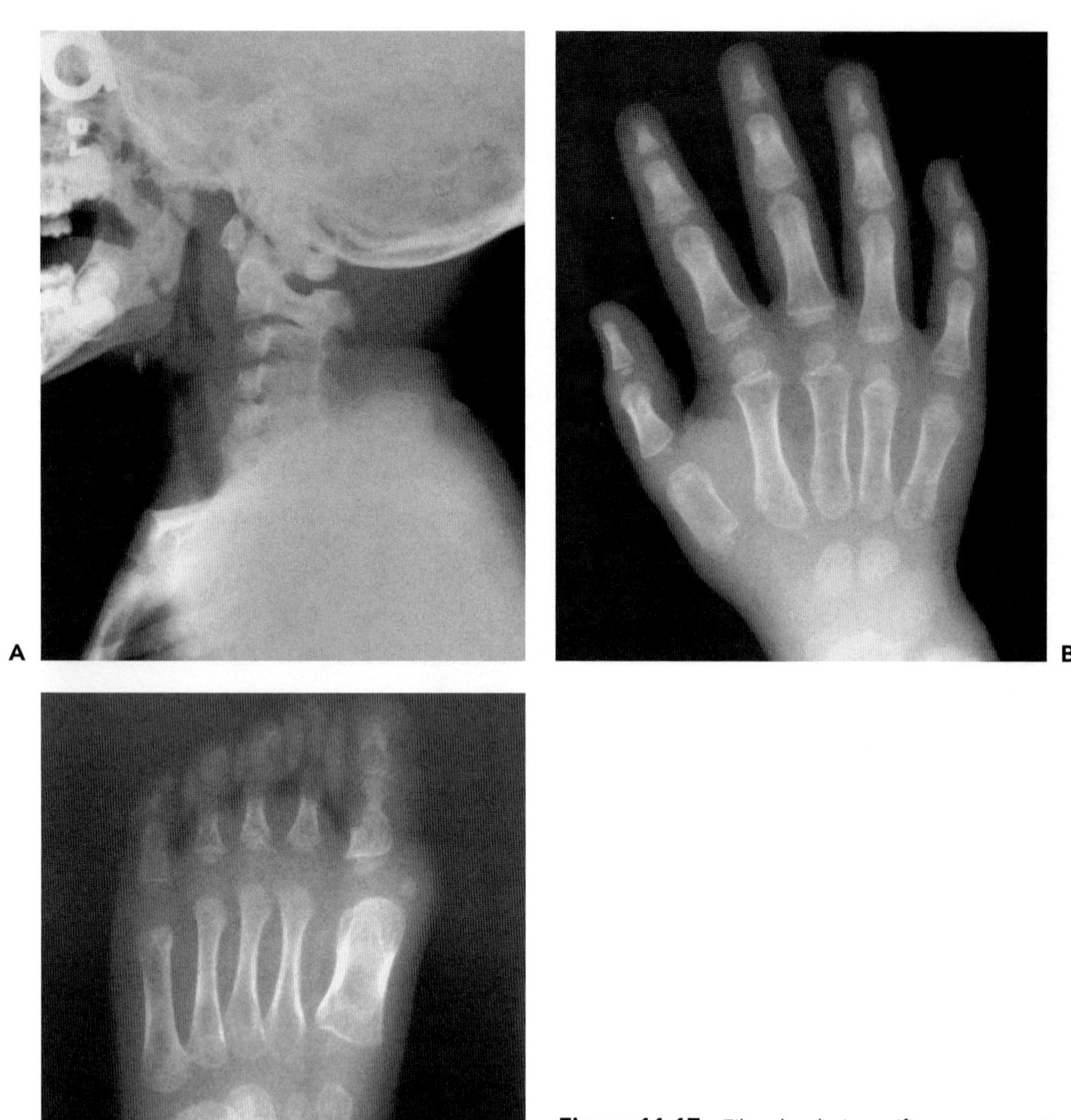

Figure 11.17 Fibrodysplasia ossificans progressiva: Radiographic features in a girl 2.5 years of age, presenting with a supraclavicular soft tissue mass. **A:** Lateral radiograph of the neck shows fusion of the posterior elements with a decreased anteroposterior (AP) dimension to the vertebral bodies. **B:** AP radiograph of the hand shows characteristic hypoplasia of the thumb. The middle phalanx of the little finger is only mildly affected. **C:** Characteristic hypoplasia is seen in the great toe.

Soft tissue osteoma (osteoma of soft parts) is an extremely rare tumor. Until the newer reports of cases in the hip and thigh (71–73), virtually all reported cases were in the head, usually in the posterior tongue or in the skin (74–76). Clinically, patients with soft tissue osteoma present with a slow-growing, hard, palpable mass, occasionally with associated pain (71–73). Simple excision is curative.

The cause of soft tissue osteoma is unknown. It may represent the end result of a post-traumatic ossifying lesion (71); however, others note it is likely not just the result of soft tissue trauma but probably a monoclonal proliferation of benign osteoid-producing osteoblasts (71). The designation of *osteoma* is used by some investigators to describe mature bone unassociated with other identifiable components (77).

Histologically, these extremity lesions are not difficult to diagnose (78). Soft tissue osteoma consists of mature lamellar bone; a well-defined haversian system, with bone marrow; and myxoid, vascular, and fibrous connective tissue between bone trabeculae (71,72). The lesion has a predominantly collagenous capsule blending into benign hyaline cartilage. Lesions lack the atypia and hypercellularity seen in malignancy, as well as the zonal pattern found in myositis ossificans (72,78).

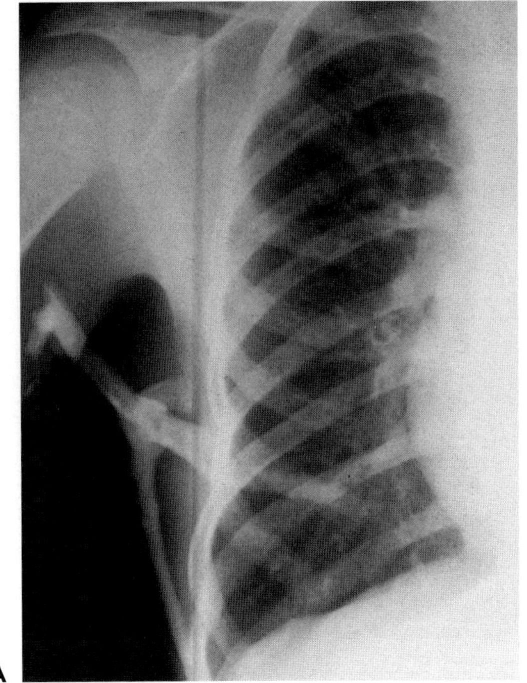

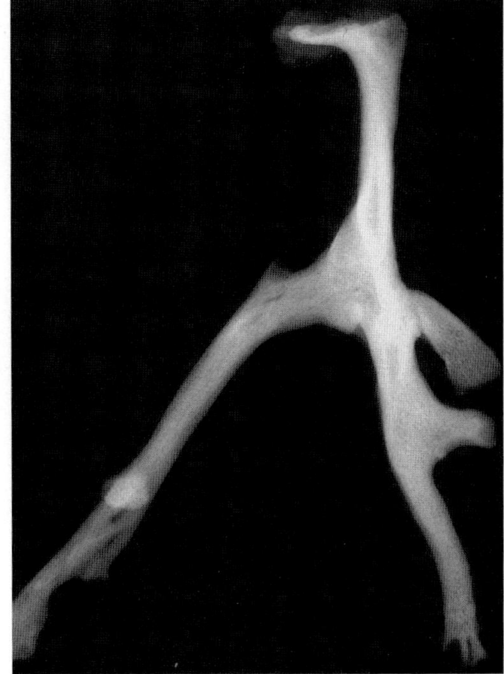

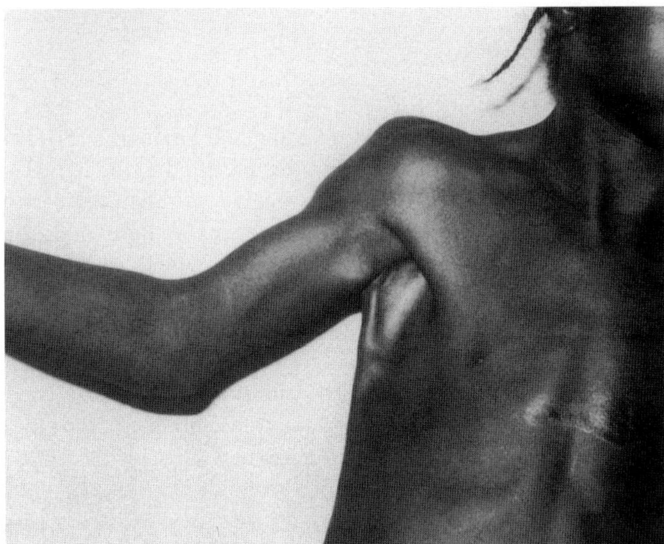

Figure 11.18 Fibrodysplasia ossificans progressiva: Radiographic features in a girl 9 years of age. **A:** Anteroposterior (AP) radiograph of the right shoulder and chest shows a well-defined osseous bar between the humerus and chest wall. **B:** Specimen radiograph of the excised specimen shows the nature of the mature bone. **C:** Clinical photograph shows the prominent osseous bar in the axilla. (*continued*)

Imaging of Osteoma

> ### KEY CONCEPTS
> - Radiographs and CT show a densely ossified mass unattached to the adjacent bone.
> - Bone scintigraphy shows intense focal tracer accumulation.
> - MR imaging demonstrates areas of mixed signal intensity, as well as signal voids on T1- and T2-weighted spin-echo MR images, consistent with cortical bone and areas of fatty and hematopoietic marrow.

Radiographs and CT depict a densely ossified mass, unattached to the adjacent bone. Bone scintigraphy shows an intense focal tracer accumulation, greater than that of adjacent bone (Fig. 11.20). MR imaging, reported in a single patient, demonstrated areas of mixed signal intensity, as well as signal voids on T1- and T2-weighted spin-echo MR images, consistent with cortical bone and areas of fatty and hematopoietic marrow (71).

Chondroma

Soft tissue chondroma is a small, benign, usually well-defined nodule of cartilage that is unattached to bone and is composed predominantly of adult-type hyaline cartilage. Synonyms are *extraskeletal chondroma* and *chondroma of soft parts* (78). Soft tissue chondromas are distinct from other

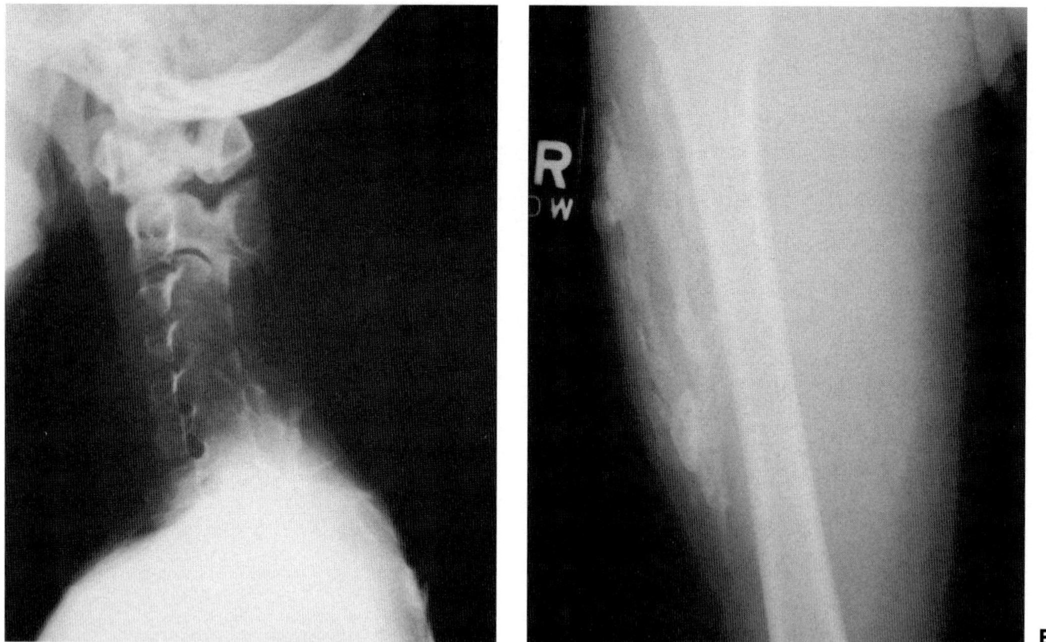

Figure 11.18 *(continued)*   **D:** Lateral cervical radiograph shows fusion of the posterior elements with a decreased AP dimension to the vertebral bodies. **E:** AP radiograph of the thigh also shows extensive bone formation.

> ### KEY CONCEPTS
> - Chondroma is a small, usually well-defined nodule of cartilage that is unattached to bone.
> - It represents approximately 1.5% of all benign soft tissue tumors.
> - Patients are evenly distributed between the second and seventh decades of life.
> - More than 80% of cases occur in the hands and feet.
> - Patients usually present with a slowly growing, painless soft tissue mass.
> - Local excision is the treatment of choice; recurrence is not uncommon.

lesions containing cartilage, such as lipomas with metaplastic cartilage, cartilage associated with synovial chondromatosis, and the cartilage found in myositis ossificans (79). Weiss and Goldblum (79) note that the origin of this lesion remains a matter of conjecture, being possibly neoplastic or metaplastic.

Over a 10-year period, 276 cases of soft tissue chondroma were diagnosed in the Department of Soft Tissue Pathology at the AFIP, representing approximately 1.5% of all benign soft tissue tumors (2). Patients ranged in age from less than 1 year to more than 85 years (mean approximately 44 years), with a relatively even distribution between the second and seventh decades of life. In the AFIP study, approximately 82% of lesions occurred in the hands and feet (54% and 28%, respectively). This compares well with Chung and Enzinger's (80) initial report in which 84% of lesions occurred in the hands and feet (64% and 20%, respectively). Almost all lesions occur in the extremities. There was a slight male predominance (1.2:1) in the 273 cases in which gender was stated. These demographics are comparable to those in the literature (29,41,42).

Patients usually present with a slowly growing soft tissue mass, occasionally with pain or tenderness (81). Lesions are typically well-demarcated and lobulated, rarely exceeding 3 cm in greatest dimension (79,80). They may be firmly attached to tendons or associated with the tendon sheath, joint capsule, or periosteum (80), and a synovial origin is suggested for some (82). Recurrence is not uncommon, with recurrence rates reported to be 15% to 25% (77,80,82). Local excision appears to be the treatment of choice (80).

Soft tissue chondromas are discrete, lobulated masses predominantly composed of adult hyaline cartilage (78), and all lesions display at least focal areas of hyaline cartilage formation. Regions of calcification and ossification may be identified within the hyaline cartilage, and approximately a third of lesions exhibit extensive microscopic calcification (78). Lesions appear to arise de novo without any apparent precursor (77). Myxoid change, sometimes extensive, may also be seen, as may regions of increased cellularity and cytologic atypia (77). Similar areas in intraosseous lesions would require a designation of chondrosarcoma. However, extraskeletal chondromas of the hands and feet displaying a similar degree of atypia

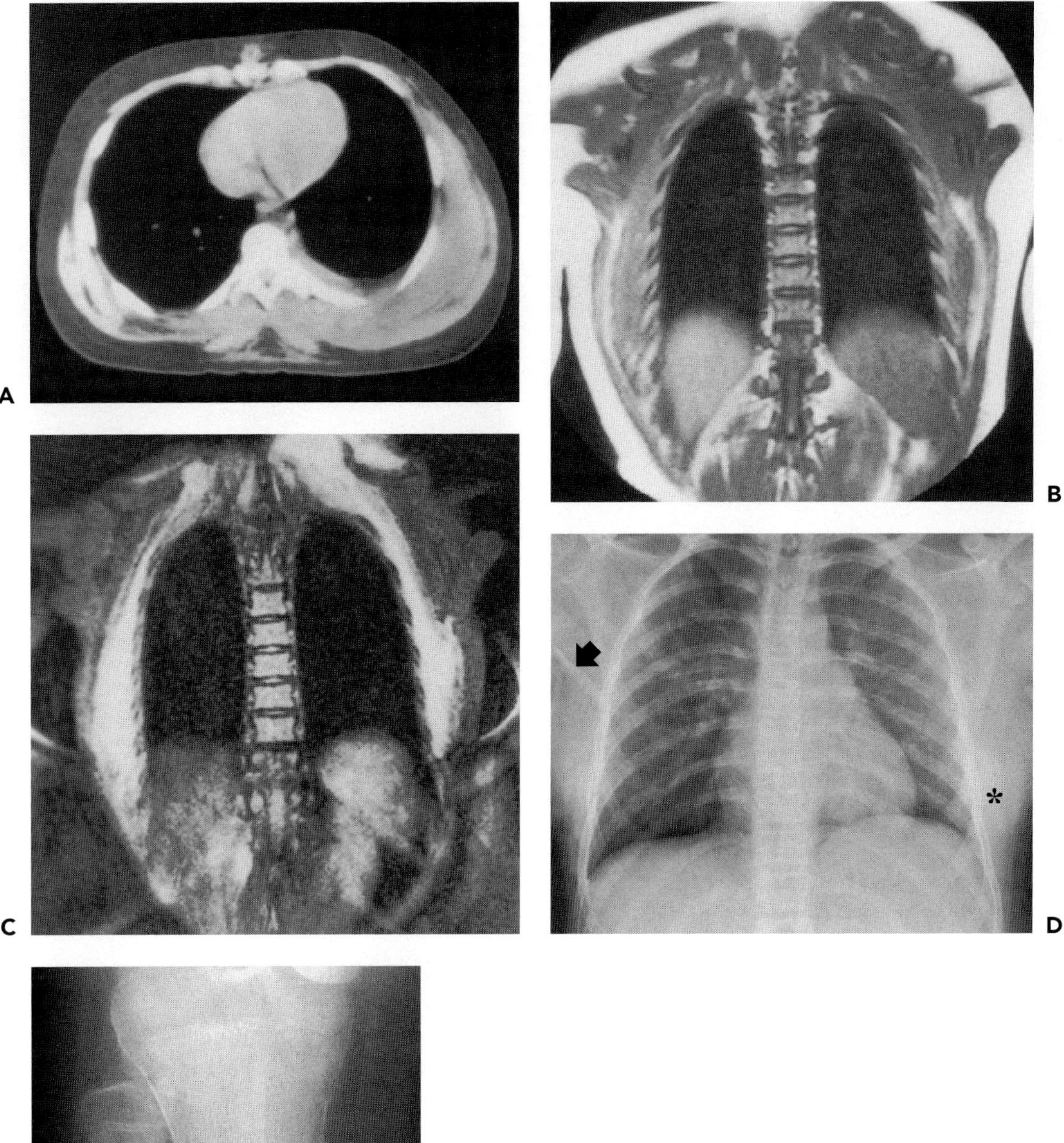

Figure 11.19 Fibrodysplasia ossificans progressiva: Imaging features in a girl 12 years of age, presenting with a large painful swelling over the chest wall. **A:** Axial contrast-enhanced CT scan shows a large, poorly defined masslike swelling involving the left chest wall. **B,C:** Coronal T1-weighted (TR/TE; 533/20) **(B)** spin-echo and short-tau recovery (STIR) (TR/TE/TI; 2000/30/100) **(C)** images of the chest show marked abnormal signal intensity along the chest walls, extending into the left neck. There is no discrete focal mass. **D:** Corresponding chest radiograph shows poorly defined soft tissue mass adjacent to the left lower chest (*asterisk*), with well-defined ossification on the right (*arrow*). **E:** Radiograph of the proximal tibia showing an osseous excrescence simulating a small osteochondroma.

failed to metastasize or behave aggressively (77,83,84). Accordingly, Reiman and Dahlin (77) note that a relatively well-defined extraskeletal cartilage lesion of the hands and feet should almost always be regarded as benign, in that metastases were not identified even in cases of alleged chondrosarcoma. Extraskeletal chondroma may also simulate extraskeletal myxoid chondrosarcoma. The latter, however, is more cellular, larger, and tends to be deep-seated in the large muscles of the upper and lower extremities and in the pelvic and shoulder girdles (80). Histologically, soft tissue chondroma and periosteal chondroma are similar; therefore, the distinction is best made based on clinical and radiologic features.

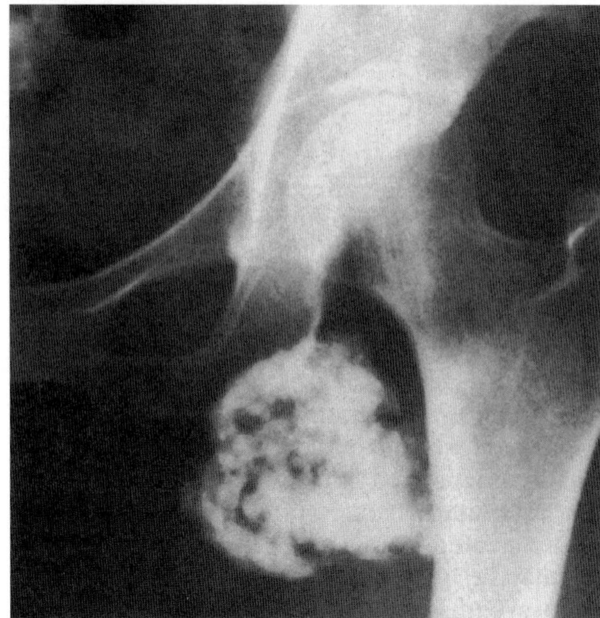

A

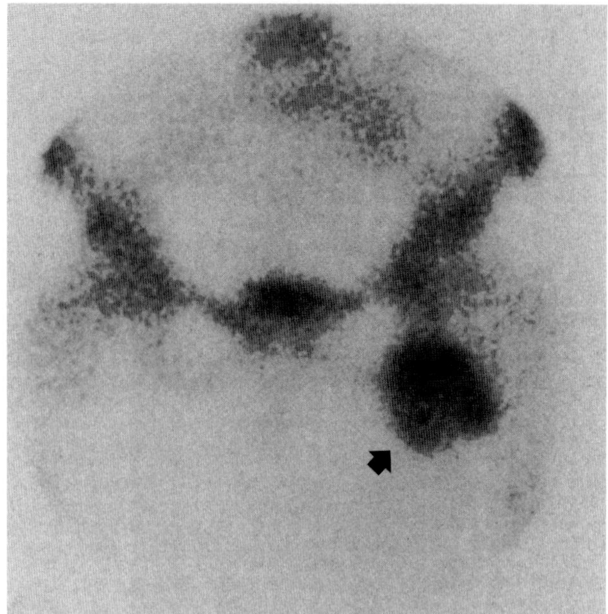

B

Figure 11.20   Osteoma of soft tissue: Radiographic and imaging features in a woman 56 years of age. **A:** Anteroposterior (AP) radiograph shows a densely mineralized mass in the soft tissue adjacent to the femur. **B:** Technetium-99m scintigraph shows markedly increased focal tracer accumulation within the lesion (*arrow*).

Imaging of Chondroma

> **KEY CONCEPTS**
> - Radiographs reveal a well-demarcated extraskeletal soft tissue mass.
> - Calcification is seen in 33% to 70% of lesions.
> - MR imaging shows high signal intensity on T2-weighted spin-echo MR images with intermediate signal intensity on T1-weighted images.
> - Calcification within lesions show decreased signal intensity on all MR pulse sequences.

There is scant literature on the radiologic appearance of soft tissue chondroma. Radiographs reveal a well-demarcated, extraskeletal soft tissue mass (85). Calcification is seen in 33% to 70% (80,82,86) of cases in the larger series (80,82,85,87,88). Mineralization may be central or peripheral (85); however, the majority of finger lesions calcify less often (87). The mineralization may have a ringlike appearance characteristic of cartilage. Ossification and peripheral rim calcification may also be seen (81). Adjacent bone may show evidence of remodeling secondary to the adjacent soft tissue mass (Fig. 11.21) (80).

Soft tissue chondromas image similarly to other hyaline cartilage tumors, showing high signal intensity on T2-weighted spin-echo MR images, with intermediate signal intensity on T1-weighted images, and corresponding areas of decreased signal intensity on both pulse sequences when significant calcification is seen (86–89). The high signal intensity of hyaline cartilage is presumably related to the high water content in relation to the mucopolysaccharide component (Figs. 11.22 and 11.23) (90).

MALIGNANT LESIONS

Malignant extraskeletal osseous and cartilaginous tumors of the extremities are relatively rare. The World Health Organization (WHO) currently classifies only extraskeletal osteosarcoma in this category. We also include two lesions that are currently classified as tumors of uncertain differentiation: ossifying fibromyxoid tumor of soft parts and extraskeletal chondrosarcoma. Although this grouping conflicts with that of the WHO, it is useful to radiologists for purposes of differential diagnosis.

Ossifying Fibromyxoid Tumor

Ossifying fibromyxoid tumor of soft tissue is a rare tumor of unknown differentiation, which was first described by Enzinger and colleagues (91) in 1989, in a report of 59 cases collected in consultation at the AFIP over a 25-year period. This lesion is included in this section because of its propensity to demonstrate an incomplete shell of mature bone in its capsular region (91). Ossifying fibromyxoid tumor was initially considered benign, to at most low-grade malignant, with one patient in the initial report having three recurrences as well as a metastasis to the opposite thigh (91). A newer review of four large

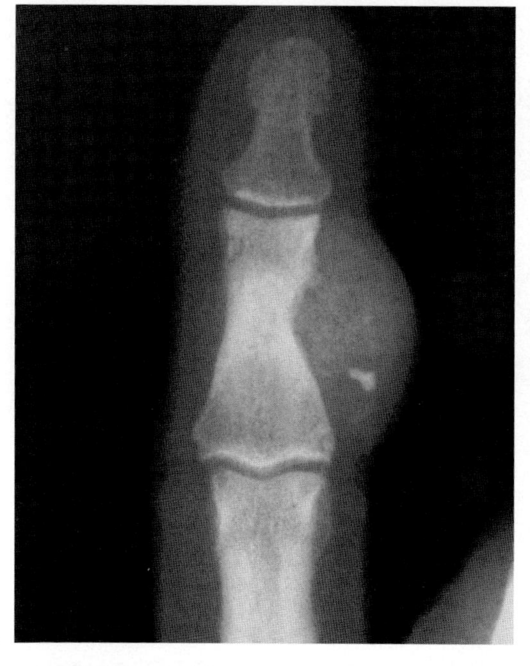

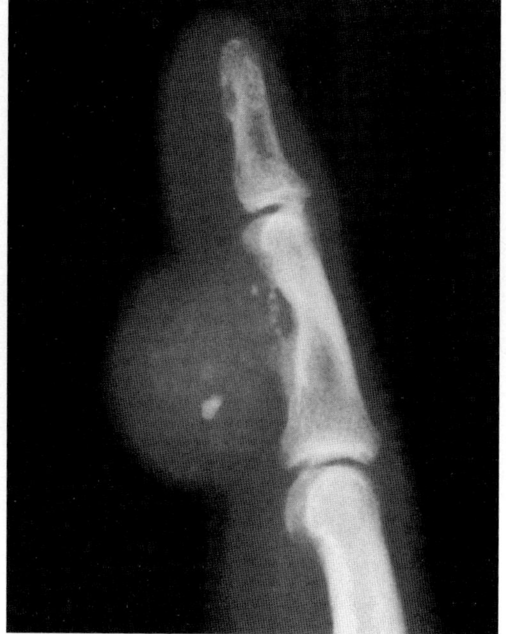

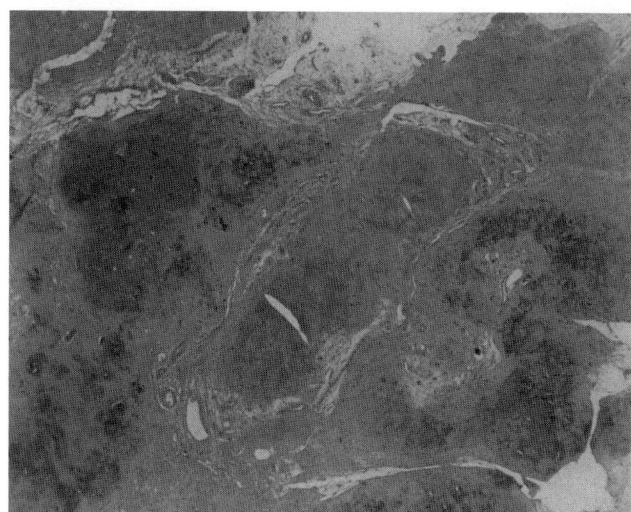

Figure 11.21 Soft tissue chondroma: Typical radiographic features in a man 59 years of age. **A,B:** Anteroposterior **(A)** and lateral **(B)** radiographs of the finger show a soft tissue mass with central punctate calcification and secondary pressure erosion of the adjacent middle phalanx. **C:** Low-power photomicrograph shows a lobulated mass of cellular hyaline cartilage, with areas of calcification.

KEY CONCEPTS

- Ossifying fibromyxoid tumor is a rare tumor of unknown differentiation.
- Initially it was considered benign, or at most low-grade malignant.
- It is now considered to have intermediate malignant potential.
- Men are affected more frequently than women.
- Lesions are almost always seen in adults.
- Patients present with a slowly growing, small, painless, extremity mass.
- Wide surgical excision remains the treatment of choice.
- Recurrence is common, reported in 17% to 27% of patients.

published studies established an overall metastatic rate of 5%, indicating the lesion should be considered "of intermediate malignancy" (92). To date, more than 120 cases have been reported (92).

Men are affected more frequently than women, and lesions are almost always seen in adults (92–94). Rare cases are reported in children, with the youngest reported case in a boy 3 weeks of age presenting with a nasal mass (95,96).

Clinically, lesions present as slowly growing, small, painless, well-circumscribed soft tissue masses (median, 4 cm) in the subcutis or muscle, with skin involvement noted in an estimated 10% of cases. Approximately 63% to 70% of lesions are located in the extremities, with the lower extremity involved somewhat more frequently. It is less frequently found in the trunk (16% to 19%) and the head and neck (9% to 13%) (1,92,97).

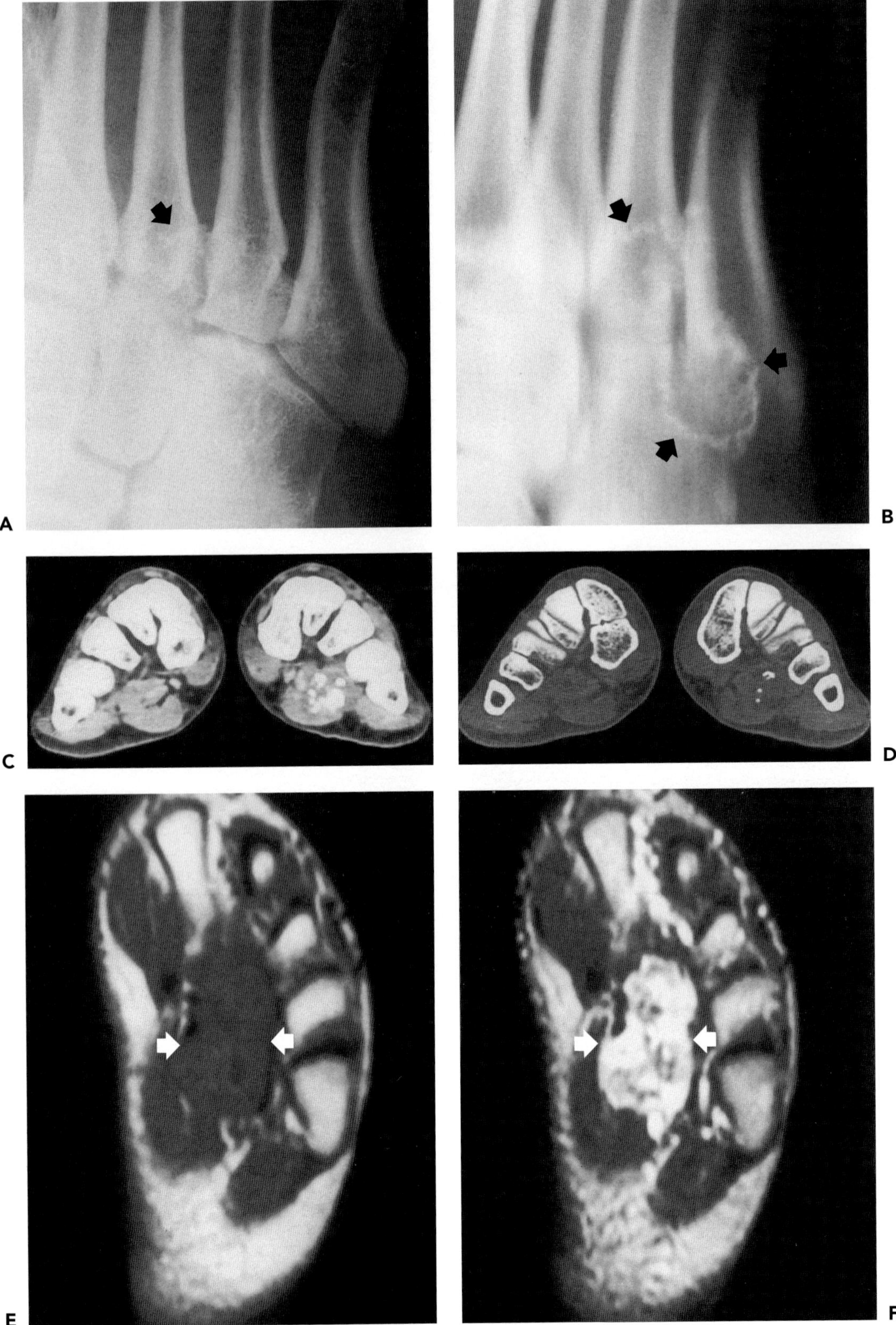

Figure 11.22 Soft tissue chondroma: Typical imaging features in the foot of a man 39 years of age. **A:** Oblique radiograph of the foot shows subtle calcifications (*arrow*) at the base of the fourth metacarpal. **B:** Linear tomogram shows this to better advantage (*arrows*). **C,D:** Coronal CT scans displayed at soft tissue **(C)** and bone **(D)** windows show the calcified mass in the plantar aspect of the foot. **E,F:** Axial T1-weighted (TR/TE; 600/20) **(E)** and T2-weighted (TR/TE; 1900/80) **(F)** spin-echo MR images show a well-defined, inhomogeneous mass (*arrows*). The areas of decreased signal intensity on both pulse sequences correspond to calcification.

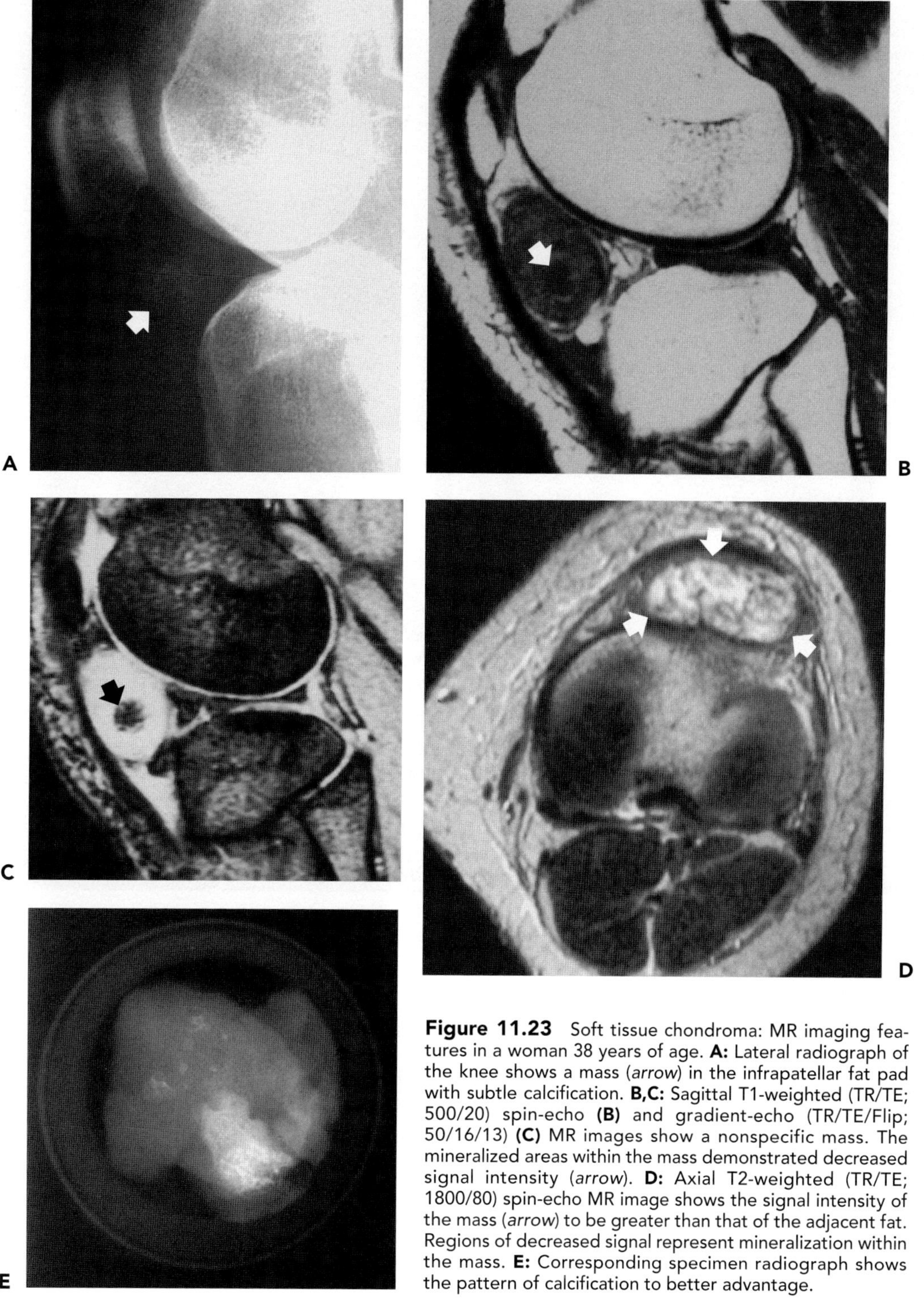

Figure 11.23 Soft tissue chondroma: MR imaging features in a woman 38 years of age. **A:** Lateral radiograph of the knee shows a mass (*arrow*) in the infrapatellar fat pad with subtle calcification. **B,C:** Sagittal T1-weighted (TR/TE; 500/20) spin-echo **(B)** and gradient-echo (TR/TE/Flip; 50/16/13) **(C)** MR images show a nonspecific mass. The mineralized areas within the mass demonstrated decreased signal intensity (*arrow*). **D:** Axial T2-weighted (TR/TE; 1800/80) spin-echo MR image shows the signal intensity of the mass (*arrow*) to be greater than that of the adjacent fat. Regions of decreased signal represent mineralization within the mass. **E:** Corresponding specimen radiograph shows the pattern of calcification to better advantage.

Wide surgical excision remains the treatment of choice. Recurrence is common, reported in 17% to 27% of patients. When present, metastases are most common to the lungs (92). Soft tissue metastases may also be seen but are less common (38%) (92).

Microscopically, the tumor is partly lobulated, and is composed of small, round cells with vesicular nuclei and indistinct cytoplasm (91). Cells are typically arranged in a cord- or nestlike pattern within a myxoid matrix, with transitions toward hyaline fibrosis and focal osteoid formation. The lesion is surrounded by a collagenous, well-formed capsule that contains trabecular bone in 80% of cases. Although the histogenesis is uncertain, investigations suggest the tumor has a schwannian differentiation, based on its frequent expression of nerve sheath markers (98,99).

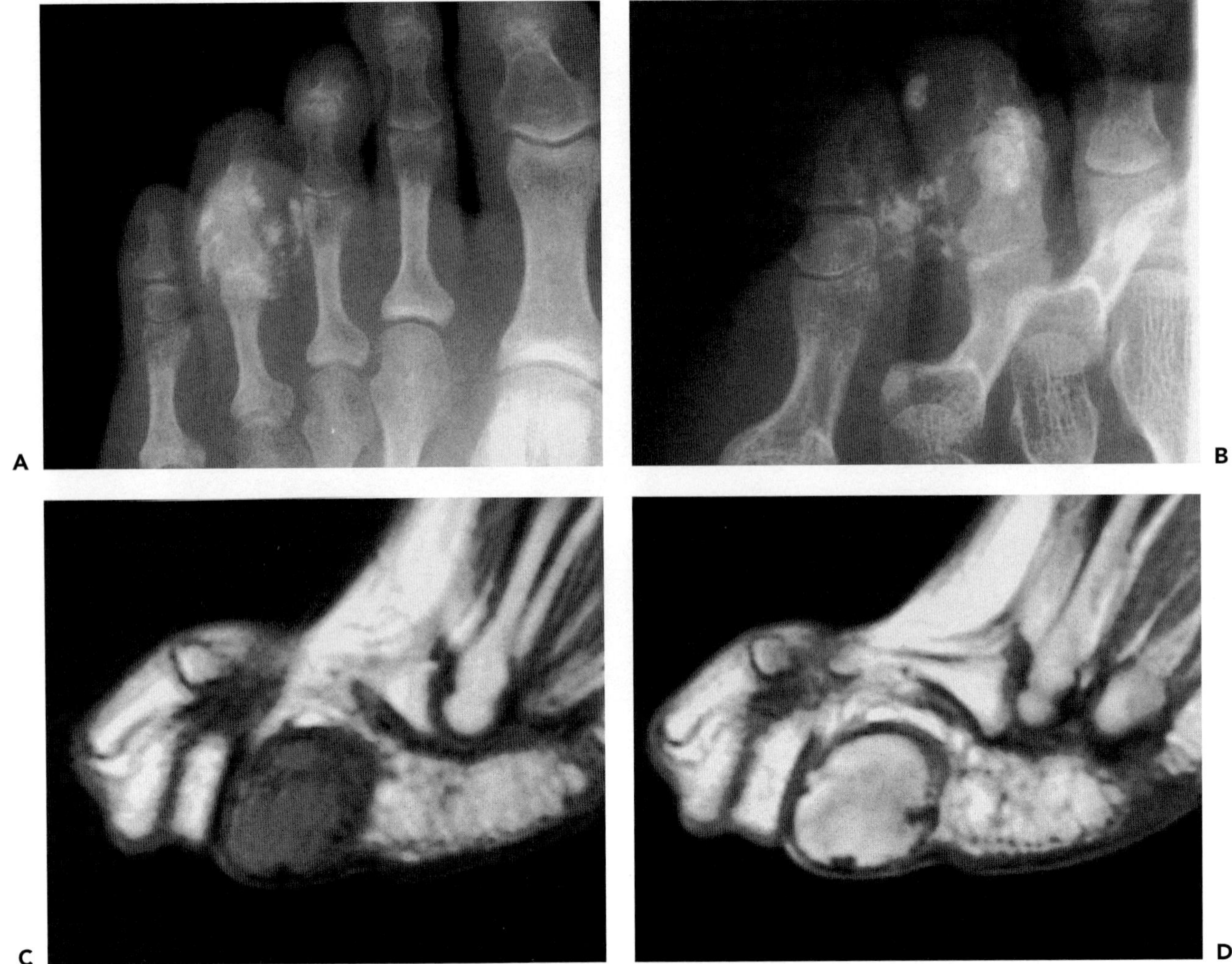

Figure 11.24   Ossifying fibromyxoid tumor: Typical imaging features in a man 46 years of age with a long-standing, slowly growing, soft tissue mass. **A,B:** Anteroposterior **(A)** and oblique **(B)** radiographs of the fourth toe show a mass with numerous foci of mineralization. **C,D:** Sagittal T1-weighted (TR/TE; 450/15) spin-echo MR images of the toe preceding **(C)** and following **(D)** contrast administration show intense minimally heterogeneous enhancement. Note prominent areas of decreased signal associated with the capsule representing ossification. (*continued*)

Imaging of Ossifying Fibromyxoid Tumor

> **KEY CONCEPTS**
> - Radiographs show a wide spectrum, from a nonmineralized to an extensively mineralized mass.
> - Scintigraphy shows a marked focal radiotracer.
> - On CT scanning, the lesion shows variable amounts of irregular mature lamellar bone formation.
> - MR imaging findings vary with the amount of ossification present:
>   - Nonmineralized regions show a nonspecific, heterogeneous signal intensity.
>   - Areas of high signal intensity similar to that of fat may be noted on T1-weighted images.
>   - Densely mineralized areas show signal voids.

There is scant literature documenting the radiographic and imaging appearance of ossifying fibromyxoid tumor.

Radiographic data were available on only nine patients in the initial report, and of those, only two were noted to have solid, patchy or linear, soft tissue densities with an incomplete ring or shell-like pattern of mineralization (Fig. 11.24) (91). Other reports showed a radiographic spectrum, from lesions that are not mineralized, to those that demonstrate focal areas of irregular bone formation, to those that are extensively mineralized (91,100–102).

Technetium methylene diphosphonate (MDP) scintigraphy demonstrates marked focal radiotracer accumulation within the tumor (100,103). On CT scanning, the lesion shows variable amounts of irregular, mature, lamellar bone formation. MR imaging findings also vary depending on the amount of ossification present, with densely mineralized areas showing signal voids (Fig. 11.24). Nonmineralized regions show a nonspecific, heterogeneous signal intensity as well as enhancement following gadolinium administration (95,100,102,103). Areas of high signal intensity similar to

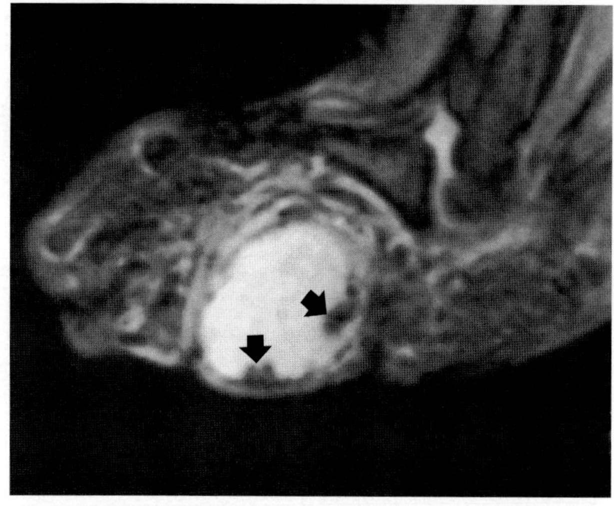

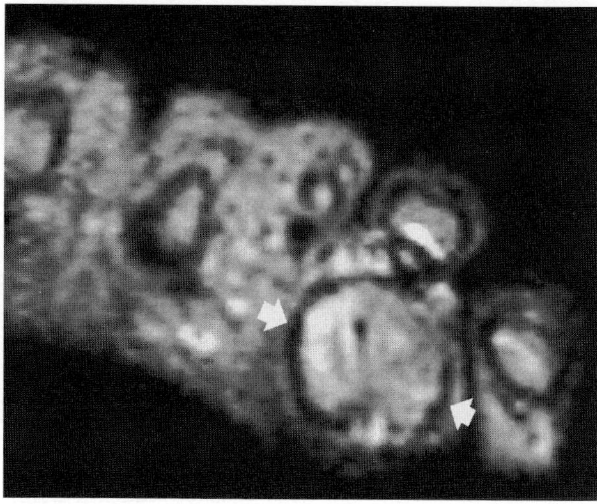

Figure 11.24 *(continued)* **E:** Sagittal gradient-echo (TR/TE/Flip; 450/12/15) MR image shows areas of decreased signal (*arrows*) from ossification associated with the capsule. **F:** Axial conventional T2-weighted (TR/TE; 2500/90) spin-echo MR image shows the mass (*arrows*) to have a nonspecific signal intensity with prominent decreased signal from the capsule. **G:** Specimen radiograph shows numerous foci of ossification.

that of fat were noted on T1-weighted images, correlating to fatty marrow between osseous trabeculae (103).

Extraskeletal Osteosarcoma

Extraskeletal osteosarcoma is the only malignancy retained by the WHO as a chondro-osseous tumor (104). Extraskeletal myxoid chondrosarcoma has been reclassified as a lesion of uncertain differentiation. Despite its name, extraskeletal myxoid chondrosarcoma shows little evidence of cartilage differentiation (1).

> *KEY CONCEPTS*
> - Extraskeletal osteosarcoma is a malignant mesenchymal neoplasm that produces osteoid and/or bone.
> - It is located in the soft tissue without attachment to bone or periosteum.
> - By definition, no other lines of differentiation may be present.

Extraskeletal osteosarcoma is a malignant mesenchymal neoplasm that produces osteoid and/or bone and is located in the soft tissue without attachment to bone or periosteum (76,105). Some extraskeletal osteosarcomas

may also contain chrondoblastic and fibroblastic components in addition to neoplastic bone (104). By definition, no other lines of differentiation may be present (104).

Clinical Features

> *KEY CONCEPTS*
> - Extraskeletal osteosarcoma is relatively rare.
> - It represents approximately 1% of soft tissue sarcomas and 4% of all osteosarcomas.
> - It is a tumor of adults, with more than 94% of patients older than 30 years.
> - The thigh is the single most common location (42%), followed by the upper extremity (12% to 23%) and retroperitoneum (8% to 17%).
> - It is typically a high-grade malignancy.
> - Local recurrence and metastases occur in 80% to 90% of patients.

Extraskeletal osteosarcoma is relatively rare, comprising approximately 1% of soft tissue sarcomas and approximately 4% of all osteosarcomas (104–107). In a 10-year review of malignant soft tissue tumors, extraskeletal osteosarcoma was diagnosed in 79 (0.6%) of 12,370 soft tissue sarcomas seen in consultation at the AFIP, within the Department of Soft Tissue Pathology (108).

Extraskeletal osteosarcoma is a tumor of adults, with a mean age of approximately 50 years at presentation (77, 105–108). More than 94% of patients are older than 30 years (77,107,108). This is in contradistinction to conventional intraosseous osteosarcoma, which is most common in the first two decades of life. There is a slight male predominance in most series (77,105–107). Tumors are most common in the lower extremity, accounting for more than half the cases, with the thigh the single most common location, comprising up to 42% of lesions. This is followed by the upper extremity (12% to 23%) and retroperitoneum (8% to 17%) (77,106–108).

Patients typically present with an enlarging soft tissue mass; pain and tenderness are noted in a quarter to a half of all patients (77,106). Extraskeletal osteosarcoma is a well-documented sequela of radiation. Approximately 4% to 13% of reported cases develop in this manner (77,106,107,109), having had a history of radiation 2 to 40 years prior to clinical presentation (77,106,109). Malignant fibrous histiocytoma (undifferentiated pleomorphic sarcoma), however, is the most common postradiation sarcoma, representing more than two-thirds of 52 cases reported by Laskin et al. (109), with extraskeletal osteosarcoma representing 13% and fibrosarcoma 11%. A history of trauma is reported in approximately 12% to 31% (6,105–107) of cases of extraskeletal osteosarcoma; however, the role of trauma in the development of extraskeletal osteosarcoma is unclear.

Extraskeletal osteosarcoma is reported to develop in myositis ossificans and at the site of previous intramuscular injection (110); however, histological documentation of preexisting myositis ossificans is available in only a small number of cases (111). Although a few well-documented cases of malignant transformation are reported, they are likely extremely rare (104). Extraskeletal osteosarcoma is also reported following chemotherapy treatment of mediastinal nonseminomatous germ-cell tumor (112). In such cases, it is postulated that chemotherapy-resistant teratomatous elements undergo transformation; rhabdomyosarcoma is the most common sarcomatous transformation (112).

Extraskeletal osteosarcoma is typically a high-grade malignancy. Low-grade lesions are described, but they are rare (113). In a report of a case in the lower leg in 2003, Okada et al. (113) reviewed the literature and found three previously reported low-grade cases. Additionally, Funhee et al. (114) reported a unique case of a well-differentiated extraskeletal osteosarcoma associated with a lobulated fatty mass and speculated that the lesion may represent malignant transformation of metaplastic bone within a lipoma. In this case, the lesion was present for 10 years in the axilla of a woman 74 years of age.

More than 80% to 90% of patients with extraskeletal osteosarcoma develop local recurrence and metastases (77,107). The interval between removal of the primary tumor and recurrence ranges from 2 months to 10 years (77), with a median of 7 months to 1 year (77,107). The interval between first operation and metastases ranges from 1 month to 4 years. Metastases occur in up to 80% (107) of cases, the overwhelming majority to the lungs (81% to 100%). Less than a quarter of patients develop metastases to the subcutis, liver, bone, and lymph nodes (6,77,107,115,116). Overall, the prognosis is poor (77), and more than half of patients die within 2 to 3 years. Tumor size is the major predictor of patient survival. Bane et al. (106) reported eight of nine long-term survivors as patients with tumors smaller than 5 cm. In contradistinction, 14 of 16 patients with tumors 5 cm or greater were dead of disease within 5 years. Survival rates are better after wide or radical resection (115). There is no correlation between the histologic appearance of the tumor and the clinical outcome (105–107).

Tumors are typically deep-seated and often fixed to surrounding tissue (77). Superficial or subcutaneous lesions may occasionally be seen. On gross appearance the tumor may appear well-defined, although microscopically it is frequently ill-defined and infiltrative, with occasional satellite nodules (77,107). A pseudocapsule may be present, and necrosis and hemorrhage within the tumor is common (117). Microscopically, all lesions contain variable amounts of osteoid or bone; cartilage is frequently present as well. The microscopic features generally reflect those of the histologic subtypes identified in conventional osteosarcoma of bone and include osteoblastic, chondroblastic, fibroblastic, and occasionally telangiectatic types. The small cell variant is rare. It is important to emphasize that extraskeletal osteosarcoma and high-grade malignant fibrous histiocytoma (undifferentiated pleomorphic sarcoma) may be quite similar both microscopically and clinically (77,106).

The immunophenotype of extraskeletal osteosarcoma is similar to its intraosseous counterpart (104). Osteocalcin may be the most specific antigen for extraskeletal osteosarcoma and is expressed in the malignant cells and matrix in a high percentage of cases (104). The genetics of this lesion have not been extensively studied, but limited reports show no systematic genetic differences between extraosseous and osseous lesions (104).

Imaging of Extraskeletal Osteosarcoma

KEY CONCEPTS

- Radiographs demonstrate mineralization in about half of the lesions.
- Mineralization may appear as a dense, cloudlike area of increased opacity.
- Bone scintigraphy shows increased tracer accumulation.
- CT is useful to identify mineralization and necrosis.
- MR imaging most often shows a well-defined heterogeneous mass with nonspecific signal intensity.

Radiographs demonstrate variable amounts of mineralization which may appear as a dense, cloudlike area of increased opacity (Figs. 11.25 and 11.26). No calcification

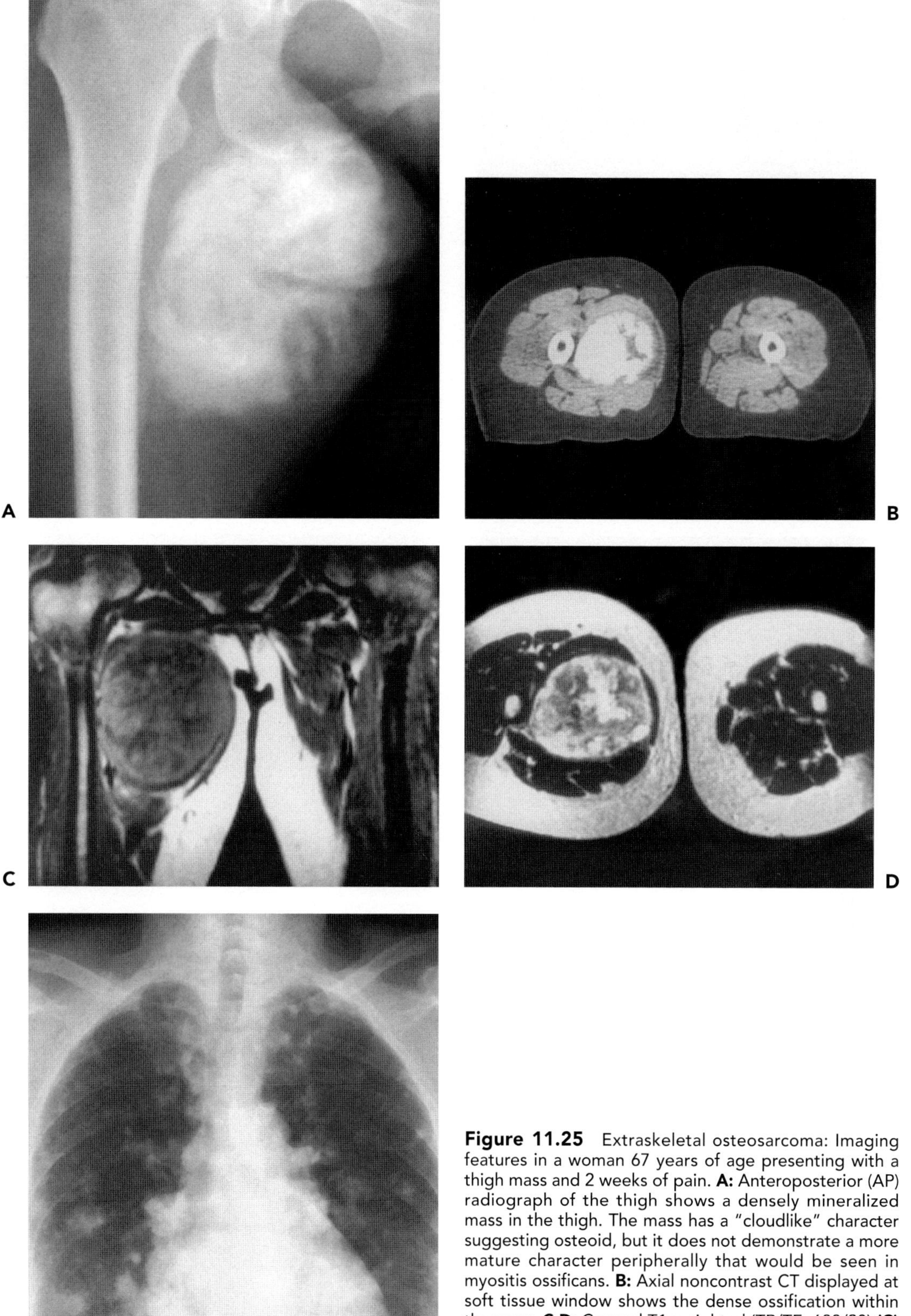

Figure 11.25 Extraskeletal osteosarcoma: Imaging features in a woman 67 years of age presenting with a thigh mass and 2 weeks of pain. **A:** Anteroposterior (AP) radiograph of the thigh shows a densely mineralized mass in the thigh. The mass has a "cloudlike" character suggesting osteoid, but it does not demonstrate a more mature character peripherally that would be seen in myositis ossificans. **B:** Axial noncontrast CT displayed at soft tissue window shows the dense ossification within the mass. **C,D:** Coronal T1-weighted (TR/TE; 600/30) **(C)** and axial T2-weighted (TR/TE; 2500/80) **(D)** spin-echo images show a well-defined, inhomogeneous, nonspecific mass. Areas of decreased signal intensity on MR correspond to dense mineralization within the mass. **E:** Chest radiograph at presentation shows multiple pulmonary metastases.

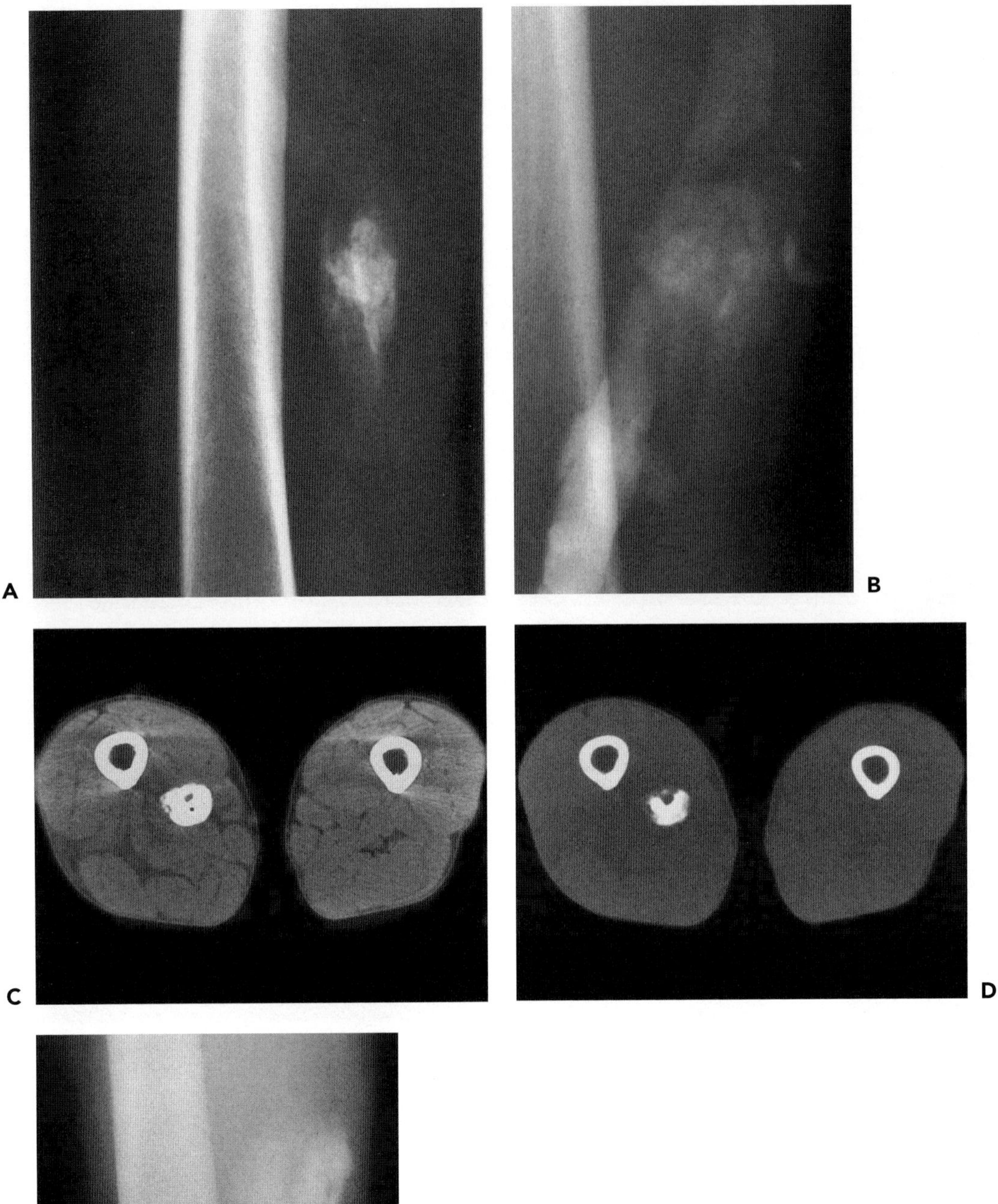

Figure 11.26 Extraskeletal osteosarcoma: Imaging features in a man 56 years of age presenting with painful swelling. **A:** Initial anteroposterior (AP) radiograph shows a densely mineralized mass in the medial thigh. The dense mineralization could suggest myositis ossificans, although an osseous character, more mature peripherally, is not present. There is a linear filling defect, corresponding to a vessel traversing the mass. **B:** Venogram shows the mass compressing the superficial femoral vein. **C,D:** Axial noncontrast CT scan at bone **(C)** and soft tissue **(D)** windows shows a densely mineralized mass in the medial aspect of the right thigh. **E:** Follow-up AP radiograph approximately 3 months later shows significant interval enlargement. (*continued*)

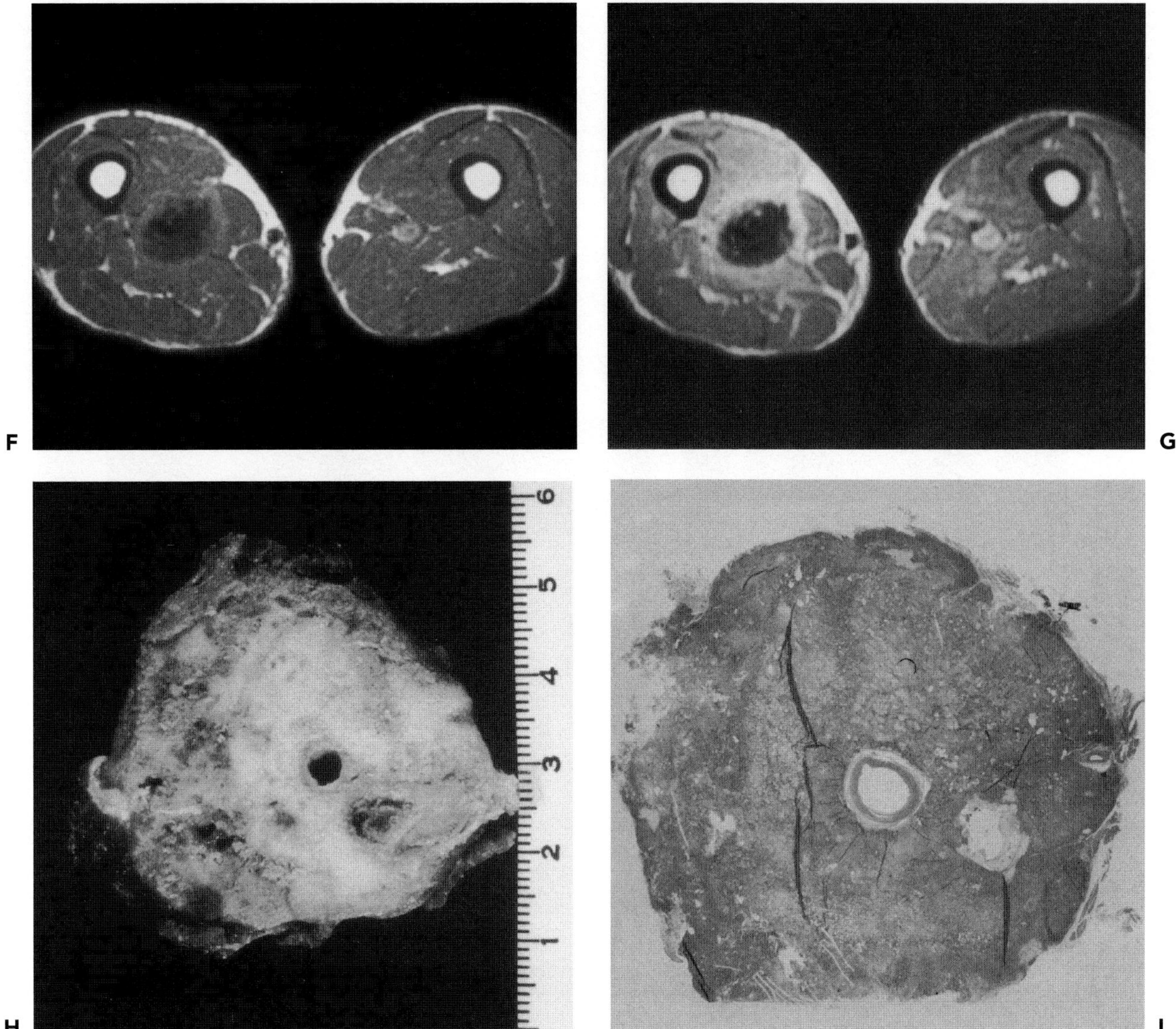

Figure 11.26 *(continued)* **F,G:** Axial T1-weighted (TR/TE; 600/20) **(F)** and T2-weighted (TR/TE; 2500/80) **(G)** spin-echo MR image shows a relatively well-defined mass with surrounding high signal intensity on the T2-weighted image, compatible with surrounding edema. There is little signal from the densely mineralized mass. **H,I:** Gross photograph **(H)** and corresponding macroscopic section **(I)** show the ossified mass encasing the superficial femoral artery and vein. (Original magnification ×1, hematoxylin and eosin.)

is seen in about half the lesions (117–119). Involvement of adjacent bone is rare (76,106).

Bone scintigraphy shows increased tracer accumulation within the mass as well as within metastases (117–119). CT is useful to identify mineralization and necrosis within the mass, and arteriography demonstrates the presence of hypervascularity. (Figs. 11.25–11.27) (76,106).

There is scant literature on the MR findings in extraskeletal osteosarcoma, with most reports consisting of isolated cases or small series. MR imaging most often shows a well-defined heterogeneous mass with a signal intensity similar to or slightly greater than that of skeletal muscle on T1-weighted images and greater than that of fat on T2-weighted spin-echo images (115,117,118). Not uncommonly, MR imaging suggests underlying hemorrhage with focal areas of high signal intensity on both T1- and T2-weighted images

(117). As with the overwhelming majority of cases, MR imaging is nonspecific and only reflects the morphology of the underlying lesion. Hemorrhagic lesions may mimic a hematoma (Fig. 11.27).

Extraskeletal Chondrosarcoma

Extraskeletal chondrosarcomas are relatively rare neoplasms, which, in general, are far less common than their intraosseous counterparts. In a 10-year review, extraskeletal chondrosarcoma was diagnosed in 263 (2.1%) of soft tissue sarcomas seen in consultation at the AFIP (108). Soft tissue chondrosarcomas are typically subdivided into myxoid, mesenchymal, and the very rare well-differentiated types. With the exception of well-differentiated chondrosarcoma, these lesions show minimal, if any, cartilage formation.

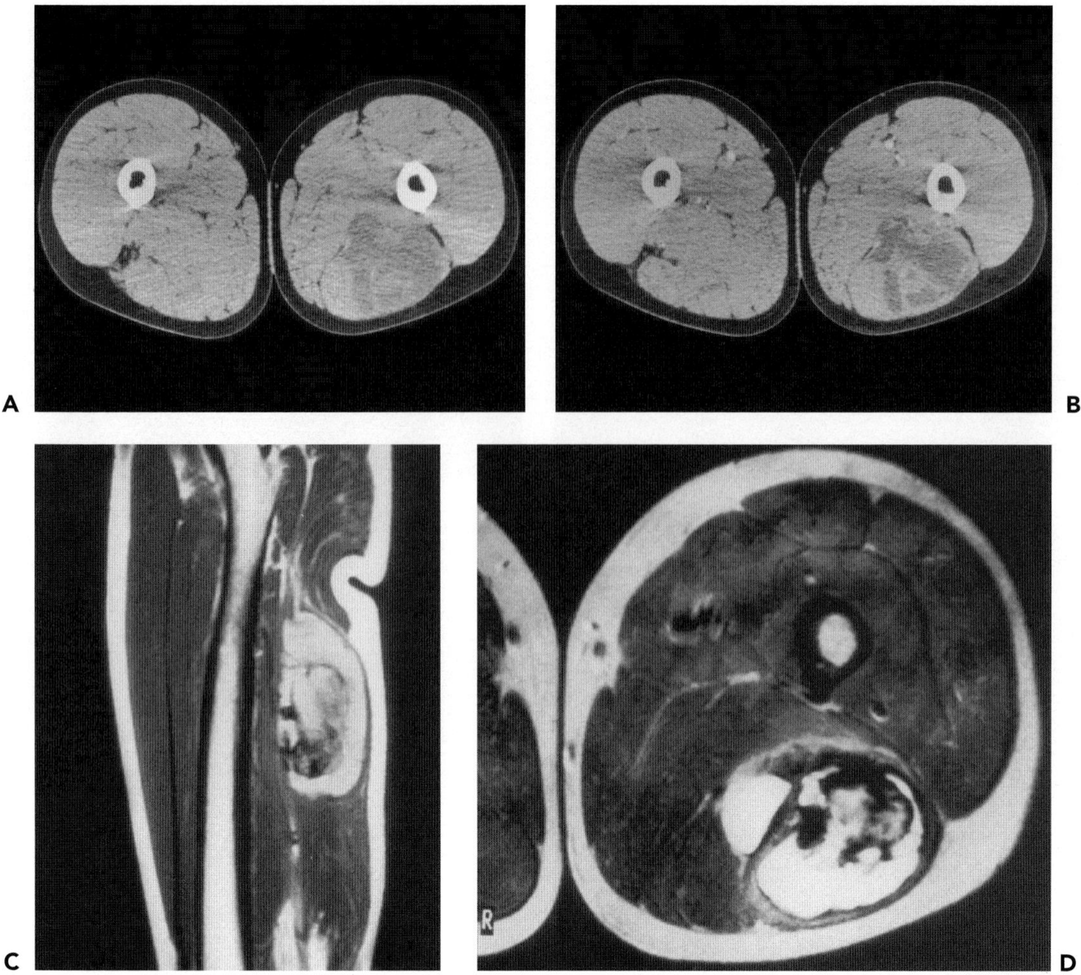

Figure 11.27 Extraskeletal osteosarcoma: CT and MR imaging features in a man 30 years of age presenting with progressive pain and swelling in the thigh. **A:** Noncontrast axial CT scan shows a mass with decreased attenuation in the posterior thigh. **B:** CT following contrast administration shows enhancement at the periphery of the mass as well as within the mass. **C,D:** Sagittal T1-weighted (TR/TE; 600/20) **(C)** and axial proton (TR/TE; 2000/50) **(D)** spin-echo MR images done 4 weeks later show evidence of subacute hematoma with hemosiderin. Follow-up incisional biopsy showed extraskeletal osteosarcoma. (*continued*)

KEY CONCEPTS

- Extraskeletal myxoid chondrosarcoma is the most common extraskeletal chondrosarcoma.
- It is a tumor of adults, with a mean age at presentation of approximately 50 years.
- It is extremely rare in patients younger than 20 years.
- Patients typically present with a slowly growing soft tissue mass.
- The vast majority of lesions are in the extremities, with the thigh the most common location.
- It is generally considered to be a low-grade sarcoma.
- Metastases are found in 40% to 45% of patients.

Extraskeletal Myxoid Chondrosarcoma

Extraskeletal myxoid chondrosarcoma is the most common extraskeletal chondrosarcoma. It is a tumor of adults with a mean age at presentation of approximately 50 years, although patients range from 4 to 92 years of age (120–123). There is a male predominance in most series that may be as high as 2:1 (120,122–124). The lesion is extremely rare in patients younger than 20 years of age (121).

Patients typically present with a slowly growing soft tissue mass. Pain or tenderness is seen in approximately a third of cases (120). The vast majority of lesions are in the extremities, with the thigh the single most common location (120,122,125). Most lesions are in the deep soft tissue, but approximately a fourth are located in the subcutis (120). Extraskeletal myxoid chondrosarcoma is generally considered a low-grade sarcoma, with a 10-year survival rate of 45% to 70% (122,124,126); however, local recurrences are common and frequently multiple (120,122). Metastases may precede detection of the primary tumor and in general are found in 40% to 46% of patients (120,122,124,126). In a report of 16 patients by McGrory et al., 3 (19%) patients presented with pulmonary metastases (126). Survival of 5 to 15 years after the development

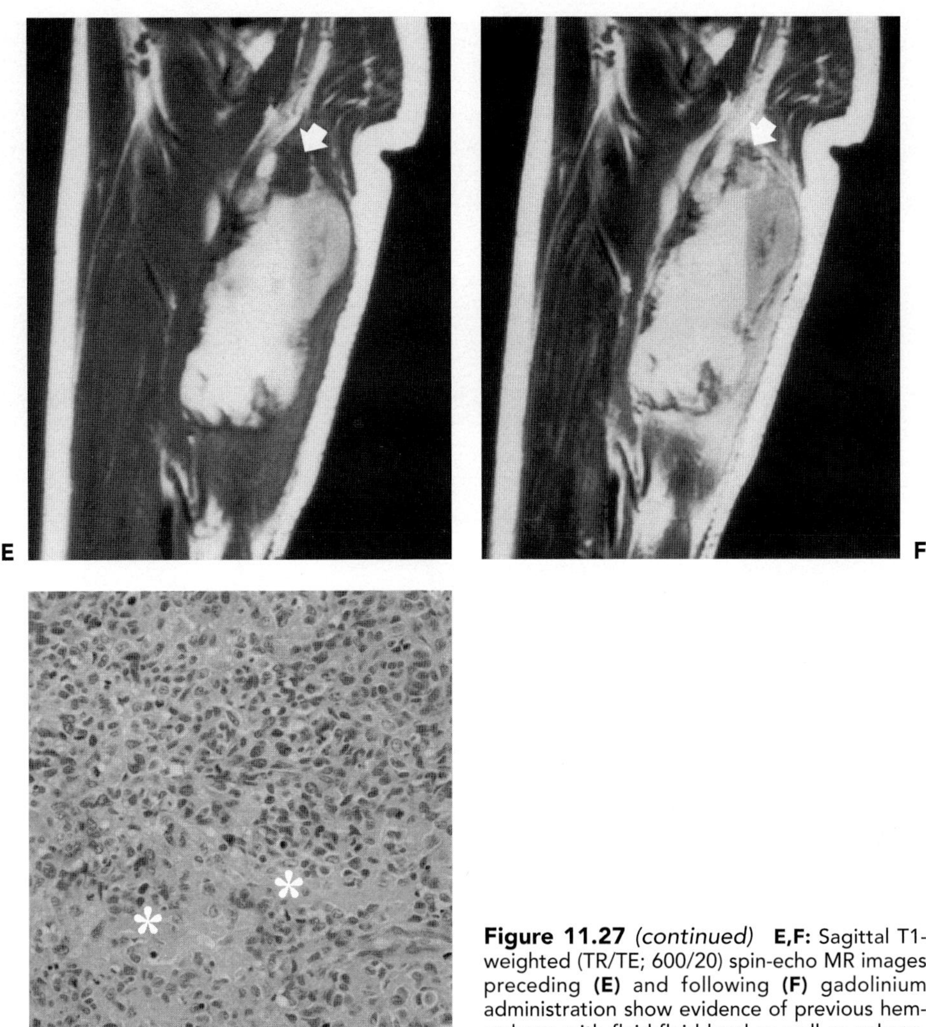

Figure 11.27 *(continued)* **E,F:** Sagittal T1-weighted (TR/TE; 600/20) spin-echo MR images preceding **(E)** and following **(F)** gadolinium administration show evidence of previous hemorrhage with fluid-fluid level as well as enhancing tumor nodule *(arrow)*. **G:** High-power photomicrograph shows lacelike osteoid *(asterisks)* and associated anaplastic cells (original magnification ×240, hematoxylin and eosin).

of metastases is not uncommon (120,122). A recent long-term study of 10 patients found 7 dead of tumor and 3 alive with metastases at 13, 14, and 16 years following diagnosis, suggesting a high potential for metastases (123).

On gross examination, the lesion is a well-defined multinodular mass with a distinctly gelatinous appearance. The lesion is usually between 4 cm and 7 cm in diameter but may be much larger, frequently with areas of cyst formation and hemorrhage (120,122). Hemorrhage may be a dominant feature, suggesting a hematoma (120). On microscopic examination, the lesions are usually surrounded by a fibrous capsule and contain fibrous septa that divide the lesion into multiple lobules. Delicate strands of small elongate-to-round chondroblasts reminiscent of those seen in fetal cartilage are suspended in an abundant myxoid matrix that possesses histochemical properties characteristic of cartilage. Foci of mature hyaline cartilage are rarely seen. Extraskeletal myxoid chondrosarcoma is characterized by a reciprocal translocation t(9;22)(q22;q12) in more than 75% of cases (127).

Imaging of Extraskeletal Myxoid Chondrosarcoma

> ### KEY CONCEPTS
> - Radiographs may demonstrate a soft tissue mass.
> - Calcification and bone formation are unusual but are occasionally seen.
> - MR imaging features are not specific:
>   - Lesions are generally intermediate to high signal intensity on T2-weighted images.
>   - Internal hemorrhage may be present.

Radiographs may demonstrate a soft tissue mass. Calcification and bone formation are usually not present, although they are occasionally seen. Soft tissue lesions are reported with a thick periosteal reaction as well as rare bone invasion (120,121,128–130).

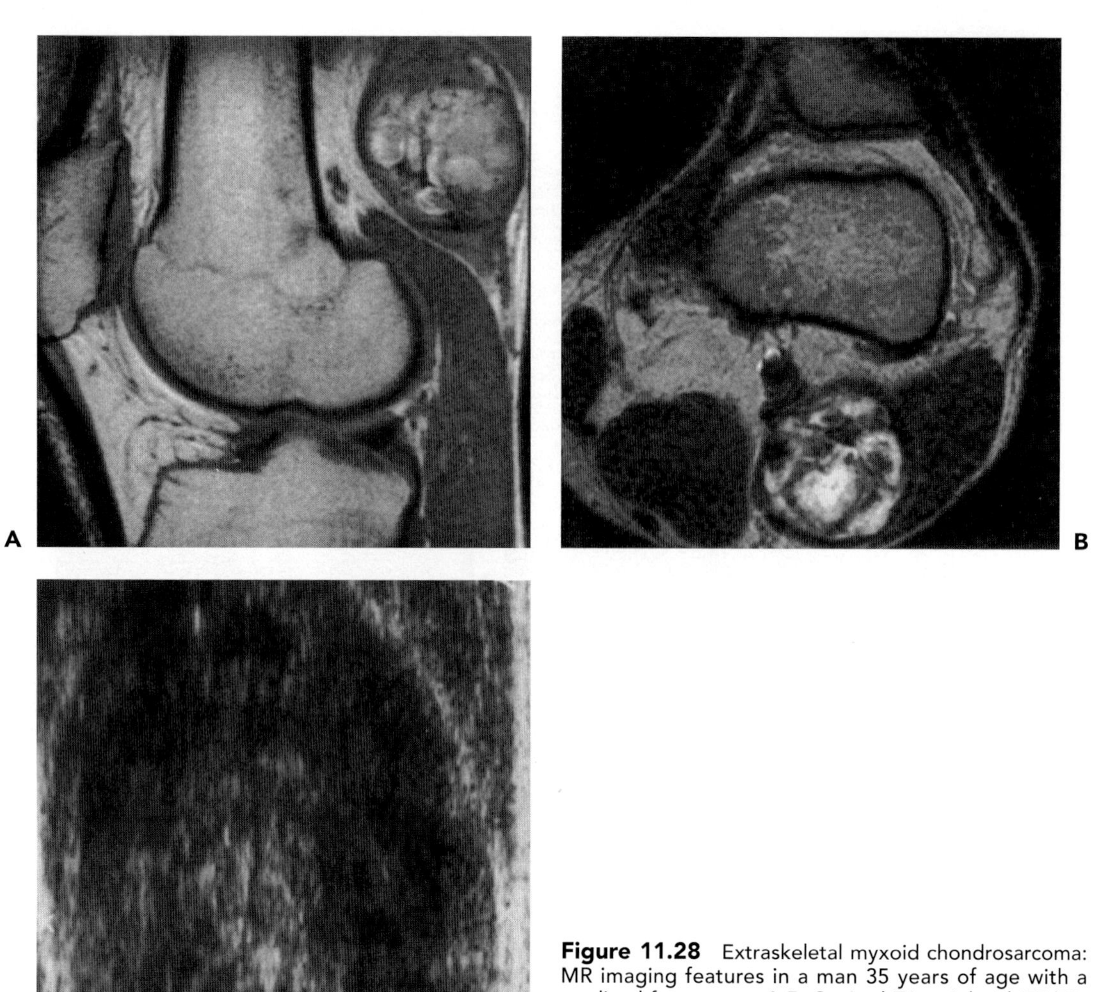

Figure 11.28 Extraskeletal myxoid chondrosarcoma: MR imaging features in a man 35 years of age with a popliteal fossa mass. **A,B:** Sagittal T1-weighted (TR/TE; 800/20) **(A)** and axial T2-weighted (TR/TE; 2000/80) **(B)** spin-echo MR images show a relatively well-defined mass in the popliteal fossa. The mass is heterogeneous, with corresponding areas of increased and decreased signal on all pulse sequences caused by subacute hemorrhage and hemosiderin. **C:** Ultrasound demonstrated a well-defined solid heterogeneous mass.

Extraskeletal myxoid chondrosarcoma shows a wide imaging spectrum. Lesions are usually a well-defined intermuscular or, less often, intramuscular soft tissue mass. As would be expected, CT and MR imaging reflect the lesions' morphology. Predominantly myxoid lesions demonstrate low attenuation on CT and very high signal intensity on T2-weighted MR images, reflective of its extremely high water content, with only mild peripheral to septal enhancement after contrast administration (131). Hemorrhagic lesions are not uncommon, and subacute hemorrhage shows increased signal intensity on all pulse sequences, characteristic of a hematoma (Figs. 11.28 and 11.29). The combination of myxoid and hemorrhagic tissue provides the variable intermediate to high signal intensity on both T1- and T2-weighted images reported with this lesion (121,128,130). We have also seen cases in which the slowly growing tumor engulfed adjacent fat, mimicking a liposarcoma (Fig. 11.30).

Extraskeletal Mesenchymal Chondrosarcoma

> **KEY CONCEPTS**
> - Approximately half of all mesenchymal chondrosarcomas arise in soft tissue.
> - Bimodal age distribution:
>   - Head and neck lesions occur primarily in the third decade of life.
>   - Deep muscle and trunk lesions occur most frequently in the fifth decade.
> - Symptoms are nonspecific with a slowly enlarging, painless soft tissue mass.

Extraskeletal mesenchymal chondrosarcoma is much less common than extraskeletal myxoid chondrosarcoma, and interestingly, approximately half of all mesenchymal chon-

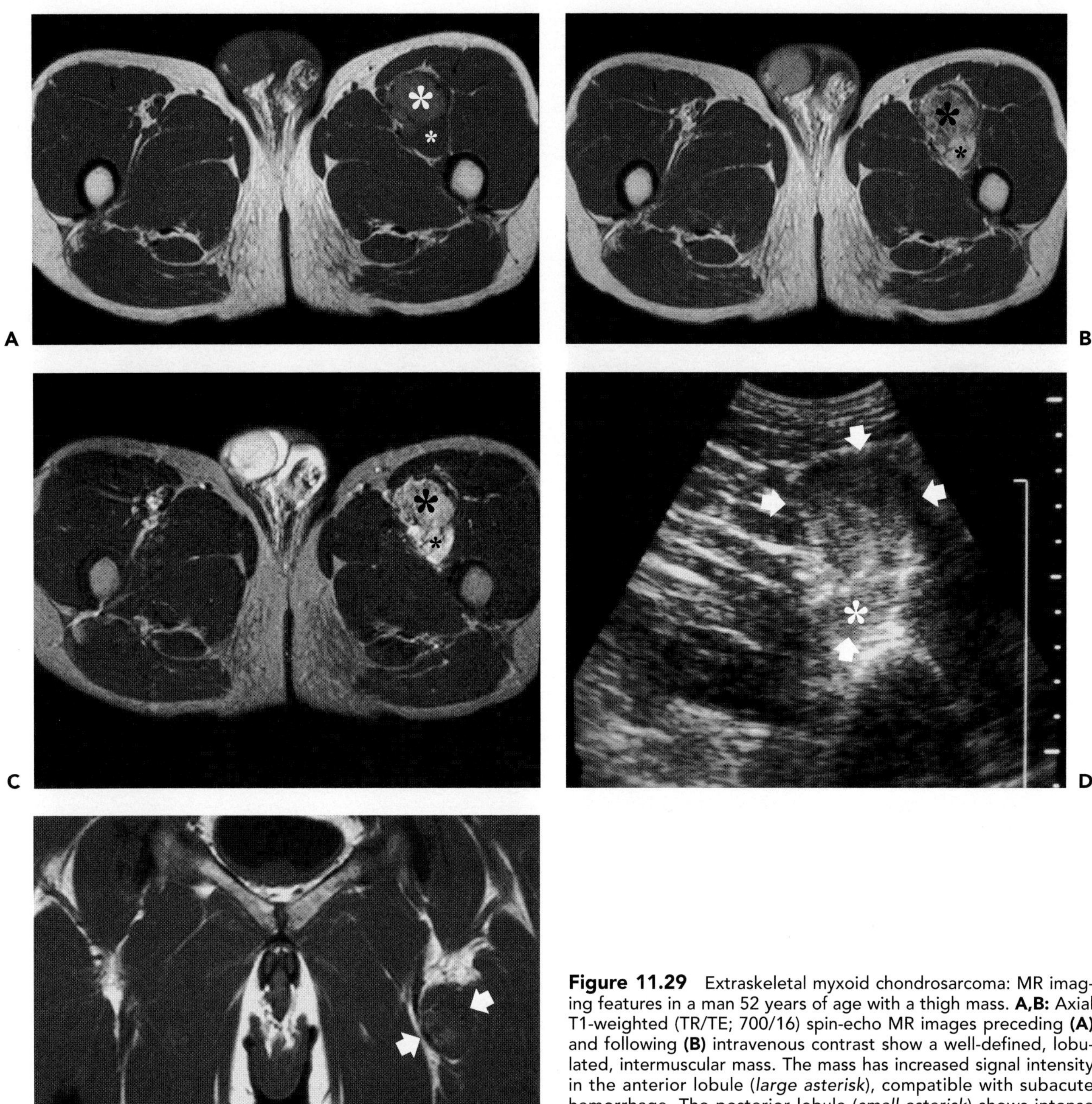

Figure 11.29 Extraskeletal myxoid chondrosarcoma: MR imaging features in a man 52 years of age with a thigh mass. **A,B:** Axial T1-weighted (TR/TE; 700/16) spin-echo MR images preceding **(A)** and following **(B)** intravenous contrast show a well-defined, lobulated, intermuscular mass. The mass has increased signal intensity in the anterior lobule (*large asterisk*), compatible with subacute hemorrhage. The posterior lobule (*small asterisk*) shows intense enhancement. **C:** Axial T2-weighted (TR/TE; 2500/80) spin-echo MR image shows the mass to be heterogeneous. **D:** The mass (*arrows*) is well-seen with ultrasound. Nonhemorrhagic tumor nodule is well-seen posteriorly (*asterisk*). **E:** Coronal T1-weighted (TR/TE; 532/16) spin-echo image shows the intermuscular location of the lesion to better advantage (*arrows*).

drosarcomas arise in soft tissue (37,132). Extraskeletal mesenchymal chondrosarcoma has a bimodal age distribution. Those occurring in the head and neck occur primarily in the third decade of life; those in the deep muscles, such as the thigh and trunk, occur most frequently in the fifth decade of life. Males and females are affected about equally (133,134).

Lesions arising in the head and neck have a propensity for the meningeal and periorbital regions. Orbital lesions may also be associated with exophthalmos, orbital pain, and visual symptoms (79). Tumors originating in the soft tissues of the extremities usually are nonspecific with a slowly enlarging painless soft tissue mass (79). The lesion has an aggressive clinical course and metastases are frequent, usually to the lungs and lymph nodes. Histologic features, such as the degree of chondroid differentiation, have little bearing on prognosis. The prognosis is generally

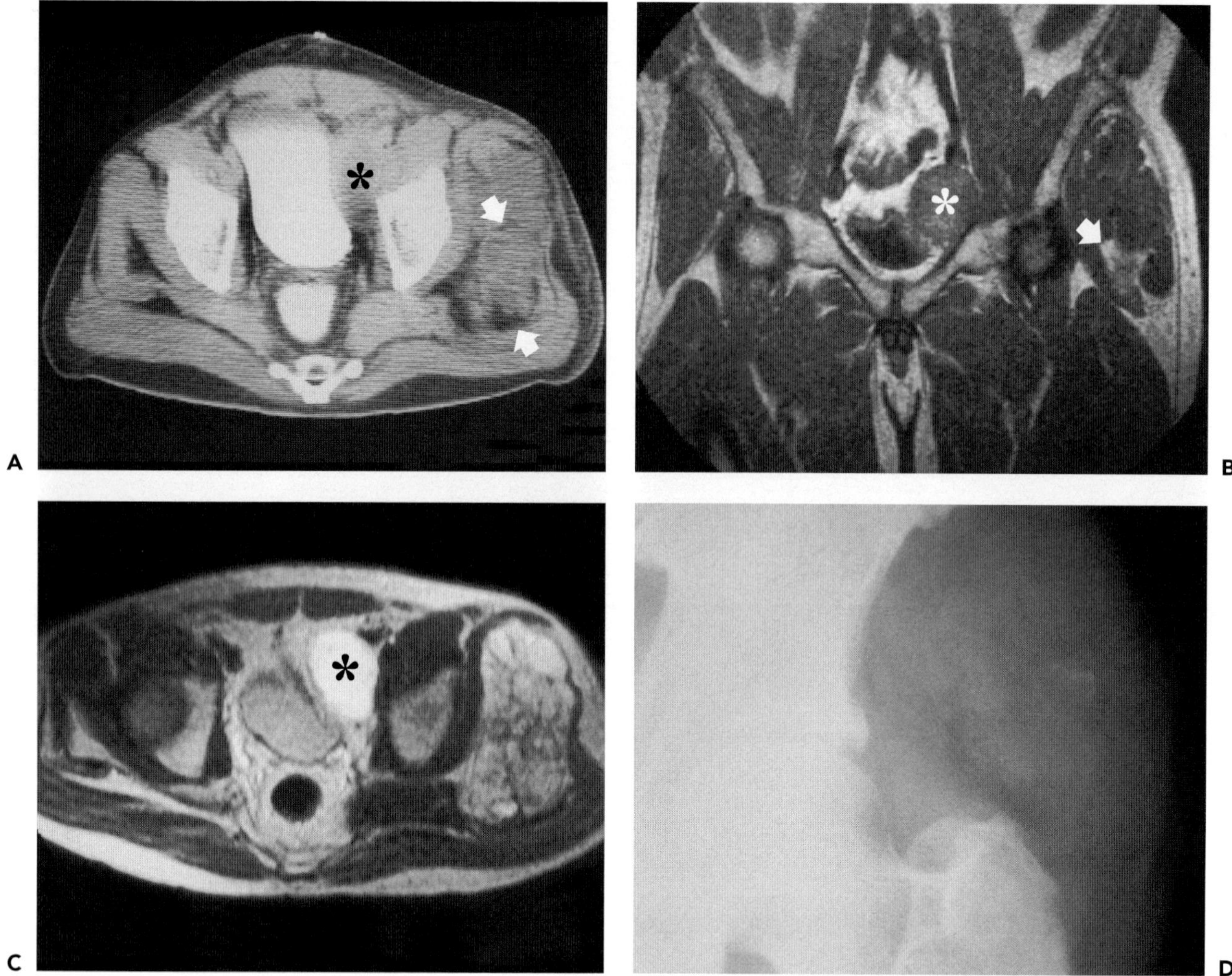

Figure 11.30 Extraskeletal myxoid chondrosarcoma: MR imaging features mimicking a liposarcoma in a man 56 years of age. **A:** Axial CT displayed at soft tissue window shows a large fat-containing mass in the left buttocks (*arrows*). The fat was engulfed by the slow-growing tumor. Note iliac nodal metastasis (*asterisk*). **B:** Coronal T1-weighted (TR/TE; 600/20) spin-echo MR image shows the mass to be relatively well-defined with fat within the tumor (*arrow*). Nodal metastasis is well seen (*asterisk*). **C:** Axial T2-weighted (TR/TE; 1500/80) spin-echo MR image shows the lesion to be well-defined with a nonspecific appearance. **D:** Anteroposterior radiograph shows small calcification within the tumor.

poor, with a 10-year survival rate approaching 25% (37,132,133).

Microscopically, mesenchymal chondrosarcoma consists of a proliferation of small primitive mesenchymal cells in which there are scattered islands of cartilage (134). A hemangiopericytomalike vascular pattern is frequently present.

Imaging of Extraskeletal Mesenchymal Chondrosarcoma

Radiographs of these lesions often demonstrate a nonspecific soft tissue mass. Areas of chondroid matrix mineralization may be apparent, and this is much more frequent in mesenchymal chondrosarcoma than in extraskeletal myxoid chondrosarcoma. In the series by Shapeero et al.,

---

KEY CONCEPTS

- Radiographs may show areas of chondroid matrix.
- Underlying bone erosion or invasion and periosteal reaction are unusual but may be seen.
- Lesions show an attenuation similar to that of skeletal muscle on CT scan.
- Intermediate signal intensity on T2-weighted MR images is observed.
- Areas of necrosis may be present.
- Intravenous contrast administration reveals prominent enhancement.

57% of seven lesions showed chondroid mineralization on radiographs or CT scanning (132). In our experience,

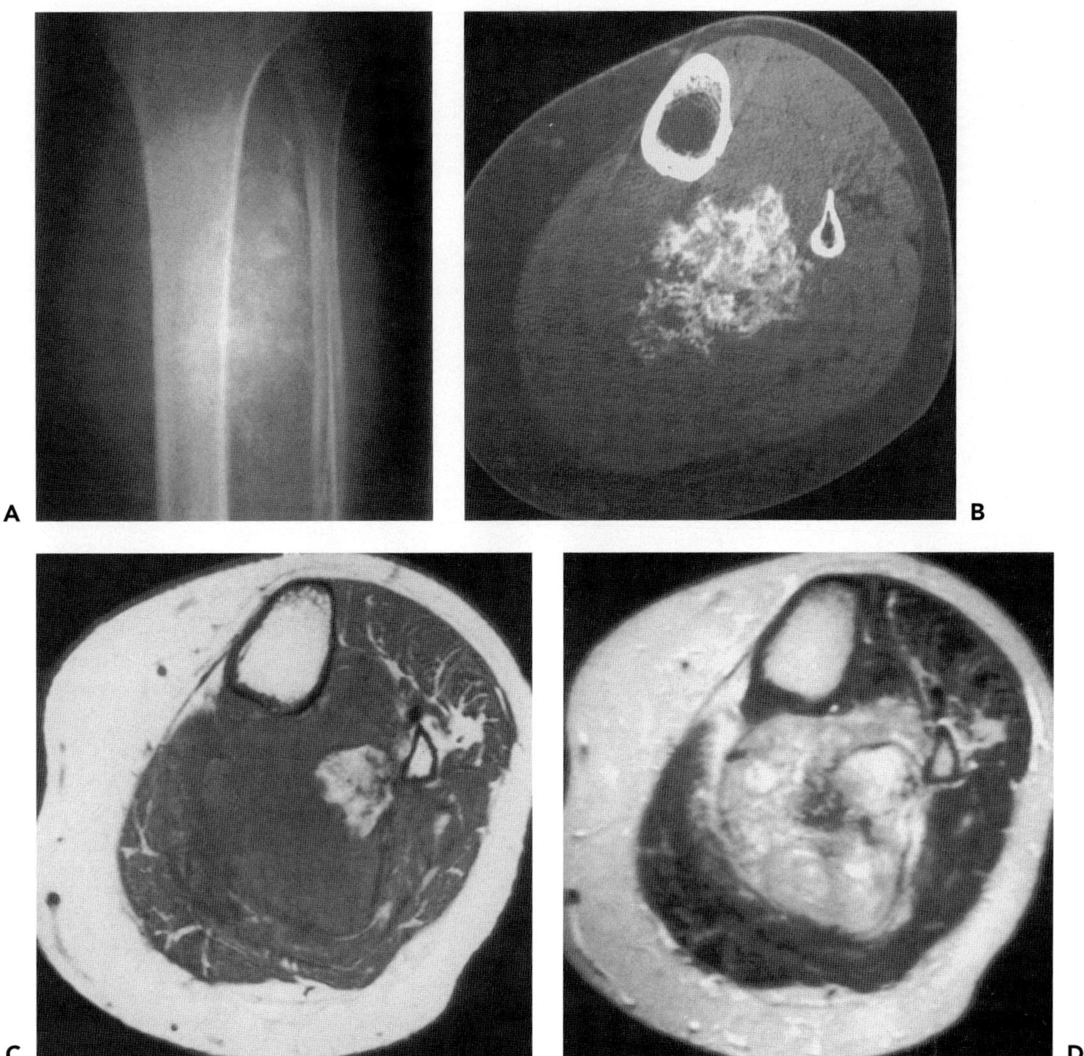

Figure 11.31 Extraskeletal mesenchymal chondrosarcoma: Typical imaging features in a woman 73 years of age. **A:** Anteroposterior radiograph demonstrates a large mineralized mass. **B:** Axial CT displayed at bone window shows the extensive mineralization within the mass. **C,D:** Axial T1-weighted (TR/TE; 700/15) **(C)** and turbo T2-weighted (TR/TE; 7000/91) **(D)** spin-echo MR images show a relatively well-defined, inhomogeneous mass, with evidence of subacute hemorrhage.

matrix mineralization is more frequent than is described in the literature (Fig. 11.31). Underlying bone erosion or invasion and periosteal reaction are unusual but may be seen (133).

Extraskeletal mesenchymal chondrosarcoma typically has lower water content than extraskeletal myxoid chondrosarcoma, caused by the intermixture of small cells and more limited cartilaginous tissue. It has similar attenuation to that of muscle on CT and typically has intermediate signal intensity on T2-weighted MR images (Fig. 11.31). Areas of necrosis may be seen and show high signal intensity on T2-weighted MR images (131). Intravenous contrast administration reveals prominent, diffuse but heterogeneous enhancement, and in our experience serpentine high-flow vessels may be seen related to the hemangiopericytoma areas which are seen histologically with extraskeletal mesenchymal chondrosarcoma.

Extraskeletal Well-Differentiated Chondrosarcoma

KEY CONCEPTS
- Extraskeletal well-differentiated chondrosarcoma is extremely rare; only a small number of cases are reported.
- Lesion is composed of lobules of well-differentiated hyaline cartilage.

The extraskeletal well-differentiated chondrosarcoma is extremely rare, and our experience is limited to only a small number of cases (135). The tumor is composed of lobules of well-differentiated hyaline cartilage. Weiss and Goldblum (79) note that the rarity of the lesion is such that lesions are more likely to represent extension or metastasis from an intraosseous lesion than a primary soft tissue tumor.

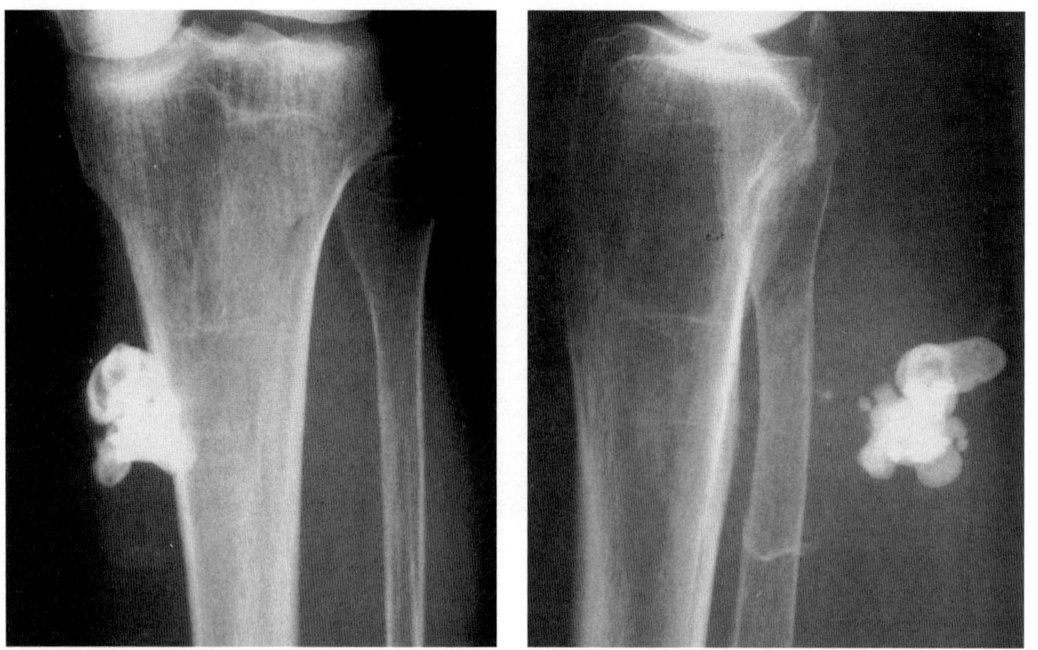

Figure 11.32 Extraskeletal well-differentiated chondrosarcoma: Radiographic features in a woman 74 years of age. **A,B:** Anteroposterior **(A)** and lateral **(B)** radiographs show a densely mineralized mass in the medial posterior soft tissues. The mass is well-defined with an osseous character.

Imaging of Extraskeletal Well-Differentiated Chondrosarcoma

Radiographs are available in two cases, showing a densely mineralized, well-defined soft tissue mass (Figs. 11.32 and 11.33). CT scan in one case showed the dense mineralization to be relatively homogeneous (Fig. 11.33). On long TR/TE spin-echo MR sequences, Cohen et al. (90) noted

> ### KEY CONCEPTS
> - Radiographs show a densely mineralized, well-defined soft tissue mass.
> - Imaging experience is limited and spectrum is not fully defined.
> - CT scan shows dense mineralization.

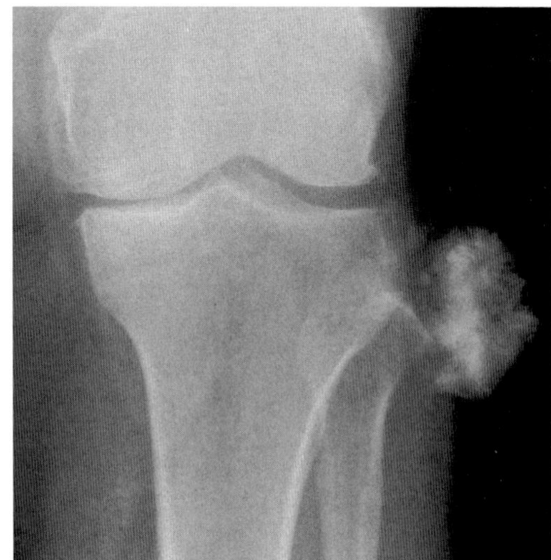
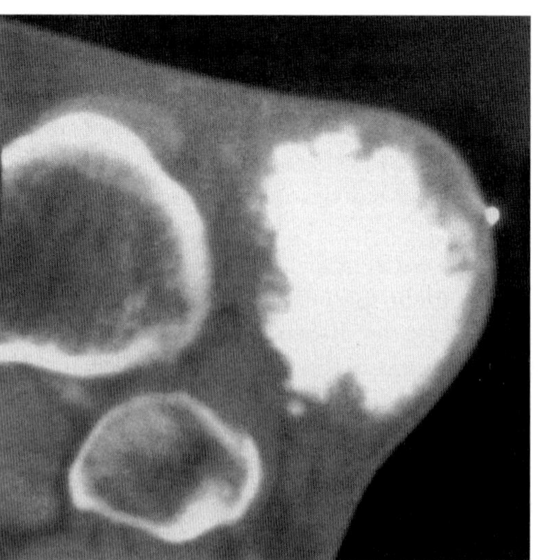

Figure 11.33 Extraskeletal well-differentiated chondrosarcoma: Radiographic and CT features in a woman 69 years of age. **A:** Anteroposterior radiograph shows a densely mineralized mass in the soft tissues adjacent to the proximal tibia. **B:** Axial CT displayed at bone window shows the dense mineralization to extend throughout the mass.

that the hyaline cartilage in a soft tissue chondrosarcoma images similar to that of its intraosseous counterpart, with varying-sized lobules of homogeneous high signal intensity. Lobules were defined by thin septa on both T1- and T2-weighted pulse sequences, with the septa composed of fibrous tissue with a cellular component. We suspect MR imaging features will also reflect the degree of tumor mineralization.

DIFFERENTIAL DIAGNOSIS

The differential diagnosis of extraskeletal osseous and cartilaginous tumors includes bone, cartilage, or calcification within other lesions. Clearly, the radiologic differentiation of an osseous matrix (characterized radiographically as "cloudlike" or "cumulus"), from a cartilaginous matrix (noted to have "arcs and rings" and "spicules and floccules") and dystrophic calcification is often best made through the retrospectoscope after a histologic diagnosis is established. The most common soft tissue sarcoma to demonstrate radiologic mineralization and the one often radiologically confused with an extraskeletal osseous or cartilaginous tumor is synovial sarcoma. As many as a third of synovial sarcomas demonstrate some internal calcification (less commonly ossification), often at the periphery of the tumor (29,57). Ossification may also be seen in soft tissue implants from giant cell tumor of bone. These implants may occur at the time of surgery or pathologic fracture (136).

Chondroid or osseous metaplasia is occasionally encountered within a lipoma, particularly if it is long standing. The term *benign mesenchymoma* is occasionally employed to describe this type of lesion (137). Similarly, chondroid and osseous metaplasia may also be seen in liposarcomas. The term *malignant mesenchymoma* is reserved to describe a small group of neoplasms that are characterized by the presence of two or more unrelated sarcomatous components. Either chondrosarcoma or osteosarcoma may make up the matrix-producing component in malignant mesenchymoma.

When mineralized juxta-articular lesions are encountered, synovial osteochondromatosis should be considered. The tophi in gout may also occasionally calcify or rarely ossify (138). Although melorrheostosis is rare, ossified soft tissue masses are a relatively common finding in melorrheostosis, noted in 8 (27%) of 30 patients reported by Murray and McCredie (139). The soft tissue masses are almost always para-articular, adjacent to areas of bone involvement, typically in regions medial to the hip and posterior to the knee (140). Mineralized juxta-articular masses may also be seen in tumoral calcinosis. These are most common in the region of the large joints, especially the hips, shoulders, and elbows (141).

Pilomatrixoma (calcifying epithelioma of Malherbe) demonstrates central mineralization in more than 80% of cases, with ossification occurring in approximately 20% of these. The lesion arises in the dermis, grows slowly, and is confined to the subcutaneous tissue, usually occurring in the face, neck, and upper extremities (65,141,142).

REFERENCES

1. Fletcher DM, Unni KK, Mertens F. Chondro-osseous tumors. In: Fletcher DM, Unni KK, Mertens F, eds. *WHO Classification of Tumors. Pathology and Genetics: Tumors of Soft Tissue and Bone.* Lyon, France: IARC Press; 2002:179.
2. Kransdorf MJ. Benign soft-tissue tumors in a large referral population: distribution of diagnoses by age, sex and location. *AJR Am J Roentgenol.* 1995;164:395–402.
3. Rosenberg AE. Myositis ossificans and fibroosseous pseudotumor of the digits. In: Fletcher DM, Unni KK, Mertens F, eds. *WHO Classification of Tumors. Pathology and Genetics: Tumors of Soft Tissue and Bone.* Lyon, France: IARC Press; 2002:52–54.
4. Weiss SW, Goldblum JR. Osseous soft tissue tumors. In: *Enzinger and Weiss's Soft Tissue Tumors.* 4th ed. St. Louis: Mosby; 2001:1389–1417.
5. Ackerman LV. Extra-osseous localized non-neoplastic bone and cartilage formation (so-called myositis ossificans). *J Bone Joint Surg Am.* 1958;40-A:279–298.
6. Hanna SL, Magill HL, Brooks MT, et al. Case of the day. Pediatric. Myositis ossificans circumscripta. *Radiographics.* 1990;10:945–949.
7. Heinrich SD, Zembo MM, MacEwen GD. Pseudomalignant myositis ossificans. *Orthopedics.* 1989;12:599–602.
8. Ogilvie-Harris DJ, Fornasier VL. Pseudomalignant myositis ossificans: heterotopic new-bone formation without a history of trauma. *J Bone Joint Surg Am.* 1980;62-A:1274–1283.
9. Parikh J, Hyare H, Saifuddin A. The imaging features of posttraumatic myositis ossificans, with emphasis on MRI. *Clin Radiol.* 2002;57(12):1058–1066.
10. Dudkiewicz I, Salai M, Chechik A. A young athlete with myositis ossificans of the neck presenting as a soft-tissue tumour. *Arch Orthop Trauma Surg.* 2001;121:234–237.
11. Sirvanci M, Ganiyusufoglu AK, Karaman K, et al. Myositis ossificans of psoas muscle: magnetic resonance imaging findings. *Acta Radiol.* 2004;45:523–525.
12. Beiner JM, Jokl P. Muscle contusion injury and myositis ossificans traumatica. *Clin Orthop.* 2002;403S:S110–119.
13. de Silva MV, Reid R. Myositis ossificans and fibroosseous pseudotumor of digits: a clinicopathological review of 64 cases with emphasis on diagnostic pitfalls. *Int J Surg Pathol.* 2003;11:187–195.
14. Heifetz SA, Galliani CA, DeRosa GP. Myositis (fasciitis) ossificans in an infant. *Pediatr Pathol.* 1992;12:223–239.
15. Nuovo MA, Norman A, Chumas J, et al. Myositis ossificans with atypical clinical, radiographic, or pathologic findings: a review of 23 cases. *Skeletal Radiol.* 1992;21:87–101.
16. Ben Hamida KS, Hajri R, Kedadi H, et al. Myositis ossificans circumscripta of the knee improved by alendronate. *Joint Bone Spine.* 2004;71:144–146.
17. Schumacher R. Myositis ossificans traumatica in young children [Letter]. *Pediatr Radiol.* 2001;31:606.
18. Hudson TM. *Radiologic-Pathologic Correlation of Musculoskeletal Lesions.* Baltimore: Williams & Wilkins; 1987:589–604.
19. Norman A, Dorfman HP. Juxtacortical circumscribed myositis ossificans: evolution and radiographic features. *Radiology.* 1979;96:301–306.
20. Goldman AB. Myositis ossificans circumscripta: a benign lesion with a malignant differential diagnosis. *AJR Am J Roentgenol.* 1976;126:32–40.
21. Drane WE. Myositis ossificans and the three-phase bone scan. *AJR Am J Roentgenol.* 1984;142:179–180.
22. Tibone J, Sakimura, Nickel VL, et al. Heterotopic ossification around the hip in spinal cord-injured patients. *J Bone Joint Surg AM.* 1978;60A:769–775.
23. Amendola MA, Glazer GM, Agha FP, et al. Myositis ossificans circumscripta: computed tomographic diagnosis. *Radiology.* 1983;149:775–779.

24. Heiken JP, Lee JKT, Smathers RL, et al. CT of benign soft-tissue masses of the extremities. *AJR Am J Roentgenol.* 1984;142:575–580.

25. Zeanah WR, Hudson TM. Myositis ossificans: radiologic evaluation of two cases with diagnostic computed tomograms. *Clin Orthop.* 1982;168:187–192.

26. Meyer CA, Kransdorf MJ, Jelinek JS, et al. Radiologic appearance of nodular fasciitis with emphasis on MR and CT. *J Comput Assist Tomogr.* 1991;15:276–279.

27. Kransdorf MJ, Meis JM, Jelinek JS. Myositis ossificans: MR appearance with radiologic-pathologic correlation. *AJR Am J Roentgenol.* 1992;157:1243–1248.

28. Yaghmai I. Myositis ossificans: diagnostic value of arteriography. *AJR Am J Roentgenol.* 1977;128:811–816.

29. De Smet AA, Norris MA, Fisher DR. Magnetic resonance imaging of myositis ossificans: analysis of seven cases. *Skeletal Radiol.* 1992;21:503–507.

30. Tsai JC, Dalinka MK, Fallon MD, et al. Fluid-fluid level: a nonspecific finding in tumors of bone and soft tissue. *Radiology.* 1990;175:779–782.

31. Gindele A, Schwamborn D, Tsironis K, et al. Myositis ossificans traumatica in young children: report of three cases and review of the literature. *Pediatr Radiol.* 2000;30:451–459.

32. Pettersson H, Eliasson J, Egund N, et al. Gadolinium-DTPA enhancement of soft tissue tumors in magnetic resonance imaging—preliminary clinical experience in five patients. *Skeletal Radiol.* 1988;17:319–323.

33. Erlemann R, Reiser MF, Peters PE, et al. Musculoskeletal neoplasms: static and dynamic Gd-DTPA-enhanced MR imaging. *Radiology.* 1989;171:767–773.

34. Nielsen GP, Fletcher CD, Smith MA, et al. Soft tissue aneurysmal bone cyst: a clinicopathologic study of five cases. *Am J Surg Pathol.* 2002;26:64–69.

35. Wang XL, Gielen JL, Salgado R, et al. Soft tissue aneurysmal bone cyst. *Skeletal Radiol.* 2004;33:477–480.

36. Lopez-Barea F, Rodriguez-Peralto JL, Burgos-Lizaldez E, et al. Primary aneurysmal cyst of soft tissue. Report of a case with ultrastructural and MRI studies. *Virchows Arch.* 1996;428:125–129.

37. Fanburg-Smith JC. Cartilage- and bone forming tumors and tumor-like lesions. In: Miettinen M, ed. *Diagnostic Soft Tissue Pathology.* New York: Churchill Livingstone; 2003:403–425.

38. Dupree WB, Enzinger FM. Fibro-osseous pseudotumor of the digits. *Cancer.* 1986;58:2103–2109.

39. Spjut HJ, Dorfman HD. Florid reactive periostitis of the tubular bone the hands and feet. A benign lesion which may simulate osteosarcoma. *Am J Surg Pathol.* 1981;5:423–433.

40. Sundaram M, Wang L, Rotman M, et al. Florid reactive periostitis and bizarre parosteal osteochondromatous proliferation: prebiopsy imaging evolution, treatment and outcome. *Skeletal Radiol.* 2001;30:192–198.

41. Schütte HE, van der Heul RO. Pseudomalignant, nonneoplastic osseous soft tissue tumors of the hand and foot. *Radiology.* 1990;176:149–153.

42. Ehara S, Nishida J, Masataka A, et al. Magnetic resonance imaging of pseudomalignant osseous tumor of the hand. *Skeletal Radiol.* 1994;23:513–516.

43. Nora FE, Dahlin DC, Beabout JW. Bizarre parosteal osteochondromatous proliferations of the hands and feet. *Am J Surg Pathol.* 1983;7:245–250.

44. Ly JQ, Bui-Mansfield LT, Taylor DC. Radiologic demonstration of temporal development of bizarre parosteal osteochondromatous proliferation. *Clin Imaging.* 2004;28:216–218.

45. Helliwell TR, O'Connor MA, Ritchie DA, et al. Bizarre parosteal osteochondromatous proliferation with cortical invasion. *Skeletal Radiol.* 2001;30:282–285.

46. Meneses MF, Unni KK, Swee RG. Bizarre parosteal osteochondromatous proliferation of bone (Nora's lesion). *Am J Surg Pathol.* 1993;17:691–697.

47. Smith NC, Ellis AM, McCarthy S, et al. Bizarre parosteal osteochondromatous proliferation: a review of seven cases. *Aust N Z J Surg.* 1996;66:694–697.

48. Bandiera S, Bacchini P, Bertoni F. Bizarre parosteal osteochondromatous proliferation of bone. *Skeletal Radiol.* 1998;27:154–156.

49. Abramovici L, Steiner GC. Bizarre parosteal osteochondromatous proliferation (Nora's lesion): a retrospective study of 12 cases, 2 arising in long bones. *Hum Pathol.* 2002;33: 1205–1210.

50. Yuen M, Friedman L, Orr W, et al. Proliferative periosteal processes of phalanges: a unitary hypothesis. *Skeletal Radiol.* 1992;21:301–303.

51. Thickman D, Bonakdar-pour A, Clancy M, et al. Fibrodysplasia ossificans progessiva. *AJR Am J Roentgenol.* 1982;139:935–941.

52. Job-Deslandre C. Inherited ossifying diseases. *Joint Bone Spine.* 2004;71:98–101.

53. Rogers JG, Geho WB. Fibrodysplasia ossificans progressiva. *J Bone Joint Surg Am.* 1979;61A:909–914.

54. Bridges AJ, Hsu KC, Singh A, et al. Fibrodysplasia (myositis) ossificans progessiva. *Semin Arthritis Rheum.* 1994;24:15–164.

55. Hagiwara H, Aida N, Machida J, et al. Contrast-enhanced MRI of an early preosseous lesion of fibrodysplasia ossificans progressive in a 21-month-old boy. *AJR Am J Roentgenol.* 2003;181: 1145–1147.

56. Mahboubi S, Glaser DL, Shore EM, et al. Fibrodysplasia ossificans progressiva. *Pediatr Radiol.* 2001;31:307–314.

57. Cadman NL, Soule EH, Kelly PJ. Synovial sarcoma: an analysis of 134 tumors. *Cancer.* 1965;18:613–627.

58. Connor JM, Evans DA. Fibrodysplasia ossificans progressiva: the clinical features and natural history of 34 patients. *J Bone Joint Surg Br.* 1982;64:76–83.

59. Baysal T, Elmali N, Kutlu R, et al. The stone man: myositis (fibrodysplasia) ossificans progressiva. *Eur Radiol.* 1998;8:479–481.

60. Herford AS, Boyne PJ. Ankylosis of the jaw in a patient with fibrodysplasia ossificans progressiva. *Oral Surg Oral Med Oral Path Radiol Endod.* 2003;96:680–684.

61. Scarlett RF, Rocke DM, Kantanie A, et al. Influenza-like viral illnesses and flare-ups of fibrodysplasia ossificans progressiva. *Clin Orthop.* 2004;423:275–279.

62. Caron KH, DiPietro MA, Aisen AM, et al. Case report. MR imaging of early fibrodysplasia ossificans progressiva. *J Comput Assist Tomogr.* 1990;14:318–321.

63. Jones G, Rocke DM. Multivariate survival analysis with double-censored data: application to the assessment of Accutane treatment for fibrodysplasia ossificans progressiva. *Stat Med.* 2002;21:2547–2562.

64. Palhares DB. Myositis ossificans progressive. *Calcif Tissue Int.* 1997;60:394.

65. Oz BB, Boneh A. Myositis ossificans progressiva: a 10-year follow-up on a patient treated with etidronate disodium. *Acta Paediatr.* 1994;83:1332–1334.

66. Forbis R, Helwig EB. Pilomatrixoma (calcifying epithelioma). *Arch Dermatol.* 1961;83:606.

67. Altschuler EL. Consideration of Rituximab for fibrodysplasia ossificans progressiva. *Med Hypotheses.* 2004;63:407–408.

68. Kan L, Hu M, Gomes WA, et al. Transgenic mice overexpressing BMP4 develop a fibrodysplasia ossificans progessiva (FOP)-like phenotype. *Am J Pathol.* 2004;165:1107–1115.

69. Fang MA, Reinig JW, Hill SC, et al. Technetium-99m MDP demonstration of heterotopic ossification in fibrodysplasia ossificans progressiva. *Clin Nucl Med.* 1986;11:8–9.

70. Guze BH, Schelbert H. The nuclear medicine bone image and myositis ossificans progressiva. *Clin Nucl Med.* 1989;14:161–162.

71. Schweitzer ME, Greenway G, Resnick D, et al. Osteoma of soft parts. *Skeletal Radiol.* 1992;21:177–180.

72. Kasper HU, Adermahr J, Dienes HP. Soft tissue osteoma: tumor entity or reactive lesion? Paraarticular soft tissue osteoma of the hip. *Histopathology.* 2004;44:91–93.

73. Holmen J, Stevens MA, El-Khoury GY. Case report: paraarticular soft-tissue osteoma of the hip. *Iowa Orthop J.* 1992;19:139–141.

74. Reiman HM, Dahlin DC. Cartilage- and bone-forming tumors of soft tissue. *Semin Diagn Pathol.* 1986;3:288–305.

75. Lekas MD, Sayegh R, Finkelstein SD. Osteoma of the base of the tongue. *Ear Nose Throat J.* 1997;76:827–828.

76. Ruggieri M, Pavone V, Smilari P, et al. Primary osteoma cutis-multiple cafe-au-lait spots and woolly hair anomaly. *Pediatr Radiol.* 1995;25:34–36.

77. Chung EB, Enzinger FM. Extraskeletal osteosarcoma. *Cancer.* 1987;60:1132–1142.

78. Nayler S, Heim S. Soft tissue chondroma. In: Fletcher DM, Unni KK, Mertens F, eds. *WHO Classification of Tumors. Pathology and Genetics: Tumors of Soft Tissue and Bone.* Lyon, France: IARC Press; 2002:180–181.

79. Weiss SW, Goldblum JR. Cartilaginous soft tissue tumors. In: *Enzinger and Weiss's Soft Tissue Tumors.* 4th ed. St. Louis: Mosby; 2001:1361–1388.

80. Chung EB, Enzinger FM. Chondroma of soft parts. *Cancer.* 1978;41:1414–1424.

81. Zlatkin MB, Lander PH, Begin LR, et al. Soft-tissue chondroma. *AJR Am J Roentgenol.* 1985;144:1263–1267.

82. Dahlin DC, Salvador AH. Cartilaginous tumors of the soft tissues of the hands and feet. *Mayo Clin Proc.* 1974;49:721–726.

83. Stout AP, Verner EW. Chondrosarcoma of the extraskeletal soft tissues. *Cancer.* 1953;6:581–590.

84. Goldenberg RR, Cohen P, Steinlauf P. Chondrosarcoma of the extraskeletal soft tissues: a report of seven cases and review of the literature. *J Bone Joint Surg Am.* 1967;49A:1487–1507.

85. Bansal M, Goldman AB, DiCarlo EF, et al. Soft tissue chondromas: diagnosis and differential diagnosis. *Skeletal Radiol.* 1993; 22:309–315.

86. Horcajadas AB, Lafuente JL, de la Cruz Burgos R, et al. Ultrasound and MR findings in tumor and tumor-like lesions of the fingers. *Eur Radiol.* 2003;13:672–685.

87. Chandramohan M, Thomas NB, Funk L, et al. MR appearance of mineralized extra skeletal chondroma: a case report and review of literature. *Clin Radiol.* 2002;57:421–423.

88. Folsom GJ, Lee DH, Lopez-Ben R, et al. Hand mass in a 15-year-old boy. *Clin Orthop.* 2003;412:269–275.

89. Varma DG, Kumar R, Carrasco H, et al. MR imaging of periosteal chondroma. *J Comput Assist Tomogr.* 1991;15:1008–1010.

90. Cohen EK, Kressel HY, Frank TS, et al. Hyaline cartilage-origin bone and soft-tissue neoplasms: MR appearance and histologic correlation. *Radiology.* 1988;167:477–481.

91. Enzinger FM, Weiss SW, Liang CY. Ossifying fibromyxoid tumor of soft parts. A clinicopathological analysis of 59 cases. *Am J Surg Pathol.* 1989;13:817–827.

92. Folpe AL, Weiss SW. Ossifying fibromyxoid tumor of soft parts: a clinicopathologic study of 70 cases with emphasis on atypical and malignant variants. *Am J Surg Pathol.* 2003;27:421–431.

94. Zamecnik M, Michal M. Low-grade fibromyxoid sarcoma: a report of eight cases with histologic, immunohistochemical, and ultrastructural study. *Ann Diagn Pathol.* 2000;4:207–217.

95. Al-Mazrou KA, Mansoor A, Payne M, et al. Ossifying fibromyxoid tumor of the ethmoid sinus in a newborn: report of a case and literature review. *Int J Pediatr Otorhinolaryngol.* 2004;68:225–230.

96. Ijiri R, Tanaka Y, Misugi K, et al. Ossifying fibromyxoid tumor of soft parts in a child: a case report. *J Pediatr Surg.* 1999;34: 1294–1296.

97. Rubin BP, Stenman G. Ossifying fibromyxoid tumor. In: Fletcher DM, Unni KK, Mertens F, eds. *WHO Classification of Tumors. Pathology and Genetics: Tumors of Soft Tissue and Bone.* Lyon, France: IARC Press; 2002:196–197.

98. Donner LR. Ossifying fibromyxoid tumor of soft parts: evidence supporting Schwann cell origin. *Hum Pathol.* 1992;23: 200–202.

99. Miettinen M. Ossifying fibromyxoid tumor of soft parts. Additional observations of a distinctive soft tissue tumor. *Am J Clin Pathol.* 1991;95:142–149.

100. Raith J, Ranner G, Schaffler G, et al. Bone scan in ossifying fibromyxoid tumor of soft parts. *Clin Nucl Med.* 1998;23: 262–264.

101. Yoshida H, Minamizaki T, Yumoto T, et al. Ossifying fibromyxoid tumor of soft parts. *Acta Pathol Jpn.* 1991;41:480–486.

102. Schaffler G, Raith J, Ranner G, et al. Radiographic appearance of an ossifying fibromyxoid tumor of soft parts. *Skeletal Radiol.* 1997;26:615–618.

103. Ogose A, Otsuka H, Morita T, et al. Ossifying fibromyxoid tumor resembling parosteal osteosarcoma. *Skeletal Radiol.* 1998;27: 578–580.

104. Rosenberg AE, Heim S. Extraskeletal osteosarcoma. In: Fletcher DM, Unni KK, Mertens F, eds. *WHO Classification of Tumors. Pathology and Genetics: Tumors of Soft Tissue and Bone.* Lyon, France: IARC Press; 2002:182–183.

105. Allan CJ, Soule EH. Osteogenic sarcoma of the somatic tissues. Clinicopathologic study of 26 cases and review of literature. *Cancer.* 1971;27:1121–1133.

106. Bane BL, Evans HL, Ro JY, et al. Extraskeletal osteosarcoma. *Cancer.* 1990;65:2762–2770.

107. Sordillo PP, Hajdu SI, Magill GB, et al. Extraosseous osteogenic sarcoma. *Cancer.* 1983;51:727–734.

108. Kransdorf MJ. Malignant soft-tissue tumors in a large referral population: distribution of diagnoses by age, sex and location. *AJR Am J Roentgenol.* 1995;164:129–134.

109. Laskin WB, Silverman TA, Enzinger FM. Postradiation soft tissue sarcomas. An analysis of 52 cases. *Cancer.* 1988;62:2330–2340.

110. Lee JH, Griffiths WJ, Bottomley RH. Extraosseous osteogenic sarcoma following an intramuscular injection. *Cancer.* 1977;40: 3097–3101.

111. Konishi E, Kusuzaki K, Murata H, et al. Extraskeletal osteosarcoma arising in myositis ossificans. *Skeletal Radiol.* 2001;30: 39–43.

112. Ulusakarya A, Terrier P, Regnard JF, et al. Extraskeletal osteosarcoma of the mediastinum after treatment of a mediastinal germ-cell tumor. *Am J Clin Oncol.* 1999;22:609–614.

113. Okada K, Ito H, Miyakoshi N, et al. A low-grade extraskeletal osteosarcoma. *Skeletal Radiol.* 2003;32:165–169.

114. Eunhee SY, Shmookler BM, Malawer MM, et al. Well-differentiated extraskeletal osteosarcoma. A soft-tissue homologue of parosteal osteosarcoma. *Arch Pathol Lab Med.* 1991;115:906–909.

115. Cook PA, Murphy MS, Innis PC, et al. Extraskeletal osteosarcoma of the hand. *J Bone Joint Surg.* 1998;80A:725–729.

116. Covello SP, Humphreys TR, Lee JB. A case of extraskeletal osteosarcoma with metastasis to the skin. *J Am Acad Dermatol.* 2003;49:124–127.

117. Varma DGK, Ayala AG, Guo S, et al. MRI of extraskeletal osteosarcoma. *J Comput Assist Tomogr.* 1993;17:414–417.

118. Doud TM, Moser RP, Giudici MAI, et al. Case report 704. Extraskeletal osteosarcoma of the thigh with several suspected skeletal metastases and extensive metastases to the chest. *Skeletal Radiol.* 1991;20:628–632.

119. Arrington ER, Eisenberg B, Orrison WW, et al. Scintigraphic appearance of uncommon soft-tissue osteogenic sarcoma metastases. *J Nucl Med.* 1990;31:679–681.

120. Enzinger FM, Shiraki M. Extraskeletal myxoid chondrosarcoma. An analysis of 34 cases. *Human Pathol.* 1972;3:421–435.

121. Whitten CG, El-Khoury GY, Benda JA, et al. Case report 829 intramuscular myxoid chondrosarcoma. *Skeletal Radiol.* 1994; 23:153–156.

122. Meis JM, Martz KL. Extraskeletal myxoid chondrosarcoma: a clinicopathologic study of 120 cases. *Lab Invest.* 1992;66:9A.

123. Saleh G, Evans HL, Ro JY, et al. Extraskeletal myxoid chondrosarcoma. A clinicopathologic study of ten patients with long term follow-up. *Cancer.* 1992;70:2827–2830.

124. Meis-Kindblom JM, Bergh P, Gunterberg B, et al. Extraskeletal myxoid chondrosarcoma: a reappraisal of its morphologic spectrum and prognostic factors based on 117 cases. *Am J Surg Pathol.* 1999;23:636–650.

125. Goldenberg RR, Cohen P, Steinlauf P. Chondrosarcoma of the extraskeletal soft tissues. *J Bone Joint Surg Am.* 1967;49A: 1487–1507.

126. McGrory JE, Rock MG, Nascimento AG, et al. Extraskeletal myxoid chondrosarcoma. *Clin Orthop.* 2001;382:185–190.

127. Sandberg AA, Bridge JA. Updates on the cytogenetics and molecular genetics of bone and soft tissue tumors: chondrosarcoma and other cartilaginous neoplasms. *Cancer Genet Cytogenet.* 2003; 143:1–31.

128. Varma DGK, Ayala AG, Carrasco CH, et al. Chondrosarcoma: MR imaging with pathologic correlation. *Radiographics.* 1992;12: 687–704.

129. Gebhardt MC, Parekh SG, Rosenberg AE, et al. Extraskeletal myxoid chondrosarcoma of the knee. *Skeletal Radiol.* 1999;28: 354–358.

130. Peterson KK, Renfrew DL, Feddersen RM, et al. Magnetic resonance imaging of myxoid containing tumors. *Skeletal Radiol.* 1991;20:245–250.

131. Murphey MD, Walker EA, Wilson AJ, et al. From the archives of the AFIP: imaging of primary chondrosarcoma: radiologic-pathologic correlation. *Radiographics.* 2003;23:1245–1278.

132. Shapeero LG, Vanel D, Couanet D, et al. Extraskeletal mesenchymal chondrosarcoma. *Radiology.* 1993;186:819–826.
133. Nakashima Y, Unni KK, Shives TC, et al. Mesenchymal chondrosarcoma of bone and soft tissue. A review of 111 cases. *Cancer.* 1986;57:2444–2453.
134. Guccion JG, Font RL, Enzinger FM, et al. Extraskeletal mesenchymal chondrosarcoma. *Arch Pathol.* 1973;95:336–340.
135. Kransdorf MJ, Meis JM. Extraskeletal osseous and cartilaginous tumors of the extremities. *Radiographics.* 1993;13:853–884.
136. Bond JR, Cooper KL. Musculoskeletal case of the day. Soft-tissue implant of giant cell tumor. *AJR Am J Roentgenol.* 1993;160:1328–1330.
137. Kransdorf MJ, Moser RP, Meis JM, et al. Fat containing soft tissue masses of the extremities. *Radiographics.* 1991;11:81–106.
138. Resnick D. Gouty arthritis. In: Resnick D, ed. *Diagnosis of Bone and Joint Disorders.* 4th ed. Philadelphia: WB Saunders; 1988:1519–1559.
139. Murray RO, McCredie J. Melorheostosis and the sclerotomes: a radiological correlation. *Skeletal Radiol.* 1979;4:57–71.
140. McLeod RA, Beabout JW, Cooper KL, et al. Case of the day. Melorheostosis. *AJR Am J Roentgenol.* 1984;142:1062–1068.
141. Martinez S, Vogler JB, Harrelson JM, et al. Imaging of tumoral calcinosis: new observations. *Radiology.* 1990;174:215–222.
142. Haller JO, Kassner EG, Ostrowitz A, et al. Pilomatrixoma (calcifying epithelioma of Malherbe): radiographic features. *Radiology.* 1977;123:151–153.

Tumors of Uncertain Histogenesis

12

BENIGN LESIONS

Tumoral Calcinosis

Tumoral calcinosis is a relatively rare disorder character-ized by the accumulation of calcium salts in the juxta-articular soft tissues (1,2). It was initially reported in 1899 by Duret, who described the process in a girl 17 years of age and her younger brother (3). The term *tumoral calcinosis* was originated by Inclan et al. in 1942 (4). Other terms for this lesion have included *calcifying bursitis, calcifying collagenolysis,* and *hip stones.* Although the cause is unclear, it is suggested that the disease is inherited in an autosomal dominant fashion with variable expressivity (5). The basic biochemical defect is unknown but likely relates to abnormal phosphate metabolism and 1,25-dihydroxyvitamin D formation in the proximal tubule of the kidney (5). As such, tumoral calcinosis may be considered a metabolic disorder, and it appears to be more metabolically active in younger patients (5). In addition to having elevated serum 1,25-dihydroxyvitamin D levels, patients may demonstrate a mild hyperphosphatemia (6).

Patients are generally young and most present in the first or second decade of life. There is no sex predilection, although there is clearly an increased incidence in blacks (3,5–7). Tumoral calcinosis is familial in approximately 33% of cases, and approximately 50% of affected children have an involved sibling (5). Lesions are more typically multiple (70% of cases) with an average of three regions per patient in the study by Martinez et al. (5). Slavin et al. (6) reported the findings in a single family, noting 68 primary lesions in seven siblings.

The juxta-articular masses are most common in the region of the large joints, particularly the hips, elbows, shoulders, scapula, and buttocks (5,6). There is less frequent involvement of the hands, feet, and knees. The lesions tend to occur in the regions known to be occupied by bursa, although no pathologic proof confirms this is the case. Martinez et al. suggested that the calcific process destroys the synovial tissue of the bursa with growth of the masses (5). The masses grow slowly and may become quite large and are often cosmetically deforming, painless, firm, and lobulated. However, because lesions begin in the extra-articular tissues, limitation of joint motion is not a prominent clinical feature. Large lesions may ulcerate and drain a chalky, milklike, gritty fluid to the skin (5). Dental, eye, bone, vascular, and skin abnormalities (pseudoxanthoma elasticum) are also described (5). Tumoral calcinosis is a diagnosis of exclusion and requires ruling out other causes of para-articular calcification, including the metastatic calcifications of renal failure, hyperparathyroidism, hypervitaminosis D, and collagen vascular disease (8). We would consider these entities as causes of secondary tumoral calcinosis.

Grossly the lesions are firm, rubbery masses extending into the adjacent muscle and tendons and may be up to 20 cm in size (usually 5 to 15 cm) (3). The mass consists of multiple small pockets of calcium salts. The calcium salts are hydroxyapatite in nature, composed of a mixture of calcium carbonate and calcium phosphate (Fig. 12.1) (3). Some lesions are also surrounded by a pseudocapsule, whereas others extend with fingerlike projections into the adjacent tissue (6). In the active phase of tumoral calcinosis, microscopy reveals areas of amorphous masses of calcified debris, surrounded by fibrous septae as a rim, containing macrophages, multinucleated osteoclastlike giant cells, and chronic inflammatory cells (Fig. 12.1) (3). These cells represent a response (similar to that seen with foreign bodies) to the calcific material. In the inactive phase, the central amorphous mass is surrounded by dense fibrous material (3).

Dietary restriction of phosphate may be useful in some patients (7), with surgical excision reserved for symptomatic lesions (5). Surgical resection is advocated when lesions are small and can be completely excised. Local recurrence is reported with incomplete resection.

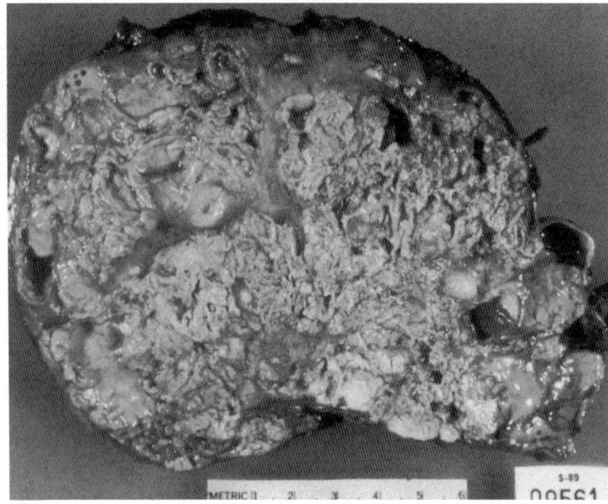

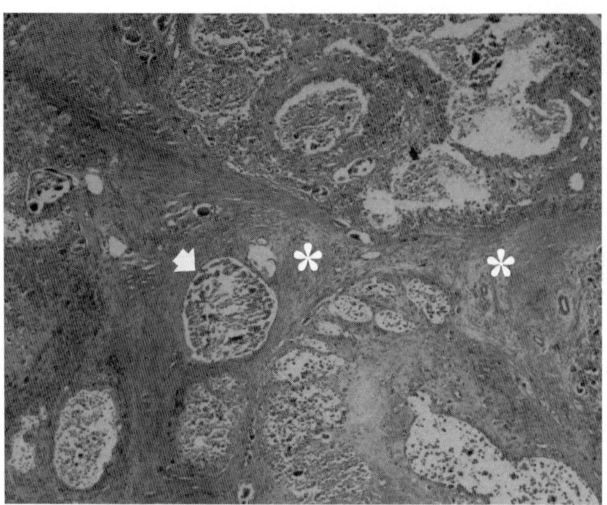

Figure 12.1 Tumoral calcinosis pathology. **A:** Gross specimen shows a multilocular mass composed of a conglomeration of pockets of calcium salts surrounded by dense collagenous tissue. **B:** Medium-power photomicrograph shows amorphous calcified material (*arrow*) separated by dense fibrous tissue (*asterisks*) with several multinucleated giant cells.

The calcified juxta-articular masses remain the radiologic hallmark of the disease. Radiographs show these as well-defined, with a lobular or multiloculated configuration, typically on the extensor surfaces of joints. Lesions are usually rounded opacities with multiple linear and curvilinear radiolucencies representing fibrous septa coursing within the lesions (Fig. 12.2) (3). These lucencies are described as having a "chicken-wire" or "cobblestone" pattern (9). Calcium fluid levels may be seen on upright films. Martinez et al. (5) believe that the identification of calcium fluid levels (sedimentation sign) indicates a metabolically active lesion with a potential to grow or diminish in response to phosphate depletion therapy. The soft tissue masses may erode the adjacent bone (8), although this is a rare manifestation. Recently described associated abnormalities include diaphyseal bone marrow lesions (diaphysitis/calcific myelitis) caused by deposition of calcium within the marrow. The diaphysitis may be associated with periosteal new bone formation (5). These osseous abnormalities are best seen on radiographs or CT scans (Fig. 12.3).

Bone scintigraphy demonstrates focally increased tracer accumulation and is the best way to detect and localize the often multifocal juxta-articular masses (5). Small lesions may not be identified on scintigraphy (5). CT imaging shows lesions to occupy the fibrofatty plane deep to the muscle (Fig. 12.4) (5). The juxta-articular masses range from uniformly calcified to predominantly cystic, with calcific walls and calcium fluid levels (similar to milk of calcium in the gallbladder) (Fig. 12.5) (5). Calcium fluid levels can also be seen in para-articular calcification related to renal failure and milk alkali syndrome. The calcified masses may demonstrate a chicken-wire pattern of low attenuation septae, similar to that seen on radiographs.

On MR imaging, tumoral calcinosis demonstrates a variable heterogeneous signal intensity (Figs. 12.2–12.4).

This varies from predominantly decreased signal intensity on all pulse sequences, caused by the calcification within the lesion, to heterogeneous increased signal intensity on T2-weighted images in those lesions with prominent fluid/inflammatory components (5,7,8). Martinez et al. (5) noted two T2-weighted MR imaging patterns: a nodular pattern with areas of alternating high and absent signal intensity and a diffuse, less intense high signal pattern (Figs. 12.2–12.4). Septal enhancement was reported by Geirnaerdt et al. (8) and was thought to correspond to vascularized tissue surrounding deposits of calcium salts (Fig. 12.2). MR imaging of diaphyseal marrow abnormalities, representing medullary calcification with periostitis, shows focal abnormal signal in the marrow, with a rind of increased signal intensity on T2-weighted images (Fig. 12.3). The involved marrow demonstrates nonspecific increased signal on T2-weighted images and decreased signal on T1-weighted images, with multiple small foci of decreased signal on all pulse sequences, representing calcific deposits (Fig. 12.3) (5).

Myxoma

Several lesions are characterized by an abundant myxoid matrix and a paucity of spindle-shaped stromal cells. These tumors, known as *myxomas*, were established as a distinctive lesion by Stout in 1948 (10), in a comprehensive report of 49 cases from the Laboratory of Surgical Pathology of Columbia University and 93 additional cases from the literature (exclusive of those within the heart). Although only 4 (3%) of the lesions in Stout's original report were intramuscular, the intramuscular myxoma is the best known of these to radiologists and the one most likely to mimic a myxoid musculoskeletal sarcoma (2,11–13). A subsequent report of

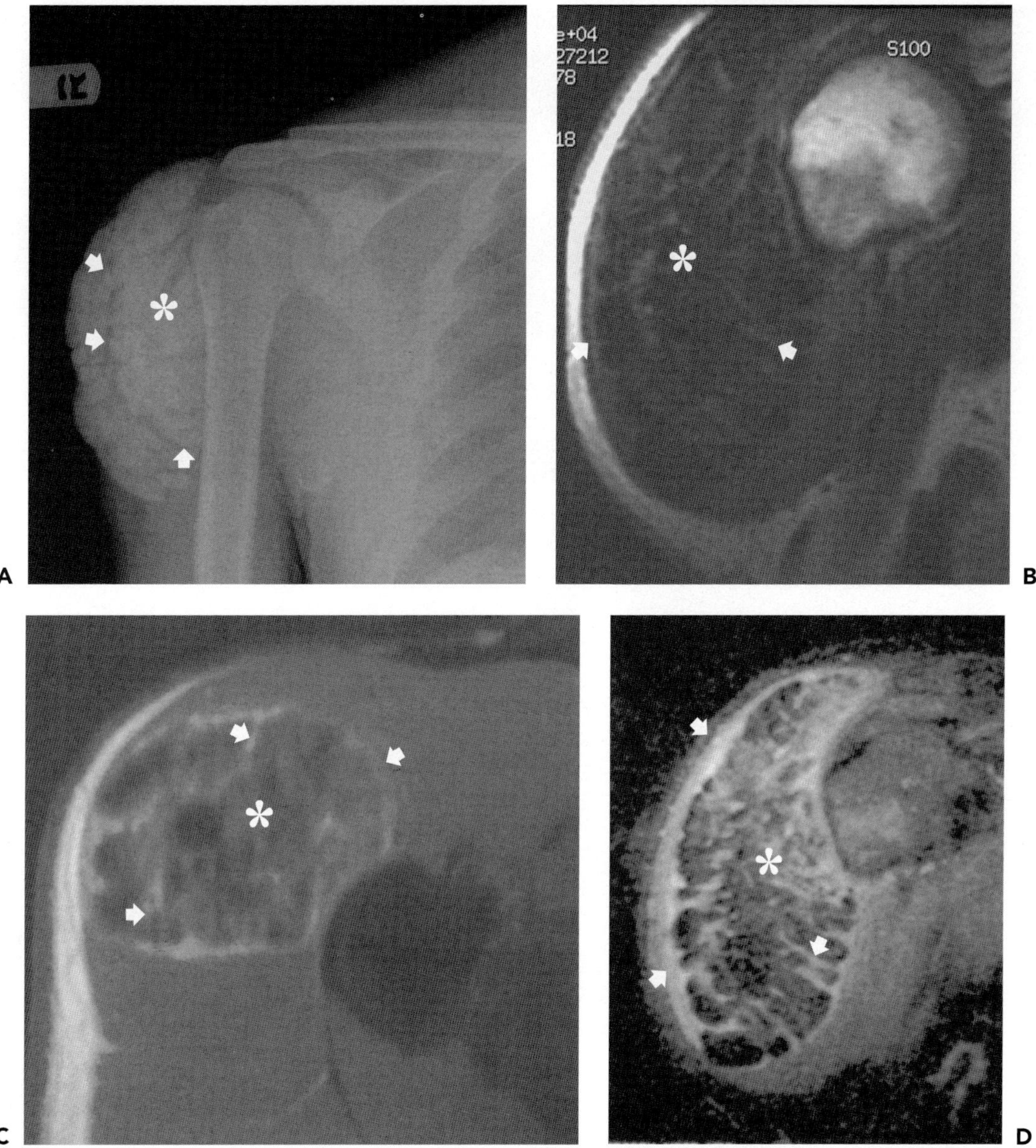

Figure 12.2 Tumoral calcinosis about the shoulder in a man 22 years of age with a nontender mass. **A:** Radiograph shows a densely calcified mass adjacent to the shoulder (*asterisk*) with radiolucent septations (*arrows*). **B–D:** Multiple MR images including coronal T1-weighted (TR/TE; 350/14) **(B)**, axial enhanced fat-suppressed T1-weighted (TR/TE; 500/13) **(C)**, and coronal fat-suppressed proton-weighted (TR/TE; 4800/28) **(D)**, image, reveal a large soft tissue mass (*asterisk*). The mass is predominantly low signal intensity on all pulse sequences with an intermediate intensity periphery and septae that reveal enhancement (*arrows*).

almost 200 myxomas of various sites from the Armed Forces Institute of Pathology (AFIP) identified 34 (17%) as intramuscular in origin (14). The reported annual incidence is 1 case per million people (2,11–13). Other locations of noncardiac myxoma, in decreasing order of frequency, include subcutaneous and aponeurotic tissue (22%), bone (18%), genitourinary tract (16%), and skin (15%) (9). We believe these figures do not reflect the distribution of lesions seen by radiologists. The study of 45 cases by Murphey et al. is probably more accurate, showing that

82% of musculoskeletal myxomas were intramuscular, 9% intermuscular, and 9% subcutaneous (15). Three of these cases were also juxta-articular (15).

The juxta-articular myxoma, also known as a periarticular myxoma, is a variant of myxoma that usually occurs around large joints, particularly the knee. The ganglion may also be classified as a myxoid lesion. Because the ganglion and juxta-articular myxoma are usually associated with joints, they are discussed in Chapter 10 on synovial tumors.

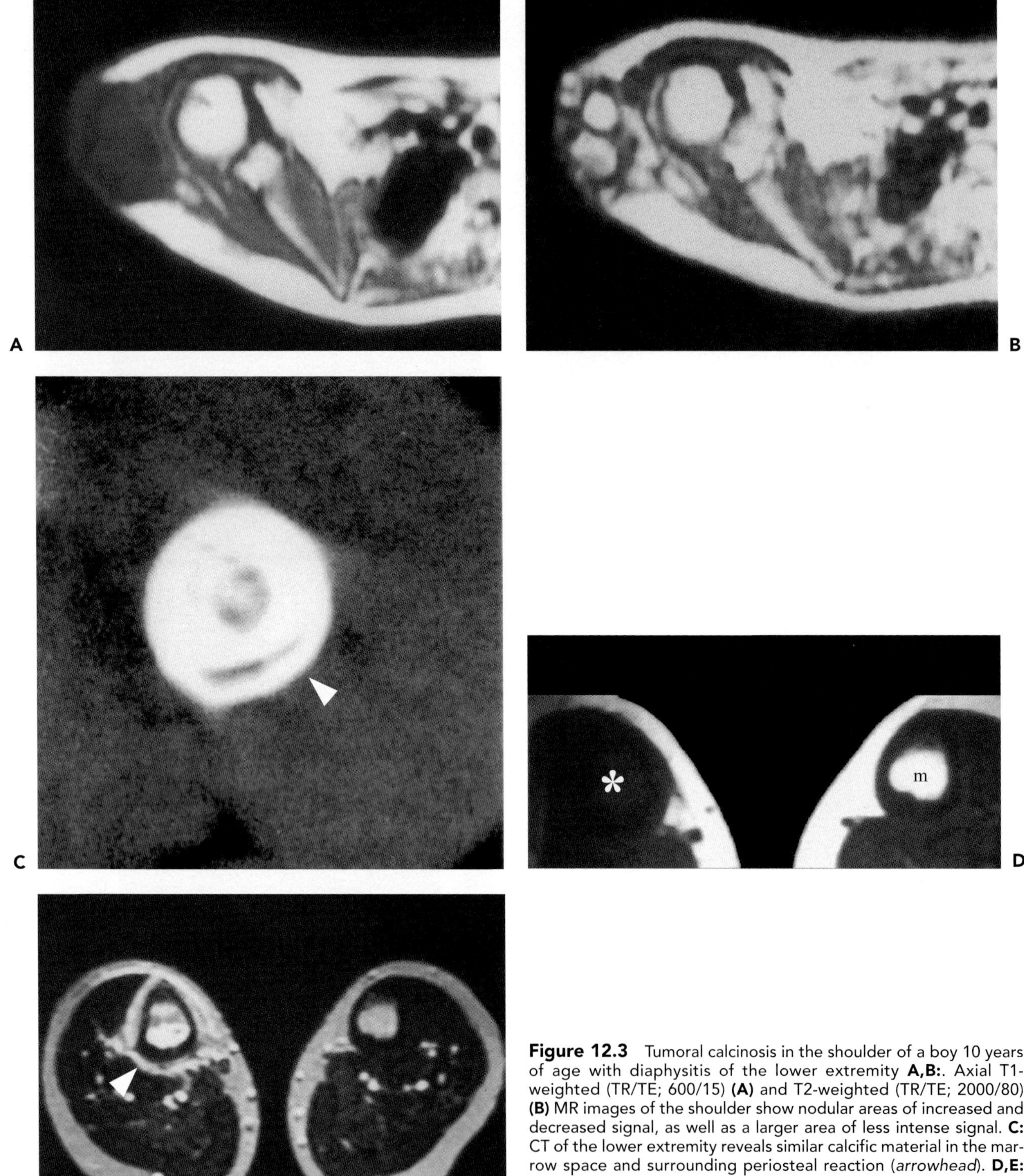

Figure 12.3   Tumoral calcinosis in the shoulder of a boy 10 years of age with diaphysitis of the lower extremity **A,B:**. Axial T1-weighted (TR/TE; 600/15) **(A)** and T2-weighted (TR/TE; 2000/80) **(B)** MR images of the shoulder show nodular areas of increased and decreased signal, as well as a larger area of less intense signal. **C:** CT of the lower extremity reveals similar calcific material in the marrow space and surrounding periosteal reaction (*arrowhead*). **D,E:** Axial T1-weighted (TR/TE; 600/20) **(D)** and T2-weighted (TR/TE; 2800/80) **(E)** MR images through the thigh show marrow replacement (*asterisk*) compared to the normal contralateral side (*m*), owing to calcific myelitis. Surrounding high signal intensity periostitis is seen (*arrowhead*) on the long TR image. (Case courtesy of Salutario Martinez, MD, Duke University.)

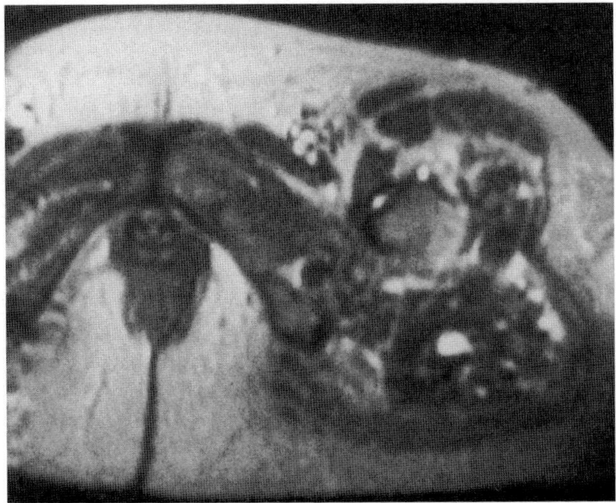

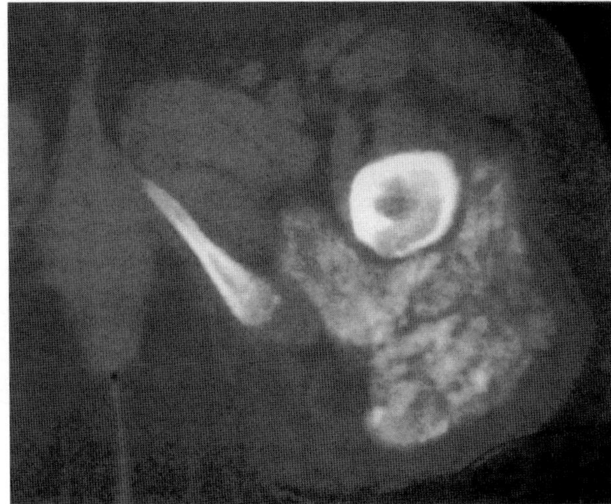

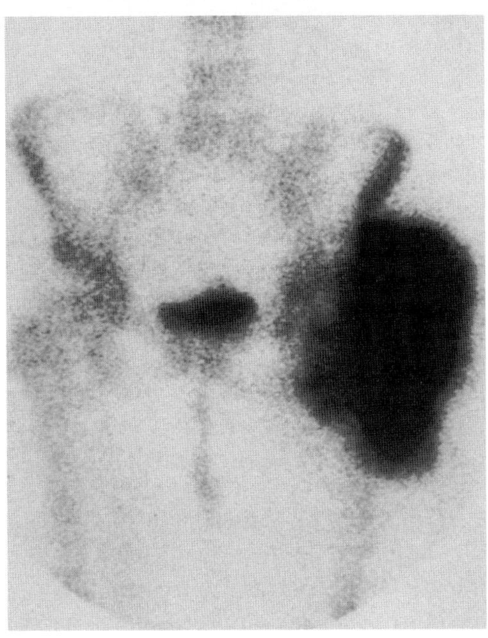

Figure 12.4   Tumoral calcinosis in the hip of a woman 53 years of age. **A:** Axial T2-weighted (TR/TE; 2000/80) MR image of the hip shows a poorly defined soft tissue mass with nodular areas of increased and decreased signal. **B:** Corresponding axial noncontrast CT scan shows the marked mineralization of the mass to better advantage. **C:** Delayed static image of the pelvis from a technetium-99m bone scan shows marked focal tracer accumulation.

Intramuscular Myxoma

In a review of 34 cases in 1965, Enzinger (14) defined intramuscular myxoma as a distinctive benign lesion, speculating that the myxoma cell is an altered fibroblast that produces excess mucopolysaccharide and is incapable of assembling mature collagen. It is a lesion usually seen in adults, with a peak presentation between the fifth and seventh decades (2,11–13). Less commonly it is seen in young adults and rarely in children (16). In most series, women are affected more commonly than men (2:1 ratio) (14,16–18). A history of trauma is elicited in fewer than 25% of patients (2,11–13).

Patients typically present with a painless, palpable mass, and less than 25% complain of pain or tenderness (14). The rate of tumor growth is variable, and there may be long intervals with no apparent clinical enlargement. Enzinger and Weiss (3) reported two cases in which the tumor was present for 13 and 15 years, respectively, with little growth after the first year.

Intramuscular myxomas are usually solitary, although multiple tumors are reported. Multiple myxomas almost always are associated with fibrous dysplasia of bone. This association is referred to as *Mazabraud syndrome* and is discussed in greater detail later in this chapter. Intramuscular myxoma is most common in the thigh, with more than 50% of lesions occurring in this location (3,14,17). Less common locations, in order of decreasing frequency, include the shoulder, buttocks, and upper arm (3).

At gross pathologic inspection, myxomas are composed of a gelatinous material and are usually 5 cm to 10 cm in size (2,11–13). Microscopically, they are hypocellular, consisting of scattered, bland spindle and stellate cells within a loose, highly myxoid, avascular stroma (19,20). Associated cystic changes may be seen (19). Although intramuscular myxoma appears well-circumscribed both

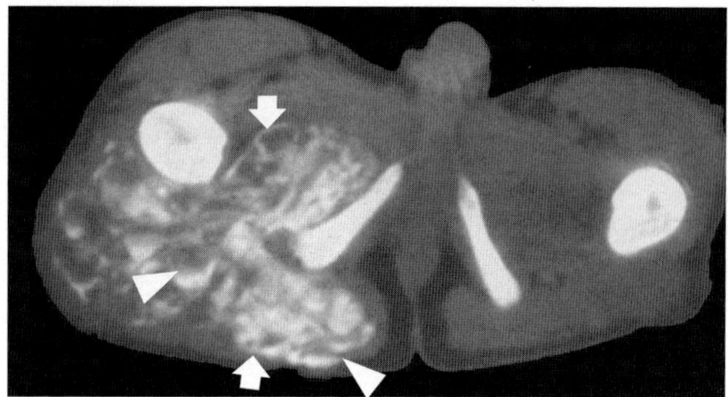

Figure 12.5 Tumoral calcinosis about the hip in a man 25 years of age. CT shows a large calcified soft tissue mass (*arrows*) with multiple calcium fluid levels (*arrowheads*).

grossly and radiographically, it has infiltrating margins on microscopy, blending imperceptibly with the adjacent muscle and fascia (19). The myxoid tissue often extends into the surrounding muscle because lesions lack a complete pseudocapsule and may result in muscle atrophy about the rim of the tumor (21). The bland appearance of the cells and the highly myxoid stroma often suggest the diagnosis of myxoid liposarcoma to the pathologist. However, the absence of a plexiform vasculature and lipoblasts is in sharp contrast to the findings in myxoid liposarcoma (19). In fact, the absence of an elaborate vasculature has suggested to many that intramuscular myxoma may not be a true neoplasm but rather a localized accumulation of reactive fibroblasts and acid mucopolysaccharide (19). However, Nielsen et al. identified more hypercellular regions (10% to 80% of the lesion volume) in 76% of cases with relatively increased vascularity (22). Mutations in the GNAS1 gene are described with myxomas similar to genetic aberrations in fibrous dysplasia (11).

Despite the occasional large size of these tumors, simple excision, even if not complete, is usually curative without recurrence (17,23–27). Nielson et al. reported no recurrences in 32 cases (22), while Ireland et al. reported only 2 local recurrences in 39 cases (5%) (16). Because of the limited growth potential, we believe observation of these lesions following biopsy may be appropriate in some patients. Metastases are not reported (25).

Radiographs may be normal (55%) or may reveal a nonspecific soft tissue mass (45%) (15). However, Ireland et al. (16) described a case of intramuscular myxoma in which the tumor was less dense than the surrounding muscle, having the radiographic appearance of a lipoma. Internal calcification is uncommonly reported (24,28). Miettinen et al. (18) reported the radiographic findings in 16 patients and found minor bone abnormalities in 14, including cortical thickening, exostoses, subchondral cysts, and supernumerary bones. We believe associated osseous findings are rare with myxoma. Bone scintigraphy

usually shows only mild or no uptake of radionuclide scintigraphy. Arteriography may reveal an avascular or hypovascular lesion.

Ultrasonography is nonspecific, showing a well-defined hypoechoic to near anechoic mass, with some internal echoes (Fig. 12.6) and increased through transmission (Fig. 12.6) (19,29,30). Small anechoic cystic areas may be seen in the majority of cases (83%) (Fig. 12.6) (15). In the study by Murphey et al. (15), Color Doppler sonography revealed lesions to be avascular or hypovascular, with surrounding vessels. No surrounding fat or edema was seen by sonography.

CT typically reveals a well-defined, homogeneous, soft tissue mass with attenuation greater than that of water and less than that of surrounding normal muscle (Figs. 12.6–12.8) (19,24,28,29,31,32). A lesion with a CT attenuation coefficient of –53 Hounsfield units, a level approaching that of fat, has also been reported (19). In this case, the low attenuation may be the result of the fat atrophy surrounding the lesion, as can be seen in 25% of cases, rather than the lesion itself (Fig. 12.8) (15). Mild enhancement following contrast, either diffuse, or septal and peripheral, is seen in 50% of cases (15).

Multiple studies (23,26,33–35) have described the MR imaging appearance of myxomas, including the largest by Murphey et al. (45 cases, 33 with MR imaging), Bancroft et al. (20 cases with MR imaging), Luna et al. (18 lesions with MR imaging), and Iwasko et al. (7 patients, 5 with MR imaging) (Figs. 12.6–12.10) (36–38). Myxomas show low (81% to 100%) to intermediate (0% to 19%) signal intensity on T1-weighted MR images (15,36–38) (Figs. 12.6, 12.7, 12.9, and 12.10). On T2-weighted MR images, all myxomas showed high signal intensity (15,36–38) (Figs. 12.6, 12.7, 12.9, and 12.10). Lesions are typically homogeneous or mildly heterogeneous, and are well-defined in 60% to 80% of cases (15,36–38) (Figs. 12.6, 12.7, 12.9, and 12.10). A small rim of fat representing atrophied surrounding muscle, as is seen pathologically, can be identified in 65% to 89% of cases (15,36–38) (Figs. 12.9 and 12.10). This fat rim is usually most prominent at the superior and inferior extent of the lesion. Surrounding high signal caused by leakage of the myxomatous tissue into surrounding muscle may be seen in 79% to 100% of myxomas (15,36–39) (Figs. 12.9 and 12.10). Following contrast administration, lesion will show mild (76%) to moderate (24%) enhancement, in either a diffuse (57%) or thick peripheral and septal (43%) pattern (Fig. 12.6). Cystic areas can be seen in 52% of myxomas by MR imaging (Fig. 12.6) (15). We believe the MR appearance of an intramuscular mass with low signal intensity on T1 weighting, high signal intensity on T2 weighting, and a peripheral rim of fat and surrounding edema is nearly pathognomonic of myxoma. These features are not apparent in other intramuscular masses (40,41). In our experience, all myxomas, regardless of location (intramuscular, subcutaneous, aponeurotic, or juxta-articular) or associated disease

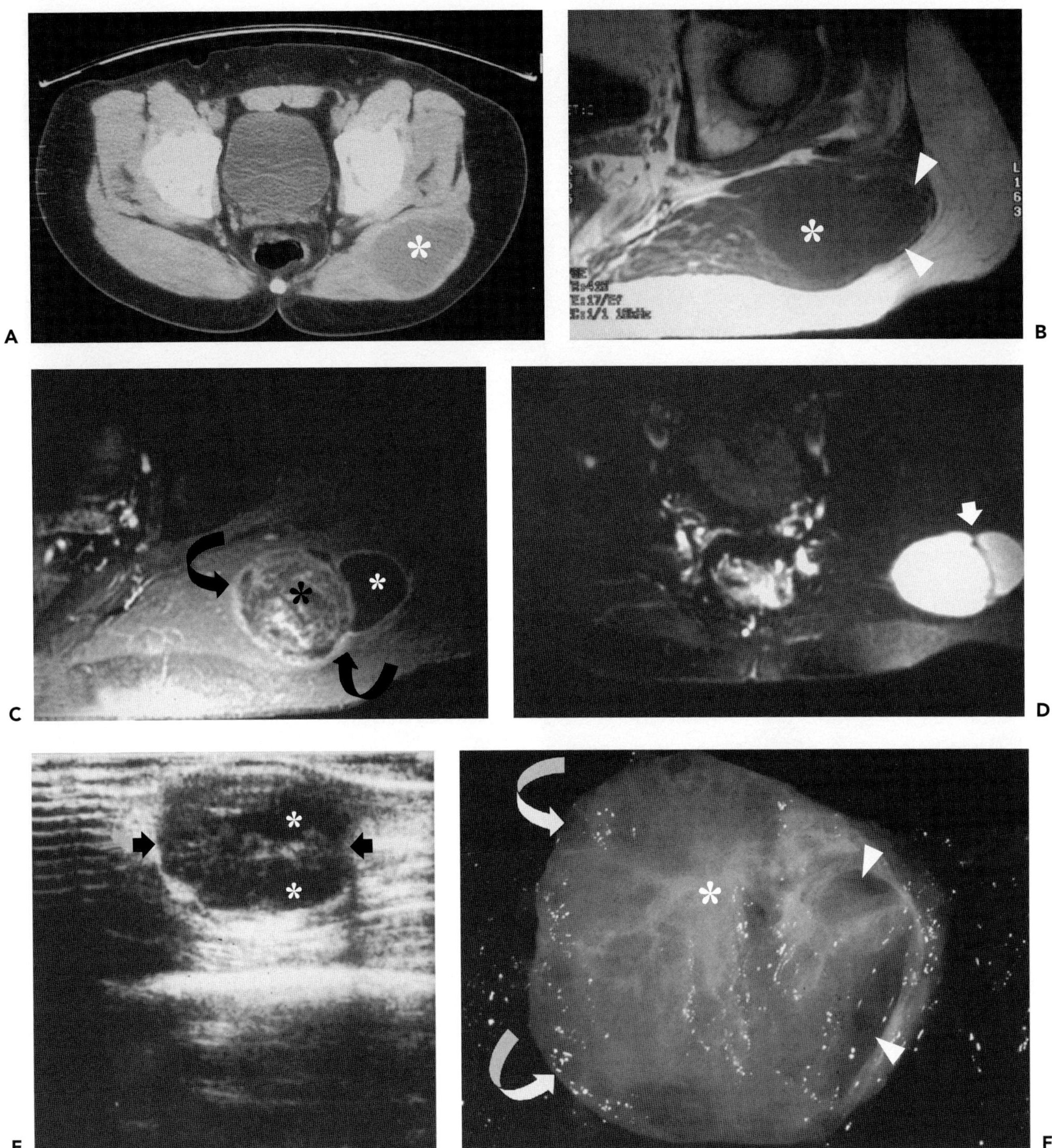

Figure 12.6 Intramuscular myxoma of the gluteal muscles in a man 40 years of age with a painless, slowly enlarging mass. **A:** CT shows a low attenuation intramuscular mass (*asterisk*). **B,C:** Axial T1-weighted (TR/TE; 416/17) spin-echo MR images preceding **(B)** and with fat-suppression following **(C)** intravenous contrast show a low-intensity intramuscular mass (*asterisk*) with an incomplete rim of fat laterally (*arrowheads*). The image after contrast shows two distinct areas with moderate diffuse enhancement of the myxoma medially (*black asterisk*) and thin peripheral enhancement of the cyst laterally (*white asterisk*). The peripheral enhancement about the entire lesion represents the pseudocapsule (*black curved arrows*). **D:** Axial fat-suppressed T2-weighted (TR/TE; 3850/135) MR image reveals diffuse high signal intensity in both components, separated by a low signal septation (*arrow*). **E:** Sonogram reveals a hypoechoic, but solid tissue mass (*arrows*) with through sound transmission and several anechoic cystic areas (*asterisk*). **F:** Sectioned gross specimen shows the myxoma (*asterisk*), the cystic component (*arrowheads*), and pseudocapsule (*white curved arrows*) corresponding to the imaging findings.

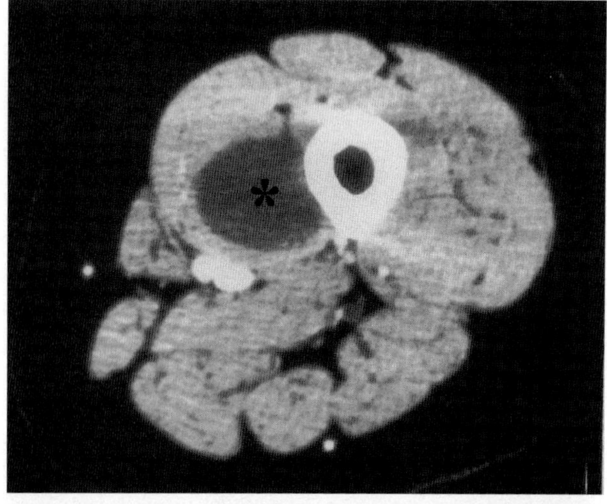

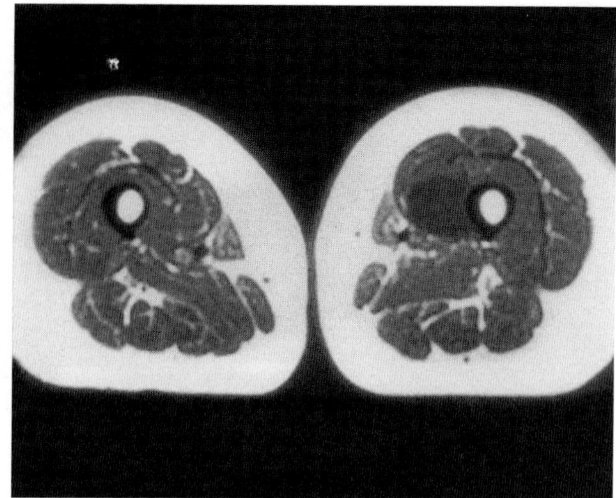

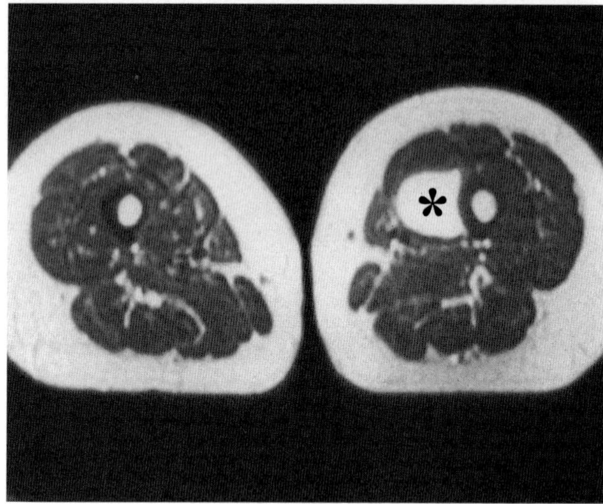

Figure 12.7   Intramuscular myxoma in a woman 58 years of age. **A:** Axial contrast-enhanced CT scan shows a well-defined mass (*asterisk*) with prominent low attenuation. **B,C:** Axial T1-weighted (TR/TE; 300/15) **(B)** and T2-weighted (TR/TE; 2500/70) **(C)** MR images of the thigh show a cystlike, intramuscular soft tissue mass (*asterisk*) in the medial aspect of the thigh, with signal characteristic similar to that of fluid.

(fibrous dysplasia), have a similar intrinsic imaging appearance (Figs. 12.11 and 12.12).

Myxoma and Fibrous Dysplasia (Mazabraud Syndrome)

The association of fibrous dysplasia with soft tissue myxoma is well established, although it is uncommon. First described by Henschen in 1926 (42), this association was emphasized by Mazabraud et al. in 1967 (43) and is often referred to as *Mazabraud syndrome* (44–51). Sundaram et al. (20) reviewed the literature through 1987 and found a total of 17 reported cases. Soft tissue myxoma is much more common with the polyostotic form of fibrous dysplasia but is reported with monostotic involvement as well (Fig. 12.11) (20). Ireland et al. (16) reported 58 patients with soft tissue myxoma, 3 of whom had multiple tumors associated with fibrous dysplasia of bone (2 of these 3 patients had polyostotic disease) (16). The myxomas occur in the vicinity of the most severely affected bones and may be multiple (20,23). Fibrous dysplasia is typically diagnosed well before the myxomas

develop. The association between these entities is suggested to be the result of a common origin for both fibrous dysplasia and myxoma (43), as well as a metabolic anomaly in the initial growth of both bone and soft tissue (52).

Malignant transformation in fibrous dysplasia is relatively uncommon, with a reported prevalence of approximately 0.5%, although two cases of malignant transformation were reported in patients with Mazabraud syndrome (53,54). This suggests that patients with fibrous dysplasia and myxomas may be at greater risk for malignant transformation than patients having fibrous dysplasia alone (53).

Subcutaneous and Aponeurotic Myxoma

As with other superficial lesions, these are typically treated on the basis of clinical findings and are rarely imaged radiologically. These lesions arise more frequently in middle-aged males. Sites of involvement include the trunk, lower extremities, and head/neck. Lesions in the eyelid region are described in association

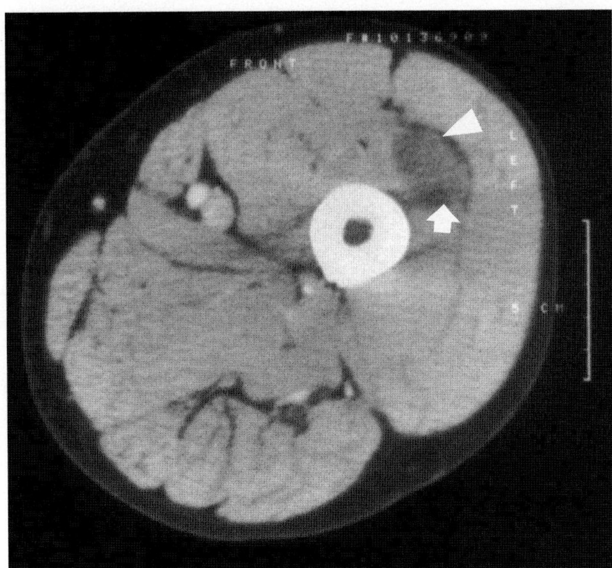
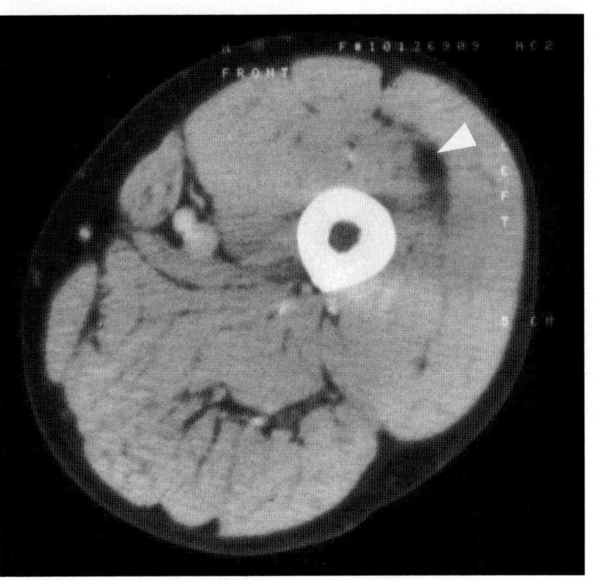

Figure 12.8 Intramuscular myxoma of the thigh in a man 66 years of age. **A,B:** CT at two different levels shows the low attenuation soft tissue mass (*arrow*) with a small rim of subtle surrounding fat (*arrowhead*).

with Carney complex (cutaneous and cardiac myxomas, spotty pigmentation, and endocrine overactivity). Subcutaneous lesions may also be referred to as superficial angiomyxoma (2,11–13,55). Subcutaneous and aponeurotic myxomas make up approximately 25% (9) of all myxomas. Digital myxomas are also described, although many of these lesions may represent mucoid cysts related to osteoarthritis. Cutaneous myxomas have an increased likelihood of local recurrence (30% to 40%) (2,11–13). The pathologic and imaging appearance of these lesions are similar to their intramuscular counterparts (Fig. 12.12).

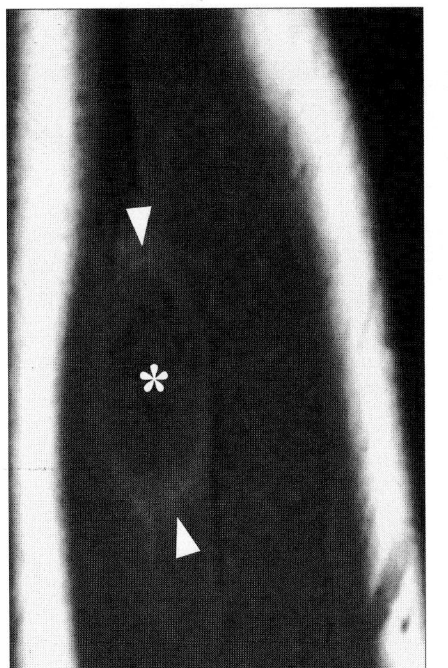
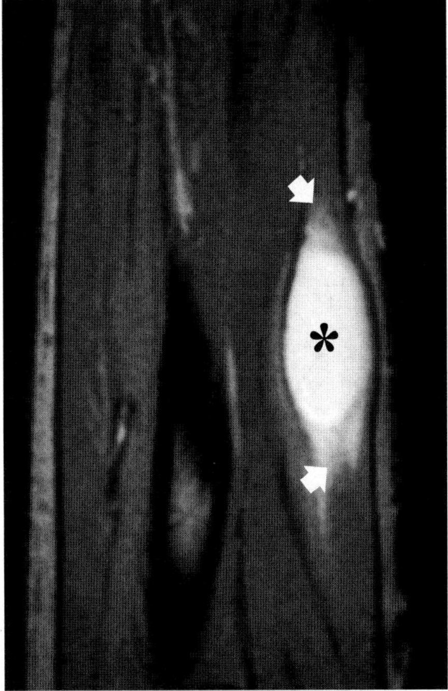

Figure 12.9 Intramuscular myxoma of the forearm in a woman 40 years of age. **A,B:** Sagittal T1-weighted (TR/TE; 600/20) **(A)** and T2-weighted (TR/TE; 2500/90) **(B)** MR images of the forearm show a well-defined cystlike mass (*asterisk*). There is a small rim of tissue with signal intensity similar to that of fat on T1-weighted image (*arrowheads*) and mild surrounding edema on T2 weighting (*arrows*), and both of these features are most prominent at the superior and inferior poles of the lesion.

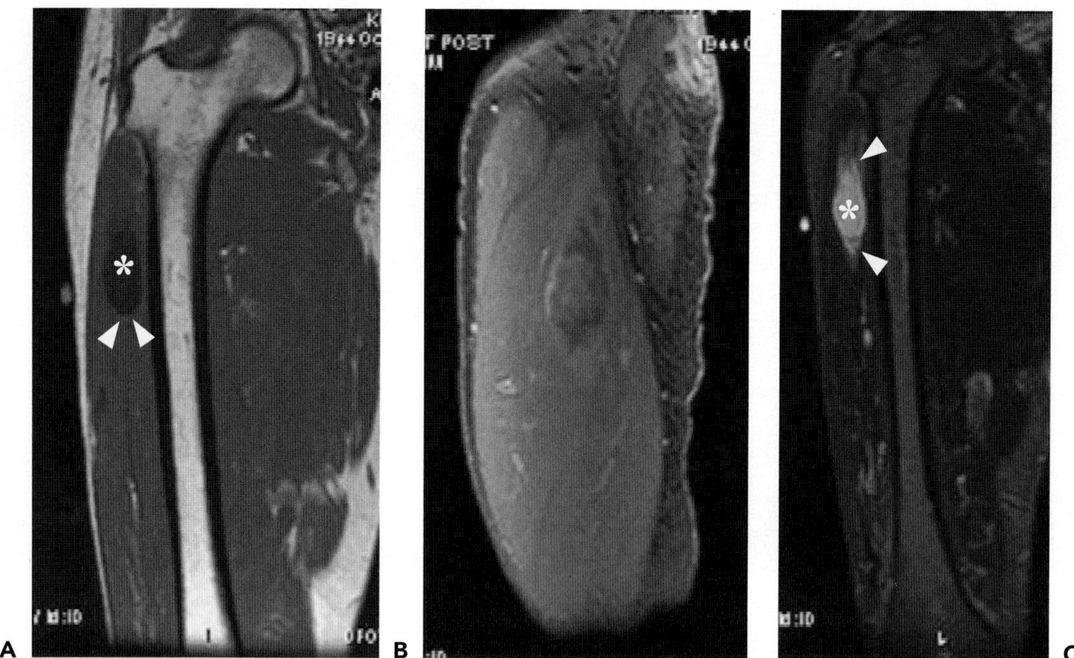

Figure 12.10   Intramuscular myxoma of the thigh in a man 60 years of age. **A–C:** Coronal T1-weighted (TR/TE; 396/8) **(A)**, sagittal enhanced fat-suppressed T1-weighted (TR/TE; 175/1.6) **(B)** and coronal T2-weighted (TR/TE; 3000/66) **(C)** MR images show an intramuscular soft tissue mass (*asterisk*). There is low signal intensity on T1-weighting and high signal intensity on T2-weighting. A small rim of signal intensity, similar to that of fat is seen about the lesion on the T1-weighted image (*arrowheads* in **A**). Note mild diffuse enhancement following contrast and mild surrounding edema on T2-weighted image (**C:** *arrowheads*).

Juxta-Articular Myxoma

The juxta-articular myxoma, also known as a *periarticular myxoma*, usually occurs around large joints (particularly the knee). Other locations include the elbow, shoulder, ankle, and hip. These lesions have some histologic features of a myxoma but are frequently associated with cystic change closely resembling ganglion. We believe that in the majority of cases, these lesions are in actuality perimeniscal or perilabral cysts rather than true myxomas. Lending further credence to this suggestion, is the high incidence of internal derangement (particularly mensical tears and osteoarthritis) in published series (11,56). In addition, the much higher recurrence rate of 34% in the study by Meis and Enzinger of juxta-articular myxoma suggests that the underlying injury was not recognized or repaired, leading to reaccumulation of the lesion (56). Because of their juxta-articular location and ganglionlike appearance, these lesions are discussed further with synovial lesions in Chapter 10 (57).

Deep Aggressive Angiomyxoma

The term *aggressive angiomyxoma* was applied to this lesion in 1983 by Steeper et al. (58). The World Health Organization (WHO) recognized this lesion as *deep aggressive angiomyxoma* (11). This lesion occurs most commonly in women in their third to sixth decade of life (peak incidence in the fourth decade). The female-to-male ratio is reported as more than 6:1 (2,11,12,59–61). Common locations include the pelvicoperineal, inguinoscrotal, and retroperitoneal regions (2,11,12,61). Aggressive angiomyxoma may be asymptomatic or cause pain and dyspareunia. Lesions may be mistaken for a Bartholin cyst because of the location.

At gross pathologic evaluation, deep aggressive angiomyxomas are often quite large (10 to 20 cm in size), lobulated, partially circumscribed, gelatinous masses (2,11,12,61). Microscopically, deep aggressive angiomyxomas are low to moderate in cellularity and composed of small, stellate, spindled cells (62). Scattered dilated vessels of variable size (from capillaries to large vessels) are usually seen in the lesion (63). The vessels are often surrounded by smooth muscle cells. Mitoses are infrequent. Cytogenetic aberrations are seen with rearrangement of 12q14–15 in various translocations (2,11,12,61,64,65).

Although wide excision is the treatment of choice for deep angiomyxoma, the large size, infiltration, and location often precludes complete removal (63,66). Thus, the local recurrence rate is high, ranging from 30% to 100% (2,11,12,61,63). Local recurrence is often adequately treated by reexcision alone without the need of adjunct therapy (63). Deep aggressive angiomyxoma has no metastatic potential.

Radiographs are usually normal or show a nonspecific soft tissue mass with displacement of pelvic structures. Angiography typically reveals a hypervascular mass. Sonography demonstrates a heterogeneous hypoechoic

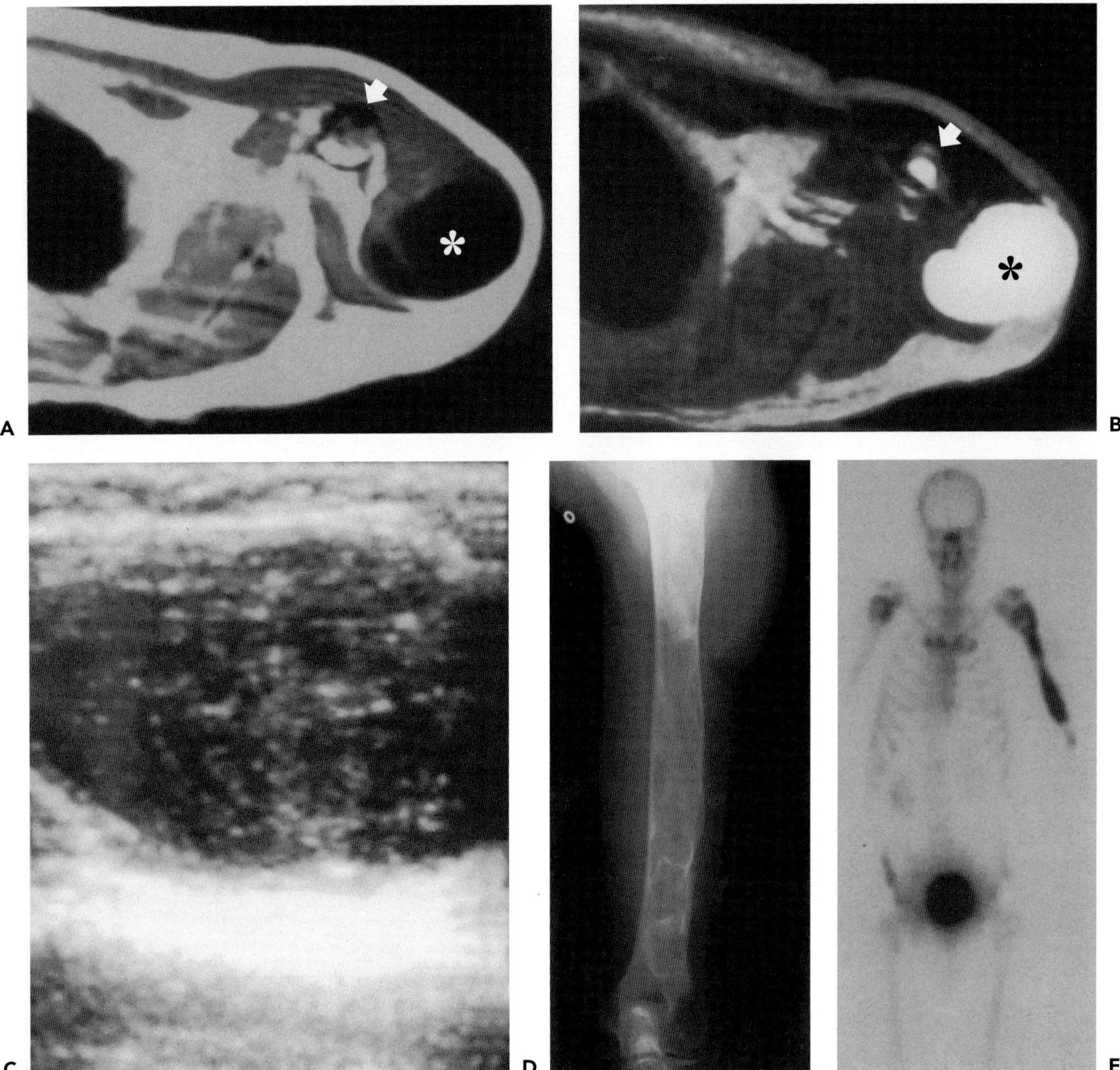

Figure 12.11 Myxoma and fibrous dysplasia (Mazabraud syndrome) in a man 55 years of age, presenting with a soft tissue mass in the shoulder. **A,B:** Axial T1-weighted (TR/TE; 600/17) **(A)** and T2-weighted (TR/TE; 2500/90) **(B)** MR images of the shoulder show a well-defined, homogeneous, intramuscular mass (*asterisk*). The signal intensity suggests that it is cystlike. Note the abnormal signal intensity in the marrow of the humerus (*arrows*). **C:** Ultrasound of the soft tissue mass shows the lesion not to be a simple cyst, with the appearance of a complex mass. **D:** Radiograph of the humerus shows changes compatible with fibrous dysplasia. **E:** Technetium-99m bone scan confirms that the fibrous dysplasia is monostotic and there is no radionuclide uptake in the myxoma.

soft tissue mass (Fig. 12.13) (67–71). Internal echogenic septae, cystic areas, and a hyperechoic rim are also described (Fig. 12.13).

CT shows a well-defined mass with attenuation lower than that of muscle (Fig. 12.14) (67,69–72). On T1-weighted MR images, deep aggressive angiomyxoma is usually low-to-intermediate in signal intensity (Figs. 12.13 and 12.14) (69,71–73). On T2-weighted MR images, these lesions reveal intermediate-to-high signal intensity, likely

because of the high water content seen histologically (Figs. 12.13 and 12.14) (69,72,73). Deep aggressive angiomyxoma is described as having a characteristic swirled or layered appearance on CT and MR imaging (Figs. 12.13 and 12.14). This appearance (83% of cases by CT or MR imaging) is seen on T2-weighted MR imaging and postcontrast CT or MR images (Figs. 12.13 and 12.14). The strands of tissue creating this swirled architecture were often best seen on contrast enhanced CT or MR imaging, and were mildly lower signal

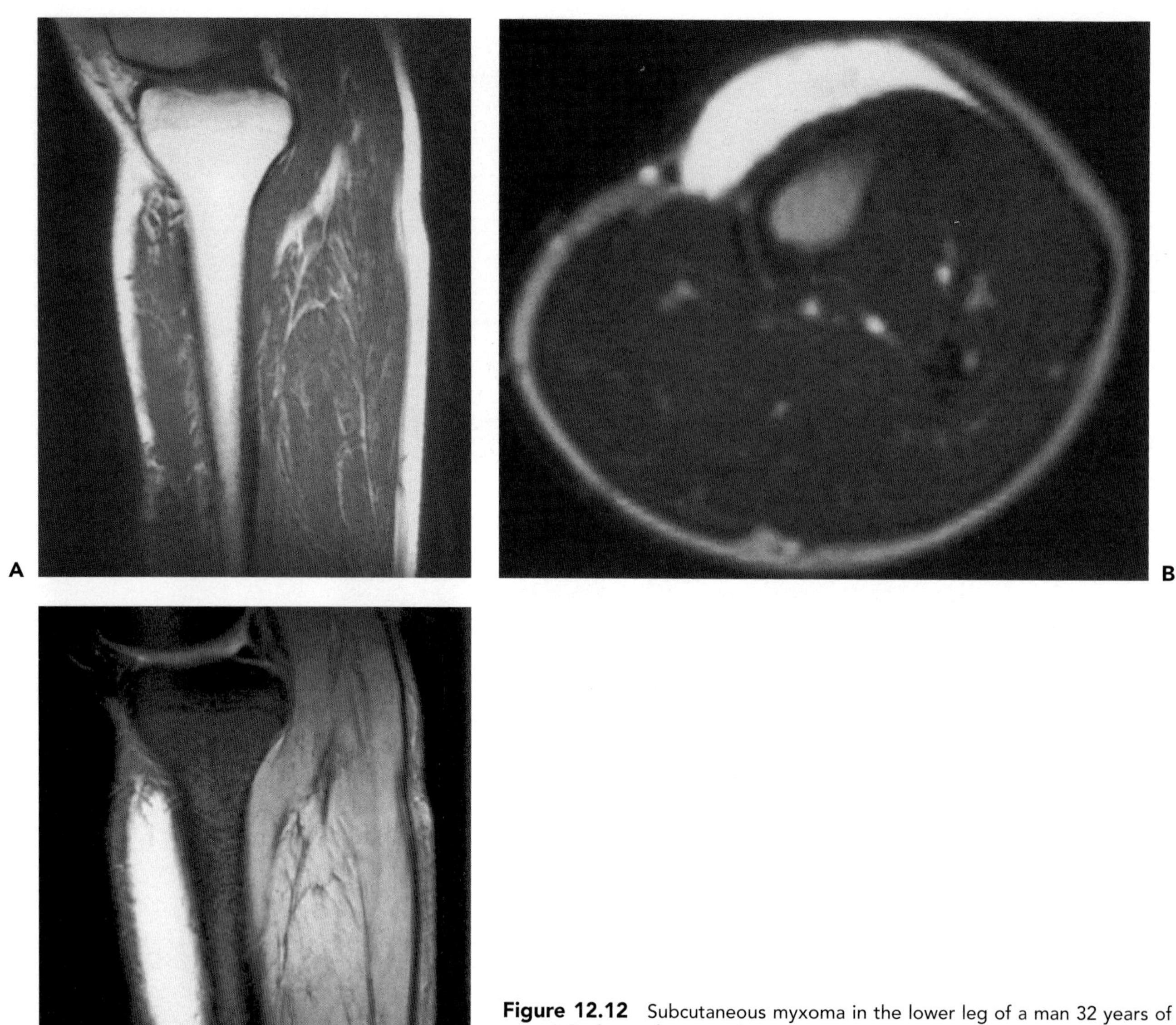

Figure 12.12 Subcutaneous myxoma in the lower leg of a man 32 years of age. **A,B:** Sagittal T1-weighted (TR/TE; 600/20) **(A)** and axial T2-weighted (TR/TE; 2500/90) **(B)** MR images show a well-defined, subcutaneous mass anterior to the tibia. The large size of the lesion precludes clearly identifying the origin in the subcutaneous tissue or aponeurosis. **C:** Corresponding sagittal gradient-echo image shows markedly increased signal intensity, similar to that seen on the T2-weighted MR image. (Case courtesy of Robert G. Dussault, MD, and Phoebe A. Kaplan, MD.)

intensity on long TR images in the study by Outwater et al. (72). Cross-sectional imaging, particularly CT or MR imaging, reveals the effect of these often large masses on surrounding pelvic structures and whether the tumor traverses the pelvic diaphragm; anatomic features that are essential in planning surgical resection.

Mixed Tumor/Myoepithelioma/Parachordoma

These tumors are grouped together currently by the WHO because of their similar epithelial and/or myoepithelial composition analogous to similar tumors that arise in the salivary glands (11). Another term for these lesions is *ectomesenchymal chondromyxoid tumor* (11,12,74,75). Adults are typically affected in the fourth to sixth decade of life

with an average of 35 years of age (11,12,74,75). However, as with many neoplasms, there is a wide age range, and 20% of patients are children younger than 10 years (11,12,74–76). A mild male predilection is reported in some series (11,12,74,75,77). Sites of involvement are most frequently the subcutaneous or deep subfascial soft tissues of the extremities (11,12,74,75). The upper extremity is more commonly affected than the lower extremity. Other involved locations include the head/neck, trunk, and rarely bone (11,12,74,75). Clinically, patients present with a nonspecific painless swelling or mass.

At gross pathologic examination these lesions are usually small (less than 3 cm) and reveal a similar spectrum as is seen in their salivary gland counterparts. Microscopically, the epithelial components of these lesions often form nests,

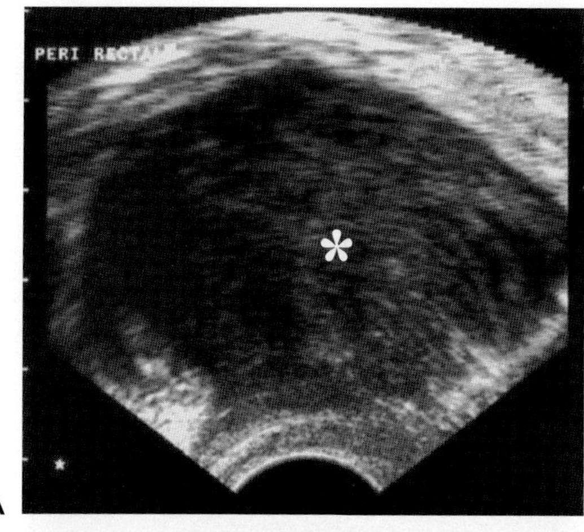

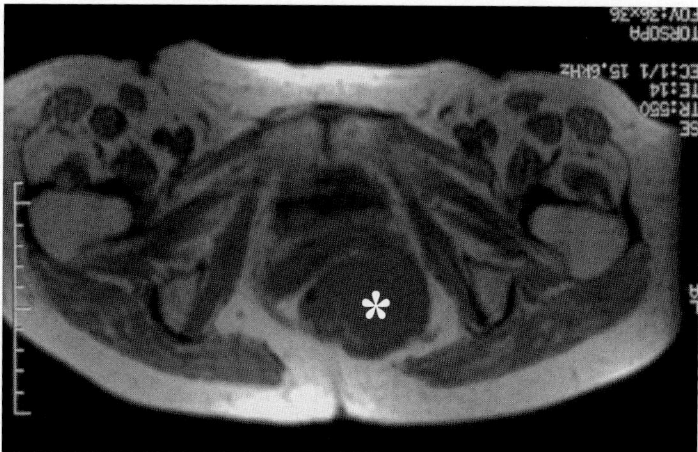

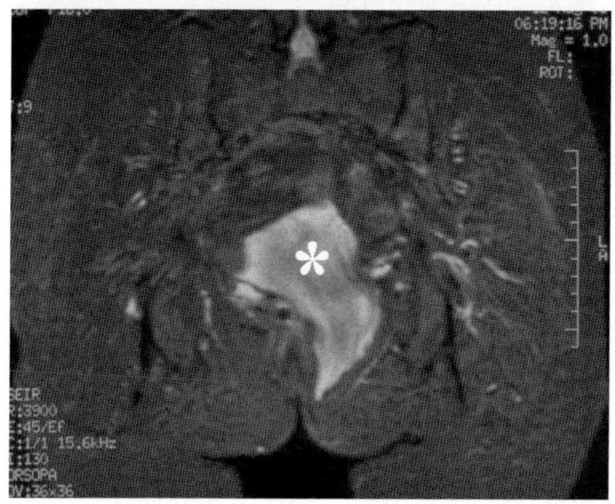

Figure 12.13 Deep aggressive angiomyxoma of the pelvis in a woman 77 years of age. **A:** Endorectal sonogram demonstrates a hypoechoic, heterogeneous, perirectal soft tissue mass (*asterisk*). **B,C:** Axial T1-weighted (TR/TE; 550/14) **(B)** and coronal short-tau inversion recovery (STIR) (TR/TE/TI; 3900/45/130) **(C)** MR images show the perivaginal soft tissue mass (*asterisk*) with low signal intensity on T1-weighting and high signal on T2-weighting. There is heterogeneity on the long TR image and a swirled/layered appearance.

cords, or ductules and are within a hyalinized-to-chondromyxoid matrix (78,79). Mitoses are scant (<2 per high-power field [HPF]) except in those unusual lesions developing frank malignancy.

The majority of mixed tumors/myoepitheliomas/parachordomas are benign and adequately treated with surgical excision alone (11,12,74,75,80,81). However, similar to salivary gland tumors, a minority of these lesions are malignant and may behave more aggressively with local recurrence (20% of cases) and distant metastases leading to patient demise (11,12,74,75). We are not aware of any features that predict the clinical behavior of these lesions.

As expected for a rare tumor located in the subcutaneous tissues, imaging of these lesions is only rarely reported (82,83). Lesions have been reported to reveal nonspecific intrinsic features on CT and MR imaging (Fig. 12.15). Heterogeneity and cystic, necrotic, or hemorrhagic areas may be apparent. Enhancement is seen following intravenous contrast administration on CT or MR imaging. Large deep-seated lesions are also described with more aggressive and invasive growth (Fig. 12.15) (82,83).

Ectopic Hamartomatous Thymoma

Ectopic hamartomatous thymoma is a unique, benign tumor that almost exclusively occurs in the superficial or deep soft tissues of the supraclavicular, suprasternal, or

presternal regions (11,84–86). This lesion affects adults (median: 43 years of age) with a marked male predilection (84,87). Clinically, patients present with a painless, long-standing, soft tissue mass (88).

At gross pathologic examination, ectopic hamartomatous thymoma is a small (1 to 3 cm), well-circumscribed but unencapsulated tumor (89). Microscopically, there is an admixture of spindle cells, epithelial islands, and fat, suggesting a branchial pouch origin (90). Small fluid-containing cysts may also be present. Surgical resection is curative (91).

Imaging of ectopic hamartomatous thymoma is only rarely reported (84). The location at a presternal or supraclavicular site is important to suggest the diagnosis (Fig. 12.16). In our experience, lesions are well-defined on MR imaging. On T1-weighted images, lesions will show an intermediate signal intensity with foci of fat, reflecting the pathologic appearance (Fig. 12.16). On T2-weighted images, these lesions may show intermediate-to-high signal intensity.

MALIGNANT LESIONS

Alveolar Soft Part Sarcoma

Alveolar soft part sarcoma is an unusual soft tissue sarcoma. It was initially described in 1951 by Smetana and

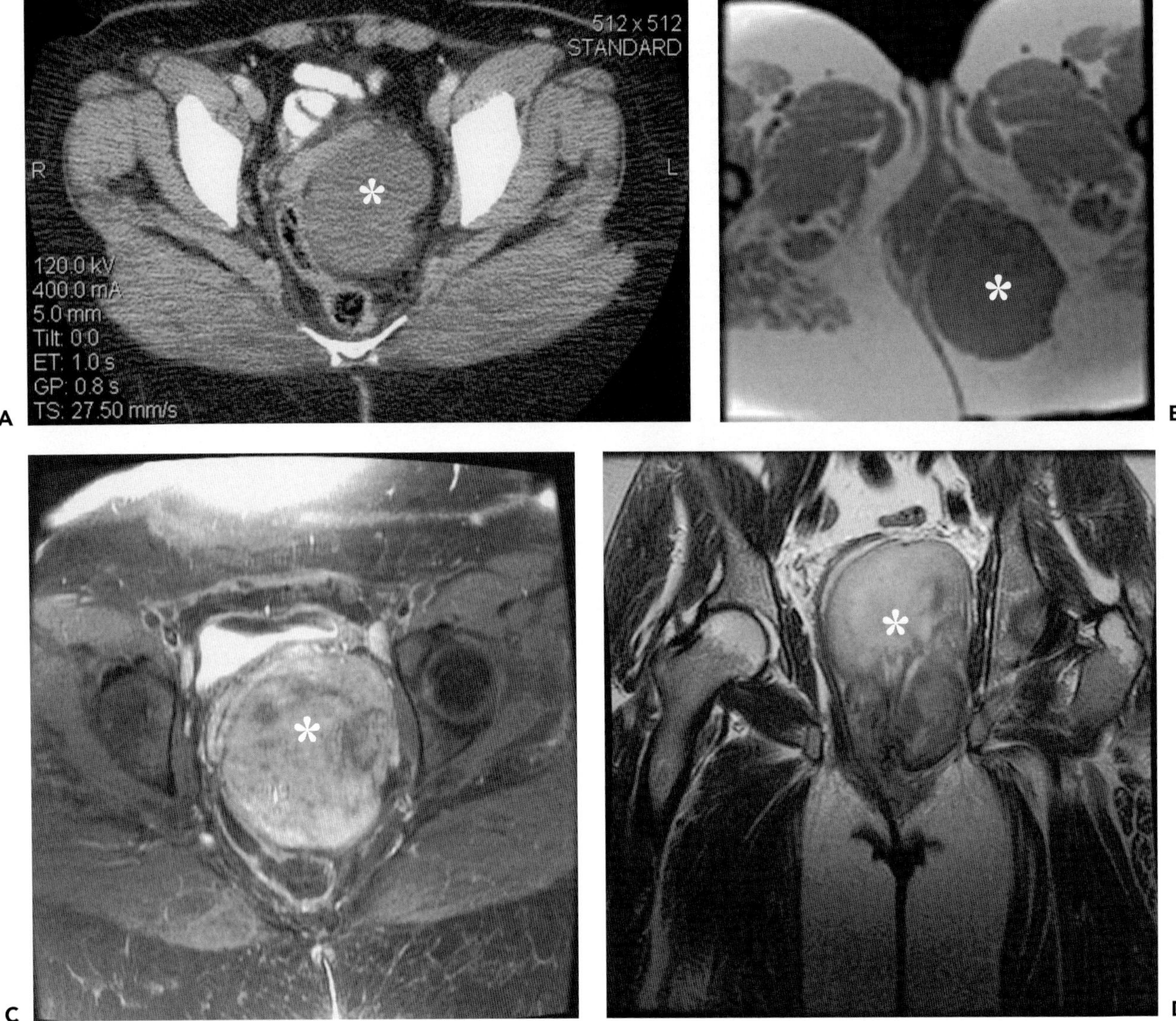

Figure 12.14   Deep aggressive angiomyxoma of the pelvis in a woman 64 years of age. **A:** CT shows a well-defined, low attenuation, soft tissue mass (*asterisk*) displacing the rectosigmoid portion of the colon. **B–D:** Multiple MR images including axial T1-weighted (TR/TE; 500/20) **(B)**, axial post-contrast fat-suppressed T1-weighted (TR/TE; 400/15) **(C)**, and coronal T2-weighted (TR/TE; 4000/60) **(D)** reveal the perirectal soft tissue mass (*asterisk*). There is low attenuation on T1-weighting, moderate diffuse enhancement and intermediate signal intensity on T2-weighting. Note swirled/layed appearance after contrast and on the long TR image.

Scott (92) and designated a malignant tumor of nonchromaffin paraganglia. The lesion was subsequently given the descriptive title *alveolar soft part sarcoma* the following year by Christopherson et al. (93).

Alveolar soft part sarcoma is a relatively rare tumor that makes up approximately 0.5% to 1.0% of all soft tissue sarcomas (11,12,75,94–97). It is most common in patients in the second through fourth decades of life (94,95,98). Most series show a female predominance in patients younger than 30 years, and a mild male predilection for patients older than 30 years (93,94). In adults, the most commonly affected site is the thigh or buttock (41% of cases). In

children and adolescents, the head and neck are most frequently affected. Other unusual locations include the calf, upper extremity, retroperitoneum, female genital tract, and stomach (11,12,75,96). Clinically, the lesion is usually identified as a slowly growing mass that may be present for months to years before the patient seeks medical attention (95,99). Tenderness to palpation is not uncommon, and the mass may be pulsatile with an associated bruit (92,100).

At gross pathologic examination, the lesion is poorly circumscribed with large areas of necrosis and hemorrhage. Large tortuous feeding vessels are typically apparent. A cytogenetic aberration of a nonbalanced translocation

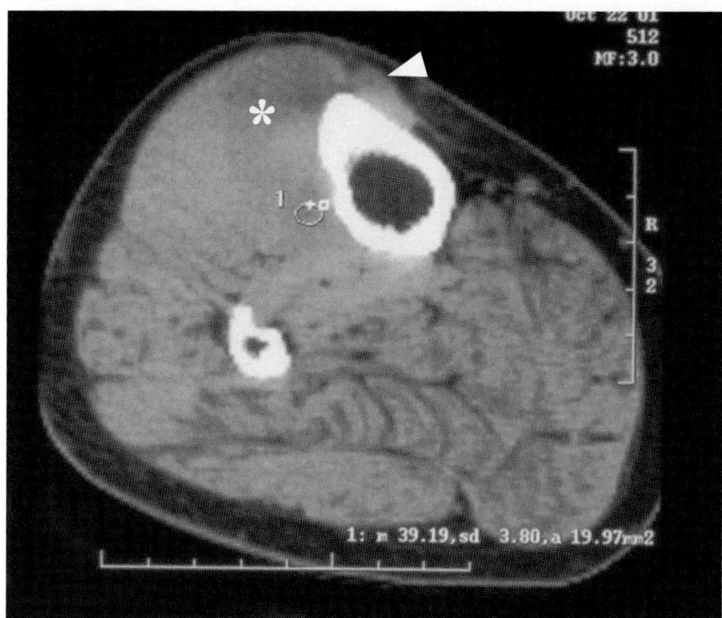
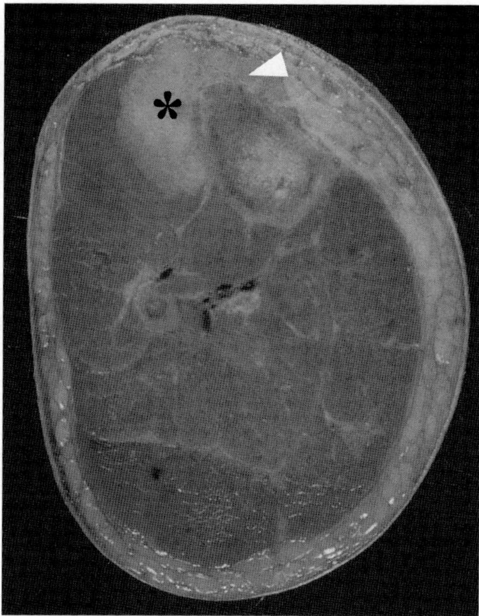

Figure 12.15   Myoepithelioma of the calf in a man 48 years of age with an enlarging mass. **A:** Axial CT precontrast shows a soft tissue mass with both subcutaneous (*arrowhead*) and intramuscular components (*asterisk*). **B:** Photograph of axially sectioned gross specimen reveals identical features as seen on the imaging with a subcutaneous lesion (*arrowhead*) invading the muscle (*asterisk*). This lesion had multiple local recurrences and was malignant myoepithelioma histologically.

t(x;17)(p11;2q25) has been identified in alveolar soft part sarcoma (11,12,75,96,101). As the name implies, the tumor is composed of nests of cells arranged in a manner similar to cells of respiratory alveoli (organoid or nesting pattern), separated by a rich vascular network (99,100, 102,103).

The prognosis of alveolar soft part sarcoma is poor (11,12,75,96). Metastases often occur early in the disease and may be the initial cause of clinical presentation despite slow tumor growth, and they are present at diagnosis in 33% of patients (11,12,75,96,104). Common metastatic sites are the lung, brain, and bone (11,12,75,96). Metastases

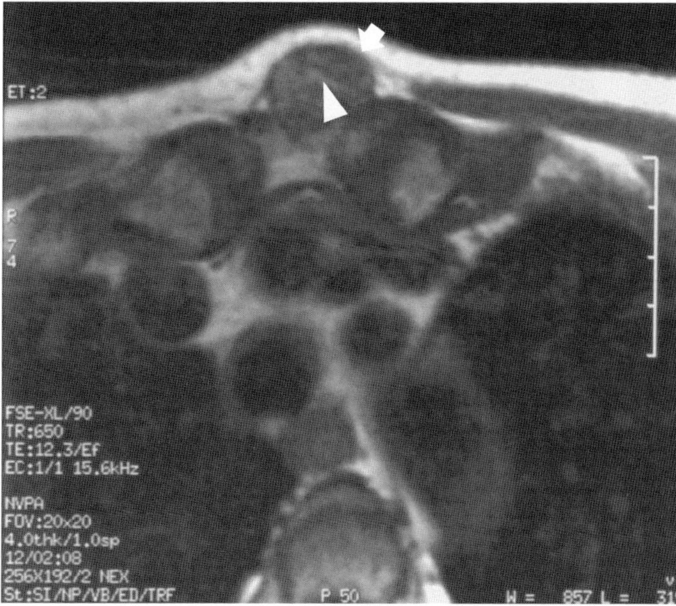
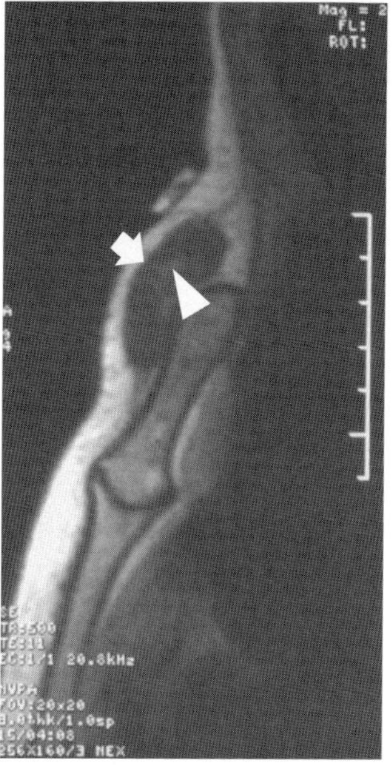

Figure 12.16   Ectopic hamartomatous thymoma in a woman 64 years of age with a presternal mass. **A,B:** Axial T1-weighted (TR/TE; 650/12) **(A)** and sagittal T1-weighted (TR/TE; 500/11) **(B)** MR images show a well-circumscribed soft tissue mass (*arrows*) with intermediate signal intensity. MR images also reveal small punctate high signal intensity areas (*arrowheads*), suggesting the presence of intermixed fat.

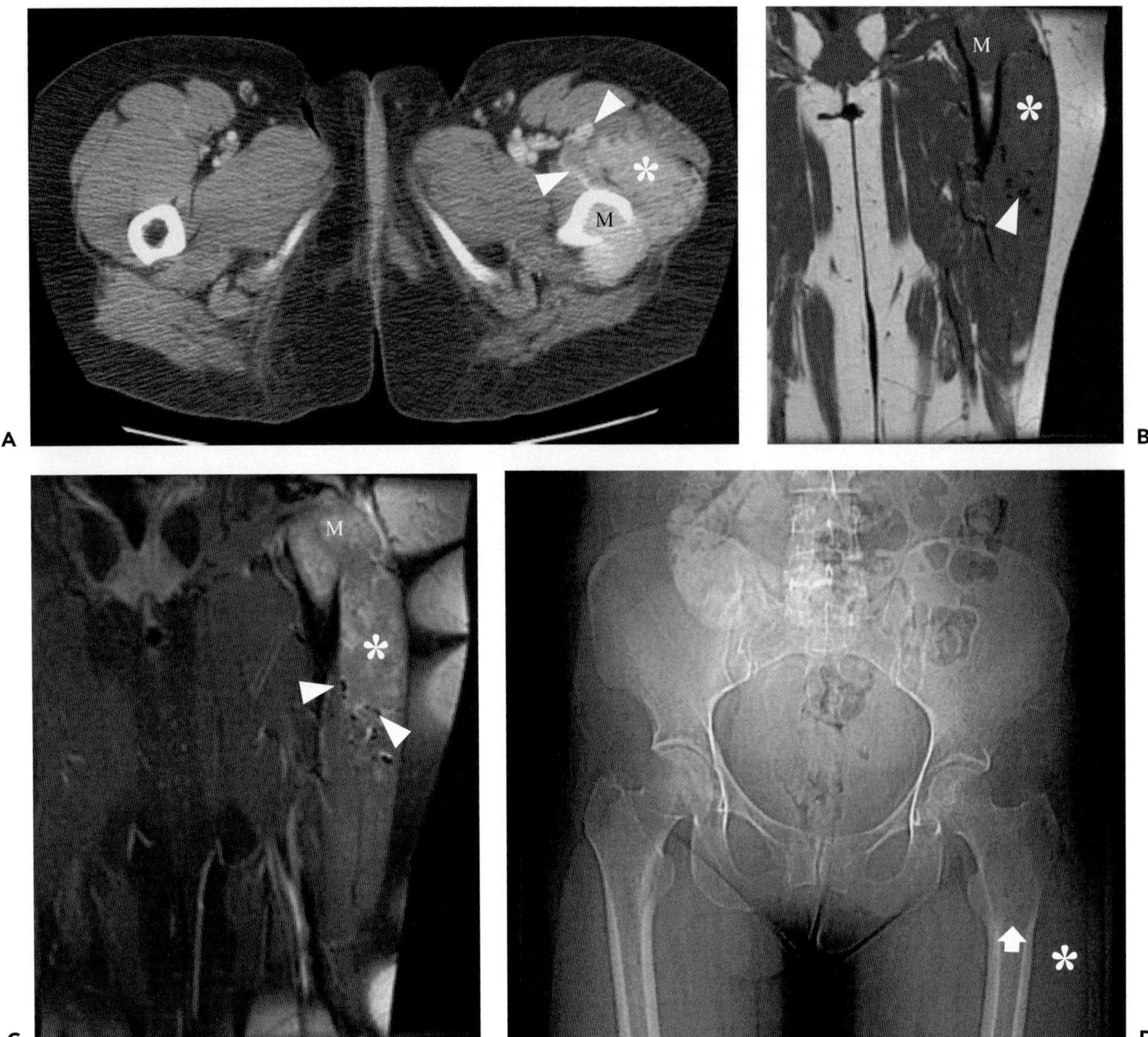

Figure 12.17 Alveolar soft part sarcoma of the proximal thigh in a woman 29 years of age with hip pain. **A:** Axial CT following intravenous contrast shows an enhancing soft tissue mass (*asterisk*) with bone marrow invasion (*M*) and large serpentine vascular structures (*arrowheads*). **B,C:** Coronal T1-weighted (TR/TE; 500/20) **(B)** and T2-weighted (TR/TE; 4500/50) **(C)** MR images reveal the soft tissue mass (*asterisk*). There is intermediate signal intensity on T1-weighting and intermediate-to-high signal intensity on T2-weighting with invasion of the femoral bone marrow (*M*). Serpentine high-flow vessels both feeding and within the lesion are also seen (*arrowheads*). **D:** Pelvis radiograph demonstrates the femoral involvement (*arrow*) and nonspecific soft tissue mass (*asterisk*). (*continued*)

may also be delayed in appearance. Treatment is radical wide resection with adjuvant radiation and chemotherapy (105). Overall survival is reported as 77% at 2 years, 60% to 67% at 5 years, but only 38% at 10 years and 15% at 20 years (97,101). Prognosis appears to be worse in older patients, lesions larger than 5 cm at presentation, and metastases at diagnosis. Interestingly, local recurrence is unusual following complete resection.

Radiographs may be normal or may demonstrate a nonspecific soft tissue mass (Fig. 12.17) (98,99). Punctate calcification may be seen (98) and was noted in 2 of 11 cases

reported by Lorigan et al. (99). Invasion of adjacent bone is uncommon but may demonstrate multiple or solitary ill-defined lytic lesions, simulating osseous metastases (Fig. 12.17) (98).

Arteriography demonstrates a vascular mass that may be markedly hypervascular, with large tortuous feeding arteries, arteriovenous shunting, numerous venous lakes, and large early draining veins (Figs. 12.18 and 12.19) (95,100,106). There may be prominent arteriovenous shunting and prolonged capillary staining (95,100,107). Ultrasonography may be useful to identify the vascular

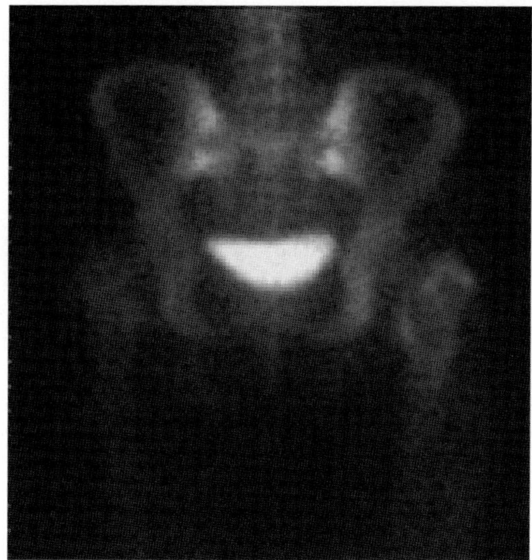 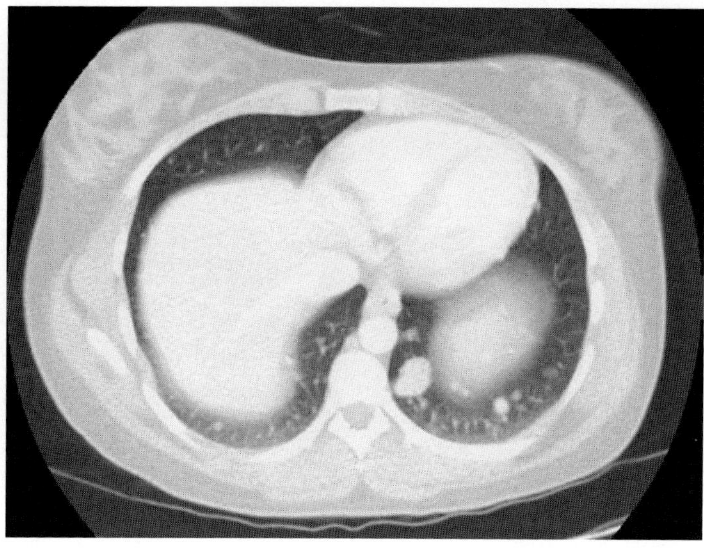

Figure 12.17 *(continued)*   **E:** Bone scintigraphy shows increased radionuclide uptake in the area of femoral involvement. **F:** Chest CT scan reveals numerous pulmonary metastases.

nature of the mass. Color Doppler examination may be particularly well-suited for this evaluation (100). Sonography is otherwise nonspecific, demonstrating a mixed echotexture or hypoechoic mass (Fig. 12.18) (100). In our anecdotal experience, technetium-99m bone scanning has shown markedly increased focal tracer accumulation on flow and blood-pool images, as well as increased radionuclide uptake on static images (Fig. 12.17).

CT demonstrates a soft tissue mass having an attenuation less than or equal to that of skeletal muscle, with margins that vary from well-defined to infiltrating (Figs. 12.17–12.19) (95,99,100). The lesion enhances markedly following contrast administration, particularly peripherally (99,100,107). Contrast enhancement may allow identification of prominent feeding vessels and draining veins (100). Central necrosis has been reported in up to 75% of cases (Figs. 12.17–12.19) (100,107).

MR imaging shows a well-defined soft tissue mass (Figs. 12.17, 12.19, and 12.20) (106,108). On T1-weighted images, the lesion demonstrates signal intensity equal to or greater than that of skeletal muscle, but less than that of subcutaneous fat (Figs. 12.17, 12.19, and 12.20) (95,99,107). Iwamoto et al. (107) reported 10 cases, noting a signal intensity greater than that of skeletal muscle on T1-weighted images in 9 (90%) cases, and similar changes were noted in 67% of lesions in the study by Suh et al. (106). Although the exact cause of the increased signal intensity is unclear, it is thought to be caused by slowly flowing blood through the extensive vascularity of the lesion or to hemorrhage (100,107). Lesions are typically heterogeneous on T2-weighted images, with a signal intensity much greater than that of fat. Serpentine flow voids, representing enlarged blood vessels, are also usually present (Figs. 12.17, 12.19, and 12.20) (95,100,106,107). These flow voids are noted to be most obvious at the margins of

the lesion (feeding vessels), but may also be present within its substance (Figs. 12.17, 12.19, and 12.20) (95,107). Marked enhancement is seen following administration of intravenous contrast (Fig. 12.18) (109).

The differential diagnosis of lesions with high-flow vascular structures as a prominent feature and solid components by cross-sectional imaging (particularly MR imaging) is limited. Lesions with this appearance include alveolar soft part sarcoma, rhabdomyosarcoma, extraskeletal Ewing sarcoma/ peripheral neuroectodermal tumor (PNET), hemangioendothelioma, hemangiopericytoma, and synovial sarcoma. It is important to understand that biopsy of these lesions may cause extensive bleeding or even exsanguination if vascular control cannot be obtained.

Epithelioid Sarcoma

Epithelioid sarcoma is a distinctive neoplasm with a remarkable predilection for the upper extremity. Initially described in 1970 by Enzinger (109,110), the lesion is often misdiagnosed and may be confused pathologically with granulomatous processes, chronic inflammation, squamous cell carcinoma, synovial sarcoma, or other malignant tumors (111).

The lesion is usually seen in young adults, with almost 75% of 241 patients reported by Chase and Enzinger presenting between 10 and 39 years of age (mean: 27 years) (94). In the decade beginning January 1, 1980, 170 cases were seen by the Department of Soft Tissue Pathology at the AFIP, with a mean of 31 years of age, and 80% presented between 15 and 54 years of age (94,109,110,112). Men are affected more commonly (1.5–2.6:1 ratio) than women (11,12,75,86,113).

Epithelioid sarcoma is most common in the distal upper extremity with approximately 60% occurring in the flexor surfaces of the finger, hand, wrist, and forearm

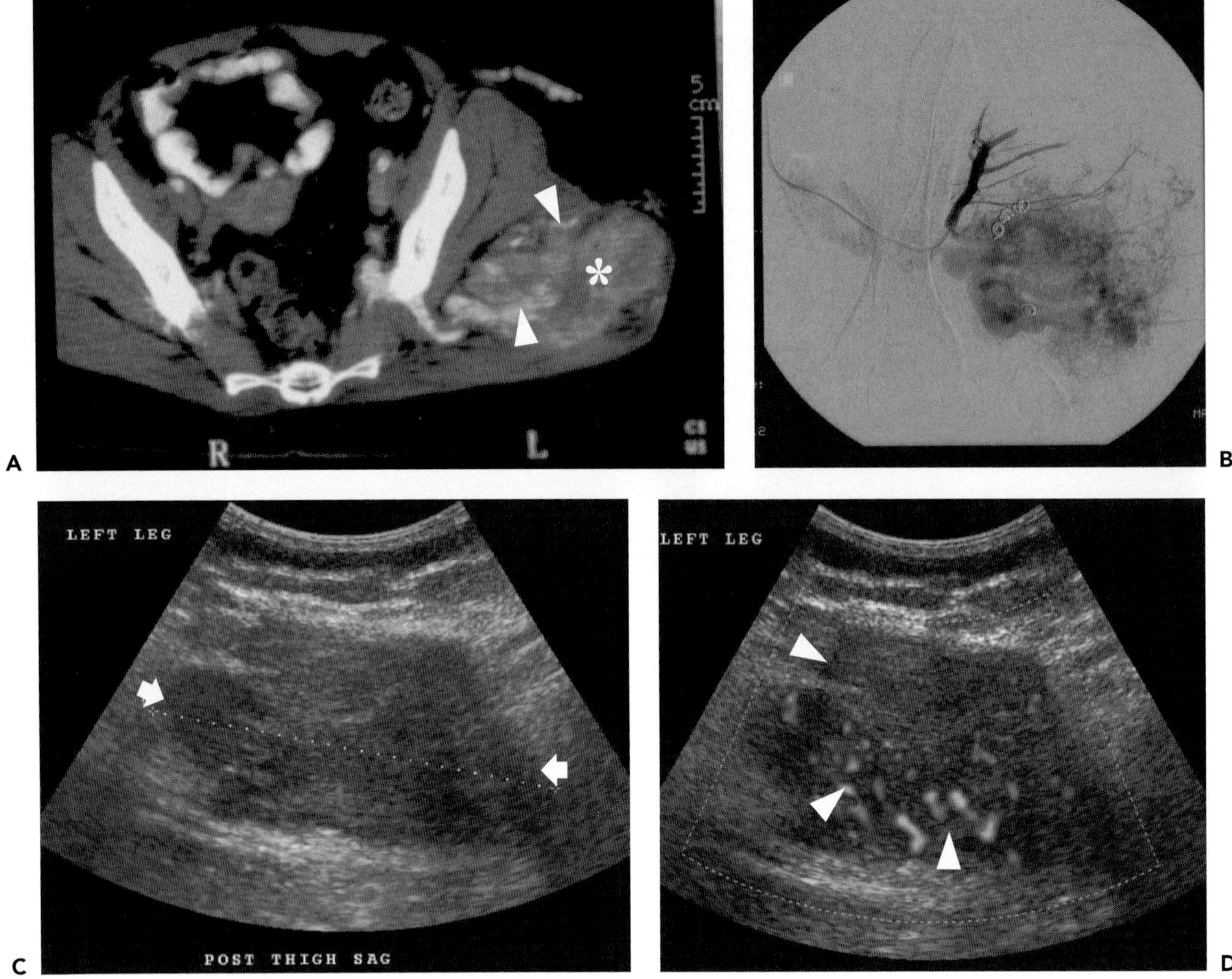

Figure 12.18 Alveolar soft part sarcoma involving the buttock in a woman 38 years of age. **A:** Axial contrast-enhanced CT scan shows a relatively well-defined soft tissue mass (*asterisk*) with serpentine enhancing vascular channels (*arrowheads*). Areas of decreased attenuation correspond to foci of necrosis within the tumor. **B:** Arterial image from a digital subtraction arteriogram shows marked vascularity to the tumor, with extensive neovascularity, tumor blush, and early draining veins. **C,D:** Sonography **(C)** and Doppler study **(D)** also reveal the soft tissue mass (*arrows*) with prominent arterial component (*arrowheads*). (*continued*)

(110–112,114,115). This distribution is confirmed by multiple reports (94). Epithelioid sarcoma is a relatively rare lesion, accounting for only approximately 1.4% of all soft tissue sarcomas, yet in the hand and wrist, it is the most common malignant tumor in the group 6 to 25 years of age, accounting for 21% to 29% of all malignant tumors (111). Locations other than the distal upper extremity include the knee/lower leg (15%), buttocks/thigh (10%), shoulder/arm (9%), and ankle/foot/toes (9%) (111). Rarely, epithelioid sarcoma affects the trunk (6%) or head/neck (4%) (111).

Patients usually present with a firm, hard, palpable mass (solitary or multiple) in the deep soft tissue, subcutaneous tissue or dermis, having a mean duration of symptoms prior to diagnosis of almost 2.5 years (111). Lesions are usually asymptomatic, with pain or tenderness seen in approximately 25% and ulceration in an estimated 10%

(110). Larger lesions and those adherent to tendons or nerves are more likely to be symptomatic (111). A history of trauma is reported in 20% to 25% of patients.

At gross pathologic evaluation, epithelioid sarcoma appears as a tan-white nonencapsulated nodule or nodules, with poorly delineated infiltrating margins and an average size of 3 cm to 6 cm. Deep-seated lesions are often larger and attached to tendons or fascia (3,111). Focal necrosis and hemorrhage may be seen (3). The nodular pattern is a conspicuous pathologic feature of the lesion (3). Areas of chronic inflammation along the tumor periphery are present in most cases. Microscopically, lesions contain a mixture of epithelioid and spindle-shaped cells with deeply eosinophilic cytoplasm, ovoid and indented nuclei, and small amounts of peripheral chromatin (18). Areas of chronic inflammation along the tumor periphery are present

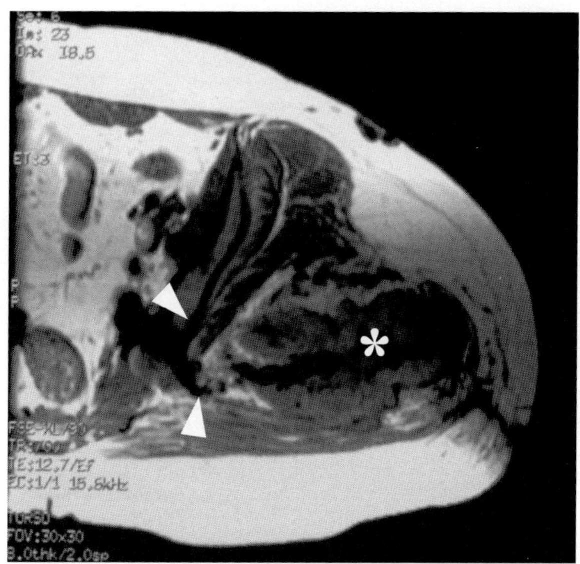

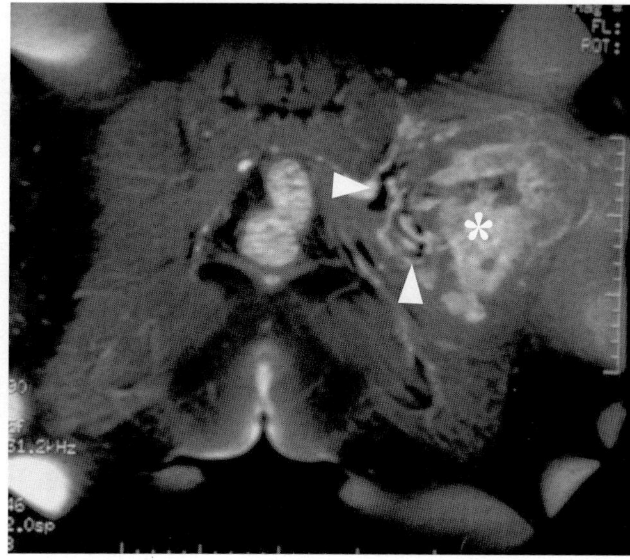

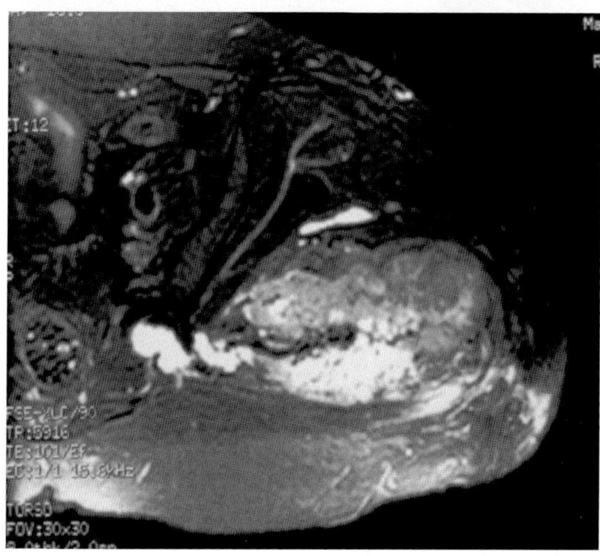

Figure 12.18 *(continued)* **E–G:** Axial T1-weighted (TR/TE; 450/10) **(E)**, coronal enhanced fat-suppressed T1-weighted (TR/TE; 400/9) **(F)**, and axial fat-suppressed proton density (TR/TE; 5216/36) **(G)**, MR images show the large buttocks mass (*asterisk*). Prominent serpentine vascular structures (*arrowheads*) are also seen (both high and low flow) in the mass as well as feeding vessels.

in most cases. Histologic feature associated with a poorer prognosis include nuclear pleomorphism and vascular or nerve invasion (111).

Chase and Enzinger (75,111) noted local tumor recurrence in 155 (77%) of 202 patients. Of patients with recurrence, most had a single recurrence, although two and three local recurrences were also seen. Metastases were found in 45%, and 32% died of their disease (75,111). Metastases are the result of lymphatic and/or hematogenous spread and are most common to lymph nodes (34%) and then, in decreasing order, to the lungs (25%), scalp (22%), bone (13%), brain (13%), liver (12%), and pleura (11%) (111). Prognosis is related to tumor size and location: the more proximal or axial the primary lesion and the larger the tumor, the worse the outcome (116). In general, the survival rate is significantly greater for superficial than for deep lesions (75,111,116). Bos et al. (116) noted that only one (11%) of nine patients with lesions greater than 3 cm at initial examination survived 10 years, whereas 34 (75%) of those with

lesions smaller than 3 cm survived 10 years. Studies have also shown an improved survival in women, with Bos et al. noting an 80% 5-year survival in women, as compared to a 40% 5-year survival in men (116). Hemorrhagic lesions may have a more aggressive course, with Romero et al. (117) noting metastases in two hemorrhagic lesions, but in only 30% of 10 nonhemorrhagic lesions. In this series, metastases appeared earlier in hemorrhagic lesions than in nonhemorrhagic lesions (5 months versus 27.6 months) (112). In reporting the results with 23 patients receiving definitive treatment at the Mayo Clinic, Sim et al. (112) noted an overall 5-year survival rate of 79% and a 10-year survival rate of 73%. This is reduced to 66% and 41%, respectively, following one or more recurrences (115).

Steinberg et al. (115) reported the surgical results in 18 patients and noted that the tumor recurred locally or metastasized after marginal excision in 11 of 12 cases, with or without radiation therapy or chemotherapy, resulting in 5 fatalities. They also noted that all 6 patients treated with

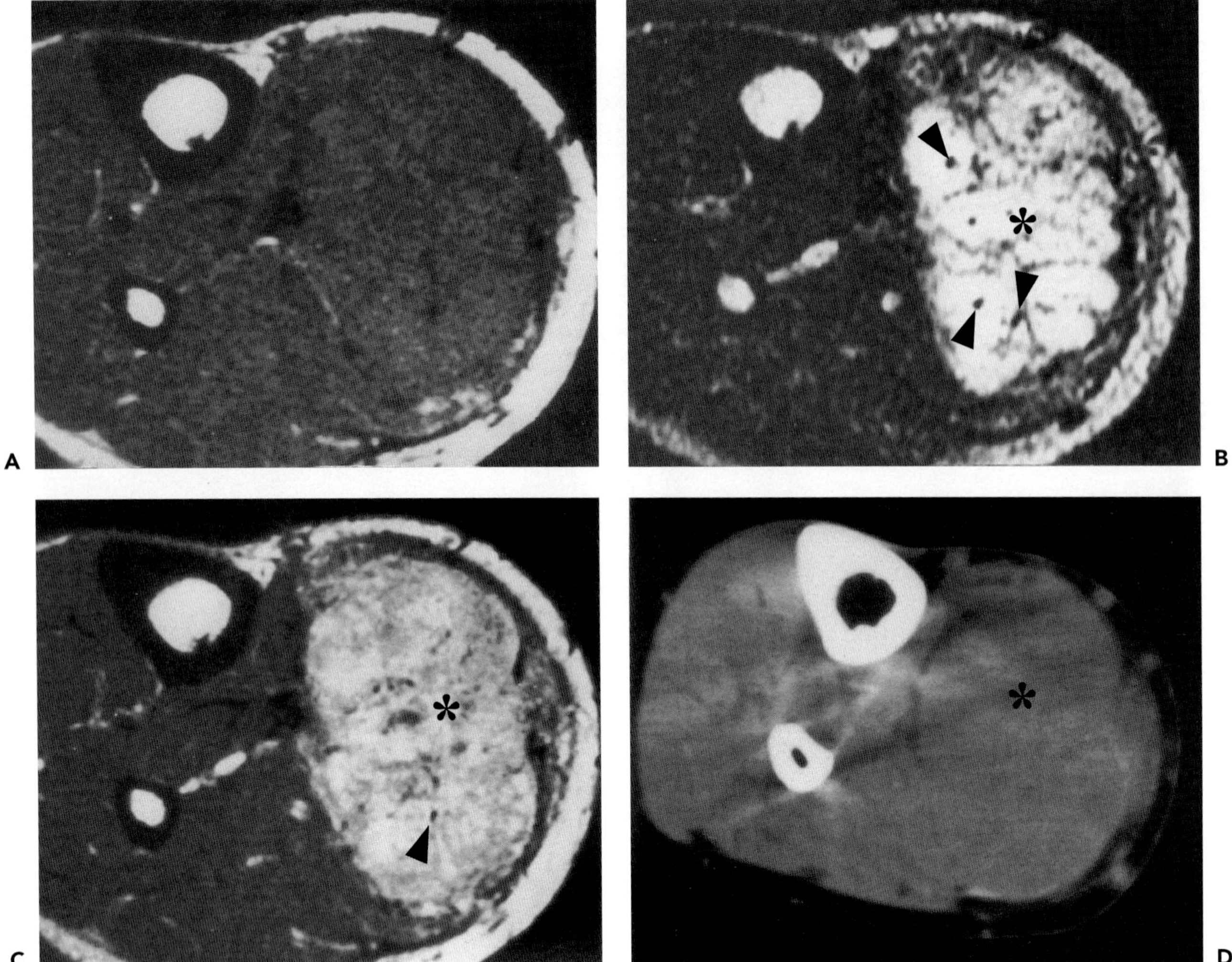

Figure 12.19 Alveolar soft part sarcoma in a man 27 years of age involving the calf. **A,B:** Axial T1-weighted (TR/TE; 400/20) **(A)** and conventional T2-weighted (TR/TE; 2000/80) **(B)** spin-echo MR images show a relatively well-defined intramuscular soft tissue mass (*asterisk*). The tumor is heterogeneous on the T2-weighted image, with a signal intensity much greater than that of fat. Circular flow voids, representing enlarged blood vessels, are well seen on the T2-weighted image B (*arrowheads*). **C:** Corresponding axial T1-weighted (TR/TE; 400/20) spin-echo MR image following contrast administration shows marked enhancement. **D:** Axial contrast-enhanced CT shows an attenuation equal to that of skeletal muscle (*asterisk*). Margins are not defined. (*continued*)

wide or radical resection survived, although 1 had local recurrence and 1 had metastases (mean follow-up: 7 years) (115). In this series, wide or radical resection proved to be effective treatment for recurrent lesions, with 5 of 7 patients surviving without further recurrence or metastases (average follow-up: 4.7 years) (112). However, overall multiple local recurrences are common. In general, wide or radical resection or amputation is indicated for this tumor because of its tendency to spread along tendon sheaths, fascial layers, and lymphatics (111). Regional lymph node dissection should also be performed.

Radiographs are often normal or may show a nonspecific soft tissue mass (Figs. 12.21 and 12.22). Chase and Enzinger (114,117) noted speckled radiographic calcification or rarely, ossification in 68 (28%) of 241 lesions

(Fig. 12.21). Calcification has also been noted in other smaller studies, although in a lower percentage of patients (8% to 19%) (118,119). Tateishi et al. reported calcification in 20% of cases by CT (118). Remodeling of the adjacent bone is infrequently reported, as direct osseous extension and periosteal reaction (118). Lo et al. (114) reported the results of lymphangiography in three patients, noting that it was unreliable in differentiating hyperplastic enlarged nodes from tumor in two patients (114).

Romero et al. (83,120–124) reviewed the MR characteristics of epithelioid sarcoma in 12 patients (Figs. 12.21–12.23). They noted that lesions generally had a nonspecific appearance. These lesions were characterized as homogeneous and isointense to muscle on T1-weighted images and heterogeneous and hyperintense to muscle on

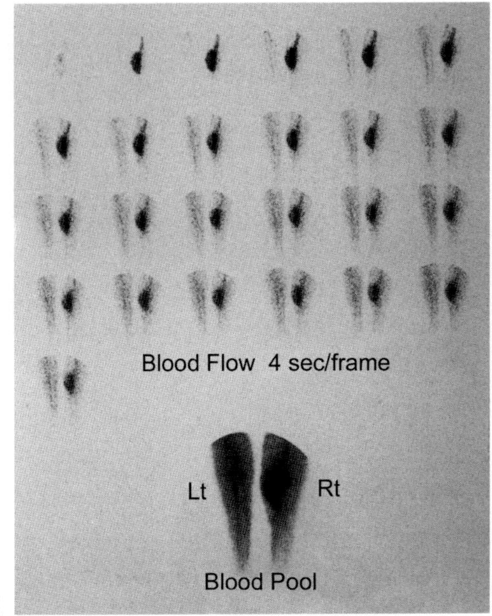

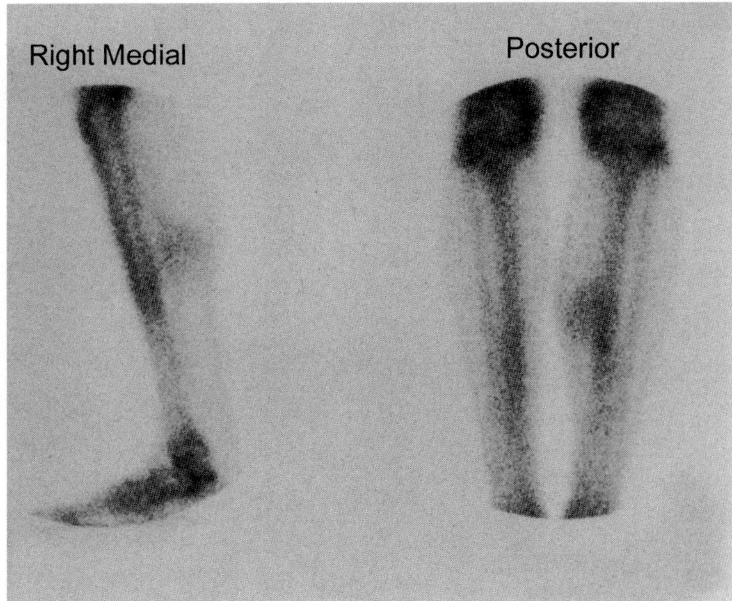

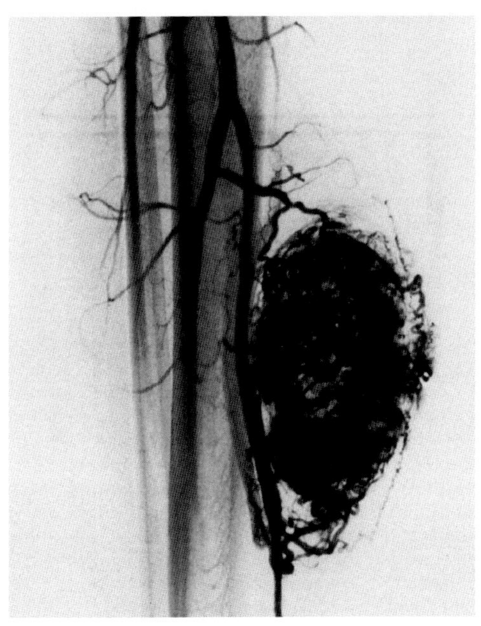

Figure 12.19 *(continued)* **E,F:** Flow and blood-pool **(E)** and delayed static **(F)** images from a technetium-99m bone scan shows marked tracer accumulation. **G:** Subtraction radiograph from an arteriogram shows a markedly hypervascular mass with large, tortuous, feeding arteries, numerous venous lakes, and large early-draining veins.

T2-weighted images (Figs. 12.21–12.23) (117). In our experience, extension along fascial planes and surrounding edema may also be seen, reflecting similar features seen pathologically; findings that are unusual in other neoplasms (Figs. 12.21–12.23). This finding was also described by Hanna et al. (125). Hanna et al. also described that two (17%) of the 12 lesions were hemorrhagic, with heterogeneous increased signal intensity on T1-weighted images (Fig. 12.22) (125). Enhancement was observed in all seven nonhemorrhagic cases following intravenous contrast administration (Fig. 12.21) (125). Prominent hemorrhagic regions with fluid levels were reported in a case by Dion et al. (124). Regional lymph node metastases should also be evaluated on CT and MR imaging. Hanna et al. showed regional metastases in 50% of their 8 cases on MR imaging (125).

Malignant Mesenchymoma

A malignant mesenchymoma historically is defined as a malignant soft tissue tumor characterized by the presence of two or more different nonepithelial tissue components in the same neoplasm (126). Fibrosarcoma or malignant fibrous histiocytoma is often present, but does not define the lesion, and two distinct malignant mesenchymal elements are required, exclusive of malignant fibrous tissue (126). The histogenesis of malignant mesenchymoma is unclear, but it likely represents differentiation of undifferentiated mesenchymal elements along multiple malignant cell lines (3).

Review of the literature shows that many of the lesions designated malignant mesenchymoma would probably

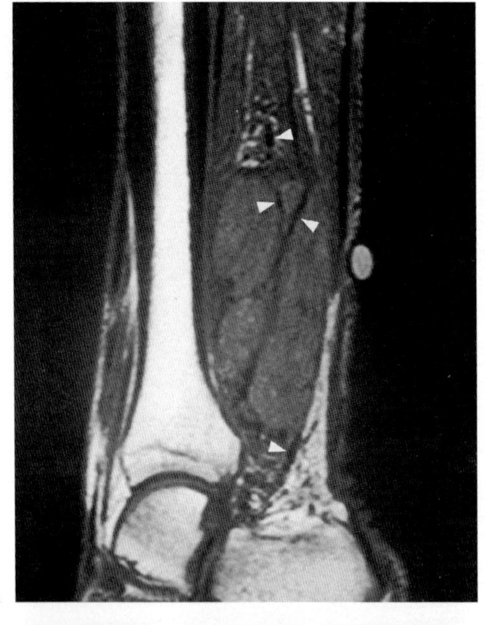

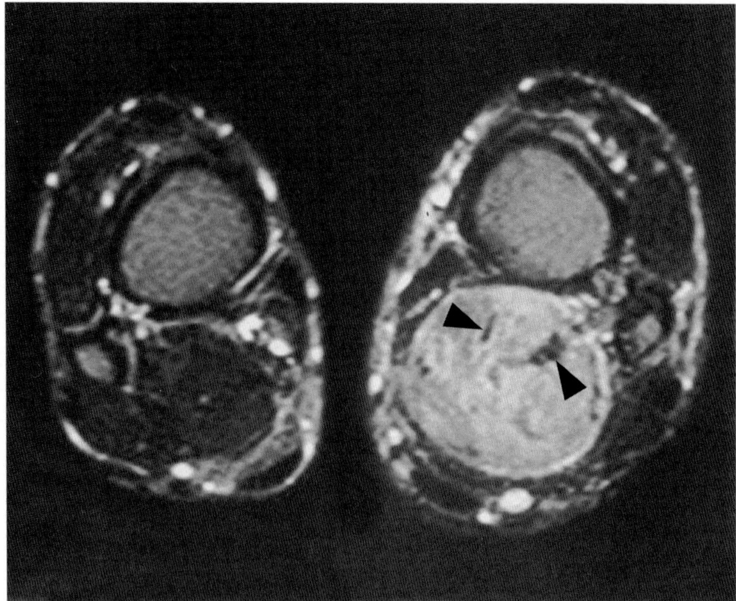

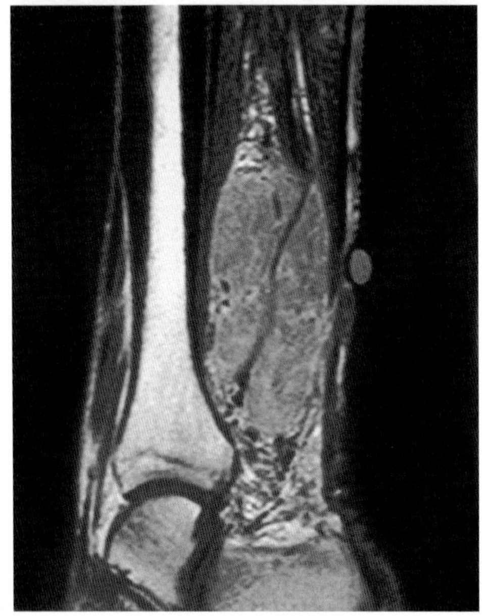

Figure 12.20 Alveolar soft part sarcoma in a man 51 years of age involving the lower calf. **A,B:** Sagittal T1-weighted (TR/TE; 500/16) **(A)** and axial T2-weighted (TR/TE; 2200/80) **(B)** spin-echo MR images show a well-defined intramuscular soft tissue mass. On the T1-weighted image **A**, the lesion shows signal intensity slightly greater than that of skeletal muscle. Note the serpentine flow voids (*arrowheads*), representing enlarged blood vessels, at the superior and inferior aspects of the lesion, as well as within the lesion. **C:** Marked enhancement, with accentuation of associated vascularity, is seen following intravenous contrast administration on the sagittal T1-weighted MR image.

not meet Stout's original diagnostic criteria (3). These lesions are divided into two groups: (a) tumors characterized by the presence of myosarcomatous (rhabdomyosarcoma or leiomyosarcoma) and liposarcomatous elements, often in addition to a fibrosarcomalike spindle cell component, and (b) tumors characterized by the presence of malignant cartilaginous or osseous tissue in addition to a clearly recognizable type of sarcoma. Today, use of the designation of *malignant mesenchymoma* has largely been abandoned by researchers and the WHO. Lesions with this intermixture of tissue are now designated by identifying the various lines of differentiation, as opposed to lumping them together as malignant mesenchymoma. The term *benign mesenchymoma* is used by some soft tissue pathologists to describe a lipoma with cartilage or osseous metaplasia, but this term has also largely been discarded (127).

The imaging appearance of the mesenchymoma (both benign and malignant) is usually nonspecific. MR and CT imaging may reflect the pattern of tumor differentiation and may demonstrate areas of fat, mineralization, and other tissue (Fig. 12.24).

Desmoplastic Small Round Cell Tumor

Desmoplastic small round cell tumor is a malignant tumor that was recognized as a distinct entity by Gerald et al. in 1991 (11,12,74,75). Synonymous terms for this lesion include *intra-abdominal desmoplastic round cell tumor, intra-abdominal desmoplastic round cell tumor with*

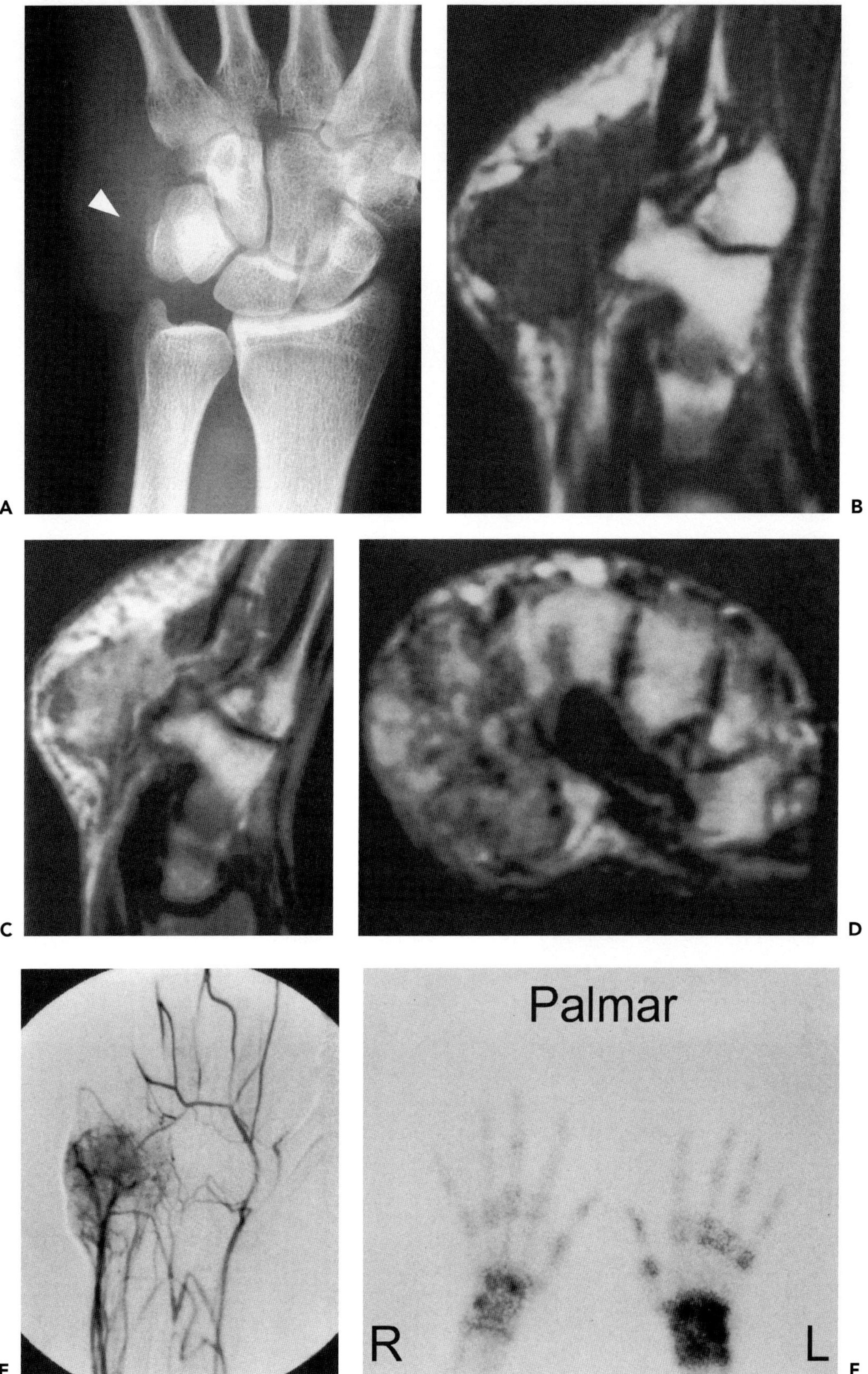

Figure 12.21 Epithelioid sarcoma involving the hand in a man 21 years of age. **A:** Hand radiograph shows a mass in the hypothenar region with subtle calcification (*arrowhead*). **B,C:** Sagittal T1-weighted (TR/TE; 350/15) spin-echo MR images preceding **(B)** and immediately following **(C)** intravenous contrast administration show marked heterogeneous enhancement. The lesion has a signal intensity similar to that of skeletal muscle on precontrast image and is relatively well-delineated from adjacent subcutaneous fat, but not from skeletal muscle. **D:** Axial T2-weighted (TR/TE; 1800/90) MR image shows marked heterogeneity of the lesion, but otherwise nonspecific appearance. Mild surrounding edema is present. **E:** Late arterial phase image from a digital subtraction arteriogram shows prominent tumor blush and early draining veins. **F:** Delayed static image from a technetium-99m bone scan shows diffuse increased tracer accumulation around the wrist, likely caused by hyperemia.

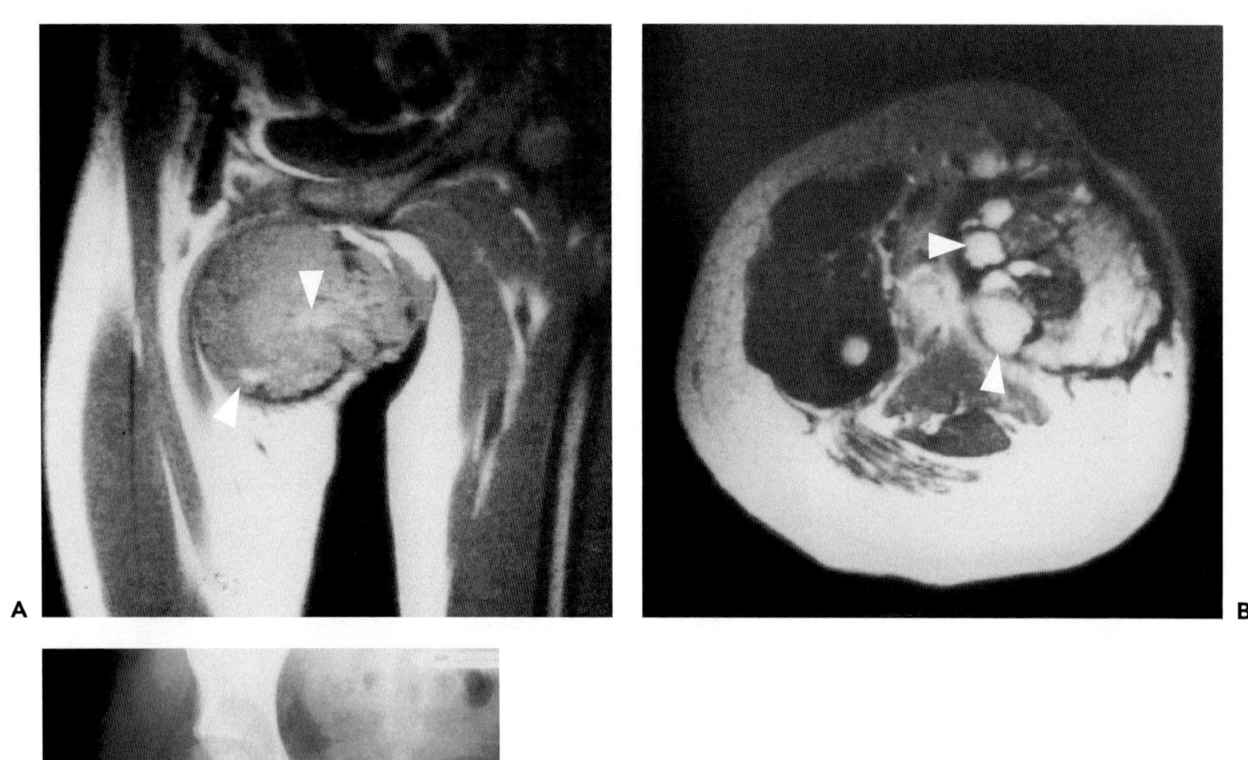

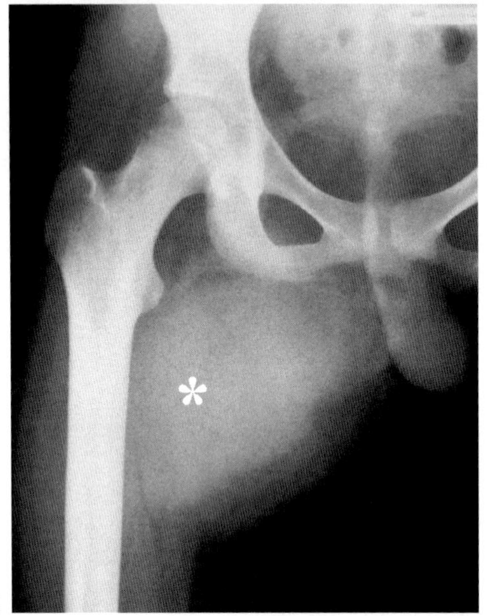

Figure 12.22 Epithelioid sarcoma in a girl 15 years of age in the subcutaneous tissue of the proximal thigh. **A,B:** Coronal T1-weighted (TR/TE; 800/15) **(A)** and axial T2-weighted (TR/TE; 2100/80) **(B)** MR images show a well-defined subcutaneous, heterogeneous mass in the medial aspect of the thigh with areas of hemorrhage (*arrowheads*). **C:** Hip radiograph shows a nonspecific soft tissue mass (*asterisk*).

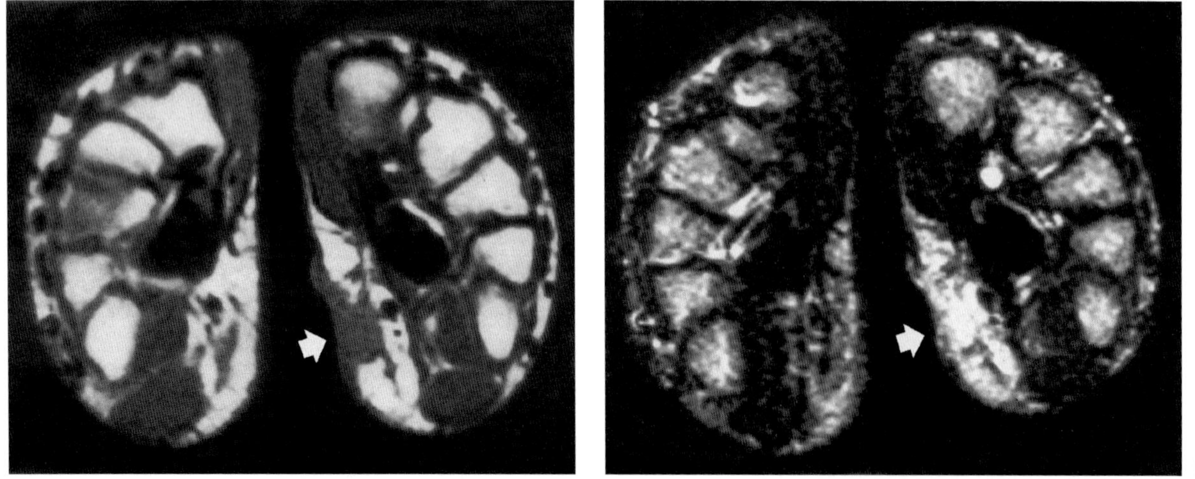

Figure 12.23 Epithelioid sarcoma in a woman 23 years of age involving the foot. **A,B:** Axial T1-weighted (TR/TE; 800/20) **(A)** and T2-weighted (TR/TE; 2200/80) **(B)** MR images show a subcutaneous mass (*arrow*). On the T2-weighted image **(B)**, the lesion is heterogeneous, with a signal intensity higher than that of subcutaneous fat. Margins are well-delineated on the T1-weighted image but there is mild surrounding edema on the long TR image.

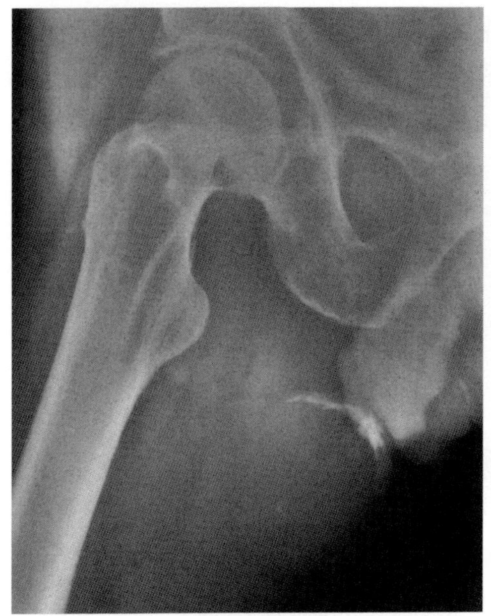

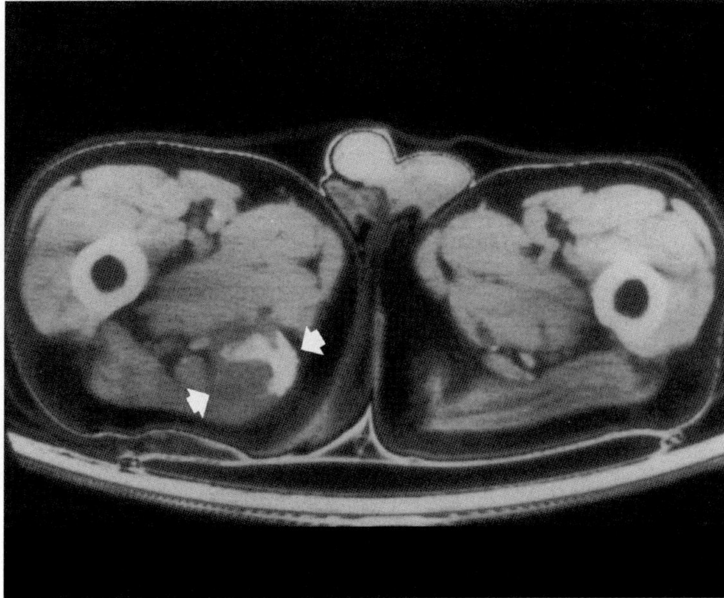

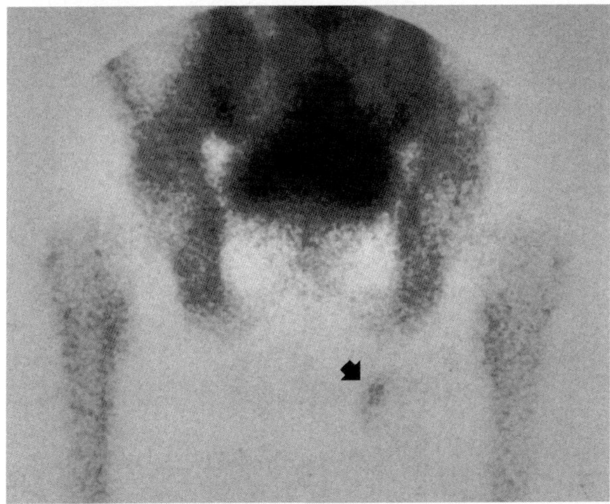

Figure 12.24 Malignant mesenchymoma in the thigh of a man 74 years of age. **A:** Hip radiograph shows a soft tissue mass with peripheral calcification. **B:** Axial noncontrast CT shows a nonspecific soft tissue mass with dense mineralization (*arrows*). **C:** Posterior view from a technetium-99m bone scan shows focal tracer accumulation within a portion of the soft tissue mass (*arrow*).

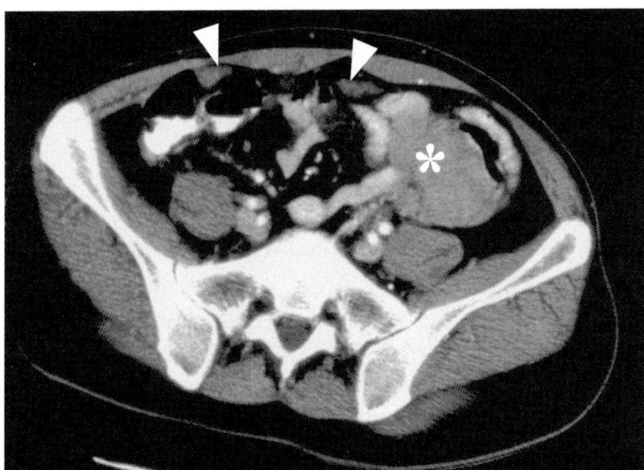

Figure 12.25 Desmoplastic small round cell tumor of the abdomen in a man 37 years of age. Axial CT shows a heterogeneous intra-abdominal soft tissue mass (*asterisk*) with several small serosal implants as well (*arrowheads*).

divergent differentiation, polyphenotypic small round cell tumor, malignant small cell epithelial tumor of the peritoneum, and *intra-abdominal neuroectodermal tumor of childhood* (127–129). Young patients are affected, typically 15 to 35 years of age (mean: 22 years), although there is a wide age range (11,12,74,75). There is a male predilection (3–5:1 ratio) (11,12,130–132). Lesion location is most frequently the abdominal or pelvic peritoneum. Other reported sites of origin include the paratesticular region, ovary, pleura, parotid, hand, and central nervous system (133,134). Clinical symptoms are usually abdominal distention or fullness, a palpable mass, pain, constipation, bowel obstruction, ascites, difficulty with urination or obstruction, and impotence (135,136).

At gross pathologic evaluation, desmoplastic small round cell tumors are often large (usually 2 to 15 cm) with multiple nodules along the peritoneal surfaces. Microscopically,

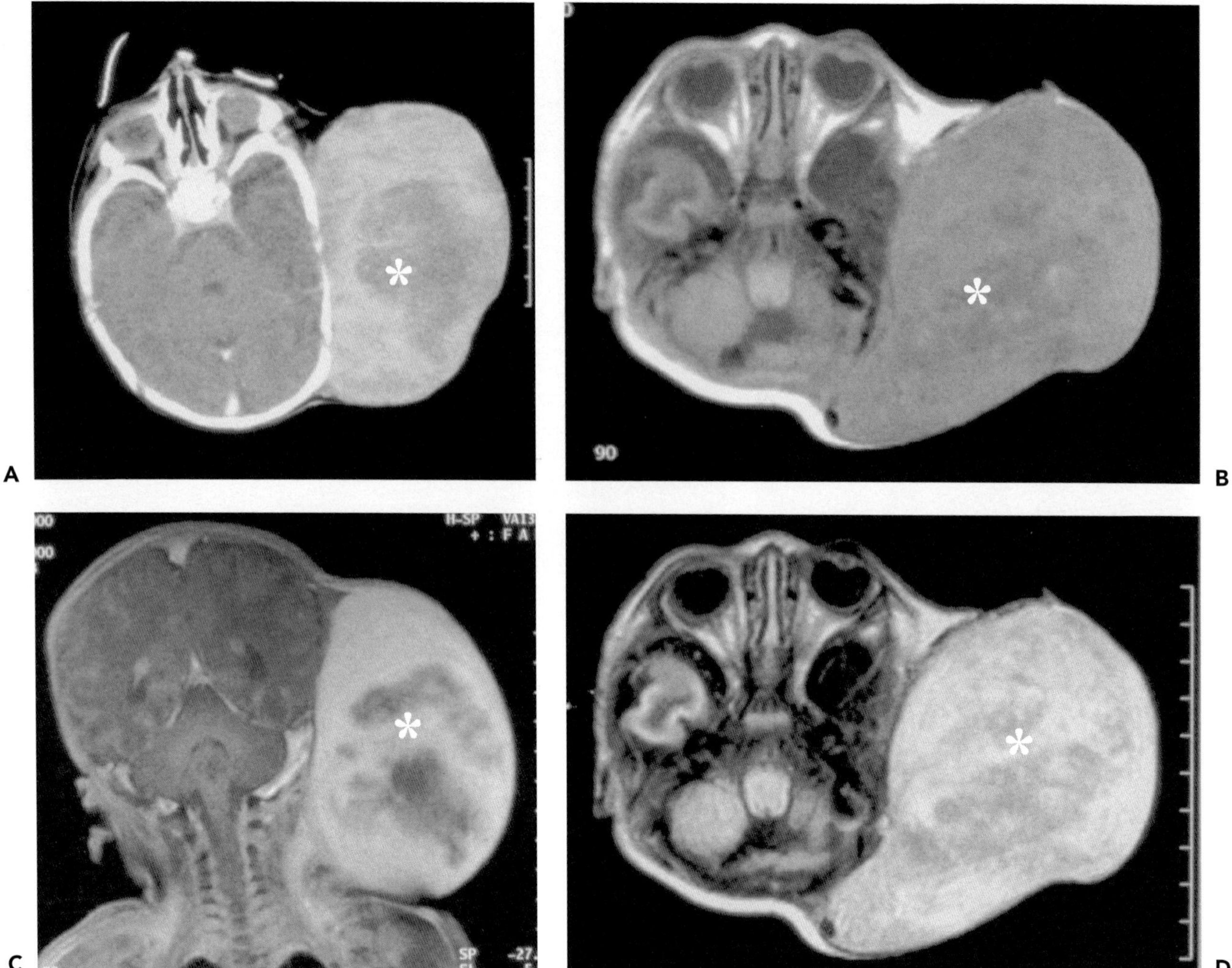

Figure 12.26 Extrarenal rhabdoid tumor in a man 21 years of age involving the head and neck. **A:** Axial CT shows a large soft tissue mass (*asterisk*) adjacent to the calvarium with central lower attenuation resulting from necrosis. **B–D:** Axial T1-weighted (TR/TE; 763/17) **(B)**, enhanced fat-suppressed coronal T1-weighted (TR/TE; 511/17) **(C)** and axial T2-weighted (TR/TE; 7000/105) **(D)** MR imges show a large heterogeneous soft tissue mass (*asterisk*). The lesion is intermediate signal intensity on T1-weighting and high signal intensity on T2-weighting. There is moderate diffuse enhancement except for central areas of necrosis.

these lesions are composed of nests of small round cells within a hypervascular, desmoplastic stroma (137–140). Necrosis is common. Desmoplastic small round cell tumors are characterized by a specific cytogenetic aberration consisting of the t(11;22) (p13;q12) translocation (141–145).

These highly aggressive tumors demonstrate a very poor prognosis despite multimodal therapy, including surgery, chemotherapy, and radiation therapy (146,147). Surgical excision often consists of debulking of the tumor because of its large size and location. Multiple series show mortality rates ranging from 41% to 75%. Newer multimodal therapies have improved 3-year survival to 58%. Metastases most commonly affect the lymph nodes, liver, spleen, lung, pleura, and bone.

Radiographs of desmoplastic round cell tumors usually demonstrate displacement of normal abdominal or pelvic structures without other abnormality. Sonography is described as demonstrating well-defined, hypoechoic soft tissue masses. CT shows multiple peritoneal soft tissue masses without an apparent visceral origin (Fig. 12.25) (146,148,149). In the study by Pickhardt et al., there was an average of 4.4 masses per patient with an average size of 5 cm (Fig. 12.25) (146,147). Areas of low attenuation, representing necrosis are common (75% to 78% of cases) (146,147). Small foci of calcification (22% of cases) may also be seen on CT (146,148,149). The primary site is usually dominant in size compared to the other peritoneal lesions on CT of MR imaging (Fig. 12.25). MR imaging reveals soft tissue masses that are low-to-intermediate signal intensity on T1-weighting and heterogeneous high signal intensity on T2-weighting (150). Areas of cyst formation and fluid levels, representing hemorrhage, were described in the study by Tateishi et al. (150). Heterogeneous mild-to-moderate contrast enhancement may be seen on CT or MR imaging, with nonenhancing central areas resulting from necrosis (146–150). Metastases to the liver, which may show calcification (50% of cases), bone, and pleura, may also be seen (11,12,74,75).

Extrarenal Rhabdoid Tumor

Extrarenal rhabdoid tumor is a rare, malignant tumor occurring in a site outside the kidney. These tumors show histologic similarity to lesions arising in the kidney (sarcomatous variant of Wilm tumor) (151). The age group affected is wide, although the vast majority of lesions occur in infants and children (152–154). Congenital and familial cases are also described (11,12, 74,75,155–159). Extrarenal rhabdoid tumors in the soft tissue are most frequently deep-seated, affecting the trunk (29%), extremities (25%), head and neck (15%, particularly the paraspinal area), and the abdomen, pelvis, and retroperitoneum (20%) (155–159). Guillou et al. described a proximal type epithelioid sarcoma with rhabdoid features that likely represents a variant of extrarenal rhabdoid tumor (160). Cutaneous lesions are also described. The clinical presentation is usually that of a rapidly growing soft tissue mass. Coexistent PNET of the central nervous system has also been reported (161,162).

At gross pathologic examination, extrarenal rhabdoid tumors are usually smaller than 5 cm and nonencapsulated. Microscopically, lesions consist of sheets of discohesive large polygonal cells. Mitoses are frequent, as is hemorrhage and necrosis. Extrarenal rhabdoid tumors frequently demonstrate cytogenetic aberrations with deletion at 22q11 and translocations at chromosome 22 (11,151,155).

The prognosis of extrarenal rhabdoid tumors is dismal. Despite multimodal aggressive therapy (surgical excision and chemotherapy), 5-year survival is less than 50%. Metastatic sites include the lungs, regional lymph nodes, and serosal surfaces.

Imaging of extrarenal rhabdoid tumors is only rarely reported (11,151,155). We would expect cross-sectional imaging to depict a soft tissue mass with nonspecific intrinsic features (Fig. 12.26). However, as with other soft tissue malignancies, imaging is helpful in the staging of these lesions.

REFERENCES

1. Miettinen M. Cartilage- and bone-forming tumor and tumor-like lesions. In: *Diagnostic Soft Tissue Pathology.* New York: Churchill Livingstone, 2003;403–425.
2. Enzinger F, Weiss SW. Benign soft tissue tumors and pseudotumors of miscellaneous type. In: Weiss SW, Goldblum JR, eds. *Soft Tissue Tumors.* 4th ed. St. Louis: Mosby; 2001:1419–1483.
3. Enzinger F, Weiss S, Goldblum J. *Enzinger and Weiss's Soft Tissue Tumors.* 4th ed. St. Louis: Mosby; 2001.
4. Inclan A, Leon P, Camejo M. Tumoral calcinosis. *JAMA.* 1942;21:490–495.
5. Martinez S, Vogler JB III, Harrelson JM, et al. Imaging of tumoral calcinosis: new observations. *Radiology.* 1990;174:215–222.
6. Slavin RE, Wen J, Kumar D, et al. Familial tumoral calcinosis. A clinical, histopathologic, and ultrastructural study with an analysis of its calcifying process and pathogenesis. *Am J Surg Pathol.* 1993;17:788–802.
7. Chew FS, Crenshaw WB. Idiopathic tumoral calcinosis. *AJR Am J Roentgenol.* 1992;158:330.
8. Geirnaerdt MJ, Kroon HM, van der Heul RO, et al. Tumoral calcinosis. *Skeletal Radiol.* 1995;24:148–151.
9. Steinbach LS, Johnston JO, Tepper EF, et al. Tumoral calcinosis: radiologic-pathologic correlation. *Skeletal Radiol.* 1995;24:573–578.
10. Stout A. Myxoma, the tumor of primitive mesenchyme. *Ann Surg.* 1948;127:706–719.
11. Fletcher C, Unni K, Mertens F. *World Health Organization Classification of tumors. Pathology and Genetics of Tumors of Soft Tissue and Bone.* Lyon, France: IARC Press; 2002.
12. Kempson R, Fletcher C, Evans H, Hendrickson M, et al. Tumors of uncertain differentiation and those in which differentiation is nonmesenchymal. In: Rosai J, ed. *Tumors of the Soft Tissues.* 3rd ed. Bethesda, MD: Armed Forces Institute of Pathology; 2001:419–501.
13. Miettinen M. Benign fibroblastic and myofibroblastic proliferations. In: *Diagnostic Soft Tissue Pathology.* New York: Churchill Livingstone; 2003:143–172.
14. Enzinger FM. Intramuscular myxoma: a review and follow-up study of 34 cases. *Am J Clin Pathol.* 1965;43:104–113.
15. Murphey MD, McRae GA, Fanburg-Smith JC, et al. Imaging of soft-tissue myxoma with emphasis on CT and MR and comparison of radiologic and pathologic findings. *Radiology.* 2002;225:215–224.
16. Ireland DC, Soule EH, Ivins JC. Myxoma of somatic soft tissues. A report of 58 patients, 3 with multiple tumors and fibrous dysplasia of bone. *Mayo Clin Proc.* 1973;48:401–410.
17. Kindblom LG, Stener B, Angervall L. Intramuscular myxoma. *Cancer.* 1974;34:1737–1744.
18. Miettinen M, Hockerstedt K, Reitamo J, et al. Intramuscular myxoma—a clinicopathological study of twenty-three cases. *Am J Clin Pathol.* 1985;84:265–272.
19. Kransdorf MJ, Moser RP Jr, Jelinek JS, et al. Intramuscular myxoma: MR features. *J Comput Assist Tomogr.* 1989;13:836–839.
20. Sundaram M, McDonald DJ, Merenda G. Intramuscular myxoma: a rare but important association with fibrous dysplasia of bone. *AJR Am J Roentgenol.* 1989;153:107–108.
21. Caraway NP, Staerkel GA, Fanning CV, et al. Diagnosing intramuscular myxoma by fine-needle aspiration: a multidisciplinary approach. *Diagn Cytopathol.* 1994;11:255–261.
22. Nielsen GP, O'Connell JX, Rosenberg AE. Intramuscular myxoma: a clinicopathologic study of 51 cases with emphasis on hypercellular and hypervascular variants. *Am J Surg Pathol.* 1998;22:1222–1227.
23. Abdelwahab AF, Kenan S, Hermann G, et al. Intramuscular myxoma: magnetic resonance features. *Br J Radiol.* 1992;65:485–490.
24. Ekelund L, Herrlin K, Rydholm A. Computed tomography of intramuscular myxoma. *Skeletal Radiol.* 1982;9:14–16.
25. Hashimoto H, Tsuneyoshi M, Daimaru Y, et al. Intramuscular myxoma. A clinicopathologic, immunohistochemical, and electron microscopic study. *Cancer.* 1986;58:740–747.
26. Shugar JM, Som PM, Meyers RJ, et al. Intramuscular head and neck myxoma: report of a case and review of the literature. *Laryngoscope.* 1987;97:105–107.
27. Silver WP, Harrelson JM, Scully SP. Intramuscular myxoma: a clinicopathologic study of 17 patients. *Clin Orthop.* 2002; 403:191–197.
28. McCook TA, Martinez S, Korobkin M, et al. Intramuscular myxoma. Radiographic and computed tomographic findings with pathologic correlation. *Skeletal Radiol.* 1981;7:15–19.
29. Pettersson H, Hudson TM, Springfield DS, et al. Cystic intramuscular myxoma. Report of a case. *Acta Radiol Diagn (Stockh).* 1985;26:425–426.
30. Fornage BD, Romsdahl MM. Intramuscular myxoma: sonographic appearance and sonographically guided needle biopsy. *J Ultrasound Med.* 1994;13:91–94.

31. Fontana M, Capanna R, Gigli F. Intramuscular myxoma: value of MR imaging. *Eur Radiol.* 1993;3:258–260.

32. Lindahl S, Markhede G, Berlin O. Computed tomography of lipomatous and myxoid tumors. *Acta Radiol Diagn (Stockh).* 1985;26:709–713.

33. Ly JQ, Bau JL, Beall DP. Forearm intramuscular myxoma. *AJR Am J Roentgenol.* 2003;181:960.

34. Schwartz HS, Walker R. Recognizable magnetic resonance imaging characteristics of intramuscular myxoma. *Orthopedics.* 1997;20: 431–435.

35. Abdelwahab IF, Kenan S, Hermann G, et al. Intramuscular myxoma of the left forearm. *Bull Hosp Jt Dis.* 1993;53:15–17.

36. Bancroft LW, Kransdorf MJ, Menke DM, et al. Intramuscular myxoma: characteristic MR imaging features. *AJR Am J Roentgenol.* 2002;178:1255–1259.

37. Iwasko N, Steinbach LS, Disler D, et al. Imaging findings in Mazabraud's syndrome: seven new cases. *Skeletal Radiol.* 2002;31: 81–87.

38. Luna A, Martinez S, Bossen E. Magnetic resonance imaging of intramuscular myxoma with histological comparison and a review of the literature. *Skeletal Radiol.* 2005;34:19–28.

39. Nishimoto K, Kusuzaki K, Matsumine A, et al. Surrounding muscle edema detected by MRI is valuable for diagnosis of intramuscular myxoma. *Oncol Rep.* 2004;11:143–148.

40. May DA, Good RB, Smith DK, et al. MR imaging of musculoskeletal tumors and tumor mimickers with intravenous gadolinium: experience with 242 patients. *Skeletal Radiol.* 1997; 26:2–15.

41. Peterson KK, Renfrew DL, Feddersen RM, et al. Magnetic resonance imaging of myxoid containing tumors. *Skeletal Radiol.* 1991;20:245–250.

42. Henschen F. Fall von Ostitis Fibrosa mit multiplen tumoren in der umghebenden muskulatur. *Veh Dtsch Ges Pathol.* 1926;21: 93–97.

43. Mazabraud A, Semat P, Roze R. Apropos of the association of fibromyxomas of the soft tissues with fibrous dysplasia of the bones [in French]. *Presse Med.* 1967;75:2223–2228.

44. Aoki T, Kouho H, Hisaoka M, et al. Intramuscular myxoma with fibrous dysplasia: a report of two cases with a review of the literature. *Pathol Int.* 1995;45:165–171.

45. Cabral CE, Guedes P, Fonseca T, et al. Polyostotic fibrous dysplasia associated with intramuscular myxomas: Mazabraud's syndrome. *Skeletal Radiol.* 1998;27:278–282.

46. Court-Payen M, Ingemann Jensen L, Bjerregaard B, et al. Intramuscular myxoma and fibrous dysplasia of bone—Mazabraud's syndrome. A case report. *Acta Radiol.* 1997;38: 368–371.

47. Delabrousse E, Couvreur M, Bartholomot B, et al. [Mazabraud syndrome: a case diagnosed with MRI] Article in French. *J Radiol.* 2001;82:165–167.

48. Fujii K, Inoue M, Araki Y, et al. Multiple intramuscular myxomas associated with polyostotic fibrous dysplasia. *Eur J Radiol.* 1996;22:152–154.

49. Gober GA, Nicholas RW. Case report 800: skeletal fibrous dysplasia associated with intramuscular myxoma (Mazabraud's syndrome). *Skeletal Radiol.* 1993;22:452–455.

50. Walker RE, Schwartz RK, Gale DR. Musculoskeletal case of the day. Mazabraud's syndrome (intramuscular myxomas associated with fibrous dysplasia of bone). *AJR Am J Roentgenol.* 1999;173: 797,800–802.

51. Kransdorf MJ, Murphey MD. Diagnosis please. Case 12: Mazabraud syndrome. *Radiology.* 1999;212:129–132.

52. Wirth WA, Leavitt D, Enzinger FM. Multiple intramuscular myxomas. Another extraskeletal manifestation of fibrous dysplasia. *Cancer.* 1971;27:1167–1173.

53. Witkin GB, Guilford WB, Siegal GP. Osteogenic sarcoma and soft tissue myxoma in a patient with fibrous dysplasia and hemoglobins. *Clin Orthop.* 1986;204:245–252.

54. Lopez-Ben R, Pitt MJ, Jaffe KA, et al. Osteosarcoma in a patient with McCune-Albright syndrome and Mazabraud's syndrome. *Skeletal Radiol.* 1999;28:522–526.

55. Carney JA. Carney complex: the complex of myxomas, spotty pigmentation, endocrine overactivity, and schwannomas. *Semin Dermatol.* 1995;14:90–98.

56. Meis JM, Enzinger FM. Juxta-articular myxoma: a clinical and pathologic study of 65 cases. *Hum Pathol.* 1992;23:639–646.

57. King DG, Saifuddin A, Preston HV, et al. Magnetic resonance imaging of juxta-articular myxoma. *Skeletal Radiol.* 1995;24: 145–147.

58. Steeper TA, Rosai J. Aggressive angiomyxoma of the female pelvis and perineum. Report of nine cases of a distinctive type of gynecologic soft-tissue neoplasm. *Am J Surg Pathol.* 1983;7:463–475.

59. Hong RD, Outwater E, Gomella LG. Aggressive angiomyxoma of the perineum in a man. *J Urol.* 1997;157:959–960.

60. Iezzoni JC, Fechner RE, Wong LS, et al. Aggressive angiomyxoma in males. A report of four cases. *Am J Clin Pathol.* 1995;104: 391–396.

61. Miettinen M. Gynecologic stomal tumors. In: *Diagnostic Soft Tissue Pathology.* New York: Churchill Livingstone; 2003; 271–285.

62. Granter SR, Nucci MR, Fletcher CD. Aggressive angiomyxoma: reappraisal of its relationship to angiomyofibroblastoma in a series of 16 cases. *Histopathology.* 1997;30:3–10.

63. Begin LR, Clement PB, Kirk ME, et al. Aggressive angiomyxoma of pelvic soft parts: a clinicopathologic study of nine cases. *Hum Pathol.* 1985;16:621–628.

64. Smith HO, Worrell RV, Smith AY, et al. Aggressive angiomyxoma of the female pelvis and perineum: review of the literature. *Gynecol Oncol.* 1991;42:79–85.

65. Tsang WY, Chan JK, Lee KC, et al. Aggressive angiomyxoma. A report of four cases occurring in men. *Am J Surg Pathol.* 1992;16: 1059–1065.

66. Steiner E, Schadmand-Fischer S, Schunk K, et al. Perineal excision of a large angiomyxoma in a young woman following magnetic resonance and angiographic imaging. *Gynecol Oncol.* 2001;82:568–570.

67. Catalano O. Case report: aggressive angiomyxoma of the pelvic soft tissues: US and CT findings. *Clin Radiol.* 1998;53:782–783.

68. Cesarani F, Garretti L, Denegri F, et al. Sonographic appearance of aggressive angiomyxoma of the bladder. *J Clin Ultrasound.* 1999;27:399–401.

69. Chien AJ, Freeby JA, Win TT, et al. Aggressive angiomyxoma of the female pelvis: sonographic, CT, and MR findings. *AJR Am J Roentgenol.* 1998;171:530–531.

70. De la Ossa M, Castellano-Sanchez A, Alvarez E, et al. Sonographic appearance of aggressive angiomyxoma of the scrotum. *J Clin Ultrasound.* 2001;29:476–478.

71. Yaghoobian J, Zinn D, Ramanathan K, et al. Ultrasound and computed tomographic findings in aggressive angiomyxoma of the uterine cervix. *J Ultrasound Med.* 1987;6:209–212.

72. Outwater EK, Marchetto BE, Wagner BJ, et al. Aggressive angiomyxoma: findings on CT and MR imaging. *AJR Am J Roentgenol.* 1999;172:435–438.

73. Kobayashi Y, Minami M, Ohtomo K, et al. MR imaging and CT appearances of aggressive angiomyxoma. *AJR Am J Roentgenol.* 1997;169:1752–1753.

74. Miettinen M. *Small Round Cell Tumors.* New York: Churchill Livingstone; 2003.

75. Enzinger F, Weiss SW. Malignant soft tissue tumors of uncertain type. In: *Soft Tissue Tumors.* 4th ed. St. Louis: Mosby; 2001; 1483–1572.

76. Dabska M. Parachordoma: a new clinicopathologic entity. *Cancer.* 1977;40:1586–1592.

77. Karabela-Bouropoulou V, Skourtas C, Liapi-Avgeri G, et al. Parachordoma. A case report of a very rare soft tissue tumor. *Pathol Res Pract.* 1996;192:972–978; discussion 979–981.

78. Imlay SP, Argenyi ZB, Stone MS, et al. Cutaneous parachordoma. A light microscopic and immunohistochemical report of two cases and review of the literature. *J Cutan Pathol.* 1998;25: 279–284.

79. Ishida T, Oda H, Oka T, et al. Parachordoma: an ultrastructural and immunohistochemical study. *Virchows Arch A Pathol Anat Histopathol.* 1993;422:239–245.

80. Fisher C, Miettinen M. Parachordoma: a clinicopathologic and immunohistochemical study of four cases of an unusual soft tissue neoplasm. *Ann Diagn Pathol.* 1997;1:3–10.

81. Folpe AL, Agoff SN, Willis J, et al. Parachordoma is immunohistochemically and cytogenetically distinct from axial chordoma

and extraskeletal myxoid chondrosarcoma. *Am J Surg Pathol.* 1999;23:1059–1067.

82. Abe S, Imamura T, Harasawa A, et al. Parachordoma with multiple metastases. *J Comput Assist Tomogr.* 2003;27:634–638.

83. Hanley SD, Alexander N, Henderson DW, et al. Epithelioid sarcoma of the forearm. *Australas Radiol.* 1996;40:254–256.

84. Fetsch JF, Weiss SW. Ectopic hamartomatous thymoma: clinicopathologic, immunohistochemical, and histogenetic considerations in four new cases. *Hum Pathol.* 1990;21:662–668.

85. Zhao C, Yamada T, Kuramochi S, et al. Two cases of ectopic hamartomatous thymoma. *Virchows Arch.* 2000;437:643–647.

86. Miettinen M. Soft tissue tumors with epithelial differentiation. In: *Diagnostic Soft Tissue Pathology.* New York: Churchill Livingstone; 2003:463–487.

87. Henderson CJ, Gupta L. Ectopic hamartomatous thymoma: a case study and review of the literature. *Pathology.* 2000;32:142–146.

88. Saeed IT, Fletcher CD. Ectopic hamartomatous thymoma containing myxoid cells. *Histopathology.* 1990;17:572–574.

89. Rosai J, Limas C, Husband EM. Ectopic hamartomatous thymoma. A distinctive benign lesion of lower neck. *Am J Surg Pathol.* 1984;8:501–513.

90. Michal M, Zamecnik M, Gogora M, et al. Pitfalls in the diagnosis of ectopic hamartomatous thymoma. *Histopathology.* 1996;29:549–555.

91. Eulderink F, de Graaf PW. Ectopic hamartomatous thymoma located presternally. *Eur J Surg.* 1998;164:629–630.

92. Smetana HF, Scott WF Jr. Malignant tumors of nonchromaffin paraganglia. *Mil Surg.* 1951;109:330–349.

93. Christopherson WM, Foote FW Jr, Stewart FW. Alveolar soft-part sarcomas; structurally characteristic tumors of uncertain histogenesis. *Cancer.* 1952;5:100–111.

94. Kransdorf MJ. Malignant soft-tissue tumors in a large referral population: distribution of diagnoses by age, sex, and location. *AJR Am J Roentgenol.* 1995;164:129–134.

95. Temple HT, Scully SP, O'Keefe RJ, et al. Clinical presentation of alveolar soft-part sarcoma. *Clin Orthop.* 1994;300:213–218.

96. Miettinen M. Miscellaneous soft tissue tumors of unknown histogenesis. In: *Diagnostic Soft Tissue Pathology.* New York: Churchill Livingstone; 2003:489–503.

97. Lieberman PH, Brennan MF, Kimmel M, et al. Alveolar soft-part sarcoma. A clinico-pathologic study of half a century. *Cancer.* 1989;63:1–13.

98. Hermann G, Abdelwahab IF, Klein MJ, et al. Case report 796. Alveolar soft part sarcoma. *Skeletal Radiol.* 1993;22:386–389.

99. Lorigan JG, O'Keeffe FN, Evans HL, et al. The radiologic manifestations of alveolar soft-part sarcoma. *AJR Am J Roentgenol.* 1989;153:335–339.

100. Daly BD, Cheung H, Gaines PA, et al. Imaging of alveolar soft part sarcoma. *Clin Radiol.* 1992;46:253–256.

101. Auerbach HE, Brooks JJ. Alveolar soft part sarcoma. A clinicopathologic and immunohistochemical study. *Cancer.* 1987;60:66–73.

102. Evans HL. Alveolar soft-part sarcoma. A study of 13 typical examples and one with a histologically atypical component. *Cancer.* 1985;55:912–917.

103. Foschini MP, Eusebi V. Alveolar soft-part sarcoma: a new type of rhabdomyosarcoma? *Semin Diagn Pathol.* 1994;11:58–68.

104. Nakashima Y, Kotoura Y, Kasakura K, et al. Alveolar soft-part sarcoma. A report of ten cases. *Clin Orthop.* 1993;294:259–266.

105. Pappo AS, Parham DM, Cain A, et al. Alveolar soft part sarcoma in children and adolescents: clinical features and outcome of 11 patients. *Med Pediatr Oncol.* 1996;26:81–84.

106. Suh JS, Cho J, Lee SH, et al. Alveolar soft part sarcoma: MR and angiographic findings. *Skeletal Radiol.* 2000;29:680–689.

107. Iwamoto Y, Morimoto N, Chuman H, et al. The role of MR imaging in the diagnosis of alveolar soft part sarcoma: a report of 10 cases. *Skeletal Radiol.* 1995;24:267–270.

108. Aluigi P, Sangiorgi L, Picci P. Alveolar soft part sarcoma. *Skeletal Radiol.* 1996;25:400–402.

109. Enzinger FM. Epithelioid sarcoma. A sarcoma simulating a granuloma or a carcinoma. *Cancer.* 1970;26:1029–1041.

110. Dobyns JH. Epithelioid sarcoma. In: Bogumill G, Fleeger E, eds. *Tumors of Hand and Upper Limb.* London: Churchill Livingstone; 1993:286–295.

111. Chase DR, Enzinger FM. Epithelioid sarcoma. Diagnosis, prognostic indicators, and treatment. *Am J Surg Pathol.* 1985;9:241–263.

112. Sim FH, Pritchard DJ, Reiman HM, et al. Soft-tissue sarcoma: Mayo Clinic experience. *Semin Surg Oncol.* 1988;4:38–44.

113. Halling AC, Wollan PC, Pritchard DJ, et al. Epithelioid sarcoma: a clinicopathologic review of 55 cases. *Mayo Clin Proc.* 1996;71:636–642.

114. Lo HH, Kalisher L, Faix JD. Epithelioid sarcoma: radiologic and pathologic manifestations. *AJR Am J Roentgenol.* 1977;128:1017–1020.

115. Steinberg BD, Gelberman RH, Mankin HJ, et al. Epithelioid sarcoma in the upper extremity. *J Bone Joint Surg Am.* 1992;74:28–35.

116. Bos GD, Pritchard DJ, Reiman HM, et al. Epithelioid sarcoma. An analysis of fifty-one cases. *J Bone Joint Surg Am.* 1988;70:862–870.

117. Romero JA, Kim EE, Moral IS. MR characteristics of epithelioid sarcoma. *J Comput Assist Tomogr.* 1994;18:929–931.

118. Tateishi U, Hasegawa T, Kusumoto M, et al. Radiologic manifestations of proximal-type epithelioid sarcoma of the soft tissues. *AJR Am J Roentgenol.* 2002;179:973–977.

119. Nakashima H, Katagiri H, Sugiura H, et al. Epithelioid sarcoma mimicking a primary osseous multifocal scapula lesion. *Skeletal Radiol.* 2002;31:430–433.

120. Hurtado RM, McCarthy E, Frassica F, et al. Intraarticular epithelioid sarcoma. *Skeletal Radiol.* 1998;27:453–456.

121. Oto A, Meyer J. MR appearance of penile epithelioid sarcoma. *AJR Am J Roentgenol.* 1999;172:555–556.

122. von Hochstetter AR, Cserhati MD. Epithelioid sarcoma presenting as chronic synovitis and mistaken for osteosarcoma. *Skeletal Radiol.* 1995;24:636–638.

123. Yamato M, Nishimura G, Yamaguchi T, et al. Epithelioid sarcoma with unusual radiological findings. *Skeletal Radiol.* 1997;26:606–610.

124. Dion E, Forest M, Brasseur JL, et al. Epithelioid sarcoma mimicking abscess: review of the MRI appearances. *Skeletal Radiol.* 2001;30:173–177.

125. Hanna SL, Kaste S, Jenkins JJ, et al. Epithelioid sarcoma: clinical, MR imaging and pathologic findings. *Skeletal Radiol.* 2002;31:400–412.

126. Massengill AD, Seeger LL, Eckardt JJ. The role of plain radiography, computed tomography, and magnetic resonance imaging in sarcoma evaluation. *Hematol Oncol Clin North Am.* 1995;9:571–604.

127. Gerald WL, Miller HK, Battifora H, et al. Intra-abdominal desmoplastic small round-cell tumor. Report of 19 cases of a distinctive type of high-grade polyphenotypic malignancy affecting young individuals. *Am J Surg Pathol.* 1991;15:499–513.

128. Basade MM, Vege DS, Nair CN, et al. Intra-abdominal desmoplastic small round cell tumor in children: a clinicopathologic study. *Pediatr Hematol Oncol.* 1996;13:95–99.

129. Fukunaga M, Endo Y, Takaki K, et al. Postmenopausal intra-abdominal desmoplastic small cell tumor. *Pathol Int.* 1996;46:281–285.

130. Cummings OW, Ulbright TM, Young RH, et al. Desmoplastic small round cell tumors of the paratesticular region. A report of six cases. *Am J Surg Pathol.* 1997;21:219–225.

131. Parkash V, Gerald WL, Parma A, et al. Desmoplastic small round cell tumor of the pleura. *Am J Surg Pathol.* 1995;19:659–665.

132. Sabate JM, Torrubia S, Roson N, et al. Intra-abdominal desmoplastic small round-cell tumor: a rare cause of peritoneal malignancy in young people. *Eur Radiol.* 2000;10:817–819.

133. Amato RJ, Ellerhorst JA, Ayala AG. Intraabdominal desmoplastic small cell tumor. Report and discussion of five cases. *Cancer.* 1996;78:845–851.

134. Kretschmar CS, Colbach C, Bhan I, et al. Desmoplastic small cell tumor: a report of three cases and a review of the literature. *J Pediatr Hematol Oncol.* 1996;18:293–298.

135. Leuschner I, Radig K, Harms D. Desmoplastic small round cell tumor. *Semin Diagn Pathol.* 1996;13:204–212.

136. Ordonez NG. Desmoplastic small round cell tumor: I: a histopathologic study of 39 cases with emphasis on unusual histological patterns. *Am J Surg Pathol.* 1998;22:1303–1313.

137. Gerald WL, Rosai J, Ladanyi M. Characterization of the genomic breakpoint and chimeric transcripts in the EWS-WT1 gene fusion of desmoplastic small round cell tumor. *Proc Natl Acad Sci U S A.* 1995;92:1028–1032.

138. Lae ME, Roche PC, Jin L, et al. Desmoplastic small round cell tumor: a clinicopathologic, immunohistochemical, and molecular study of 32 tumors. *Am J Surg Pathol.* 2002;26:823–835.

139. Liu J, Nau MM, Yeh JC, et al. Molecular heterogeneity and function of EWS-WT1 fusion transcripts in desmoplastic small round cell tumors. *Clin Cancer Res.* 2000;6:3522–3529.

140. Rodriguez E, Sreekantaiah C, Gerald W, et al. A recurring translocation, t(11;22)(p13;q11.2), characterizes intra-abdominal desmoplastic small round-cell tumors. *Cancer Genet Cytogenet.* 1993;69:17–21.

141. Kurre P, Felgenhauer JL, Miser JS, et al. Successful dose-intensive treatment of desmoplastic small round cell tumor in three children. *J Pediatr Hematol Oncol.* 2000;22:446–450.

142. Kushner BH, LaQuaglia MP, Wollner N, et al. Desmoplastic small round-cell tumor: prolonged progression-free survival with aggressive multimodality therapy. *J Clin Oncol.* 1996;14:1526–1531.

143. Quaglia MP, Brennan MF. The clinical approach to desmoplastic small round cell tumor. *Surg Oncol.* 2000;9:77–81.

144. Lal DR, Su WT, Wolden SL, et al. Results of multimodal treatment for desmoplastic small round cell tumors. *J Pediatr Surg.* 2005;40:251–255; discussion 255.

145. Schwarz RE, Gerald WL, Kushner BH, et al. Desmoplastic small round cell tumors: prognostic indicators and results of surgical management. *Ann Surg Oncol.* 1998;5:416–422.

146. Outwater E, Schiebler ML, Brooks JJ. Intraabdominal desmoplastic small cell tumor: CT and MR findings. *J Comput Assist Tomogr.* 1992;16:429–432.

147. Pickhardt PJ, Fisher AJ, Balfe DM, et al. Desmoplastic small round cell tumor of the abdomen: radiologic-histopathologic correlation. *Radiology.* 1999;210:633–638.

148. Dao HN, Dachman AH. CT findings of regression in intraabdominal desmoplastic small-cell tumor. *Clin Imaging.* 1995;19:244–246.

149. Varma DG, McDaniel K, Ordonez NG, et al. Primary malignant small round cell tumor of the abdomen: CT findings in five cases. *AJR Am J Roentgenol.* 1992;158:1031–1034.

150. Tateishi U, Hasegawa T, Kusumoto M, et al. Desmoplastic small round cell tumor: imaging findings associated with clinicopathologic features. *J Comput Assist Tomogr.* 2002;26:579–583.

151. Hosli I, Holzgreve W, Danzer E, et al. Two case reports of rare fetal tumors: an indication for surface rendering? *Ultrasound Obstet Gynecol.* 2001;17:522–526.

152. Hsueh C, Kuo TT. Congenital malignant rhabdoid tumor presenting as a cutaneous nodule: report of 2 cases with review of the literature. *Arch Pathol Lab Med.* 1998;122:1099–1102.

153. Proust F, Laquerriere A, Constantin B, et al. Simultaneous presentation of atypical teratoid/rhabdoid tumor in siblings. *J Neurooncol.* 1999;43:63–70.

154. White FV, Dehner LP, Belchis DA, et al. Congenital disseminated malignant rhabdoid tumor: a distinct clinicopathologic entity demonstrating abnormalities of chromosome 22q11. *Am J Surg Pathol.* 1999;23:249–256.

155. Kent AL, Mahoney DH Jr, Gresik MV, et al. Malignant rhabdoid tumor of the extremity. *Cancer.* 1987;60:1056–1059.

156. Kodet R, Newton WA Jr, Sachs N, et al. Rhabdoid tumors of soft tissues: a clinicopathologic study of 26 cases enrolled on the Intergroup Rhabdomyosarcoma Study. *Hum Pathol.* 1991;22:674–684.

157. Parham DM, Weeks DA, Beckwith JB. The clinicopathologic spectrum of putative extrarenal rhabdoid tumors. An analysis of 42 cases studied with immunohistochemistry or electron microscopy. *Am J Surg Pathol.* 1994;18:1010–1029.

158. Tsokos M, Kouraklis G, Chandra RS, et al. Malignant rhabdoid tumor of the kidney and soft tissues. Evidence for a diverse morphological and immunocytochemical phenotype. *Arch Pathol Lab Med.* 1989;113:115–120.

159. Wick MR, Ritter JH, Dehner LP. Malignant rhabdoid tumors: a clinicopathologic review and conceptual discussion. *Semin Diagn Pathol.* 1995;12:233–248.

160. Guillou L, Wadden C, Coindre JM, et al. "Proximal-type" epithelioid sarcoma, a distinctive aggressive neoplasm showing rhabdoid features. Clinicopathologic, immunohistochemical, and ultrastructural study of a series. *Am J Surg Pathol.* 1997;21:130–146.

161. Handgretinger R, Kimmig A, Koscielnak E, et al. Establishment and characterization of a cell line (Wa-2) derived from an extrarenal rhabdoid tumor. *Cancer Res.* 1990;50:2177–2182.

162. Newsham I, Daub D, Besnard-Guerin C, et al. Molecular sublocalization and characterization of the 11;22 translocation breakpoint in a malignant rhabdoid tumor. *Genomics.* 1994;19:433–440.

Masses That May Mimic Soft Tissue Tumors

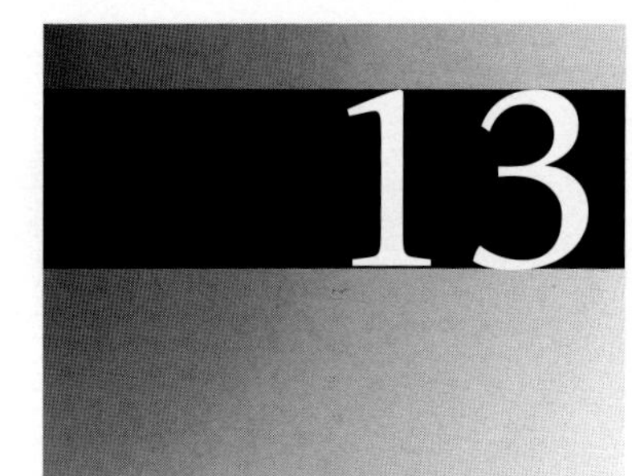

There are a large number of tumorlike lesions of soft tissue. Many of these have a clinical presentation simulating that of a soft tissue neoplasm. The lesions presented here are not an all-inclusive, comprehensive review of tumorlike masses, but merely our experience with lesions that may clinically present as musculoskeletal tumors. For organizational purposes, we have classified these into broad categories: inflammatory lesions, crystal deposition disease, masslike lesions, and traumatic lesions.

INFLAMMATORY/INFECTIOUS LESIONS

Soft tissue inflammatory/infectious diseases are relatively common. They demonstrate a wide spectrum of clinical and radiologic features and in many cases may simulate a soft tissue mass. These diseases are usually classified in the following categories: cellulitis, abscess, myositis, fasciitis, lymphedema, and lymphangitis. In general, these entities are not rigorously defined, nor do they form a continuum. In many cases, various inflammatory processes may coexist with one another, such as an abscess with associated cellulitis. For the purpose of this review, they are discussed separately.

Cellulitis

In general, the term *cellulitis* is used to describe an infection of the skin and subcutaneous tissue without gross suppuration (1). Cellulitis is sometimes used to denote specifically hemolytic group A *Streptococcus* infection because this infection behaves somewhat differently from other pyogens, spreading between cells and tissue planes; however, more

<table>
<tr><td>

KEY CONCEPTS

- Cellulitis is an infection of the skin and subcutaneous tissue without gross suppuration.
- Associated abscess, ascending lymphangitis, regional lymph node involvement, osteomyelitis, and pyoarthrosis may also be seen.
- Radiographs typically show soft tissue swelling and edema with obliteration of the adjacent fascial planes.
- Imaging studies show strandlike or reticulated areas of abnormal fluidlike signal within the subcutaneous fat.
- Contrast-enhanced MR imaging is generally not required but makes associated complications more conspicuous.

</td></tr>
</table>

commonly the term *cellulitis* is used to denote any poorly defined soft tissue pyogenic process (2). Clinically, cellulitis is usually relatively well-demarcated, with the area of involvement being hot, red, and painful (3). Associated abscess, ascending lymphangitis, regional lymph node involvement, osteomyelitis, and pyoarthrosis may also be seen (3,4).

Soft tissue cellulitis is typically the result of direct contamination following local trauma. Any disruption of the skin surface can lead to secondary infection, particularly in immunocompromised individuals (5). Nonpenetrating trauma may cause soft tissue infection, but the mechanism is unclear.

The diagnosis of cellulitis is made clinically. Imaging is usually used to assess the extent of the disease and to identify associated complications (6). Uncomplicated cellulitis is treated medically.

Radiographs typically show soft tissue swelling and edema with obliteration of the adjacent fascial planes (Fig. 13.1)

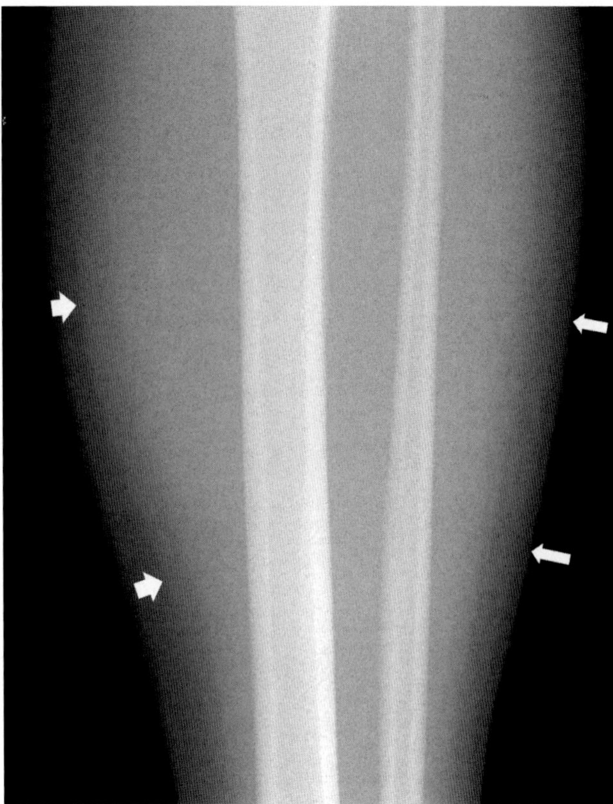

Figure 13.1 Cellulitis: Radiographic features in a woman 40 years of age. Anteroposterior radiograph of the lower leg shows soft tissue swelling and edema in the lateral aspect of the lower leg (*long arrows*), with obliteration of the adjacent fascial plane. Note well-defined margin between the muscle and subcutaneous fat medially (*short arrows*).

(5,7). When soft tissue air is present, it demonstrates radiolucent streaks. Osseous erosions may be present, but infection usually does cause pressure erosions, in contradistinction to neoplasm.

Beauchamp et al. (1) reviewed the computed tomography (CT) appearance of soft tissue infection and inflammation. They noted that in cellulitis, CT demonstrates increased attenuation in the involved subcutaneous fat, with loss of the well-defined margin between muscle and fat (1). The overlying skin may be thickened and asymmetric enhancement may be seen following contrast administration (1). On MR imaging, cellulitis demonstrates strandlike or reticulated areas of abnormal fluidlike signal within the subcutaneous fat. This is often pronounced in areas adjacent to the muscular fascia (Fig. 13.2). Contrast-enhanced MR imaging is generally not required; however, enhanced imaging makes associated fluid collections and abscesses more conspicuous (8). The appearance of cellulitis is indistinguishable from that of noninfectious edema (4). Sonography shows diffuse thickening of the skin and subcutaneous tissue without a focal fluid collection. The subcutaneous tissue is heterogeneous and dissected by anechoic strands in a reticular pattern (9).

Abscess

KEY CONCEPTS

- An abscess is a localized collection of pus confined to a specific space.
- A phlegmon refers to focal inflammatory process without liquefaction.
- CT scanning shows a fluid attenuation mass with associated inflammation.
- MR imaging shows a well-demarcated, fluidlike collection; signal intensity varies depending on the amount of internal proteinaceous debris, necrosis, foreign matter, and so on.
- Foreign matter, such as wood or plastic, within an abscess, produces a signal void on MR imaging.
- Ultrasonography is especially useful for diagnosis and guidance for percutaneous aspiration and/or drainage.

An *abscess*, in contrast to cellulitis, is defined as a localized collection of pus confined to a specific space, tissue, or organ (a focal collection of necrotic tissue, white cells, and bacteria) (1,2). An abscess may, with time, become walled off by highly vascularized connective tissue (1) and may be associated with diffuse inflammation.

An abscess may arise within the soft tissue as a result of penetrating trauma, hematogenous dissemination, or contamination from an adjacent septic focus, such as an infected joint (10). In the acute phase, the term *phlegmon* is more appropriate, indicating inflammation of connective tissue. When the process involves muscle, the term *infectious myositis* may be used (10). Although a phlegmon may resolve, it may also become walled off and undergo liquefaction, forming an abscess (10).

Radiographs may be unremarkable (10), but more often they show soft tissue swelling and edema with obliteration of the adjacent fascial planes (5,7). When soft tissue air is present, it may show radiolucent streaks or a mottled appearance (Fig. 13.3) (11). Dystrophic calcification may be identified in the wall of a chronic abscess (11). Periosteal reaction may also be seen in adjacent osseous structures (11).

On CT, an abscess presents as a fluid attenuation mass. The margins vary from well-defined to infiltrating, depending on the causative organism and the degree of associated inflammation; the greater the associated inflammation, the greater the distortion of normal muscle anatomy and fascial planes. The CT attenuation of an abscess varies as a function of its composition. Gas may occasionally be present, depending on the underlying causative organism. Following contrast enhancement, the capsule, which is highly vascularized, will usually enhance (Fig. 13.4) (1).

An abscess is more readily detected on MR imaging than on CT scanning because of the greater lesion conspicuity. MR imaging is also more accurate in the detection of soft

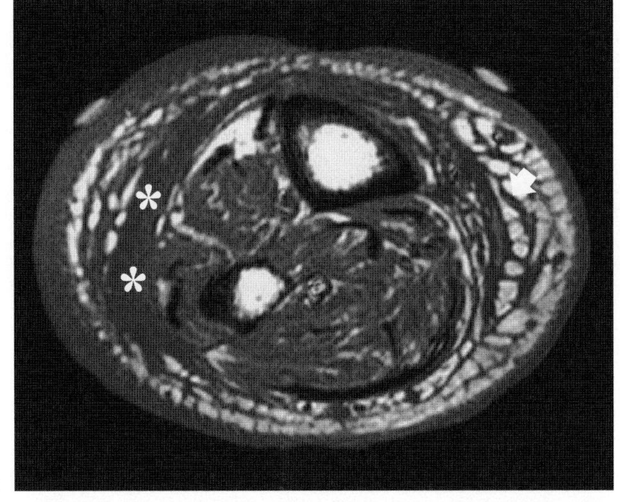
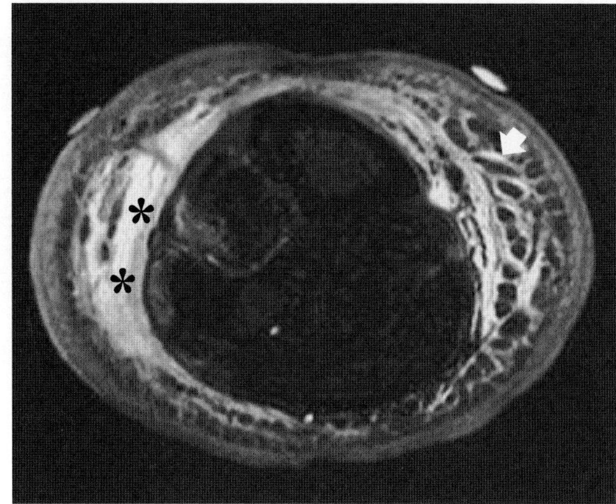
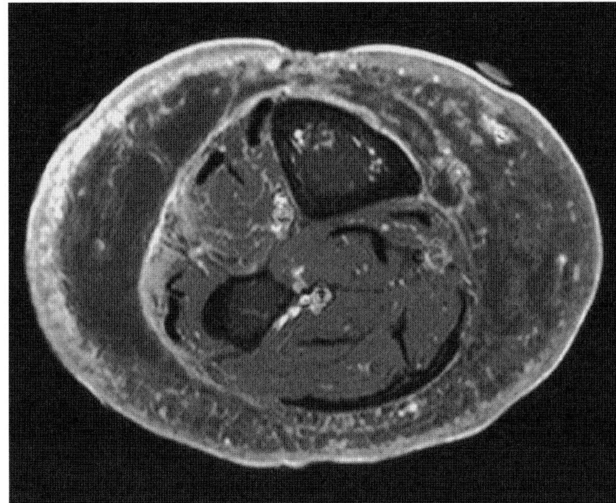

Figure 13.2 Cellulitis: MR imaging features in a man 71 years of age following traumatic laceration of the lower leg. **A,B:** Axial T1-weighted (TR/TE; 460/17) **(A)** spin-echo and short-tau inversion recovery (STIR) (TR/TE/TI; 5990/86/160) **(B)** MR images show prominent skin thickening, reticulated areas of abnormal fluidlike signal within the subcutaneous fat (*arrow*) and edema adjacent to the muscular fascia (*asterisks*). **C:** Corresponding axial enhanced fat-suppressed T1-weighted (TR/TE; 484/17) spin-echo MR image shows enhancement in the skin and adjacent tissue with scant enhancement of the edema.

tissue abscess than a technetium-99m methylene diphosphonate bone scan, indium-111-labeled leukocyte scintigraphy, and gallium-67 scintigraphy (12,13). More importantly, scintigraphy cannot always adequately differentiate between cellulitis and a soft tissue abscess (13).

On MR imaging, a soft tissue abscess appears as a well-demarcated collection of increased signal intensity on T2-weighted pulse sequences and decreased signal intensity on T1-weighted images (12). The internal portion of the lesion is usually relatively homogeneous, although homogeneity and signal intensity vary depending on the amount of internal proteinaceous debris, necrosis, foreign matter, gas, and the like (4). The lesion is surrounded by a rind of variable signal intensity, which shows marked enhancement following intravenous gadolinium administration (Fig. 13.5) (4). This pattern of enhancement is not surprising because the wall of an abscess cavity may contain highly vascularized connective tissue. The wall will also demonstrate increased signal intensity on T1-weighted images, greater than that of muscle, also reflecting its rich vascularity. Although air is readily demonstrated on CT scanning, gas-containing lesions may also be identified on

MR imaging with the use of gradient echo imaging because of the greater magnetic susceptibility and "blooming" associated and soft tissue air (Fig. 13.6) (14).

A discrete abscess can be differentiated from a diffuse inflammatory process (phlegmon) in that the latter shows poorly defined increased signal intensity on T2-weighted images, with indistinct margins (an edema pattern), but no focal fluid collection. This edema pattern is frequently seen in association with an abscess.

Foreign matter, such as wood or plastic, within an abscess, produces a signal void on MR imaging (15,16), whereas metallic foreign matter, even when minute, may produce significant artifact (Fig. 13.7), depending on the type of metal. Although foreign matter may be associated with abscess formation, it may be encased in granulation tissue with associated inflammation (15). In such cases, MR imaging reveals a signal void corresponding to the foreign body itself, with surrounding high signal on T2-weighted images. When the foreign body is long and thin, such as a splinter or toothpick, a "target" appearance may be present (15,16), with the wood showing a decreased signal intensity (16). The amount and size of the surrounding

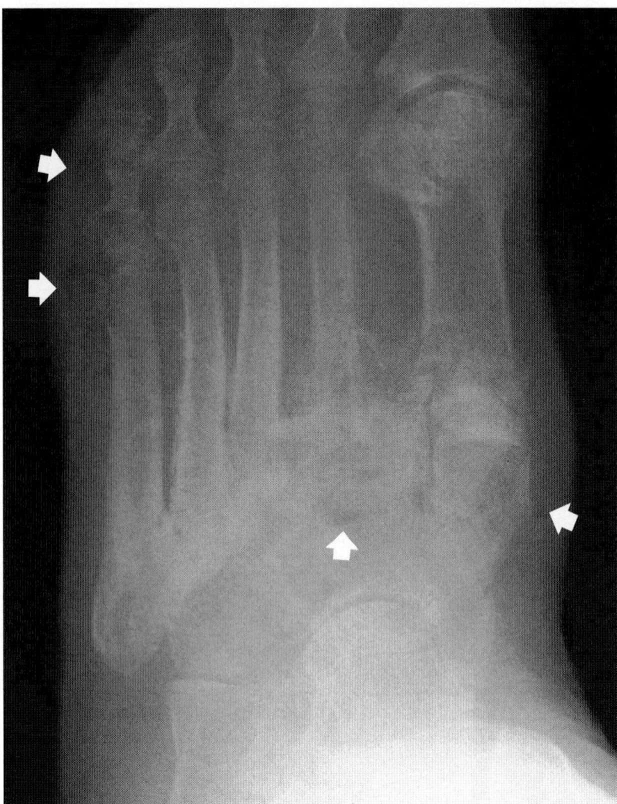

Figure 13.3 Abscess: Radiographic features in a man 77 years of age with an infected neuropathic foot. Oblique radiograph of the foot shows marked neuropathic arthropathy with multiple air densities (*arrows*).

granulation tissue and inflammation are quite variable, ranging from a diffuse swelling to a small region immediately around the foreign body (15) (Fig. 13.8).

We find ultrasonography to be very useful in identifying discrete focal fluid collections as well as in localizing foreign matter within abscess cavities (Fig. 13.9) (16). Ultrasonography is also useful in providing guidance for percutaneous aspiration and/or drainage of abscess cavities (17). Intramuscular and subcutaneous abscesses show a variable internal echo texture, depending on the internal composition (10,17). This texture varies from anechoic in liquefied abscess cavities to variable amounts of internal echoes from associated debris, necrosis, foreign matter, and gas. In general, on ultrasonography, lesions are elliptical or spherical and posterior acoustic enhancement is characteristic (11,17). The margins are variable, from irregular or poorly defined to relatively sharp, and they may merge with adjacent cellulitis or may be outlined by a hypoechoic/anechoic rim (9,17). The vascularized tissue in the abscess wall typically demonstrates hyperemia on Doppler ultrasound (11). Cellulitis, in contrast, is generally a poorly defined process with somewhat diffusely decreased echogenicity. An abscess may be indistinguishable sonographically from a liquefied hematoma or rarely may be confused with a neoplasm. Consequently, close clinical correlation is essential.

Lymphedema and Lymphangitis

KEY CONCEPTS

- Lymphedema is the accumulation of interstitial fluid as a result of stasis of lymph caused by obstruction, destruction, or hypoplasia of lymph vessels.
- Lymphangitis is a nonsuppurative infection of the lymphatics.
- Hereditary lymphedema is characterized by an autosomal dominant pattern of inheritance.
- Hereditary lymphedema is typically subdivided into three types by age of onset:
  - Congenital onset (Milroy disease)
  - Peripubetal onset (Meige disease or lymphedema praecox)
  - Late onset, usually after 35 years of age (lymphedema tarda)
- Secondary lymphedema is the result of lymphatic obstruction.
- On MR imaging, lymphedema causes a honeycomb appearance of the subcutaneous connective tissue with thickening of the overlying skin.

Lymphedema is defined as the accumulation of interstitial fluid as a result of stasis of lymph caused by obstruction, destruction, or hypoplasia of lymph vessels (1). The term *lymphangitis* is used to designate a nonsuppurative infection of the lymphatics (1). Lymphangitis may be associated with cellulitis.

Hereditary lymphedema is uncommon (18,19). It typically affects the lower extremities and is characterized by an autosomal dominant pattern of inheritance with reduced penetrance and variable expression (19). Autosomal recessive and X-linked forms of congenital lymphedema are also described (19). Hereditary lymphedema is typically subdivided into three types by age of onset: congenital onset (Milroy disease); peripubetal onset (Meige disease or lymphedema praecox); and late onset, usually after 35 years of age (lymphedema tarda) (19,20). In a study of 98 families with 572 affected persons, the age of onset was known in 456. Of this group, 183 (40%) had congenital onset, 240 (53%) had lymphedema praecox, and 33 (7%) had lymphedema tarda (19). Although it is convenient to use this classification scheme, age of onset of the noncongenital forms is variable, with lymphedema praecox usually appearing between 10 and 25 years of age and lymphedema tarda appearing as late as 55 years of age.

Secondary lymphedema, far more common than primary lymphedema, is the result of lymphatic obstruction. Although there are a variety of causes, the most common in developed countries is previous treatment of malignancy which has resulted in interference of limb lymphatic drainage (18). Other causes, such as parasitic infection, are

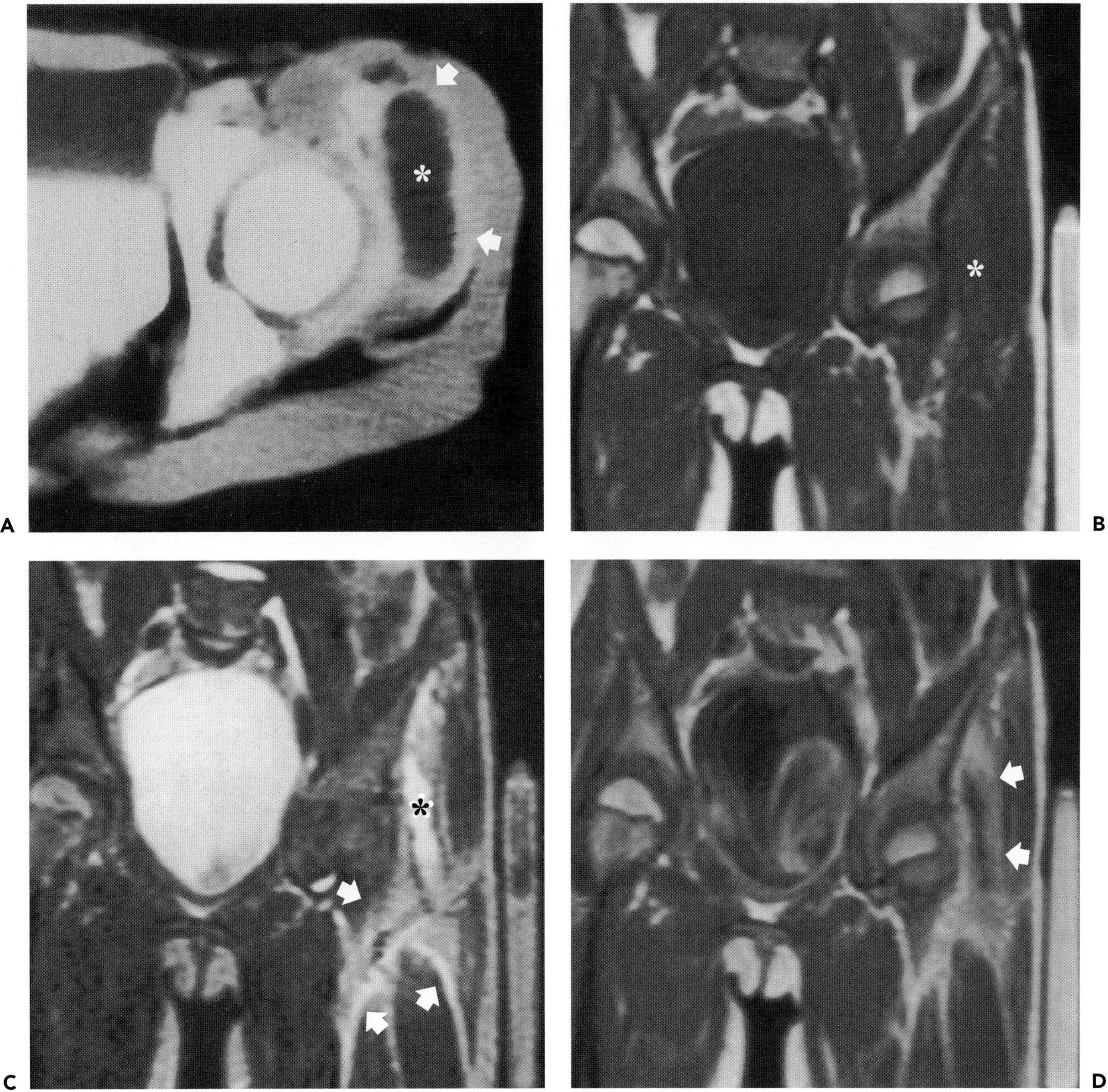

Figure 13.4   Abscess: Typical imaging features in the hip of a girl 8 years of age. **A:** Axial contrast-enhanced CT scan shows the abscess (*asterisk*) to have an attenuation similar to that of fluid. Note enhancement of the abscess wall (*arrows*). **B,C:** Coronal T1-weighted (TR/TE; 400/20) **(B)** and T2-weighted (TR/TE; 1800/80) **(C)** spin-echo MR images of the thigh show a poorly defined mass adjacent to the left hip (*asterisk*). The ill-defined distribution of signal abnormality on T2-weighted image (*arrows*) is compatible with that of associated edema. Note fluid in fascial planes. **D:** Coronal T1-weighted image following gadolinium administration shows enhancement of the abscess wall (*arrows*) and surrounding edema.

rare in the United States. Patients with chronic lymphedema are at risk for the development of angiosarcoma (21). This situation is reviewed in Chapter 5.

MR imaging is especially useful in evaluating lymphedema by identifying any underlying cause, as well as accurately assessing its extent (18). On MR imaging, lymphedema causes a honeycomb appearance of the subcutaneous connective tissue, with thickening of the overlying skin (1). This is seen as strands of increased attenuation on CT imaging and T1 and T2 prolongation on MR imaging. The subjacent muscle and fascia are normal, whereas the overlying skin may be thickened (Fig. 13.10) (1). The MR imaging appearance of lymphedema may be strikingly similar to that seen with cellulitis (Fig. 13.2).

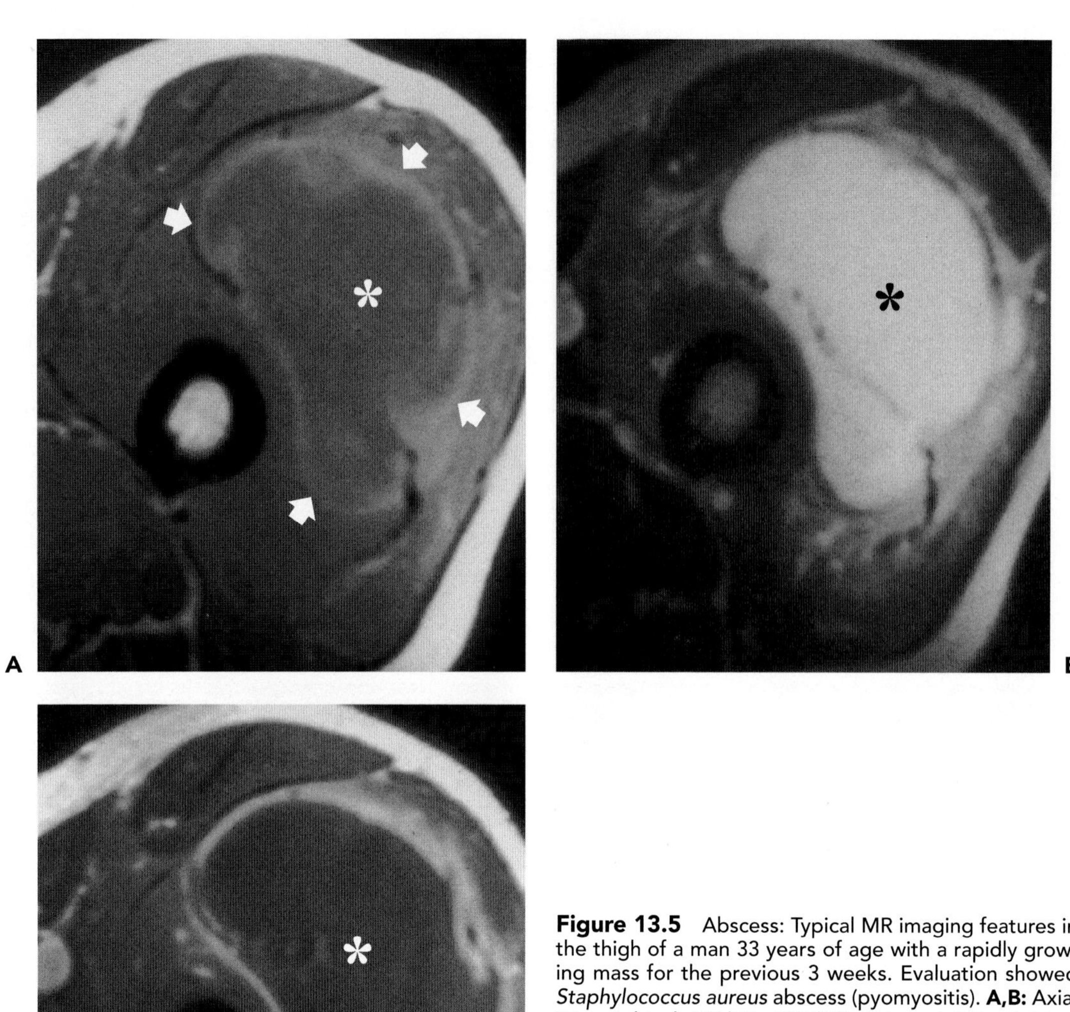

Figure 13.5 Abscess: Typical MR imaging features in the thigh of a man 33 years of age with a rapidly growing mass for the previous 3 weeks. Evaluation showed *Staphylococcus aureus* abscess (pyomyositis). **A,B:** Axial T1-weighted (TR/TE; 522/25) **(A)** and T2-weighted (TR/TE; 2303/90) **(B)** spin-echo MR images show a well-defined, relatively homogeneous mass in the anterior compartment of the left thigh (*asterisk*). The mass shows a signal intensity very slightly less than that of the surrounding muscle and greater than that of fat on corresponding T2-weighted images. There is some heterogeneous, as well as diffuse increased signal intensity in the entire anterior compartment, suggesting diffuse muscle edema. Note slight increased T1-weighted signal intensity within the wall of the abscess (*arrows* in **A**). **C:** Axial T1-weighted (TR/TE; 522/25) spin-echo MR image following intravenous gadolinium administration shows a rind of uniform peripheral enhancement.

Fasciitis

> ### KEY CONCEPTS
> - Fasciitis is an inflammatory process predominantly confined to the fascia.
> - Necrotizing fasciitis is a rapidly progressive, life-threatening fasciitis characterized by necrosis and suppuration.
> - On MR imaging, fasciitis shows thickening of the deep fascia with a nonspecific signal intensity.
> - Absence of enhancement following contrast administration is indicative of tissue necrosis.

The term *fasciitis* is used when an inflammatory process is predominantly confined to the fascia, initially sparing the subjacent muscle (1). With increasing inflammation, the adjacent tissue becomes involved. The term *necrotizing fasciitis* is used for extensive fasciitis in which the infection is rapidly progressive, life-threatening and characterized by necrosis and suppuration (22,23).

The distinction between infective fasciitis and early necrotizing fasciitis may be extremely difficult (22,23). The clinical presentation and physical findings in both diseases are similar; however, the treatments are quite different (23). Infective fasciitis is readily treated with antibiotics without debridement, whereas necrotizing fasciitis requires prompt surgical intervention (23) with a 24% to 75% mortality rate (22,23).

A history of local trauma is usually present in both necrotizing and nonnecrotizing fasciitis (22). Patients

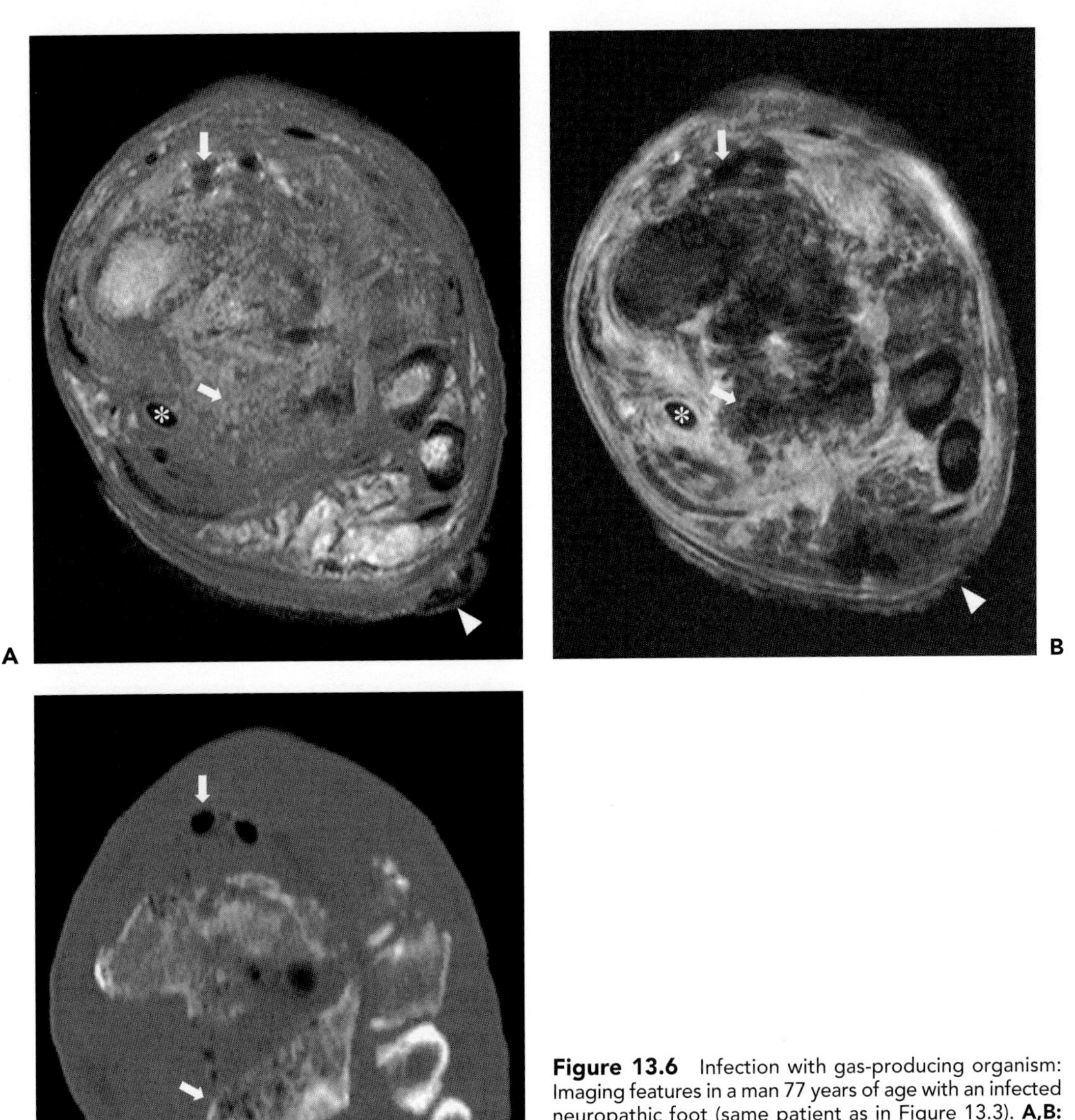

Figure 13.6 Infection with gas-producing organism: Imaging features in a man 77 years of age with an infected neuropathic foot (same patient as in Figure 13.3). **A,B:** Coronal T1-weighted (TR/TE; 712/17) spin-echo **(A)** and gradient-echo (TR/TE; 463/56) **(B)** MR images show "blooming" to multiple soft tissue and intraosseous air densities (*arrows*). Signal loss from tendons (*asterisk*) is unchanged. Note cutaneous ulcer along lateral margin of foot (*short arrow*). **C:** Corresponding CT scan shows air densities (*arrows*) to better advantage. No ulcer (*arrowhead*) along margin of foot.

are often immunocompromised, with an increased incidence in patients with diabetes mellitus, chronic renal failure, and human immunodeficiency virus (HIV) infection, although it may also be seen in healthy individuals (22). Affected individuals typically have a fever and increased leukocyte count indicative of an underlying infection. The most commonly implicated causative organisms are *Streptococcus pyogenes* and *Staphylococcus aureus* (23). Less commonly, anaerobic organisms may be seen (23).

On MR imaging, non-necrotizing soft tissue infection demonstrates thickening of the subcutaneous tissues with or without fluid collections within the subcutis and super-ficial fascia (22). With fasciitis, there is thickening of the deep fascia, with a nonspecific signal intensity showing decreased signal intensity on T1-weighted images and high signal intensity on fluid-sensitive sequences (22,23) (Figs. 13.11 and 13.12). Absence of enhancement following contrast administration is indicative of tissue necrosis and is a useful sign in suggesting the diagnosis of necrotizing fasciitis (23) (Figs. 13.13 and 13.14). The sensitivity and specificity of MR imaging in this diagnosis is reported to be 89% to 100% and 46% to 86%, respectively (22,24,25). When no deep fascial involvement is seen, fasciitis can be excluded (26); however caution is required in that involvement in early findings may be quite subtle.

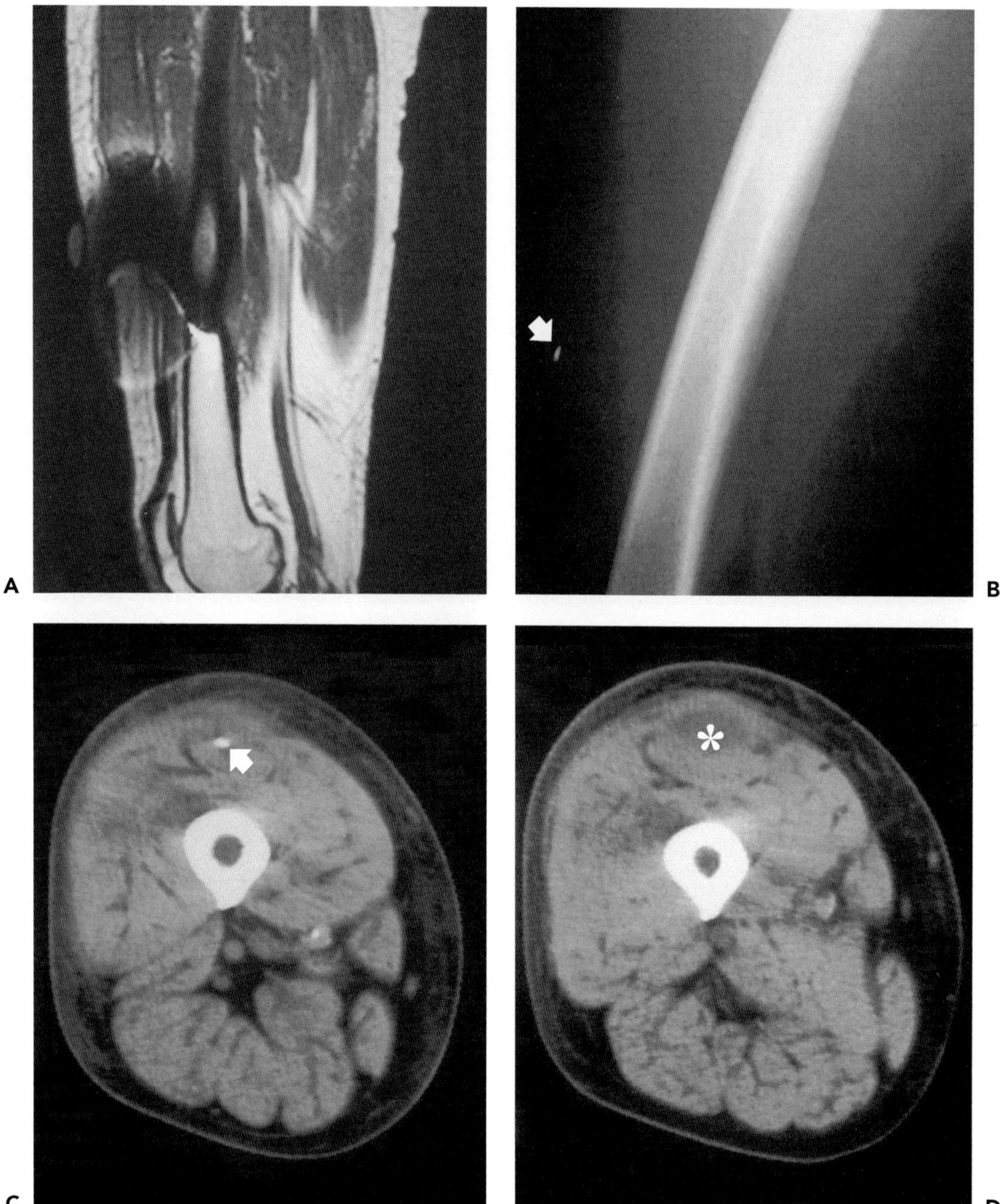

Figure 13.7   Abscess associated with metallic foreign body: Imaging findings in a man 48 years of age with recent onset of pain and tenderness in the thigh. **A:** Sagittal T1-weighted (TR/TE; 500/16) spin-echo MR image shows a marked metallic artifact. On questioning, the patient remembered a penetrating injury 30 years earlier. **B:** Lateral radiograph shows a metallic foreign body (*arrow*) in the anterior soft tissues. **C:** Axial noncontrast CT scan shows a metallic foreign body in the anterior soft tissues (*arrow*), with poor delineation of the fat planes and increased attenuation of the adjacent subcutaneous fat, compatible with associated inflammatory change. **D:** Axial noncontrast CT scan just proximal to **C** shows an ill-defined area of decreased attenuation (*asterisk*), compatible with an intramuscular abscess. (*continued*)

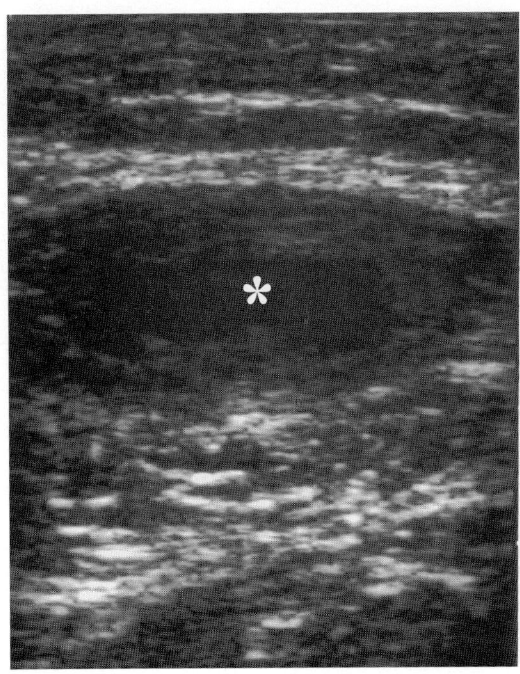

E

Figure 13.7 (*continued*)   **E:** Sonogram shows the abscess cavity (*asterisk*) to better advantage.

Myositis

> ### KEY CONCEPTS
> - Myositis is inflammation of the skeletal muscle and may be infectious or noninfectious.
> - Pyomyositis is used to denote a primary bacterial infection involving skeletal muscle.
> - CT criteria for pyomyositis include:
>   - Enlarged muscle(s) with heterogeneous attenuation.
>   - Rim-enhancing central fluid collection.
>   - Associated cellulitis.
> - MR criteria for pyomyositis include:
>   - Abnormal signal intensity of involved muscle(s) on T1-weighted images with central decreased signal and higher signal intensity rim.
>   - Enhancing rim following gadolinium administration.
>   - Increased signal intensity on T2-weighted images in the affected muscle(s).
>   - Central fluidlike signal.
>   - Associated skin thickening, subcutaneous fat stranding, and swelling of fascial planes.

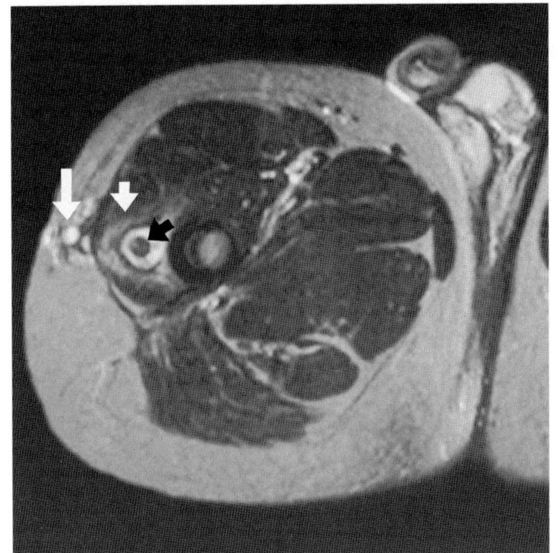

A

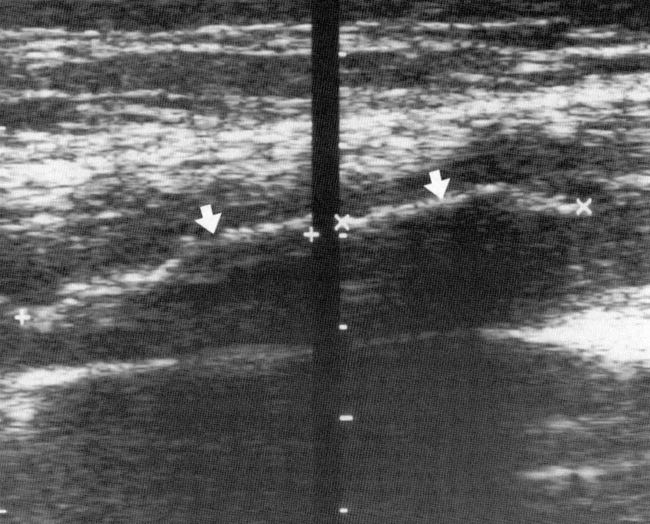

B

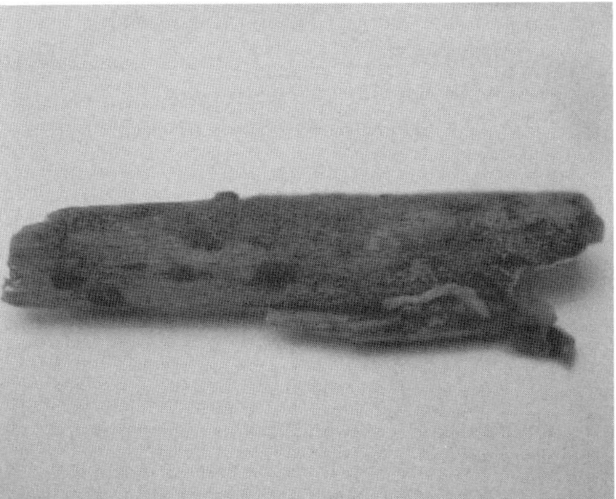

C

Figure 13.8   Wooden foreign body: MR imaging "target" sign in a man 49 years of age who fell off a roof into a hedge and subsequently developed a draining sinus tract. **A:** Axial T2-weighted (TR/TE; 2716/80) spin-echo MR image shows the draining sinus tract (*long white arrow*) extending through the subcutaneous tissue. Note "target" appearance of the foreign body (*short black arrow*) as well as associated inflammation (*short white arrow*). **B:** Sonogram shows acoustic shadowing from leading edge (*arrows*) of the wooden foreign body. **C:** Photograph of the wooden foreign body (twig) removed from the vastus lateralis muscle.

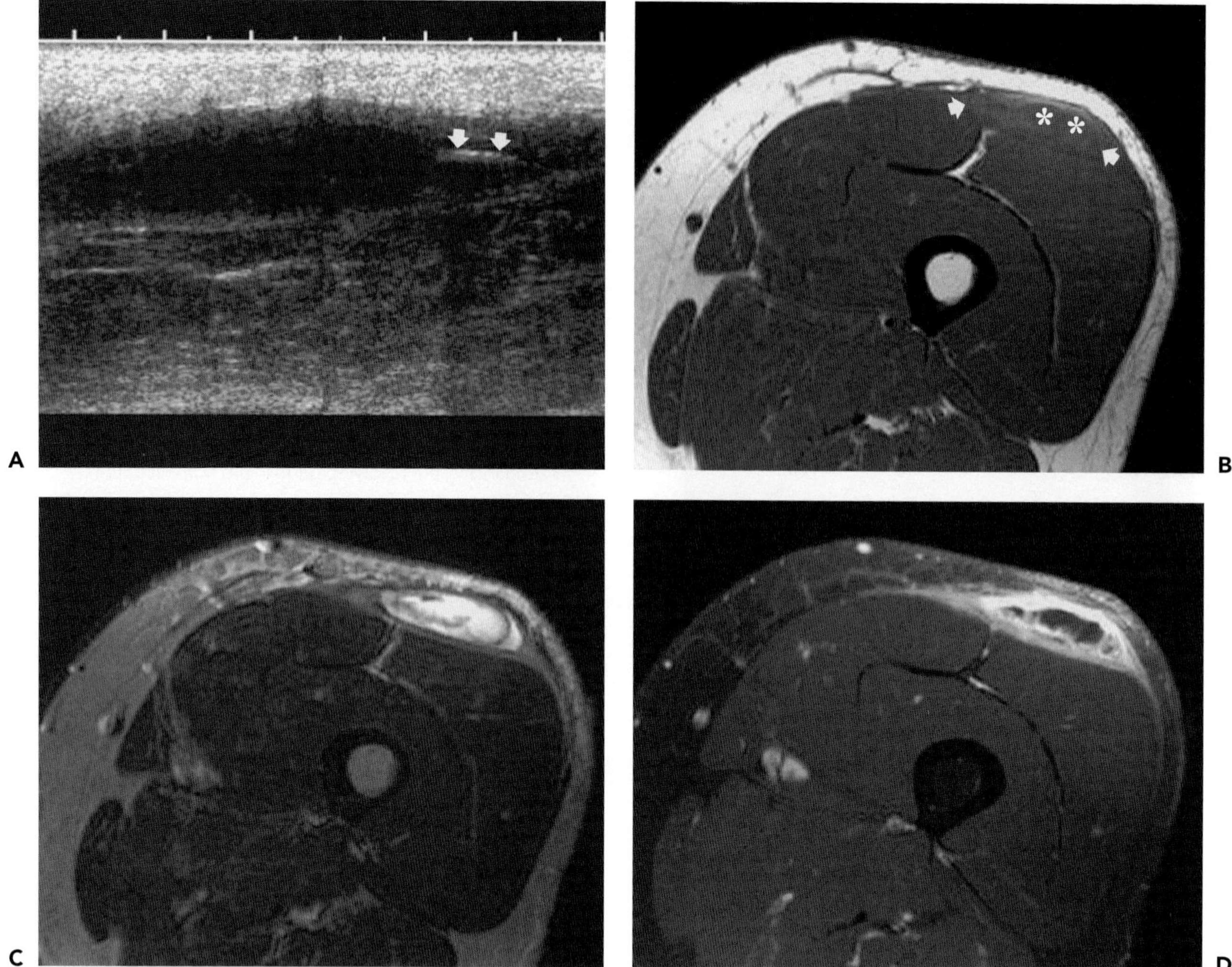

Figure 13.9   Abscess: Ultrasound and MR imaging of an abscess with occult foreign body in the thigh of a man 32 years of age with a remote history of puncture injury. **A:** Sonogram shows an abscess in the thigh with a well-defined foreign body (*arrows*) adjacent to the medial aspect of the lesion. **B,C:** Coronal T1-weighted (TR/TE; 500/12) **(B)** and T2-weighted (TR/TE; 2246/80) **(C)** spin-echo MR images show an abscess (*asterisks*) in the anterior thigh. Note increased signal intensity in the fibrovascular wall in **B** (*arrows*). **D:** Axial, fat-suppressed, T1-weighted (TR/TE; 480/12) spin-echo MR image following intravenous gadolinium administration shows marked enhancement of the wall. Foreign body, which was readily seen on sonography, was not identified on MR imaging.

Myositis is inflammation of the skeletal muscle. It may be infectious or noninfectious and may become focally necrotic (myonecrosis) (Fig. 13.15) (1). The term *pyomyositis* is used to denote a primary bacterial infection involving skeletal muscle, often the result of *Staphylococcus aureus* in about 90% of cases (27). The remaining 10% of cases are the result of varied species of *Streptococcus* (27). Pyomyositis is also referred to as *tropical pyomyositis* because it is endemic in warm climates (27).

Patients with pyomyositis usually have concurrent diseases such as diabetes, HIV infection, connective tissue disorder, previous malignancy, or a condition requiring long-term steroid use (27). These likely produce some degree of immunosuppression, which increases susceptibility to infection as a result of minor trauma (27). Symptoms

include diffuse pain, progressive erythema, swelling, and edema, with or without fever (27). With time there is progressive induration, swelling, pain, and possible extension into adjacent bone or joints (27). Septicemia and death are reported in as many as 1.8% of patients (28).

Gordon et al. developed CT and MR criteria for pyomyositis. CT criteria include: (a) enlarged muscle(s) with heterogeneous attenuation and a central fluid collection with rim enhancement, and (b) associated findings of cellulitis, including skin thickening, stranding of the subcutaneous fat, blurring of the fat and fascial planes, and distention of subcutaneous veins (27). MR criteria for pyomyositis consist of: (a) slightly increased signal intensity of involved muscle(s) on T1-weighted images, with a central area of decreased signal or signal intensity similar

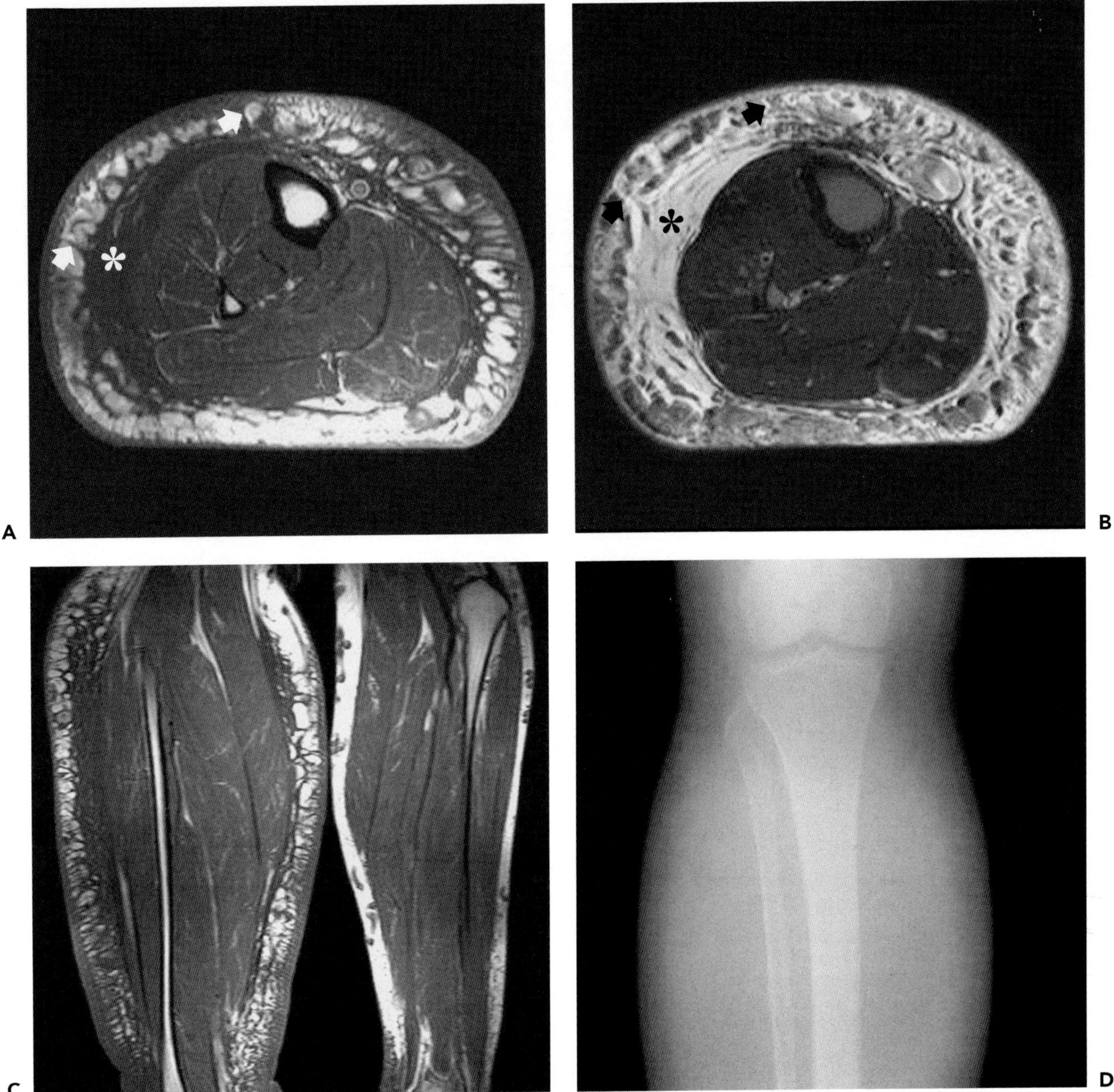

Figure 13.10   Lymphedema: MR imaging in a man 37 years of age with congenital lymphedema (Milroy disease). **A,B:** Axial T1-weighted (TR/TE; 500/15) **(A)** and T2-weighted (4127/80) **(B)** spin-echo MR images show a honeycomb appearance of the subcutaneous connective tissue (*arrows*) with thickening of the overlying skin. Note prominent fluid collection adjacent to fascia (*asterisk*). **C:** Coronal T1-weighted (TR/TE; 636/15) spin-echo MR image shows similar findings. Contralateral lower leg is normal. **D:** Anteroposterior radiograph shows the skin thickening and reticulated opacity of subcutaneous edema.

to or less than that of normal skeletal muscle and a higher signal intensity rim, (b) abscess rim enhancement following gadolinium administration, (c) increased signal intensity on T2-weighted images in the affected muscle(s) with central fluid collection, and surrounding thin rim of decreased signal (corresponding to a rim of increased signal on T1-weighted images), (d) associated skin thickening, subcutaneous fat stranding, and swelling of fascial planes,

and (e) fluid in the joint distal to the affected muscle(s) (Fig. 13.5). Fleckenstein et al. found similar MR findings in patients with myositis and acquired immunodeficiency syndrome, with the exception of normal subcutaneous tissues (29).

On power Doppler ultrasound, an abscess shows an absence of flow centrally and hyperemia in the surrounding tissue (30). Ultrasound may be quite helpful in

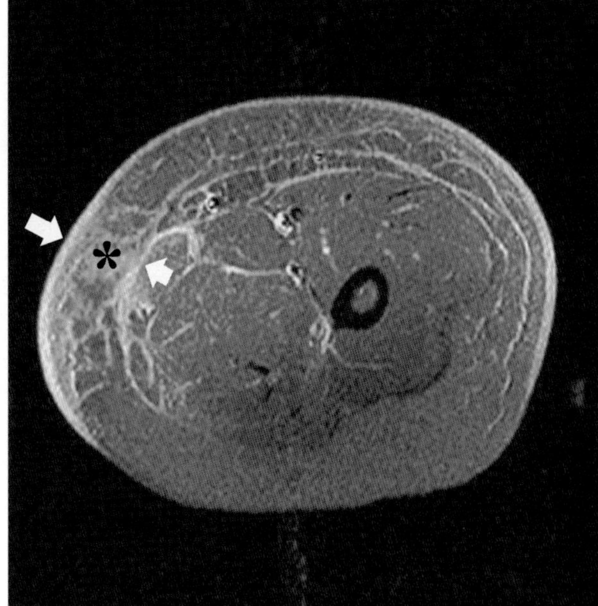 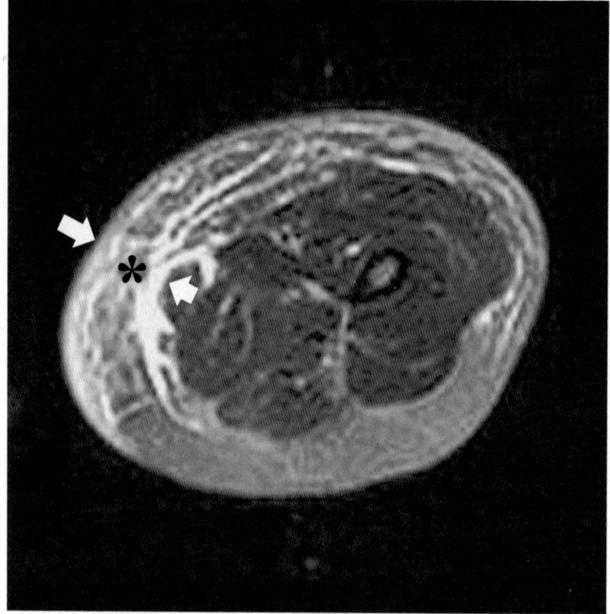

Figure 13.11 Non-necrotizing fasciitis with associated cellulitis: MR imaging features in a woman 22 years of age presenting with rapidly progressive pain and swelling in the proximal medial thigh. **A:** Axial fat-suppressed T1-weighted (TR/TE; 659/12) MR image following gadolinium administration shows cellulitis with enhancement of the skin (*long arrow*) and subcutaneous tissue (*asterisk*). Associated fasciitis is seen with thickening and enhancement of the deep fascia (*short arrow*). Note subtle enhancement of muscle deep to the fascial indicative of myositis. **B:** Axial T2-weighted (TR/TE; 4000/91) spin-echo MR image shows similar findings with high signal in the affected areas.

distinguishing between an inflammatory and noninflammatory collection. In addition to diagnosis, ultrasound is quite useful to guide aspiration of drainage.

The idiopathic inflammatory myopathies are a group of disorders that includes polymyositis, dermatomyositis, and inclusion body myositis (31). They are characterized by edema within and around muscle, subcutaneous reaction, muscle calcification, and fatty infiltration of muscle (31). Patients are usually diagnosed clinically, presenting with proximal limb or neck weakness, sometimes associated with muscle pain. Characteristic laboratory results include elevated serum creatine kinase, aldolase, lactic dehydrogenase, and transaminases, as well as a characteristic electromyogram (32). When imaging is performed, it is typically not for diagnosis but rather to establish the extent of muscle involvement, determine the result of therapy, or identify a suitable biopsy location (33) (Fig. 13.16). Lesions are typically multiple and bilaterally symmetric.

Cat-Scratch Disease

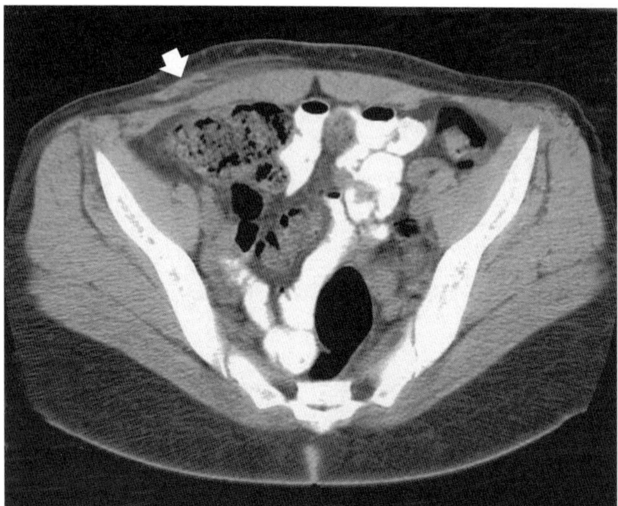

Figure 13.12 Non-necrotizing fasciitis with associated cellulitis: CT imaging features in a woman 34 years of age presenting with right lower quadrant pain. Axial noncontrast CT scan shows fascial thickening (*arrow*), with poorly localized increased attenuation in the adjacent tissue.

KEY CONCEPTS
- Benign regional lymphadenitis is associated with exposure to cats.
- It is caused by infection from *Bartonella henselae*, a gram-negative bacillus.
- Most patients are young; two-thirds of cases occur in individuals between 5 and 21 years of age.
- Single node involvement is seen in 44% to 85% of patients.
- MR imaging shows a regional lymphadenopathy with surrounding edema.

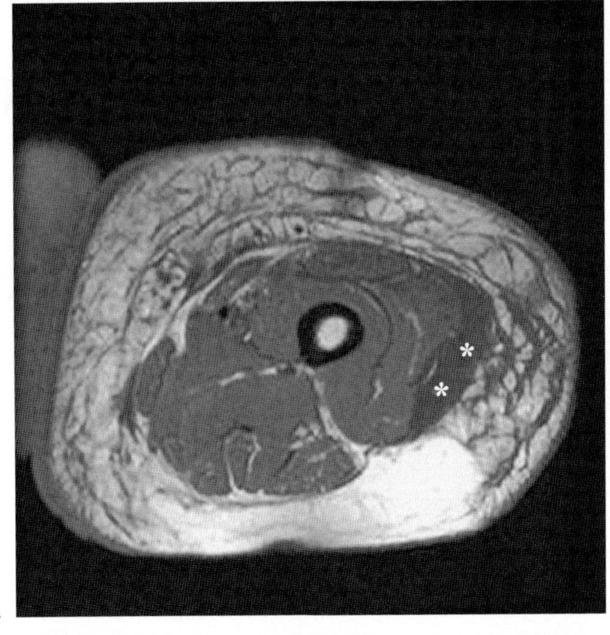

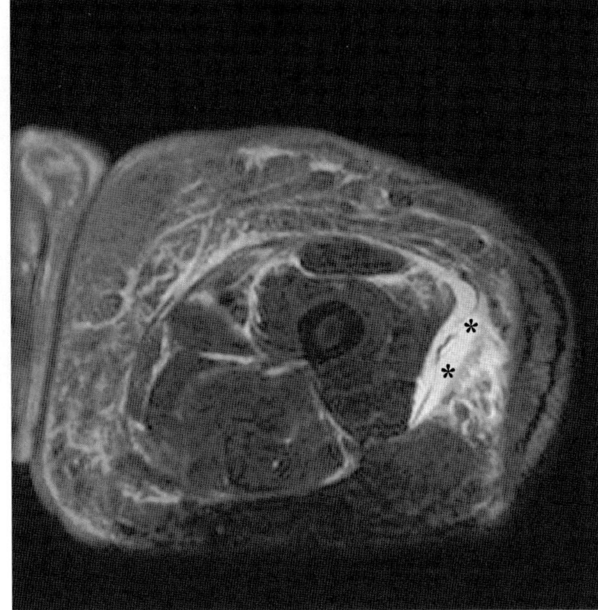

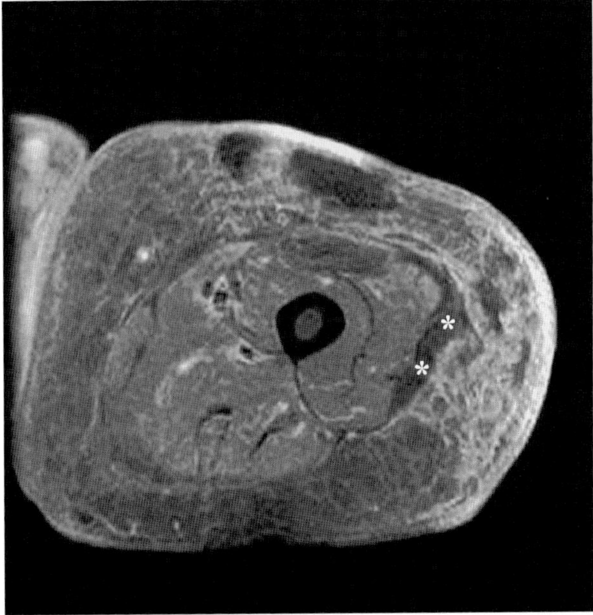

Figure 13.13 Necrotizing fasciitis: MR imaging findings in a man 51 years of age with diabetes and rapidly progressing pain and swelling in the thigh. **A,B:** Axial T1-weighted (TR/TE; 716/15) **(A)** and fat-suppressed T2-weighted (TR/TE; 6566/105) **(B)** spin-echo MR images show changes of cellulitis with extensive abnormal signal (*asterisks*) centered on the fascia. Note abnormal signal in adjacent muscle indicative of associated myositis. **C:** Axial T1-weighted (TR/TE; 650/15) spin-echo MR image following intravenous gadolinium administration shows nonenhancing tissue laterally (*asterisks*) and anteriorly. Necrosis was identified at surgery.

Cat-scratch disease is a benign regional lymphadenitis associated with exposure to cats, cat scratches, or both (34). It is caused by infection from *Bartonella henselae*, a gram-negative bacillus (35). In the healthy host, the disease is usually self-limiting and resolves spontaneously within weeks to months (34). Although the condition was first described by Parinaud in 1889 (36), the cat was not identified as the carrier until 1931 (34).

Most patients are young, with approximately two-thirds of cases seen in individuals between 5 and 21 years of age (34). More than 90% of patients have a history of exposure to cats (34). Infection may manifest itself with nonpruritic papules or pustules within 3 to 10 days following exposure and typically resolves within days to weeks. Regional lym-

phadenopathy in the draining nodes develops within 3 to 4 weeks (34). This is most common in the epitrochlear region, neck, and groin (34). Nodes typically range in size from 1 to 5 cm (35).

Single node involvement is seen in 44% to 85% of patients (37,38). Multiple node involvement at a single site is seen in 24% of cases (37), and disseminated disease occurs in approximately 5% to 10% of cases (39). The adenopathy typically resolves in 3 months but may persist for as long as 1 year (37). The disease is self-limiting, and antibiotic treatment does not alter the course of the disease in noncompromised hosts (34). Bone lesions are quite rarely reported, occurring in 0.2% of patients (40). Bone lesions are typically lytic, but periosteal reaction

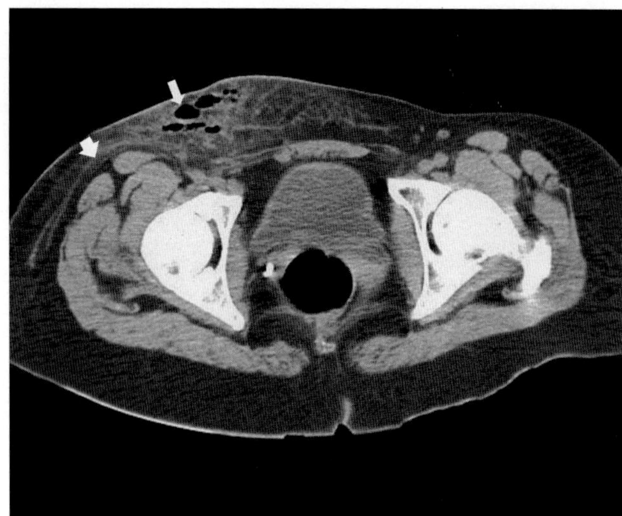

Figure 13.14 Necrotizing fasciitis: CT imaging features in a woman 40 years of age. Axial noncontrast CT scan shows fascial thickening (*short arrow*) with reticulated and poorly localized increased attenuation in the adjacent tissue, compatible with cellulitis and fasciitis. Note air (*long arrow*) secondary to tissue necrosis.

and associated sclerosis may be seen (35). These osseous lesions are usually not contiguous with the involved node (41).

MR imaging shows a regional lymphadenopathy, with nodes appearing as mildly heterogeneous masses and associated surrounding edema (Fig. 13.17) (34). The signal intensity of the lesions is similar to that of skeletal muscle on T1-weighted images and equal to or greater than that of fat on T2-weighted images (34). There is mild enhancement of the lymph nodes, often peripherally, as well as of the surrounding edema following contrast administration (Figs. 13.18 and 13.19) (34). CT demonstrates a soft tissue mass corresponding to involved lymph nodes. Low attenuation may be noted centrally, caused by necrosis (34,42). Radiographs may be unremarkable or may reveal a nonspecific soft tissue mass.

Hydatid Disease

KEY CONCEPTS
- Hydatid disease is caused by *Echinococcus granulosus*.
- Soft tissue involvement is unusual, accounting for approximately 1% to 2% of cases.
- Multivesicular lesions are considered to be characteristic of hydatid disease, with a large cyst and multiple daughter cysts.
- MR imaging is usually superior to ultrasonography in suggesting a vesicular structure.
- The multilocular pattern and regular enhancing rim are considered distinctive features of hydatid disease.

Hydatid disease is caused by *Echinococcus granulosus*. Although infrequent in the United States, it is common in many parts of the world. The vast majority of lesions involve the liver and lungs, with only 10% to 15% involving other organs (43). Soft tissue involvement is unusual, accounting for approximately 0.8% to 2.3% of reported cases, and it is predominantly intramuscular (44,45), although Chevalier et al. (46) reported a patient with subcutaneous involvement.

Hydatid cysts are classified on their imaging appearance into four types (44):

Type I: These appear as a well-defined, anechoic mass with or without hydatid sand and septa.
Type II: These are cysts in conjunction with daughter cyst(s) and matrix.
Type III: These lesions represent dead cysts and demonstrate calcified walls.
Type IV: These are cysts complicated by rupture and superinfection.

The contractility of skeletal muscle and the presence of lactic acid within muscle make it a difficult place for hydatid cysts to grow (44). The propensity of soft tissue lesions to occur in the neck and trunk may relate to the increased vascularity and decreased activity of these areas (44). Type I, II, and III cysts are described in soft tissue (44).

Patients with soft tissue involvement present with a palpable mass (45). There is a marked lower extremity prevalence (45). Martin et al. described three cases in the soft tissue and noted that the radiologic findings were similar to those described in the liver (45). Multivesicular lesions are considered to be characteristic of hydatid disease, with the presence of a large cyst and multiple daughter cysts (45). This pattern of multivesicular lesions was seen in two of their three cases and considered diagnostic. The third patient's lesion imaged as a solid mass and mimicked a soft tissue tumor. In the evaluation of soft tissue lesions, MR imaging is usually superior to ultrasonography in suggesting a vesicular structure. The multilocular pattern and regular enhancing rim are considered distinctive features of hydatid disease (Figs. 13.20 and 13.21) (46,48).

CRYSTAL DEPOSITION DISEASES

The diagnosis of the vast majority of crystal deposition diseases is made clinically, although this is not invariably the case, and patients may come to medical attention for the evaluation of a "soft tissue mass." This is especially the case in calcium hydroxyapatite disease, which is typically monoarticular, and the calcification may suggest a mineralized soft tissue mass. Less commonly, patients with tophaceous gout and rarely pseudogout (calcium pyrophosphate dihydrate crystal deposition disease) may present for the evaluation of a soft tissue mass.

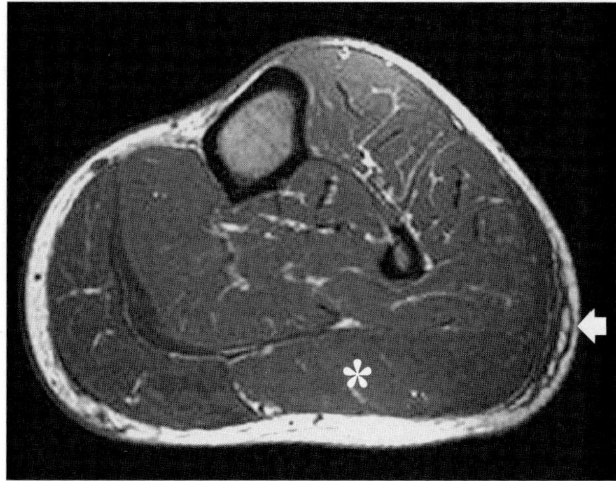

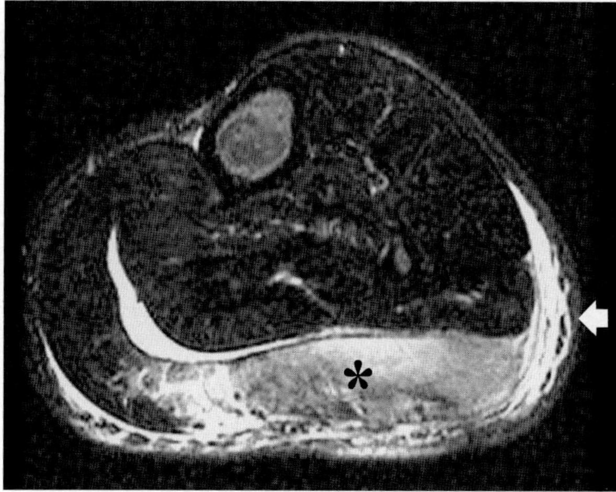

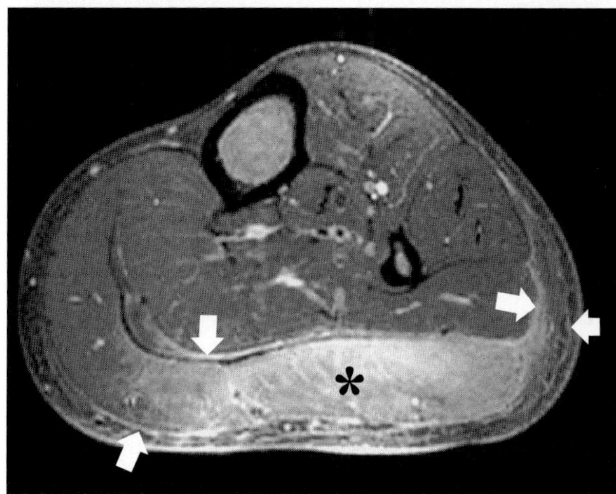

Figure 13.15 Inflammatory myositis: MR imaging features in a man 69 years of age with lymphoma and myelodysplastic syndrome presenting with pain, fever, and a swollen red lower leg. **A,B:** Axial T1-weighted (TR/TE; 450/14) **(A)** spin-echo and short-tau inversion recovery (STIR) (TR/TE/TI; 4467/105/150) **(B)** MR images of the lower leg show abnormal signal within the muscle (*asterisk*), most prominently in the lateral head of the gastrocnemius muscle. Note associated cellulitis (*arrow*) and fluid between the gastrocnemius and soleus muscles and adjacent to the fascia. **C:** Axial fat-suppressed T1-weighted (TR/TE; 700/14) spin-echo MR image shows enhancement of the abnormal muscle (*asterisk*). Note cellulitis laterally (*arrow*) and enhancing fascia (*long arrows*), compatible with associated fasciitis.

Calcium Hydroxyapatite Disease (Calcific Tendinitis)

Recurrent, painful, calcific deposits in tendons and periarticular soft tissues are frequent, but it was not until relatively recently that these were identified as hydroxyapatite crystals (49). The ability of these crystals to cause bursitis and other periarticular inflammatory diseases is well-established (49). The following discussion focuses on manifestations of calcium hydroxyapatite disease, which may suggest a soft tissue mass. This typically occurs when calcific deposits form in a masslike manner within a tendon (calcific tendinitis), which does not insert in the juxta-articular region.

The origin of calcific tendonitis is unknown, but hypoxia in the critical (relatively avascular) zone of the tendon is the suggested cause (50). The hypoxia may be followed by fibrocartilaginous metaplasia with subsequent calcification (50,51). The calcification is irritating to the surrounding soft tissue, resulting in pain and inflammation. Synonyms include *calcifying peritendonitis, peri-*

arthritis calcarea, peritendonitis, and *calcareus tendonitis* (49,52).

Calcific tendonitis is most common in the shoulder, in the distal supraspinatus tendon (50), with this location accounting for approximately 60% of cases (52).

KEY CONCEPTS

- After the shoulder, the wrist and the hip (gluteus maximus) are the next most common locations of calcium hydroxyapatite disease.
- Radiographs show amorphous soft tissue calcification that may taper away from the bone, simulating a "comet tail."
- Bone erosions can appear aggressive radiologically and suggest a neoplasm.
- Bone scintigraphy shows increased tracer accumulation.
- MR imaging is variable, depending on the amount of associated inflammation.
- Calcification usually images as a signal void on all MR imaging pulse sequences.

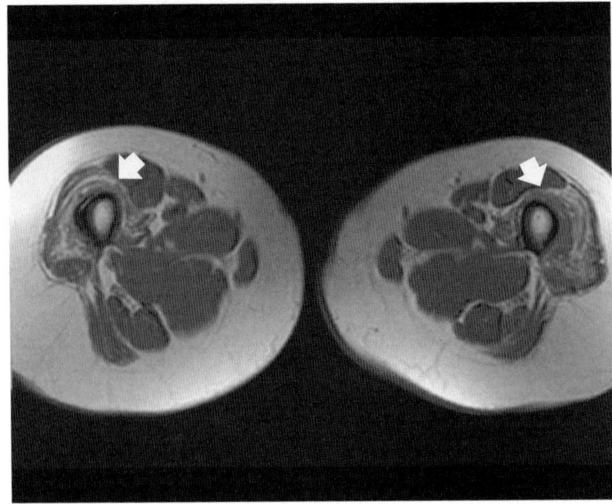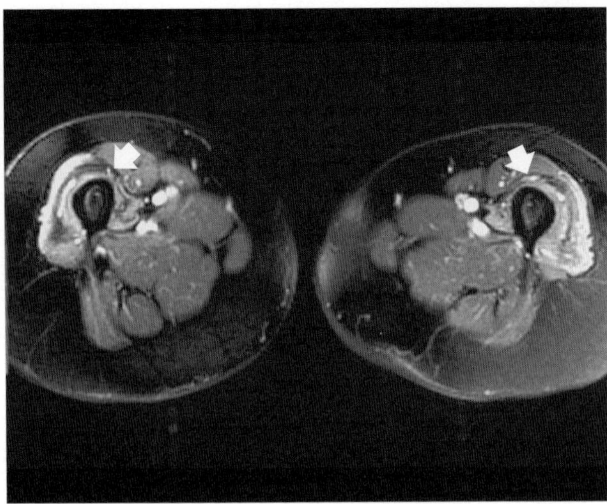

Figure 13.16   Inflammatory myositis: MR imaging features in a woman 67 years of age with inclusion body myositis. **A,B:** Axial T1-weighted (TR/TE; 616/17) **(A)** and fat-suppressed T2-weighted (TR/TE; 4000/105) **(B)** spin-echo MR images show relatively symmetric atrophy and abnormal signal most prominently in the vastus lateralis and vastus intermedius muscles (*arrows*). The MR imaging findings were not specific but served to direct biopsy, which allowed definitive diagnosis.

The wrist and hip (gluteus maximus) are the next most common locations, accounting for approximately 14% and 12% of cases, respectively (52). Clinically, patients present with localized pain and point tenderness over the lesion (50,52). Calcific tendonitis is most common between 40 and 70 years of age, with men and women affected equally (53). Patients are usually treated with nonsteroidal anti-inflammatory medication. Calcific tendonitis may also be treated with fluoroscopically guided lavage and aspiration (54,55). With this technique, the calcifications are injected under local anesthesia using fluoroscopic guidance. Calcifications are injected with saline, or a mixture of saline and lidocaine, and then aspirated. This is repeated until the aspirate is free of calcific particles (54). Fine-needle aspiration technique with triamcinolone injection also shows good results (55).

Grossly, the lesion appears as a white, pastelike material. The focal calcific deposits are separated from each other by strands of fibrocartilaginous tissue (56). Diffraction studies on the calcific deposits show them to be hydroxyapatite crystals (56).

Radiographs show amorphous soft tissue calcification. Calcifications are usually poorly defined in the early phase of the disorder, becoming progressively more rounded and dense (57). Calcifications may remain stable with time, enlarge, or resorb (57). When present, the soft tissue calcification tapers away from the bone, simulating a "comet tail" and suggesting the distribution of a tendon (Fig. 13.22) (50). The comet-tail appearance is seen in about half of cases (58). Cortical bone erosion, although unusual, is reported (Fig. 13.23) (50,58,59). Bone erosions can appear aggressive radiologically, suggesting a neoplasm, and they are most frequent in the proximal humerus and femoral diaphysis (58). Although erosions limited to the cortex are most common, marrow involvement is seen in 36% of patients with osseous involvement.

Bone scintigraphy shows increased tracer accumulation (50). CT scanning shows a calcified nodule (Fig. 13.23). The density and margins of the nodule may vary with its age. Pope and Keats (53) reported three cases of calcific tendinitis in the vastus lateralis muscle and noted that in the acute phase (2 weeks after onset of complaints), the calcification was ill-defined and associated with edema in the surrounding muscle. After several months, calcification was denser and more sharply defined, with mild edema. At 1 year, calcification was less dense. MR imaging findings vary with the degree of inflammation. When significant inflammation is present, it demonstrates areas of ill-defined fluidlike signal without a focal mass. The tendon calcification images as a signal void on all pulse sequences (Fig. 13.22) (53).

Gout

Gout is a metabolic disease characterized by hyperuricemia and develops as a result of either overproduction and/or decreased renal excretion of uric acid (60). Soft tissue involvement is usually seen in patients with focal deposits of monosodium urate, termed *tophi* (60). Tophi usually do not appear until several years after the initial gouty episode. Rarely, soft tissue tophi occur in the absence of articular disease (60). We have encountered patients occasionally presenting with a soft tissue mass that was presumed to be neoplastic but was actually

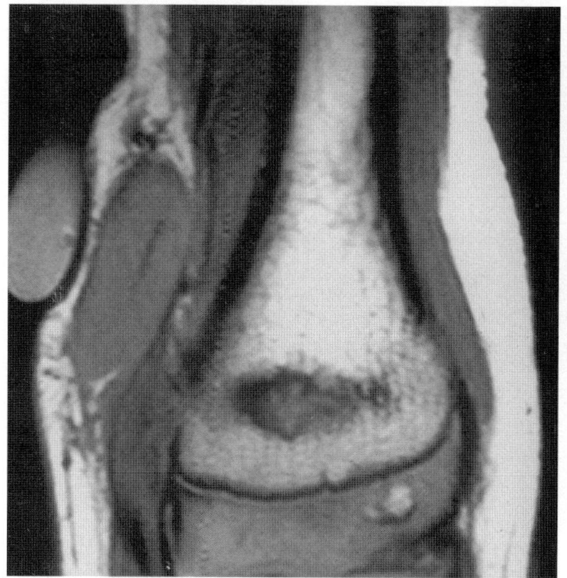

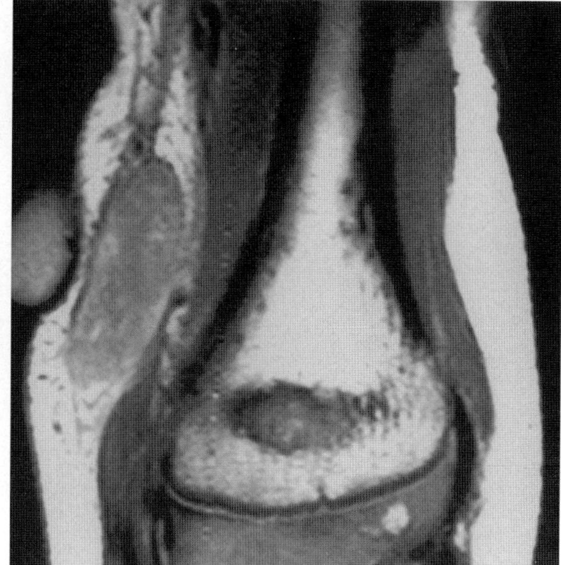

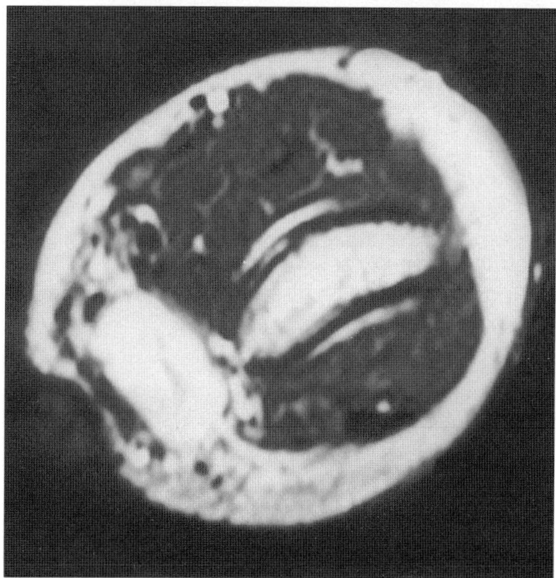

Figure 13.17 Cat-scratch disease: MR imaging findings of epitrochlear lymphadenopathy in a girl 4 years of age. **A,B:** Coronal T1-weighted (TR/TE; 650/20) spin-echo MR images preceding **(A)** and following **(B)** contrast administration show a large epitrochlear node with surrounding edema. The node shows mild heterogeneous enhancement. **C:** Axial T2-weighted (TR/TE; 2000/80) spin-echo MR image shows the node to be mildly heterogeneous, with a signal intensity slightly greater than that of subcutaneous fat. Note associated edema.

KEY CONCEPTS

- Soft tissue tophi usually do not appear until several years after the initial gouty episode.
- Soft tissue tophi rarely occur in the absence of articular disease.
- Radiographs of gouty tophi usually reveal a juxta-articular, lobulated, soft tissue mass.
- Calcification of the mass may be seen, although it is unusual.
- On T1-weighted images, tophi show an intermediate signal intensity.
- Signal intensity on T2-weighted imaging is variable, but typically demonstrates persistent low-to-intermediate signal intensity.
- Enhancement associated with tophi reflects the surrounding granulation tissue.

tophaceous gout or, less commonly, tophaceous pseudo-gout (see later).

Pathologically, gouty tophi are aggregations of urate crystals and a proteinaceous matrix, surrounded by an intense inflammatory reaction (61). Urate crystals show strong negative birefringence as opposed to calcium pyrophosphate dihydrate (CPPD), which reveals weak positive features under polarized light. Gouty tophi may be seen around joints, including feet, hands, ankles, elbows, knees, spine, and the acromioclavicular joint (61–63, 64–67), and they also have a predilection for the olecranon and prepatellar regions.

Radiographs of gouty tophi usually reveal a lobulated juxta-articular soft tissue mass (60). Calcification of the mass may be seen, although it is uncommon, and typically seen to better advantage on CT images, which can also detect the associated soft tissue mass (Fig. 13.24).

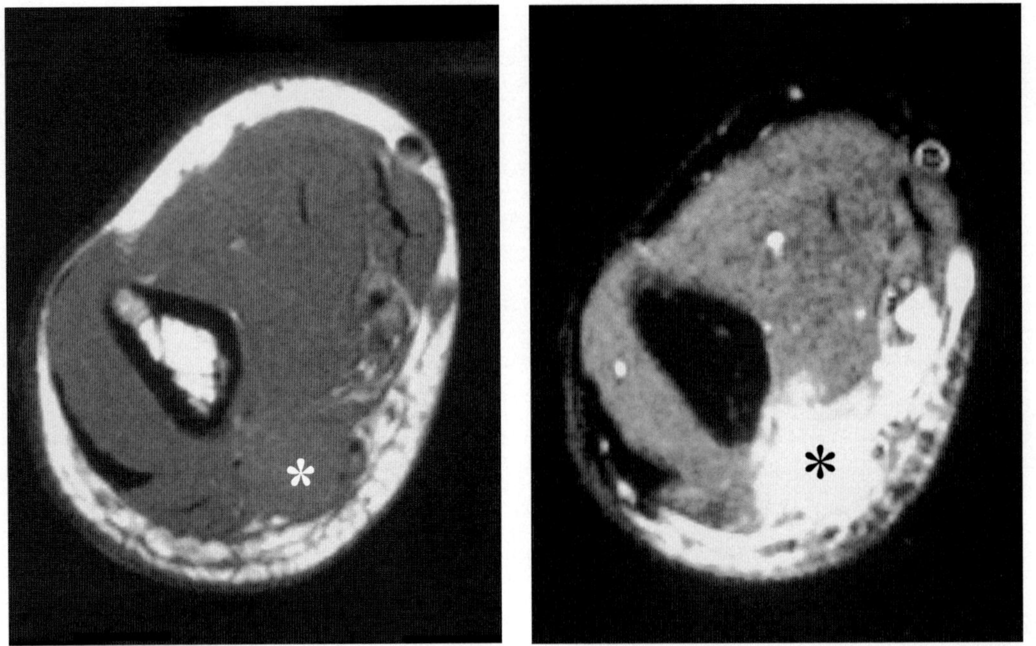

Figure 13.18   Cat-scratch disease: MR imaging findings of edema and lymphadenopathy in a boy 14 years of age. **A,B:** Axial T1-weighted (TR/TE; 480/15) **(A)** spin-echo and short-tau inversion recovery (STIR) (TR/TE/TI; 3220/22/150) **(B)** MR spin-echo MR images show enlarged epitrochlear lymphadenopathy (*asterisk*) with prominent associated edema.

Long-standing tophi cause pressure erosions on the adjacent bone. On T1-weighted images, tophi show an intermediate signal intensity. The signal intensity on T2-weighted imaging is variable but typically demonstrates persistent intermediate-to-low signal intensity in both noncalcified and calcified gouty tophi (Figs. 13.25 and 13.26) (61,68,69). The relatively decreased signal intensity in gouty tophi is likely from the presence of urate crystals and fibrous tissue (61). An increased signal intensity may be seen on fat-suppressed fluid-sensitive images (70), and also is noted on conventional T2-weighted images, but is uncommon (69). The intense enhancement associated with tophi reflects the surrounding granulation tissue and increased vascularity of the affected synovium (61). Homogeneous enhancement within the tophi has also reported (69).

Tophaceous Pseudogout (Calcium Pyrophosphate Dihydrate Crystal Deposition Disease)

Calcium pyrophosphate dihydrate (CPPD) crystal deposition disease is the most common crystalline arthropathy and is characterized by the deposition of crystals in the articular and juxta-articular tissues (71). CPPD crystal deposition disease is quite common, reported with a frequency of 1 in 1,000, and a prevalence in patients 85 years and older approaching 45% (72). In contrast, the tophaceous form of pseudogout is rare (73). Rather than being a generalized process as seen in the conventional form of the disease, the tophaceous form is distinctive and may be a local

> **KEY CONCEPTS**
> - CPPD crystal deposition disease is the most common crystalline arthropathy.
> - Tophaceous pseudogout is a distinctive form and may be a local process seen without associated chondrocalcinosis.
> - Radiographically, tophaceous pseudogout may resemble tumoral calcinosis, appearing as a lobular, well-defined, extensively mineralized, soft tissue mass.
> - MR imaging shows an intermediate signal intensity on T1-weighted images and a decreased-to-intermediate signal intensity on T2-weighted images.

process that need not be seen in association with chondrocalcinosis (74).

In the cervical spine, CPPD crystal deposition is seen around the atlantoaxial joint and may present as an extra-axial mass at the craniovertebral junction causing cord compression associated with chondrocalcinosis, subchondral cyst formation, osseous erosions, and odontoid fractures (72,75). Kakitsubata et al. (75) reviewed nine patients with type 2 odontoid fractures and found evidence of CPPD crystal deposition disease in all cases. Subchondral cyst formation and osseous erosions were also seen to varying degrees, in all patients.

Histologically, the lesion is characterized by chondroid metaplasia accompanied by massive CPPD deposition and foreign body reaction (74). Radiographically, tophaceous pseudogout may resemble tumoral calcinosis (73),

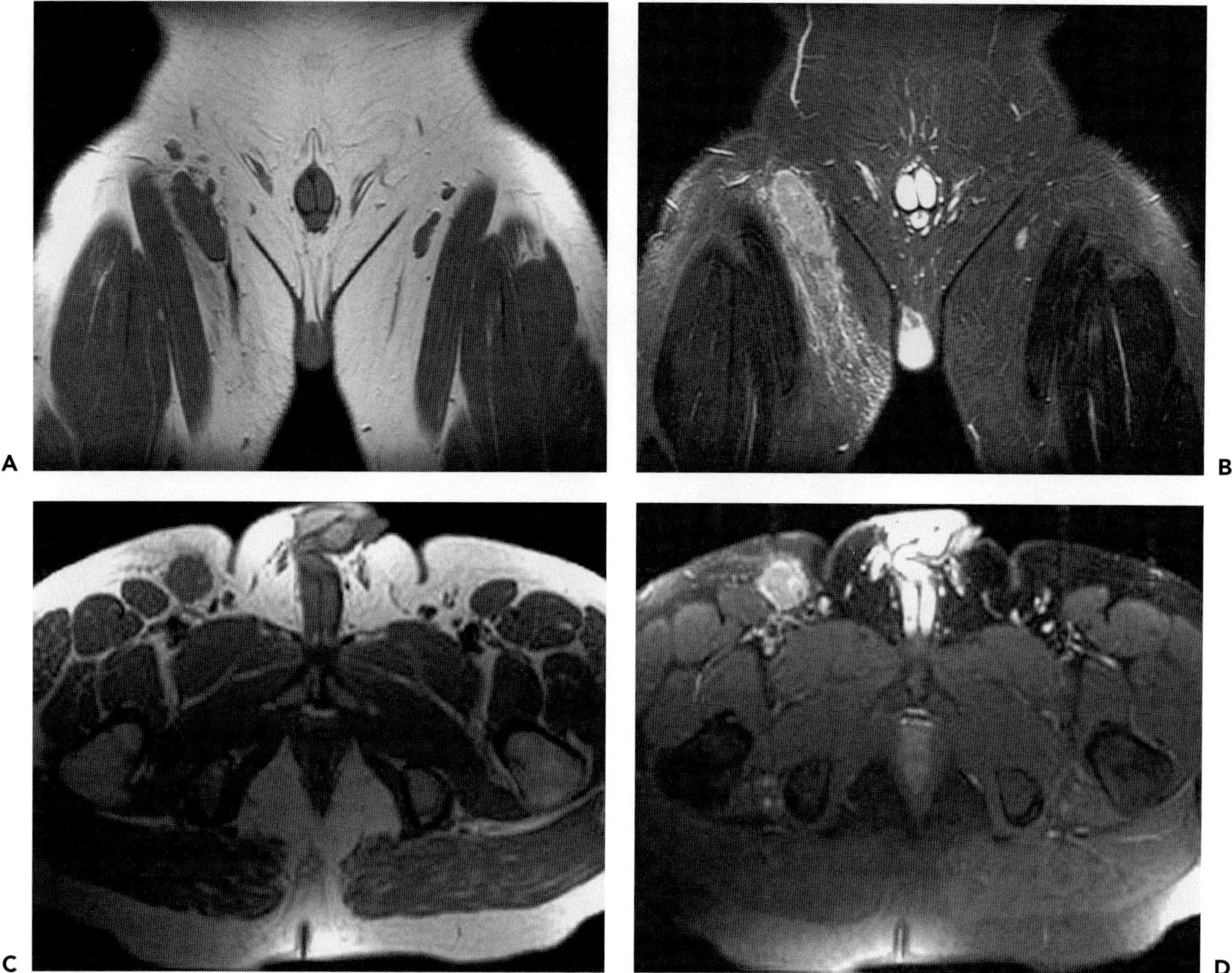

Figure 13.19 Cat-scratch disease: MR imaging findings of groin lymphadenopathy in a man 26 years of age, with a rapidly growing, painful groin mass. **A,B:** Coronal T1-weighted (TR/TE; 750/17) **(A)** and T2-weighted (TR/TE; 5950/68) **(B)** spin-echo MR images show a nodal mass in the right groin with prominent associated edema. **C,D:** Axial T1-weighted (TR/TE; 600/15) spin-echo images preceding **(C)** and with fat-suppression following **(D)** contrast administration show a large right inguinal node with surrounding edema. The node shows mild heterogeneous enhancement.

appearing as a lobular, well-defined, extensively mineralized, soft tissue mass (Fig. 13.27). Osseous remodeling is also reported (74). On MR imaging, limited reports show the lesion to have an intermediate signal intensity on T1-weighted images and a decreased-to-intermediate signal intensity on T2-weighted images, although high signal intensity has also been reported (Fig. 13.28) (71,72). MR imaging signal intensity is affected by the degree of mineralization of the mass.

TUMORLIKE LESIONS

Amyloid

Amyloid deposition can occur throughout the musculoskeletal system, including bone, disc space, and soft tissues. Involvement in the soft tissues occurs primarily in the tenosynovium, capsule, ligaments, and tendons. Deposition in the soft tissues is more common in secondary than in

---

KEY CONCEPTS

- Amyloid deposition may be primary or secondary.
- Soft tissue involvement is more common in secondary than in primary amyloidosis.
- CT and MR imaging of tenosynovial amyloid deposition is seen as thickening around a joint.
- Extrinsic erosion of bone is not infrequent.
- MR imaging signal intensity is similar to that of muscle on T1-weighted images and shows low-to-intermediate signal intensity on T2-weighted MR pulse sequences.

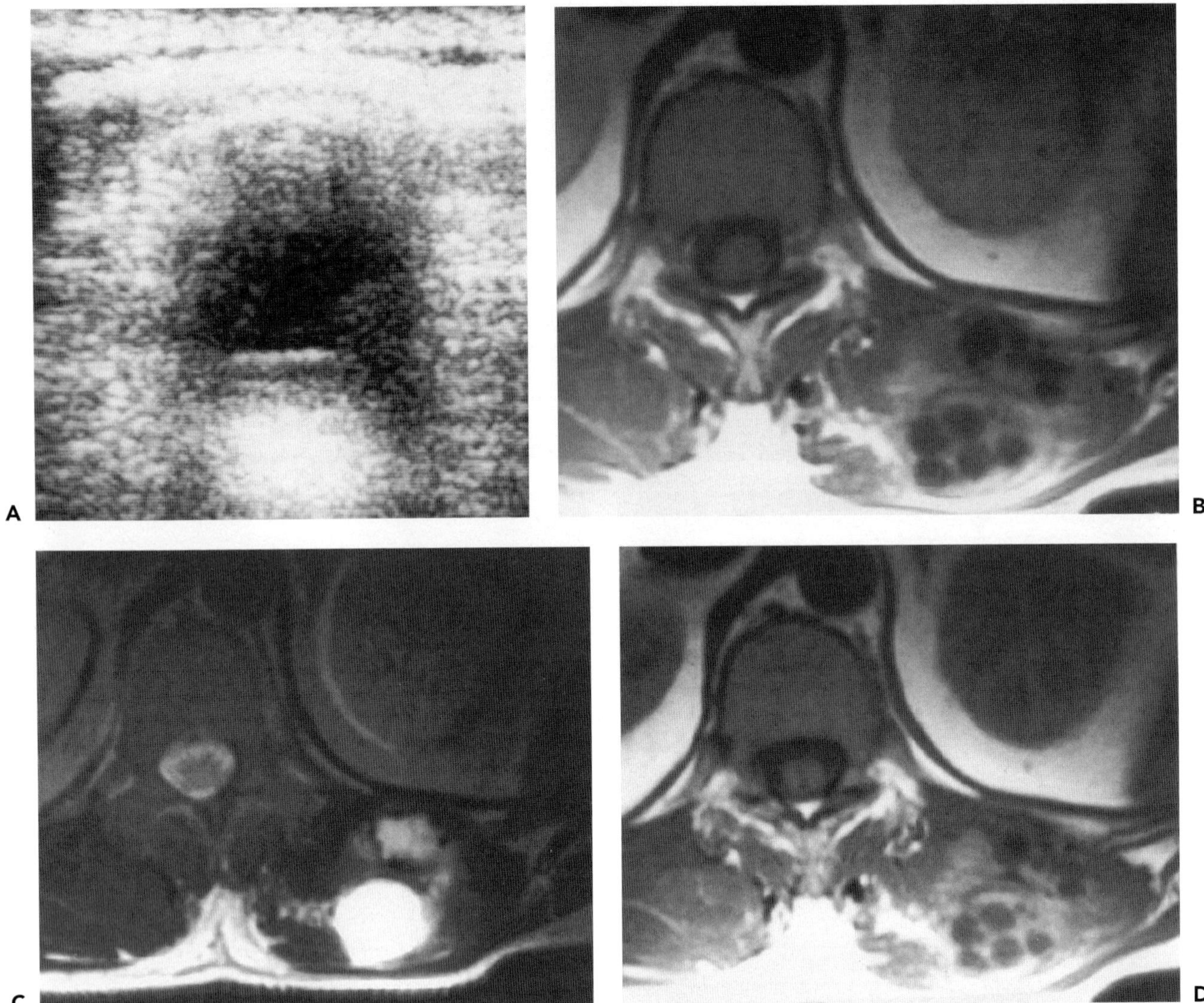

Figure 13.20 Hydatid disease, caused by *Echinococcus granulosus*: Imaging features in a man 40 years of age presenting with a paraspinal mass. **A:** Ultrasonography shows a complex paraspinal mass. **B,C:** Axial T1-weighted (TR/TE; 600/15) **(B)** and T2-weighted (TR/TE; 2200/80) **(C)** spin-echo MR images show a multivesicular paraspinal lesion. MR is superior to ultrasonography in delineating the vesicular nature of the lesion. **D:** Postgadolinium T1-weighted (TR/TE; 600/15) spin-echo MR image shows minimal enhancement.

primary amyloidosis. Secondary amyloidosis is associated with chronic inflammatory diseases and multiple myeloma (5% to 10% of patients) (76). The most frequent type of secondary amyloidosis is associated with chronic renal failure, particularly, although not exclusively, in patients undergoing hemodialysis. Tenosynovial deposition of amyloid is most common in the shoulder and hip. Indeed, Camacho et al. showed an incidence of 71% and 35%, respectively, in these two joints in a group of 88 patients (77). Involvement is usually polyarticular. Deposition in the carpal tunnel, with median nerve compression, occurs in 2% to 31% of patients with chronic renal failure (76). Unlike idiopathic carpal tunnel syndrome, which shows a predominance in women and in the right hand, no such predilection is seen in patients with amyloid deposition.

Pathologically, secondary amyloid associated with chronic renal failure is caused by deposition of β2-microglobulin, a different protein than is seen in primary amyloidosis (78). Amyloid has a similar appearance to collagen histologically, and can be identified on Congo red stain with characteristic birefringence. In addition, specific immunohistochemical stains are available to identify the β2-microglobulin.

CT and MR imaging of tenosynovial deposition of amyloid is seen as capsular thickening around a joint. In locations such as the carpal tunnel, it is often prominent and extensive (79–82). Extrinsic erosion of bone is not infrequent, with punched-out lesions apparent on radiographs, particularly in the hips and shoulders. CT shows the thickening to be of soft tissue attenuation, whereas the

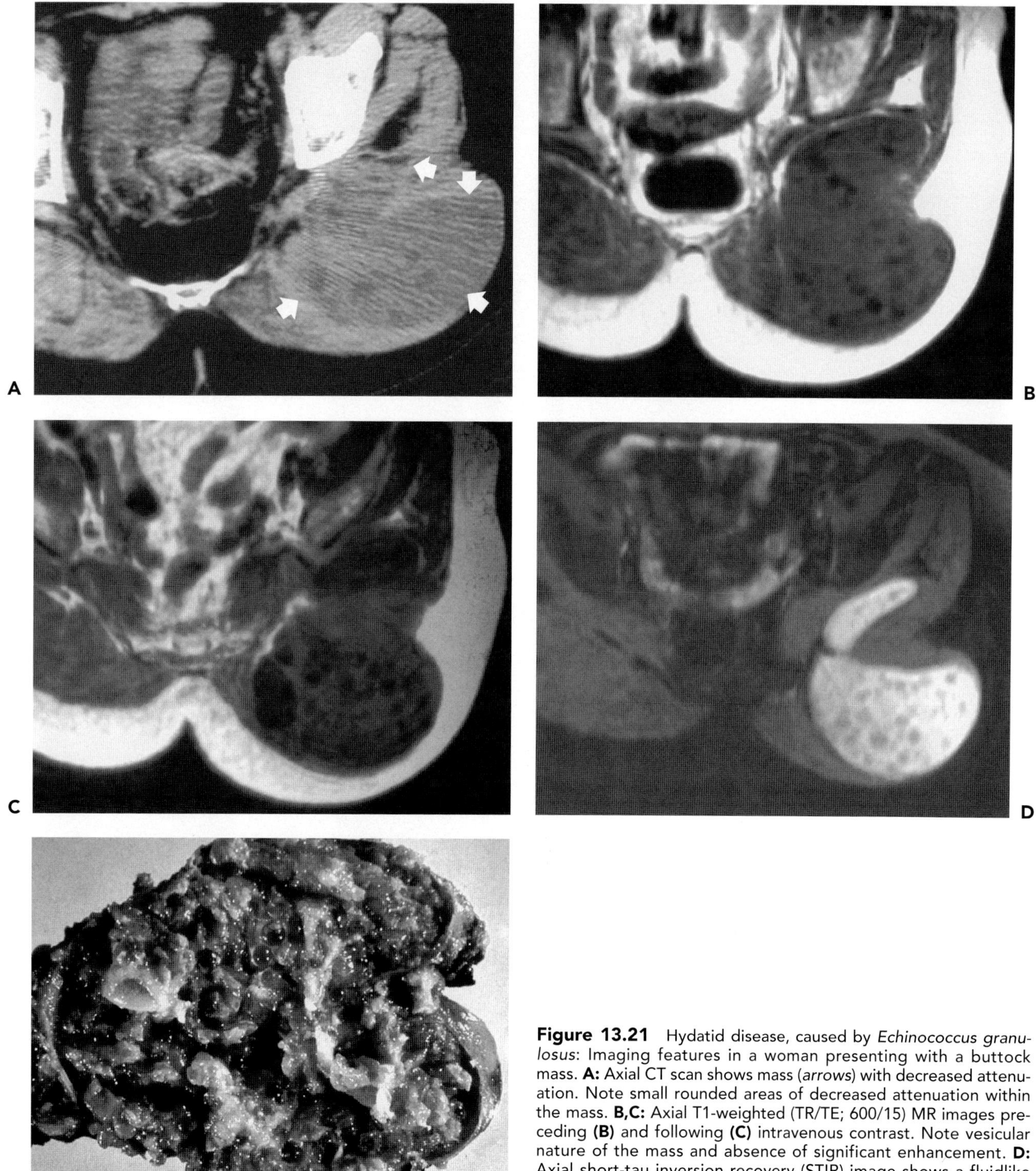

Figure 13.21 Hydatid disease, caused by *Echinococcus granulosus*: Imaging features in a woman presenting with a buttock mass. **A:** Axial CT scan shows mass (*arrows*) with decreased attenuation. Note small rounded areas of decreased attenuation within the mass. **B,C:** Axial T1-weighted (TR/TE; 600/15) MR images preceding (**B**) and following (**C**) intravenous contrast. Note vesicular nature of the mass and absence of significant enhancement. **D:** Axial short-tau inversion recovery (STIR) image shows a fluidlike signal to the mass with multiple, small, internal nodules. **E:** Photograph of the resected specimen shows the complex internal architecture with multiple "daughter cysts" and matrix.

signal intensity is similar to that of muscle on T1-weighted MR images. However, the most characteristic imaging appearance is the low-to-intermediate signal intensity on T2-weighted MR pulse sequences (Fig. 13.29) (61). This appears to reflect the collagenlike pathology of amyloid.

Small focal areas of fluid with high signal on long TR MR images are also frequent. Amyloid deposition within a joint can simulate pigmented villonodular synovitis, although the polyarticular involvement typifies the former disease as opposed to monoarticular changes in the latter.

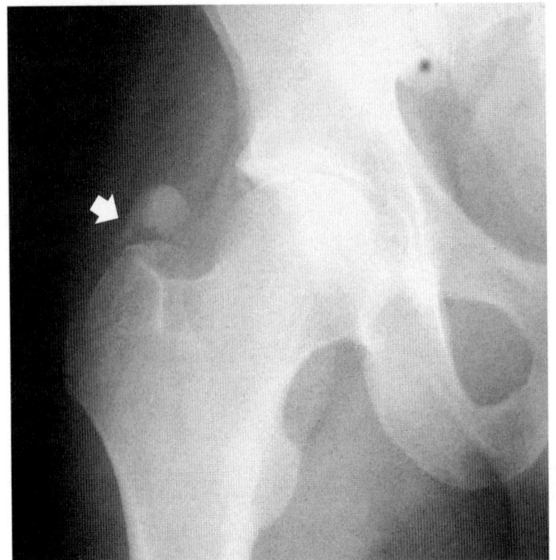

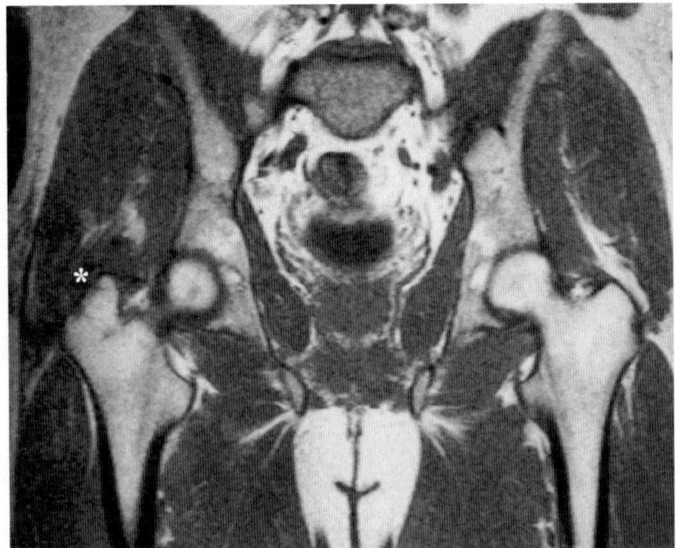

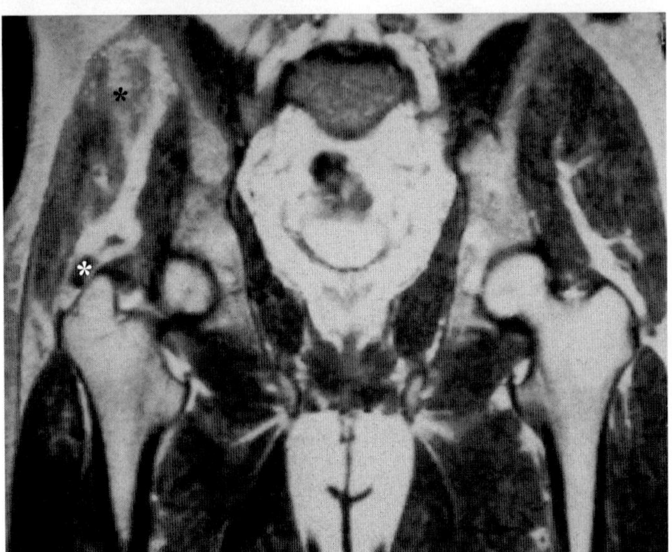

Figure 13.22 Calcium hydroxyapatite disease: MR imaging features in the hip of a man 30 years of age. **A:** Anteroposterior (AP) radiograph of the right hip shows a globular area of calcification adjacent to the greater trochanter. The calcification tapers away from the bone with a "comet tail" (*arrow*). **B,C:** Coronal T1-weighted (TR/TE; 400/15) **(B)** and turbo T2-weighted (TR/TE; 3600/90) **(C)** spin-echo MR images show a poorly defined area of abnormal signal adjacent to the greater trochanter and extending superiorly, with diffuse abnormal signal in the gluteus medius muscle (*black asterisk* in **C**). The area of decreased signal intensity (*white asterisk*) corresponds to the calcification seen in **A**.

In our experience, enhancement of amyloid disposition can be seen following intravenous contrast injection on MR imaging.

Aneurysm and Pseudoaneurysm

Peripheral aneurysms, especially when large, may mimic a soft tissue tumor. Defined as a dilatation of the wall of a vessel, an aneurysm may be true or false. A true aneurysm contains all three layers of the arterial wall (intima, media, and adventitia), whereas a false or pseudoaneurysm contains only adventitia, and is often considered to be analogous to an intramural hematoma.

The popliteal artery is the most frequently affected by peripheral aneurysm (83,84). Typically arteriosclerotic, up to 75% are bilateral, and 45% are associated with

KEY CONCEPTS

- A true aneurysm contains all three layers of the arterial wall.
- A false or pseudoaneurysm wall contains only adventitia.
- The popliteal artery is the most frequently affected peripheral artery.
- Pseudoaneurysms are usually the result of injury to the arterial wall.
- MR imaging in uncomplicated aneurysm cases reveals dilatation of the vessel, with a persistent flow signal void.
- Pseudoaneurysms typically show a more complex signal intensity, with areas of increased and decreased signal intensity.
- Distinction between an aneurysm with extensive thrombus and a pseudoaneurysm may be difficult.

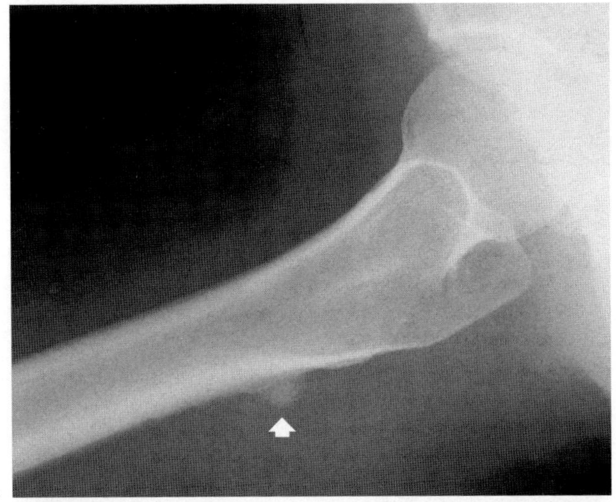

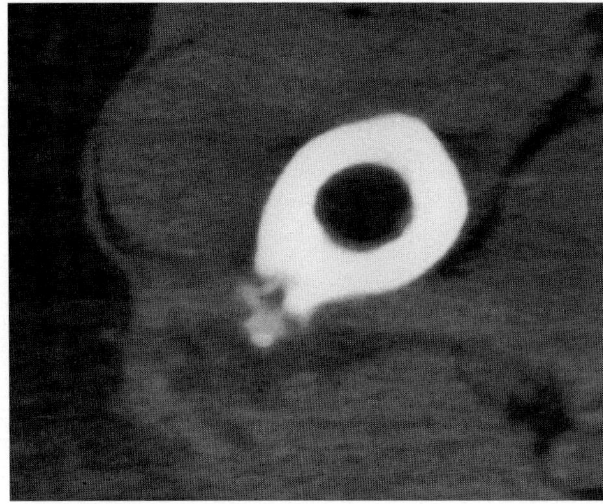

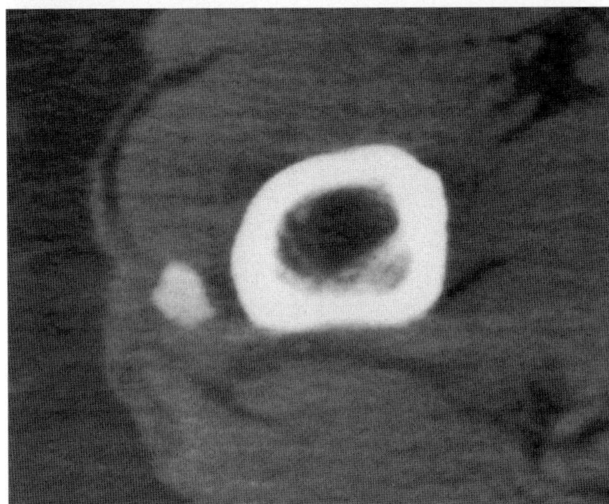

Figure 13.23 Calcium hydroxyapatite disease: Radiographic and CT features in a woman 46 years of age, with a history of thigh pain. **A:** Frog-leg lateral radiograph of the right hip shows a focal area of calcification (*arrow*) adjacent to the lateral aspect of the proximal femur. **B:** Axial noncontrast CT scan shows calcification immediately adjacent to the posterolateral aspect of the femur with associated bone erosion. Note the absence of an associated mass. **C:** Image just cranial to **B** shows the homogeneous character of the calcification.

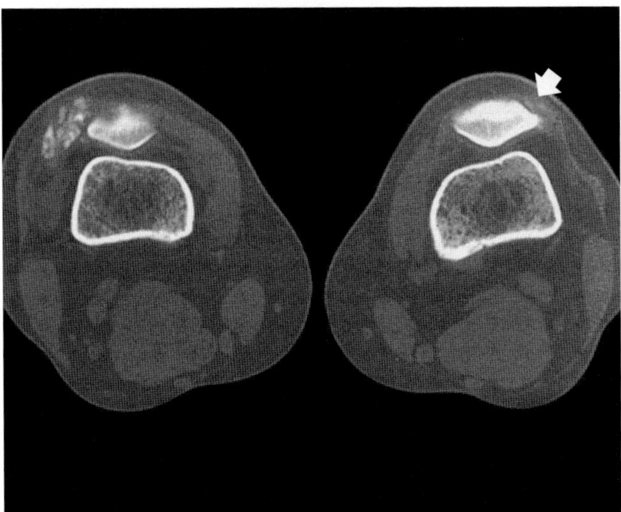

Figure 13.24 Gout: CT findings in a man 38 years of age. Axial noncontrast CT displayed on bone window shows an amorphously mineralized soft tissue mass with associated erosion in the right patella. A subtle lesion is seen adjacent to the left patella (*arrow*).

another aneurysm, especially of the abdominal aorta (83). Patients are generally older men, in the fifth and sixth decades (83,84). As many as half of patients may be asymptomatic. When symptoms are present, they may suggest vascular occlusive disease, including claudication, rest pain, ulceration, and venous obstruction (83–85). Lesions are usually smaller than 5 cm, although aneurysms up to 22 cm have been reported (83,85). Aneurysms may be complicated by extensive arteriosclerotic disease and internal thrombus.

Pseudoaneurysms are usually the result of injury to the arterial wall, with extravasation of blood and hematoma formation. The hematoma may compress and seal the injury (86). Lesions may remain stable for years, and symptoms may relate to the overall size of the lesion (86). Peripheral embolization is unusual (86). The diagnosis may be difficult in patients without a history of previous surgery, arteriography, or trauma.

Radiographs reveal a nonspecific soft tissue mass. Curvilinear calcifications may be present, although the

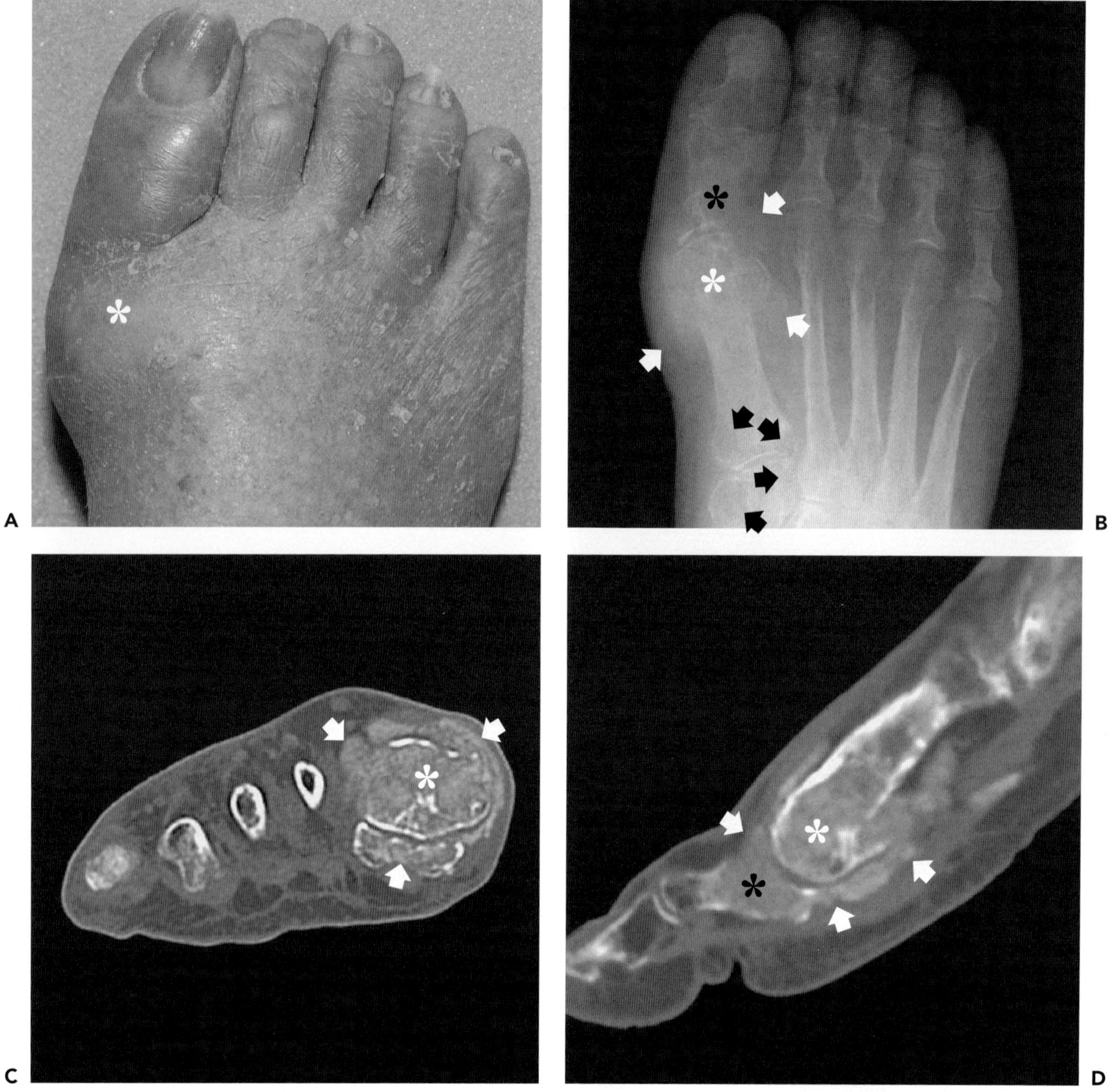

Figure 13.25 Gout: Imaging features in a woman 78 years of age presenting with a long-standing foot mass. **A:** Photograph of foot with mass (*asterisk*). Patient had no history of gout. **B:** Anteroposterior radiograph of the forefoot shows the mass (*white arrows*) and extension into the first metatarsal head (*white asterisk*). Note involvement of the base of the proximal phalynx (*black asterisk*) as well as subtle erosions at the base of the first metatarsal (*black arrows*). **C,D:** Axial **(C)** and reformatted sagittal **(D)** CT scans show the mass (*arrows*) and extensive osseous extension (*white asterisk*). Involvement of the proximal phalynx base (*black asterisk*) is well-demonstrated on sagittal image **D.** (*continued*)

frequency of calcification is unknown (83). MR imaging in uncomplicated cases reveals dilation of the vessel, with a persistent flow signal void. Frequently, MR imaging demonstrates a complex mass; signal intensities vary with the size and morphology of the aneurysm and the relative amounts of residual lumen, turbulent flow, atheromatous plaque, fibrosis, subacute blood, and hemosiderin-laden tissue. Lesions are typically well-defined, with a round-to-elliptical shape. Infiltration of tissue planes beyond the aneurysm may be seen with leaking aneurysms (84). On conventional spin-echo MR imaging, aneurysms show a variable signal intensity on the basis of blood flow, showing

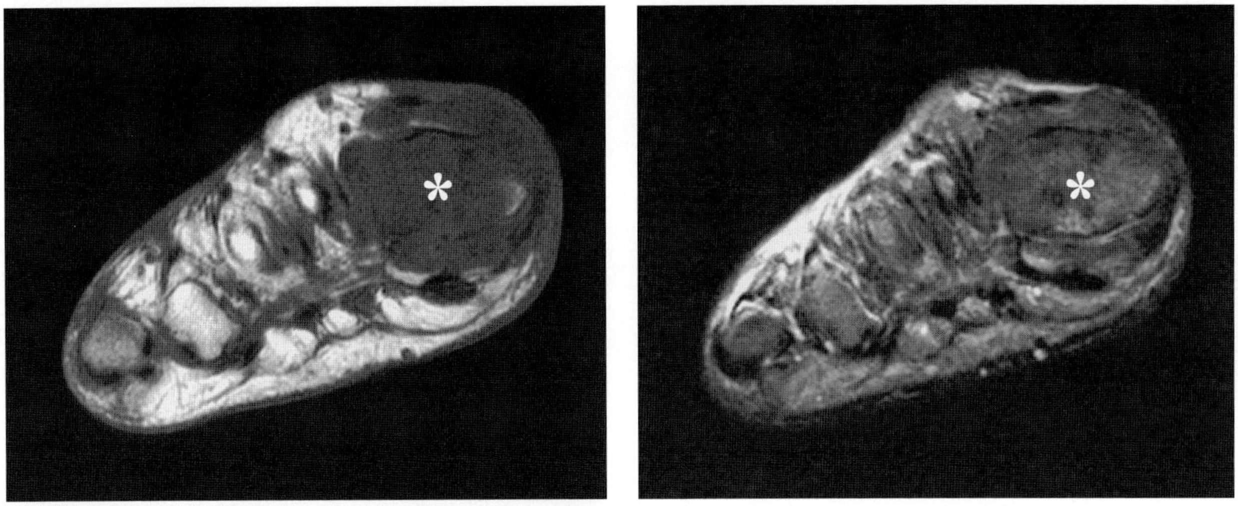

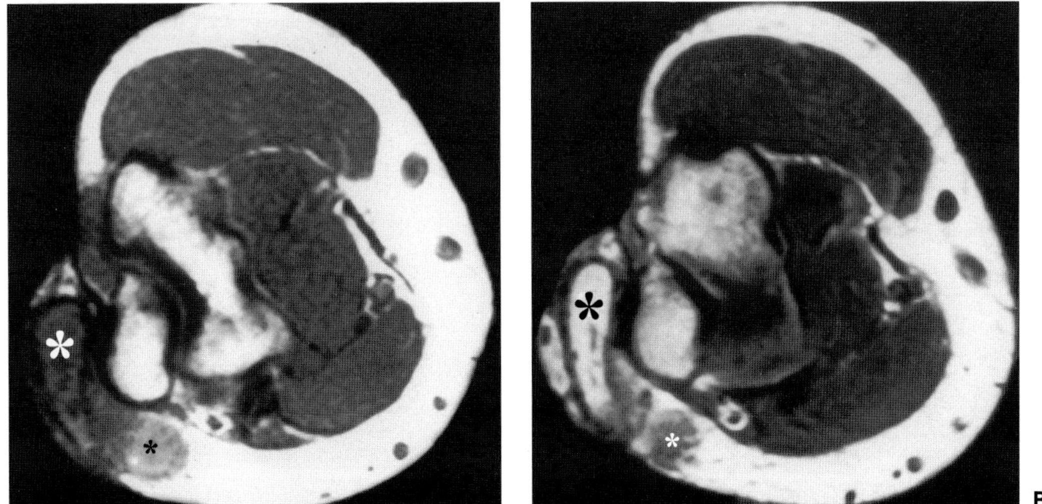

Figure 13.25 *(continued)* **E,F:** Axial T1-weighted (TR/TE; 606/17) **(E)** and T2-weighted (TR/TE; 2350/80) **(F)** spin-echo MR images show the mass (*asterisk*) with an intermediate signal intensity. **G:** Axial, fat-suppressed, T1-weighted (TR/TE; 574/14) spin-echo MR image following intravenous gadolinium administration shows nonenhancing tissue centrally (*asterisk*) with peripheral enhancement (*arrows*).

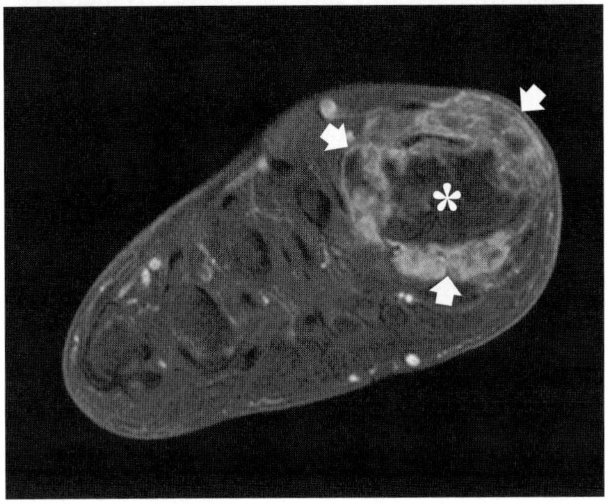

Figure 13.26 Gout: MR imaging features in a man 42 years of age with a mass adjacent to the olecranon. **A,B:** Axial T1-weighted (TR/TE; 600/20) **(A)** and T2-weighted (TR/TE; 200/80) **(B)** spin-echo MR images show an intermediate signal intensity mass (*small asterisk*) adjacent to the olecranon bursa. Note fluid in the olecranon bursa (*large asterisk*).

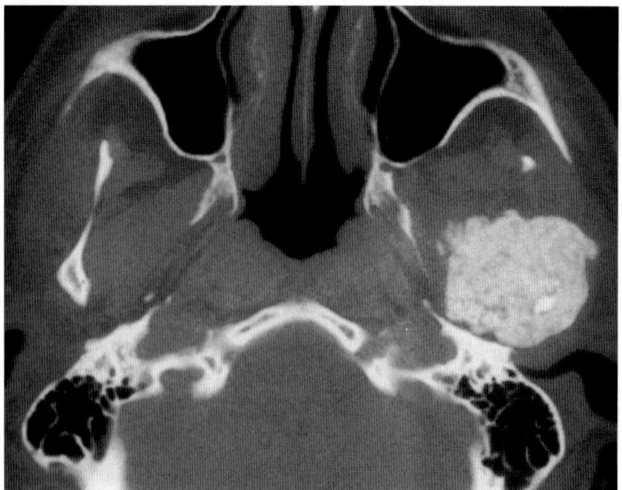

Figure 13.27 Tophaceous pseudogout: CT imaging features in a man 57 years of age. Axial noncontrast CT of the temporomandibular joint displayed on bone window shows a densely mineralized mass. The character of the lesion simulates that of tumoral calcinosis.

flow void in areas of rapidly flowing blood and increased signal in areas of slowly flowing blood (Fig. 13.30). Pseudoaneurysms are usually elliptical soft tissue masses adjacent to the involved vessel. Pseudoaneurysms typically show a more complex signal intensity, with areas of increased and decreased signal intensity on all pulse sequences, corresponding to subacute blood and hemosiderin-laden tissue (Figs. 13.31 and 13.32). Gradient-echo images may be very useful in identifying hemosiderin-laden tissue. A flow void from the native vessel may be seen within or at the periphery of the mass. It has been our experience that the imaging distinction between an aneurysm with extensive thrombus and a pseudoaneurysm may be difficult.

CT scanning of aneurysms shows a well-defined, homogeneous, low-attenuation mass (Fig. 13.32) (87). Curvilinear calcification may be identified in the vessel wall. Subacute hemorrhage in pseudoaneurysms reveals decreased attenuation, typically at the periphery of the lesion, a distribution opposite to that of the central necrosis and hemorrhage seen in high-grade sarcomas (Fig. 13.30).

An aneurysm should be considered in the differential diagnosis when a mass is identified in the popliteal fossa region (or other area adjacent to vessels) and imaging shows a complex structure, especially with a lamellated appearance. Bilotta et al. (84) note that complete encasement (i.e., the vessel in the center of a soft tissue mass) or obliteration of the popliteal vessels by a tumor is rare, and this finding should suggest an aneurysm.

Adventitial Cystic Disease

Adventitial cystic disease is a rare cause of lower extremity claudication, resulting from the formation of cystic collections of mucinous material within the adventitia of the popliteal artery, subsequently narrowing the arterial lumen (88–90). It is included here because it may appear as a soft tissue mass on MR imaging (88). Physical exam

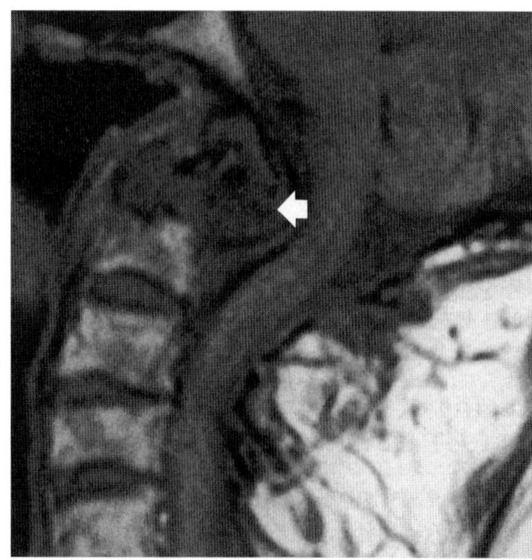

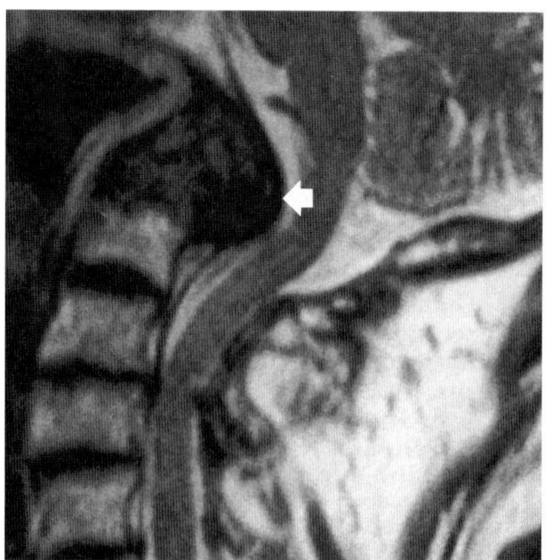

Figure 13.28 Tophaceous pseudogout: MR imaging features in a man 56 years of age, with a traumatic type 2 odontoid fracture and a retro-ondontoid mass. **A,B:** Sagittal T1-weighted (TR/TE; 705/15) **(A)** and fast T2-weighted (TR/TE; 4282/94) **(B)** spin-echo MR images show a lobulated mass (*arrow*) with a low-to-intermediate signal intensity that compresses the cord. (Courtesy of Donald Resnick, MD, La Jolla, California, from reference 72.)

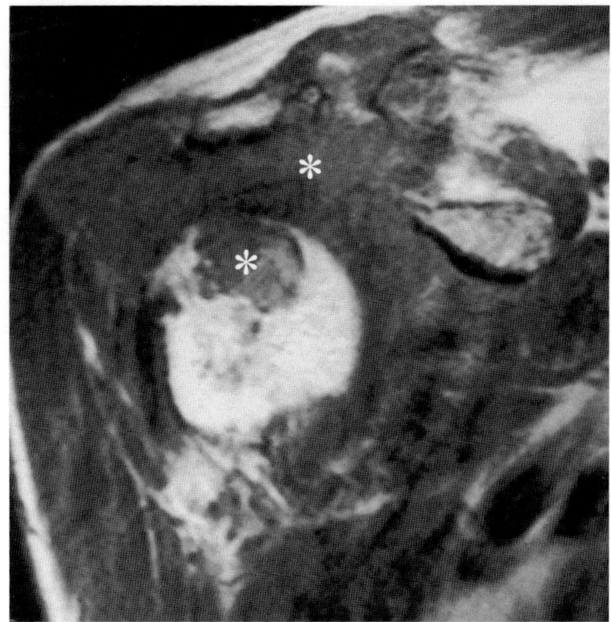
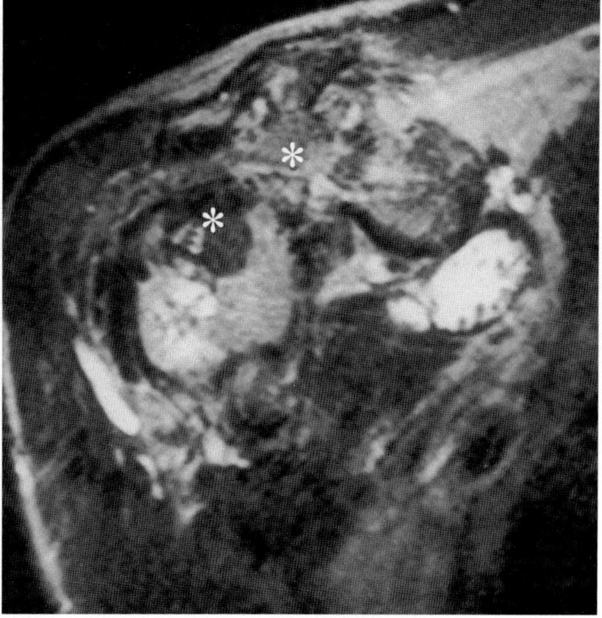

Figure 13.29 Secondary amyloidosis: MR imaging features in the shoulder of a man 52 years of age with long-standing chronic renal failure. **A,B:** Coronal T1-weighted (TR/TE; 533/20) **(A)** and T2-weighted (TR/TE; 2000/80) **(B)** spin-echo MR images show a large, lobulated mass (*asterisks*) extrinsically eroding bone. The mass displays a low-to-intermediate signal intensity on both T1- and T2-weighted spin-echo MR images. Associated joint fluid as well as fluid in the subacromial/subdeltoid bursa is seen. This appearance mimics that of pigmented villonodular synovitis.

KEY CONCEPTS

- Adventitial cystic disease results from the formation of cystic collections of mucinous material within the arterial adventitia.
- Any peripheral artery can be affected; however, the disorder has a striking proclivity for the popliteal artery.
- MR imaging demonstrates aggregates of multiple small, round or oval masses originating in the wall of the involved peripheral artery.
- Individual intramural masses show homogenous low signal intensity on T1-weighted images and high signal intensity on T2-weighted or fluid-sensitive sequences.
- Angiography demonstrates the extrinsic, intramural nature of the stenosis.

may demonstrate a soft tissue mass, and in the setting of a younger patient with no evidence of arteriosclerosis, clinicians often focus on the soft tissue mass, questioning a soft tissue sarcoma or a popliteal cyst rather than a vascular cause. The basis of adventitial cystic disease is unknown, but possible causes are repetitive adventitial trauma, myxoid degeneration, and inclusion of rests of mucus-secreting cells in the adventitia (89,90).

Any peripheral artery can be affected; however, adventitial cystic disease has a striking proclivity for the popliteal

artery. The disorder usually afflicts young to middle-aged men, in the third through fifth decades, without evidence of atherosclerosis or other systemic vascular disease (90–92). Affected patients typically present with sudden onset of rapidly progressive calf claudication and lower extremity pain.

Lesions are typically small and unilateral, involving the adventitia (89). Long-standing lesions may become large enough to present as a soft tissue mass. They may occasionally extend into the media or produce popliteal artery thrombosis (89). The cystic lesions contain glycoproteins, hyaluronic acid, and hydroxyproline and may rarely rupture spontaneously (89). Surgery is usually curative. Percutaneous ultrasound-guided cyst aspiration is an effective alternative to surgery in patients who do not have thrombotic occlusion (89,93).

MR imaging demonstrates aggregates of multiple small round or oval masses, originating in the wall of the involved peripheral artery, with larger lesions having a multilobulated appearance. The individual intramural masses demonstrate homogenous low signal intensity on T1-weighted images and high signal intensity on T2-weighted or fluid-sensitive sequences, consistent with a cystlike character. Following gadolinium administration, lesions typically do not enhance; however, mild peripheral enhancement may be seen (92,94). The multilobulated cystic masses compromise the arterial lumen to varying

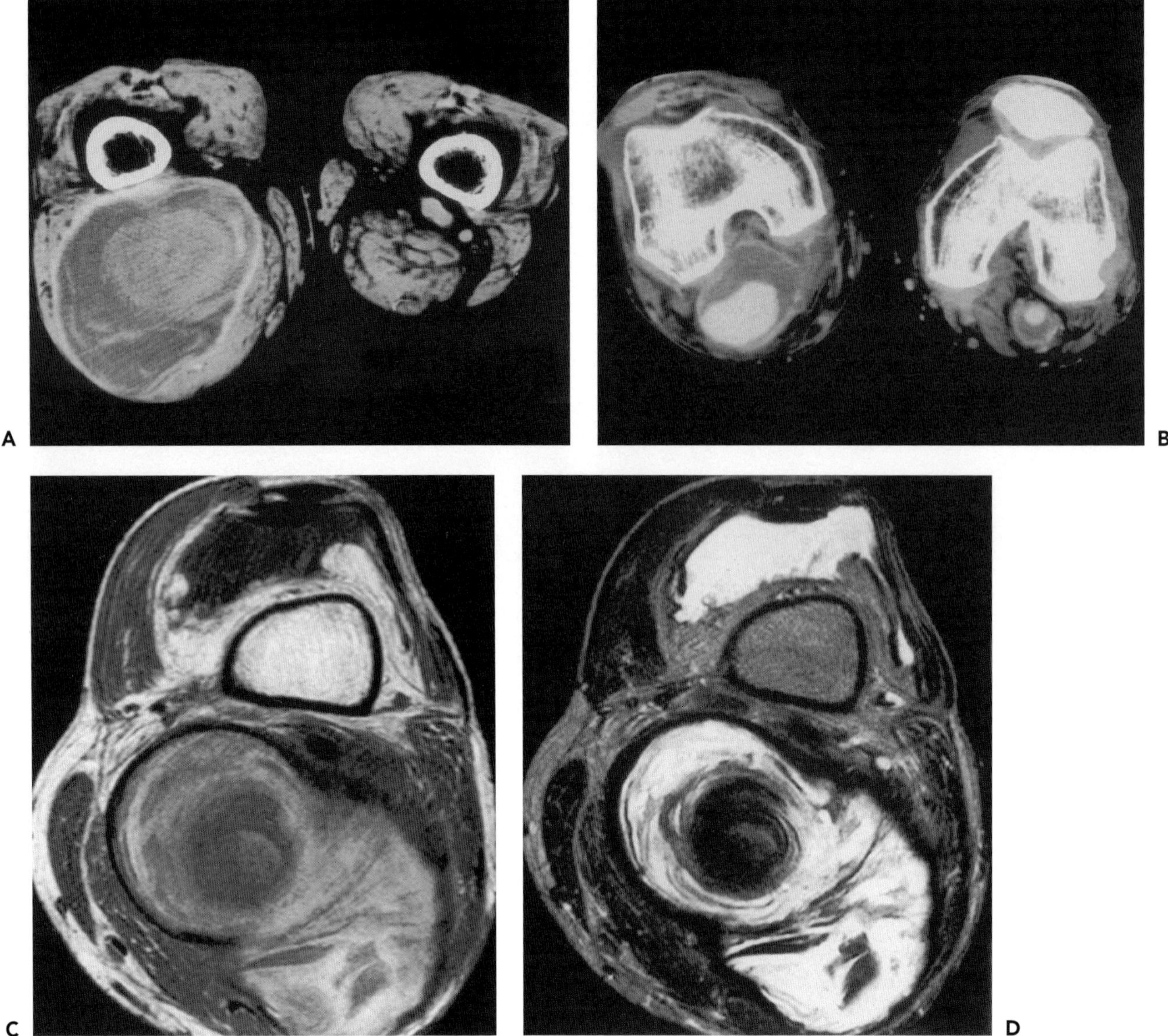

Figure 13.30 Aneurysm and pseudoaneurysm: Imaging features in a man 62 years of age with a "slowly growing" mass in the popliteal fossa for several years. He had no history of previous surgery. **A:** Axial contrast-enhanced CT scan through the midportion of the mass shows a complex appearance with a central area of relatively increased attenuation. The fluidlike decreased attenuation is peripheral, a pattern that would be unlikely with a necrotic tumor. **B:** Axial CT scan inferior to **A** shows the associated aneurysm as well as an aneurysm of the contralateral popliteal artery. **C,D:** Axial T1-weighted (TR/TE; 800/16) **(C)** and T2-weighted (TR/TE; 2344/80) **(D)** spin-echo MR images show a complex mass. The corresponding areas of decreased and increased signal intensity correspond to hemosiderin and subacute blood, respectively. Note the more pronounced signal loss on the T2-weighted image. (*continued*)

degrees, which range from minimal eccentric indentation, to cresentic stenosis, to complete occlusion.

MR and conventional catheter angiography demonstrate the degree of luminal compromise and the extrinsic intramural nature of the stenosis. Stenosis is usually focal and relatively smoothly tapered, and in the popliteal artery, it is at the level of the femoral condyles (Figs. 13.33 and 13.34) (89). The stenosis may show an hourglass, curvilinear, or spiral configuration without poststenotic dilation, or there may be complete occlusion (91). The stenosis may extend for several centimeters. The lesion shows a decreased attenuation on CT scanning, with rim enhancement following contrast administration (90,91).

Sonography demonstrates multilobulated collections of small rounded or oval anechoic or hypoechoic masses arising in the walls of the affected arteries. Crescentic indentation upon the anechoic lumina of the vessels is

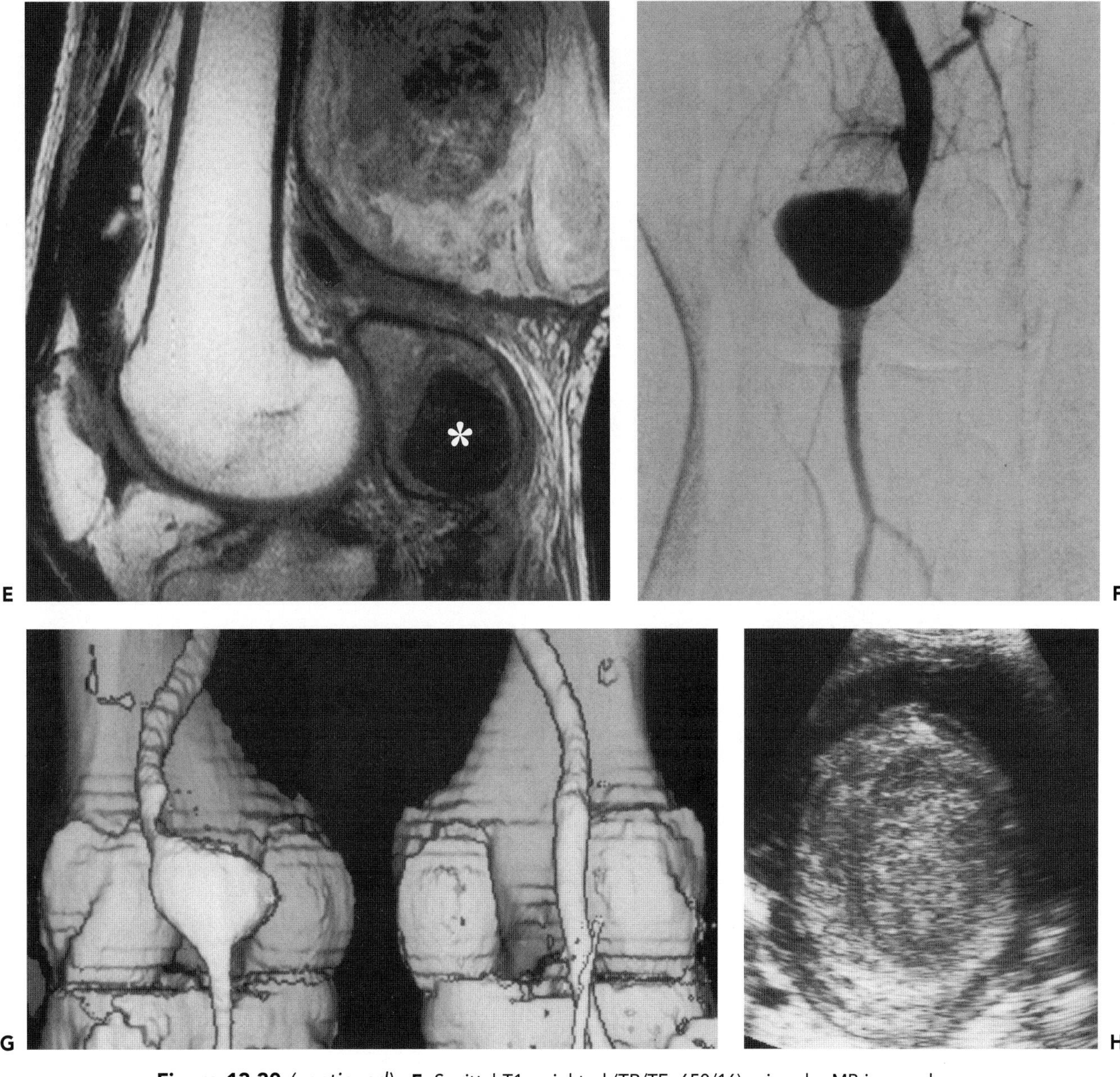

Figure 13.30 *(continued)* **E:** Sagittal T1-weighted (TR/TE; 650/16) spin-echo MR image shows the flow void of the popliteal artery aneurysm (*asterisk*) inferiorly, with the large pseudoaneurysm above it. **F:** Digital subtraction arteriogram shows the focal popliteal artery aneurysm, although the pseudoaneurysm shows no flow. **G:** Corresponding three-dimensional reformatted CT scan shows a similar appearance. **H:** Ultrasonography of the popliteal fossa pseudoaneurysm shows a complex mass, with an appearance similar to that seen on CT. *(continued)*

seen with eccentric narrowing or occlusion by the cystic masses (Fig. 13.34). Low-level echoes may be seen within the masses, indicative of debris within the contents of the cysts (92).

Castleman Disease

Castleman disease is a rare lymphoproliferative disorder also known as *angiomatoid lymphoid hamartoma, angiofollicular hyperplasia, giant lymph node hyperplasia,* and *follicular lymphoreticuloma* (95,96). It was originally described by Castleman et al. in 1956 (97), who reported 13 patients with enlarged mediastinal lymph nodes resembling thymic tumors radiologically, grossly, and even microscopically. The cause remains unknown, although it is thought to be either infectious, hamartomatous, or inflammatory (95,98).

There are two histologic variations: the hyaline vascular variant accounts for approximately 90% of cases, and the plasma cell variant accounts for the remaining 10%

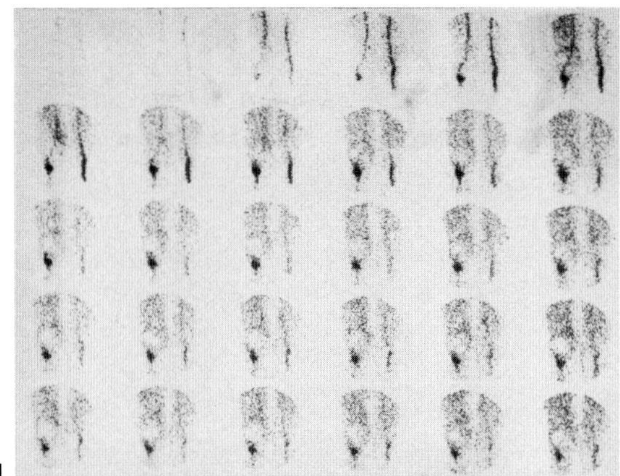

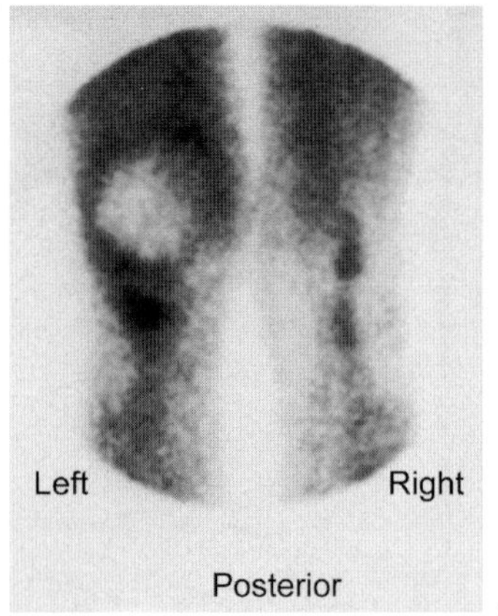

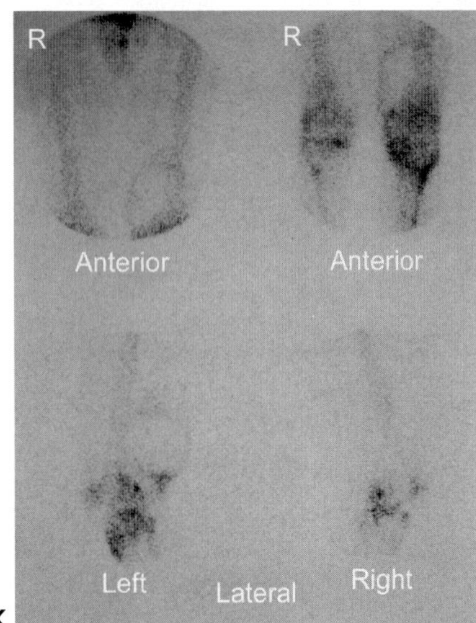

Figure 13.30 *(continued)* **I,J:** Flow **(I)** and blood-pool **(J)** images from a technetium-99m bone scintigram show increased tracer accumulation within the aneurysm, with no tracer identified in the pseudoaneurysm. **K:** Delayed static images show the prominent photopenic area of the pseudoaneurysm.

KEY CONCEPTS

- Castleman disease is a rare lymphoproliferative disorder also known as *angiofollicular hyperplasia*.
- Two histologic variations include:
  - Hyaline vascular variant, which accounts for approximately 90% of cases.
  - Plasma cell variant, which accounts for the remaining 10% of cases.
- Patients typically present with an asymptomatic, solitary, mediastinal mass.
- Constitutional symptoms may be seen in approximately half of patients with the plasma cell variant.
- Hyaline vascular subtype is usually a solitary mass; the plasma cell variety may be multifocal.
- CT scanning in patients with typical thoracic disease usually show a rounded solitary mass.
- Prominent homogeneous contrast enhancement is characteristically seen on CT.
- MR imaging shows the lesion to have a nonspecific appearance.

(95,98,99). The former consists of small lymphoreticular follicles distributed in a hypervascular, hyalinized stroma, whereas the latter consists of larger lymphoreticular nodules, separated by sheets of plasma cells, in a less vascular stroma (95,100).

Both men and women are affected about equally (96,99). Patients range in age from the first through the sixth decade (96). Approximately 70% of patients with the hyaline vascular type are younger than 30 years (99). Patients typically present with an asymptomatic solitary mediastinal mass. However, symptoms may occur if the mass compresses adjacent structures. The mediastinum accounts for 40% to 70% of cases (95). Approximately 30% of cases are extrathoracic, and an estimated 10% to 40% are cervical (99,101). Cervical lesions tend to occur laterally and may simulate lymphadenopathy (95). Other sites include the abdomen, pelvis, axilla, retroperitoneum, and mesentery (95,101). Constitutional symptoms, such as fever, sweating, and fatigue, may be seen in approximately half of patients with the plasma cell variant (98,101). There is also an association with hypergammaglobulinemia and

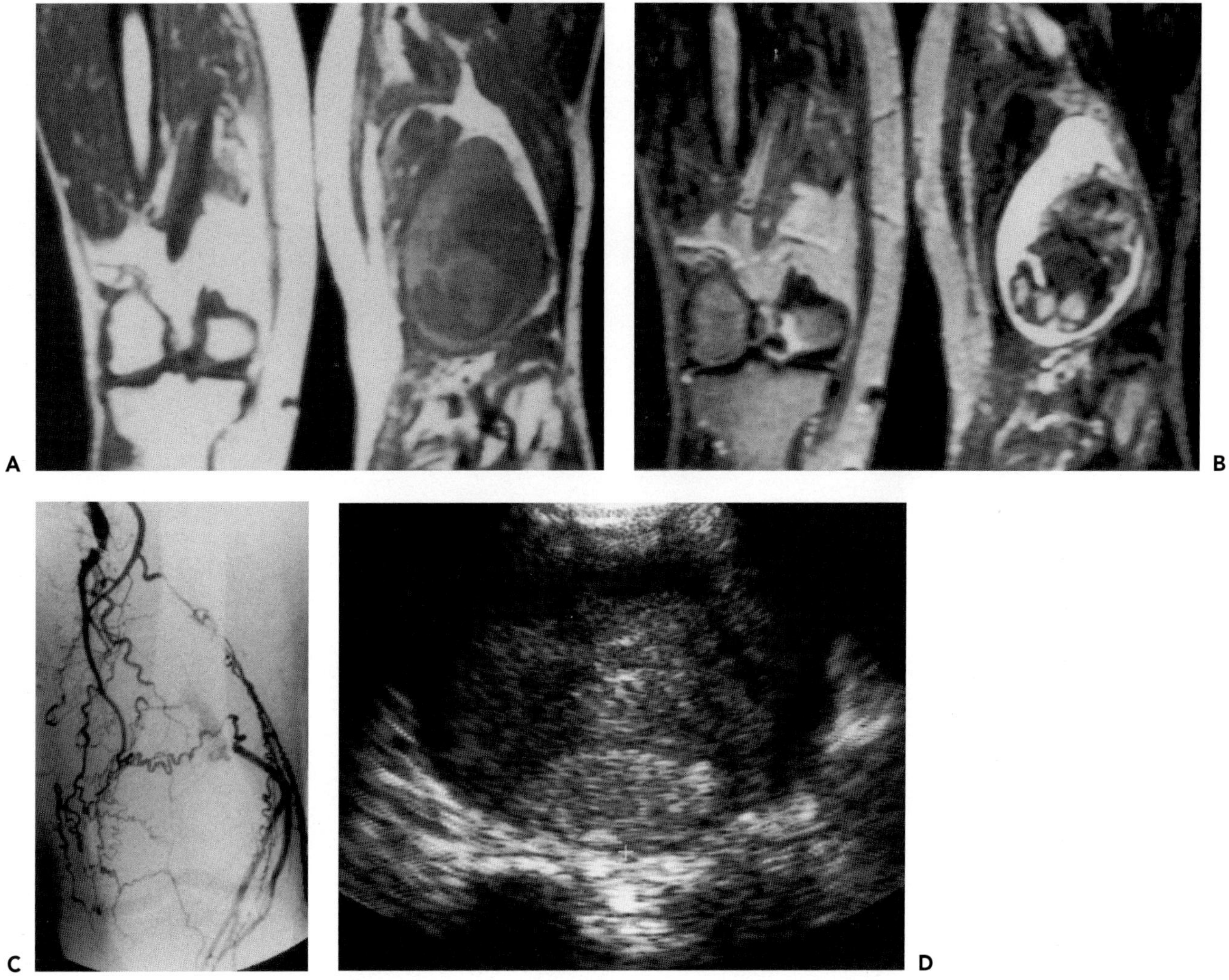

Figure 13.31 Pseudoaneurysm: Imaging features in a man 65 years of age with a popliteal fossa mass. **A,B:** Coronal T1-weighted (TR/TE; 650/20) **(A)** and T2-weighted (TR/TE; 2000/80) **(B)** spin-echo MR images show a well-defined mass with a complex pattern of signal intensities, compatible with subacute and chronic hemorrhage. **C:** The arteriogram shows an occluded distal superficial femoral and popliteal arteries, with multiple collateral vessels displaced by the pseudoaneurysm. **D:** A popliteal fossa sonogram shows a complex mass.

hypoalbuminemia (98,101). Whereas lesions of the hyaline vascular subtype are usually solitary masses, lesions of the plasma cell variety may be multifocal (101).

There have been numerous reports of Castleman disease with systemic manifestations similar to those of a multicentric lymphoproliferative disorder (102,103). This is seen with both histologic subtypes but is more common in the plasma cell variant (102). These cases are characterized by an aggressive clinical course, multifocal lymphadenopathy, hepatosplenomegaly, and abnormal liver and renal function. There is an association with malignancy, usually lymphoma, although other malignancies are reported (102). This phenomenon has led to a distinction between the aggressive multicentric form, which may be fatal, and the localized form, which may

be an incidental finding (103). The multicentric form is usually seen in older men, with a mean age of 57 years (103).

CT scanning in patients with typical thoracic disease usually shows rounded, solitary mediastinal or hilar masses (104). Pleural disease may present as a well-defined interlobular mass or as a large pleural effusion (104). Following contrast administration, CT demonstrates homogeneous contrast enhancement or multicentric ring enhancement (95,99,100,103). In the abdomen and pelvis, a single, well-defined enhancing mass is also most frequently seen (105). Although the histologic basis for the enhancement pattern is unknown (Fig. 13.35), the pattern of enhancement is considered to be characteristic (104,106). Lesions larger than 5 cm may

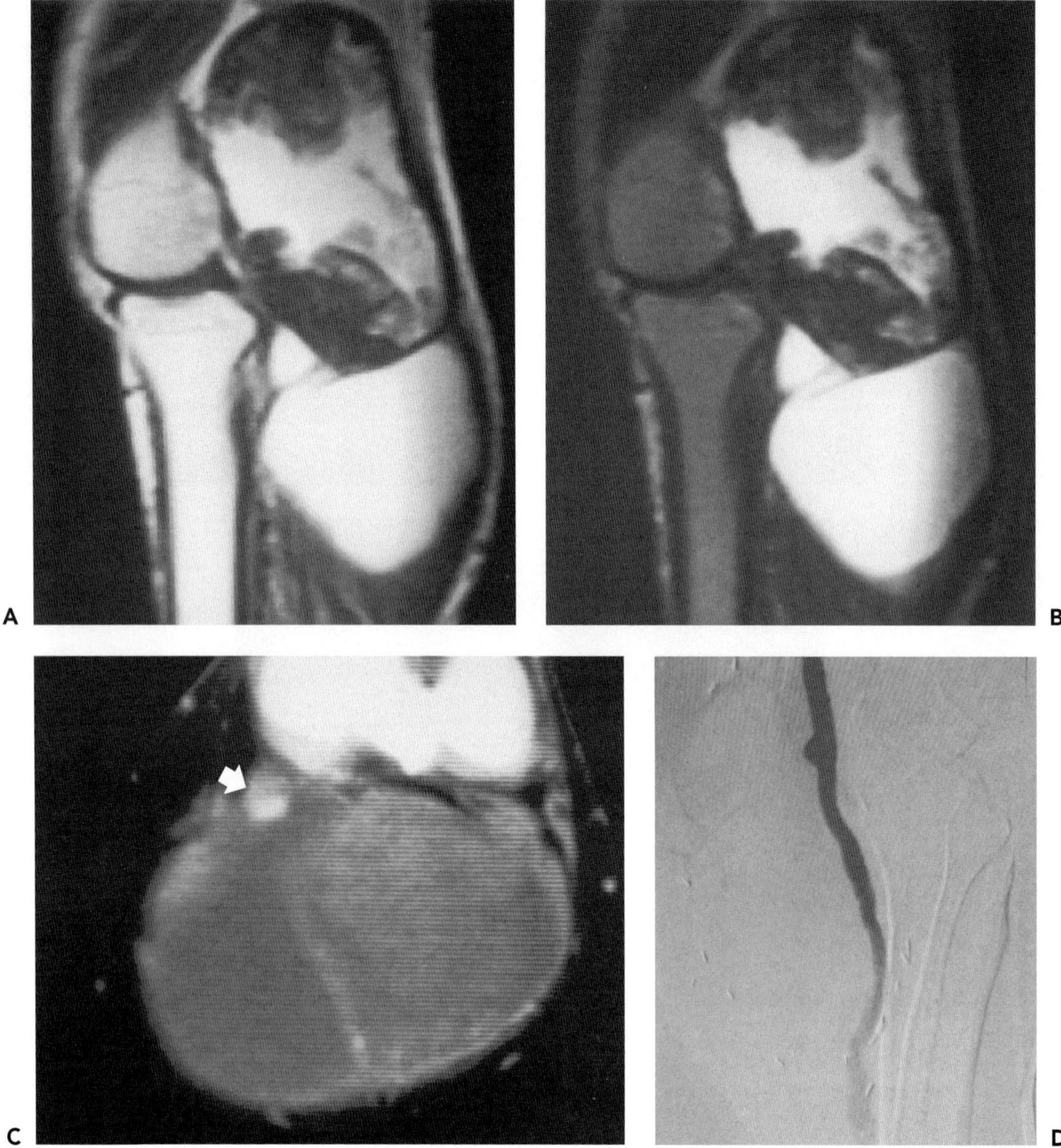

Figure 13.32 Pseudoaneurysm: Imaging features in a man 68 years of age with a "slowly grow-ing" mass in the popliteal fossa. Patient had a history of previous bypass surgery. **A,B:** Sagittal T1-weighted (TR/TE; 700/32) **(A)** and T2-weighted (TR/TE; 2000/80) **(B)** spin-echo MR images show a well-defined mass with a complex pattern of signal intensities, and corresponding areas of increased and decreased signal intensity on all pulse sequences, compatible with subacute and chronic hemor-rhage. Note the debris in the dependent portion of the lesion. **C:** Axial contrast-enhanced CT shows a complex mass with both solid and cystic components. Note the enhancing vessel anteromedially (*arrow*). **D:** An arteriogram shows an intact femoral popliteal graft. Note multiple vascular clips from previous surgery.

show heterogeneous enhancement with areas of decreased attenuation caused by necrosis and degeneration (104,105). Calcification within the lesion is noted (107,108), and dense calcification is reported more frequently in retroperitoneal lesions (103). Calcification is seen in approx-imately one-third to one-half of abdominal and pelvic lesions and is described as having an arborizing pattern that appears to radiate from the center of the mass (105,109,110).

The plasma cell variant shows multifocal lymphadenopathy as well as hepatosplenomegaly and is indistinguishable from adenopathy of other causes (Fig. 13.36).

Limited experience with MR imaging shows the lesion to have a nonspecific appearance. Most lesions are isoin-tense or slightly hyperintense to skeletal muscle on T1-weighted images and heterogeneously hyperintense on long TR images and enhanced T1-weighted images

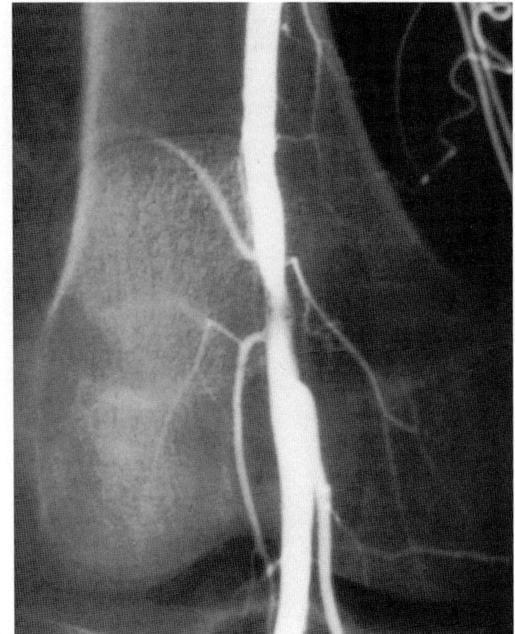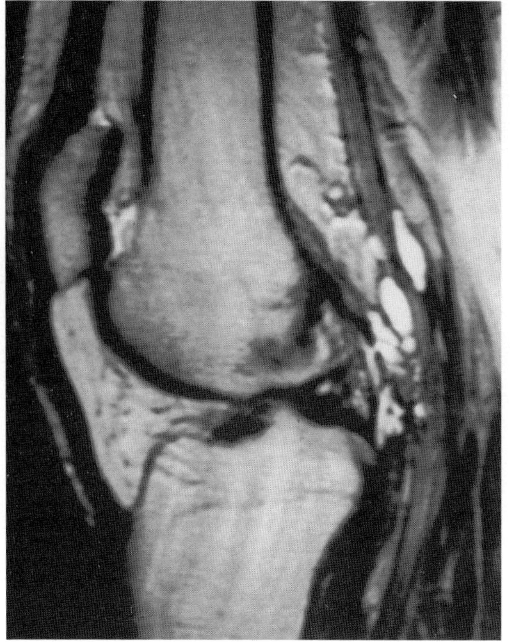

Figure 13.33 Adventitial cystic disease: Arteriographic and MR imaging features in a man 62 years of age. **A:** Arteriogram of the popliteal artery shows relatively smoothly tapered stenosis, without poststenotic dilation, at the level of the femoral condyles. **B:** Sagittal turbo T2-weighted (TR/TE; 4000/85) spin-echo MR image shows small oval masses eccentrically compressing the popliteal artery. The masses have a signal intensity identical to that of fluid.

(104,111,112). Debatin et al. (101) reported a case of Castleman disease of the adrenal gland and noted the lesion to be well-defined and homogeneous, with a signal hypointense to that of liver on T1-weighted images and uniformly hyperintense on T2-weighted images. Dense mineralization within the mass causes a heterogeneous appearance, with areas of decreased signal intensity (103). Luburich et al. (113) reported a case in the pelvis in which the lesion showed a signal intensity slightly more than that of skeletal muscle on T1-weighted images and similar to that of fat on T2-weighted images, with streaks of decreased signal on all pulse sequences.

At angiography, the mass is hypervascular, with large feeding vessels and a capillary blush (86,113). Ultrasonography demonstrates uniform hypoechogenicity (102). Sonography reveals a hypoechoic mass with prominent flow on power Doppler evaluation (104,110).

Hematoma

The MR appearance of a hematoma is variable and a function of the age of the lesion (114). Extracranial hematomas are usually classified by age as *acute, subacute,* or *chronic,* although these terms are not rigorously defined. In general usage, the term *acute hematoma* is used for a lesion hours to days old. A subacute hematoma is one that is 1 week to approximately 3 months old, and a chronic hematoma is one older than 3 months (115,116).

The MR imaging of extracranial hematomas was well-described by Rubin et al. (116) in a report of 20 cases. On spin-echo MR imaging, an acute hematoma shows a

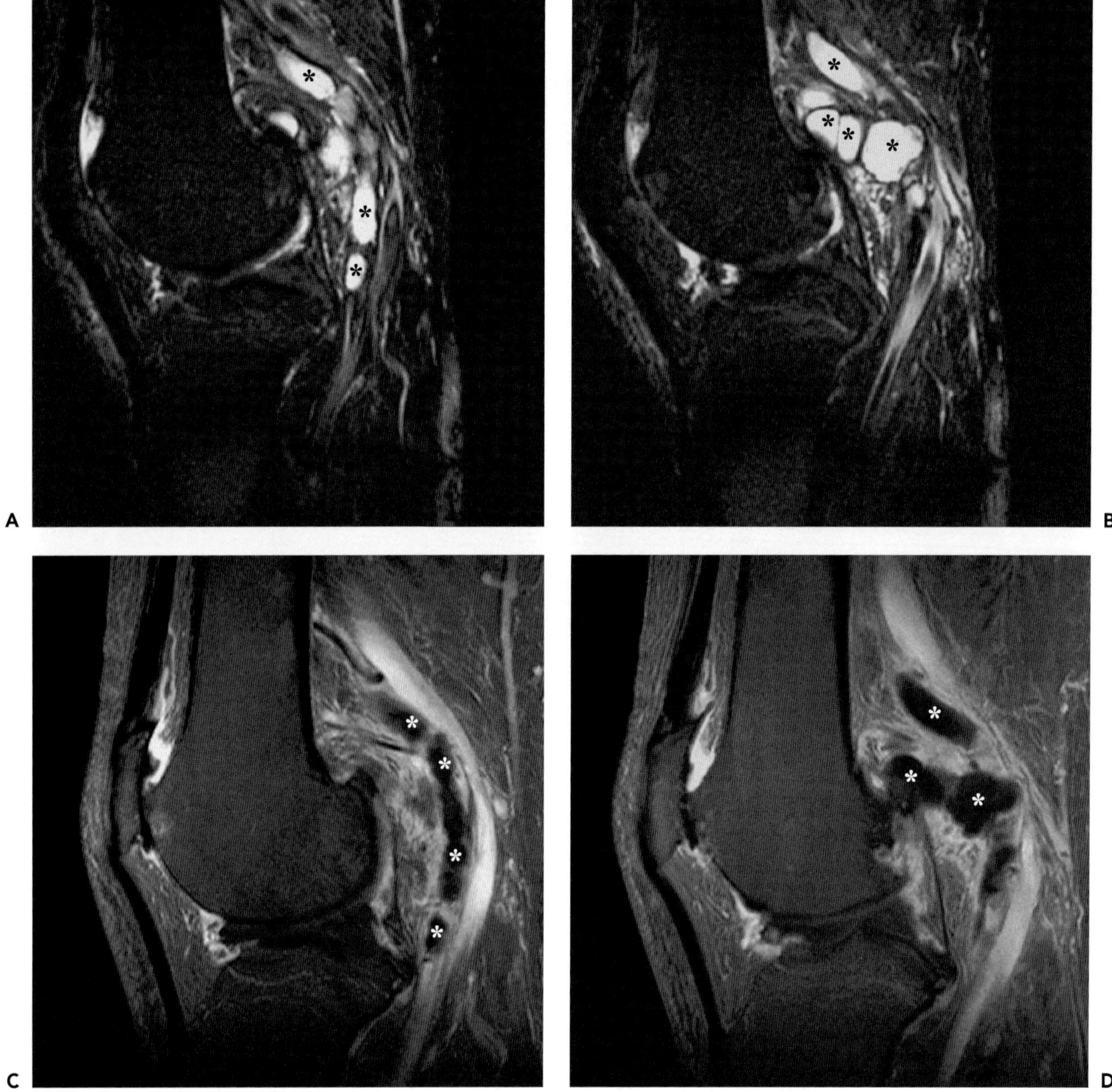

Figure 13.34 Adventitial cystic disease: Arteriographic and MR imaging features in a man 50 years of age. **A,B:** Sagittal short-tau inversion recovery (STIR) MR images through the popliteal artery **(A)** and lateral to the popliteal artery **(B)** show innumerable cysts (*asterisks*) of variable size. **C,D:** Corresponding sagittal, fat-suppressed, T1-weighted spin-echo MR images following contrast administration also show multiple cysts (*asterisks*) of variable sizes. Note enhancement around the cysts. (*continued*)

signal intensity relatively similar to that of skeletal muscle on T1-weighted images, varying from slightly hyperintense to hypointense. A decreased signal intensity, less than that of skeletal muscle, is seen on T2-weighted images (Fig. 13.37). Acute hematomas are typically homogeneous, although considerable variability and a heterogeneous appearance may be seen; in addition, adjacent edema may be a prominent feature (Fig. 13.38).

Subacute hematomas (approximately 1 week to 3 months old) demonstrate homogeneous increased signal on both T1- and T2-weighted spin-echo MR images (Fig. 13.39). Early subacute lesions show an intermediate intensity center with a high signal intensity periphery (Fig. 13.40). A rind of decreased signal intensity caused by the accumulation of hemosiderin-laden macrophages may be seen and was noted in 9 (56%) of 16 subacute hematomas reviewed by Rubin et al. (116).

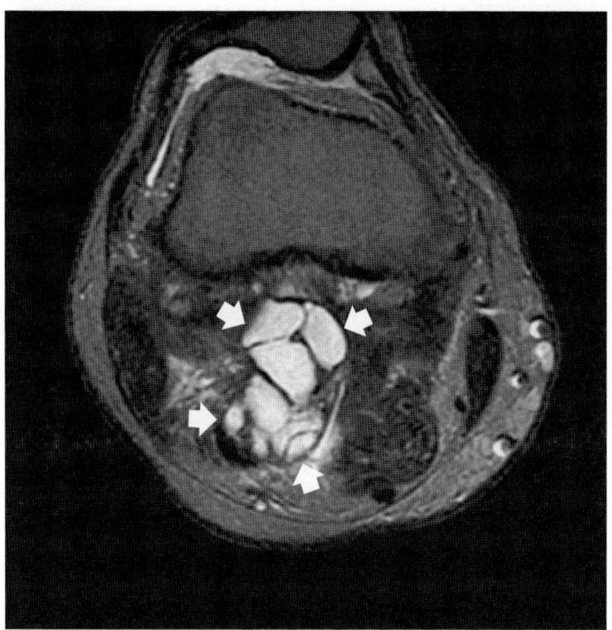

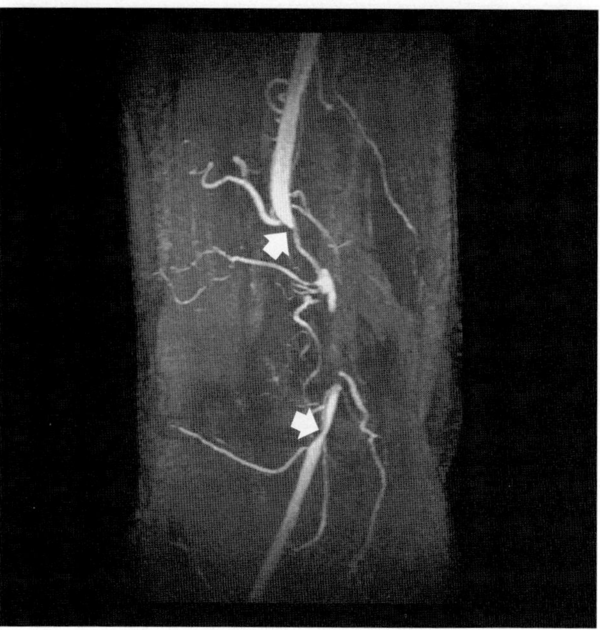

Figure 13.34 *(continued)* **E:** Axial T2-weighted spin-echo MR image through the popliteal artery shows multiple cysts *(arrows)* giving a masslike contour. **F:** MR arteriogram of the popliteal artery shows segmental occlusion with rounded and cresentic margins *(arrows)*, consistent with extrinsic occlusion.

Chronic hematomas reveal increased signal intensity on all spin-echo MR pulse sequences, similar to that seen in subacute lesions. The rind of hemosiderin-laden tissue may be quite extensive, and eventually the lesion shows a signal intensity less than that of skeletal muscle on all pulse sequences (Fig. 13.40). The time sequence for this is not established (Fig. 13.39).

The CT appearance of hematoma is also variable. Early lesions show increased attenuation compared with that of skeletal muscle (Figs. 13.38 and 13.40), whereas subacute to chronic lesions demonstrate an attenuation equal to or less than that of skeletal muscle (Fig. 13.39) (115).

Care must be taken during imaging to differentiate a malignant soft tissue tumor with hemorrhage from a

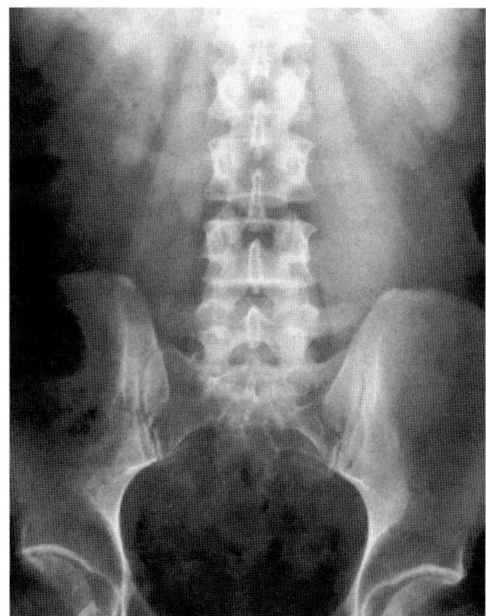

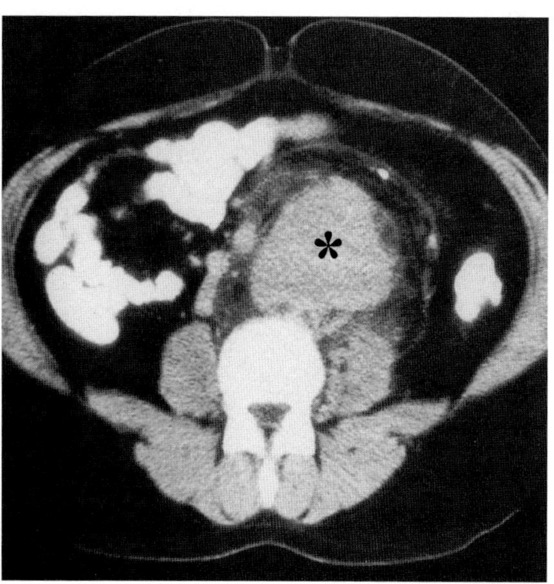

Figure 13.35 Castleman disease: Hyaline vascular variant in a man 39 years of age presenting with left flank pain. **A:** Kidney-ureter-bladder film shows loss of definition of the left psoas margin. **B:** Axial contrast-enhanced CT scan shows a large retroperitoneal mass *(asterisk)* displacing the left ureter and great vessels. A retroperitoneal sarcoma or lymphoma could have a similar appearance.

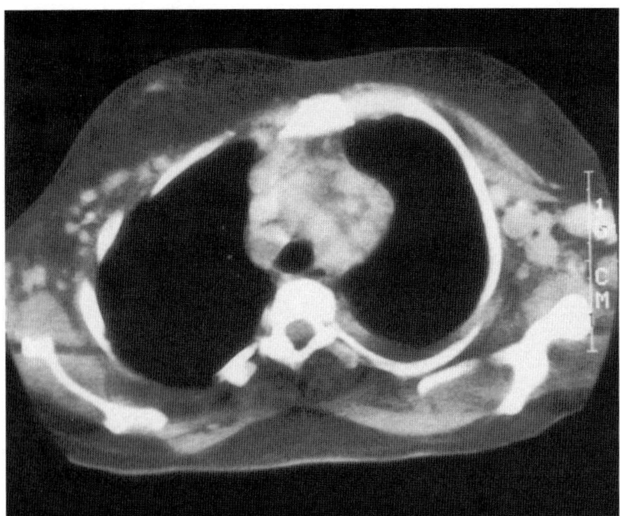

Figure 13.36 Castleman disease: Plasma cell variant in a woman 36 years of age presenting with generalized lymphadenopathy, fatigue, weight loss, and malaise. Axial contrast-enhanced CT shows axillary and mediastinal adenopathy. Lymphoma or adenopathy from various causes could have a similar appearance.

hematoma. The presence of a tumor nodule or rim of tumor may be helpful in distinguishing a simple hematoma from a hemorrhagic neoplasm (114). Gadolinium-enhanced imaging is also useful in these circumstances to identify an underlying tumor nodule. This differentiation is often difficult because hematomas may organize, resulting in a complex appearance with enhancing fibrovascular tissue (Fig. 13.41). Nevertheless, careful clinical correlation is needed, as is a healthy dose of skepticism. A history of

"spontaneous hematoma" should always initiate a vigilant search for a hemorrhage associated with a neoplasm. If imaging is inconclusive, close follow-up is essential. Lenchik et al. (117) studied the CT scans of 44 patients with abnormalities of the iliopsoas compartment (15 neoplasms, 21 abscesses, and 8 hematomas), to identify findings that would be useful to differentiate these processes. They noted that these processes could not be reliably distinguished on the basis of CT imaging findings. The most reliable CT feature for a hematoma was involvement of the entire muscle. The most reliable feature of neoplasm was irregular margins, but this was also common in abscesses and hematomas. Clinical enlargement of a soft tissue mass may be the result of necrosis and hemorrhage within a tumor (118). This enlargement is more common in large, high-grade sarcomas and may occur spontaneously, or as a result of chemotherapy (118). The differentiation between tumor growth and hemorrhage is especially important in patients undergoing chemotherapy to establish clinical response.

The term *Morel-Lavallée lesion* is applied to a special form of chronic hematoma. The lesion, typically seen in the proximal thigh and trochanteric region, is thought to be the result of traumatic separation of the subcutaneous fibrofatty tissue from the adjacent fascia, causing disruption of the rich vascular plexus involving the fascia in this area (119–121). These lesions are prone to rebleed, and long-standing lesions are typically encapsulated with serosanguinous fluid containing blood and lymph (119).

Clinically, the lesion may present as a slowly enlarging soft tissue mass, long after the initiating traumatic injury

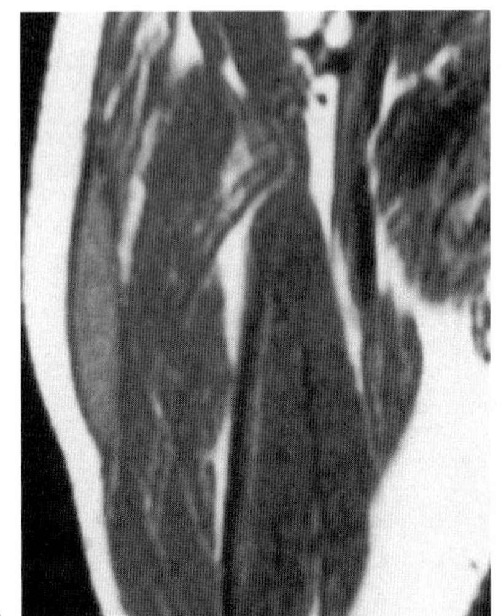

A

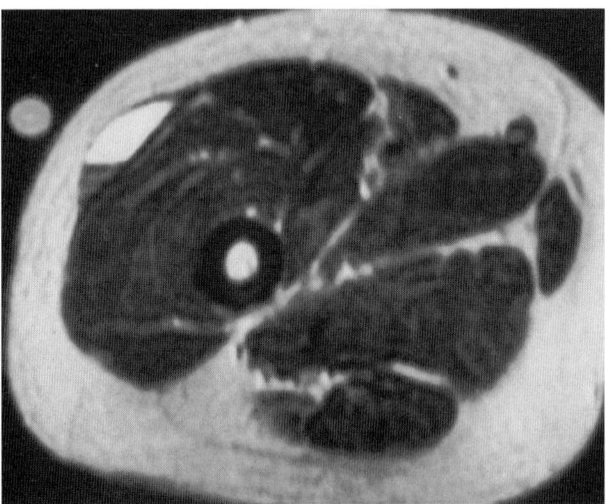

B

Figure 13.37 Hematoma: Imaging features of acute hematoma in the tensor fascia sheath of a man 59 years of age. **A:** Coronal T1-weighted (TR/TE; 500/20) spin-echo MR image shows a well-defined, homogeneous mass with a signal intensity slightly greater than that of skeletal muscle. The shape of the lesion, conforming to that of the fascial plane, is quite atypical for a tumor. **B:** Axial T2-weighted (TR/TE; 2200/80) spin-echo MR image shows a fluid–fluid level not visible on the corresponding T1-weighted image. The dependent aspect shows a signal intensity similar to that of skeletal muscle, with the remainder showing a signal intensity greater than that of fat.

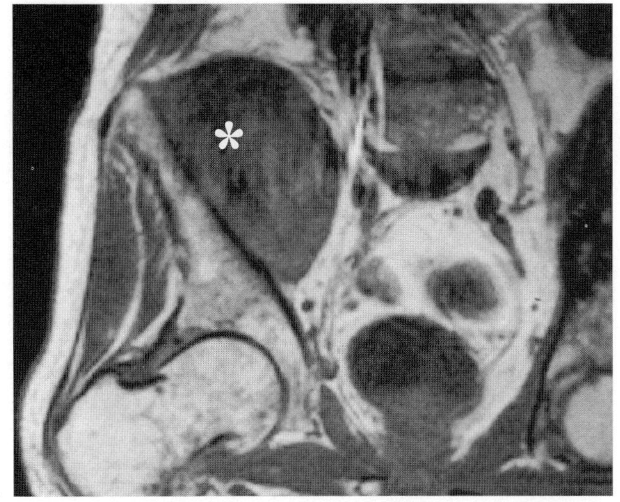

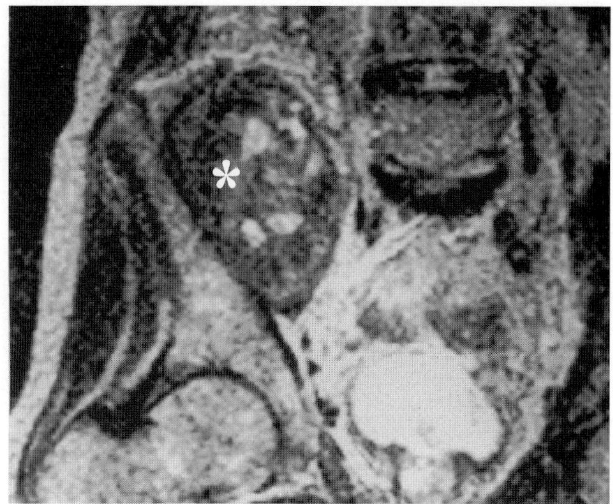

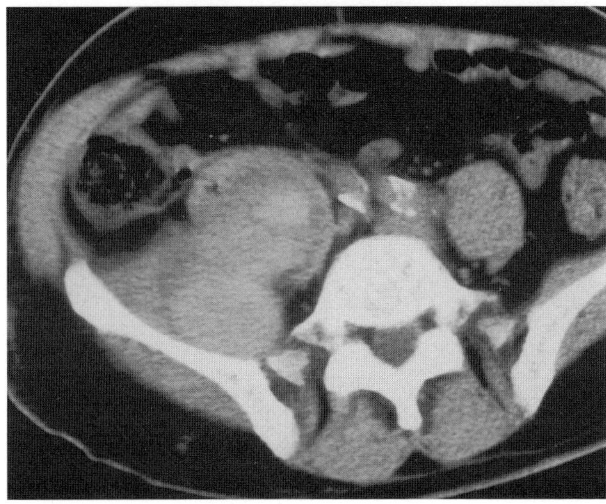

Figure 13.38 Hematoma: Imaging features of acute hematoma in the pelvis of a man 70 years of age on warfarin. **A,B:** Coronal T1-weighted (TR/TE; 600/15) **(A)** and T2-weighted (TR/TE; 2000/80) **(B)** spin-echo MR images show a poorly defined, heterogeneous mass (*asterisk*) in the right iliopsoas. The signal intensity is similar to that of skeletal muscle on the T1-weighted image and relatively similar to that of fat on the T2-weighted image. **C:** Axial noncontrast CT shows an ill-defined mass with areas of attenuation less than and greater than that of skeletal muscle.

has been forgotten. Delays in clinical presentation of weeks to years are not uncommon (119,122). Mellado et al. (119) noted three MR imaging patterns in patients with Morel-Lavallée lesions, reflecting the character of the lesion contents. Lesions consisting of serosanguinous fluid or seroma show imaging characteristics similar to those of fluid, with a partial or complete surrounding hypointense rim, showing homogeneous hypointense signal on T1-weighted images and hyperintense signal on T2-weighted images. Lesions may also show hyperintense signal intensity on both T1-weighted and T2-weighted images, surrounded by a hypointense peripheral ring that reflects subacute blood with peripheral hemosiderin. The final pattern shows a heterogeneous hyperintensity on T1-weighted and T2-weighted images, also having a peripheral rim of decreased signal intensity that correlates with varying amounts of hemosiderin, granulation tissue, necrotic debris, fibrin, and chronic organizing hematoma. Varying enhancements following contrast administration reflects associated inflammatory change and hematoma organization (Fig. 13.42).

Melorheostosis

KEY CONCEPTS

- Melorheostosis is a relatively rare bone dysplasia.
- Radiographs show characteristic undulated cortical thickening having a classic "flowing candle wax" appearance.
- Soft tissue masses are also a recognized feature, occurring in about 30% of cases.
- Mineralized soft tissue masses are frequent and easily recognized on radiographs or CT.
- Nonmineralized soft tissue masses have a CT attenuation similar to that of muscle.
- On MR imaging, nonmineralized components may show focal areas with adipose tissue characteristics or reveal intermediate signal intensity on T1-weighted MR images and high signal on T2 weighting.
- Gadolinium-enhanced MR images may show marked uptake of contrast within the nonmineralized soft tissue components.

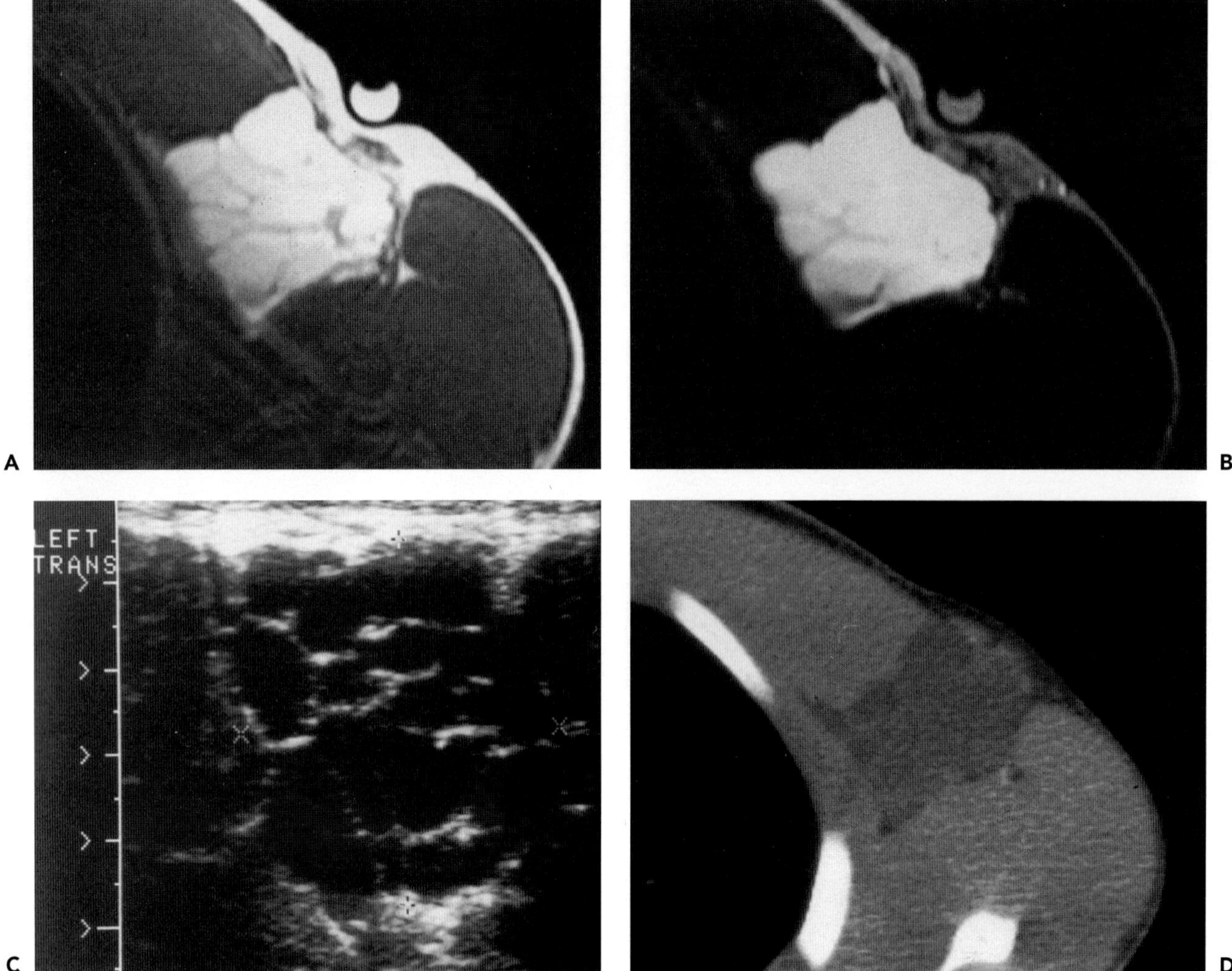

Figure 13.39   Hematoma: Imaging features of a subacute hematoma in the axilla of a boy 17 years of age. **A:** Axial T1-weighted (TR/TE; 600/20) spin-echo MR image shows a well-defined, lobulated mass, with signal intensity similar to that of subcutaneous fat. **B:** Corresponding T2-weighted (TR/TE; 2000/80) spin-echo MR image shows a similar configuration, with signal intensity greater than that of fat and compatible with that of subacute blood. **C:** Ultrasonography shows a cystic mass with multiple septations. **D:** Axial noncontrast CT scan shows a well-defined mass with homogeneously decreased attenuation.

Melorheostosis is a relatively rare bone dysplasia that was originally described by Leri and Joanny in 1922 (123). Osseous manifestations are frequently characteristic, with radiographs showing undulated cortical thickening having a classic "flowing candle wax" appearance (123–129). Patients are often symptomatic, with pain, contractures, and limited range of motion. The lower limb is most frequently affected in a sclerotomal pattern (osseous distribution of a spinal sensory nerve), usually involving multiple contiguous osseous sites.

Soft tissue masses are a recognized feature of melorheostosis. Murray and McCredie reported soft tissue masses in 27% of their 30 patients with melorheostosis (124). The soft tissue masses are often, but not invariably, associated with areas of characteristic cortical thickening. There may

also be associated fibrosis and resulting joint contracture. Desmoid tumors, as well as lymphatic and vascular anomalies and neoplasms, are also described in patients with melorheostosis (125,130).

Pathologically, the soft tissue masses have a varied composition, although osseous and chondroid elements are the most prominent components (128). In addition, fibrolipomatous and vascular tissues are also frequently present (125).

Treatment of these soft tissue masses is based on the clinical assessment. Symptomatic lesions, particularly those causing joint contractures, are usually excised. Recurrence is infrequent.

The appearance of the soft tissue masses associated with melorheostosis on imaging is variable. Mineralized soft

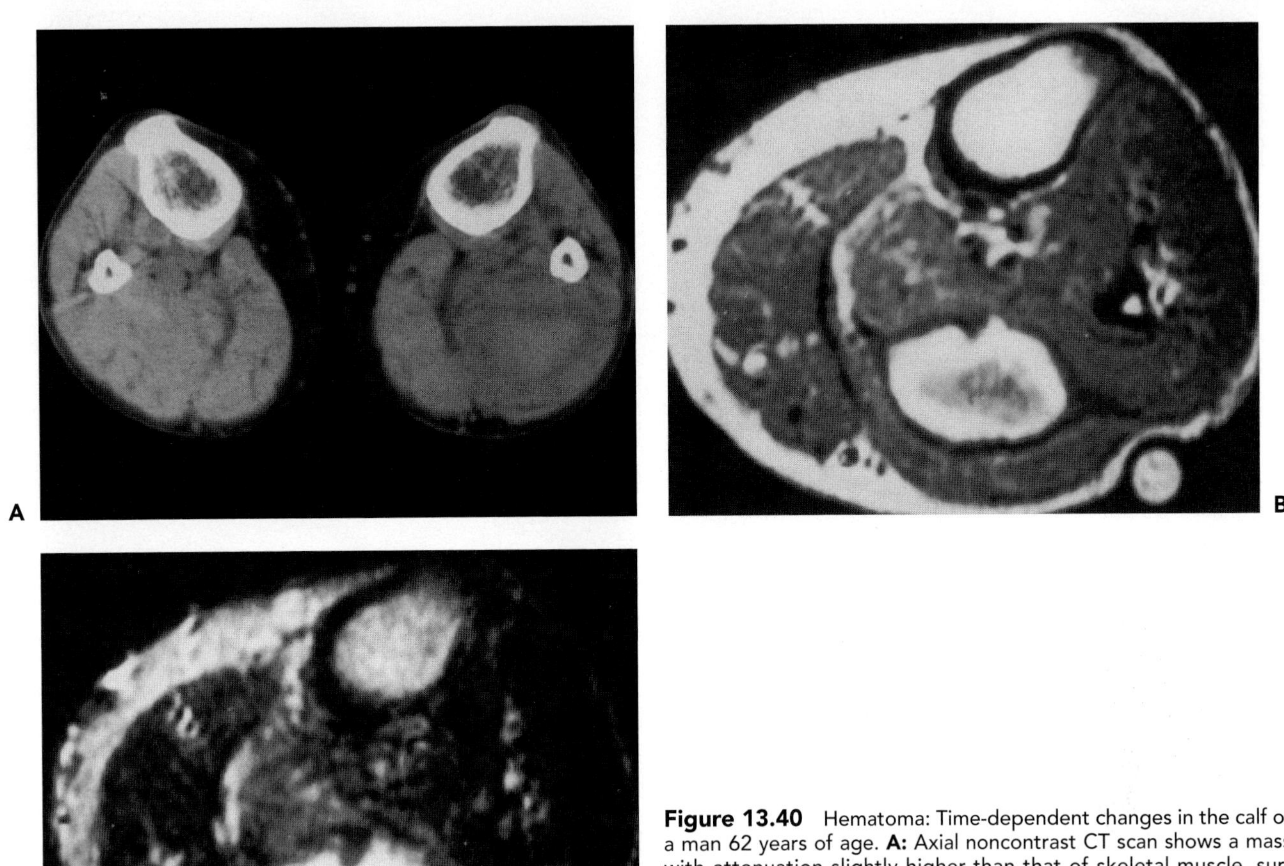

Figure 13.40 Hematoma: Time-dependent changes in the calf of a man 62 years of age. **A:** Axial noncontrast CT scan shows a mass with attenuation slightly higher than that of skeletal muscle, surrounded by a rind of decreased attenuation. **B,C:** Axial T1-weighted (TR/TE; 800/20) **(B)** and T2-weighted (TR/TE; 2500/80) **(C)** spin-echo MR images done 17 days later show a well-defined mass. On T1-weighted images, the lesion shows a signal intensity similar to that of subcutaneous fat, with an intermediate-intensity center and a rind of decreased signal. The signal intensity is much greater than that of fat on the T2-weighted image. (*continued*)

tissue masses are easily recognized on radiographs or CT scanning, and show markedly increased uptake of radionuclide on bone scintigraphy (123–129). Nonmineralized soft tissue masses associated with melorheostosis are more difficult to assess, and, if not recognized as a manifestation of the disease, may be confused with a more ominous process (131). Judkiewicz et al. (131) reviewed the imaging findings in 17 patients with melorheostosis. Soft tissue masses were noted in 9 patients (53%), 5 of which had CT scans that showed the lesions to be prominently mineralized in 80%.

MR imaging of mineralized regions, as expected, shows low signal intensity on all pulse sequences (Fig. 13.43) (124–128,131). CT of nonmineralized components reveals a soft tissue mass of similar attenuation to that of muscle. The soft tissue masses are heterogeneous on all MR pulse sequences. Nonmineralized components, in our experience, may show focal areas of adipose tissue characteristics or reveal intermediate signal intensity on T1-weighted MR images and high signal on T2 weighting,

presumably corresponding to vascularized fibrous tissue with relatively low collagen content. Gadolinium-enhanced MR images may show uptake of contrast within the nonmineralized components of the soft tissue mass that can be dramatic (Fig. 13.44). Perhaps the most important aspect of these soft tissue manifestations of melorheostosis for radiologists is their recognition as a component of this disease rather than other neoplastic lesions. This can be a particular dilemma if characteristic radiographs are not available for review or MR imaging is the first radiologic study, because the pathognomonic cortical thickening may not be as apparent on advanced imaging.

Retroperitoneal Fibrosis

Retroperitoneal fibrosis is a disease characterized by fibrosis localized to the lower aorta and common iliac arteries (132). As many as 15% of patients have associated fibrotic processes, most commonly mediastinal fibrosis, Riedel

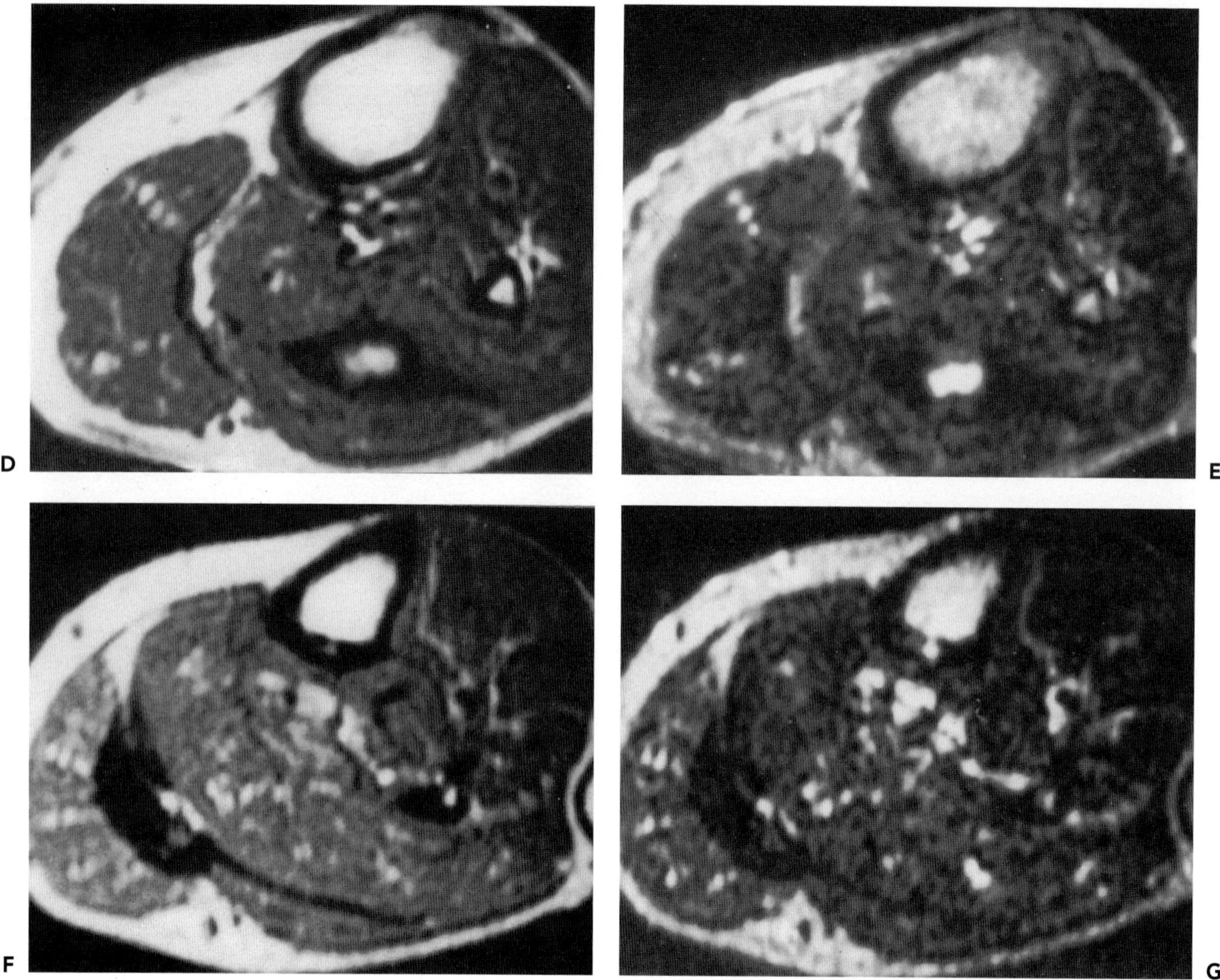

Figure 13.40 *(continued)* **D,E:** Axial T1-weighted (TR/TE; 800/20) **(D)** and T2-weighted (TR/TE; 1800/80). **(E)** spin-echo MR images done approximately 3 months later show the mass to be considerably smaller, with a prominent rind of decreased signal on all pulse sequences. **F,G:** Axial T1-weighted **(F)** and T2-weighted **(G)** images at the lower aspect of the mass show it to have a crescent shape with decreased signal intensity on all pulse sequences.

KEY CONCEPTS

- Retroperitoneal fibrosis is characterized by fibrosis localized to the lower aorta and common iliac arteries.
- Symptoms are often vague and nonspecific; the ureters are the most commonly affected structures.
- Retroperitoneal fibrosis may be detected in the workup of patients with newly diagnosed renal failure.
- The classic triad identified on excretory urogram (EXU) includes upper ureteral dilatation, medial deviation of the ureters, and smooth, extrinsic ureteral compression in the lower lumbar region.
- Imaging shows a retroperitoneal mass beginning below the aortic bifurcation and extending cephalad.
- On CT scanning, the attenuation of the lesion is similar to that of adjacent muscle.
- On MR imaging, the signal intensity is equal to or less than that of skeletal muscle.
- Contrast enhancement varies with the maturity of the lesion, with early lesions enhancing more.

fibrosing thyroiditis, sclerosing cholangitis, and fibrotic orbital pseudotumor (133). Retroperitoneal fibrosis is idiopathic in approximately two-thirds of cases and is sometimes referred to as *Ormond disease*, for John K. Ormond, the urologist who established the disease as a distinct clinical entity in 1948 (132). The remaining cases are typically associated with ergot-derivative medications, retroperitoneal hemorrhage, or tumor-stimulated desmoplastic response (132). The idiopathic form of retroperitoneal fibrosis occurs around areas of severe arteriosclerotic plaque, and it is postulated that the disease develops in response to leakage of ceroid from the atheroma into the periaortic tissue (132). Identifiable causes include methysergide, bromocriptine, β-blockers, methyldopa, hydralazine, retroperitoneal fluid collections, surgery, radiation therapy, and desmoplastic response to carcinoma of the breast, lung, gastrointestinal tract, and genitourinary tract (134).

Patients are usually between 30 and 60 years of age. Males outnumber females in the idiopathic forms 2:1, with

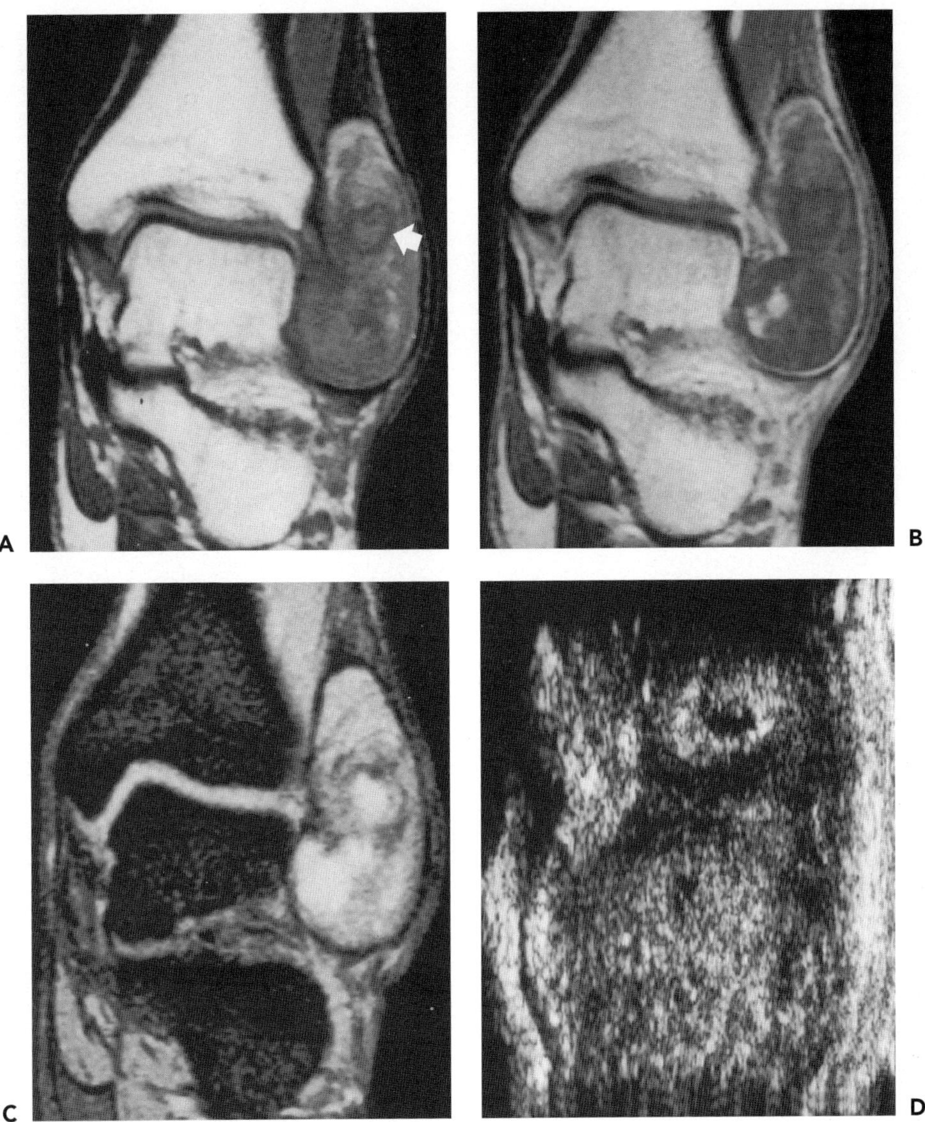

Figure 13.41 Hematoma: Organizing hematoma in a boy 17 years of age with previous injury and acute swelling 10 weeks earlier. **A,B:** Coronal T1-weighted (TR/TE; 600/15) spin-echo MR images preceding **(A)** and following **(B)** intravenous contrast show a heterogeneous mass with peripheral, and some central, enhancement. Note the ringlike area of decreased signal intensity (*arrow* in **A**). **C:** Coronal gradient-echo (TR/TE/Flip; 500/12/15) MR image shows heterogeneous increased signal intensity. The ringlike area shows the effect of hemosiderin with "blooming." **D:** Corresponding sonogram shows a predominantly solid mass.

this ratio reversed for cases associated with methysergide (132). Men and women are affected equally in cases associated with malignancy (132). Symptoms are often vague, nonspecific and related to the organ system affected by the fibrosis. The ureters are the most commonly affected structures, and retroperitoneal fibrosis is frequently detected in the evaluation of patients with newly diagnosed renal failure (135). Other structures secondarily involved include the inferior vena cava, gonadal veins, lymphatics, and even arteries (132). Lesions tend to develop at the level of the midureters, drawing them medially (136). The classic triad identified on excretory urography includes upper ureteral dilatation, medial deviation of the ureters, and smooth

extrinsic ureteral compression in the lower lumbar region. Bilateral ureteral involvement is seen in two-thirds of cases in adults and in an estimated one-half of cases in children (132).

Treatment is directed at identifying and removing the causative agent. Cessation of drug therapy usually results in regression and resolution of ureteral obstruction (132). Retroperitoneal fibrosis secondary to perianeurysmal fibrosis is treated by aneurysm repair and ureterolysis (132). Idiopathic disease is treated with ureterolysis, with or without corticosteroid therapy (132).

Lesions are gray-white in color with a woody consistency on gross examination (132). Histologic evaluation

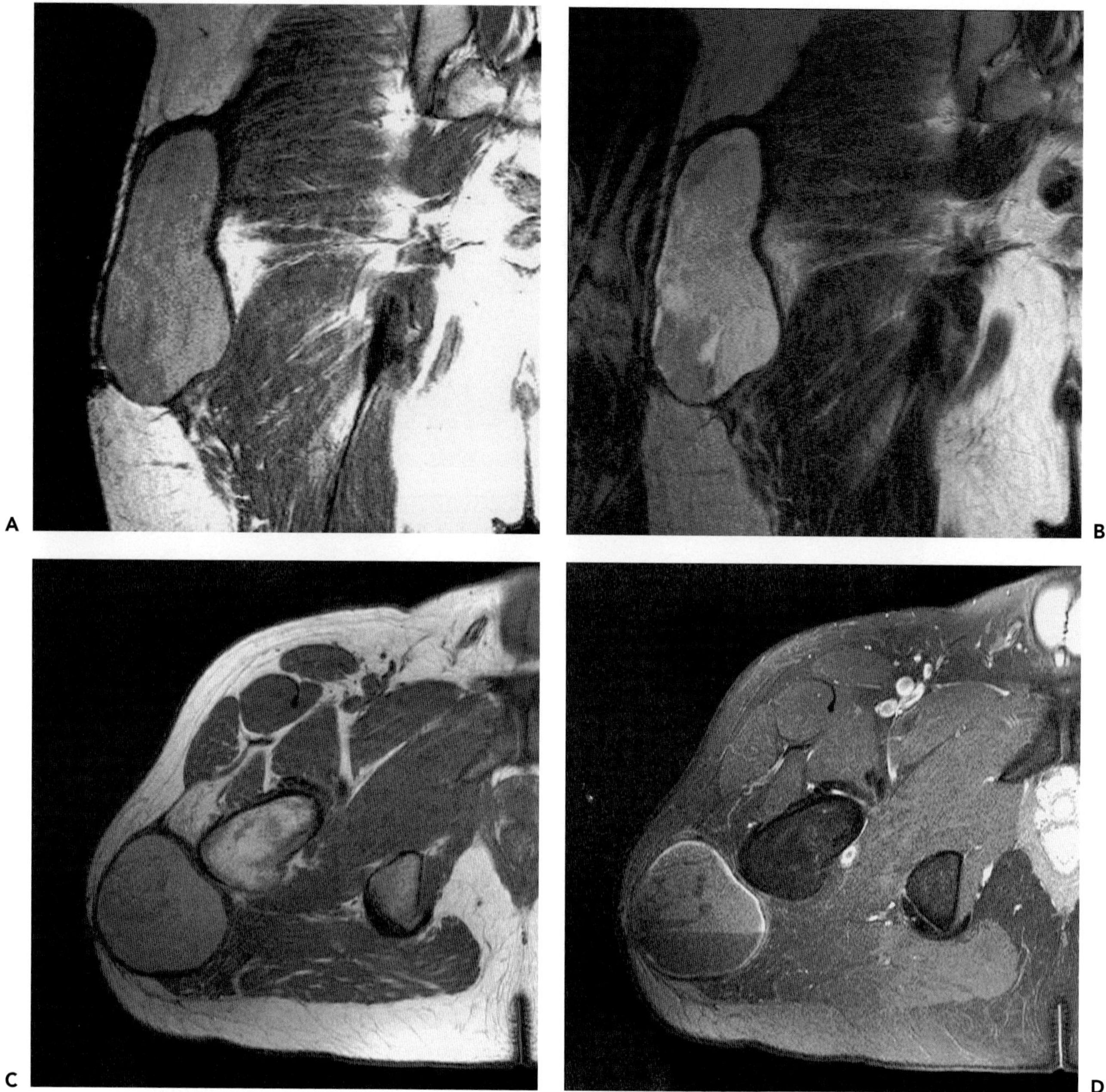

Figure 13.42 Morel-Lavallée lesion: MR imaging features in a man 30 years of age, with a history of motor vehicle accident and soft tissue mass in the hip. **A,B:** Coronal T1-weighted (TR/TE; 653/15) **(A)** and turbo T2-weighted (TR/TE; 4460/81) **(B)** spin-echo MR images show a well-defined mass associated with the fascia. The lesion has a rind of decreased signal intensity and is heterogeneous with signal intensity hyperintense to that of skeletal muscle on T1-weighted images and hyperintense to that of fat on T2-weighted images. **C:** Axial T1-weighted (TR/TE; 637/17) spin-echo MR image shows the lesion's association with the fascia lata. Note peripheral rind of decreased signal intensity. **D:** Enhanced, fat-suppressed, T1-weighted (TR/TE; 672/17) spin-echo image shows enhancing rind and fluid–fluid level not appreciated in **C**. (*continued*)

shows diffuse or localized fibroblastic proliferation, bands of hyalinized collagen, and lymphocytic and plasmacytic infiltrates (137). Mature lesions show increased hyalinized collagen and decreased cellular activity (132). The chronic inflammation and repair are retractile processes, accounting for the lack of mass effect on the encased structures (136).

CT and MR imaging reveal a retroperitoneal mass that begins below the level of the aortic bifurcation and spreads cephalad along the anterior surface of the spine, toward the renal hila (132). The process ultimately encases the aorta and inferior vena cava and entraps the ureters (132,138). It can extend inferiorly to involve the rectosigmoid, bladder, and pelvic organs (132). The lesion may be localized or extensive,

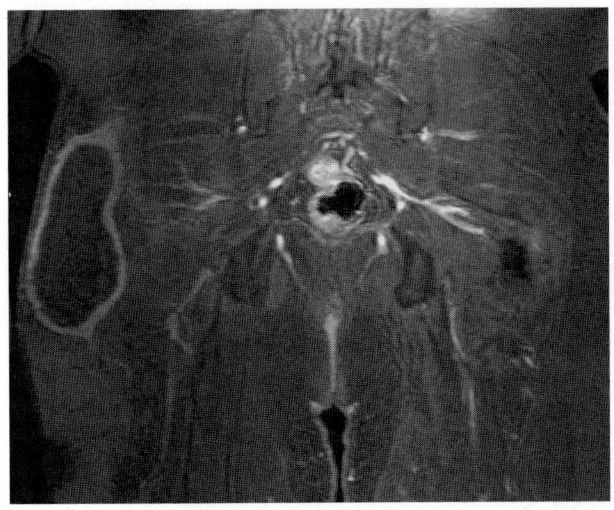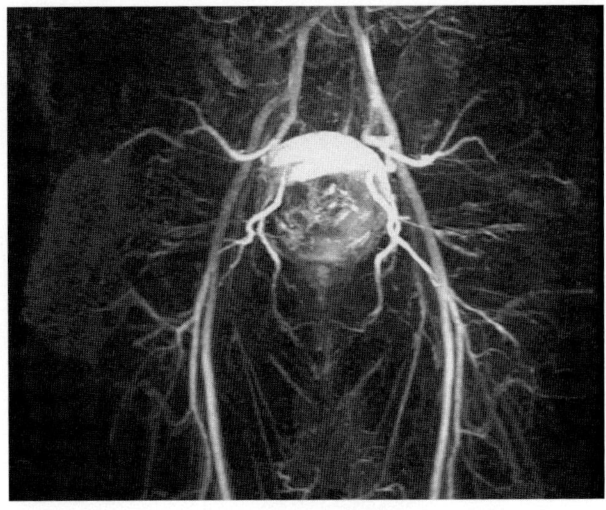

Figure 13.42 *(continued)* **E,F:** Coronal volume acquisition MR angiography source **(E)** and maximum-intensity project (MIP) **(F)** images show the lesion to be avascular with an enhancing rind.

well-defined or poorly defined, midline or asymmetric (132). Mulligan et al. (138) reviewed the MR and CT findings in five patients and noted an irregular, scalloped border in all patients. On CT, the attenuation of the lesion is similar to that of adjacent muscle (Figs. 13.45 and 13.46) (132). On T1-weighted spin-echo MR images, lesions show a signal intensity equal to or less than that of skeletal muscle. The signal intensity on T2-weighted images is variable, ranging from heterogeneous high signal intensity to low signal intensity (132,134,139), most typically similar to or less than that of fat (Figs. 13.45 and 13.46) (132,139). High signal intensity lesions on T2-weighted images are associated with malignant retroperitoneal fibrosis and idiopathic retroperitoneal fibrosis with associated inflammatory edema (134). Low signal intensity lesions on T2-weighted images are typically long standing (132). Contrast enhancement varies with the maturity of the lesion, with early lesions enhancing to a greater degree (140).

Sonography demonstrates a smoothly marginated hypoechoic/anechoic mass anterior to the lower lumbar spine or sacrum (132). Retroperitoneal fibrosis may be difficult to distinguish from a retroperitoneal tumor or adenopathy. The pattern of growth of retroperitoneal fibrosis is one that encases the aorta and inferior vena cava, rather than displaces them forward, as in lymphoma and malignant adenopathy (136,141). This is presumed to be because of the position of lymph nodes, which lie posterior to the aorta and inferior vena cava.

Soft Tissue Implant in Giant Cell Tumor

Soft tissue implants in giant cell tumor of bone are rare complications, presumed to be caused by seeding at the time of surgery (142), pathologic fracture (143), or direct tumor extension. The incidence is unknown. Cooper et al. (142) reported 17 cases (1.5%) from a group of approximately 1,100 giant cell tumors. The time interval between initial pre-

sentation and resection of the soft tissue implant varied between 1 year and 5 years, 10 months. All cases reported by Cooper et al. had at least one interosseous recurrence. Tumor cell metaplasia is thought to be the cause of the characteristic bone production in the soft tissue implants that is seen radiographically (142,143). Soft tissue implants may occur without radiologically apparent ossification, although histologic examination may reveal ossification (142,143). The soft tissue implants may vary in size from small nodules measuring a few millimeters, to masses as large as 13 cm (142).

The peripheral ossification in soft tissue implants in giant cell tumor may mimic myositis ossificans and, when occurring around a joint, synovial chondromatosis. The ossification in giant cell implants, however, is fine and delicate in appearance and does not show rapid maturation. The history of previous giant cell tumor of bone and the continued growth with time allow differentiation.

Radiographs show a soft tissue mass with peripheral ossification. This may vary from a thin osseous shell to a thick rind. In 1 of 17 cases reported by Cooper et al. (142), ossification was located centrally within the mass. There are no characteristic imaging features. In our limited experience, MR imaging is nonspecific, but the superior resolution allows delineation of the soft tissue mass (Fig. 13.47). The delicate ossification seen on radiographs is not apparent on MR imaging. CT is ideal to identify the ossification in the nodules, but is also otherwise nonspecific (Fig. 13.48).

Lymphoma

KEY CONCEPTS

- Primary lymphoma of soft tissue of any histologic subtype is extremely rare.
- Patients with lymphoma may present with a palpable mass that simulates a soft tissue sarcoma.
- MR imaging appearance of lymphoma is not specific.

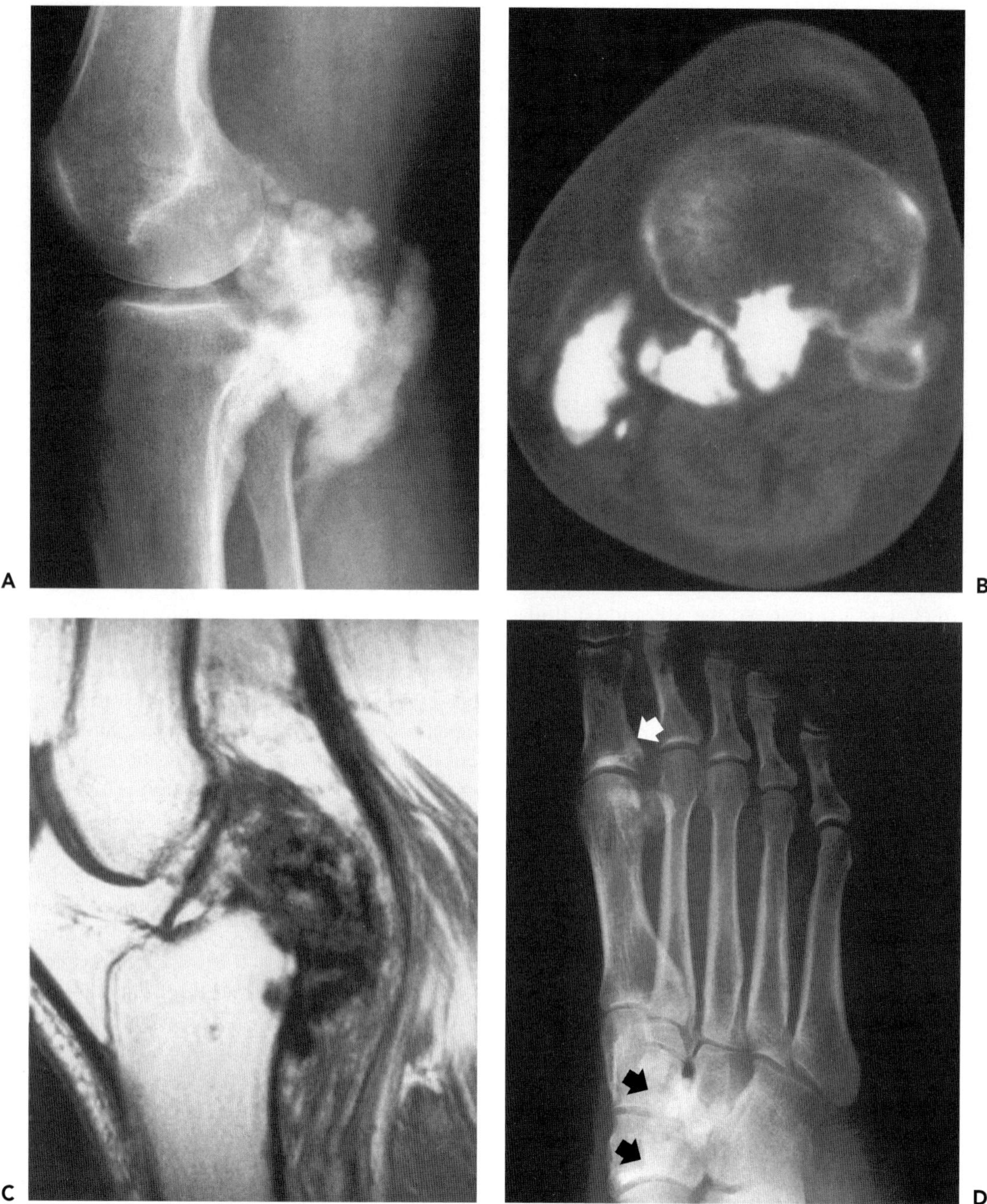

Figure 13.43 Melorheostosis: Imaging features in the popliteal fossa of a man 41 years of age. **A:** Lateral radiograph shows a densely mineralized mass. Bone involvement is not appreciated, and differential diagnosis includes a densely mineralized soft tissue mass, including synovial sarcoma and soft tissue osteosarcoma. **B:** Axial noncontrast CT shows the mass as well as bone involvement. **C:** Sagittal T1-weighted spin-echo MR image shows the densely mineralized mass as well as subtle bone involvement. **D:** Radiograph of the foot shows multiple bone involvement (*arrows*) in the typical sclerotome distribution.

Although lymphoma may involve any organ or system, true primary lymphoma of soft tissue of any histologic subtype is extremely rare (144). Consequently, it is mentioned only in passing. Lymphoma is traditionally classified into Hodgkin disease and non-Hodgkin lymphoma. Classification is essential to establish the natural history of the disease, determine its prognosis, and allow institution of appropriate therapy.

Patients with lymphoma may present with a palpable mass, simulating a soft tissue sarcoma. Imaging evaluation with positron emission tomography (PET) or MR imaging in these cases usually, although not invariably, shows abnormalities in the adjacent osseous structures or lymph nodes, suggesting the diagnosis or at least allowing multifocal lymphoma to be included in the differential diagnosis (Fig. 13.49) (145–147). Clearly, lymphoma may rarely

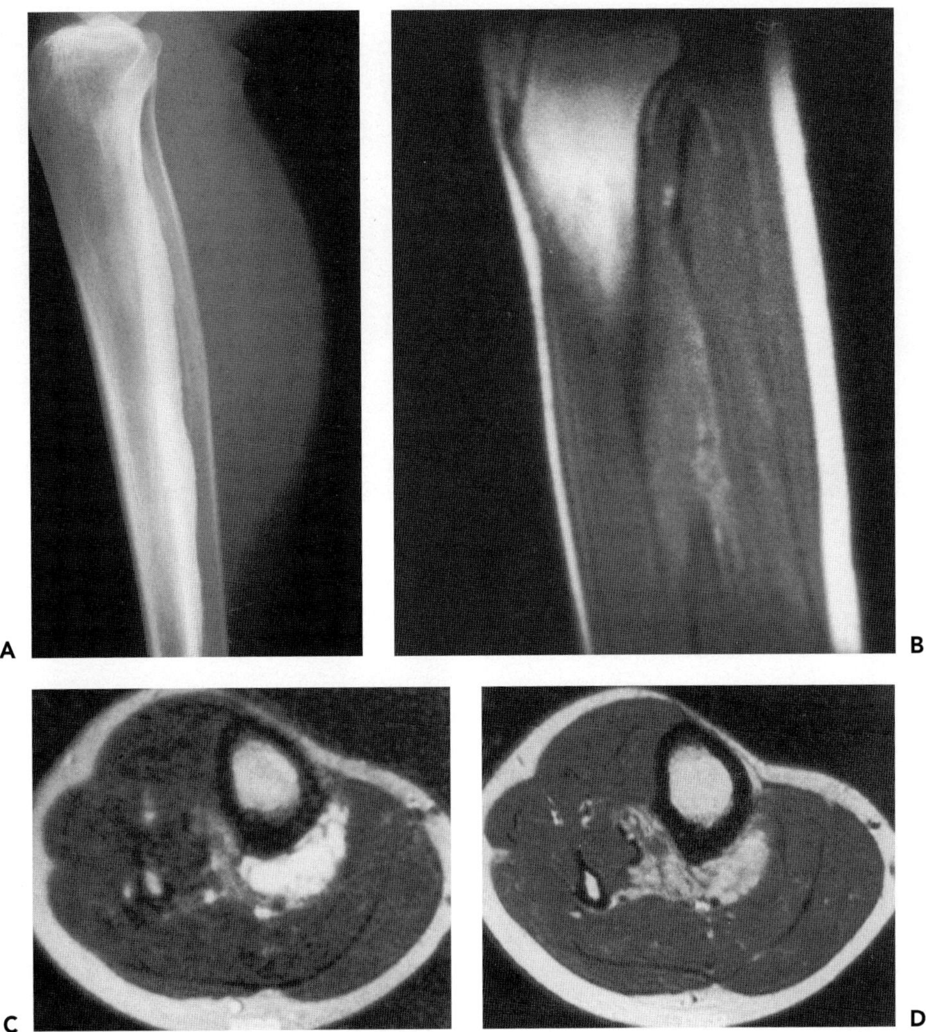

Figure 13.44 Melorheostosis of the lower leg in a woman 21 years of age. **A:** Lateral radiograph shows a densely mineralized mass flowing along the posterior aspect of the tibia. **B,C:** Sagittal T1-weighted (TR/TE; 600/20) **(B)** and axial T2-weighted (TR/TE; 2433/80) **(C)** spin-echo MR images show a prominent, nonmineralized mass with intermediate signal intensity on T1-weighted MR images and high signal intensity on T2 weighting, and an infiltrating pattern of growth. **D:** Axial gadolinium-enhanced T1-weighted (TR/TE; 567/20) spin-echo MR image shows marked heterogeneous enhancement.

present as an isolated soft tissue or subcutaneous mass (Figs. 13.50 and 13.51) (144,145,148). The imaging appearance in such cases is nonspecific.

POST-TRAUMATIC LESIONS

Calcific Myonecrosis

Calcific myonecrosis is an unusual late complication of trauma in which a single muscle or muscle group undergoes necrosis, liquefaction, and peripheral calcification (149,150). O'Keefe et al. (150) reviewed the literature in 1995 and noted a total of 15 reported cases, including 3 of their own, all involving the leg. Calcific myonecrosis is likely the result of a severe ischemic injury and subsequent acute compartment syndrome (150). There also appears to be an association with peripheral nerve injury (149).

> **KEY CONCEPTS**
> - Calcific myonecrosis is an unusual late complication of trauma in which a single muscle or muscle group undergoes necrosis, liquefaction, and peripheral calcification.
> - Calcific myonecrosis is likely the result of acute compartment syndrome.
> - Radiographs reveal a fusiform mass with plaquelike calcifications.
> - Calcifications are typically thin and linear and organized around the periphery of the lesion.
> - CT and MR imaging reflects the underlying pathophysiology.

Ectopic calcification as a late manifestation of compartment syndrome was previously reported (151), and only

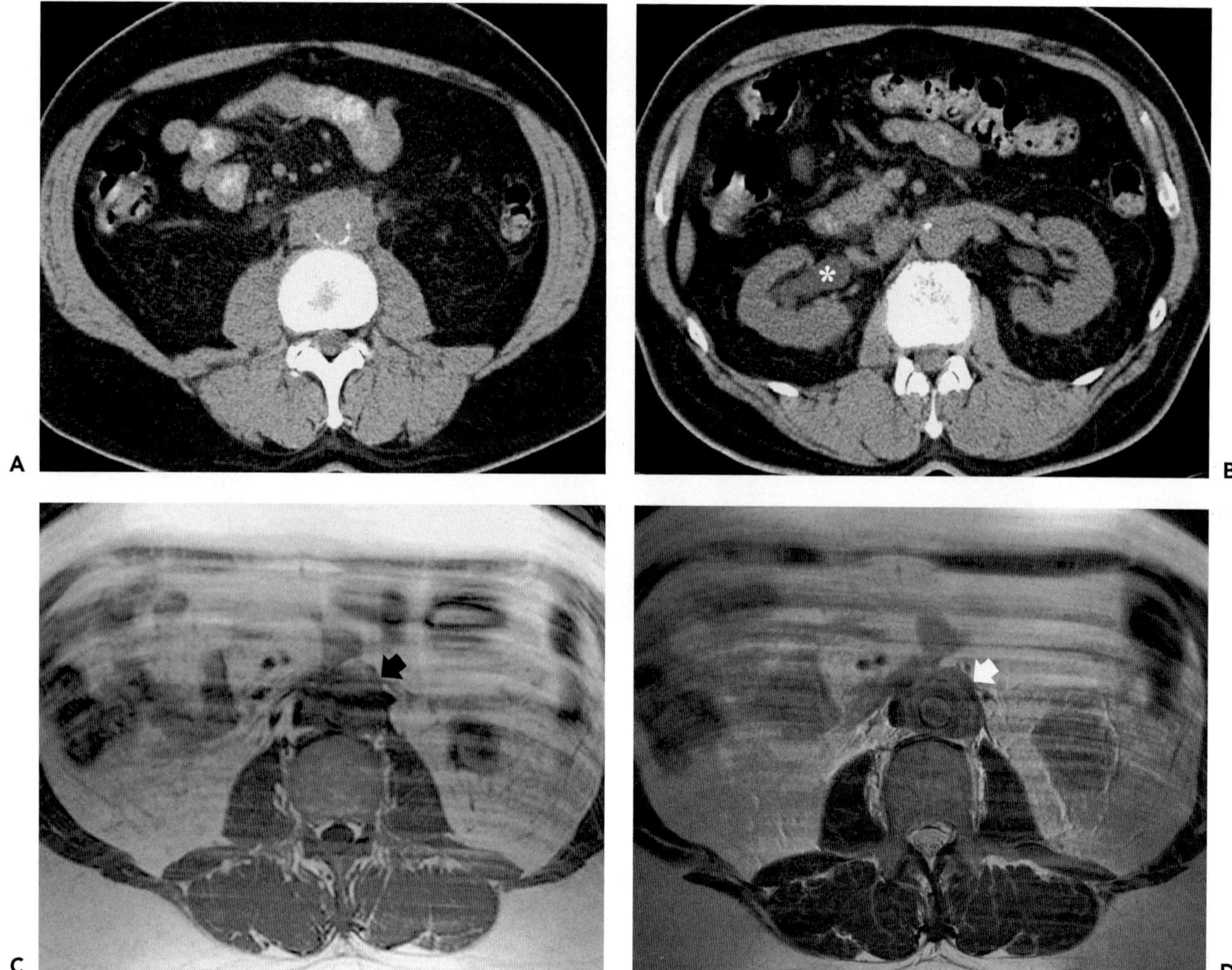

Figure 13.45 Retroperitoneal fibrosis: Imaging features in a man 67 years of age presenting with back and flank pain. **A:** Unenhanced axial CT scan shows a soft tissue mass encasing the aorta. **B:** Unenhanced CT scan at the level of the kidneys shows mildly hydronephrotic right kidney (*asterisk*). **C,D:** Axial T1-weighted **(C)** and fast T2-weighted **(D)** spin-echo MR images show a mass (*arrow*) encompassing the aorta. The mass shows a signal intensity similar to that of muscle and is well-delineated from the adjacent fat. (*continued*)

two cases of calcific myonecrosis have occurred in the absence of recognized vascular injury to the leg.

Patients at time of diagnosis in reported cases range from 34 to 80 years of age (mean: 59 years), with presentation 22 years to more than 60 years following the initial traumatic event (150,152). The lesion typically affects a single muscle or compartment, although it may involve all compartments of the leg (149,150). It is important to establish the diagnosis radiologically. Chronic infection with draining sinuses was reported in 4 (27%) of 15 patients following surgery, 1 of which eventually required leg amputation (149,150).

Grossly, the calcific myonecrosis shows central areas of necrosis and cystic change, filled with debris (150,152). The lesion walls contain needlelike, elongated, calcified fragments of necrotic tissue that correspond to the plaque-like calcifications identified on radiologic evaluation

(150). Microscopic evaluation of the wall demonstrates fibrous tissue with hemosiderin-laden macrophages, whereas the central cystic area contains necrotic skeletal muscle, acellular amorphous debris, and evidence of organizing thrombus (150).

Radiographs reveal a fusiform mass with plaquelike calcifications (149–151). The calcifications are typically thin and linear and organized around the periphery of the lesion (150). The adjacent bone may show remodeling (pressure erosion) secondary to a long-standing mass (150). CT scanning shows a mass with a rimlike peripheral calcification that may follow fascial planes (Fig. 13.52) (151). A low-attenuation center (149) may show punctate calcifications.

MR imaging has a nonspecific signal intensity and reflects the pathophysiology of the underlying compartment syndrome. The MR appearance varies from that of a homogeneous mass, imaging similar to fluid, with foci of

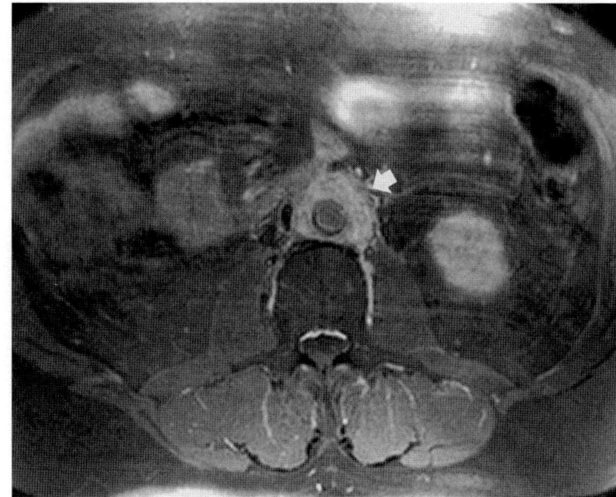

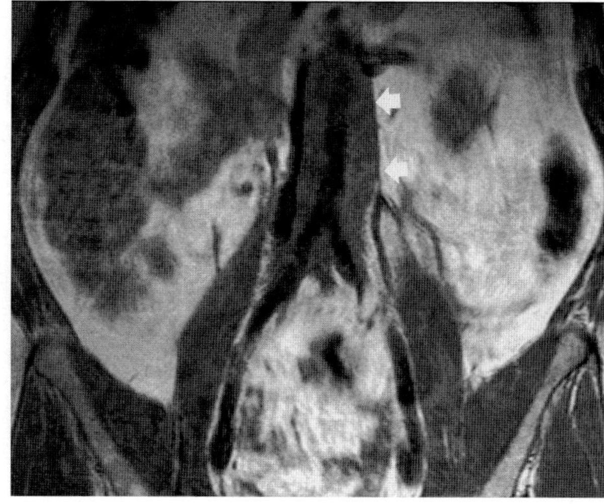

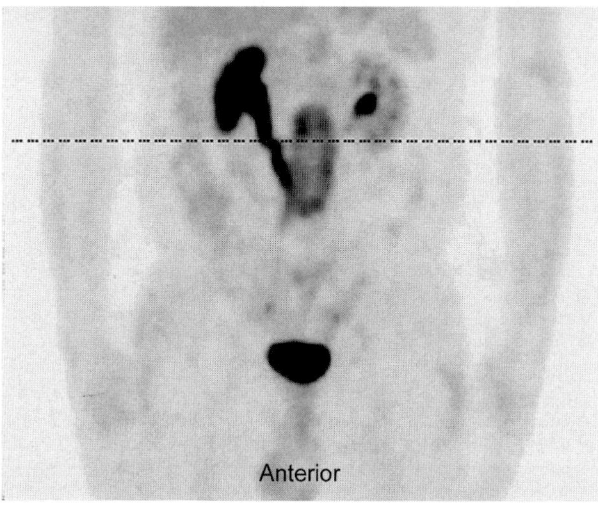

Figure 13.45 *(continued)* **E:** Corresponding axial fat-suppressed T1-weighted spin-echo MR image following contrast administration shows the mass (*arrow*) to enhance significantly. **F:** Coronal unenhanced T1-weighted spin-echo image shows the longitudinal extent of the mass (*arrows*). **G:** Anterior image from positron emission tomography (PET) scan shows the mass to be hypermetabolic. Note hydronephrotic right kidney.

decreased signal at its periphery, representing calcification (149), to an irregularly shaped heterogeneous mass with areas of intermediate and high signal intensity on T2-weighted images (Fig. 13.52) (151). The surrounding muscle is atrophic and fatty replaced. No enhancement occurs following gadolinium administration (151).

Focal Myositis

KEY CONCEPTS

- Focal myositis is a pseudotumor of soft tissue; subclinical injury is the suspected cause.
- Approximately one-third of patients with focal myositis subsequently developed polymyositis.
- The lesion is typically confined to a single muscle or muscle group.
- MR imaging shows a heterogeneous mass with variable signal intensity on T2-weighted images and extensive surrounding edema.

Focal myositis is a pseudotumor of soft tissue, first described in 1977 by Heffner et al. (153), based on a review of 16 cases. The lesion typically occurs in the soft tissue of the extremities, and is relatively rare. Although the cause is unknown, subclinical injury was initially suspected. That same year, Cumming et al. (154) reported three similar patients, two of whom subsequently developed a diffuse myopathy consistent with polymyositis. In 1993, Flaisler et al. reported a case of focal myositis in the lower leg and reviewed the 39 previously reported cases (155), noting that approximately one-third of patients with focal myositis subsequently developed polymyositis, with clinical symptoms including generalized weakness, fever, myalgia, weight loss, and elevation of creatine phosphokinase (CPK). They suggest that focal myositis is a localized form of polymyositis in some cases, and that because the entities are histologically identical, follow-up is necessary to distinguish the two conditions. Patients with recurrent focal myositis affecting multiple discrete muscle groups without subsequent development of polymyositis are also reported, as are those demonstrating metachronous, symmetric involvement (156).

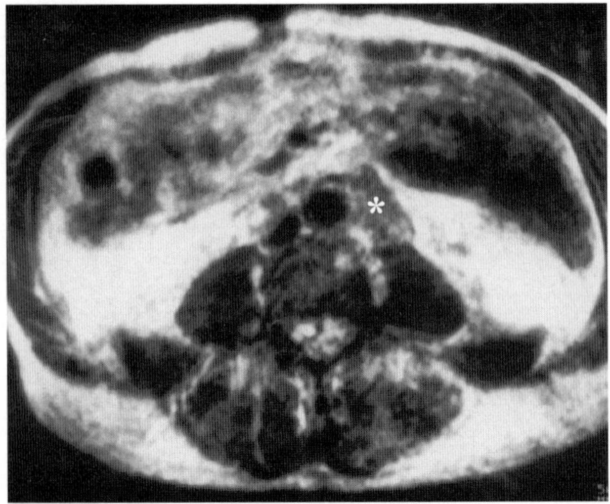

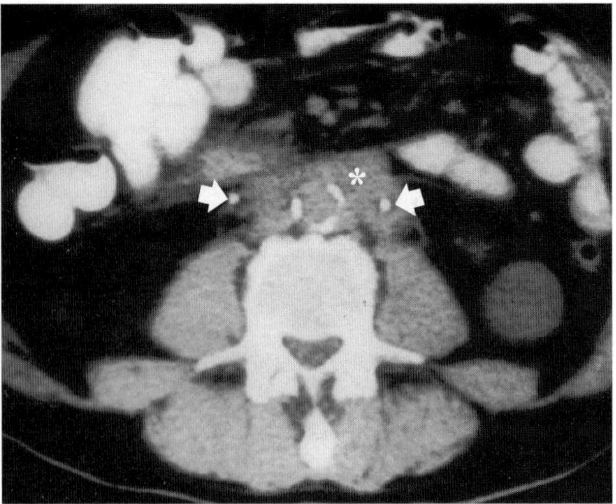

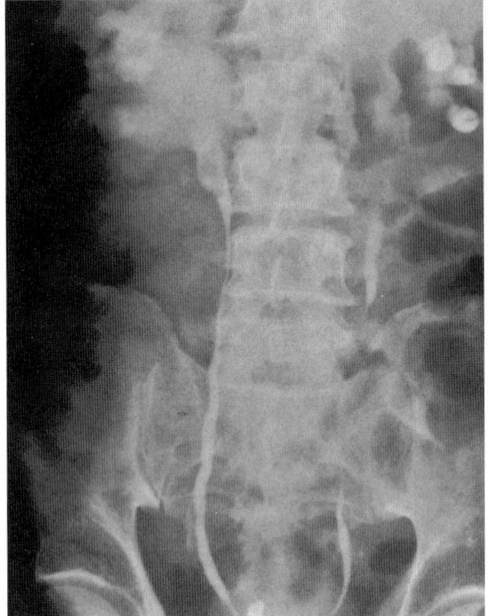

Figure 13.46   Retroperitoneal fibrosis: Imaging features in a man 62 years of age presenting with marked renal failure. **A:** Axial T2-weighted (TR/TE; 2250/80) spin-echo MR image shows a mass (*asterisk*) encompassing the ureters and great vessels. The mass shows a signal intensity slightly greater than that of skeletal muscle and is well-delineated from the adjacent fat. **B:** Corresponding axial contrast-enhanced CT shows a nonspecific mass (*asterisk*) encasing the great vessels and ureters. The ureters (*arrows*) are well-delineated with contrast. **C:** Radiographs from a retrograde pyelogram shows medial displacement of the ureters as well as bilateral hydronephrosis.

Focal myositis can occur in children or adults (range: 7 to 70 years of age), with patients presenting with a localized intramuscular soft tissue mass, which may be rapidly enlarging over a period of weeks (153,155,157,158). The lesion is typically confined to a single muscle, although multiple muscle involvement may be seen (153,155). Males and females are affected equally (153,158,159). Lesions are most common in the lower extremity, with approximately 50% occurring in the thigh and 25% occurring in the lower leg (153,159).

Pain is the most common clinical symptom, seen in more than half of patients (153). The clinical course is benign, with spontaneous regression and no recurrence following excision (158,159); however, a clinical course characterized by debilitating pain may be seen (156). Extensive time required for spontaneous resolution and the painful nature of the lesion may justify surgical excision (158).

Histologically, there is lymphocytic infiltration of the perimysial and endomysial spaces, scattered muscle fiber necrosis and regeneration, and interstitial fibrosis (153). Hemorrhage, necrosis, or calcification is not seen (153,159). Arteriography is reported to be normal, without neovascularity (159). Our experience with the imaging appearance of this lesion is limited to a few cases, and the spectrum of findings is unknown.

There is scant literature describing the imaging appearance of focal myositis. On CT, focal myositis shows a nonspecific appearance, with the lesions demonstrating an attenuation less than or similar to that of skeletal muscle. The affected muscle is enlarged, with poorly defined margins and loss of the tissue planes between muscles (160,161). Moskovic et al. (162) reported two patients with calf lesions showing ill-defined fatty infiltration of the gastrocnemius and soleus muscles, without a discrete mass. This pattern likely reflects diffuse fatty replacement. MR imaging characteristics are not well-characterized, but are described on the basis of isolated cases as heterogeneous, and with variable signal intensity on T2-weighted

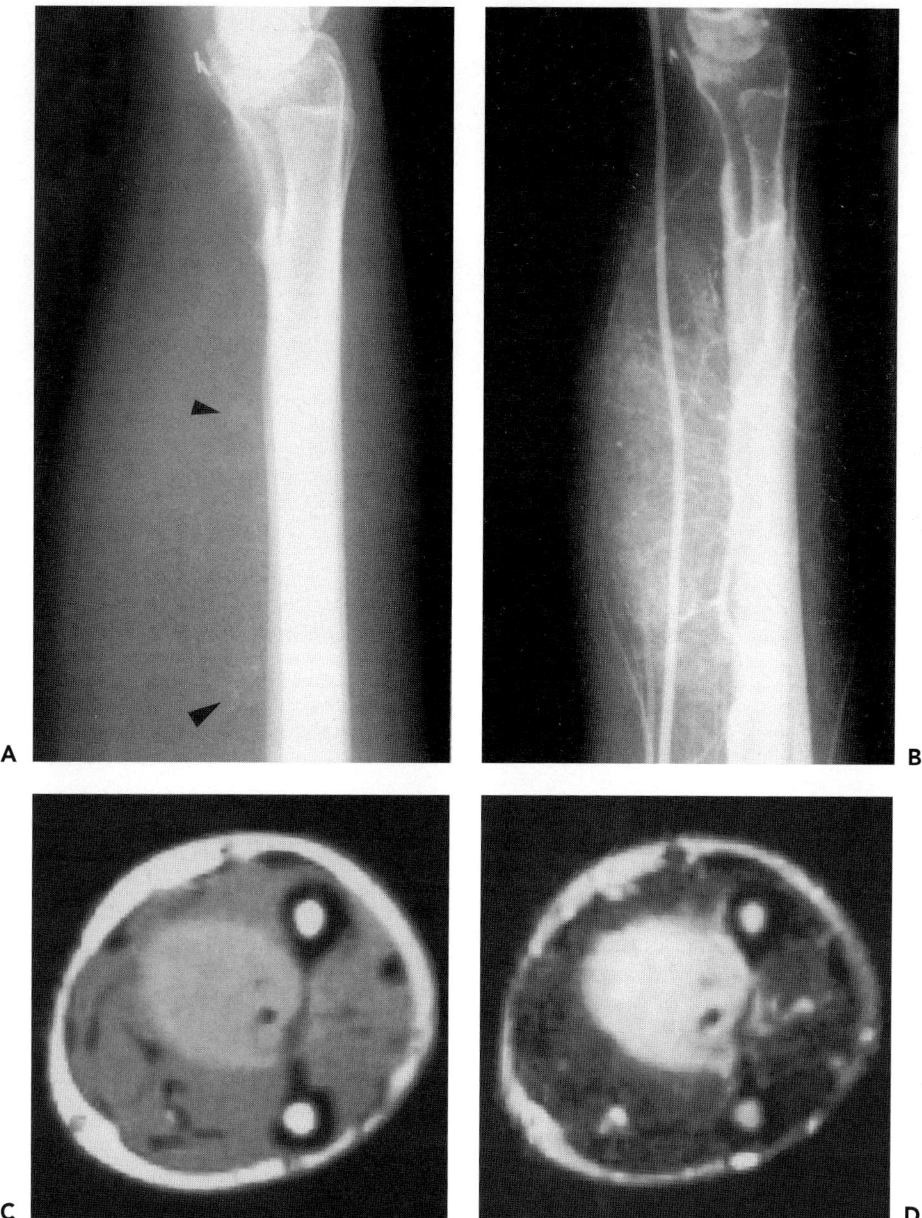

Figure 13.47 Soft tissue implant in a giant cell tumor: Radiographic, arteriographic, and MR imaging features in a woman 29 years of age with previous local recurrence. **A:** Lateral radiograph of the forearm and wrist shows a poorly defined soft tissue mass with delicate ossification (*arrowheads*). **B:** Corresponding arteriogram shows a markedly hypervascular mass. **C,D:** Axial T1-weighted (TR/TE; 500/17) **(C)** and T2-weighted (TR/TE; 2100/90) **(D)** spin-echo MR images show a well-defined mass. The hyperintensity on the T1-weighted image likely reflects its hypervascularity.

images, which may involve a single muscle or muscle group (155,160,163). There may be extensive surrounding edema (156,160). A focal mass may be seen as well, with the lesion enhancing less than the surrounding edema (Fig. 13.53).

Hoffa Disease

Hoffa disease is a term used to describe anterior knee pain thought to be caused by impingement of the infrapatellar

---

KEY CONCEPTS

- Hoffa disease refers to anterior knee pain thought to be caused by impingement of the infrapatellar fat pad.
- It is thought to be the result of chronic minor trauma with inflammation, hypertrophy, and fibrosis of the infrapatellar fat pad, which is pinched between the tibia and femur during extension.
- Edematous fat is replaced by scar that may contain islands of cartilage and bone.

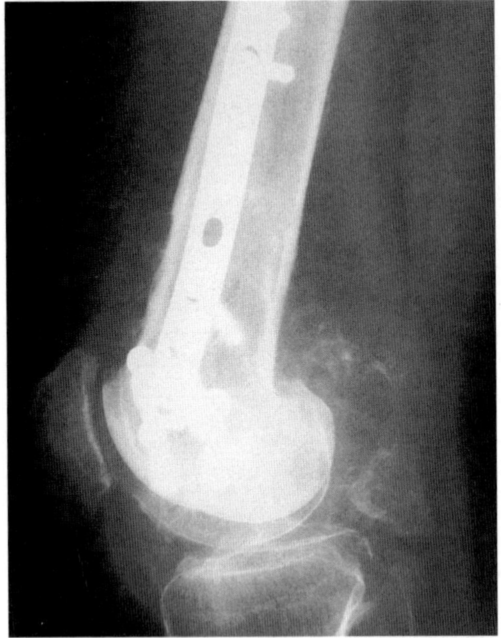
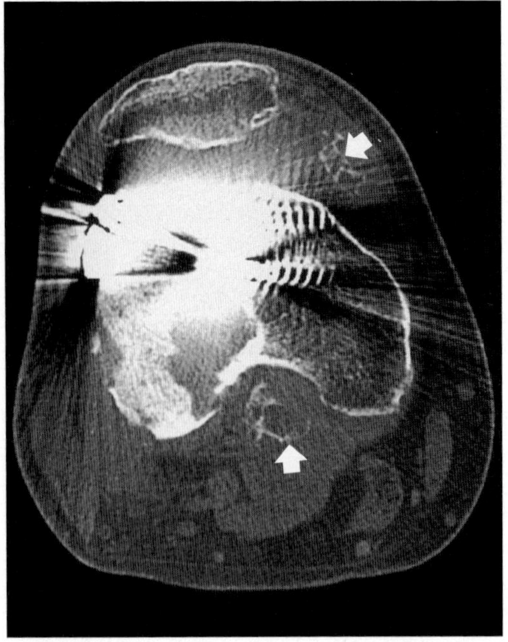

Figure 13.48   Soft tissue implant in a giant cell tumor: CT features in a man 36 years of age with previous local recurrence. **A:** Lateral radiograph of the knee shows multiple masses with peripheral ossification. **B:** Axial noncontrast CT displayed at bone window shows resorption of a femoral allograft and multiple tumor nodules with ossification (*arrows*).

fat pad (164). Initially described by Albert Hoffa in 1904 (164) with a report of 20 cases, it is now thought to be the result of chronic minor trauma with inflammation, hypertrophy, and fibrosis of the infrapatellar fat pad, which is pinched between the tibia and femur during extension (165).

Patients are usually in the fourth decade of life (166), presenting with pain and tenderness localized to the anterior knee (167). An effusion may be present, as may a decreased range of motion (165). On physical examination, the patient experiences pain at terminal extension with pressure on the fat pad (Hoffa sign) (165,167). Initially pain occurs from mechanical pressure on the edematous adipose tissue (165). This is followed by replacement of the edematous fat by scar tissue, which may contain islands of cartilage and bone (165). The identification of cartilage and bone led some investigators to suggest that an ossifying chondroma of the infrapatellar fat pad may represent the end result of Hoffa disease (165).

Treatment consists of conservative therapy, including nonsteroidal anti-inflammatory medication and physical therapy (165). Operative intervention for resection of the infrapatellar fat pad is reserved for patients not responding to conservative therapy (167).

Radiographs may be normal or may show soft tissue swelling in the region of the infrapatellar fat pad. Calcification and ossification may occasionally be seen (Fig. 13.54). (See discussion of soft tissue chondroma in Chapter 11.)

CUTANEOUS (SKIN) LESIONS

The wide variety of cutaneous tumors are typically small, and they are diagnosed and treated without radiologic imaging. On rare occasions, however, these lesions may become quite large and may mimic a soft tissue mass. The following lesions reflect our experience with those cutaneous appendage tumors that may present clinically as musculoskeletal lesions.

Epidermal Inclusion Cyst (Infundibular Cyst)

> **KEY CONCEPTS**
> - Epidermal inclusion cysts may occur anywhere, but are most common in the head, neck, and trunk.
> - On CT and MR imaging, the lesion appears as a small, well-defined, subcutaneous mass.
> - The character of the lesion varies with the contents of the cyst.
> - Large lesions may show dependent debris.

The epidermal inclusion cyst, also known as an infundibular cyst, is a simple epithelial cyst lined with infundibular or epidermislike cells that keratinize (168). The majority form as a result of progressive cystic ectasia of the infundibulum of the hair follicle, as a result of mechanical obstruction, scarring, or inflammation (168). In this

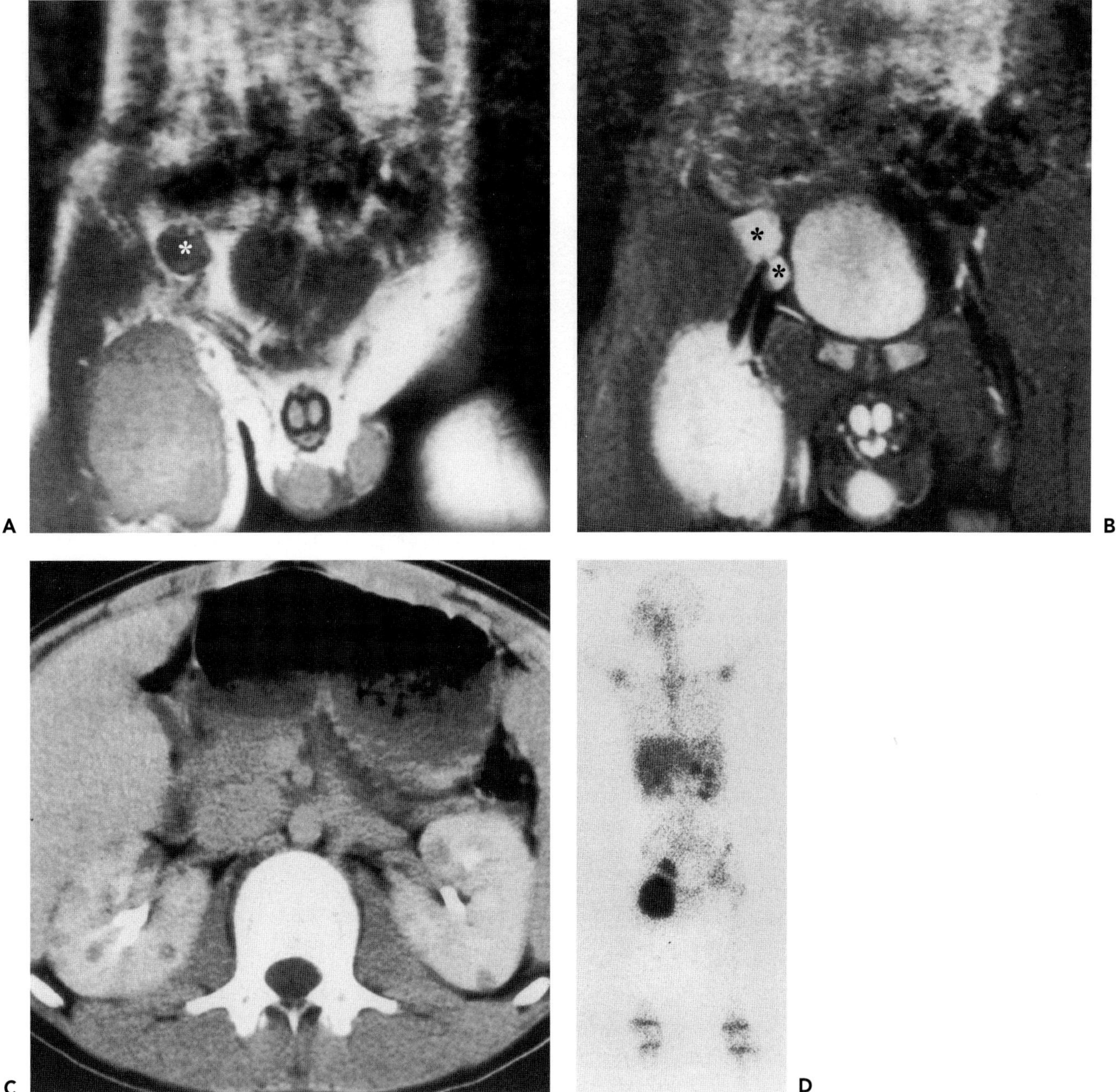

Figure 13.49   Lymphoma: Imaging features (small noncleaved cell, pleomorphic type) in a boy 13 years of age presenting as a soft tissue mass. **A,B:** Coronal T1-weighted (TR/TE; 600/30) spin-echo **(A)** and short-tau inversion recovery (STIR) (TR/TE/TI; 2500/30/150) **(B)** images show a large, well-defined, homogeneous mass in the right groin. Note small adjacent nodes (*asterisks*). **C:** Axial contrast-enhanced CT shows lesions in both kidneys. **D:** Whole-body image from a gallium-67 scan shows abnormal tracer accumulation in the mass, inguinal nodes, and kidneys.

sense, most are retention cysts rather than inclusion cysts (168).

Lesions may occur anywhere, but they are most common in the head, neck, and trunk (168). They are typically small subcutaneous or cutaneous nodules, less than 5 cm in size (168). Cysts are filled with loosely packed lamellae of keratin (168). The walls of the cyst resemble follicular infundibular epithelium (168). Cyst walls may rupture, with secondary foreign body–type reaction, granulomatous reaction, granulation tissue, or abscess formation (168).

On CT and MR imaging, the lesion appears as a small, well-defined subcutaneous mass (Fig. 13.55). The character of the lesion varies with the contents of the cyst, and large lesions may show dependent debris (Figs. 13.56 and 13.57).

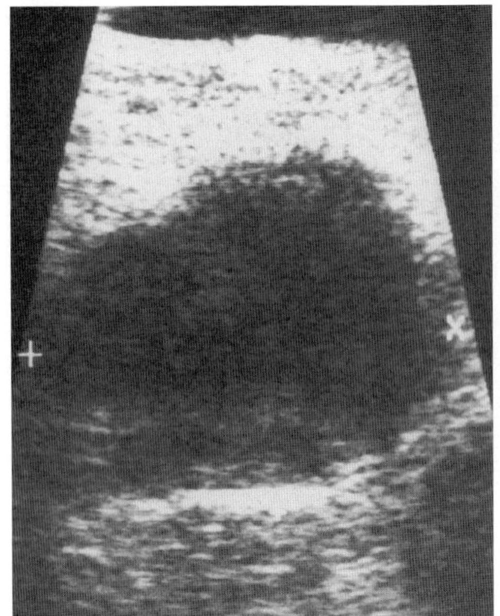
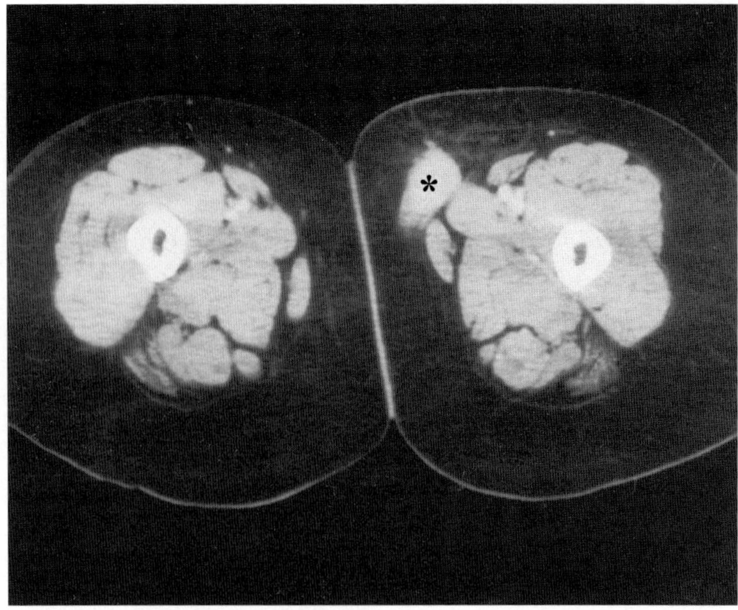

Figure 13.50 Lymphoma: CT and ultrasound features (diffuse, mixed small cell cleaved, and large cell with sclerosis) in a man 45 years of age presenting as a mildly tender soft tissue mass. The mass remained stable in size over 6 months of observation. **A:** Ultrasonography of the thigh shows a well-defined hypoechoic mass. **B:** Axial contrast-enhanced CT shows a well-defined, homogeneous mass (*asterisk*) in the anterior thigh. No adenopathy was noted.

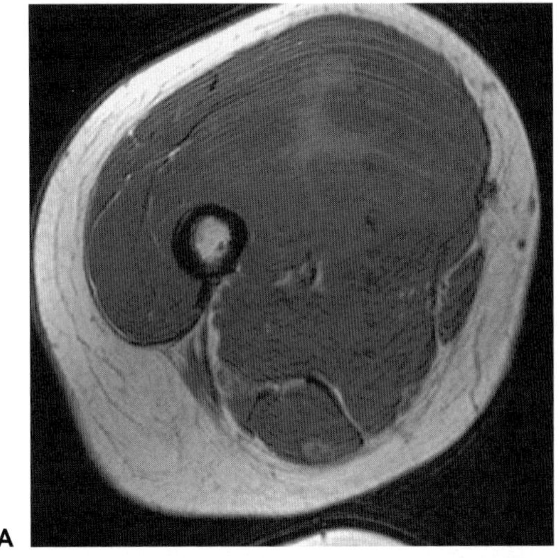
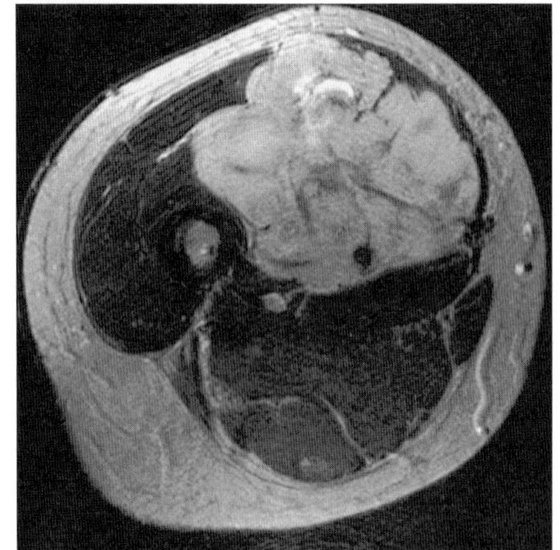
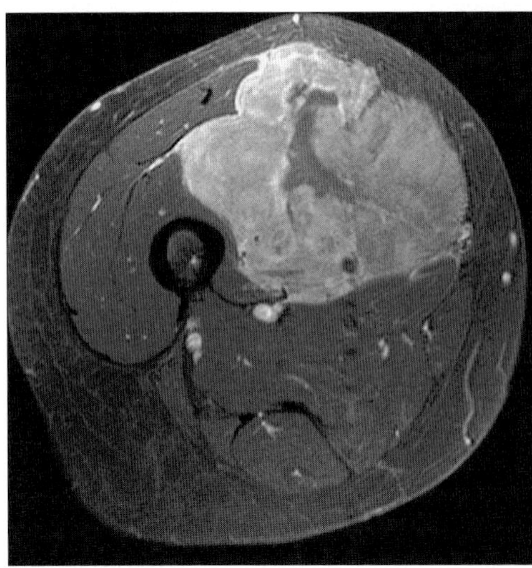

Figure 13.51 Lymphoma: MR features (large B-cell type) in a woman 53 years of age presenting with leg pain and mass. **A,B:** Axial T1-weighted (TR/TE; 677/17) **(A)** and T2-weighted (TR/TE; 2430/83) **(B)** spin-echo MR images show a large, relatively well-defined mass involving multiple muscles in the anterior compartment. The mass shows an area of increased signal intensity in **(A)** compatible with hemorrhage. On T2-weighted images the lesion shows predominantly intermediate signal intensity. **C:** Axial fat-suppressed T1-weighted (TR/TE; 692/17) spin-echo MR image following gadolinium administration shows intense enhancement, except for the hemorrhagic area.

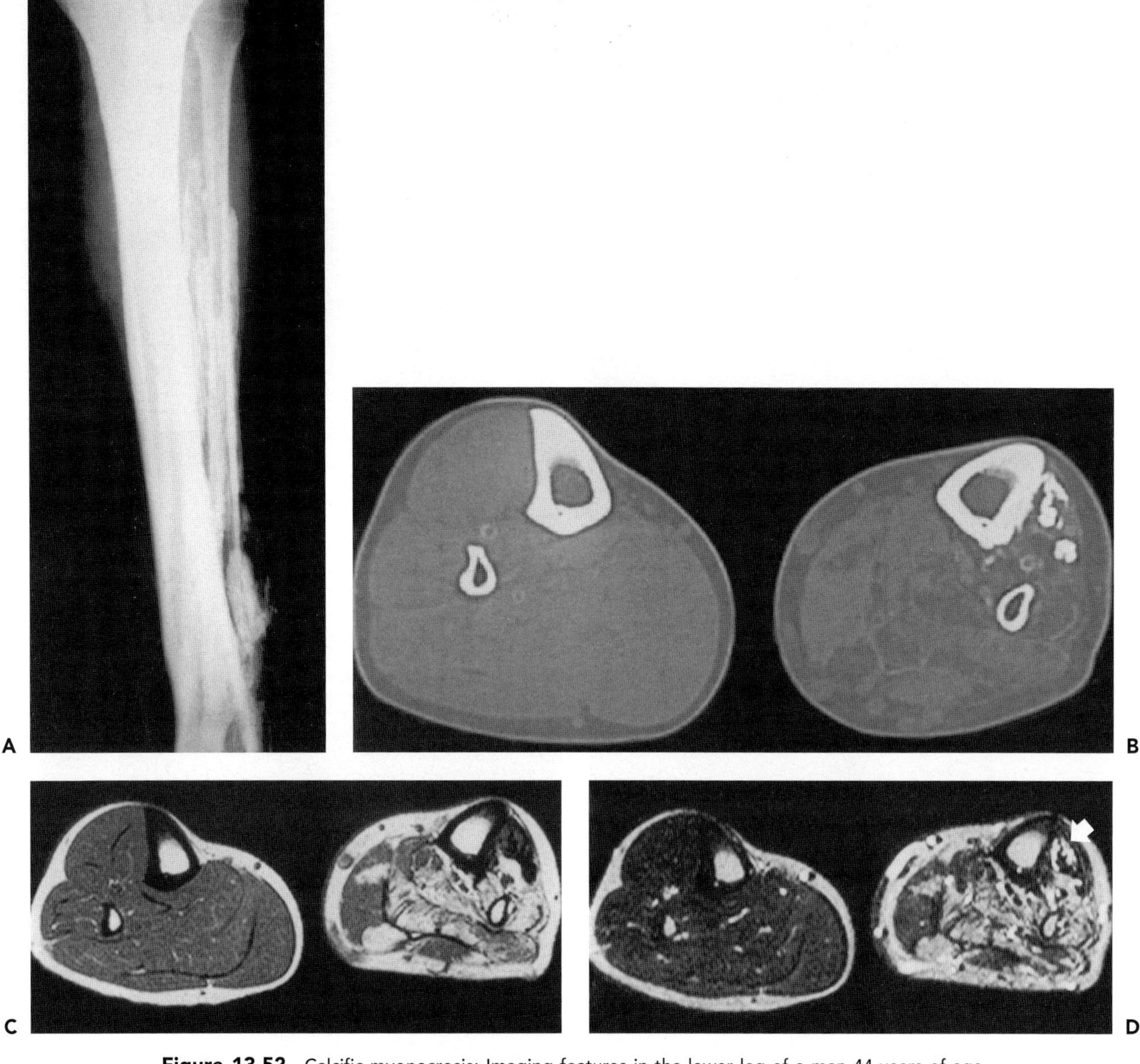

Figure 13.52 Calcific myonecrosis: Imaging features in the lower leg of a man 44 years of age with a remote history of lower extremity trauma and compartment syndrome on the left. **A:** Anteroposterior radiograph reveals a fusiform mass with linear plaquelike calcifications. Deformity is present that is compatible with remote trauma. **B:** Axial noncontrast CT displayed on bone window shows the plaque calcification to better advantage. **C,D:** Corresponding axial T1-weighted (TR/TE; 700/16) **(C)** and T2-weighted (TR/TE; 2350/80) **(D)** spin-echo MR images show marked atrophy of the left lower leg with fatty overgrowth. There is a small fluidlike focus (*arrow* in **D**).

Granuloma Annulare

Granuloma annulare is an uncommon, benign, inflammatory dermatosis characterized by the formation of dermal papules that have a tendency to form rings (169,170). Although the cause is unknown, some evidence suggests it can be a postviral phenomenon and can be accompanied by immune complex deposition in at least some cases (171). There are several clinically distinct forms. The subcutaneous form is the most frequently encountered by radiologists because the lesion presents as a subcutaneous mass; other forms include the localized and generalized forms (169). The localized form is the most common type and presents as a nodular, ringed skin eruption, typically on the dorsum of the hands and feet, forearms, arms, legs, and thighs (172). It is a disease of children and young adults, with two-thirds of patients presenting by 30 years of age (173). The generalized form is similar and differs only in its wide spread distribution. Approximately 15% of patients with granuloma annulare have more than 10 lesions (172). Patients with the generalized form are usually younger than 10 or older than 40 years (172).

The subcutaneous form differs from other forms of granuloma annulare in that it is seen almost exclusively in

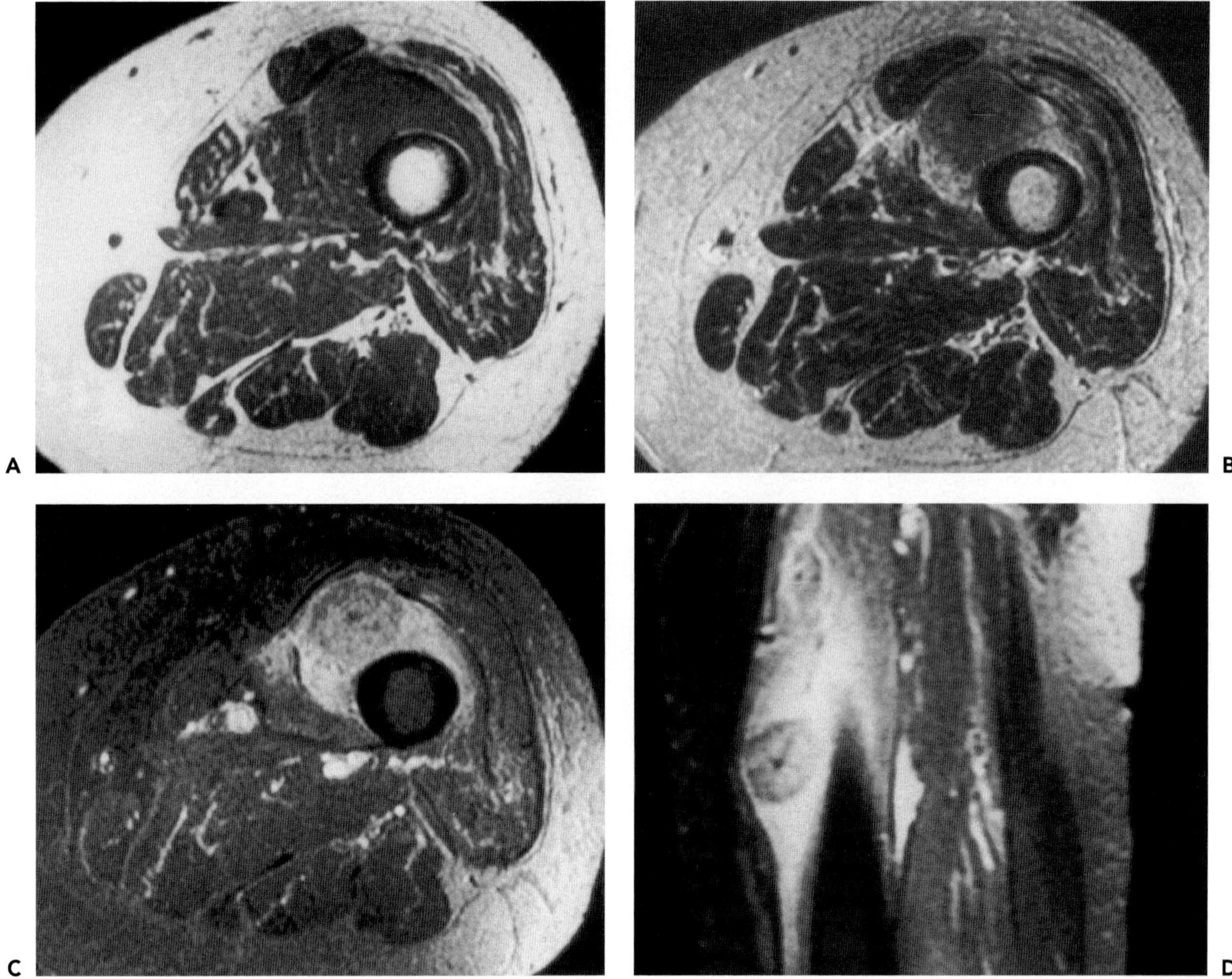

Figure 13.53 Focal myositis: MR imaging features in the thigh of a woman 75 years of age. **A,B:** Axial T1-weighted (TR/TE; 588/11) **(A)** and turbo T2-weighted (TR/TE; 3600/102) **(B)** spin-echo MR images of the thigh show a poorly defined mass. The mass has a signal intensity similar to that of skeletal muscle on the T1-weighted image and a signal intensity between that of skeletal muscle and that of fat on the fast spin-echo T2-weighted image. There is surrounding edema. **C,D:** Fat-suppressed, axial T1-weighted (TR/TE; 550/11) **(C)** and sagittal (TR/TE; 533/10) **(D)** spin-echo MR images show heterogeneous enhancement to the mass, with greater enhancement of the surrounding edema.

KEY CONCEPTS

- Granuloma annulare is an uncommon, benign, inflammatory dermatosis.
- The subcutaneous form is the form most frequently encountered by radiologists.
- The subcutaneous form is seen almost exclusively in children.
- CT shows a soft tissue mass with a variable attenuation relative to that of skeletal muscle.
- MR imaging reveals a subcutaneous mass with indistinct margins, decreased signal intensity on T1-weighted images, and decreased to intermediate signal intensity on T2-weighted images.
- Enhancement following contrast administration may be seen on CT and MR imaging.

children (169,173). This form has also been termed *deep granuloma annulare* and *subcutaneous palisading granuloma* (173). The lesion is histologically indistinguishable from the subcutaneous nodules seen in rheumatoid arthritis and may also be referred to as *pseudorheumatoid nodule* or *benign rheumatoid nodule* (173,174). A fine-needle aspirate may be inadequate for diagnosis and may lead to a mistaken diagnosis of sarcoma (169).

Patients typically present with a rapidly growing, painless, solitary subcutaneous nodule (169). Multiple subcutaneous nodules may be seen (175). Lesions are most common in the pretibial region but may be seen in the scalp, foot, and ankle (169,173). The typical clinical course is one of spontaneous regression over months to years, with local and distal recurrence common (169). The treatment is local excision, although resection following initial biopsy is gen-

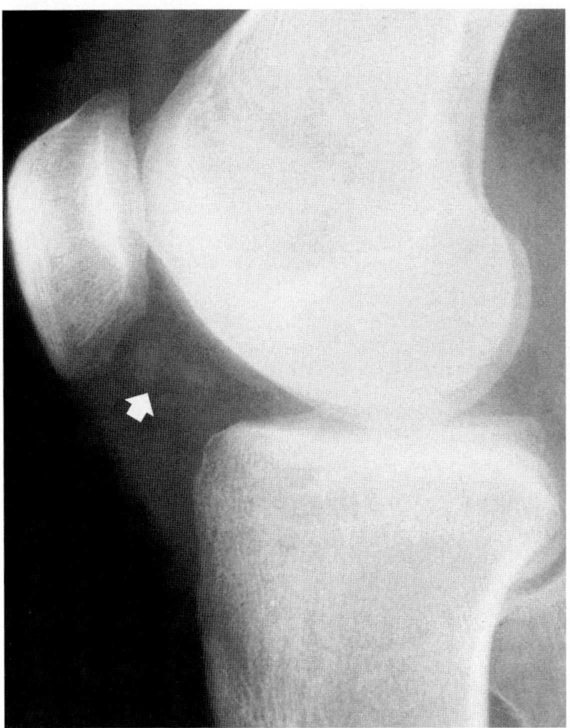

Figure 13.54   Hoffa disease: Radiographic features in a man 46 years of age. Lateral radiograph shows soft tissue swelling in the region of the infrapatellar fat pad with calcification (*arrow*).

erally not required, in view of the natural history, and may be reserved for lesions that are symptomatic (such as lesions that interfere with shoe ware) (169). Davids et al. (169) reported subcutaneous granuloma annulare in 12 children and noted subsequent lesions in 9 (75%), these being local recurrence and/or distant lesions. Three patients (25%) subsequently developed the generalized form of granuloma

annulare. In contrast to other varieties of granuloma annulare, the subcutaneous form has no associated connective tissue disorders or rheumatologic conditions (169).

Radiographs may show evidence of a subcutaneous mass without bone involvement, calcification, or ossification (Fig. 13.58) (169,173). CT shows a soft tissue mass with a variable attenuation relative to that of skeletal muscle; enhancement following contrast administration is typically seen (173). The lesion is usually not well-delineated from subcutaneous fat and adjacent muscle. MR imaging reveals a subcutaneous mass with indistinct margins, decreased signal intensity on T1-weighted images, and decreased-to-intermediate signal intensity on T2-weighted images (Figs. 13.58 and 13.59) (176,177). On ultrasonography, the lesion is hypoechoic to subcutaneous fat (169).

Pilomatrixoma

> ### KEY CONCEPTS
> - Pilomatrixoma is also known as *calcifying epithelioma of Malherbe.*
> - The lesion arises in the dermis from cells that normally differentiate toward hair matrix cells.
> - The face, neck, and upper extremities are most commonly affected.
> - Calcification, which is more typically central, is seen in approximately 84% of lesions.
> - Ossification occurs in an estimated 20% of these and is more typically peripheral.
> - MR imaging shows an intermediate signal intensity on T1-weighted and fast spin-echo T2-weighted images.
> - Slight heterogeneous enhancement follows contrast administration.

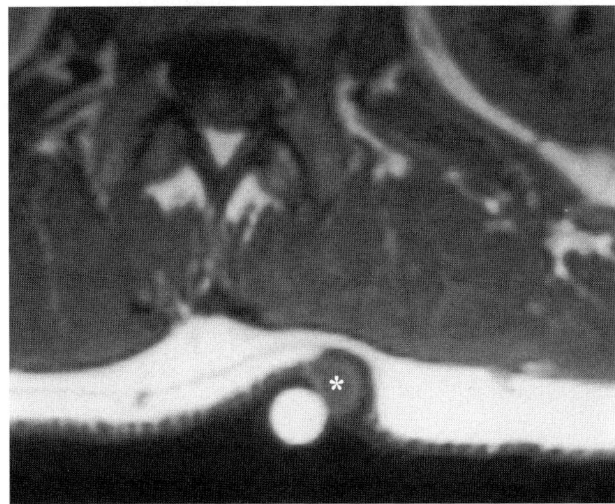

A

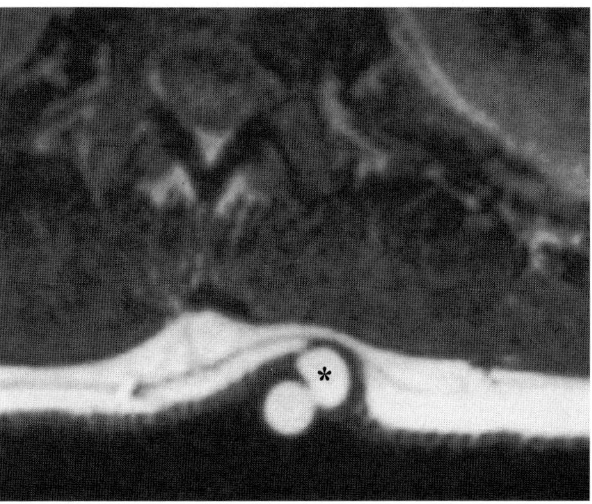

B

Figure 13.55   Inclusion cyst (infundibular cyst): Imaging features in the back of a man 33 years of age. **A,B:** Axial T1-weighted (TR/TE; 600/20) **(A)** and T2-weighted (TR/TE; 1700/80) **(B)** spin-echo MR images of the back show a small, homogeneous, cystlike mass (*asterisk*) in the subcutaneous adipose tissue. A lipid marker overlies the lesion. (Case courtesy of James S. Jelinek, MD, Washington, DC.)

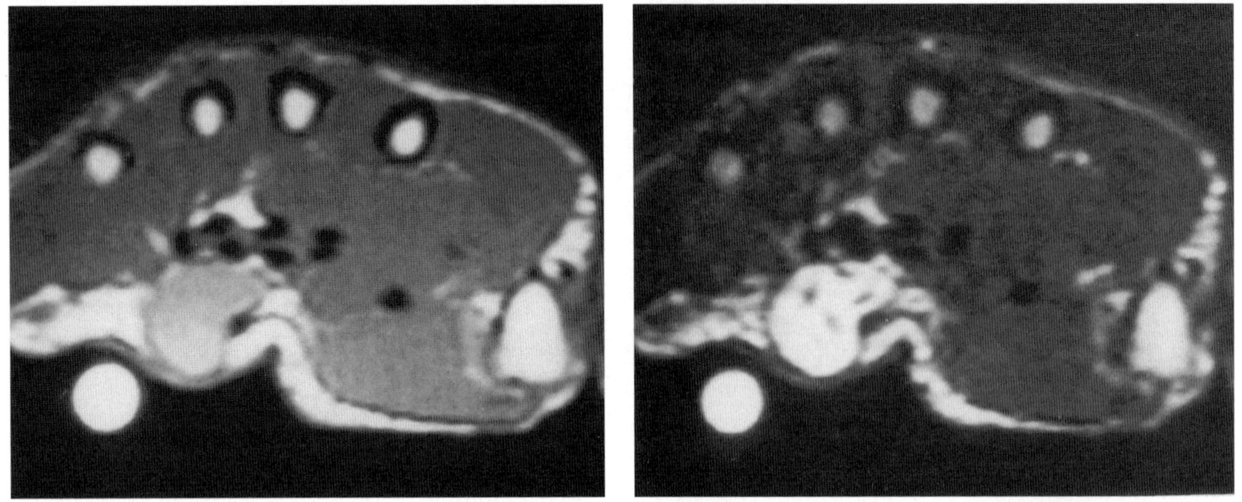

Figure 13.56 Inclusion cyst (infundibular cyst): Imaging features in a man 58 years of age. **A,B:** Axial T1-weighted (TR/TE; 600/20) **(A)** and T2-weighted (TR/TE; 2000/80) **(B)** spin-echo MR images show a nonspecific, well-defined mass in the subcutaneous adipose tissue of the palm. The lesion is heterogeneous on the T2-weighted image, with focal internal areas of decreased signal.

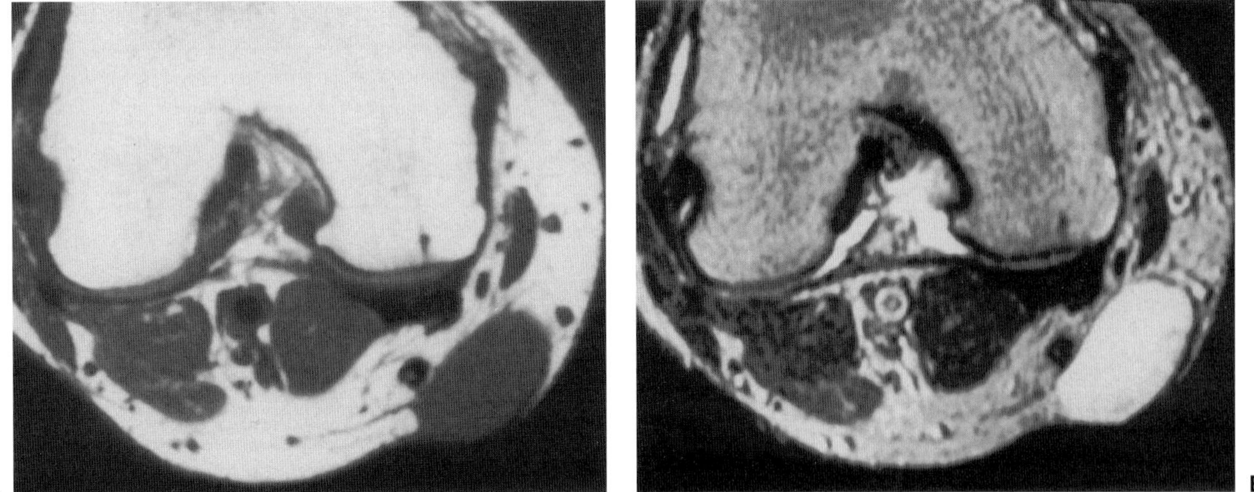

Figure 13.57 Inclusion cyst (infundibular cyst): Imaging features in a man 45 years of age, with a history of a mass for approximately 30 years. **A,B:** Axial T1-weighted (TR/TE; 600/20) **(A)** and T2-weighted (TR/TE; 2500/80) **(B)** spin-echo MR images of the knee show a nonspecific well-defined mass in the subcutaneous adipose tissue. The lesion is heterogeneous on the T2-weighted image, with debris in the dependent aspect.

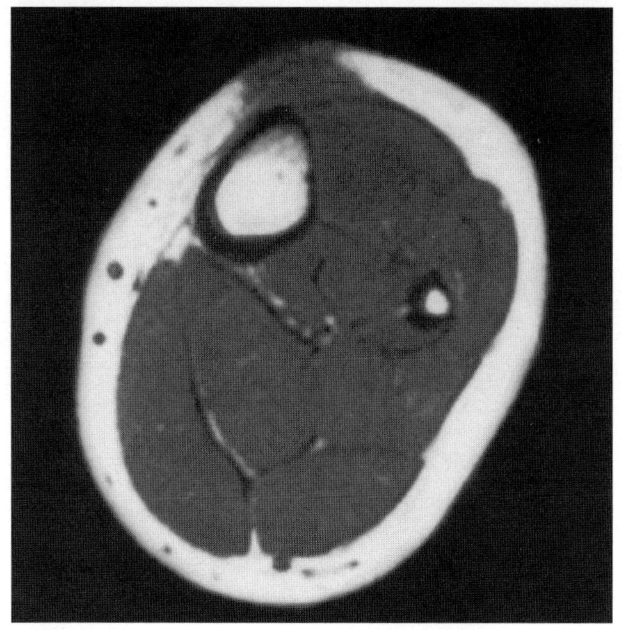

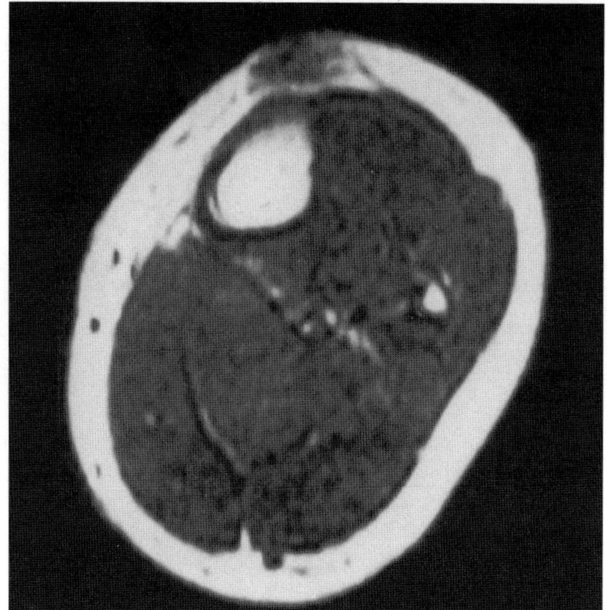

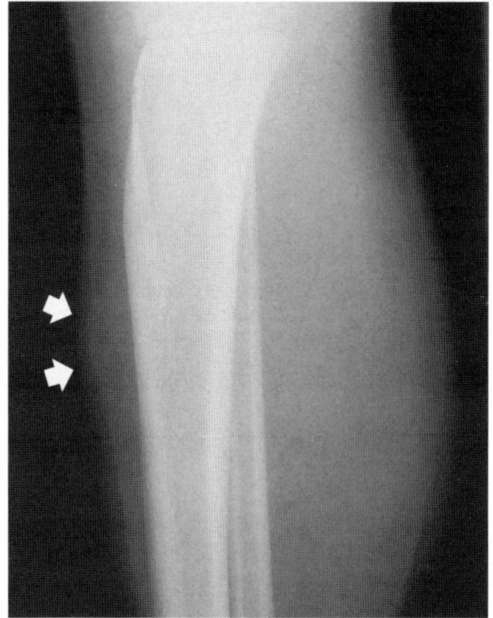

Figure 13.58 Granuloma annulare: MR imaging features in the lower leg of a girl 5 years of age. **A,B:** Axial T1-weighted (TR/TE; 500/20) **(A)** and T2-weighted (TR/TE; 2000/80) **(B)** spin-echo MR images show a mass in the anterior subcutaneous tissue of the lower leg. The lesion has a decreased signal intensity on all pulse sequences with a somewhat indistinct margin. **C:** Lateral radiograph shows the lesion in the anterior subcutaneous tissue. (Case courtesy of Joseph A. Utz, MD, Jacksonville, FL.)

Pilomatrixoma, also known as *calcifying epithelioma of Malherbe,* was initially described by Malherbe in 1880 as a benign calcifying tumor thought to arise from skin appendages (178). The lesion arises in the dermis from primitive cells that normally differentiate toward hair matrix cells (179,180).

Most patients are young, with a peak incidence between 10 and 15 years of age (178). Approximately 40% occur in children younger than 10 years (179,181). The face, neck, and upper extremities are most commonly affected (178,181,182). Tumors are small, usually less than 3 cm in diameter (168,178), grow slowly, and are confined to the subcutaneous tissue (Fig. 13.60) (179). Females are affected more commonly than males by a ratio of approxi-

mately 1.5:1 (178). Approximately 2% to 3% of tumors are multiple (178,181).

Local excision is usually curative, and recurrence is rare (178). Aggressive local behavior is only rarely reported (182,183). Distant metastases are not identified (178,182), and bone invasion is exceedingly rare, with only a single reported case (178). These aggressive lesions are termed *pilomatrix carcinoma* or *calcifying epitheliocarcinoma of Malherbe* (183). Clinically, they are more common in men and occur in an older age group (183).

Microscopy shows differentiation toward hair matrix (178). The tumor consists of sheets and bands of epithelial cells in a connective tissue stroma (179). Shadow cells (which are histochemically similar to inner root

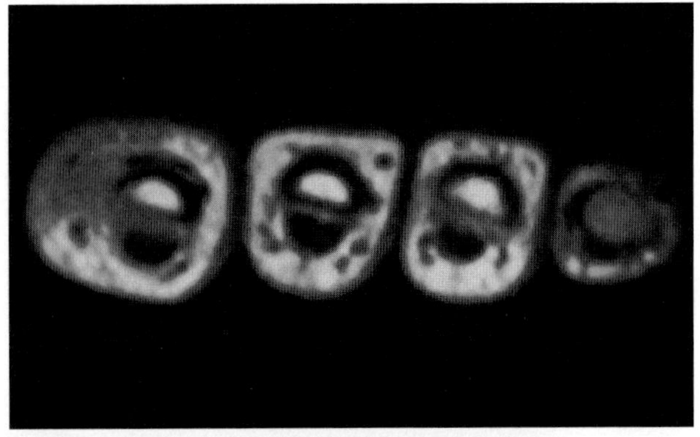 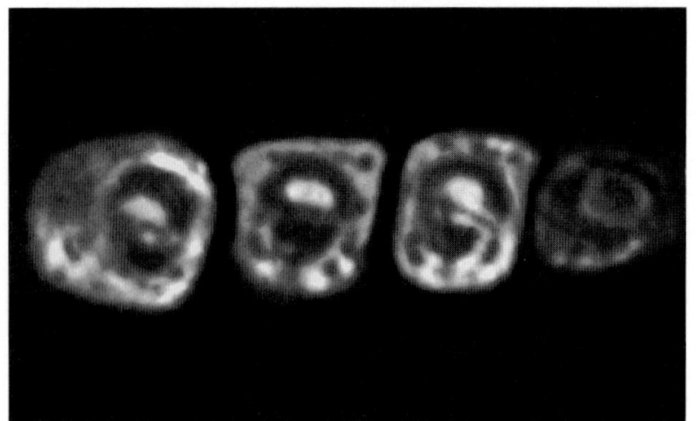

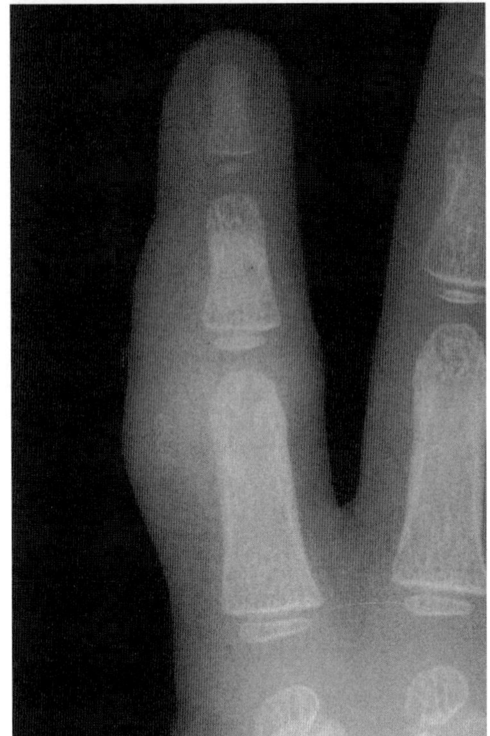

Figure 13.59 Granuloma annulare: MR imaging features in the hand of a girl 2 years of age. **A,B:** Axial T1-weighted (TR/TE; 660/15) **(A)** and T2-weighted (TR/TE; 2415/90) **(B)** spin-echo MR images of the fingers show a poorly defined mass in the radial soft tissues of the index finger, with decreased signal intensity on all pulse sequences. **C:** Radiograph of the hand shows the lesion in the ulnar aspect of the index finger.

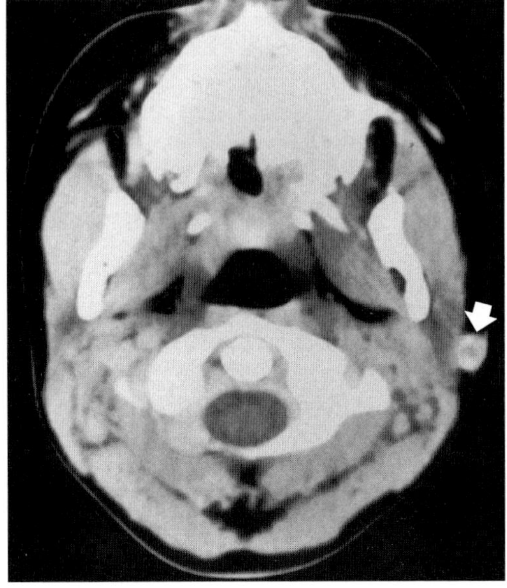 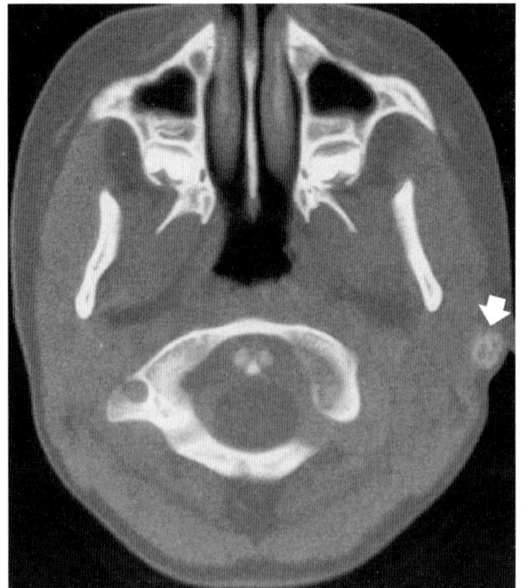

Figure 13.60 Pilomatrixoma: CT features in the neck of a boy 7 years of age. **A,B:** Axial contrast-enhanced CT scans displayed on soft tissue **(A)** and bone **(B)** windows show a calcified mass with delicate ossification, more prominent peripherally.

sheath keratin), occur within nests of basophilic cells (179).

Calcification, which is more typically central, is seen in approximately 84% of lesions (180). The calcification is described as homogeneous speckles or sandlike. Ossification occurs in an estimated 20% of these and is more typically peripheral (180). Lesions are subcutaneous with a well-defined, sharp margin (Fig. 13.60) (179,181). Limited MR imaging data notes the nonmineralized portions of the lesion to have an intermediate signal intensity on T1-weighted and fast spin-echo T2-weighted images, with slight heterogeneous enhancement following contrast administration (181).

REFERENCES

1. Beauchamp NJ, Scott WW, Gottlieb LM, et al. CT evaluation of soft tissue and muscle infection and inflammation: a systemic compartmental approach. *Skeletal Radiol.* 1995;24:317–324.
2. Robbins SL. *Pathology of Disease.* Philadelphia: WB Saunders, 1974:55–105.
3. Finch R. Skin and soft-tissue infection. *Lancet.* 1988;2:164–167.
4. Hopkins KL, Li KCP, Bergman G. Gadolinium-DTPA-enhanced magnetic resonance imaging of musculoskeletal infectious processes. *Skeletal Radiol.* 1995;24:325–330.
5. Resnick D. Osteomyelitis, septic arthritis, and soft tissue infection: mechanisms and situations. In: Resnick D, ed. *Diagnosis of Bone and Joint Disorders.* Philadelphia: WB Saunders, 2002: 2377–2480.
6. Restrepo CS, Lemos DF, Gordillo H, et al. Imaging findings in musculoskeletal complications of AIDS. *Radiographics.* 2004; 24:1029–1049.
7. Johnston C, Keogan MT. Imaging features of soft-tissue infections and other complications in drug users after direct subcutaneous injection ("skin popping"). *AJR Am J Roentgenol.* 2004; 182:1195–1202.
8. Miller TT, Randolph DA, Staron RB, et al. Fat-suppressed MRI of musculoskeletal infection: fast T2-weighted techniques versus gadolinium-enhanced T1-weighted images. *Skeletal Radiol.* 1997;26:654–658.
9. Loyer EM, Dubrow RA, David CL, et al. Imaging of superficial soft-tissue infections: sonographic findings in cases of cellulitis and abscess. *AJR Am J Roentgenol.* 1996;166:149–152.
10. Struk DW, Munk PL, Lee MJ, et al. Imaging of soft tissue infections. *Radiol Clin North Am.* 2001;39:277–303.
11. Chau CLF, Griffith JF. Musculoskeletal infections: ultrasound appearances. *Clin Radiol.* 2005;60:149–159.
12. Beltran J, Noto AM, McGhee RB, et al. Infections of the musculoskeletal system: high-field-strength MR imaging. *Radiology.* 1987;164:449–454.
13. Beltran J, McGhee RB, Shaffer PB, et al. Experimental infections of the musculoskeletal system: evaluation with MR imaging and Tc-99m MDP and Ga-67 scintigraphy. *Radiology.* 1988;167: 167–172.
14. Mirowitz SA. Fast scanning and fat-suppression MR imaging of musculoskeletal disorders. *AJR Am J Roentgenol.* 1993;161: 1147–1157.
15. Monu JUV, McManus CM, Ward WG, et al. Soft-tissue masses caused by long-standing foreign bodies in the extremities. *AJR Am J Roentgenol.* 1995;165:395–397.
16. Peterson JJ, Bancroft LW, Kransdorf MJ. Wooden foreign bodies: imaging appearance. *AJR Am J Roentgenol.* 2002;178:557–562.
17. Vincent LW. Ultrasound of soft tissue abnormalities of the extremities. *Radiol Clin North Am.* 1988;26:131–144.
18. Witte CL, Witte MH, Unger EC, et al. Advances in imaging of lymph flow disorders. *Radiographics.* 2000;20:1697–1719.
19. Levinson KL, Feingold E, Ferrell RE, et al. Age of onset in hereditary lymphedema. *J Pediatr.* 2003;142:704–708.
20. Evans AL, Bell R, Brice G, et al. Identification of eight novel VEGFR-3 mutations in families with primary congenital lymphoedema. *J Med Genet.* 2003;40:697–703.
21. Schindera ST, Streit M, Kaelin U, et al. Stewart-Treves syndrome: MR imaging of a postmastectomy upper-limb chronic lymphedema with angiosarcoma. *Skeletal Radiol.* 2005;34: 156–160.
22. Arslan A, Pierre-Jerome C, Borthne A. Necrotizing fasciitis: unreliable MRI findings in the preoperative diagnosis. *Eur J Radiol.* 2000;36:139–143.
23. Brothers TE, Tagge DU, Stutley JE, et al. Magnetic resonance imaging differentiates between necrotizing and non-necrotizing fasciitis of the lower extremity. *J Am Coll Surg.* 1998;187: 416–421.
24. Schmid MR, Kossmann T, Duewell S. Differentiation of necrotizing fasciitis and cellulitis using MR imaging. *AJR Am J Roentgenol.* 1998;170:615–620.
25. Hopkins KL, King CP, Bergman G. Gadolinium-DTPA-enhanced magnetic resonance imaging of musculoskeletal infectious processes. *Skeletal Radiol.* 1995;24:325–330.
26. Loh NN, Chen IY, Cheung LP, et al. Deep fascial hyperintensity in soft-tissue abnormalities as revealed by T2-weighted MR imaging. *AJR Am J Roentgenol.* 1997;168:1301–1304.
27. Gordon BA, Martinez S, Collins AJ. Pyomyositis. Characteristics at CT and MR imaging. *Radiology.* 1995;197: 279–286.
28. Taylor J, Templeton A, Henderson B. Pyomyositis: a clinical-pathological study based on 19 autopsy cases, Mulago Hospital 1964–1968. *East Afr Med J.* 1979;3–501.
29. Fleckenstein JL, Burns DK, Murphy FK, et al. Differential diagnosis of bacterial myositis in AIDS: evaluation with MR imaging. *Radiology.* 1991;179:653–658.
30. Robben SGF. Ultrasound of musculoskeletal infections in children. *Eur J Radiol.* 2004;14:L65-L77.
31. Adams EM, Chow CK, Premkumar A, et al. The idiopathic inflammatory myopathies: spectrum of MR imaging findings. *Radiographics.* 1995;15:563–574.
32. Plootz PH, Leff RL, Miller FW. Inflammatory and metabolic myopathies. In: Schumacher HR, ed. *Primer on the Rheumatic Diseases.* 10th ed. Atlanta: Arthritis Foundation; 1993:127–131.
33. Schweiter ME, Fort J. Cost-effectiveness of MR imaging in evaluating polymyositis. *AJR Am J Roentgenol.* 1995;165:1469–1471.
34. Dong PR, Seeger LL, Yao L, et al. Uncomplicated cat-scratch disease: findings at CT, MR imaging, and radiography. *Radiology.* 1995;195:837–839.
35. Hopkins KL, Simoneaux SF, Patrick LE, et al. Imaging manifestations of cat-scratch disease. *AJR Am J Roentgenol.* 1996;166: 435–438.
36. Parinaud H. Conjonctivite infectieuse paraissant transmise à l'homme par les animaux. *Soc Ophthalmol Paris.* 1889;2:29–31.
37. Margileth AM. Dermatologic manifestations and update of cat-scratch disease. *Pediatr Dermatol.* 1988;5:1–9.
38. Margileth AM. Cat scratch disease: nonbacterial regional lymphadenitis: the study of 145 patients and a review of the literature. *Pediatrics.* 1968;42:803–818.
39. Margileth AM. Cat scratch disease. *Adv Pediatr Infect Dis.* 1993;8:1–21.
40. Carithers HA. Cat-scratch disease. *Am J Dis Child.* 1985;139: 1124–1133.
41. Muszynski MJ, Eppes S, Riley HD. Granulomatous osteolytic lesion of the skull associated with cat-scratch disease. *Pediatr Infect Dis J.* 1987;6:199–201.
42. Fox BC, Gurtler RA. Cat-scratch disease mimicking rhabdomyosarcoma. *Orthop Rev.* 1993;11:1148–1149.
43. Beggs I. The radiology of hydatid disease. *AJR Am J Roentgenol.* 1985;145:639–648.
44. Polat P, Kantarci M, Alper F, et al. Hydatid disease from head to toe. *Radiographics.* 2003;23:475–494.
45. Martin J, Marco V, Zidan A, et al. Hydatid disease of the soft tissues of the lower limb: findings in three cases. *Skeletal Radiol.* 1993;22:511–514.
46. Chevalier X, Rhamouni A, Bretagne S, et al. Hydatid cyst of the subcutaneous tissues without other involvement. *AJR Am J Roentgenol.* 1994;163:645–646.

48. Pedrosa I, Saiz A, Arrazola J, et al. Hydatid disease: radiologic and pathologic features and complications. *Radiographics.* 2000;20:795–817.
49. Resnick D. Calcium hydroxyapatite crystal deposition disease. In Resnick D, ed. *Diagnosis of Bone and Joint Disorders.* 4th ed. Philadelphia: WB Saunders, 2002:1619–1657.
50. Hayes CW, Rosenthal DI, Plata MJ, et al. Calcific tendinitis in unusual sites associated with cortical bone erosion. *AJR Am J Roentgenol.* 1987;149:967–970.
51. Uhthoff HK. Calcifying tendonitis, an active cell-mediated calcification. *Virchows Arch.* 1975;366:51–58.
52. Berney JW. Calcifying peritendinitis of the gluteus maximus tendon. *Radiology.* 1972;102:517–518.
53. Pope TL, Keats TE. Case report 733. Calcific tendinitis of the origin of the medial and lateral heads of the rectus femoris muscle and the anterior iliac spine (AIIS). *Skeletal Radiol.* 1992;21: 271–272.
54. Farin PU, Jaroma H, Soimakallio S. Rotator cuff calcifications: treatment with US-guided technique. *Radiology.* 1995;195:841–843.
55. Aina R, Cardinal E, Bureau NJ, et al. Calcific shoulder tendinitis: treatment with modified US-guided fine-needle technique. *Radiology.* 2001;221:455–461.
56. Uhthoff HK, Sarkar K, Maynard JA. Calcifying tendonitis. A new concept of its pathogenesis. *Clin Orthop.* 1976;118: 164–168.
57. Ramon FA, Degryse HR, De Schepper AM, et al. Calcific tendinitis of the vastus lateralis muscle. A report of three cases. *Skeletal Radiol.* 1991;20:21–23.
58. Flemming DJ, Murphey MD, Shekitka KM, et al. Osseous involvement in calcific tendonitis: a retrospective review of 50 cases. *AJR Am J Roentgenol.* 2003;181:965–972.
59. Cahir J, Saifuddin A. Calcific tendonitis of pectoralis major: CT and MRI findings. *Skeletal Radiol.* 2005;34:234–238.
60. Resnick D. Gouty arthritis. In: Resnick D, ed. *Diagnosis of Bone and Joint Disorders.* 4th ed. Philadelphia: WB Saunders, 2002: 1519–1559.
61. Narvaez JA, Narvaez J, Ortega R, et al. Hypointense synovial lesions on T2-weighted images: differential diagnosis with pathologic correlation. *AJR Am J Roentgenol.* 2003;181: 761–769.
62. Leisen JCC, Austad ED, Bluhm GB, et al. The tophus in calcium pyrophosphate deposition disease. *JAMA.* 1980;244:1711–1712.
63. Schumacher HR, Bonner H, Thompson JJ, et al. Tumor-like soft tissue swelling of the distal phalanx due to calcium pyrophosphate dihydrate crystal deposition. *Arthritis Rheum.* 1984;27: 1428–1433.
64. El-Khoury GY, Foucar E, Blair WF, et al. Case report 364. *Skeletal Radiol.* 1986;15:313–316.
65. Lambert RGW, Becker EJ, Pritzker KPH. Case report 597. *Skeletal Radiol.* 1990;19:139–142.
66. Ruiz ME, Erickson SJ, Carrera GF, et al. Monarticular gout following trauma: MR appearance. *J Comput Assist Tomogr.* 1993; 17: 151–153.
67. Recht MP, Seragini FC, Kramer J, et al. Isolated or dominant lesions of the patella in gout: report of seven patients. *Skeletal Radiol.* 1994;23:113–116.
68. Llauger J, Palmer J, Roson N, et al. Nonseptic monoarthritis: imaging features with clinical and histopathologic correlation. *Radiographics.* 2000;20:S263–S278.
69. Yu JS, Chung C, Recht M, et al. MR imaging of tophaceous gout. *AJR Am J Roentgenol.* 1997;168:523–527.
70. Chen C, Chen CK, Yeh L, et al. Intra-abdominal gout mimicking pelvic abscess. *Skeletal Radiol.* 2005;34:229–233.
71. Abreu M, Johnson K, Chung CB, et al. Calcification in calcium pyrophosphate dihydrate (CPPD) crystalline deposits in the knee: anatomic, radiographic, MR imaging, and histologic study in cadavers. *Skeletal Radiol.* 2004;33:392–398.
72. Rivera-Sanfeliz G, Resnick D, Haghighi P, et al. Tophaceous pseudogout. *Skeletal Radiol.* 1996;25:699–701.
73. Leisen J. Calcium pyrophosphate diahydrate deposition disease: tumorous form. *AJR Am J Roentgenol.* 1982;138:962.
74. Ling D, Murphy WA, Kyriakos M. Tophaceous pseudogout. *AJR Am J Roentgenol.* 1982;138:162–165.
75. Kakitsubata Y, Boutin RD, Theodorou DJ, et al. Calcium pyrophosphate dihydrate crystal deposition in and around the atlantoaxial joint: association with type 2 odontoid fractures in nine patients. *Radiology.* 2000;216:213–219.
76. Resnick D. Plasma cell dyscrasias and dysgammaglobulinemias. In: Resnick D, ed. *Diagnosis of Bone and Joint Disorders.* 4th ed. Philadelphia: WB Saunders, 2002:2188–2232.
77. Camacho CR, Meléndez AT, Brewster DC, et al. Radiological findings of amyloid arthropathy in long-term hemodialysis. *Eur J Radiol.* 1992;2-4:305–308.
78. Casey TT, Stone WJ, DiRaimondo CR, et al. Tumoral amyloidosis of bone of beta-2-microglobulin origin in association with long-term hemodialysis: a new type of amyloid disease. *Hum Pathol.* 1986;17:731–738.
79. Cobby MJ, Adler RS, Swartz R, et al. Dialysis-related amyloid arthropathy: MR findings in four patients. *AJR Am J Roentgenol.* 1991;157:1023–1027.
80. Ross LV, Ross GJ, Mesgar Z, et al. Hemodialysis-related amyloidomas of bone. *Radiology.* 1991;178:263–265.
81. Arthanasou NA, Ayers D, Ruiney AJ. Joint and systemic distribution of dialysis amyloid. *Q J Med.* 1991;287:205–214.
82. Bardin T, Kuntz D, Zingraff J, et al. Synovial amyloidosis in patients undergoing long-term hemodialysis. *Arthritis Rheum.* 1985;28:1052–1058.
83. Ross GJ, Ross LV, Hartz WH, et al. Case report 723. Popliteal artery aneurysm. *Skeletal Radiol.* 1992;21:190–193.
84. Bilotta W, Walker H, McDonald DJ, et al. Case report 651. Thrombosed, leaking popliteal aneurysm. *Skeletal Radiol.* 1991; 20:71–72.
85. Szilagyi DE, Schwartz RL, Reddy DJ. Popliteal arterial aneurysms. *Arch Surg.* 1981;116:724–728.
86. Ludwig WD, Yuh WTC, Montgomery WJ. MR imaging of post-traumatic pseudoaneurysm of the deep femoral artery. *J Comput Assist Tomogr.* 1987;116:1093–1095.
87. Fujimoto H, Yasuda S, Kashimada A, et al. Diagnosis of aneurysm of superior thyroid artery by CT and MR imaging. *Acta Radiol.* 1992;33:420–422.
88. Saeed M, Wolf YG, Dilley RB. Adventitial cystic disease of the popliteal artery mistaken for an endoluminal lesion. *J Vasc Interv Radiol.* 1993;4:815–818.
89. Lossef SV, Rajan S, Calcagno D, et al: Spontaneous rupture of an adventitial cyst of the popliteal artery: confirmation with MR imaging. *J Vasc Interv Radiol.* 1992;3:95–97.
90. Deutsch AL, Hyde J, Miller SM, et al: Cystic adventitial degeneration of the popliteal artery: CT demonstration and directed percutaneous therapy. *AJR Am J Roentgenol.* 1985;145:117–118.
91. Wilbur AC, Woelfel GF, Meyer JP, et al. Adventitial cystic disease of the popliteal artery. *Radiology.* 1985;155:63–64.
92. Peterson JJ, Kransdorf MJ, Bancroft LW, et al. Imaging characteristics of cystic adventitial disease of the peripheral arteries: presentation as soft-tissue masses. *AJR Am J Roentgenol.* 2003;180: 621–625.
93. Do DD, Braunschweig M, Baumgartner I, et al. Adventitial cystic disease of the popliteal artery: percutaneous US-guided aspiration. *Radiology.* 1997;203:743–746.
94. Elias DA, White LM, Rubenstein JD, et al. Clinical evaluation and MR imaging features of popliteal artery entrapment and cystic adventitial disease. *AJR Am J Roentgenol.* 2003; 180:627–632.
95. Chaloupka JC, Castillo M, Hudgins P. Castleman disease in the neck: atypical appearance on CT. *AJR Am J Roentgenol.* 1990; 154: 1051–1052.
96. Tung KSK, McCormack LJ. Angiomatous lymphoid hamartoma. Report of five cases with a review of the literature. *Cancer.* 1967;21:525–536.
97. Castleman B, Iverson L, Menendez VP. Localized mediastinal lymph-node hyperplasia resembling thymoma. *Cancer.* 1956;9: 822–830.
98. Keller A, Hochholzer L, Castleman B. Hyaline-vascular and plasma-cell types of giant lymph node hyperplasia of the mediastinum and other locations. *Cancer.* 1971;29:670–683.
99. Koslin B, Berland LL, Sekar C. Cervical Castleman disease: CT study with angiographic correlation. *Radiology.* 1986;160: 213–214.

100. Onik G, Goodman PC. CT of Castleman disease. *AJR Am J Roentgenol.* 1983;140:691–692.
101. Debatin JF, Spritzer CE, Dunnick NR. Castleman disease of the adrenal gland: MR imaging features. *AJR Am J Roentgenol.* 1991;157:781–783.
102. Libson E, Fields S, Strauss S, et al. Widespread Castleman disease: CT and US findings. *Radiology.* 1988;166:753–755.
103. Bartkowski DP, Ferrigni RG. Castleman's disease: an unusual retroperitoneal mass. *J Urol.* 1988;139:118–120.
104. Ko SF, Hsieh MJ, Ng SH, et al. Imaging spectrum of Castleman's disease. *AJR Am J Roentgenol.* 2004;182:769–775.
105. Meador TL, McLarney JK. CT features of Castleman disease of the abdomen and pelvis. *AJR Am J Roentgenol.* 2000;175:115–118.
106. Pickhardt PJ, Bhalla S. Unusual nonneoplastic peritoneal and subperitoneal conditions: CT findings. *Radiographics.* 2005;25: 719–730.
107. Rahmouni A, Golli M, Mathieu D, et al. Castleman disease mimicking liver tumor: CT and MR features. *J Comput Assist Tomogr.* 1992;16:699–703.
108. Moon WK, Im JG, Han MC. Castleman's disease of the mediastinum: MR imaging features. *Clin Radiol.* 1994;49:466–468.
109. Goodman K, Baim RS, Clair MR, et al: Angiomatous lymphoid hamartoma of the pelvis. Characteristic calcification and computed tomographic appearance. *Radiology.* 1983;146:728.
110. Bui-Mansfield LT, Chew FS, Myers CP. Angiofollicular lymphoid hyperplasia (Castleman disease) of the axilla. *AJR Am J Roentgenol.* 2000;174:1060.
111. Khan J, von Sinner W, Akhtar M, et al. Castleman's disease of the chest. Magnetic resonance imaging features. *Chest.* 1994;105: 1608–1610.
112. Ecklund K, Hartnell GG. Mediastinal Castleman disease: MR and MRA features. *J Thorac Imaging.* 1994;9:156–159.
113. Luburich P, Nicolau C, Ayuso MC, et al. Pelvic Castleman disease: CT and MR appearance. *J Comput Assist Tomogr.* 1992;16: 657–659.
114. Sundaram M, McLeod RA. MR imaging of tumor and tumor-like lesions of bone and soft tissue. *AJR Am J Roentgenol.* 1990; 155:817–824.
115. Unger EC, Glazer HS, Lee JKT, et al. MRI of extracranial hematomas: Preliminary observations. *AJR Am J Roentgenol.* 1986;146:403–407.
116. Rubin JI, Gomori JM, Grossman RI, et al. High-field MR imaging of extracranial hematomas. *AJR Am J Roentgenol.* 1987;148: 813–817.
117. Lenchik L, Dovgan DJ, Kier R. CT of the iliopsoas compartment: value in differentiating tumor, abscess and hematoma. *AJR Am J Roentgenol.* 1994;162:83–86.
118. Panicek DM, Casper ES, Brennan MF, et al. Hemorrhage simulating tumor growth in malignant fibrous histiocytoma at MR imaging. *Radiology.* 1991;181:398–400.
119. Mellado JM, Perez del Palomar L, Diaz L, et al. Long-standing Morel-Lavallée lesions of the trochanteric region and proximal thigh: MRI features in five patients. *AJR Am J Roentgenol.* 2004;182:1289–1294.
120. Parra JA, Fernández MA, Encinas B, et al. Morel-Lavallée effusions in the thigh. *Skeletal Radiol.* 1997;26:239–241.
121. Sterling A, Butterfield WC, Bonner R Jr, et al. Post-traumatic cysts of soft tissue. *J Trauma.* 1977;17:392–396.
122. Kuklo TR, Murphey MD, Islinger RB, et al. Pseudotumors presenting in nonhemophiliacs. *Orthopedics.* 2001;24:483–486.
123. Leri A, Joanny L. Une affection non décrite de os. Hyperostose "en coulée" sur toute à la longeur d'un membre oru "melorheostose." *Bull Mem Soc Med Hop Paris.* 1922;46:1141–1145.
124. Murray RO, McCredie J. Melorheostosis and the sclerotomes: a radiological correlation. *Skeletal Radiol.* 1979;4:57–71.
125. Garver P, Resnick D, Haghighi P, et al. Melorheostosis of the axial skeleton with associated fibrolipomatous lesions. *Skeletal Radiol.* 1982;9:41–44.
126. Morris JM, Samilson RL, Corley CL. Melorheostosis: review of the literature and report of an interesting case with nineteen-year follow-up. *J Bone Joint Surg Am.* 1963;45:1191–1203.
127. Campbell CJ, Papademetriou T, Bonfiglio M. Melorheostosis. A report of the clinical, roentgenographic, and pathological findings in fourteen cases. *J Bone Joint Surg Am.* 1968;50:1281–1304.
128. Yu JS, Resnick D, Vaughan LM, et al. Melorheostosis with an ossified soft tissue mass: MR features. *Skeletal Radiol.* 1995;24: 367–370.
129. McCleod RA, Beabout JW, Cooper KL, et al. Case of the day: melorheostosis. *AJR Am J Roentgenol.* 1984;142:1062–1063.
130. Kalbermatten NT, Vock P, Rüfenacht D, et al. Progressive melorheostosis in the peripheral and axial skeleton with associated vascular malformations: imaging findings over three decades. *Skeletal Radiol.* 2001;30:48–52.
131. Judkiewicz AM, Murphey MD, Resnik CS, et al. Advanced imaging of melorheostosis with emphasis on MRI. *Skeletal Radiol.* 2001;30:447–453.
132. Amis ES. Retroperitoneal fibrosis. *AJR Am J Roentgenol.* 1991; 157: 321–329.
133. Stewart TW, Friberg TR. Idiopathic retroperitoneal fibrosis with diffuse involvement: further evidence of systemic idiopathic fibrosis. *South Med J.* 1984;77:1185–1187.
134. Barrett RL, Horrow MH, Gubernick JA, et al. US case of the day. Retroperitoneal fibrosis with perirenal involvement. *Radiographics.* 1995;15:1024–1026.
135. Lalli AF. Retroperitoneal fibrosis and inapparent obstructive uropathy. *Radiology.* 1977;122:339–342.
136. Degesys GE, Dunnick NR, Silverman PM, et al. Retroperitoneal fibrosis: use of CT in distinguishing among possible causes. *AJR Am J Roentgenol.* 1986;146:57–60.
137. Enzinger FM, Weiss SW. *Soft Tissue Tumors.* 3rd ed. St. Louis: Mosby, 1995:201–229.
138. Mulligan SA, Holley HC, Koehler RE, et al. CT and MR imaging in the evaluation of retroperitoneal fibrosis. *J Comput Assist Tomogr.* 1989;13:277–281.
139. Hricak H, Higgins CB, Williams RD. Nuclear magnetic resonance imaging in retroperitoneal fibrosis. *AJR Am J Roentgenol.* 1983;141:35–38.
140. Rubenstein WA, Gray G, Auh YH, et al. CT of fibrous tissues and tumors with sonographic correlation. *AJR Am J Roentgenol.* 1986;147:1067–1074.
141. Fagan CJ, Larrieu AJ, Amparo EG. Retroperitoneal fibrosis: ultrasound and CT features. *AJR Am J Roentgenol.* 1979;133: 239–243.
142. Cooper KL, Beabout JW, Dahlin DC. Giant cell tumor: ossification in soft-tissue implants. *Radiology.* 1984;153:597–602.
143. Bond JR, Cooper KL. Musculoskeletal case of the day. Soft-tissue implant of giant cell tumor. *AJR Am J Roentgenol.* 1993;160: 1328–1330.
144. Lattes R. *Tumors of the Soft Tissue.* Washington, DC: Armed Forces Institute of Pathology; 1982.
145. Lee HJ, Im JG, Goo JM, et al. Peripheral T-cell lymphoma: spectrum of imaging findings with clinical and pathologic features. *Radiographics.* 2003;23:7–28.
146. Metser U, Goor O, Lerman H, et al. PET-CT of extranodal lymphoma. *AJR Am J Roentgenol.* 2004;182:1579–1586.
147. Guermazi A, Brice P, de Kerviler E, et al. Extranodal Hodgkin disease: spectrum of disease. *Radiographics.* 2001;21: 161–179.
148. Nelson MC, Petrik JH, Lack EE, et al. Lymphocyte-predominant Hodgkin disease manifest as a subcutaneous arm mass. *AJR Am J Roentgenol.* 1990;155:658–659.
149. Janzen DL, Connell DG, Vaisler BJ. Calcific myonecrosis of the calf manifesting as an enlarging soft-tissue mass: imaging features. *AJR Am J Roentgenol.* 1993;160:1072–1074.
150. O'Keefe RJ, O'Connell JX, Temple HT, et al. Calcific myonecrosis. A late sequela to compartment syndrome. *Clin Orthop.* 1995;318: 205–213.
151. Viau MR, Pedersen HE, Salciccioli GG, et al. Ectopic calcification as a late sequela of compartment syndrome. *Clin Orthop.* 1983; 176:178–180.
152. Broder MS, Worrell RV, Shafi NQ. Cystic degeneration and calcification following ischemic paralysis of the leg. *Clin Orthop.* 1977;122:193–195.
153. Heffner RR, Armbrustmacher VW, Earle KM. Focal myositis. *Cancer.* 1977;40:301–306.
154. Cumming WJK, Weiser R, Teoh R, et al. Localized nodular myositis: a clinical pathological variant of polymyositis. *Q J Med.* 1977;46:531–546.

155. Flaisler F, Blin D, Asencio G. Focal myositis: a localized form of polymyositis? *J Rheumatol.* 1993;20:1414–1426.

156. Kransdorf MJ, Temple HT, Sweet DE. Focal myositis. *Skeletal Radiol.* 1998;27:283–287.

157. Plotz PH, Leff RL, Miller FW. Inflammatory and metabolic myopathies. In: Schumacher HR, Klippel JH, Koopman WJ, eds. *Primer on the Rheumatic Diseases.* 10th ed. Atlanta: Arthritis Foundation; 1993:127–131.

158. Maguire JK, Milford LW, Pitcock JA. Focal myositis in the hand. *J Hand Surg.* 1988;13A:140–142.

159. Liefeld PA, Ferguson AB, Fu FH. Focal myositis: a benign lesion that mimics malignant disease. *J Bone Joint Surg Am.* 1982;64:1371–1373.

160. Naughton M, Jessop JD, Williams BD. Idiopathic recurrent non-suppurative focal myositis: a report of two cases. *Br J Rheumatol.* 1993;32:1101–1104.

161. Caldwell CJ, Swash M, van der Walt JD, et al. Focal myositis: a clinicopathological study. *Neuromuscul Disord.* 1995;5:317–321.

162. Moskovic E, Fisher C, Westbury G. Focal myositis, a benign inflammatory pseudotumor: CT. *Br J Radiol.* 1991;64:489–493.

163. Finger DR, Dennis GJ. Focal myositis [letter]. *J Rheumatol.* 1995;22:188–189.

164. Hoffa A. Influence of adipose tissue with regard to the pathology of the knee joint. *JAMA.* 1904;41:795–796.

165. Krebs VE, Parker RD. Arthroscopic resection of an extrasynovial ossifying chondroma of the infrapatellar fat pad: end-stage Hoffa's disease. *Arthroscopy* 1994;10:301–304.

166. DesMarchais J, Gagnon PA. Hoffa's disease (proceedings and reports of councils and associations). *J Bone Joint Surg Br.* 1974;56:586.

167. Ogilvie-Harris DJ, Giddens J. Hoffa's disease: arthroscopic resection of the infrapatellar fat pad. *Arthroscopy* 1994;10:184–187.

168. Murphy GF, Elder DE. *Atlas of Tumor Pathology. Non-Melanocytic Tumors of the Skin.* Washington, DC: Armed Forces Institute of Pathology; 1991.

169. Davids JR, Kolman BH, Billman GF, Krous HF. Subcutaneous granuloma annulare: recognition and treatment. *J Pediatr Orthop.* 1993;13:582–586.

170. Calista D, Landi G. Disseminated granuloma annulare in acquired immunodeficiency syndrome: case report and review of the literature. *Cutis.* 1995;55:158–160.

171. Person JR. Generalized granuloma annulare, mononucleosis and positive rheumatoid factor. *Int J Dermatol.* 1995;34:40–41.

172. Dahl MV. Granuloma Annulare. In: Fitzpatrick TB, Eisen AZ, Wolff K, et al, eds. *Dermatology in General Medicine.* 3rd ed. New York: McGraw-Hill; 1993:1187–1191.

173. Argent JD, Fairhurst JJ, Clarke NMP. Subcutaneous granuloma annulare: four cases and review of the literature. *Pediatr Radiol.* 1994;24:527–529.

174. Yu GV, Farrer AK. Benign rheumatoid nodule versus subcutaneous granuloma annulare: a diagnostic dilemma. Are they the same entity? *J Foot Ankle Surg.* 1994;33:156–166.

175. Minifee PK, Buchino JJ. Subcutaneous palisading granulomas (benign rheumatoid nodules) in children. *J Pediatr Surg.* 1986;21:1078–1080.

176. Kransdorf MJ, Murphey MD, Temple HT. Subcutaneous granuloma annulare: radiologic appearance. *Skeletal Radiol.* 1998;27:266–270.

177. DeMaeseneer M, Vande Walle H, Lenchik J, et al. Subcutaneous granuloma annulare: MR imaging findings. *Skeletal Radiol.* 1998;27:215–217.

178. Wickremaratchi T, Collins CMP. Pilomatrixoma or calcifying epithelioma of Malherbe invading bone. *Histopathology.* 1992;21:79–81.

179. Haller JO, Kassner EG, Ostrowitz A, et al. Pilomatrixoma (calcifying epithelioma of Malherbe): radiographic features. *Radiology.* 1977;123:151–153.

180. Forbis R, Helwig EB. Pilomatrixoma (calcifying epithelioma). *Arch Dermatol.* 1961;83:606–618.

181. Ichikawa T, Nakajima Y, Fujimoto H, et al. Giant calcifying epithelioma of Malherbe (pilomatrixoma): imaging features. *Skeletal Radiol.* 1997;26:602–605.

182. Veliath AJ, Reddy KS, Gomathinayagam D. Malignant pilomatrixoma. Report of a case. *Acta Radiol Oncol.* 1984;23:429–431.

183. Sloan JB, Sueki H, Jaworsky C. Pigmented malignant pilomatrixoma: report of a case and review of the literature. *J Cutan Pathol.* 1992;19:240–246.

Compartmental Anatomy

The radiologic staging of a soft tissue tumor is a vital part of a patient's evaluation (1,2). As previously noted in Chapter 3, accurate staging is essential to determine appropriate clinical treatment and prognosis. Complete staging typically requires information that is not available at the time of initial patient presentation, such as tumor grade and presence or absence of metastases. The local extent of disease, however, is a critical part of tumor staging and is accurately defined at initial patient presentation with MR imaging (2). Inherent in the determination of local extent for staging is the concept of *anatomic compartment*.

Anatomic compartments are defined by natural barriers that prevent the spread of tumor (3). These barriers include major fascial septae, periosteum, cortical bone, joint articular cartilage, and joint capsules (3). Lesions that are confined to a specific anatomic space by these barriers are considered to be *intracompartmental*. This designation has clinical implications in that intracompartmental lesions are lower stage than similar grade extracompartmental lesions and generally have an improved prognosis. *Extracompartmental* lesions are those that have spread beyond the compartment of origin. Mechanisms of extracompartmental spread include direct tumor extension, contamination from hemorrhage, or inappropriate open or percutaneous biopsy (3,4).

Accurate delineation of the local extent and tumor compartment is essential not only in local staging, but also in planning definitive surgery, as well as in planning surgical or percutaneous biopsy. As a general rule, image-guided biopsy is usually done using the shortest path between the skin and the lesion, avoiding vital structures such as vessels and nerves (3). The biopsy of musculoskeletal lesions and specifically soft tissue tumors, however, has additional requirements, and it is essential that the biopsy needle path not violate any uninvolved compartment, neurovascular structure, or joint (3). Definitive surgery includes complete removal of the biopsy needle tract, which is considered to be contaminated tissue, and consequently, the biopsy needle tract should ideally be made in the same location as the incision for definitive surgery (3).

As radiologists, we are often called on to perform image-guided biopsies. To ensure optimum patient care, biopsy of a soft tissue tumor should never be undertaken without prior consultation from the surgeon who will do the definitive surgery (5,6). Accordingly, percutaneous biopsy should be planned as carefully as the definitive surgery (5). In a landmark study done by Mankin et al. in 1982, members of the Musculoskeletal Tumor Society reported the accuracy of diagnosis and incidence of complications associated with biopsy (5). This study of 329 patients noted that the optimum treatment plan had to be altered as a result of biopsy-related problems in 18.2% of patients, unnecessary amputation was performed as a result of problems with biopsy in 4.5%, and the prognosis and outcome were adversely affected in 8.5%. A similar study was performed in 1992 involving 597 patients and showed almost identical results (7). Although these studies did not specifically address percutaneous image-guided biopsies, they serve as a poignant reminder of the potential harm of inappropriate biopsy, such as violating compartmental anatomy or crossing tissue planes that will compromise subsequent definitive surgery.

This chapter reviews the anatomic compartments of the musculoskeletal system. This knowledge is required for the local staging of soft tissue tumors and for the planning and performing of percutaneous image-guided biopsy.

GENERAL PRINCIPLES OF COMPARTMENTAL ANATOMY

Skin and subcutaneous fat: The skin and subcutaneous fat contain no barriers to tumor spread and therefore are considered to be a single compartment. They are separated from the deeper structures by thick fascia (3).

Muscle: A lesion confined to a single muscle is intracompartmental. A lesion that extends beyond the muscle of origin, however, may still be intracompartmental if it does not violate the barriers defined for that specific anatomic location (3).

Joint: Each joint is considered to be a distinct compartment (3).

Bone: Each bone is considered to be a distinct compartment. The space between the bone and the adjacent soft tissue is termed the *parosseous* tissue, and it is also considered a compartment (3).

Vessels and nerves: Neurovascular structures are not considered to be specific compartments, but they may be a path of tumor spread (3). As such, they must be specifically addressed during staging and biopsy planning.

Specific Compartments

Upper Extremity

Upper Arm

The soft tissues of the upper arm are divided into two compartments: anterior and posterior (Fig. 14.1) (8). Other comparts associated with the upper arm include the periscapular compartment (infraspinatus, teres minor and rhomboid muscles). The supraspinatus and deltoid muscles are their own separate compartments (3).

Anterior compartment: Biceps, brachialis, coricobrachialis, and brachioradialis muscles.

Posterior compartment: Triceps muscle.

Periscapular compartment: Infraspinatus, teres minor, rhomboid muscle.

Other: Supraspinatus and deltoid muscles are separate compartments.

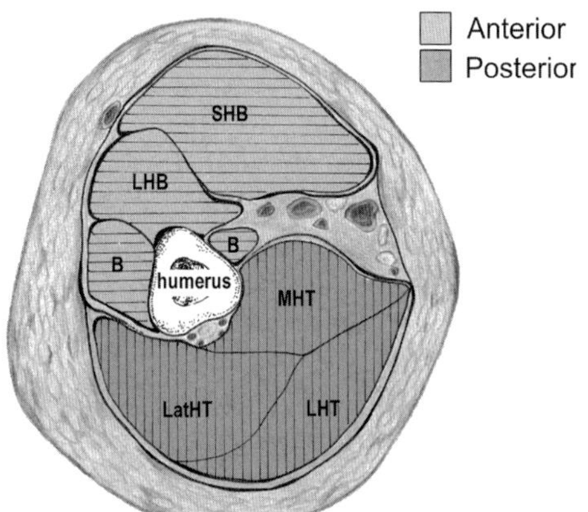

Figure 14.1 Upper arm compartmental anatomy. *Anterior compartment:* Long head biceps (*LHB*), short head biceps (*SHB*), and brachialis (*B*) muscles. *Posterior compartment:* Lateral head triceps (*LatHT*), medial head triceps (*MHT*), and long head triceps (*LHT*) muscles.

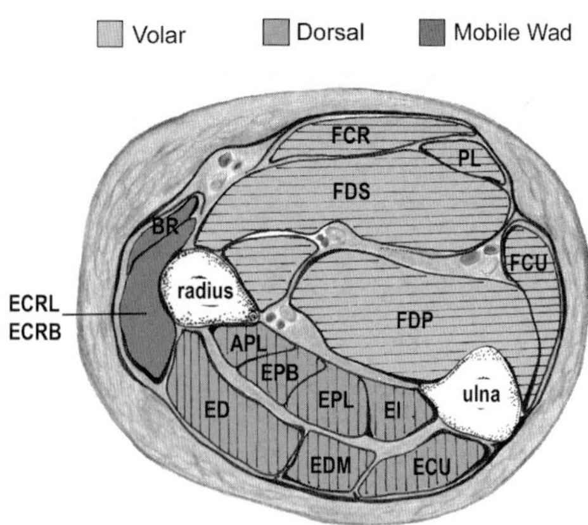

Figure 14.2 Forearm compartmental anatomy. *Volar compartment:* The deep group consists of the flexor digitorum profundus (*FDP*), flexor pollicis longus, and the pronator quadratus muscles. The superficial group includes the flexor carpi ulnaris (*FCU*), palmaris longus (*PL*), flexor carpi radialis (*FCR*), and flexor digitorum superficialis (*FDS*) muscles. *Dorsal compartment:* The muscles of the dorsal compartment are also subdivided into deep and superficial groups. The deep group consists of the abductor pollicis longus (*APL*), extensor pollicis brevis (*EPB*), extensor pollicis longus (*EPL*) and extensor indices (*EI*) muscles. The superficial compartment includes the extensor digitorum (*ED*), extensor digiti minimi (*EDM*), and extensor carpi ulnaris (*ECU*) muscles. *Mobile wad compartment:* Extensor carpi radialis brevis (*ECRB*), extensor carpi radialis longus (*ECRL*), and brachioradialis (*BR*) muscles.

Forearm

The forearm is divided into three compartments: volar, dorsal, and mobile wad (Fig. 14.2) (8).

Volar compartment: The muscles of the volar compartment are further subdivided into deep and superficial groups (8). The deep group consists of the flexor digitorum profundus, flexor pollicus longus, and the pronator quadratus muscles. The superficial group includes the flexor carpi ulnaris, palmaris longus, flexor carpi radialis, flexor digitorum superficialis, and pronator teres (8).

Dorsal compartment: The muscles of the dorsal compartment are also subdivided into deep and superficial groups (8). The deep group consists of the supinator abductor pollicis longus and the extensor pollicis longus and brevis, and extensor indices muscles (8). The superficial compartment includes the extensor digitorum, extensor digiti minimi, and extensor carpi ulnaris muscles (8).

Mobile wad compartment: Extensor carpi radialis brevis and longus and brachioradialis muscles.

Pelvis

Each muscle of the pelvis is considered to be a separate compartment (3).

Lower Extremity

Thigh

The thigh has three anatomic compartments: anterior, posterior, and medial (Fig. 14.3) (3,9). The groin (inguinal and femoral triangle) and popliteal fossa are considered to be extracompartmental (3,9).

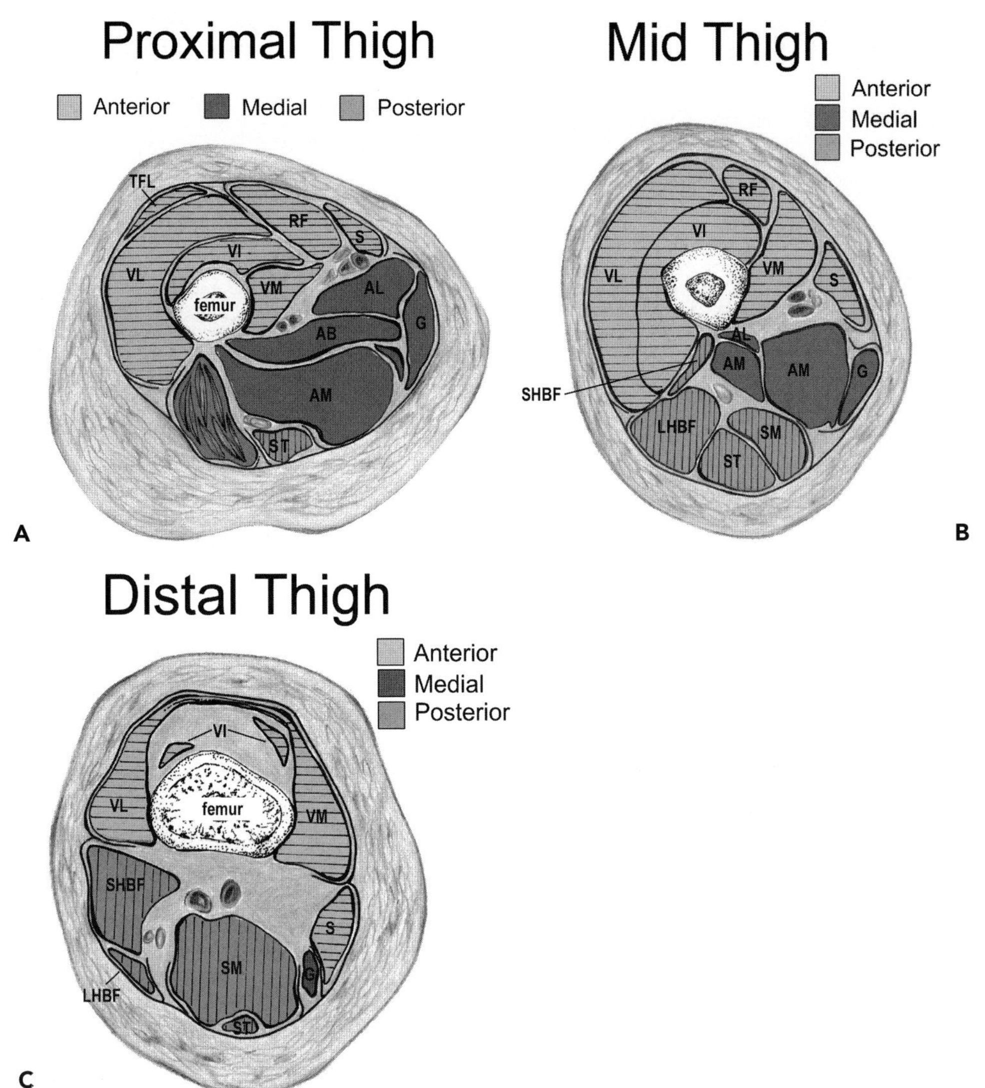

Figure 14.3 Thigh compartmental anatomy: Proximal **(A)**, mid **(B)**, and distal **(C)** thigh. *Anterior compartment:* The anterior compartment includes the sartorius (*S*), tensor fascia latae (*TFL*), rectus femoris (*RF*), vastus medialis (*VM*), vastus intermedius (*VI*), and vastus lateralis (*VL*) muscles. *Posterior compartment:* The posterior compartment consists of the hamstring muscles; the semimembranosus (*SM*), semitendinosus (*ST*), and long head (*LHBF*) and short head (*SHBF*) biceps femoris muscles. *Medial compartment:* The medial compartment consists of the gracilis (*G*), adductor longus (*AL*), adductor brevis (*AB*), and adductor magnus (*AM*) muscles.

Anterior compartment: The anterior compartment includes the sartorius, iliotibial tract and tensor fascia lata, and the quadriceps muscles (rectus femoris, vastus medialis, vastus lateralis, and vastus intermedius muscles). The vastus intermedius muscle is sometimes considered to be a separate compartment (3).

Posterior compartment: The posterior compartment consists of the hamstring muscles; the semimembranosus, semitendinosus, and biceps femoris muscles. The sciatic nerve is within the posterior compartment.

Medial compartment: The medial compartment consists of the gracilis and adductor muscles (adductor longus, brevis, and magnus muscles).

Lower Leg

The lower leg is divided into four compartments: anterior, lateral, superfical posterior, and deep posterior (Fig. 14.4) (3,9). The ankle and dorsum of the foot are considered to be extracompartmental (3).

Anterior compartment: The muscles of the anterior compartment include the tibialis anterior, extensor hallucis longus, and extensor digitorum longus. The anterior compartment includes the anterior tibial artery and vein as well as the deep peroneal nerve (3).

Lateral compartment: The lateral compartment is made up of the peroneal muscles. It also includes the common and superficial peroneal nerves (3).

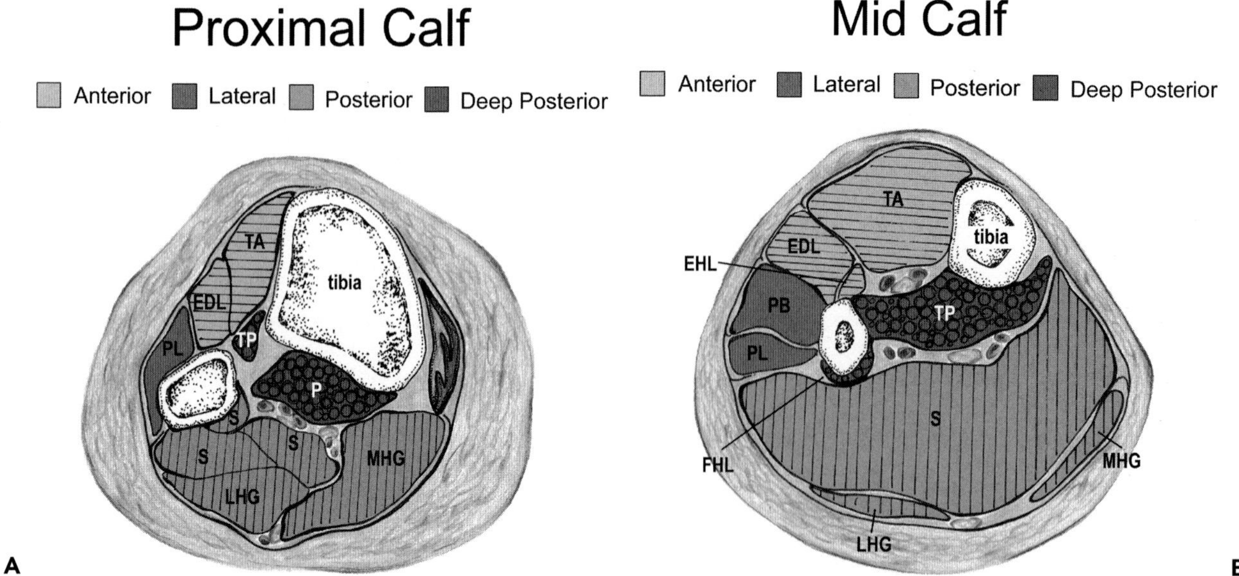

Figure 14.4   Lower leg compartmental anatomy: Proximal **(A)** and mid **(B)** lower leg. *Anterior compartment:* The muscles of the anterior compartment include the tibialis anterior (*TA*), extensor hallucis longus (*EHL*), and extensor digitorum longus (*EDL*) muscles. *Lateral compartment:* The lateral compartment is made up of the peroneal brevis (*PB*) and peroneal longus (*PL*) muscles. *Superficial posterior compartment:* This compartment contains the medial head gastrocnemius (*MHG*) and lateral head (*LHG*) gastrocnemius and soleus (*S*) muscles. *Deep posterior compartment:* The deep posterior compartment includes the tibialis posterior (*TP*), flexor hallucis longus (*FHL*), and popliteus (*P*) muscles.

Superficial posterior compartment: This compartment contains the gastrocnemius and soleus muscles, as well as the sural nerve (3).

Deep posterior compartment: The deep posterior compartment includes the tibialis posterior, flexor hallucis longus, and flexor digitorum longus muscles. It also includes the posterior tibial and peroneal arteries and posterior tibial nerve (3).

Foot

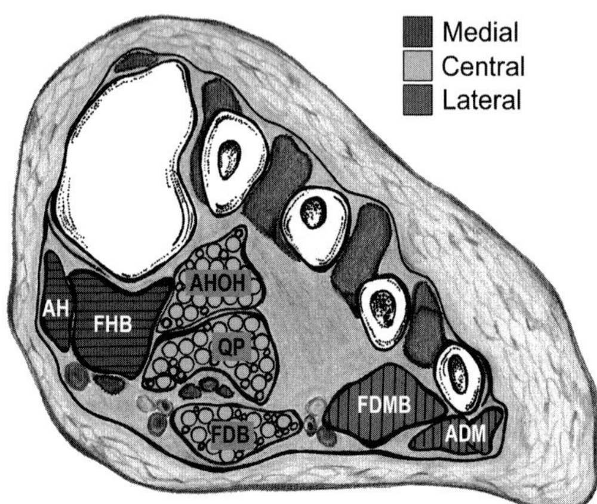

Figure 14.5   Foot compartmental anatomy. *Medial compartment:* The medial compartment contains the abductor hallucis (*AH*) and flexor hallucis brevis (*FHB*) muscles. *Central compartment:* The central compartment includes the flexor digitorum brevis (*FDB*), quadratus plantae (*QP*), and adductor hallucis oblique head (*AHOH*) muscles. *Lateral compartment:* The lateral compartment contains the abductor (*ADM*) and flexor digiti minimi brevis (*FDMB*) muscles.

Foot

The plantar aspect of the foot is divided into three compartments: medial, lateral, and central (Fig. 14.5) (9). The dorsum of the foot and ankle are considered extracompartmental.

Medial compartment: The medial compartment contains the abductor hallucis and flexor hallucis brevis muscles (9).

Central compartment: The central compartment includes the flexor digitorum brevis, quadratus plantae lumbrical, and adductor hallucis muscles (9).

Lateral compartment: The lateral compartment contains the abductor and flexor digiti minimi muscles.

REFERENCES

1. Enneking WF, Spanier SS, Goodman MA. A system for the surgical staging of musculoskeletal sarcoma. *Clin Orthop.* 1980;153:106–120.
2. Peabody TD, Simon MA. Principles of staging soft-tissue sarcomas. *Clin Orthop.* 1993;289:19–31.
3. Anderson MW, Temple HT, Dussault RG, et al. Compartmental anatomy: relevance to staging and biopsy of musculoskeletal tumors. *AJR Am J Roentgenol.* 1999;173:1663–1671.
4. Peabody TD, Gibbs CP, Simon MA. Evaluation and staging of musculoskeletal neoplasms. *J Bone Joint Surg Am.* 1998;80:1204–1218.
5. Mankin HJ, Lange TA, Spanier SS. The hazards of biopsy in patients with malignant primary bone and soft-tissue tumors. *J Bone Joint Surg Am.* 1982;64:1121–1127.
6. Shives TC. Biopsy of soft-tissue tumors. *Clin Orthop.* 1993;289: 32–35.
7. Mankin HJ, Mankin CJ, Simon MA. The hazards of biopsy, revisited: members of the Musculoskeletal Tumor Society. *J Bone Joint Surg Am.* 1996;78:656–663.
8. Boles CA, Kannam S, Cardwell AB. The forearm: anatomy of muscle compartments and nerves. *AJR Am J Roentgenol.* 2000;174:151–159.
9. Toomayan GA, Robertson F, Major NM. Lower extremity compartmental anatomy: clinical relevance to radiologists. *Skeletal Radiol.* 2005;34:30–313.

Index

Note: An *f* following page numbers refer to figures, and a *t* refers to tables.